MW00769185

CONCISE LEARNING AND MEMORY: THE EDITOR'S SELECTION

CONCISE LEARNING AND MEMORY: THE EDITOR'S SELECTION

Editor
John H. Byrne
Department of Neurobiology & Anatomy, The University of Texas Medical School at Houston, Houston, Texas, USA

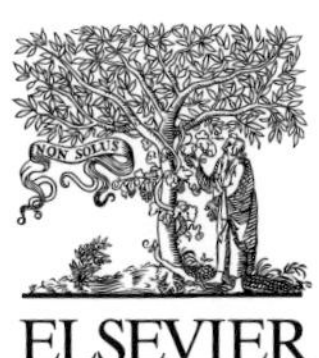

AMSTERDAM BOSTON HEIDELBERG LONDON NEW YORK OXFORD
PARIS SAN DIEGO SAN FRANCISCO SINGAPORE SYDNEY TOKYO

Academic Press is an imprint of Elsevier
32 Jamestown Road, London, NW1 7BY, UK
525 B Street, Suite 1900, San Diego, CA 92101-4495, USA

First edition 2009

British Library Cataloguing in Publication Data
A catalogue record for this book is available from the British Library

Library of Congress Catalog Number: 2008933909

ISBN: 978-0-12-374627-6

For information on all Academic Press publications
visit our website at www.elsevierdirect.com

Printed and bound in Slovenia

09 10 11 12 13 10 9 8 7 6 5 4 3 2 1

Contents

Contributors

K. L. Agster
Brown University, Providence, RI, USA

J. B. Aimone
Salk Institute for Biological Studies, La Jolla CA, USA

E. G. Antzoulatos
The University of Texas Medical School at Houston, Houston, TX, USA

B. W. Balleine
University of California, Los Angeles, CA, USA

D. A. Balota
Washington University, St. Louis, MO, USA

J. L. Banko
Vanderbilt University Medical Center, Nashville, TN, USA

M. F. Bear
Massachusetts Institute of Technology, Cambridge, MA, USA

R. S. Blumenfeld
University of California at Davis, Davis, CA, USA

M. E. Bouton
University of Vermont, Burlington, VT, USA

R. D. Burwell
Brown University, Providence, RI, USA

J. H. Byrne
The University of Texas Medical School at Houston, Houston, TX, USA

C. A. Chapleau
University of Alabama at Birmingham, Birmingham, AL, USA

J. Chin
Gladstone Institute of Neurological Disease and University of California, San Francisco, CA, USA

K. M. Christian
National Institutes of Health, Bethesda, MD, USA

J. H. Coane
Washington University, St. Louis, MO, USA

J. M. Ellenbogen
Beth Israel Deaconess Medical Center, Brigham and Women's Hospital, Harvard Medical School, Boston, MA, USA

A. N. Eslick
Duke University, Durham, NC, USA

L. K. Fazio
Duke University, Durham, NC, USA

D. Fioravante
The University of Texas Medical School at Houston, Houston, TX, USA

F. H. Gage
Salk Institute for Biological Studies, La Jolla CA, USA

S. E. Gathercole
University of York, York, UK

P. E. Gold
University of Illinois at Urbana-Champaign, Champaign, IL, USA

M. K. Goode
Washington University, St. Louis, MO, USA

E. L. Grigorenko
Yale University, New Haven, CT, USA

C. Hansel
Erasmus University Medical Center, Rotterdam, The Netherlands

S. Jessberger
Salk Institute for Biological Studies, La Jolla CA, USA

J. E. LeDoux
New York University, New York, NY, USA

J. M. Levenson
University of Wisconsin School of Medicine and Public Health, Madison, WI, USA

F. D. Lorenzetti
The University of Texas Medical School at Houston, Houston, TX, USA

E. J. Marsh
Duke University, Durham, NC, USA

A. Martin
National Institute of Mental Health, Bethesda, MD, USA

K. B. McDermott
Washington University, St. Louis, MO, USA

J. L. McGaugh
University of California at Irvine, Irvine, CA, USA

R. R. Miller
State University of New York at Binghamton, Binghamton, NY, USA

S. B. Moldakarimov
Salk Institute for Biological Studies, La Jolla, CA, USA

R. Mozzachiodi
The University of Texas Medical School at Houston, Houston, TX, USA

L. Mucke
Gladstone Institute of Neurological Disease and University of California, San Francisco, CA, USA

E. J. Nestler
The University of Texas Southwestern Medical Center, Dallas, TX, USA

R. J. Nudo
University of Kansas Medical Center, Kansas City, KS, USA

S. B. Ostlund
University of California, Los Angeles, CA, USA

M. G. Packard
Texas A&M University, College Station, TX, USA

J. D. Payne
Beth Israel Deaconess Medical Center, Harvard Medical School, Harvard University, Boston, MA, USA

A. M. Poulos
University of California, Los Angeles, CA, USA

L. Pozzo-Miller
University of Alabama at Birmingham, Birmingham, AL, USA

C. Ranganath
University of California at Davis, Davis, CA, USA

E. D. Roberson
Gladstone Institute of Neurological Disease and University of California, San Francisco, CA, USA

H. L. Roediger, III
Washington University, St. Louis, MO, USA

E. T. Rolls
University of Oxford, Oxford, UK

B. Roozendaal
University of California at Irvine, Irvine, CA, USA

K. Rosenblum
Department of Neurobiology and Ethology, Mount Carmel, University of Haifa, Haifa, Israel

S. J. Sara
Collège de France, Paris, France

D. L. Schacter
Harvard University, Cambridge, MA, USA

G. E. Schafe
Yale University, New Haven, CT, USA

T. J. Sejnowski
Salk Institute for Biological Studies and University of California at San Diego, La Jolla, CA, USA

Y. Shrager
University of California at San Diego, La Jolla, CA, USA

W. K. Simmons
National Institute of Mental Health, Bethesda, MD, USA

L. R. Squire
University of California at San Diego, La Jolla, CA, USA

W. D. Stevens
Harvard University, Cambridge, MA, USA

R. Stickgold
Beth Israel Deaconess Medical Center, Harvard Medical School, Boston, MA, USA

J. D. Sweatt
University of Alabama at Birmingham, Birmingham, AL, USA

K. K. Szpunar
Washington University, St. Louis, MO, USA

R. F. Thompson
University of Southern California, Los Angeles, CA, USA

G. P. Urcelay
State University of New York at Binghamton, Binghamton, NY, USA

M. P. Walker
Beth Israel Deaconess Medical Center, Harvard Medical School, Boston, MA, USA

E. J. Weeber
Vanderbilt University Medical Center, Nashville, TN, USA

N. M. White
McGill University, Montreal, Canada

G. S. Wig
Harvard University, Cambridge, MA, USA

C. A. Winstanley
University of British Columbia, Vancouver, Canada

N. E. Winterbauer
University of California, Los Angeles, CA, USA

M. A. Wood
University of California at Irvine, Irvine, CA, USA

A. M. Woods
University of Vermont, Burlington, VT, USA

F. M. Zaromb
Washington University, St. Louis, MO, USA

INTRODUCTION

This single volume contains selected papers from the four volume *Learning and Memory: A Comprehensive Reference* (ISBN: 978-0-12-370504-4, and online at ScienceDirect.com). The goal of the *Comprehensive Reference* was to present an overview of the important and current topics of interest in scientific approaches to the study of learning and memory, covering a wide territory in depth. The *Comprehensive Reference* was divided into four volumes, resulting in *Learning Theory and Behavior* edited by Randolf Menzel; *Cognitive Psychology of Memory* edited by Henry Roediger III; *Memory Systems* edited by Howard Eichenbaum; and *Molecular Mechanisms of Memory* edited by David Sweatt. The goal for this new single volume, however, was to select major aspects of the field of learning and memory represented by the *Comprehensive Reference* and to present them in a form that is accessible for researchers and students as a reference or textbook. The original four volumes were transformed into a single volume with one-sixth of the original material organized by theme. While an attempt was made to cover the field in as much depth and breadth as possible, the editor regrets having to leave out many stellar chapters from the *Comprehensive Reference.*

The volume begins with an introduction to the types of memory and their presently used definitions. The chapter by Roediger, Zaromb, and Goode provides a lexicon of the primary terms that readers will encounter in subsequent chapters. This set of definitions is essential for navigation through the volume as precise definitions for different types of memory are not universally agreed upon, and, in some cases, authors use different descriptors for phenomena that seem identical (e.g., declarative memory and explicit memory). The second chapter, "Declarative Memory System: Amnesia" by Squire and Shrager nicely complements the first chapter, albeit from a different perspective. Although it may seem odd to have a chapter on amnesia at the beginning of the book, studies of amnesia have provided key insights in defining and describing different memory systems. Additionally, this chapter introduces the readers to the anatomy of the different memory systems. The concept of multiple parallel memory systems is continued in the next chapter by White, and also contains a review of theories of learning (e.g., S-S *vs.* S-R), reinforcers, and learning paradigms, completing the general introduction to memory.

The next five chapters comprise a thorough description of the different memory systems. Stevens, Wig, and Schacter focus on priming, which is a major form of implicit memory, and introduces the readers to the technique of functional magnetic resonance imaging (fMRI), a technique that has become a major tool for identifying which regions of the brain are involved in different memory processes. In the next chapter, Balota and Coane tackle the field of semantic memory, including the relationship between semantic and episodic memory, and emphasize the major themes at the center of research on what it means "to know something." Martin and Simmons continue with what is known about the locations in the brain for semantic memories, including more examples illustrating the power of fMRI. Szpunar and McDermott give a report on the history of episodic memory, the present knowledge of the anatomy of the episodic memory system, and describe the phenomenon of "mental time travel." They also address the intensely debated issue of whether episodic memory is a uniquely human phenomenon. Finally, Gathercole provides an introduction to the major alternative theoretical approaches to the study of working memory, including a discussion of working memory in learning during human development.

The anatomy of two brain structures critical for memory is the topic of the next two chapters as knowledge of the anatomy and microcircuitry is essential for understanding the analyses of memory mechanisms.

Ranganath and Blumenfeld present a framework for understanding the role of different prefrontal regions of the brain in memory processes including working memory, while Burwell and Agster present an overview of the functional anatomy of structures that support episodic memory in the mammalian brain (hippocampal formation and parahippocampal region). The hippocampus has become a focus of intense investigation by cellular neurobiologists interested in memory mechanisms both because the anatomy is well described and because physiological measures can be made on acute brain slices.

Following the description of memory systems and their anatomy, the focus moves to changes at the cell level and mechanisms implicated in various examples of learning and memory. Sweatt describes the cellular phenomenon of long-term potentiation (LTP), an enduring enhancement of synaptic transmission produced by a brief burst of neuronal activity, while Hansel and Bear review the opposite phenomenon, long-term depression (LTD). Both LTP and LTD are widely regarded as candidates for mechanisms underlying memory. One way in which the changes in synaptic efficacy associated with LTP and LTD might be expressed is through changes in the structure of the synapse. The chapter by Chapleau and Pozzo-Miller discusses the evidence for activity-dependent structural plasticity of dendritic spines in the hippocampus and introduces the reader to progress in understanding the cellular mechanisms underlying memory disorders, such as those associated with Rett syndrome. Mozzachiodi and Byrne discuss the evidence that learning paradigms, as well as patterns of electrical stimulation of neurons and neural pathways, produce persistent changes in intrinsic neuronal excitability, showing that changes in synaptic strength are not the exclusive means for the expression of neuronal plasticity associated with learning and memory.

Although some "memories" might be localized in a single cell or synapse or a very small group of cells, most memories (particularly complex memories) are more likely to be distributed over many neurons and synapses, and theories and models about how these systems operate need to be developed. Moldakarimov and Sejnowski provide an overview of basic learning rules and they give examples of learning algorithms used in neural network models, including those that combine several types of plasticity. Rolls describes a quantitative computational theory of hippocampal function and then compares it with other models.

The next eight chapters review the substantial progress that has been made in analyzing examples of nondeclarative (procedural) learning in a variety of different model systems. Packard reviews the basic neurobiology of procedural learning including the role for dorsal striatal dopamine, acetylcholine, and glutamate in memory consolidation underlying stimulus-response learning. Several invertebrates have proven to be extremely useful model systems for gaining insights into the neural and molecular mechanisms of simple forms of procedural learning. Indeed, the pioneering discoveries of Eric Kandel using the marine mollusk *Aplysia* were recognized by his receiving the Nobel Prize in Physiology or Medicine in 2000. Fioravante et al. and Lorenzetti and Byrne describe work on *Aplysia* that has provided mechanistic insights into simple forms of nonassociative learning (habituation and sensitization) and forms of associative learning (classical and operant conditioning). Poulos, Christian, and Thompson review the tremendous progress made in understanding the neural systems and mechanisms underlying associative learning of discrete motor responses (e.g., eyeblink reflexes) and conditioned fear. Schafe and Le Doux expand the discussion of neural and molecular mechanisms of fear, including the more complex aspects of fear learning and the fear learning system in human beings. Rosenblum describes taste behavior and the associated molecular and cellular mechanisms of learning and remembering taste, and presents the current working model of taste memory formation, consolidation, and retention. The importance of reinforcement/reward in learning is introduced by Ostlund, Winterbauer and Balleine as they describe a theory of a reward system in which associations and memories guide choices and anticipation in a manner more complex than simple Pavlovian conditioning. Winstanley and Nestler describe the neural circuitry of reward and the role of dopamine and intracellular signaling pathways. In the final chapter on nondeclarative learning, Nudo reviews nonhuman primate neurophysiology and the human neuroimaging studies that demonstrate the distributed network in the brain that underlies different aspects of motor learning.

The next three chapters deal with the consolidation of memory and memory modulation. Payne, Ellenbogen, Walker, and Stickgold provide a thorough and up-to-date review of the role of sleep in the consolidation of memory. McGaugh and Roozendaal review animal research and human research on how stress hormones, activated by emotional arousal, can modulate (depress) the consolidation of memory and recent experiences. They also review evidence that a coordinated modulatory system serves to regulate the strength of memories in relation to their emotional significance, and to review evidence that stress hormones influence memory retrieval and working memory. On the other side, Gold discusses drugs that can enhance or strengthen memories.

The next group of chapters examines aspects of the fragility of memories. Bouton and Woods discuss extinction (decrease in learned behavior) and reviews the literature from both classical and operant conditioning, as well as evidence for extinction as context-dependent learning rather than forgetting. Sara reviews the literature on the intriguing phenomenon known as reconsolidation in which a memory becomes fragile when it is recalled. When memory fails, is it because the memory is lost or because it is present but cannot be accessed? In the next chapter, Urcelay and Miller review the retrieval process. Finally, there is the issue of false memories, which is reviewed by Marsh, Eslick, and Fazio. An understanding of false memories not only provides insights into the normal memory process, but also has fundamental implications for eyewitness suggestibility in criminal cases.

While fragility of memory is universal, certain diseases rob of us our memory along with our knowledge of who we are. Chin, Roberson, and Mucke provide a comprehensive review of the molecular mechanisms underlying Alzheimer's disease, which primarily affects the elderly. Developmental disorders also affect memory systems. Grigorenko reviews developmental learning disabilities along with possible correlates and interventions. Banko and Weeber describe the progress being made in understanding Angelman Syndrome, a specific developmental disorder which affects memory. They describe the implications of CaMKII misregulation as a molecular cause as well as the potential mechanisms underlying CaMKII dysfunction. Levenson and Wood extend the discussion of mechanisms of Rett syndrome from the earlier chapter by Chapleau and Pozzo-Miller. They also explore the hypothesis that regulation of chromatin structure through epigenetic mechanisms represents a unique molecular substrate for long-term information storage. How are memory systems formed? Does learning involve the synthesis of new neurons? Can damaged memory systems be replaced with new neurons? These are some of the key questions for the future. In the final chapter, Jessberger, Aimone, and Gage describe the phenomenon of neurogenesis, a process that has only been recognized relatively recently as occurring throughout life.

It is hoped that this volume will be extremely useful as an introduction to the field of study of learning and memory, and that the shortened version will be appropriate as a textbook for upper division and graduate students. The *Comprehensive Reference* is always available as a resource for students and scientists, but this shorter volume should be more available for everyone's book shelf. Again, the editor thanks all of the contributors for their terrific contributions to the *Comprehensive Reference*, and regrets that only a subset can be included here.

John H. Byrne

1 A Typology of Memory Terms

H. L. Roediger, III, F. M. Zaromb, and M. K. Goode, Washington University in St. Louis, St. Louis, MO, USA

1.1 Introduction

The English language provides us with the term memory to denote several interrelated ideas, such as 'the power of the mind to remember things' or 'something remembered from the past; a recollection' (both quotes are from the Oxford American Dictionary). These definitions of memory are fine for everyday conversation and communication, but scientists interested in studying the biochemical, neural, or psychological underpinnings of this topic have found the need to describe many distinctions about memory that laypeople do not use. Such a need is further underscored by a growing interest in interdisciplinary approaches to the study of human memory (*See* Chapter 9) and in adapting cognitive research paradigms to the study of nonhuman animal learning, an area that has developed largely in isolation of the human memory research tradition (e.g., Wright, 1998; Wright and Roediger, 2003). This chapter is intended to explain the meaning of some of the most popular terms that have been contributed to the literature.

We aim to paint with a fairly broad brush and not to get involved in matters such as whether one term (say, implicit memory) is to be preferred to another term (indirect memory), although buckets of ink have been spilt on these matters. Rather, we intend to provide general definitions and meanings of terms without defending them as theoretically critical (or not). In this sense, the chapter is descriptive rather than theoretical, although we fully understand that by choosing one's terms and their definitions, one implicitly adopts a theory.

How many types of memory are there? In the early 1970s, Tulving wrote: "In a recent collection of essays edited by Norman (1970) one can count references to some 25 or so categories of memory, if one is willing to assume that any unique combination of an adjectival modifier with the main term refers to something other than any of the references of other such unique combinations" (Tulving, 1972: 382). Tulving added two more terms (episodic memory and semantic memory) in that chapter. Yet more important for present purposes, Tulving continued to keep a list of memory terms as he encountered them. Thirty-five years later, Tulving (2007) wrote another chapter entitled "Are there 256 different kinds of memory?" which was the number of combinations of the adjective + memory sort that he had collected by that time. The list goes from abnormal memory (at the beginning), through terms such as diencephalic memory and false memory, then on to rote memory and sensory memory, and finally, at the end of the list, to working memory. (There are 250 others.)

We hasten to add that we are not going to cover 256 kinds of memory in this chapter. We aim to provide a lexicon of some of the primary terms that readers will find in the four volumes of *Learning and Memory: A Comprehensive Reference.* We have tried to weave the terms together in a loose sort of story, so as not to provide just a glossary with a long list of terms and definitions. The story is one conception of the varieties of memory provided elsewhere (Roediger et al., 2002). We try to give a verbal definition of each type of memory we chose to include, as well as a practical example of how the type of memory might operate in a person or other animal, and we usually point to a paradigm by which this type of memory is studied, to provide kind of an operational definition.

The reader will notice that in some cases the same memory term (e.g., episodic memory) may refer to a process, entity (e.g., memory trace), system, mental state of awareness, or type of cognitive task, depending on the context. Such linguistic flexibility can easily lead to confusion, so we attempt to distinguish among different uses of each term where appropriate. The index of the book can be used to glean other uses of the term. In addition, semantic confusion can easily arise from the types of metaphors employed to describe a memory concept. Most cognitive psychologists use a spatial metaphor in which memories are conceived as physical entities stored in a mind space, and the act of remembering involves searching through the mind's space in order to retrieve the objects of memory (e.g., Roediger, 1980; Tulving, 2000; *See* Chapter 31). In contrast, others have proposed nonspatial metaphors that make analogies to concepts such as strength – memories are comparable to muscles whose strengths are directly related to performance on memory tasks (e.g., Hull, 1943); construction – the act of remembering involves constructing memories from available information (e.g., Bartlett, 1932); depth of processing – memory is a by-product of the level of perceptual analysis (Craik and Tulving, 1975); or auditory resonance – memories are like notes played on piano keys or individual tuning forks resonating (e.g., Wechsler, 1963; Ratcliff, 1978), to list but a few. To reiterate, we do not mean to provide exhaustive coverage, but rather to paint with broad strokes and to represent the way memory terms are used by cognitive psychologists and others.

We begin with consideration of some general distinctions made among types of memory. We then turn to the idea that it is useful to catalog memories by their time course in the system (from brief sensory memories, to short-term conscious memories, to various sorts of long-term memory). Most work has been devoted to the various types of long-term memory that have been described, so this is the focus of the next section of the chapter. Inevitably, given our organization, there is a bit of repetition because we needed to cover the same term (say, episodic memory) in more than one context.

1.2 Broad Distinctions

This section of the chapter is devoted to consideration of several broad distinctions among forms of memory. We consider the issue of explicit and implicit memory, conscious and unconscious forms of memory, voluntary and involuntary retention, intentional and incidental learning and retrieval, declarative and procedural memory, and retrospective and prospective memory.

1.2.1 Explicit and Implicit Memory

Explicit memory refers to cases of conscious recollection. When we remember our trip to Paris or recognize that some words occurred in a recent list, these are instances of explicit memory. In cases of explicit retention, people respond to a direct request for information about their past, and such tests are called explicit memory tests. On the other hand, on tests of implicit memory, people are asked to perform some task, and the measure of interest is how some prior experience affects the task. For example, take the simple case of the word elephant appearing in a long list of words. If subjects are given a recognition test in which they are instructed to identify words studied in the list (and to reject nonstudied words), then their choice of elephant as a studied word would represent an instance of explicit retention. However, if a different group of subjects were given the same set of words to study and then were given a word stem completion test (with instructions to say the first word that comes to mind to the word stem ele_______), then this would constitute a test of implicit memory. The relevant measure on this test is priming, the greater probability of completing the stem with elephant rather than other plausible words (element, elegant, electricity, etc.) when the word has been studied than when it has not been studied. For example, the probability of producing elephant to the word stem might be 10% if the word had not been studied in the list and 40% when it had been studied, which would constitute a 30% priming effect. One reason for believing that these two measures represent different forms of memory is that they can be dissociated by many experimental (and subject) variables.

Graf and Schacter (1985) introduced the terms explicit and implicit memory to the field. Explicit retention refers to most typical measures of retention that psychologists have used over the years (recall, recognition, and their variations), whereas implicit memory refers to transfer measures when people may not be aware of using memory at all (Jacoby, 1984). Some writers prefer the terms direct and indirect memory for this contrast, because explicit tests measure memory directly, whereas implicit tests are indirect measures. Schacter (1987) offers a fine historical review of concepts related to implicit memory.

1.2.2 Conscious and Unconscious Forms of Memory

Conscious and unconscious forms of memory refer to the mental states of awareness associated with remembering the past. Attempts to describe human memory in relation to consciousness hearken back to the early introspective tradition of experimental psychology and the writings of Wilhelm Wundt, Edward Titchener, and William James (e.g., James, 1890/1950), as well as the psychoanalytic tradition and especially the well-known writings of Sigmund Freud (e.g., Freud, 1917/1982). Less well known is the fact that in the very first experiments on memory, Ebbinghaus (1885/1964) devised a relearning/savings technique for measuring memory that could detect unconscious knowledge. In fact, Ebbinghaus preferred savings measures over the merely introspective techniques of recall and recognition, because these latter tests cannot, almost by definition, measure memories that are not conscious (Slamecka, 1985).

In contemporary studies of memory, conscious recollection refers to the subjective awareness of remembering information encountered in the past, a process that is likened to the experience of mentally traveling back in time (Tulving, 1985). Tulving has also termed this state of awareness autonoetic (self-knowing) consciousness. In contrast, a noetic (knowing) state of consciousness is the type of awareness associated with retrieving previously learned information, such as a geographical, historical, or personal fact, without recollecting details about the place and time in which that information was originally acquired. For example, noetic consciousness might characterize the experience of a person being asked to name the capital of Canada and who, after thinking for a bit, responds “Ottawa” without remembering when he or she last encountered or originally learned this fact. Autonoetic consciousness, on the other hand, is reflected by the person’s ability to think back to and re-experience an episode, such as a visit to Ottawa.

Conscious recollection may be intentional and effortful, or it may occur without the intent to explicitly remember information relevant to a given memory task, as is the case with involuntary conscious recollection (e.g., Richardson-Klavehn et al., 1996). This term refers to the fact that one may suddenly be remembering some event from the past without ever having tried to do so. In some cases of patients with damage to the frontal lobes, they may experience confabulation, or the experience of conscious recollection occurring for events that never occurred. The patients believe they are having memories, but in many cases the events are preposterous and could not have occurred. Such cases are extremely rare yet do occur.

Unconscious retention may be observed in performance on tests of implicit memory where individuals indirectly demonstrate their prior exposure to the test material under conditions in which they do not consciously recognize the material. Tulving has referred to the state of awareness associated with unconscious retention as anoetic consciousness. Unconscious retention also occurs when subjects show savings in retention without being able to recollect the experience that gave rise to the savings, as Ebbinghaus (1885/1964) first pointed out.

1.2.3 Voluntary and Involuntary Retention

Voluntary retention refers to deliberate, willful recollection, whereas involuntary or incidental retention refers to recollection that occurs without conscious effort. Involuntary retention, as the name implies, refers to memories that arise in consciousness unbidden, with no conscious effort to recollect. For example, in studies of autobiographical memory (memory for events in one's life), voluntary recollections may be assessed by asking individuals to remember personal events in response to queries (e.g., recall a memory from your past that is associated with an automobile). The naturalistic study of involuntary memories can be achieved by asking individuals to keep a diary and jotting down memories that seem to come out of the blue, as it were, wherever and whenever they occur (e.g., Berntsen and Rubin, 2002; Rubin and Berntsen, 2003).

It should be noted, though, that acts of voluntary or involuntary recollection may not be entirely pure, and one may influence the other. For instance, a person's attempt to remember the details of a baseball game that occurred years ago might be influenced by his inadvertently remembering details of a more recent game. Or when engaging in a test of implicit memory, such as completing word fragments, a person might become aware of the fact that some of the target words were encountered during the study phase and, therefore, might intentionally think back to the study phase to help complete the test word fragments (Jacoby, 1991). In addition, as previously mentioned, one might experience involuntary conscious recollection whereby thoughts of a past event come to mind automatically, and it might take further reflection to realize how the memory came to mind (Richardson-Klavehn et al., 1996).

1.2.4 Intentional and Incidental Learning and Retrieval

1.2.4.1 Intentional and incidental learning

Intentional and incidental learning refer to whether or not people intend to learn material to which they are exposed. Of course, as we go about the world watching TV, driving, or reading the paper, we rarely say to ourselves: I need to remember this commercial on TV. Educational systems provide the main form of relentless intentional learning, although of course we all sometimes try to remember the name of a new acquaintance or the name of a book or movie someone recommended. In the laboratory, intentional or incidental learning is manipulated by instructions to subjects. In an intentional learning situation, an individual studies certain materials with the express purpose of remembering them at some later point in time. In an incidental learning task, the same materials might be provided but with an orienting task to induce some sort of processing of the material but without any instructions concerning a later memory test. For example, in a standard levels-of-processing manipulation (e.g., Craik and Tulving, 1975), a person might be shown a list of words and asked to judge whether each word (e.g., BEAR) is presented in capital letters (graphemic or structural processing), whether it rhymes with a certain word like chair (phonemic processing), or whether it fits into a certain category such as animals (semantic processing). Subjects in incidental learning conditions would be told that the researchers are interested in studying the speed with which people can make such decisions. In the intentional learning conditions, they would be told the same rationale, but would also be told that their memory for the words will be tested later.

The natural expectation is that material studied under intentional learning conditions is better retained than under incidental learning conditions, and this outcome is sometimes obtained (Postman, 1964). However, at least when semantic orienting tasks are used, the differences between incidental and intentional learning conditions are surprisingly slight and often there is no difference at all (Craik and Tulving, 1975; Hyde and Jenkins, 1969).

1.2.4.2 Intentional and incidental retrieval

Just as intentionality can be manipulated during study of materials, so can it be manipulated during testing. In fact, the distinction already drawn between explicit and implicit memory tests can be cast in this light. Explicit tests require intentional retrieval, but implicit tests reveal incidental retrieval (Jacoby, 1984). Under intentional retrieval conditions, a person is asked to engage in conscious, deliberate recollection of a past event (e.g., recalling a word from a previously studied list that completes a word stem). By contrast, incidental retrieval involves giving people the same word stem with the instruction to write the first word that comes to mind. Incidental retrieval is indexed by priming, the better performance in completing the stem with the target word relative to a control condition in which the word had not been studied.

As noted, the comparison between intentional and incidental retrieval is not necessarily a pure one, because performance on explicit memory tests may be affected by incidental retrieval just as performance on implicit memory tests can be influenced by intentional retrieval (Jacoby, 1991). Several solutions exist for attempting to gain leverage on this issue. Schacter and his colleagues (1989) proposed the retrieval intentionality criterion to test for the contamination of incidental retrieval measures by conscious recollection. The basic idea is to compare incidental and intentional recollection, holding all other study and test conditions constant. If performance differs markedly between the two tests when all conditions are held constant except for instructions just prior to the test, then one can have greater confidence that they measure intentional (conscious) and incidental (automatic or unconscious) retrieval. Roediger et al. (1992) crossed intentional and incidental study and test conditions with other variables and showed that incidental tests reflected quite different patterns of performance from the intentional tests. Jacoby (1991) proposed a different method, the process dissociation procedure, to separate conscious from unconscious influences during retrieval. Although providing the details of his ingenious method is outside the scope of this chapter, his method has proved extraordinarily useful in separating conscious from unconscious (or automatic) cognitive processes.

1.2.5 Declarative and Nondeclarative Memory

Declarative memory and nondeclarative memory (sometimes referred to as procedural memory) are terms that have gained prominence following their use by Squire (1982), although the original distinction was proposed by Ryle (1949). Ryle distinguished between declarative knowledge (knowing that) and procedural knowledge (knowing how). For example, we know that Washington, D.C., is the capital of the United States, but we know how to tie our shoes.

More recently, Squire has proposed declarative memory as an overarching category that includes episodic memory (remembering specific events of the past) as well as semantic memory (general knowledge). Declarative memory processes rely upon the hippocampus and related structures in the medial-temporal lobe including the perirhinal, entorhinal, and parahippocampal cortices. As it has been extended, the term declarative memory has become a bit of a misnomer, because the concept is often applied to infrahuman species that are not prone to making declarations. (Ryle tied his distinction specifically to linguistic usage so that people would know that such and such occurred.)

Procedural memory was originally intended to cover motor skills, such as tying shoes, riding a bicycle, or typing (Ryle, 1949), but it was broadened to cover mental as well physical procedures. For example, the mental processes involved in multiplying 24×16 are examples of mental procedures that can be studied. As Squire (1992) developed his theory, the term procedural memory became broader and covered such topics as priming on implicit memory tests, classical conditioning of responses, and habituation. Because of these and other uses, the broader term nondeclarative memory came into use. It refers both to traditional procedural tasks and to others such as priming and skill learning. The distinction between declarative and nondeclarative types of memory rests partly on evidence that different brain structures are involved in various forms of memory. The evidence supporting the differences between the different forms of memory has come both from studies of human amnesic patients with damage to the medial-temporal lobes and in animals where such alterations can be achieved experimentally (e.g., Squire, 1992).

As noted, the term declarative memory originally referred to memories that could be verbally stated (Ryle, 1949). This term has also been broadened so that it now includes many other kinds of memory, including spatial memory, some types of long-term visual memory, and any other form of memory subserved by the hippocampal complex. Nondeclarative memories include all other types, whether they involve memories for physical movements and actions, priming, or skills.

Tulving (1985) has proposed a somewhat different schematic arrangement of episodic, semantic, and procedural memory systems. In Tulving's scheme, procedural memory is phylogenetically oldest and is shared among all organisms. Semantic memory grows out of (and depends upon) procedural memory. Episodic memory is evolutionarily most recent and, according to Tulving, only humans have this form of memory (see Tulving, 2005, for further elaboration). Different forms of consciousness are proposed for the three systems: anoetic (non-knowing) for procedural memory, noetic (knowing) for semantic memory, and autonoetic (self-knowing) for episodic memory. Tulving proposes that a critical function of autonoetic consciousness is planning for the future, which brings us to another critical distinction.

1.2.6 Retrospective and Prospective Memory

The vast majority of memory research deals with the ability to remember past events when given specific cues (as in explicit memory tests of recall or recognition) or with the effects of past experience on current behavior (priming on implicit memory tests). All tests that fall into these categories assess retrospective memory: memory for the past or effects of past experience on current behavior. In the past 2 decades, researchers have examined memory for intentions to be performed in the future, or prospective memory. Strictly speaking, prospective memory is retrospective in nature: it involves remembering a past intention. A prospective memory task differs from a retrospective memory tasks in that there is usually no explicit cue to elicit recall of the intention. Instead, a prospective memory task requires that subjects must use an environmental cue to know when to retrieve the intention, so it is a curious mix of incidental and intentional retrieval. We face prospective memory tasks all the time, whenever we need to remember to perform some act in the future. Prospective memory tasks can be classified as cue-based or event-based when some cue should remind us to perform an action (e.g., pass along a message to a friend when we see her) or time-based (e.g., remembering to take out the trash Tuesday evenings). Both cue-based and time-based prospective memory tasks have been investigated in naturalistic settings and in the laboratory. Retrieval of prospective memories may sometimes involve monitoring and may sometimes be spontaneous and effortless (Einstein and McDaniel, 2005).

We turn next to categorizations of memory based on (roughly) the time they persist, starting with varieties of short-term memory.

1.3 Types of Short-Term Memory

Information from the external world is believed to be represented in various storage systems that, roughly speaking, hold information for fractions of a second, seconds, or much longer. Atkinson and Shiffrin's (1969, 1971) influential theory, shown in **Figure 1**, provides one conceptualization. Our treatment here provides some amendments to their original theory.

1.3.1 Sensory Memories

The border between perceiving and remembering is blurred. There is no good answer to the question: When does perception end and memory begin? Even the operations in the two types of experiments are similar. When stimuli are presented rapidly to the visual or auditory system and some report or judgment is made quickly afterward, the experiment is referred to as one of perception. If the report or judgment is delayed after presentation, the study is usually called a memory experiment. Sensory memories are the brief holding systems for information presented to the various sensory systems; the information is thought to be held briefly in each system as it undergoes further processing.

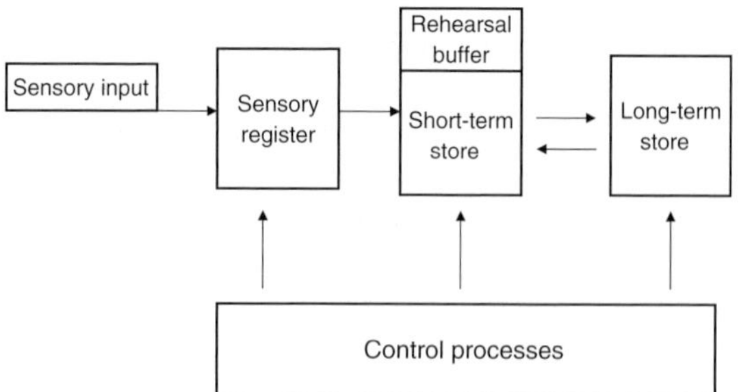

Figure 1 Simplified version of the original multi-store memory model of Shiffrin and Atkinson. Information is conceived as being transmitted through various memory stores. Adapted from Shiffrin RM and Atkinson RC (1969) Storage and retrieval processes in long-term memory. *Psychol. Rev.* 76: 179–193; used with permission of the American Psychological Association.

Sperling (1960) identified a rapidly fading store of visual information that he called precategorical visual storage. The term precategorical was in the title, because Sperling's evidence convinced him that the information was held in a relatively raw form, before linguistic categorizations had been applied. Somewhat later, other researchers proposed a system of precategorical acoustic storage, the auditory equivalent of Sperling's visual store (Crowder and Morton, 1969). These two sensory stores have been studied quite thoroughly by many researchers, but the names they are given in the literature today have been changed to iconic and echoic memory (following Neisser's (1967) suggested terminology). Iconic memory refers to the visual store, whereas echoic memory is used for auditory storage. Echoic storage seems to persist longer than iconic storage, although the decay characteristics of both systems have been debated and depend on such factors as stimulus intensity and the technique used to measure loss of information over time.

Researchers assume that similar storage systems exist for the other senses, but touch is the only sense that has been studied in this regard (and rather sporadically). The close association between smell and taste makes such studies difficult, although longer-term olfactory memory, in particular, has been well studied.

1.3.2 Short-Term Storage

Short-term memory (or short-term storage; the two are often used interchangeably) refers to retention of information in a system after information has been categorized and reached consciousness. In fact, contents of short-term memory are sometimes equated with the information of which a person is consciously aware. Information can be continually processed in short-term storage (e.g., via rehearsal or subvocal repetition). If a person is distracted, information is rapidly lost from this store.

Many different techniques have been developed to study aspects of short-term memory, but all have in common that subjects are given relatively brief numbers of items (often digits or words) and are asked to recall or recognize them later (often after some brief interfering task). Another term used for short-term memory is primary memory, owing to a distinction introduced by William James (1890/1950) between primary and secondary memory (reintroduced to the field much later by Waugh and Norman, 1965). Primary memory is what can be held in mind at once, whereas secondary memory referred to all other kinds of long-term memory. The terms short-term memory and long-term memory seem to have become accepted today.

1.3.3 Working Memory

Working memory is a term for the type of memory used to hold information for short periods of time while it is being manipulated (Baddeley, 2001). Working memory encompasses short-term memory, which in Baddeley's theory refers only to the short-term passive storage of information. Working memory also adds the concept of a central executive that functions to manipulate information in working memory and three separate storage components: the phonological loop, visuospatial sketchpad, and episodic buffer (see **Figure 2**). To test the short-term memory of humans, tasks that require short-term storage of information (such as digits in a digit span task) are used. On the other hand, working memory tests use tasks that require both short-term storage and manipulation of information (such as the operation span task, in which

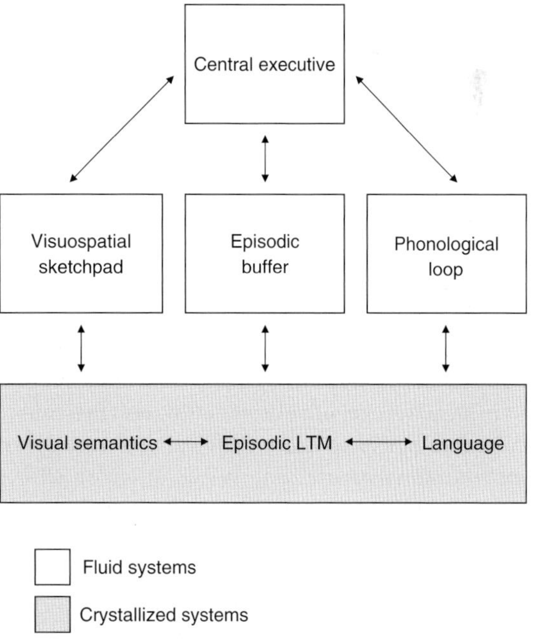

Figure 2 Baddeley's updated working memory model. Working memory is conceived as having separate storage components and a central executive process. LTM, long-term memory. Adapted from Baddeley A (2001) Is working memory still working? *Am. Psychol.* 56: 849–864; used with permission.

subjects solve simple arithmetic problems while also being given words to remember (*See* Chapter 8).

Three different storage systems are believed to constitute working memory. The phonological loop is involved in subvocal rehearsal and storage of auditory information (or written visual information) and is the most-studied component of working memory. The phonological loop is responsible for subvocal rehearsal and is used to account for many different empirical findings, such as the word length effect, or the finding that longer words are recalled less well than shorter words (because they take longer to rehearse).

The visuospatial sketchpad is similar to the phonological loop, except it maintains visual and spatial information, rather than acoustic information. The visual and spatial components of the sketchpad are at least partially separable, because one can observe dissociations between performance on visual working memory tasks and spatial working memory tasks (Baddeley, 2001). Most of the work on the visuospatial sketchpad up to now has focused on dissociating it from the other components of working memory.

The episodic buffer is the newest component of working memory, proposed only recently by Baddeley (2000) to explain several experimental findings. The episodic buffer is much like the phonological loop or the visuospatial sketchpad: It is a short-term store of information, although it is assumed to be able to store information of different modalities. Any information that is retrieved from long-term episodic memory (see section titled 'Episodic memory') is temporarily stored and manipulated in the episodic buffer.

The central executive component of working memory controls the subsystems. Some critics have complained that the concept is underspecified and that the concept is used to explain findings not well handled by the basic model. However, the executive component has much in common with other proposals of a central executive attention system that is used to explain how people can divide attention to different sources of information, switch attention among sources or tasks, or focus attention exclusively on one task.

1.3.4 Long-Term Working Memory

Long-term working memory extends the concept of working memory to account for a person's ability to readily access and utilize information stored in long-term memory. The concept of long-term working memory is particularly useful in explaining how skilled readers have the ability to easily read and comprehend texts. Indeed, the act of reading seems to require much more capacity and flexibility than the proposal for short-term or working memory can offer. A skilled reader must keep in mind words from previous sentences, paragraphs, or pages of text and readily access prior background knowledge in order to quickly and fluently process upcoming words and understand the text as a whole (e.g., Ericsson and Kintsch, 1995).

The concept of long-term working memory is also used to describe the superior mnemonic skills of experts functioning within their domain of expertise. For instance, chess masters demonstrate a remarkable ability to quickly encode and accurately remember the positions of every piece on a chess board sampled from the middle of a game, or to readily call to mind moves played in thousands of previous games in order to decide how to make the next move in a game. While researchers have attempted to explain the superior memory capacity of experts in their domain within the limits of short-term memory (Chase and Simon, 1973), evidence suggests that expert memory performance is mediated by long-term memory (e.g., Chase and Ericsson, 1982; Charness, 1991).

In contrast to the limited, fixed capacity of short-term working memory, the capacity of long-term term working memory is assumed to be flexible and may even be expanded through training. Thus, according to Ericsson and Kintsch (1995), long-term working memory is not a general cognitive ability, but rather a specialized ability that is acquired through the development of expertise for specific domains of knowledge. On the other hand, long-term working memory still depends upon the maintenance and utilization of a few retrieval cues in working memory that are, in turn, linked to retrieval structures stored in long-term memory.

1.4 Varieties of Long-Term Memory

Long-term memory is one of the most abused terms in psychology (and there is great competition for this honor). The reason is that the term is made to cover nearly every kind of memory not covered in the previous section. The term is used to refer to retention of words from the middle of a list presented 15 s previously to recollection of early childhood memories.

Not surprisingly, there exist various ways of carving up this huge subject. One is by type of material and mode of presentation, with the primary distinctions being among verbal memory, visual/spatial memory, and olfactory memory. Relatedly, learning of motor skills (sometimes called procedural memory, as discussed in the section 'Declarative and nondeclarative memory') is another critical and somewhat separate topic, sometimes called kinesthetic memory.

Another set of distinctions, which cut across those above, are among types of declarative (or perhaps explicit) memory: Episodic memory, autobiographical memory, semantic memory, and collective memory. We begin discussing specific codes thought to underlie long-term memory and then turn to the various types of explicit, declarative memory that have been proposed.

1.4.1 Code-Specific Forms of Retention

As humans possess multiple senses, there are multiple ways to sense new information and to encode that information. Raw sensory information comes in as visual, auditory, or olfactory information, as well as in other modalities. However, memories for tastes have not been much studied and because smell so greatly affects taste, separating these modalities would be difficult. Haptic memory, referring to memory for skin sensations, is also not much studied, although kinesthetic memory (for muscular movements) is a well-studied area. Studying memory for information presented in different sensory modalities has revealed both similarities and remarkable differences in how modality affects memory performance.

1.4.1.1 Visual–spatial memory

Memory for scenes and spatial relationships is often referred to as visual–spatial memory or just spatial memory. This type of memory is responsible for humans navigating around town in a car and for squirrels finding buried caches of acorns. Although spatial memory and episodic memory both rely on the hippocampus and surrounding areas, some theorists have argued that spatial memory is different from episodic memory and other relational (semantic) memory systems because it requires the formation of mental maps (O'Keefe and Nadel, 1978). On the other hand, Mackintosh (2002) argued that spatial learning is no different than other types of associative learning.

1.4.1.2 Imagery

Information presented either in events or pictures or words may be represented in the spatial system in imaginal form. One may see a butterfly and remember its appearance using this imaginal coding, or one may hear the word butterfly and be asked to form an image of the named insect. Converting verbal memories to images aids their memorability, either because the image is a deeply meaningful form (Nelson, 1979) or because coding information in verbal and imaginal codes provides additional retrieval routes to the information (Paivio, 1986).

1.4.1.3 Olfactory memory

Olfactory memory is more difficult to study than visual or auditory memory. Due to limitations of human olfaction, memory for odors has generally been tested with recognition tests, not with recall tests (see Herz and Engen, 1996, for a review). Olfactory memories seem to differ in some ways from other forms of memory, such as a tendency of smells to be particularly evocative of emotional memories. Indeed, the olfactory nerve is only two synapses away from the amygdala (responsible for certain types of emotions) and three synapses away from the hippocampus (which is critical for long-term memory). Olfactory memory is similar to auditory and visual memory in that performance on recognition tests decreases as the distracter set increases and as distracter similarity to targets increases. However, olfactory memory does differ from other kinds of memory in two respects. First, olfactory memory is highly resistant to forgetting: Multiple studies have shown that recognition performance for odors in a laboratory preparation is only about 5% less after 1 year than after a 30-s delay. Related to this remarkably flat forgetting curve is the finding that olfactory memory is highly resistant to retroactive interference. Proactive interference reduces olfactory memory performance greatly.

1.4.1.4 Skill learning

Perhaps the largest subset of different kinds of memory is the broad class of memories classified as types of kinesthetic memory or skill learning or procedural memory (the last of which was described earlier). Kinesthetic memories are those involved in motor skills: The swing of a baseball bat, how to keep a hula hoop going, and so on through hundreds of other examples. These are motor skills, the classic type of procedural memory. However, many other types of skill learning exist. There is verbal skill learning, such as learning to read distorted or inverted text (Kolers and Roediger, 1984) – learning of grammars, both real ones and artificial ones – and even the skillful learning of what items belong in what categories. Although a review of the various kinds of skill learning is beyond the scope of this article (see Gupta and Cohen, 2002), we can briefly point out one of the most consistent findings across the procedural learning literature: Skill learning is highly specific and transfer is often quite narrow, for example, learning to read inverted (upside down) text does not aid in learning to read backward text (Kolers and Roediger, 1984; Healy, 2007).

1.4.1.5 Verbal memory

Doubtless the greatest form of memory recoding and storage for human beings is based on language. People can remember events as verbal information even if they were originally presented in a different form (visual, auditory, or even olfactory or kinesthetic). Psychologists have long believed in the primacy of verbal coding, and Glanzer and Clark (1964) even proposed a verbal loop hypothesis, which theorized that all human experience is recoded into language. Subsequent research indicates that this hypothesis was a bit overstated and other forms of coding exist, but nonetheless verbal coding and verbal memories are critically important in human cognition. Verbal recoding can be impaired by instructing subjects to perform some irrelevant verbalization such as repeating nonsense words while being exposed to nonverbal information, a technique known as articulatory suppression.

1.4.2 Forms of Explicit Memory

We have covered these earlier in the 'Broad distinctions' section, but review them again here in more detail and provide more detailed examples of tasks used to study these forms of memory.

1.4.2.1 Episodic memory

Episodic memory refers to memory for particular events situated in space and time, as well as the underlying cognitive processes and neural mechanisms involved in remembering those events. A key ingredient of episodic memory that distinguishes it from other forms of memory is the retrieval of information regarding the spatial and/or temporal context in which the remembered event occurred. As previously mentioned, episodic memory is also associated with autonoetic consciousness, considered by some researchers to be an evolutionarily advanced, unique human capacity (e.g., Wheeler, 2000; Tulving, 2002, 2005).

One can point to a wide variety of examples of episodic memory, ranging from remembering what a friend wore at a party the night before to individual words studied in a list moments ago. In most contexts, episodic memory is synonymous with explicit memory, although the former term is usually used to represent a memory system and the latter term to designate types of tests that are used. Many tests have been designed to measure certain aspects of episodic memory in the lab, including free recall (recall of a set of material in any order), serial recall (recall of events in order), cued recall (recall of events given specific cues), recognition judgments (recognizing studied material intermixed with nonstudied material), source judgments (recognizing the source of presented material, such as whether it was presented auditorily or visually). Subjects may also be asked to make judgments of the recency of an event, its frequency of occurrence, or of some other quality. In addition, subjects can be asked to make metamemory judgments, or judgments about their memories. For example, a student might be asked to rate how confident he or she is in the accuracy of his/her recollections. Similarly, individuals might be asked to judge whether they can remember the moment an event occurred or the context in which it occurred or whether they only just know that they were previously encountered but cannot remember the context (Tulving, 1985). These remember/know judgments (with remember judgments reflecting episodic recollection) have been much studied.

1.4.2.2 Autobiographical memory

Autobiographical memory refers to memory for one's personal history (Robinson, 1976). Examples might include memories for experiences that occurred in childhood, the first time learning to drive a car, or even one's Social Security number or home address. Brewer (1986) divided autobiographical memories into categories of personal memories, autobiographical facts, and generic personal memories. Personal memories are memories for specific events in one's life that are accompanied by imagery. As such, personal autobiographical memories are thought by some to be the real-world analog to episodic memories as studied in the lab, because they are the episodes of one's life as dated in space and time. On the other hand, autobiographical facts are facts about the person that are devoid of personally experienced temporal or spatial context information. For example, you know when and where you were born, but you cannot remember the event. Finally, generic personal memory refers to more abstract knowledge about oneself (what you are like) or to acquired procedural knowledge such as knowledge of how to ride a bicycle, ski, or play a musical instrument. Despite the conceptual overlap across classification schemes, a unique feature of autobiographical memory is that it must directly relate to oneself or one's sense of personal history.

A variety of techniques have been used to examine autobiographical memory. One approach is to simply ask people to report the most important personal events of their life (e.g., Fitzgerald, 1988; Berntsen and Rubin, 2002; Rubin and Berntsen, 2003) or to report self-defining memories (e.g., Conway et al., 2004). Another frequently used method is to ask people to describe for each of a given set of cue words the first personal memory that comes to mind, e.g., being given the word window and asked to retrieve a discrete event from your past involving a window. This task is known as the Galton-Crovitz cueing technique after its inventor (Galton, 1879) and its first modern proponent (Crovitz and Schiffman, 1974).

Many studies have plotted the temporal distribution of autobiographical memories across the life span, as described more fully by Conway. Briefly, such distributions usually exhibit three striking features (Rubin et al., 1986; Janssen et al., 2005). The first is that people tend to recall very little from the first few years of their life. This is referred to as childhood amnesia. Second, people tend to recall quite a few events from early adulthood, roughly the ages 15–25. This effect is called the reminiscence bump. Finally, most reported events are recalled from the last few years, which (like many other examples of good recall of recent information) is known as the recency effect.

Due to the personal nature of autobiographical memory, researchers have difficulty comparing what a person remembers to what actually occurred. Researchers overcome this challenge in one of several ways. One approach is to have subjects keep a diary for a length of time (e.g., days, months, years) and to record events that occurred to them at regular intervals or in response to specific cues. In addition to providing descriptions of the events that occurred, subjects might also record other accompanying details such as the exact time or location of the event and its emotional valence, salience, or distinctiveness. In turn, the diary entries are treated as the to-be-remembered stimuli in subsequent tests of memory. Moreover, as previously mentioned, the diary method is also used to capture involuntary recollections of personal events that are extremely difficult to elicit in laboratory settings. Such involuntary recollections tend to come out of the blue in response to environmental cues such as specific smells, words, or objects (e.g., Berntsen, 1996).

Another method is to assess individuals' recollections for specific historical events (e.g., the German occupation and liberation of Denmark during World War II) and then to compare the recollections with objective records of what occurred at the time, such as weather reports, newspapers, or radio broadcasts (Berntsen and Thomsen, 2005). Numerous studies of flashbulb memories (vivid recollections that surround a salient personal experience) focus on personal recollections surrounding unexpected, momentous, or emotionally charged events of public or personal significance, such as the assassination of President John F. Kennedy, the explosion of the space shuttle Challenger, or the more recent terrorist attacks on New York's World Trade Center (Brown and Kulik, 1977; Neisser and Harsh, 1993; Talarico and Rubin, 2003). However, it still remains unclear how reliable such memories are, what types of events induce flashbulb memories, and whether they really differ from memories for emotionally charged stimuli or circumstances.

1.4.2.3 Semantic memory

Semantic memory broadly refers to a person's general knowledge of the world. Of course, this is a vast store of information. Examples of semantic memory range from knowledge of words and their meanings, all kinds of concepts, general schemas or scripts that organize knowledge, and also specific facts about the world, such as the capital of France or famous battles in World War II.

It is reasonable to assume that when information is first learned, it is accompanied by information regarding the time and place of the learning episode. Over time and with repeated presentations of the same information, the accompanying episodic information may be lost or detached, and what remains is semantic memory. Still the distinction between episodic and semantic memory can easily blur. If someone asks about what you learned during a recent lecture, your response will likely reflect the influence of both episodic and semantic memory: Your reliance on temporal or contextual cues to remember particular points made during the lecture would reflect episodic memory. In contrast, how you choose to reconstruct, organize, interpret, or paraphrase knowledge garnered from the lecture would reflect the influence of semantic memory.

In addition to tests of explicit and implicit memory, a variety of cognitive tests are designed to measure the contents and organization of semantic memory. These tasks might involve naming as many members of a category or words that start with a given letter that come to mind, providing word definitions, answering general knowledge questions. Other measures are designed to capture the psychological representations of word meanings by having individuals provide quantitative ratings of individual words along a variety of semantic dimensions (e.g., Osgood et al., 1957).

One of the most powerful tools for studying semantic memory is the word-priming technique in which individuals are asked to make lexical decisions (word–nonword decisions) for pairs of stimuli that might be semantically related or unrelated. For example, individuals are faster and more accurate at identifying a word (doctor) if it is was preceded by a related word (nurse) relative to an unrelated word (shoe). Indeed, comparisons in the response times for items that are semantically related versus unrelated to current or previously encountered stimuli have inspired and helped to distinguish among competing theories of how knowledge is mentally represented and accessed (e.g., Collins and Quillian, 1969; Meyer and Schvaneveldt, 1971; Collins and Loftus, 1975; Neely, 1977; *See* Chapter 5).

1.4.2.4 Collective memory

Collective memory is conceptualized in a variety of ways. In a literal sense, collective memory refers to remembering that occurs within any social context. When employees at a company meeting attempt to recall what was discussed during a previous meeting, they are engaging in a collaborative recall effort. In general, social situations can influence what individuals remember or choose to report of the past. A given social setting can dictate what sorts of recollections are most appropriate or commensurate with individual goals of communication. For instance, it is very tempting to highlight or embellish certain details of a remembered event in order tell a more entertaining story. And in turn, an individual can influence what other individuals of a group remember of the past. Studies of collaborative recall typically involve having a group of people study lists of words, pictures, or prose passages and then asking them to recall the previously studied materials either individually or in collaboration with the rest of the group (Weldon, 2000).

Work in this area has shown that collaborative recall can increase the amount of previously studied information recalled as compared to individual recall performance, but that collaborative recall tends to reduce or inhibit the amount of information recalled per individual within a group (e.g., Weldon and Bellinger, 1997). Furthermore, collaborative recall can induce recall errors, as erroneous information supplied by one member of a group is accepted and later remembered by other members of the group (e.g., Roediger et al., 2001; Meade and Roediger, 2002).

Collective memory also refers to a representation of the past that is shared by members of broader social groups defined by nationality, religion, ethnicity, or age cohort. Such a conception of collective memory is shared across the fields of psychology, anthropology, and sociology, as may be seen in the writings of Wilhelm Wundt (1910/1916), Sir Frederic Bartlett (1932), and the French sociologists Maurice Halbwachs (1950/1980) and Emile Durkheim (1915). Carl Jung (1953) used the notion of a collective unconscious in a similar sense. One commonly held assumption is that remembering is shaped by active participation within the life of a particular group. Thus, group characteristics may bias the recollections of individual group members. For instance, Russian and American high school students are likely to tell strikingly different versions of the history of World War II, with each group recalling and weaving together a different set of key events in their narratives (Wertsch, 2002). Despite the widespread use of the term collective memory, both in public discussions of how groups remember historical events such as the Vietnam War or the Holocaust and across academic disciplines, there is still little agreement as to its definition or methods of study.

In contemporary memory research, studies of collective memory bear resemblance to those of autobiographical memory in the sense that remembering one's personal history may be heavily influenced by one's cultural background. For instance, numerous studies of flashbulb memories have examined individual recollections for major historical events such as the assassinations of President John F. Kennedy, Martin Luther King, Jr., and the fall of the Berlin Wall in 1989. Some of these studies have shown striking differences in recollections across groups.

Berntsen and Thomsen (2005) examined Danes' memories for the German invasion of Denmark in 1940 and their liberation in 1945. Interestingly, they found that individuals who had ties to the Danish resistance had more vivid and accurate memories than those who did not. A key difference between autobiographical and collective memory might, therefore, lie in the impact of group identification on memory and the extent to which remembering in general is socially framed.

1.5 Conclusions

This chapter has surveyed some of the most common terms and distinctions among types of memory. Although we have considered only a fraction of the 256 types that Tulving (2007) identified in his (semi-serious) essay, we believe we have hit upon the great majority in contemporary use. Most of the terms used in this chapter were not used by researchers 50 years ago. We hazard the guess that someone examining the field in 50 more years might have an even greater variety of items to review, even if the serious contenders do not quite approach 256.

References

Atkinson RC and Shiffrin RM (1971) The control of short-term memory. *Sci. Am.* 225: 82–90.

Baddeley A (2000) The episodic buffer: A new component of working memory? *Trends Cogn. Sci.* 4: 417–423.

Baddeley A (2001) Is working memory still working? *Am. Psychol.* 56: 849–864.

Bartlett FC (1932) *Remembering: A Study in Experimental and Social Psychology*. Cambridge: Cambridge University Press.

Berntsen D (1996) Involuntary autobiographical memories. *Appl. Cogn. Psychol.* 10: 435–454.

Berntsen D and Rubin DC (2002) Emotionally charged autobiographical memories across the life span: The recall of happy, sad, traumatic, and involuntary memories. *Psychol. Aging* 17: 636–652.

Berntsen D and Thomsen DK (2005) Personal memories for remote historical events: Accuracy and clarity of flashbulb memories related to World War II. *J. Exp. Psychol. Gen.* 134: 242–257.

Brewer WF (1986) What is autobiographical memory? In: Rubin DC (ed.) *Autobiographical Memory*, pp. 25–49. Cambridge: Cambridge University Press.

Brown R and Kulik J (1977) Flashbulb memories. *Cognition* 5: 73–99.

Charness N (1991) Expertise in chess: The balance between knowledge and search. In: Ericsson KA and Smith J (eds.) *Toward a General Theory of Expertise: Prospects and Limits*, pp. 39–63. Cambridge: Cambridge University Press.

Chase WG and Ericsson KA (1982) Skill and working memory. In: Bower GH (ed.) *The Psychology of Learning and Motivation,* vol. 16, pp. 1–58. New York: Academic Press.

Chase WG and Simon HA (1973) The mind's eye in chess. In: Chase WG (ed.) *Visual Information Processing*, pp. 215–281. New York: Academic Press.

Collins AM and Loftus EF (1975) A spreading activation theory of semantic processing. *Psychol. Rev.* 82: 407–428.

Collins AM and Quillian MR (1969) Retrieval time from semantic memory. *J. Verb. Learn. Verb. Behav.* 8: 240–248.

Conway MA, Singer JA, and Tagini A (2004) The self and autobiographical memory: Correspondence and coherence. *Soc. Cogn.* 22: 491–529.

Craik FIM and Tulving E (1975) Depth of processing and the retention of words in episodic memory. *J. Exp. Psychol. Gen.* 104: 268–294.

Crovitz HF and Schiffman H (1974) Frequency of episodic memories as a function of their age. *Bull. Psychon. Soc.* 4: 517–518.

Crowder RG and Morton J (1969) Precategorical acoustic storage (PAS). *Percept. Psychophys.* 5: 365–373.

Durkheim E (1915) *Elementary Forms of the Religious Life*. New York: Macmillan.

Ebbinghaus H (1885/1964) *Memory: A Contribution to Experimental Psychology*. New York: Dover.

Einstein GO and McDaniel MA (2005) Prospective memory: Multiple retrieval processes. *Curr. Dir. Psychol. Sci.* 14: 286–290.

Ericsson KA and Kintsch W (1995) Long-term working memory. *Psychol. Rev.* 102: 211–245.

Fitzgerald JM (1988) Vivid memories and the reminiscence phenomenon: The role of a self narrative. *Hum. Dev.* 31: 261–273.

Freud S (1917/1982) An early memory from Goethe's autobiography. In: Neisser U (ed.) *Memory Observed: Remembering in Natural Contexts*, pp. 289–297. New York: Freeman.

Galton F (1879) Psychometric experiments. *Brain* 2: 149–162.

Glanzer M and Clark WH (1964) The verbal-loop hypothesis: Conventional figures. *Am. J. Psychol.* 77: 621–626.

Graf P and Schacter DL (1985) Implicit and explicit memory for new associations in normal and amnesic subjects. *J. Exp. Psychol. Learn. Mem. Cogn.* 11: 501–518.

Gupta P and Cohen NJ (2002) Theoretical and computational analysis of skill learning, repetition priming, and procedural memory. *Psychol. Rev.* 109: 401–448.

Halbwachs M (1950/1980) *The Collective Memory*, Ditter FJ Jr and Ditter VY (trans.) New York: Harper and Row.

Healy AF (2007) Transfer: Specificity and generality. In: Roediger HL, Dudai Y, and Fitzpatrick SM (eds.) *Science of Memory: Concepts*, pp. 271–282. New York: Oxford University Press.

Herz RS and Engen T (1996) Odor memory: Review and analysis. *Psychon. Bull. Rev.* 3: 300–313.

Hull CL (1943) *Principles of Behavior*. New York: Appleton-Century-Crofts.

Hyde TS and Jenkins JJ (1969) Differential effects of incidental tasks on the organization of recall of a list of highly associated words. *J. Exp. Psychol.* 82: 472–481.

Jacoby LL (1984) Incidental versus intentional retrieval: Remembering and awareness as separate issues. In: Squire LR and Butters N (eds.) *Neuropsychology of Memory*, pp. 145–156. New York: Guilford Press.

Jacoby LL (1991) A process dissociation framework: Separating automatic from intentional uses of memory. *J. Mem. Lang.* 30: 513–541.

James W (1890/1950) *The Principles of Psychology*, vol. 1. New York: Henry Holt and Co.

Janssen SMJ, Chessa AG, and Murre JMJ (2005) The reminiscence bump in autobiographical memory: Effects of age, gender, education, and culture. *Memory* 13: 658–668.

Jung CG (1953) Read H, Fordham M, and Adler G (eds.) *The Collected Works of CG Jung,* vol. 9, Part I. New York: Pantheon Books.

Kolers PA and Roediger HL (1984) Procedures of mind. *Jo. Verb. Learn. Verb. Behav.* 23: 425–449.
Mackintosh NJ (2002) Do not ask whether they have a cognitive map, but how they find their way about. *Psicologica* 23: 165–185.
Meade ML and Roediger HL (2002) Explorations in the social contagion of memory. *Mem. Cogn.* 30: 995–1009.
Meyer DE and Schvaneveldt RW (1971) Facilitation in recognizing pairs of words: Evidence of a dependence between retrieval operations. *J. Exp. Psychol.* 90: 227–234.
Neely JH (1977) Semantic priming and retrieval from lexical memory: Roles of inhibitionless spreading activation and limited-capacity attention. *J. Exp. Psychol. Gen.* 106: 226–254.
Neisser U and Harsh N (1993) Phantom flashbulbs: False recollections of hearing the news about Challenger. In: Winograd E and Neisser U (eds.) *Affect and Accuracy in Recall: Studies of "Flashbulb" Memories*, pp. 9–31. New York: Cambridge University Press.
Neisser U (1967) *Cognitive Psychology*. East Norwalk, CT: Appleton-Century-Crofts.
Nelson DL (1979) Remembering pictures and words: Appearance, significance, and name. In: Cermak LS and Craik FIM (eds.) *Levels of Processing in Human Memory*, pp. 45–76. Hillsdale, NJ: Erlbaum.
Norman DA (ed.) (1970) *Models of Human Memory*. New York: Academic Press.
O'Keefe J and Nadel L (1978) *The Hippocampus as a Cognitive Map*. New York: Oxford University Press.
Osgood CE, Suci GJ, and Tannenbaum PH (1957) *The Measurement of Meaning*. Urbana, IL: University of Illinois Press.
Paivio A (1986) *Mental Representations: A Dual Coding Approach*. New York: Oxford University Press.
Postman L (1964) Short-term memory and incidental learning. In: Melton AW (ed.) *Categories of Human Learning*, pp. 145–201. New York: Academic Press.
Ratcliff R (1978) A theory of memory retrieval. *Psychol. Rev.* 85: 59–108.
Richardson-Klavehn A, Gardiner JM, and Java RI (1996) Memory: Task dissociation, process dissociations and dissociations of consciousness. In: Underwood GDM (ed.) *Implicit Cognition*, pp. 85–158. Oxford: Oxford University Press.
Robinson JA (1976) Sampling autobiographical memory. *Cogn. Psychol.* 8: 578–595.
Roediger HL (1980) Memory metaphors in cognitive psychology. *Mem. Cogn.* 8: 231–246.
Roediger HL, Weldon MS, Stadler ML, and Riedgler GL (1992) Direct comparison of two implicit memory tests: Word fragment and word stem completion. *J. Exp. Psychol. Learn. Mem. Cogn.* 18: 1251–1269.
Roediger HL, Meade ML, and Bergman ET (2001) Social contagion of memory. *Psychon. Bull. Rev.* 8: 365–371.
Roediger HL, Marsh EJ, and Lee SC (2002) Varieties of memory. In: Pashler H and Medin D (eds.) *Steven's Handbook of Experimental Psychology,* 3rd edn. Hoboken, NJ: John Wiley and Sons.
Rubin DC and Berntsen D (2003) Life scripts help to maintain autobiographical memories of highly positive, but not highly negative, events. *Mem. Cogn.* 31: 1–14.
Rubin DC, Wetzler SE, and Nebes RD (1986) Autobiographical memory across the adult life span. In: Rubin DC (ed.) *Autobiographical Memory*, pp. 202–221. Cambridge: Cambridge University Press.
Ryle G (1949) *The Concept of Mind*. New York: Barnes and Noble.
Schacter DL (1987) Implicit memory: History and current status. *J. Exp. Psychol. Learn. Mem. Cogn.* 13: 501–518.
Schacter DL, Bowers J, and Booker J (1989) Intention, awareness, and implicit memory: The retrieval intentionality criterion. In: Lewandowsky S, Dunn J, and Kirsner K (eds.) *Implicit Memory: Theoretical Issues*, pp. 47–65. Hillsdale, NJ: Lawrence Erlbaum Associates.
Shiffrin RM and Atkinson RC (1969) Storage and retrieval processes in long-term memory. *Psychol. Rev.* 76: 179–193.
Slamecka NJ (1985) Ebbinghaus: Some associations. *J. Exp. Psychol. Learn. Mem. Cogn.* 11: 414–435.
Sperling G (1960) The information available in brief visual presentation. *Psychol. Monogr.* 11: 29.
Squire LR (1982) The neuropsychology of human memory. *Annu. Rev. Neurosci.* 5: 241–273.
Squire LR (1992) Declarative and nondeclarative memory: Multiple brain systems supporting learning and memory. *J. Cogn. Neurosci.* 4: 232–243.
Talarico JM and Rubin DC (2003) Confidence, not consistency, characterizes flashbulb memories. *Psychol. Sci.* 14: 455–461.
Tulving E (1972) Episodic and semantic memory. In: Tulving E and Donaldson W (eds.) *Organization of Memory*, pp. 381–403. New York: Academic Press.
Tulving E (1985) Memory and consciousness. *Can. J. Psychol.* 26: 1–12.
Tulving E (2000) Concepts of memory. In: Tulving E and Craik FIM (eds.) *The Oxford Handbook of Memory*, pp. 33–43. New York: Oxford University Press.
Tulving E (2002) Episodic memory: From mind to brain. *Annu. Rev. Psychol.* 54: 1–25.
Tulving E (2005) Episodic memory and autonoesis: Uniquely human? In: Terrace H and Metcalfe J (eds.) *The Missing Link in Cognition: Origins of Self-Reflective Consciousness*, pp. 3–56. New York: Oxford University Press.
Tulving E (2007) Are there 256 kinds of memory? In: Nairne J (ed.) *The Foundations of Remembering: Essays in Honor of Henry L Roediger III*, pp. 39–52. New York: Psychology Press.
Waugh NC and Norman DA (1965) Primary memory. *Psychol. Rev.* 72: 89–104.
Weldon MS (2000) Remembering as a social process. In: Medin DL (ed.) *The Psychology of Learning and Motivation,* vol. 40, pp. 67–120. San Diego: Academic Press.
Weldon MS and Bellinger KD (1997) Collective memory: Collaborative and individual processes in remembering. *J. Exp. Psychol. Learn. Mem. Cogn.* 23: 1160–1175.
Wechsler DB (1963) Engrams, memory storage, and mnemonic coding. *Am. Psychol.* 18: 149–153.
Wertsch JV (2002) *Voices of Collective Remembering*. Cambridge: Cambridge University Press.
Wheeler MA (2000) Episodic memory and autonoetic awareness. In: Tulving E and Craik FIM (eds.) *The Oxford Handbook of Memory*, pp. 597–608. New York: Oxford University Press.
Wright AA (1998) Auditory and visual serial position functions obey different laws. *Psychon. Bull. Rev.* 5: 564–584.
Wright AA and Roediger HL (2003) Interference processes in monkey auditory list memory. *Psychon. Bull. Rev.* 10: 696–702.
Wundt W (1910/1916) *Elements of Folk Psychology*, Schaub EL (trans.). New York: Macmillan.

2 Declarative Memory System: Amnesia

L. R. Squire and Y. Shrager, University of California at San Diego, San Diego, CA, USA

2.1 Introduction

Memory is not a single entity but is composed of several separate systems (*See* Chapters 1, 3; Squire, 1992; Schacter and Tulving, 1994). Long-term memory can be divided into several parallel memory systems. The major distinction is between declarative and nondeclarative memory. Declarative memory refers to conscious knowledge of facts and events. Nondeclarative memory refers to a collection of nonconscious knowledge systems that provide for the capacity of skill learning, habit formation, the phenomenon of priming, and certain other ways of interacting with the world. The terms 'explicit memory' and 'implicit memory' are sometimes used as well and have approximately the same meanings as declarative and nondeclarative memory, respectively.

The brain is organized such that declarative memory is a distinct and separate cognitive function, which can be studied in isolation from perception and other intellectual abilities. Significant information about how memory is organized has come from the study of patients with memory disorders (amnesia) and from animal models of amnesia. Amnesia (neurological amnesia and functional amnesia) refers to difficulty in learning new information or in remembering the past.

Neurological amnesia is characterized by a loss of declarative memory. It occurs following brain injury or disease that damages the medial temporal lobe or diencephalon. Neurological amnesia causes severe difficulty in learning new facts and events (anterograde amnesia). Patients with neurological amnesia also typically have some difficulty remembering facts and events that were acquired before the onset of amnesia (retrograde amnesia).

Functional amnesia is rarer than neurological amnesia and can occur as the result of an emotional trauma. It presents as a different pattern of anterograde and retrograde memory impairment than neurological amnesia. Functional amnesia is characterized by a profound retrograde amnesia with little or no anterograde amnesia. In some cases, patients fully recover. Functional amnesia is a psychiatric disorder, and no particular brain structure or region is known to be damaged.

2.2 Etiology of Neurological Amnesia

Neurological amnesia results from a number of conditions including Alzheimer's disease or other dementing illnesses, temporal lobe surgery, chronic alcohol abuse, encephalitis, head injury, anoxia, ischemia, infarction, and the rupture and repair of an anterior communicating artery aneurism. The common factor in all of these conditions is the disruption of normal function in one of two areas of the brain – the medial aspects of the temporal lobe, and the diencephalic midline. Bilateral damage results in global amnesia, and unilateral damage results in material-specific amnesia. Specifically, left-sided damage affects memory for verbal material, while right-sided damage affects memory for nonverbal material (e.g., memory for faces and spatial layouts).

2.3 Anatomy

Well-studied cases of human amnesia and animal models of amnesia provide information about the neural connections and structures that are damaged. In humans, damage limited to the hippocampus itself is sufficient to cause moderately severe amnesia. For example, in one carefully studied case of amnesia (patient R.B.), the only significant damage was a bilateral lesion confined to the CA1 field of the hippocampus (Zola-Morgan et al., 1986). The severity of memory impairment is exacerbated by additional damage outside of the hippocampus. Thus, severe amnesia results when damage extends beyond CA1 to the rest of the hippocampus and to the adjacent cortex. (Animal studies later elucidated the critical anatomical components of this memory system; see following.) One well-studied case (H.M.) had surgery in 1953 to treat severe epilepsy. Most of the hippocampus and much of the surrounding medial temporal lobe cortices were removed bilaterally (the entorhinal cortex and most of the perirhinal cortex). Although the surgery was successful in reducing the frequency of H.M.'s seizures, it resulted in a severe and persistent amnesia.

It is also possible through structural magnetic resonance imaging (MRI) to detect and quantify the neuropathology in amnesic patients. Many patients with restricted hippocampal damage have an average reduction in hippocampal volume of about 40%. Two such patients whose brains were available for detailed, postmortem neurohistological analysis (patients L.M. and W.H.) proved to have lost virtually all the neurons in the CA fields of the hippocampus. These observations suggest that a reduction in hippocampal volume of approximately 40%, as estimated from MRI scans, likely indicates the near complete loss of hippocampal neurons (Rempel-Clower et al., 1996). The amnesic condition is associated with neuronal death and tissue collapse, but the tissue does not disappear altogether because fibers and glia remain. In patients with larger lesions of the medial temporal lobe, volume reduction as measured by MRI is more dramatic. For example, patient E.P., who became amnesic as a result of viral encephalitis, has damage to all of the perirhinal cortex, all of the entorhinal cortex, virtually all of the hippocampus, and most of the parahippocampal cortex (Stefanacci et al., 2000).

As questions about amnesia and the function of medial temporal lobe structures have become more specific, it has become vital to obtain detailed, quantitative information about the damage in the patients being studied. In addition, single-case studies are not nearly as useful as group studies involving well-characterized patients. In the case of patients with restricted hippocampal damage, one can calculate the volume of the hippocampus itself as a proportion of total intracranial volume. One can also calculate the volumes of the adjacent medial temporal lobe structures (the perirhinal, entorhinal, and parahippocampal cortices) in proportion to intracranial volume. Last, when there is extensive damage to the medial temporal lobe, it is important to calculate the volumes of lateral temporal cortex and other regions that might be affected. It is important to characterize patients in this way in order to address the kinds of questions now being pursued in studies of memory and the brain.

Functional MRI (fMRI) of healthy individuals who are engaged in learning and remembering allows one to ask what brain areas are associated with these memory processes. The same tasks that are administered to amnesic patients can also be administered to healthy individuals while their brain activation is measured. fMRI reveals activation during these tasks of learning and remembering in the same structures that, when damaged, cause amnesia.

To understand the anatomy of human amnesia, and ultimately the anatomy of normal memory, animal models of human amnesia have been established in the monkey (**Figure 1**) and in the rodent. An animal

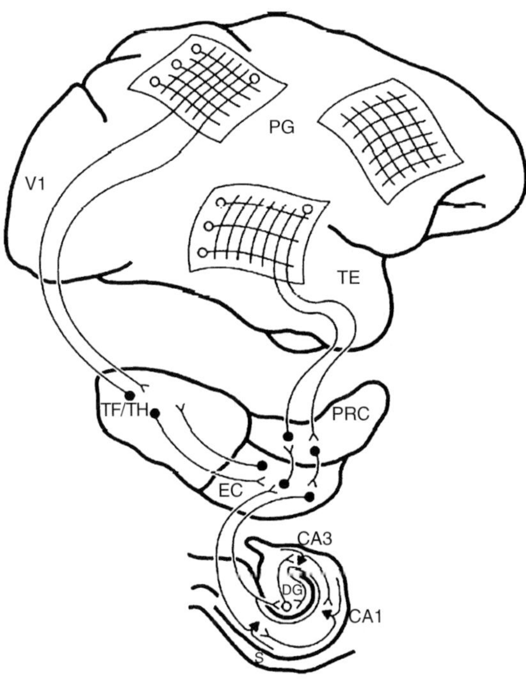

Figure 1 Schematic drawing of primate neocortex together with the structures and connections in the medial temporal region important for establishing long-term memory. The networks in the cortex show putative representations concerning visual object quality (in area TE) and object location (in area PG). If this disparate neural activity is to cohere into a stable, long-term memory, convergent activity must occur along projections from these regions to the medial temporal lobe. Projections from neocortex arrive initially at the parahippocampal gyrus (TF/TH) and perirhinal cortex (PRC) and then at entorhinal cortex (EC), the gateway to the hippocampus. Further processing of information occurs in the several stages of the hippocampus, first in the dentate gyrus (DG) and then in the CA3 and CA1 regions. The fully processed input eventually exits this circuit via the subiculum (S) and the entorhinal cortex, where widespread efferent projections return to neocortex. The hippocampus and adjacent structures are thought to support the stabilization of representations in distributed regions of neocortex (e.g., TE and PG) and to support the strengthening of connections between these regions. Subsequently, memory for a whole event (e.g., a memory that depends on representations in both TE and PG) can be revivified even when a partial cue is presented. Damage to the medial temporal lobe system causes anterograde and retrograde amnesia. The severity of the deficit increases as damage involves more components of the system. Once sufficient time has passed, the distributed representations in neocortex can operate independently of the medial temporal lobe. (This diagram is a simplification and does not show diencephalic structures involved in memory function.)

model of human amnesia was established in the monkey in the early 1980s (Mishkin, 1982; Squire and Zola-Morgan, 1983). Following lesions of the bilateral medial temporal lobe or diencephalon, memory impairment is exhibited on the same kinds of tasks of new learning ability that human amnesic patients fail. The same animals succeed at tasks of motor skill learning. They also do well at learning pattern discriminations, which share with motor skills the factors of incremental learning and repetition over many trials.

Systematic and cumulative work in monkeys, using the animal model, succeeded in identifying the system of structures in the medial temporal lobe essential for memory (Squire and Zola-Morgan, 1991). The important structures are the hippocampal region (hippocampus proper, dentate gyrus, and subicular complex) and adjacent, anatomically related structures (entorhinal cortex, perirhinal cortex, and parahippocampal cortex). The amygdala, although critical for aspects of emotional learning (Davis, 1994; LeDoux, 1996) and for the enhancement of declarative memory by emotion (Adolphs et al., 1997), is not a part of the declarative memory system itself. The consistency between the available neuroanatomical information from humans and the findings from monkeys have considerably illuminated the description of memory impairment and its anatomical basis. These lines of work have also made it possible to pursue parallel studies in simpler animals like rats and mice. As a result, one can now study memory in rodents and have some confidence that what one learns will be relevant to the human condition.

Anatomical connections from different parts of the neocortex enter the medial temporal lobe at different points (Suzuki and Amaral, 1994a,b), which raises the question of whether these medial temporal lobe structures play different roles in declarative memory. For example, visual association cortex projects more strongly to the perirhinal cortex than to the parahippocampal cortex, whereas the parietal cortex projects to the parahippocampal cortex but not to the perirhinal cortex. Further, the hippocampus lies at the end of the medial temporal lobe system and is a recipient of convergent projections from each of the structures that precedes it in the hierarchy. The possibility that different medial temporal lobe structures make different contributions to memory has been addressed in a number of studies in monkeys, comparing performance on memory tasks following damage to different components of the medial temporal lobe. This work has shown that the severity of memory impairment depends on the locus and extent of damage within the medial temporal lobe memory system. Damage limited to the hippocampal region causes significant memory impairment, but damage to the adjacent cortex increases the severity of memory impairment. It is also important to note that the discovery that larger medial temporal lobe lesions produce more severe amnesia than smaller lesions is compatible with the idea that structures within the medial temporal lobe might make qualitatively different contributions to memory function. Indeed, damage to the perirhinal cortex especially impairs object recognition, whereas damage to the parahippocampal cortex especially impairs spatial memory.

Another important brain area for memory is the diencephalon. The important structures include the mediodorsal thalamic nucleus, the anterior thalamic nucleus, the internal medullary lamina, the mamillary nuclei, and the mammillo-thalamic tract. Monkeys with medial thalamic lesions exhibit an amnesic disorder, and monkeys with mammillary nucleilesious exhibit a modest impairment. Because diencephalic amnesia resembles medial temporal lobe amnesia in the pattern of sparing and loss, these two regions likely form an anatomically linked, functional system.

2.4 The Nature of Amnesia

Amnesic individuals exhibit significant memory impairment. Yet, despite their memory deficit, patients have intact ability for some forms of new learning and memory (see section 2.5.2). Also, they have intact immediate memory and memory for a great deal of information from the past, especially childhood. In addition, patients with neurological amnesia can have intact intelligence test scores, intact language and social skills, and intact perceptual abilities. In fact, amnesic patients can appear quite normal on casual observation. It is only when one interrogates their capacity for new learning of conscious knowledge that the impairment becomes evident.

2.4.1 Impairment in Declarative Memory

It is important to appreciate that amnesic patients are not impaired at all kinds of long-term memory. The major distinction is between declarative and nondeclarative memory. Declarative memory is the kind of memory impaired in amnesia. Declarative memory refers to the capacity to remember the facts and events of everyday life. It is the kind of memory that is meant when the term 'memory' is used in ordinary language. Declarative memory can be brought to mind as a conscious recollection. Declarative memory provides a way to model the external world, and in this sense it is either true or false. The stored representations are flexible in that they are accessible to multiple response systems and can guide successful performance under a wide range of test conditions. Last, declarative memory is especially suited for rapid learning and for forming and maintaining associations between arbitrarily different kinds of material (e.g., learning to associate two different words).

2.4.2 Anterograde Amnesia

Amnesia is characterized especially by profound difficulty in new learning, and this impairment is referred to as anterograde amnesia. Amnesia can occur as part of a more global dementing disorder that includes other cognitive deficits such as impairments in language, attention, visuospatial abilities, and general intellectual capacity. However, when damage is restricted to the medial temporal lobe or midline diencephalon, amnesia can also occur in the absence of other cognitive deficits and without any change in personality or social skills. In this more circumscribed form of amnesia, patients have intact intellectual functions and intact perceptual functions, even on difficult tests that require the ability to discriminate between highly similar images containing overlapping features (Levy et al., 2005; Shrager et al., 2006). In some patients with memory impairment, visual perceptual deficits have been described (Lee et al., 2005a,b). In these cases, damage might extend laterally, beyond the medial temporal lobe, and quantitative brain measurements are needed in order to understand what underlies these deficits. Thus, present data support the idea that declarative memory is separable from other brain functions.

Amnesic patients are impaired on tasks of new learning, regardless of whether memory is tested by free (unaided) recall, recognition (e.g., presenting an item and asking whether it was previously encountered or not), or cued recall (e.g., asking for recall of an item when a hint is provided). For instance, in a standard test of free recall, participants are read a short prose passage containing 21 segments. They are then asked to recall the passage immediately and after a 12-min delay. Amnesic patients with damage to the medial temporal lobe do well at immediate recall but are impaired at the delay, usually recalling zero segments (Squire and Shimamura, 1986). Amnesic patients are also impaired on recognition tests, where a list of words is presented and participants try to decide (yes or no) if each word had been presented in a recent study list (Squire and Shimamura, 1986). Last, in a cued recall task, individuals study a list of word pairs, such as ARMY–TABLE. During test, they are presented with one word from each pair (ARMY), and they are asked to recall the word that was paired with it (TABLE). Amnesic patients are impaired on this task as well.

The memory impairment in amnesia involves both difficulty in learning factual information (semantic memory) as well as difficulty in learning about specific episodes and events that occurred in a certain time and place (episodic memory). The term 'semantic memory' is often used to describe declarative memory for organized world knowledge (Tulving, 1983). In recalling this type of information, one need not remember any particular past event. One needs only to know about certain facts. Episodic memory, in contrast, is autobiographical memory for the events of one's life (Tulving, 1983). Unlike semantic memory, episodic memory stores spatial and temporal landmarks that identify the particular time and place when an event occurred. Both episodic memory and semantic memory are declarative.

Formal experiments have compared directly the ability to accomplish fact learning (or semantic memory ability) and event learning (or episodic memory ability). In one experiment, amnesic patients were taught new factual knowledge in the form of three-word sentences (e.g., MEDICINE cured HICCUP). Then, during testing, sentence fragments were presented with the instruction to complete each fragment with a word that had been studied (e.g., MEDICINE cured ______). The amnesic patients were similarly impaired on tests of fact memory (what word completed the sentence fragment) and on tests of event memory (what specific events occurred during the testing session) (Hamann and Squire, 1995). Taken together, the data favor the view that episodic memory and semantic memory are similarly impaired in amnesia (Squire and Zola, 1998). Semantic knowledge is thought to accumulate in cortical storage sites as a consequence of experience and with support from the medial temporal lobe. In contrast, episodic memory is thought to require these cortical sites and the medial temporal lobes to work together with the frontal lobes in order to store when and where a past experience occurred (Janowsky et al., 1989).

Last, the memory deficit in amnesia is global and encompasses all sensory modalities (e.g., visual, auditory, olfactory). That is, memory is impaired regardless of the kind of material that is presented and the sensory modality in which information is presented. For example, recognition memory of amnesic patients was assessed for line drawings of objects (visual), designs (visual), and odors (olfactory) (Levy et al., 2004). The patients were impaired on all three tasks, showing that their impairment spans the visual and olfactory domains. Formal experiments have also demonstrated recognition memory impairment for auditory stimuli.

2.4.3 Remembering versus Knowing and Recollection versus Familiarity

Remembering (R) is meant to refer to the circumstance when an item elicits a conscious recollection that includes information about the context in which the item was learned. Knowing (K) is meant to refer to a circumstance when an item appears familiar, but memory for the original learning context is not available (Tulving, 1985). Thorough studies of healthy individuals indicate that in practice, remembering and knowing responses are closely related to the strength of a memory and that items given K responses are often items for which information is also available about the original learning context (Wixted and Stretch, 2004). In any case, formal studies show that both R and K responses are impaired in amnesia. In one such experiment, amnesic patients and control participants were given a recognition test 10 min after studying words. For each word, participants indicated whether they remembered it (R) or whether they knew that the word was presented but had no recollection about it (K). The patients were impaired for both R and K responses, and they performed like a control group that was tested after 1 week. That is, the patients were similarly impaired for R and K responses (Knowlton and Squire, 1995; also see Manns et al., 2003). Accordingly, the evidence suggests that remembering and knowing are two different expressions of declarative memory.

A distinction closely related to remembering and knowing is recollection and familiarity. Recollection involves remembering the contextual associations of the original learning experience, whereas familiarity does not require any recollection of the original experience. It has sometimes been proposed that recollection relies on the hippocampus, while familiarity can be supported by the adjacent cortex within the medial temporal lobe. In this view, patients with damage limited to the hippocampus should be selectively, or disproportionately, impaired at recollecting information and less impaired at recognizing material when it can be supported by familiarity.

An alternative view is that recognition decisions are based on a unidimensional strength-of-memory variable that combines estimates of recollection and familiarity. Thus, as in the case of remembering and knowing, a capacity for recollection is likely to be associated with strong memories and familiarity with weaker memories (Wixted, 2007). In one study, patients with hippocampal damage were impaired on a recognition memory test, where they gave confidence judgments (scale of 1–6). The results indicated that both processes, recollection and familiarity, were operative in the absence of the hippocampus (Wais et al., 2006). Last, electrophysiological recordings from patients being evaluated for epilepsy surgery found neurons in the hippocampus that responded to familiar images during a recognition test. These familiarity signals were present even when recollection failed (i.e., there was a familiarity signal in the hippocampus regardless of whether any recollection had occurred) (Rutishauser et al., 2006).

2.4.4 Retrograde Amnesia

In addition to impaired new learning, damage to the medial temporal lobe also impairs memories that were acquired before the onset of amnesia. This type of memory loss is referred to as retrograde amnesia. Retrograde amnesia is usually temporally graded. That is, information acquired in the distant past (remote memory) is spared relative to more recent memory (Ribot, 1881). The extent of retrograde amnesia can be relatively short and encompass only 1 or 2 years, or it can be more extensive and cover decades. Even then, memories for the facts and events of childhood and adolescence are typically intact. Indeed, severely amnesic patients can produce detailed autobiographical narratives of their early life. These memories were indistinguishable from the memories of healthy individuals with respect to the number of details, the duration of the narratives, and the number of prompts needed to begin a narrative (Bayley et al., 2003, 2005b).

The severity and extent of retrograde amnesia is determined by the locus and extent of damage. Patients with restricted hippocampal damage have limited retrograde amnesia covering a few years prior to the onset of amnesia. Patients with large medial temporal lobe damage have extensive retrograde amnesia covering decades. When damage occurs beyond the brain system that supports declarative memory, which can result from conditions such as encephalitis and head trauma, retrograde amnesia sometimes can be ungraded and extensive and include the facts and events of early life.

Because the study of human retrograde amnesia is based almost entirely on findings from retrospective tests, the clearest data about retrograde amnesia gradients come from studies using experimental animals, where the delay between initial learning and a lesion can be manipulated directly. Findings from such studies make three important points. First, temporal gradients of retrograde amnesia can occur within long-term memory. That is, retrograde amnesia does not reflect simply the vulnerability of a short-term memory that has not yet been converted into a long-term memory. Second, after a lesion, remote memory can be even better than recent memory. Third, lesions can spare old weak memories while disrupting strong recent ones, showing that it is the age of the memory that is critical.

These same points can be illustrated by a study of rabbits given trace eyeblink conditioning. Trace conditioning is a variant of classical conditioning in which the condition stimulus (CS), such as a tone, is presented and terminated, and then a short interval (e.g., 500 ms) is imposed before the presentation of the unconditioned stimulus (US). In normal rabbits, forgetting occurs gradually after training, and retention of the conditioned response is much poorer

30 days after training than after only 1 day. Nevertheless, complete aspiration of the hippocampus 1 day after training abolished the strong 1-day-old memory, whereas the same lesion made 30 days after training had no effect on the weaker 30-day-old memory (Kim et al., 1995).

The sparing of remote memory relative to more recent memory illustrates that the brain regions damaged in amnesia are not the permanent repositories of long-term memory. Instead, memories undergo a process of reorganization and consolidation after learning, during which time the neocortex becomes more important. During the process of consolidation, memories are vulnerable if there is damage to the medial temporal lobe or diencephalon. After sufficient time has passed, storage and retrieval of memory no longer require the participation of these brain structures. Memory is at that point supported by neocortex. The areas of neocortex important for long-term memory are thought to be the same regions that were initially involved in the processing and analysis of what was to be learned. Thus, the neocortex is always important, but the structures of the medial temporal lobe and diencephalon are also important during initial learning and during consolidation.

2.4.5 Spatial Memory

Since the discovery of hippocampal place cells in the rodent (O'Keefe and Dostrovsky, 1971), an influential idea has been that the hippocampus creates and uses spatial maps and that its predominant function is to support spatial memory (O'Keefe and Nadel, 1978). Discussions of amnesia have therefore focused especially on the status of spatial memory. It is clear that spatial memory is impaired in human amnesia. Amnesic patients are impaired on tests that assess their knowledge of the spatial layout of an environment, and they are also impaired when asked to navigate to a destination in a virtual environment (Maguire et al., 1996; Spiers et al., 2001). Similarly, the noted patient H.M. was impaired at recalling object locations (Smith, 1988). It is also clear, though, that amnesic patients are impaired on memory tests that have no obvious spatial component, such as recall or recognition of items (Squire and Shimamura, 1986). Furthermore, formal experiments that directly compared spatial and nonspatial memory in amnesic patients showed that the patients were similarly impaired on tests of spatial memory and tests of nonspatial memory. There was no special difficulty with the test of spatial memory (Cave and Squire, 1991).

As is the case with nonspatial memory, remote spatial knowledge is intact. One well-studied patient with large medial temporal lobe lesions and severe amnesia (E.P.) was able to mentally navigate his childhood neighborhood, use alternate and novel routes to describe how to travel from one place to another, and point correctly to locations in the neighborhood while imagining himself oriented at some other location (Teng and Squire, 1999). These findings show that the medial temporal lobe is not needed for the long-term storage of spatial knowledge and does not maintain a spatial layout of learned environments that is necessary for successful navigation. Accordingly, the available data support the view that the hippocampus and related medial temporal lobe structures are involved in learning new facts and events, both spatial and nonspatial. Further, these structures are not repositories of long-term memory, either spatial or nonspatial.

2.5 Spared Learning and Memory Abilities

It is a striking feature of amnesia that many kinds of learning and memory are spared. Memory is not a unitary faculty of the mind but is composed of many parts that depend on different brain systems. Amnesia impairs only long-term declarative memory and spares immediate and working memory, as well as nondeclarative memory. Immediate memory and working memory can be viewed as a collection of temporary memory capacities that operate shortly after material is presented. Nondeclarative memory refers to a heterogeneous collection of abilities, all of which afford the capacity to acquire knowledge nonconsciously. Nondeclarative memory includes motor skills, perceptual and cognitive skills, priming, adaptation-level effects, simple classical conditioning, habits, and phylogenetically early forms of experience-dependent behavior like habituation and sensitization. In these cases, memory is expressed through performance rather than recollection.

2.5.1 Immediate and Working Memory

Amnesic patients have intact immediate memory. Immediate memory refers to what can be held actively in mind beginning the moment that information is received. It is the information that forms the focus of current attention and that occupies the current stream of thought. The capacity of immediate memory is quite limited. This type of memory is reflected, for example, in the ability to repeat back a short string of digits. Intact immediate memory explains why amnesic patients can carry on a conversation and appear quite normal to the casual observer. Indeed, if the amount of material to be remembered is not too large (e.g., a three-digit number), then patients can remember the material for minutes, or as long as they can hold it in mind by rehearsal. One would say in this case that the patients have carried the contents of immediate memory forward by engaging in explicit rehearsal. This rehearsal-based activity is referred to as working memory, and it is independent of the medial temporal lobe system (*See* Chapter 8). The difficulty for amnesic patients arises when an amount of information must be recalled that exceeds immediate memory capacity (typically, when a list of eight or more items must be remembered) or when information must be recalled after a distraction-filled interval or after a long delay. In these situations, when the capacity of working memory is exceeded, patients will remember fewer items than their healthy counterparts.

The intact capacity for immediate and working memory was well illustrated by patient H.M. when he was asked to remember the number 584. H.M. was left to himself for several minutes, and he was able to retain this information by working out mnemonic schemes and holding the information continuously in mind. Yet, only a minute or two later, after his attention had been directed to another task, he could not remember the number or any of his mnemonic schemes for holding the number in mind.

2.5.2 Nondeclarative Memory

Nondeclarative memory refers to a collective of nonconscious knowledge systems, but it is not itself a brain-systems construct. Rather, the term encompasses several different kinds of memory. Nondeclarative forms of memory have in common the feature that memory is nonconscious. Memory is expressed through performance and does not require reflection on the past or even the knowledge that memory is being influenced by past events.

The following examples illustrate that nondeclarative memory is distinct from declarative memory. It is spared in amnesia, and it operates outside of awareness. Nondeclarative forms of memory depend variously on the neostriatum, the amygdala, and the cerebellum and on processes intrinsic to neocortex (**Figure 2**).

2.5.2.1 Motor skills and perceptual skills

One can learn how to ride a bicycle but be unable to describe what has been learned, at least not in the same sense that one might recall riding a bicycle on a particular day with a friend. This is because the learning of motor skills is largely nondeclarative, and amnesic

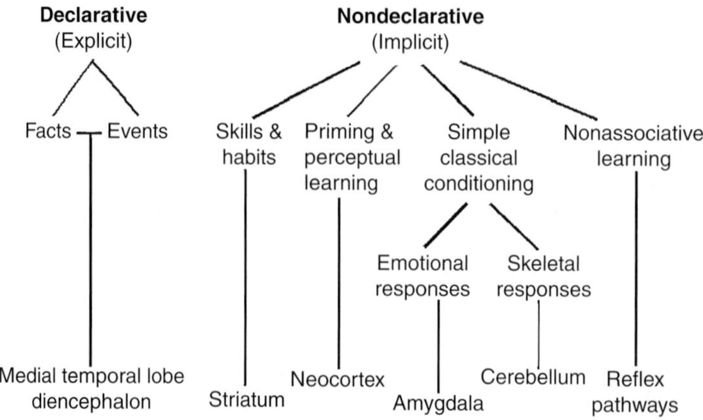

Figure 2 Classification of mammalian long-term memory systems. The taxonomy lists the brain structures thought to be especially important for each form of declarative and nondeclarative memory. In addition to the central role of the amygdala in emotional learning, it is also able to modulate the strength of both declarative and nondeclarative learning.

patients can learn these skills at a normal rate. In one experiment, amnesic patients and control participants performed a serial reaction-time task, in which they responded successively to a sequence of four illuminated spatial locations. The task was to press one of four keys as rapidly as possible as soon as the location above each key was illuminated. The amnesic patients learned the sequence, as did the normal participants, as measured by their decreased reaction times for pressing a key when it was illuminated. When the sequence was changed, the reaction times increased for both groups. Strikingly, the amnesic patients had little or no declarative knowledge of the sequence, though they had learned it normally (Reber and Squire, 1994).

Perceptual skills are also often intact in amnesic patients. These include such skills as reading mirror-reversed print and searching a display quickly to find a hidden letter. In formal experiments, amnesic patients acquired perceptual skills at the same rate as individuals with intact memory, even though the patients did not remember what items were encountered during the task and sometimes did not remember the task itself. For example, amnesic patients learned to read mirror-reversed words at a normal rate and then retained the skill for months. Yet, after they had finished the mirror-reading task, they could not remember the words that they had read, and in some cases they could not remember that they had ever practiced the mirror-reading skill on a previous occasion (Cohen and Squire, 1980).

2.5.2.2 Artificial grammar learning

Another kind of learning that is intact in amnesia is the learning of artificial grammars. In an artificial grammar–learning task, participants are presented with a series of letter strings that are generated according to a rule system that specifies what letter sequences are permissible. After viewing these letter strings, participants are told for the first time that the letter strings were formed according to a set of rules and that their task is to decide for a new set of letter strings whether each one is formed by the same set of rules as the set they had just studied. Even though individuals often report that they are simply guessing, they are able to classify new letter strings as grammatical or nongrammatical. Amnesic patients classify items as grammatical or nongrammatical as well as healthy individuals, despite being impaired at recognizing the letter strings that were used during the initial training (Knowlton et al., 1992; Knowlton and Squire, 1994, 1996).

2.5.2.3 Category learning

In tasks involving category learning, participants are exposed to several exemplars of a single category. Then, participants try to classify new items according to whether they are or are not members of that category. In addition, participants identify the prototype, or central tendency of the category, as a member of the learned category more readily than the items used during training, even when the prototype itself was not presented. Amnesic patients are also able to classify items according to a learned category, despite a severe deficit in recognizing the items that were used to train the category (Knowlton and Squire, 1993). In one experiment, amnesic patients and control participants were shown a series of dot patterns formed by distorting a randomly generated pattern that was defined arbitrarily as the prototype of the category. Having seen a series of dot patterns, all of which were distortions of an underlying prototype, participants then were able to discriminate new dot patterns that belonged to the training category from other dot patterns that did not. Amnesic patients performed as well as control participants, even though the patients were severely impaired at recognizing which dot patterns had been presented for training. It is worth noting that it has been suggested that a model assuming a single memory system was able to account for the dissociation between categorization and recognition (Nosofsky and Zaki, 1998).

2.5.2.4 Priming

Priming refers to an improved ability to identify or produce a word or other stimulus as a result of its prior presentation. The first encounter with an item results in a representation of that item, and that representation then allows it to be processed more efficiently than items that were not encountered recently. For example, suppose that line drawings of a dog, hammer, and airplane are presented in succession, with the instruction to name each item as quickly as possible. Typically, about 800 ms are needed to produce each name aloud. If in a later test these same pictures are presented intermixed with new drawings, the new drawings will still require about 800 ms to name, but now the dog, hammer, and airplane are named about 100 ms more quickly. The improved naming time occurs independently of whether one remembers having seen the items earlier. Amnesic patients exhibit this effect at full strength, despite having poor memory of seeing the items earlier.

The dissociation between intact priming and impaired recognition memory in amnesic patients can be particularly compelling. One study investigated priming in patient E.P., who is so severely amnesic that he exhibits no detectable declarative memory (Hamann and Squire, 1997). E.P. sustained complete bilateral damage to the medial temporal lobe as the result of herpes simplex encephalitis. Two tests of priming were given. In one of the priming tests, word stem completion, participants were shown a short word list, which included, for example, the words MOTEL and ABSENT. Then, they were shown the fragments MOT___ and ABS___, with instructions to form the first word that comes to mind. Participants had a strong tendency (30–50%) to produce the words that were recently presented. (The probability was about 10% that participants would produce these words if they had not been presented recently.) In addition, two parallel tests of recognition memory for words were given: alternative forced-choice and yes–no recognition. E.P. performed entirely normally on the two priming tests but performed at chance (50%) on the recognition tests.

In another experiment, participants saw words slowly clearing from a mask. They tried to identify each word as quickly as possible and then make a recognition judgment (old/new) about whether the word had been presented in a preceding study phase. Amnesic patients exhibited intact fluency (the tendency to label those words that were identified more quickly as old) and intact priming, but their recognition was impaired (Conroy et al., 2005). These results support the idea that priming depends on brain structures independent of the medial temporal lobe, and they show that the combined effects of priming and fluency are not sufficient to increase recognition performance.

2.5.2.5 Adaptation-level effects

Adaptation-level effects refer to the finding that experience with one set of stimuli influences how a second set of stimuli is perceived (e.g., their heaviness or size). For example, experience with light-weighted objects subsequently causes other objects to be judged as heavier than they would be if the light-weighted objects had not been presented. Amnesic patients show this effect to the same degree as healthy individuals, even when they experience the first set of objects with one hand and then make judgments with the other hand. However, they have difficulty remembering their prior experience accurately (Benzing and Squire, 1989).

2.5.2.6 Classical conditioning

Classical conditioning refers to the development of an association between a previously neutral stimulus (CS) and an unconditioned stimulus (US), and is a quintessential example of nondeclarative memory. One of the best-studied examples of classical conditioning in humans is delay conditioning of the eyeblink response. It is reflexive and automatic and depends solely on structures below the forebrain, including the cerebellum and associated brainstem circuitry (Thompson and Krupa, 1994). In a typical conditioning procedure, a tone repeatedly precedes a mild airpuff directed to the eye. After a number of pairings, the tone comes to elicit an eyeblink in anticipation of the airpuff. Amnesic patients acquire and retain the tone–airpuff association at the same rate as healthy individuals. In both groups, awareness of the temporal contingency between the tone and the airpuff is unrelated to successful conditioning.

In trace conditioning, a brief interval of 500–1000 ms is interposed between the CS and the US. This form of conditioning requires the hippocampus (McGlinchey-Berroth et al., 1997). Formal experiments suggest that trace conditioning is hippocampus dependent because it requires the acquisition and retention of conscious knowledge during the course of the conditioning session (Clark and Squire, 1998). Only those who became aware of the CS-US relationship acquired differential trace conditioning. There was a correlation between measures of awareness taken after the conditioning and trace conditioning performance itself, whereas there was no correlation between awareness and conditioning performance on a delay conditioning task.

2.5.2.7 Habit learning

Habit learning refers to the gradual acquisition of associations between stimuli and responses, such as learning to make one choice rather than another. Habit learning depends on the neostriatum (basal ganglia). Many tasks can be acquired either declaratively, through memorization, or nondeclaratively as a habit. For example, healthy individuals will solve many trial-and-error learning tasks quickly by simply engaging declarative memory and memorizing which responses are correct. In this circumstance, amnesic patients are disadvantaged. However, tasks can also be constructed that defeat memorization strategies, for example, by making the outcomes on each trial probabilistic. In such a case, amnesic patients and healthy individuals learn at the same gradual rate (Knowlton et al., 1992).

It is also true that severely amnesic patients who have no capacity for declarative memory can gradually acquire trial-and-error tasks, even when the task can be learned declaratively by healthy individuals. In this case they succeed by engaging habit memory. This situation is nicely illustrated by the eight-pair concurrent discrimination task, which requires individuals to learn the correct object in each of eight object pairs. Healthy individuals can learn all eight pairs in one or two test sessions. Severely amnesic patients acquire this same task over many weeks, even though at the start of each session they cannot describe the task, the instructions, or the objects. It is known that this task is acquired at a normal (slow) rate by monkeys with medial temporal lobe lesions, and that monkeys with lesions of the neostriatum (basal ganglia) are impaired. Thus, humans appear to have a robust capacity for habit learning that operates outside of awareness and independently of the medial temporal lobe structures that are damaged in amnesia (Bayley et al., 2005a).

2.6 Functional Amnesia

Functional amnesia, also known as dissociative amnesia, is a dissociative psychiatric disorder that involves alterations in consciousness and identity. Although no particular brain structure or brain system is implicated in functional amnesia, the cause of the disorder must be due to abnormal brain function of some kind. Its presentation varies considerably from individual to individual, but in most cases functional amnesia is preceded by physical or emotional trauma and occurs in association with some prior psychiatric history. Often, the patient is admitted to the hospital in a confused or frightened state. Memory for the past is lost, especially autobiographical memory and even personal identity. Semantic or factual information about the world is often preserved, though factual information about the patient's life may be unavailable. Despite profound impairment in the ability to recall information about the past, the ability to learn new information is usually intact. The disorder often clears, and the lost memories return. Sometimes, the disorder lasts longer, and sizable pieces of the past remain unavailable.

2.7 Summary

The study of amnesia has helped to understand the nature of memory disorders and has led to a better understanding of the neurological foundations of memory. Experimental studies in patients, neuroimaging studies of healthy volunteers, and related studies in experimental animals continue to reveal insights about what memory is and how it is organized in the brain. As more is learned about the neuroscience of memory, and about how memory works, more opportunities will arise for achieving better diagnosis, treatment, and prevention of diseases and disorders that affect memory.

References

Adolphs R, Cahill L, Schul R, and Babinsky R (1997) Impaired declarative memory for emotional material following bilateral amygdala damage in humans. *Learn. Mem.* 4(3): 291–300.

Bayley PJ, Frascino JC, and Squire LR (2005a) Robust habit learning in the absence of awareness and independent of the medial temporal lobe. *Nature* 436: 550–553.

Bayley PJ, Gold JJ, Hopkins RO, and Squire LR (2005b) The neuroanatomy of remote memory. *Neuron* 46(5): 799–810.

Bayley PJ, Hopkins RO, and Squire LR (2003) Successful recollection of remote autobiographical memories by amnesic patients with medial temporal lobe lesions. *Neuron* 38(1): 135–144.

Benzing WC and Squire LR (1989) Preserved learning and memory in amnesia: Intact adaptation-level effects and learning of stereoscopic depth. *Behav. Neurosci.* 103(3): 538–547.

Cave CB and Squire LR (1991) Equivalent impairment of spatial and nonspatial memory following damage to the human hippocampus. *Hippocampus* 1: 329–340.

Clark RE and Squire LR (1998) Classical conditioning and brain systems: The role of awareness. *Science* 280(5360): 77–81.

Cohen NJ and Squire LR (1980) Preserved learning and retention of pattern-analyzing skill in amnesia: Dissociation of knowing how and knowing that. *Science* 210(4466): 207–210.

Conroy MA, Hopkins RO, and Squire LR (2005) On the contribution of perceptual fluency and priming to recognition memory. *Cogn. Affect. Behav. Neurosci.* 5(1): 14–20.

Davis M (1994) The role of the amygdala in emotional learning. *Int. Rev. Neurobiol.* 36: 225–266.

Hamann SB and Squire LR (1995) On the acquisition of new declarative knowledge in amnesia. *Behav. Neurosci.* 109: 1027–1044.

Hamann SB and Squire LR (1997) Intact perceptual memory in the absence of conscious memory. *Behav. Neurosci.* 111: 850–854.

Janowsky JS, Shimamura AP, and Squire LR (1989) Source memory impairment in patients with frontal lobe lesions. *Neuropsychologia* 27(8): 1043–1056.

Kim JJ, Clark RE, and Thompson RF (1995) Hippocampectomy impairs the memory of recently, but not remotely, acquired trace eyeblink conditioned responses. *Behav. Neurosci.* 109(2): 195–203.

Knowlton BJ, Ramus SJ, and Squire LR (1992) Intact artificial grammar learning in amnesia: Dissociation of classification learning and explicit memory for specific instances. *Psychol. Sci.* 3: 172–179.

Knowlton BJ and Squire LR (1993) The learning of categories: Parallel brain systems for item memory and category knowledge. *Science* 262(5140): 1747–1749.

Knowlton BJ and Squire LR (1994) The information acquired during artificial grammar learning. *J. Exp. Psychol. Learn. Mem. Cogn.* 20(1): 79–91.

Knowlton BJ and Squire LR (1995) Remembering and knowing: Two different expressions of declarative memory. *J. Exp. Psychol. Learn. Mem. Cogn.* 21(3): 699–710.

Knowlton BJ and Squire LR (1996) Artificial grammar learning depends on implicit acquisition of both abstract and exemplar-specific information. *J. Exp. Psychol. Learn. Mem. Cogn.* 22(1): 169–181.

LeDoux JE (1996) *The Emotional Brain*. New York: Simon and Schuster.

Lee AC, Buckley MJ, Spiers H, et al. (2005a) Specialization in the medial temporal lobe for processing of objects and scenes. *Hippocampus.* 15(6): 782–797.

Lee AC, Bussey TJ, Murray EA, et al. (2005b) Perceptual deficits in amnesia: Challenging the medial temporal lobe 'mnemonic' view. *Neuropsychologia.* 43(1): 1–11.

Levy DA, Hopkins RO, and Squire LR (2004) Impaired odor recognition memory in patients with hippocampal lesions. *Learn. Mem.* 11(6): 794–796.

Levy DA, Shrager Y, and Squire LR (2005) Intact visual discrimination of complex and feature-ambiguous stimuli in the absence of perirhinal cortex. *Learn. Mem.* 12(1): 61–66.

Maguire EA, Burke T, Phillips J, and Staunton H (1996) Topographical disorientation following unilateral temporal lobe lesions in humans. *Neuropsychologia* 34: 993–1001.

Manns JR, Hopkins RO, Reed JM, Kitchener EG, and Squire LR (2003) Recognition memory and the human hippocampus. *Neuron* 37(1): 171–180.

McGlinchey-Berroth R, Carrillo MC, Gabrieli JD, Brawn CM, and Disterhoft JF (1997) Impaired trace eyeblink conditioning in bilateral, medial-temporal lobe amnesia. *Behav. Neurosci.* 111(5): 873–882.

Mishkin M (1982) A memory system in the monkey. *Philos. Trans. R. Soc. Lond. B Biol. Sci.* 298: 83–95.

Nosofsky RM and Zaki SR (1998) Dissociation between categorization and recognition in amnesic and normal individuals: An exemplar-based interpretation. *Psychol. Sci.* 9: 247–255.

O'Keefe J and Dostrovsky J (1971) The hippocampus as a spatial map. Preliminary evidence from unit activity in the freely-moving rat. *Brain Res.* 34(1): 171–175.

O'Keefe J and Nadel L (1978) *The Hippocampus as a Cognitive Map*. Oxford: Oxford University Press.

Reber PJ and Squire LR (1994) Parallel brain systems for learning with and without awareness. *Learn. Mem.* 1(4): 217–229.

Rempel-Clower NL, Zola SM, Squire LR, and Amaral DG (1996) Three cases of enduring memory impairment after bilateral damage limited to the hippocampal formation. *J. Neurosci.* 16(16): 5233–5255.

Ribot T (1881) *Les Maladies de la Memoire* [English translation: Diseases of Memory]. New York: Appleton-Century-Crofts.

Rutishauser U, Mamelak AN, and Schuman EM (2006) Single-trial learning of novel stimuli by individual neurons of the human hippocampus-amygdala complex. *Neuron* 49(6): 805–813.

Schacter DL and Tulving E (1994) *Memory Systems.* Cambridge, MA: MIT Press.

Shrager Y, Gold JJ, Hopkins RO, and Squire LR (2006) Intact visual perception in memory-impaired patients with medial temporal lobe lesions. *J. Neurosci.* 26(8): 2235–2240.

Smith ML (1988) Recall of spatial location by the amnesic patient H.M. *Brain Cogn.* 7: 178–183.

Spiers HJ, Burgess N, Maguire EA, et al. (2001) Unilateral temporal lobectomy patients show lateralized topographical and episodic memory deficits in a virtual town. *Brain* 124: 2476–2489.

Squire LR (1992) Memory and the hippocampus: A synthesis from findings with rats, monkeys, and humans. *Psychol. Rev.* 99(2): 195–231.

Squire LR and Shimamura AP (1986) Characterizing amnesic patients for neurobehavioral study. *Behav. Neurosci.* 100(6): 866–77.

Squire LR and Zola SM (1998) Episodic memory, semantic memory, and amnesia. *Hippocampus* 8: 205–211.

Squire LR and Zola-Morgan S (1983) The neurology of memory: The case for correspondence between the findings for human and nonhuman primate. In: Deutsch JA (ed.) *The Physiological Basis of Memory*, pp. 199–267. New York: Academic Press.

Squire LR and Zola-Morgan S (1991) The medial temporal lobe memory system. *Science* 253: 1380–1386.

Stefanacci L, Buffalo EA, Schmolck H, and Squire LR (2000) Profound amnesia after damage to the medial temporal lobe: A neuroanatomical and neuropsychological profile of patient E. P. *J. Neurosci.* 20(18): 7024–7036.

Suzuki WA and Amaral DG (1994a) Perirhinal and parahippocampal cortices of the Macaque monkey: Cortical afferents. *J. Comp. Neurol.* 350: 497–533.

Suzuki WA and Amaral DG (1994b) Topographic organization of the reciprocal connections between the monkey entorhinal cortex and the perirhinal and parahippocampal cortices. *J. Neurosci.* 14: 1856–1877.

Teng E and Squire LR (1999) Memory for places learned long ago is intact after hippocampal damage. *Nature* 400: 675–677.

Thompson RF and Krupa DJ (1994) Organization of memory traces in the mammalian brain. *Annu. Rev. Neurosci.* 17: 519–549.

Tulving E (1983) *Elements of Episodic Memory*. New York: Oxford University Press.

Tulving E (1985) How many memory systems are there? *Am. Psychol.* 40: 385–398.

Wais PE, Wixted JT, Hopkins RO, and Squire LR (2006) The hippocampus supports both the recollection and the familiarity components of recognition memory. *Neuron* 49: 459–466.

Wixted JT (2007) Dual-process theory and signal-detection theory of recognition memory. *Psychol. Rev.* 114(1): 152–176.

Wixted JT and Stretch V (2004) In defense of the signal detection interpretation of remember/know judgments. *Bull. Rev.* 11(4): 616–641.

Zola-Morgan S, Squire LR, and Amaral DG (1986) Human amnesia and the medial temporal region: Enduring memory impairment following a bilateral lesion limited to field CA1 of the hippocampus. *J. Neurosci.* 6(10): 2950–2967.

3 Multiple Memory Systems in the Brain: Cooperation and Competition

N. M. White, McGill University, Montreal, Canada

3.1 Introduction

Both casual and scientific observation inform us that behavior changes with experience. This phenomenon is called learning. Its existence implies that information about experience is retained or stored in some way so it can influence future behavior. This is called memory. Learning can be observed. Memory cannot be observed but is inferred from learned behavior. Such inferences are quite common in daily life. One of their best-known applications is the inference that students have acquired certain specific memories from their performance on an examination.

Identification and description of the information stored as memory is a major subject of this chapter. Perhaps the earliest recorded example of such a description was associationism, the notion that neural representations of certain ideas and events are connected in some way. This inference was made from the observation that temporally contiguous ideas and events tend to evoke memories of each other, expressed as thoughts and behavior.

As early as 1804, Maine de Biran described how language reveals memory for several different kinds of information, including motor functions (speech), emotions and the situations that evoke them, and abstract associations among ideas and concepts (Maine de Biran, 1804). In his 1883 book, *Les Maladies de la Mémoire* (Diseases of Memory), Ribot described a series of patients with apparent damage to the cerebral cortex who had lost all personal, conscious memories and temporal information but retained normal memory for habits and skills such as handicrafts (Ribot, 1883). He suggested that personal and conscious memories are stored in the cortex, and that memories for skills and habits must be stored elsewhere in the brain. Together, these two early French authors described a basic version of the multiple memory systems idea: that different types of information are stored in different parts of the brain.

Other early evidence for localization of memory types came from observations of pathological states such as the amnesic syndromes named for Alzheimer (1987) and Korsakoff (Ljungberg, 1992), who suggested that damage to the cortex (including the hippocampus) and medial thalamus were involved in storing the memories their patients had lost.

This early evidence for the localization of memories for different kinds of information contributed to a controversial science called phrenology, the idea that the human personality could be studied by observing the shape of the head (Gall and Spurzheim, 1819). The basis of this claim was the hypothesis that individual differences in the development (i.e., size) of brain areas with different functions determines both personality and the shape of the skull that encloses them. Although the idea that skull shape is related to brain function was discredited, the concept of localization of function in the brain has become a basic principle of neuroscience. The multiple memory systems idea applies this principle to the processing and storage of different types of information.

3.2 Inferring Information Type from Learned Behavior

3.2.1 The Rigorous Study of Learning

The scientific study of memory requires a rigorous methodology for observing and recording learned behavior. The first such investigations are usually attributed to Ebbinghaus (1885). Ebbinghaus memorized lists of nonsense syllables (used because differences in the familiarity of words would have influenced learning and recall rates). He recorded the number of trials required to reach specific levels of performance and observed how this number was reduced each time the same list was rememorized (savings). By this experiment and many others, he showed that memory could be brought under experimental control and studied with precision, even though it could not be directly observed. Other researchers extended Ebbinghaus' original work (Anderson and Bower, 1979), and some began applying the principles he developed to the study of learning and memory in animals.

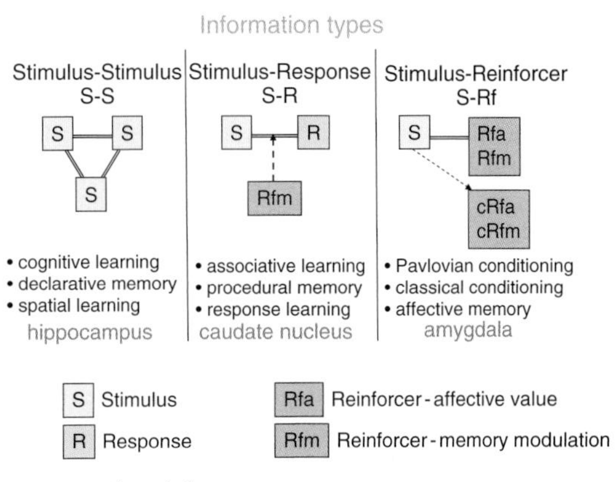

Figure 1 Information types. The headings of each column show the names of the three types of information, derived as explained in the text. Each type consists of associations in which three elements (stimuli, responses, reinforcers) are associated in different ways. The diagrams show how the elements are associated in each type of information. Below each diagram are common synonyms for each type of information used in the learning and memory literature. At the bottom of each column is the name of the brain structure central to the anatomical system thought to process each type of information.

3.2.2 Theories of Learning

During the first part of the twentieth century the behavioral investigation of learning in rats formed the basis of several major research programs which differed, sometimes radically, in the inferences they made from behavior about the kinds of information stored in memory (Hilgard and Bower, 1966). The concepts that emerged from this research (**Figure 1**) are useful starting points for describing the kinds of information stored as memory.

3.2.2.1 Stimulus-response (S-R) associations

The simplest theory, initially proposed by Thorndike (1898, 1911), was based on the observation that the probability of a stimulus evoking a response depends on the number of times the response has been made in the presence of the stimulus and followed by a reinforcer (e.g., food). Thorndike postulated that all learned behavior is the result of a series of associations or bonds between neural representations of stimuli and responses that have been strengthened, or 'stamped in' by a reinforcer. This makes the stimulus more likely to elicit the response.

The idea that behavior is based on stored stimulus-response, or S-R, associations became the foundation of an elaborate system developed by Hull (1943), whose theory predicted the probability of a response based on numerous factors, including the number of times the reinforced S-R pairing was experienced, the number of hours of food deprivation, the amount of reinforcer given, the properties of the reinforcer, how often the response had been made recently, and many others. One purpose of this complex specification was to explain behavior without considering any unobservable variables such as conscious knowledge of a situation or awareness of its emotional (or affective) content, which were considered inadmissible by the behaviorist approach to psychological investigation (Watson, 1912; Bergmann and Spence, 1964).

3.2.2.2 Stimulus-stimulus (S-S) associations

In direct contrast, Tolman (1932, 1948, 1949) argued that behavior is based on cognitive information rather than being controlled by specific response tendencies. One example of an observation leading to this inference was the partial reinforcement extinction effect (Skinner, 1938; Humphreys, 1939). One group of rats received reinforcement after every correct response they made in a learning task, another group received reinforcement after only half of their correct responses. When tested with no reinforcement (extinction), the group that had been reinforced for half of its responses kept responding longer than the group that had been reinforced for all responses. This result is the opposite of what was predicted by Hull's S-R theory, which held that the strength of a response tendency is directly related to the number of times it has been reinforced. Tolman concluded that the rats' behavior was based on their knowledge of the situation and what events they expected. The rats in the 100% group expected reinforcement for every response, so a few unreinforced responses were enough for them to detect the change in conditions and stop responding. The rats in the 50% group did not expect reinforcement for every response, so more unreinforced responses were required before they stopped.

Tolman (1932) postulated that learning consists of acquiring information about the relationships among stimuli and events. This information constitutes 'knowledge' and is represented as a series of interlocking relationships among stimuli known as stimulus-stimulus (S-S) associations (**Figure 1**). S-S associations can represent spatial relationships, leading to the concept of the spatial map (see section 3.3.4), and temporal relationships, leading to expectancy (knowing what comes next in a sequence of events).

3.2.2.3 Stimulus-reinforcer (S-Rf) associations

The third type of information was described by Pavlov (1927). Pavlov was studying the internal secretions produced by food in hungry dogs. When the dogs were repeatedly exposed to the experimental situation, the secretions began to occur in the absence of food. Accordingly, Pavlov postulated that an association was formed between the food (the unconditioned stimulus, or US) and stimuli in the experimental situation (the conditioned stimulus, or CS). This made the CS capable of eliciting conditioned responses (CR) similar to those produced by the US.

USs are events that elicit responses without previous experience. These include food, water, sexual partners, and certain aversive events. The elicited unconditioned responses (URs) include approach or withdrawal and responses of the autonomic nervous system and certain brain structures and neurotransmitters. Neutral stimuli acquire CS properties when a US occurs in their presence. The issue of whether Pavlovian learning is the result of a CS-US or a CS-UR association is controversial (e.g., Donahoe and Vegas, 2004). Reflecting this controversy, the process is often described as a CS-US/UR learning. In the multiple memory systems context, this form of learning is called stimulus-reinforcer (S-Rf) learning (**Figure 1**), because it is restricted to responses that are elicited by reinforcers.

3.2.3 Reinforcers

The events called USs in Pavlovian theory are the same ones that Thorndike labeled reinforcers. The three theories include three different functions of the responses elicited by reinforcers:

1. Reinforcers elicit internal, unobservable responses that strengthen, or modulate, S-R and S-S (Packard and Teather, 1998; Packard and Cahill, 2001) and S-Rf (White and Carr, 1985; Holahan et al., 2006) associations when their occurrence is temporally contiguous with the acquisition of the association (Thorndike, 1933; Landauer, 1969; McGaugh and Herz, 1972; White, 1989b; White and Milner, 1992) (shown as Rfm in **Figure 1**).
2. Reinforcers elicit internal, unobservable responses that are perceived as positive or negative affect (Young and Christensen, 1962; Cabanac, 1971; White, 1989b; White and Milner, 1992; Burgdorf and Panksepp, 2006) (shown as Rfa in **Figure 1**). Humans and animals can learn about these affective states and how to obtain or avoid them in, a process called instrumental learning.
3. Reinforcers elicit observable orienting and approach or withdrawal responses. Normally, stimuli that elicit approach also elicit positive affect and are sometimes called rewards. Stimuli that elicit withdrawal and also elicit negative affect are described as aversive, or as punishments. Both rewarding and aversive events strengthen or modulate memory (Huston et al., 1977; White, 1989b; Holahan et al., 2006).

Because the learning theorists used rats in their experiments, they also had to use biologically relevant reinforcers to control behavior and the information being processed and stored during the experimental trials. Although it is not necessary to use such reinforcers with humans, who can follow instructions, feedback about correct and incorrect responses is also used and has many of the same functions as biological reinforcers in rats (see Thorndike, 1933). Both instructions and feedback control human behavior and information processing in experimental trials.

3.2.4 Information Types: Relationships among Elements

Each learning theory made different inferences from observed behavior about the kinds of information processed and stored during learning, but, as illustrated in **Figure 1**, in each case the information consists of different combinations of the same three elements: stimuli, responses, and reinforcers. The information types differ in the relationships among these elements. S-S, S-R, and S-Rf associations can all be thought of as different types of information created by experience, stored in the brain, and recalled to influence behavior. Large parts of this chapter describe evidence that these types of information are processed and stored in different parts of the brain.

3.3 Localization of Information Processing

3.3.1 Early Localization Attempts

S. I. Franz (1902) was among the first to apply systematic behavioral methodology to the study of brain areas involved in memory. He reported that cats could learn a series of complex responses to escape from a box and that large lesions of various parts of the cortex had only temporary effects on this learned behavior. He concluded that there was no evidence for localization of memory functions in the brain.

Franz's student, Karl Lashley, pursued these studies, testing rats on a variety of memory tasks with similar results (Beach et al., 1960). No part of the cortex seemed more important than any other – temporary deficits in learned behavior were usually quickly reversed with additional training. Only very large lesions including most of the cortex produced permanent, although generally still partial, deficits. Lashley concluded that the memory functions of any part of the cortex could substitute for any other part, a principle he called equipotentiality. Lashley's frustration at his inability to localize and understand memory is revealed by his summary statement in a 1950 article describing a lifetime of work on the problem:

> I sometimes feel, in reviewing the evidence on the memory trace, that the necessary conclusion is that learning is just not possible. (Lashley, 1950, p. 477)

Notwithstanding their methods, Franz's and Lashley's experiments failed to localize memory functions because they assumed that a single brain structure (the cerebral cortex) processed and stored all memories. It followed from this assumption that damaging the critical structure should eliminate all forms of memory. Although the idea that different parts of the brain process different kinds of memory had been suggested, Franz and Lashley did not make use of this idea, possibly because of behaviorist strictures on the use of such unobservable entities as information types.

3.3.2 HM and the Function of the Hippocampus

In the early 1950s new clinical evidence for the localization of different types of memory in the brain emerged. A patient with intractable epilepsy, known by his initials (HM), underwent a bilateral excision of a major portion of his temporal lobes (including much of the hippocampus) as a last-chance treatment, making him perhaps the most famous patient in modern neurology (Scoville and Milner, 1957). He was given a full psychological assessment by Brenda Milner, who reported (Milner and Penfield, 1955; Milner, 1958, 1959) that he was unable to recall personal experiences or other events from the previous 20 or so years (retrograde amnesia), and that he was also unable to remember any current experience for more than a few minutes (anterograde amnesia). HM also had difficulty finding his way around, even in familiar environments.

However, HM retained other forms of memory. He was able to learn a simple maze that required him to move a stylus through a series of left and right turns on a board (Corkin, 1968; Milner et al., 1968). He performed this task accurately, while at the same time claiming he had never seen it before. This showed that the memory deficit produced by temporal lobe resection was limited to information about HM's previous experiences. The deficit did not include the information that allowed him to learn the maze, which must have been dependent on some other part of the brain.

Although Milner and her coauthors carefully described their observation that the effects of bilateral hippocampal ablation are limited specifically to memory for new ongoing experience and spatial orientation, and that other kinds of memory, including verbal abilities, emotion, and skills and habits remained normal, these distinctions were largely ignored at first.

3.3.2.1 Attempts to replicate HM's syndrome with animals

3.3.2.1.(i) Monkeys Orbach et al. (1960) proposed that a strong test of the temporal lobe memory hypothesis would be met only if temporal lobe damage impaired performance regardless of what behavioral task their monkeys were required to learn. These workers did find deficits on some memory tasks, but only with very large temporal lobe lesions.

The reasons for this (and other) failures to replicate HM's syndrome were revealed by Mahut and coworkers, who reported that monkeys with hippocampal (Mahut, 1971), fimbria-fornix, or entorhinal cortex (Mahut, 1972; Zola and Mahut, 1973) lesions were impaired on spatial tasks when no local stimuli were available to guide their behavior. In the same monkeys, nonspatial tasks were unaffected, and when small cue objects were added to spatial discrimination tasks, performance actually improved relative to that of normal controls (Killiany et al., 2005). These experiments showed that memory deficits are produced by hippocampal damage in monkeys, provided tasks requiring the use of the kind of information processed in the hippocampus are used (Mahut et al., 1981).

3.3.2.1.(ii) Rats A number of workers also tried to demonstrate the effects of hippocampal lesions on memory in rats. These studies had such limited success that several theories suggesting alternate functions for the rat hippocampus were proposed (Kimble and Kimble, 1965; Douglas and Pribram, 1966; Kimble, 1968; Isaacson and Kimble, 1972) and refuted (Nadel et al., 1975). These hypotheses did not completely reject memory-related functions but were primarily concerned with explaining the highly inconsistent effects of hippocampal lesions on the performance of various memory tasks. The inconsistency was the result of a failure to appreciate the specific type of information processed in the hippocampus and the consequent use of tasks that could be performed on the basis of some other kind of information processed in other parts of the brain.

3.3.3 Contextual Retrieval

In what is now considered a major conceptual breakthrough, Hirsh (1974) provided an explanation for the inconsistent effects of hippocampal lesions on memory tasks in rats. Hirsh pointed out that hippocampal lesions did not affect learning tasks that could be performed on the basis of a single S-R association, but they impaired performance of tasks that could not be correctly performed using this kind of information. He suggested that tasks impaired by hippocampal lesions involved acquisition of two or more S-R associations, and that the hippocampus mediated a process by which one of these was selected by the context. An example of a behavioral observation that led to the inference of this contextual retrieval process is illustrated in **Figure 2**. Rats were trained in a T-maze to turn left for food when hungry and right for water when thirsty (Hsiao and Isaacson, 1971). The choice point in the maze became a stimulus associated with two responses: the left and right turns. The deprivation state was the context that selected the appropriate S-R association. Normal rats learned to make the correct turn depending on their deprivation state. Rats with various impairments of the hippocampal system (Hirsh and Segal, 1971; Hsiao and Isaacson, 1971; Hirsh et al., 1978a,b) made one turn or the other, regardless of their deprivation state. They were unable to use the motivational context to select the correct response.

Another example is reversal learning. As shown in **Figure 3**, normal rats and rats with hippocampal lesions learned to turn left for food at similar rates. When the food was switched to the right arm of the maze, normal rats adjusted their behavior much more quickly than rats with hippocampus lesions. The normal rats were able to change the direction of their turn on the basis of new information about the location of the food obtained on the first few trials after the switch. According to Hirsh, the switch altered the context that selected the appropriate response. Hippocampectomized rats were unable to use this type of information. They had to extinguish the old S-R association and acquire a new one when the reinforcer was switched.

Hirsh's main contribution to the idea of localized memory functions based on the content of the memory was to explain it in terms of the existing animal learning literature, an area of research that was very well developed and had up to that time generally rejected or ignored this possibility. Although it took some time, "The hippocampus and contextual

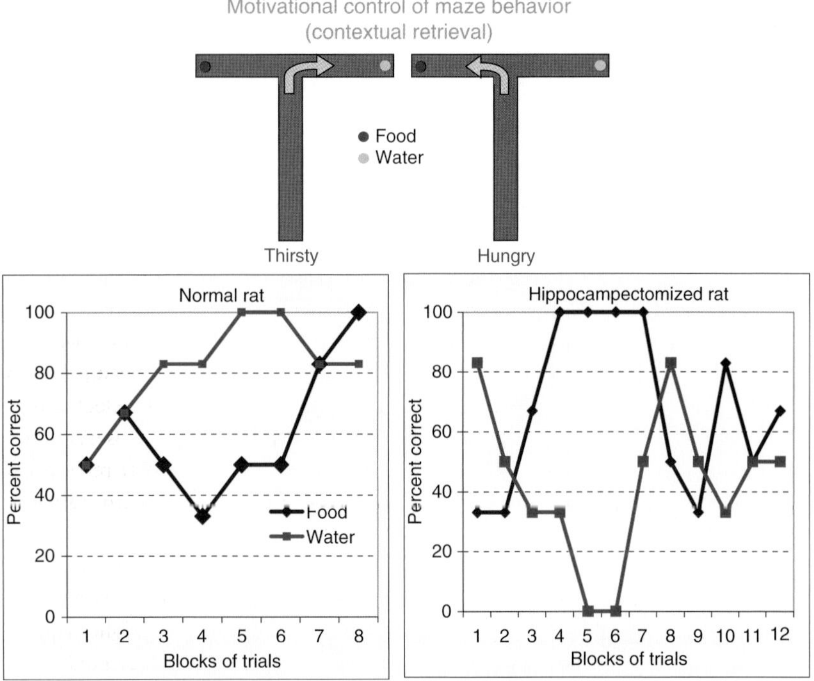

Figure 2 Motivational control of maze behavior (contextual retrieval). The figure illustrates an experiment in which rats were trained on a T-maze with food in one arm and water in the other. The rats were food or water deprived on alternate days. The graph on the left shows the behavior of a normal rat that learned to turn right for water on days when it was thirsty first (trial blocks 1–5). Between blocks 5 and 8 the rat also learned to turn left for food when hungry, while maintaining the correct response for water. This shows that the rat had learned to use its motivational state to perform the correct response at the choice point in the maze. The graph on the right shows the behavior of a hippocampectomized rat that began by learning to turn right for water. As the rat's performance on the days when it was hungry improved, its performance on thirsty days declined. After a few more trial blocks, the rat's performance when thirsty improved, whereas its performance when hungry declined. Several more such reversals were observed, suggesting that this rat was able to learn one of two simple S-R associations but was unable to use its motivational state to select between the two. Adapted from Hirsh R (1980) The hippocampus, conditional operations and cognition. *Physiol. Psychol.* 8: 175–182.

retrieval of information from memory: A theory" (Hirsh, 1974) has come to be regarded as a major turning point in research on memory.

3.3.4 Spatial Learning

In *The Hippocampus as a Cognitive Map*, O'Keefe and Nadel (1978) presented evidence that the hippocampus is the primary structure for representing and possibly storing spatial information. The two main lines of evidence for this idea were impairments in spatial learning produced by hippocampal lesions and the observation that the activity levels of certain hippocampal neurons increased whenever a rat was in a specific spatial location (O'Keefe and Dostrovsky, 1971; O'Keefe, 1976). This suggestion that the hippocampus contains information about the animal's position in space led O'Keefe and Nadel to postulate the spatial map, a neural representation of the relationships among constant features of an environment. The information in these representations can be described as consisting of a series of S-S associations. This relational information is purely descriptive, with no specific implications for behavior. O'Keefe and Nadel distinguished hippocampus-based spatial learning (also called allocentric) from taxon (or egocentric) learning, in which each environmental feature can evoke one specific response, as in the case of S-R learning. O'Keefe and Nadel did not speculate about the neural substrate for taxon learning.

The idea that the hippocampus processes information consisting of relationships among features of an environment has been extended and incorporated into the theory that the structure processes relational information of all kinds (Hirsh, 1980; Cohen and

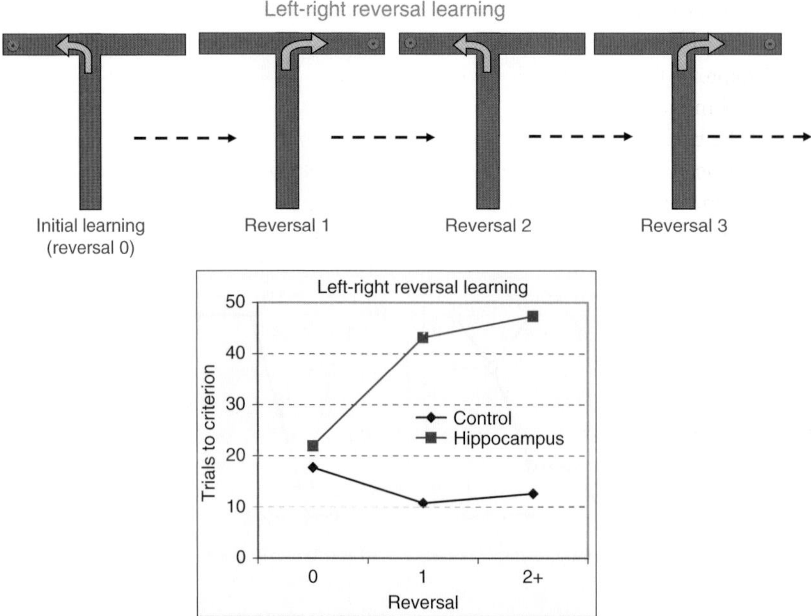

Figure 3 Effects of hippocampus lesions on reversal learning. Hungry rats learned to find food in a maze by turning left at the choice point. Both normal rats and rats with hippocampal lesions learned the initial response to criterion (five consecutive correct responses) equally well (Reversal 0). However, when the correct response was reversed, the hippocampectomized rats were severely impaired. The impairment continued on subsequent reversals. All rats were given a total of 100 trials, during which the control rats met the criterion and were reversed an average of 8.1 times. Hippocampectomized rats met the criterion and were reversed an average of 2.2 times. Adapted from Kimble DP and Kimble RJ (1965) Hippocampectomy and response preservation in the rat. *J. Comp. Physiol. Psychol.* 60: 474–476.

Eichenbaum, 1991; Eichenbaum and Cohen, 2001). This information, stored as S-S representations, can be used flexibly to produce behaviors appropriate to different circumstances. The theory that the information processed in the hippocampus is purely spatial, and the idea that it represents relationships of a more general nature including spatial have been debated (Wiener et al., 1989; Cohen and Eichenbaum, 1991; Nadel, 1991; Eichenbaum et al., 1992).

3.3.5 Memory and Habit

Mishkin et al. (1984) described an experiment in which monkeys were shown pairs of objects. Displacing one of them revealed a morsel of food. When shown the same two objects a short time later, displacing the other object revealed food. The monkeys were given a large number of trials over several days, with different pairs of objects on every trial. Normal monkeys learned this 'delayed nonmatching to sample' rule, but monkeys with hippocampal lesions were unable to do so – a deficit that is consistent with a general loss of memory for recent events. In contrast, when a large number of object pairs were presented repeatedly, normal and hippocampal monkeys learned to respond to the correct member of each pair equally well. Thus, hippocampal lesions impaired memory for novel objects seen for the first time but did not affect learning to make a consistent response to each pair of objects after repeated reinforced trials. Mishkin et al. described the latter behavior as a habit and speculated that the memory for this type of behavior might be mediated in the caudate nucleus.

3.3.6 Declarative versus Procedural Memory

Cohen and Squire (1980) trained human participants to read words in a mirror. Both normal participants and patients with amnesia resulting from medial temporal lobe dysfunction learned the mirror reading skill; they improved with practice and improved more for words that were repeated in each session than for words that were new. However, when tested shortly after a training trial, normal participants were able to remember most of the words they had just read; the amnesic patients were severely impaired.

Cohen and Squire concluded that memory for the words (declarative memory) requires a functional hippocampus (*See* Chapter 10), but that the mirror reading skill (procedural memory) must be dependent on some other part of the brain.

Declarative and procedural memory describe different kinds of remembered information, corresponding to S-S and S-R learning as described by Tolman and Thorndike, respectively, as well as to Mishkin et al.'s distinction between memory and habit, to Hirsh's descriptions of contextual memory versus S-R memory, and to O'Keefe and Nadel's concepts of the spatial map and taxon learning. These distinctions were all made by showing that hippocampal damage impairs performance on tasks requiring S-S information but has no effect on tasks that can be performed using S-R information. None of these distinctions includes evidence concerning the neural substrate of S-R information processing.

3.3.7 Double Dissociation of S-S and S-R Learning in Humans

Butters and coworkers (Martone et al., 1984; Butters et al., 1986; Heindel et al., 1989) found that patients with Korsakoff's syndrome, who are amnesic as a result of hemorrhagic lesions of medial thalamus and mammillary bodies, learned the mirror reading skill normally but were unable to recognize words they had recently read. In contrast, patients with Huntington's disease, in which neurons in the basal ganglia (including the caudate nucleus) degenerate, had the opposite pattern of disabilities: They were unable to acquire the mirror reading skill but recognized previously seen words normally.

This pattern of effects constitutes a double dissociation, in which subjects with impairments of one of two brain areas were compared on two memory tasks. Impaired function of each brain area affected only one of the two tasks, leaving performance on the other task intact. This led to the conclusion that each brain area was involved in processing the type of information required for the impaired task, but not the information required for the unimpaired task. As described in the previous section, recall of recently seen words requires declarative, or S-S, information; mirror reading is a skill that may require a complex of S-R associations.

Although there was no direct confirmation of the brain damage in these studies, they are significant because they provide evidence for the neural substrate that processes information that may include S-R information and dissociate it from S-S information processing. The studies point to the basal ganglia, specifically the caudate nucleus, as the location of S-R information processing. A number of experiments with rats are consistent with this conclusion about the caudate nucleus (Divac et al., 1967; Divac, 1968; Thompson et al., 1980; Chozick, 1983; Mitchell and Hall, 1987, 1988; Cook and Kesner, 1988; Packard and Knowlton, 2002). Phillips and Carr (1987) specifically proposed that S-R learning is mediated in the basal ganglia.

3.3.8 Dissociation of Three Information Types in Rats

Packard et al. (1989) used a double dissociation to compare the impairments in information processing capacity produced by lesions to the fimbria-fornix (a major input-output pathway of the hippocampus) and the caudate nucleus. This was extended by McDonald and White (1993) to include the amygdala in a triple dissociation of memory tasks. All three tasks were performed on an eight-arm radial maze (**Figure 4**) consisting of a center platform with eight arms radiating from it in a sunburst pattern about 1 m from the floor. Each task required the use of a different type of information.

3.3.8.1 Win-shift task – hippocampus-based S-S memory

The win-shift radial maze task (Olton and Samuelson, 1976; Olton and Papas, 1979) was used to examine S-S information processing. The maze was situated in a room with various extra-maze stimuli (or cues) that constituted a spatial environment. A small food pellet was placed at the end of each arm. Hungry rats were placed on the center platform and allowed to forage for food. Pellets consumed were not replaced, so to obtain the eight available pellets most efficiently the rat had to enter each arm once only. Second or more entries to arms were considered to be errors. Normal rats attained an average of less than one error per trial after five to seven daily trials.

To enter each arm once only, a rat must remember which arms it has entered as the trial proceeds (working memory). To do this, it must be able to discriminate the arms from each other. There is evidence that rats perform this discrimination by associating each arm with the environmental cues that are visible from it (O'Keefe and Nadel, 1978; Suzuki et al., 1980). Since all the individual cues are visible from several of the arms, no individual cue can

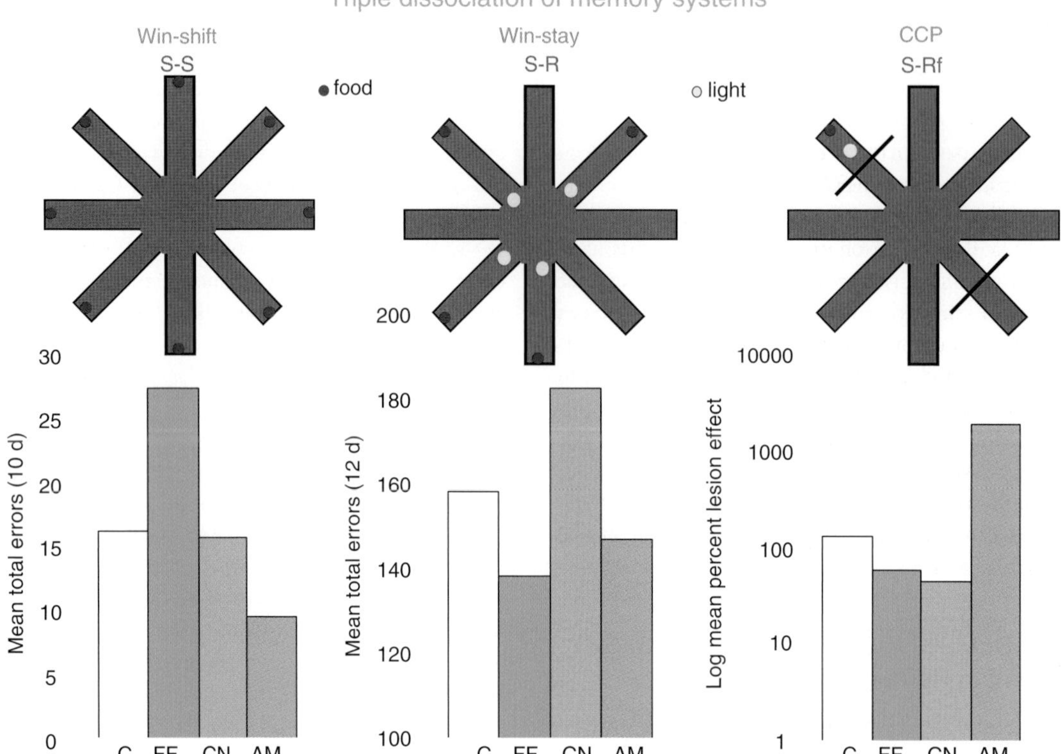

Figure 4 The triple dissociation. Three different tasks on the eight-arm radial maze are illustrated at the top. The type of information processing thought to be required to perform each task is indicated, corresponding to the information types described in **Figure 1**. As explained in the text, correct performance of the win-shift task requires rats to obtain the food pellet at the end of each arm without reentering arms. This requires spatial (or S-S) information processing. Performance of this task was impaired by lesions of fimbria-fornix (FF), but not by caudate nucleus (CN) or amygdala (AM) lesions. The win-stay task requires a simple association between a cue light and the arm entry response, reinforced by eating the food at the end of the lit arms. A different set of four arms is lit and baited on each daily trial. This is an instance of S-R information processing. Performance on this task was impaired by lesions of the caudate nucleus but not by lesions of fimbria-fornix or amygdala. The improved performance on this task produced by fimbria-fornix lesions is explained in **Figure 5**. In the conditioned cue preference (CCP) task, the rats acquire an S-Rf association between the light and the food reinforcer, causing the light to acquire conditioned stimulus properties. This results in a preference for the food-paired arm even when no food is present on the test trial. Performance on this task was impaired by lesions of the amygdala, but not by lesions of fimbria-fornix or caudate nucleus. Adapted from McDonald RJ and White NM (1993) A triple dissociation of memory systems: Hippocampus, amygdala and dorsal striatum. *Behav. Neurosci.* 107: 3–22.

identify any single arm. However, the arms can be identified by their unique locations within a spatial map of the environment. This requires relational or S-S information.

Good performance on this task requires continually updated information about the status of each arm as a trial proceeds. At the start of a trial all arm-identifying cue arrays indicate the location of a food pellet, but once an arm has been entered and the pellet consumed, the same array must indicate the absence of food. In this way information about the spatial environment is used flexibly to guide behavior according to changing conditions.

3.3.8.2 Win-stay task – caudate-based S-R memory

The win-stay task was used to study S-R information processing. The same maze was used, but the location of the food was indicated by a small light mounted at the entrance to each arm. When a hungry rat was placed on the center platform at the start of a trial, four of the arms were lit, and only those four arms contained a food pellet. The other arms were empty. Efficient performance required the rats to enter lit arms and avoid dark arms. The information required to produce this behavior is simple: When a rat approaches a lit arm (S), enters it (R), and consumes the reinforcer, the S-R association is strengthened, increasing the probability that the stimulus will elicit the response again. No spatial information or working memory is required for the win-stay task.

3.3.8.3 Conditioned cue preference task – amygdala-based S-Rf memory

The conditioned cue preference (CCP) task was used to study S-Rf information processing. The radial maze was surrounded by curtains. Hungry rats were confined on an arm with a light and a supply of food and on alternate days were confined on a different, dark arm with no food. After several days of such trials the rats were placed on the center platform of the maze and given a choice between the two arms, neither of which contained food. Normal rats spent more time on the food-paired than on the unpaired arm.

Since the rats were exposed to the food while confined on a maze arm they could not have acquired any S-R associations or instrumental responses leading to their preference for the food-paired arm. The curtains surrounding the maze and confinement in one arm at a time severely limited the rats' ability to acquire a spatial map of the environment (Sutherland and Linggard, 1982; Sutherland and Dyck, 1984; Sutherland, 1985; White and Ouellet, 1997). Therefore, the preference was probably not a result of learned information about the spatial location of food (i.e., S-S learning). The alternative is that consuming the food (US) during the training trials elicited an internal rewarding response (UR). This caused the arm cues (light or dark) in the food-paired arm to acquire CS properties. On the test trial, the CS elicited a conditioned reward response, causing the rat to remain in the food-paired arm longer than in the no-food arm. This analysis explains the preference for the food-paired arm as the product of S-Rf information processing.

3.3.8.4 Dissociation by damaging brain structures

As shown in **Figure 4**, performance on each of the three tasks was impaired by only one of the three lesions. (Performance of the win-stay task was actually improved by fimbria-fornix lesions. This phenomenon is explained in **Figure 5**.) Since the three tasks had identical sensory and motor requirements, and the same reinforcer was used for all three, the differences in the effects of the lesions were attributed to differences in the kinds of information required to perform the tasks. The effects of the lesions imply that each lesioned structure was involved in processing only one of the three kinds of information.

None of these attributions was original to the triple dissociation experiments. It was already well known that lesions of the hippocampus and related structures impair spatial learning (Hirsh and Segal, 1971; O'Keefe et al., 1975; Olton et al., 1978; Olton, 1978; Morris et al., 1982), and that Pavlovian conditioning involving S-Rf information processing is impaired by amygdala lesions (Weiskrantz, 1956; Bagshaw and Benzies, 1968; Jones and Mishkin, 1972; Nachman and Ashe, 1974; Peinado-Manzano, 1988; Everitt et al., 1989, 1991; Hatfield and Gallagher, 1995; Davis, 1997; Fanselow and Gale, 2003). There were also numerous reports of learning impairments produced by caudate nucleus lesions, but the evidence that these involved S-R learning was not clear (e.g., Gross et al., 1965; Divac et al., 1967; Divac, 1968; Kirkby, 1969; Winocur and Mills, 1969; Mitchell and Hall, 1987, 1988). The contribution of the triple dissociation experiment was to define these various tasks in terms of the kinds of information required to perform them and to show that the processing of each type of information was dependent on a different part of the brain.

3.3.8.5 Dissociation by reinforcer devaluation

Reinforcer devaluation is a procedure in which a rewarding reinforcer is paired with an aversive event, reducing the positive affective value of the reinforcer (Young and Christensen, 1962; Dickinson et al., 1983). The prototype is the conditioned taste aversion (Garcia and Koelling, 1966; Nachman and Ashe, 1974; Yamamoto and Fujimoto, 1991), in which pairing consumption of a rewarding substance such as a sugar solution with injections of lithium chloride (LiCl) (which produces gastric illness) decreases or eliminates consumption of the solution.

Yin and Knowlton (2002) used the devaluation procedure in conjunction with the CCP task on the radial maze. After CCP training the rats ate some of the same food pellets in their home cages, followed by LiCl or saline (control) injections. When tested in their home cages the rats that received LiCl ate much less than the rats that received saline, demonstrating the reduced net reward value of the food. When given a preference test on the radial maze with no food present the rats that received saline preferred their food-paired arms, but the rats that received LiCl exhibited an aversion to their food-paired arms (see **Figure 6**). This finding

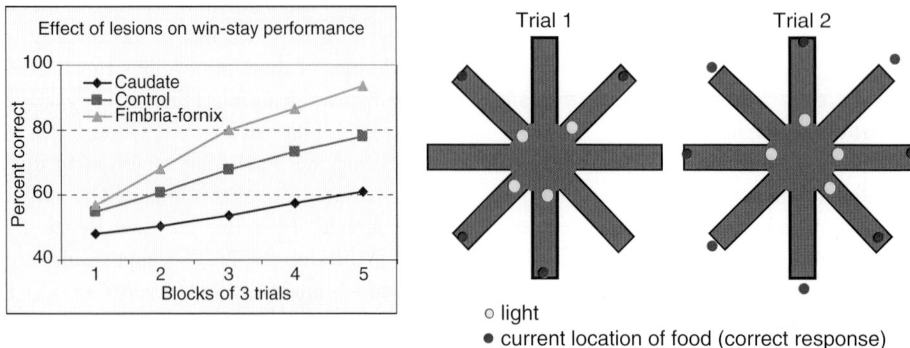

Figure 5 Fimbria-fornix lesions improve performance on the win-stay task. The graph shows the effects of lesions on performance of the win-stay task (see **Figure 4**). Compared with normal control rats, rats with caudate lesions performed poorly, suggesting that this structure is involved in processing the S-R information required for performing the task. In contrast, lesions of fimbria-fornix (part of the hippocampal system) improved win-stay performance compared with controls. The maze diagrams on the right explain this improved performance. They show two consecutive trials on the win-stay task. In both cases the arms containing food are indicated by lights at their entrances, but the food is located in different arms on the two trials. Caudate-based processing of information comprising the consistently reinforced S-R association between the lights and the arm entry response results in correct behavior on both trials. However, on Trial 1 the hippocampus system acquires information about the fixed cues in the spatial environment and about the location of food in relation to those cues. As shown in the figure, this information is incorrect on Trial 2, because a different set of four arms contains food. Therefore, any tendency to enter arms that previously contained food promoted by the hippocampal system would result in errors. Fimbria-fornix lesions eliminate this S-S information and the erroneous responses it promotes, resulting in improved performance of the S-R task. Because the information processing capacities of the two systems cause them to promote different behaviors in the same situation, the effect of fimbria-fornix lesions on win-stay performance reveals a competitive interaction between the behavioral effects of the two kinds of information processing. Adapted from Packard MG, Hirsh R, and White NM (1989) Differential effects of fornix and caudate nucleus lesions on two radial maze tasks: Evidence for multiple memory systems. *J. Neurosci.* 9: 1465–1472.

suggests that the preference for the food-paired arm was the result of a memory that involved the affective property of the reinforcer. This memory was positive in the saline-injected rats, leading to a preference for the food-paired arm. It was much less positive, even negative, in the LiCl-injected rats, leading to avoidance of the food-paired arm. This is consistent with the idea that the CCP is based on information comprising an S-Rf association.

In contrast to these findings, Sage and Knowlton (2000) found that the same devaluation procedure did not affect the performance of well-trained rats on the win-stay task, even though they stopped eating the food at the ends of the lit arms (**Figure 6**). This observation is consistent with the idea that performance on this task is unrelated to the affective value of the reinforcer, which acts simply to strengthen the caudate-based S-R association that produces the win-stay behavior.

Sage and Knowlton (2000) also found that rats trained on the win-shift task performed normally after devaluation (**Figure 6**). These rats did not completely reject the food while running the maze. Most of them ate the pellets in the first few arms entered and then stopped eating while continuing to perform correctly. This suggests that they did not spontaneously transfer the aversion from the home cage to the new situation but recalled it only after tasting the food in the new context. That this rejection of the food had little effect on the accuracy of their win-shift performance is consistent with the hypothesis that information involving the affective value of the food is not required for win-shift performance, which depends on information about the presence and absence of food in each arm as the trial progresses.

Although the devaluation data do not dissociate the neural substrates of information processing in the three tasks, they constitute evidence that S-S and S-R information can control behavior independently of the affective value of reinforcers in the situation. This contrasts with the evidence for the representation of these affective properties in S-Rf information processing.

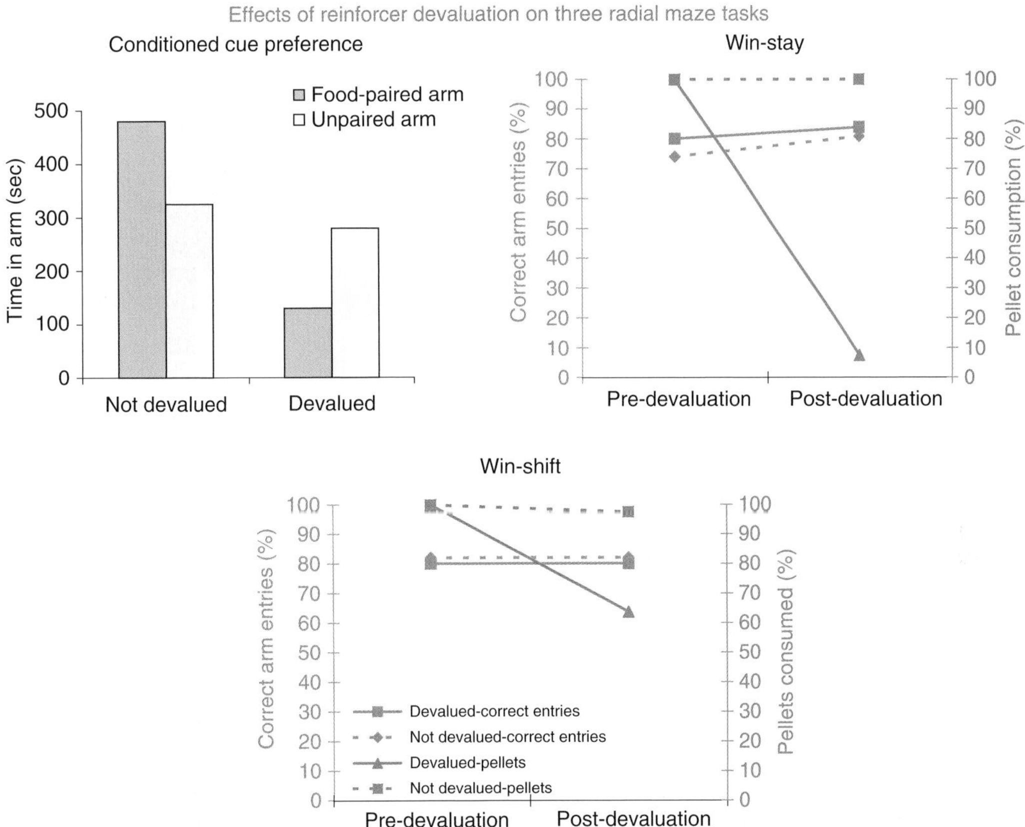

Figure 6 Effects of reinforcer devaluation on three radial maze tasks. *CCP:* The graph on the top left shows the amounts of time spent by rats in their food-paired and unpaired radial maze arms in a CCP test (see section 3.3.8.3). Rats that experienced reinforcer devaluation (explained in the text) exhibited an aversion to their food-paired arms. Rats that did not experience devaluation exhibited a normal conditioned preference for their food-paired arms. The effect of devaluation on the preference is evidence that the rats' behavior is controlled by information that includes a representation of the affective value of the reinforcer. *Win-stay:* The graph on the top right shows the percent correct responses and the percent of total food pellets available that were consumed before and after reinforcer devaluation. Before devaluation the rats ate all pellets available; after devaluation they ate very few. However, this did not affect the accuracy of their win-stay performance. This constitutes evidence that the affective value of the reinforcer is irrelevant to win-stay behavior and is consistent with the idea that the reinforcer acts to strengthen the S-R association that controls behavior in this situation. *Win-shift:* The graph on the bottom shows the percent correct responses and percent of total pellets consumed on the win-shift task before and after reinforcer devaluation. Performance was maintained after devaluation, whereas pellet consumption decreased. The pellets were not completely rejected, suggesting that a representation of the affective value of the reinforcer may have contributed to win-shift performance. However, the maintenance of accuracy shows that positive affect was not required for performance of this task, which can be produced by information about the presence and absence of food in the arms. Adapted from Sage JR and Knowlton BJ (2000) Effects of US devaluation on win-stay and win-shift radial maze performance in rats. *Behav. Neurosci.* 114: 295–306; Yin HH and Knowlton BJ (2002) Reinforcer devaluation abolishes conditioned cue preference: Evidence for stimulus-stimulus associations. *Behav. Neurosci.* 116: 174–177.

3.4 Information Processing Systems

This section describes a series of theoretical ideas that constitute a theory of multiple parallel memory systems in the brain. The ideas are suggested by the findings already described and will be useful for organizing and interpreting the literature describing dissociations among brain structures and processing of information types.

3.4.1 Systems Concept

Although the idea that different kinds of information are processed in different parts of the brain is suggested by the effects of damage to individual brain areas, the fact that no individual brain area can perform any function on its own leads naturally to the idea that information is processed in neural systems or pathways that can, in principle, be defined anatomically. The two visual systems described by Ungerleider and Mishkin (1982; Mishkin et al., 1983) are an example of anatomically defined neural systems that process different kinds of information. Both systems originate in the striate and prestriate visual cortex, making these structures parts of both pathways. A ventral path connects to inferior temporal areas; damage to structures in this pathway impairs object recognition. The dorsal path connects to inferior parietal areas; damage to this pathway impairs learning the visual location of objects. Visual information originating in striate cortex is integrated with other information at stages along each pathway. In this way the visual information comes to represent spatial relationships in one system and object properties in the other.

A similar concept can be applied to the evidence for independent processing of different types of information that is the subject of this chapter (see **Figure 7**). Information originating in the external and internal sense organs is processed and represented in the thalamus and cerebral cortex. This information is distributed to several different neural pathways or systems. It flows through the systems as neural activity, undergoing processing and modification at stages along the way. This results in the differentiation of the information into a unique representation in each system. The outputs of the systems converge to influence behavior and thought.

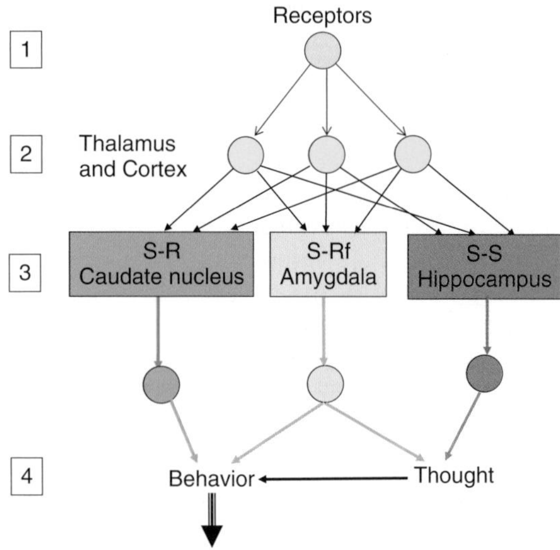

Figure 7 The multiple memory systems concept. 1. Patterns of neural activity originate in exteroceptors and interoceptors. 2. These patterns converge on thalamic and cortical areas, where they are processed and combined into activity patterns that represent the current external and internal environments. 3. These processed activity patterns are transmitted to subcortical areas, each of which is specialized to extract and represent a different kind of information contained in the activity patterns: the caudate nucleus represents reinforced stimulus-response (S-R) associations, the amygdala represents stimulus-reinforcer (S-Rf) relationships, and the hippocampus represents stimulus-stimulus (S-S) relationships. 4. The outputs of the systems converge on brain areas that mediate behavior and thought. See text for more information about the information types, how they are represented in the systems, and how the outputs of the systems interact.

3.4.1.1 Systems process incompatible information

Sherry and Shachter (1987) suggested that independent neural systems evolved to process fundamentally incompatible information. According to this idea, flexible memory for facts and unique situations and memory for stereotyped skills and habits are incompatible. This concept corresponds to the mutually exclusive involvement of the hippocampus and caudate nucleus in these types of memory. Although Sherry and Shachter did not discuss the amygdala, evidence from the triple dissociation experiment suggests that similar considerations may apply to the unique kind of information processed in that structure.

3.4.1.2 Systems are internally specialized

The information processing specialization of each system is determined at the level of its neuronal and synaptic microcircuitry. Although neural activity representing all of the elements reaches all systems, their internal specializations lead to differences in the ways they represent the relationships among the elements (**Figure 1**). There have been several attempts to describe how the internal structures of the hippocampus (Muller et al., 1996; Knierim et al., 1998; Taube, 1998; Mizumori and Leutgeb, 2001; Lever et al., 2002; Leutgeb et al., 2005; Sargolini et al., 2006), caudate nucleus (Centonze et al., 2001; Graybiel, 2001, 2004; Gurney et al., 2004), and amygdala (Pitkänen et al., 1997; Fendt and Fanselow, 1999;

Maren and Quirk, 2004; Maren, 2005; Schafe et al., 2005; Kim and Jung, 2006) process and store the information mediated in these structures.

3.4.1.3 Coherence: Some representations are better than others

Coherence is a hypothetical property of the representation of a learning situation in a neural system. The coherence of a representation reflects the degree to which all parts of the system are activated in a similar way when processing information that represents a particular situation. This is determined by the correspondence between the information content of the learning situation and the representational specialization of the system. The better the correspondence, the more coherent the representation. The coherence of the representation of a learning situation in a system is assumed to determine the degree to which the system influences behavior and/or thought when the representation is activated during recall.

The development of hippocampal place cells, which occurs during the first 10–30 min of exposure to a novel environment (O'Keefe and Dostrovsky, 1971; O'Keefe, 1976; Ferbinteanu and Shapiro, 2003; Kentros et al., 2003; Kennedy and Shapiro, 2004), may be an example of the creation of a coherent representation of a spatial map (S-S information) of the environment. Conversely, the same system is very slow to form a coherent representation of the S-R information content of a learning situation such as the win-stay task. This is suggested by the failure of rats with caudate lesions but an intact hippocampus to learn the win-stay task (see **Figure 4**). This and other evidence (see section 3.5) suggest that the caudate system acquires a coherent representation of S-R information more easily (in fewer trials) than the hippocampus system.

3.4.1.4 The learning-rate parameter

The coherence of the representation of a situation in a system usually improves with repeated exposure to the situation. One system may represent a situation coherently after only a single trial; another system may simultaneously form a representation of the same situation, but this may require many more trials to attain coherence. The amount of exposure required to form a coherent representation in a system is a learning-rate parameter. Differences in this parameter are important determinants of the interactions among the systems.

3.4.1.5 Cooperation and competition among systems

At any given point during training in any learning situation, each system has acquired a representation of the situation with some degree of coherence that determines the amplitude of its output. The fact that the systems all influence the behavior of the same animal (or person) means that these outputs must converge (**Figure 7**). The nature of the interactions among these outputs depends on the behavioral tendency promoted by the representation in each system and on the relative amplitudes of their outputs.

In some situations the outputs of the systems may promote the same behavior or different parts of a complex behavior required to perform a task. These are cooperative interactions. In other situations the outputs of the systems may promote different behaviors. This results in competitive interactions. The improvement in win-stay performance produced by fimbria-fornix lesions, explained in **Figure 5**, is thought to reflect such an interaction.

3.4.2 Information Processing and Memory

As we have seen, observation of learned behavior is a tool for studying the neural basis of information processing. The existence of a learned behavior also implies the existence of a memory for the information processed by each system. The definition of a system means that the information processed by the system must be stored somewhere within the system.

The neuroplastic processes that store representations of information processed by each system could be located in a discrete part or parts of each system, or they could be distributed throughout the systems. A single storage location (e.g., the cerebral cortex) could store and provide information to all systems. All of these possibilities may apply in various combinations at different stages of the learning process.

The idea that different kinds of information are processed in differently specialized parts of the brain means that, before the relationship between neuroplastic processes and the storage of information can be studied, it is critical to identify the type of information stored in each system. In the absence of this information, evidence for synaptic or neurophysiological changes correlated with the development of learned behavior cannot be interpreted. Accordingly, the evidence reviewed in this chapter does not pertain to memory storage mechanisms. It addresses the prior issue of localizing the processing and storage of different kinds of information.

3.4.3 Dissociations of Memory Systems

The remaining sections of this chapter focus on evidence that dissociates the information processing properties of the three proposed memory systems. As in the review of the historical development of the idea of independent memory systems, the nature of the information being processed is inferred from the ability to perform a memory task of some kind, and the anatomical focus is on the hippocampus and fimbria-fornix, the caudate nucleus, and the amygdala. Evidence for independent information processing in the three structures, taken two at a time, is described. Evidence for competition among the systems is a major feature of the review.

The review is limited to studies in which parts of the brain are functionally disabled in various ways and to studies that measure relative levels of activation in brain areas (primarily imaging studies in humans). Space limitations do not permit a consideration of neurophysiological evidence for localized processing of information types (Mizumori et al., 2004; Davis et al., 2005; Gill and Mizumori, 2006), evidence obtained by manipulations of memory consolidation (Packard and White, 1991; Packard and McGaugh, 1992; Packard et al., 1994; Packard and Teather, 1997, 1998; Packard and Cahill, 2001), or evidence that each of the three systems appear to include subsystems that probably process subtypes of information.

3.5 S-S versus S-R Information Processing

3.5.1 Studies with Rats

3.5.1.1 Competition on the radial maze

As we have already seen, lesions of the fimbria-fornix impair win-shift (S-S) but not win-stay (S-R) learning, and lesions of the caudate nucleus impair win-stay but not win-shift learning (Packard et al., 1989; McDonald and White, 1993), a double dissociation. Furthermore, as described in **Figure 5**, fimbria-fornix lesions did not just impair win-stay learning, they actually improved it so that the performance of the lesioned rats was better than that of normal controls. This observation can be explained as the result of competition between the tendency to enter lit arms, represented as S-R information in the caudate system, with a tendency to forage for food in places where it had previously been available, represented as S-S information in the hippocampus system. Disabling the hippocampus-system with fimbria-fornix lesions eliminated these errors, resulting in improved win-stay performance.

Competition between caudate-based S-R learning and spatial learning has also been demonstrated with caudate lesions (Mitchell and Hall, 1988). Rats were trained to find food in a constant arm of a radial maze. To start each trial the rat was placed in the arm immediately to the right or the arm immediately to the left of the food arm. The food remained in the same spatial location, but either a right or a left turn was required to reach it. Rats with caudate lesions made fewer erroneous turns than normal rats, suggesting that in normal rats S-R associations between local maze cues and either the left or right turn response interfered with behavior based on information about the spatial location of the food. Caudate lesions eliminated S-R learning and the erroneous responses it produced.

3.5.1.2 Cross maze

The cross maze paradigm (Tolman et al., 1946; Blodgett and McCutchan, 1947), illustrated and explained in **Figure 8**, is a simple and elegant method for distinguishing between behavior produced by processing S-S and S-R information. Although the task was originally introduced as a demonstration of learned behavior that is not dependent on S-R information, it was soon shown that both spatial (S-S) and S-R information are acquired during training (Restle, 1957). Increasing the number of training trials favors behavior controlled by S-R information; increasing the availability of spatial stimuli favors behavior controlled by S-S information

3.5.1.2.(i) Competition on the cross maze Packard and McGaugh (1996) exploited the training trial effect on this task to dissociate the caudate and hippocampal memory systems. As shown in **Figure 9**, when tested after 8 days of training, most normal rats ran to the correct spatial location of the food, indicating spatial learning, but when tested again after 8 more days of training the same rats made the turn that had been reinforced during training, which led away from the food, indicating S-R based learning.

In other groups of rats either the hippocampus or the caudate nucleus was temporarily inactivated with lidocaine during the test trials. After 8 days of

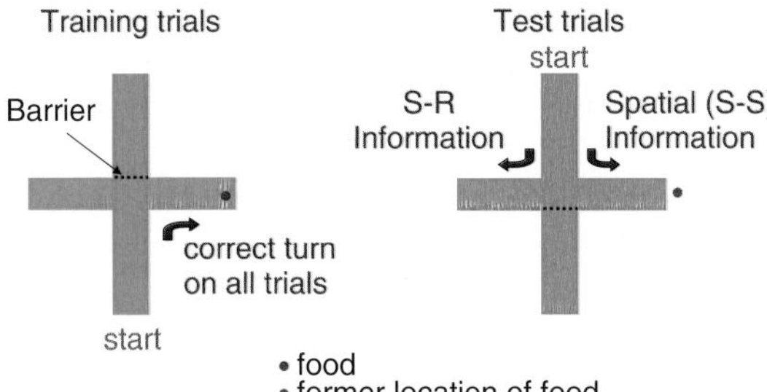

Figure 8 Use of the cross maze to distinguish between responding based on S-S and S-R information. The apparatus is a maze built in the shape of a cross. It is used with a barrier that makes it function as a T-maze. As illustrated on the left, during the training trials rats are placed into the start arm and allowed to explore until they find the food, which is available on every trial. This requires a right turn. After a number of training trials a test trial is given. As shown on the right, the barrier is moved and the rat is placed into the maze at the opposite end of the start arm. The direction of the turn the rat chooses to make on this trial indicates what kind of information was acquired during the training trials. A right turn (the response made during training), which leads away from the food location, indicates behavior controlled by an S-R association – a specific response to the choice point stimulus. A left turn, which leads toward the food location, indicates behavior controlled by an S-S association – spatial information about the location of the food.

training, the normal tendency to make the spatial response was eliminated by hippocampal inactivation, but caudate nucleus inactivation had no effect (**Figure 9**). This is consistent with other findings showing that processing spatial information requires a functional hippocampus but not a functional caudate nucleus.

After 16 days of training, the normal tendency to make the S-R response was eliminated by caudate nucleus inactivation, but hippocampal inactivation had no effect (**Figure 9**). These observations are consistent with others showing that processing S-R information requires a functional caudate nucleus but not a functional hippocampus. Taken together with the findings for 8 training days, they constitute a double dissociation of S-S and S-R information processing with respect to the hippocampus and caudate nucleus, respectively.

Perhaps the most interesting observation in this study focuses on what the rats did when an inactivation treatment impaired their normal behavior. After 8 days hippocampal inactivation resulted in a random choice of arms. This shows that no other information capable of influencing behavior had been acquired at that time.

After 16 days rats that underwent caudate inactivation made the spatial response. This shows that the hippocampus-based spatial information was not eliminated by the additional training that resulted in acquisition of caudate-based S-R information. The spatial information was still present and able to influence behavior when the caudate was inactivated.

The hippocampus system apparently acquired a coherent spatial representation of the location of the food in fewer trials than the caudate system required to acquire a coherent representation of the S-R association. Therefore, behavior was controlled by the hippocampal system after 8 days of training. When additional trials had strengthened the S-R representation sufficiently, the behavioral output of the caudate system assumed control of the rats' behavior. Inactivation of the caudate system allowed the output of the hippocampus system to reassume control. This shows that the behavioral outputs of the systems were in competition with each other.

These findings illustrate several important points. First, they show that S-R memory is inflexible, producing the same response to a stimulus regardless of conditions. In contrast, the S-S system is flexible, using sensory information at the choice point to produce an appropriate response. Second, they reveal a difference in the learning rate parameter: A coherent hippocampus-based representation of the spatial environment was acquired in fewer trials than are required for the formation of a coherent caudate-based representation of a reinforced S-R association. Finally, the pattern of effects shows that the outputs of the systems compete with each other for the control of behavior.

3.5.1.2.(ii) Dissociations in measures of neural function Using cross-maze training parameters that produced approximately equal numbers of rats that made the spatial and S-R responses on the test trial, Columbo et al. (2003) measured phosphorylated response element binding protein (pCREB) in the hippocampus and caudate nucleus 1 h after testing (as explained elsewhere, CREB has been linked to the formation of long-term memories). Increased levels of pCREB expression were found in the hippocampus but not the caudate nucleus of the rats that made the spatial response, and in the caudate but not the hippocampus of rats that made the S-R response. This double dissociation is consistent with the findings in the inactivation experiment.

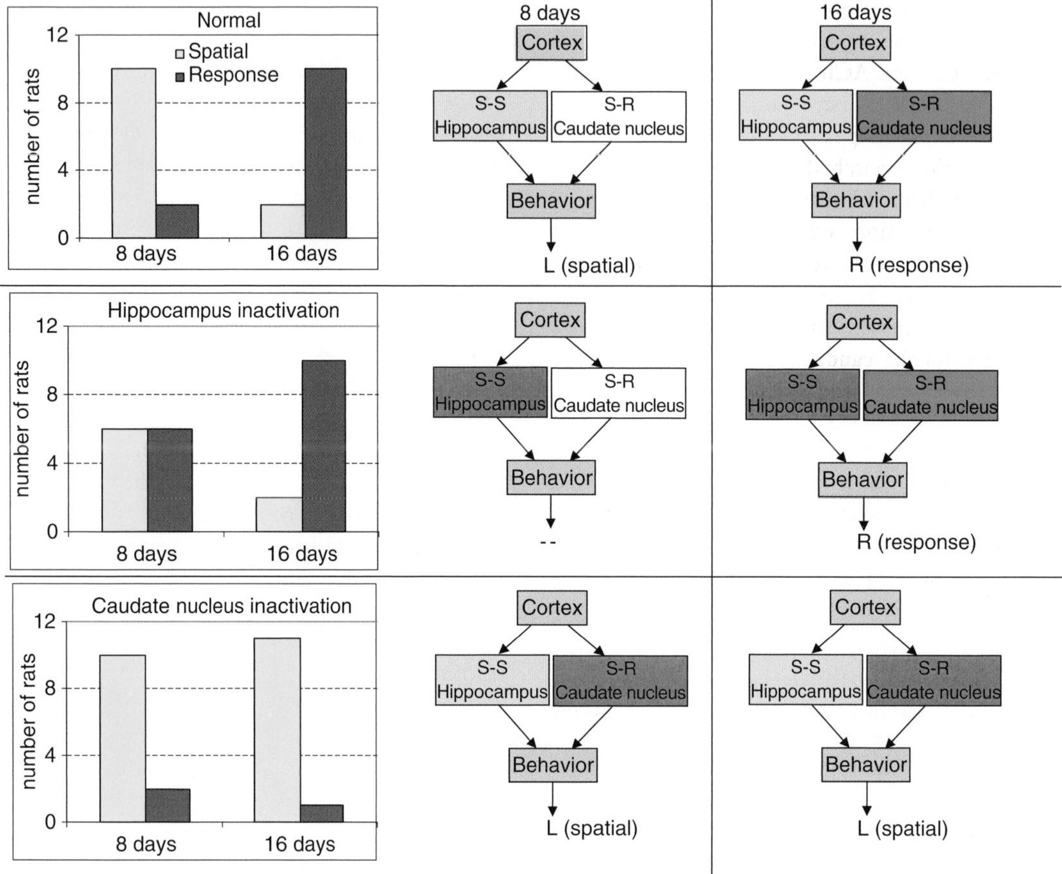

Figure 9 Dissociation and competition on the cross maze. *Top row:* normal rats. The graph shows the number of rats that turned in the direction of the food, indicating the use of spatial information, or away from the food, indicating use of S-R information on the test trials given after 8 or 16 days of training. After 8 days most rats turned toward the food as a result of hippocampus-based processing of spatial information (light green). At this time insufficient caudate-based S-R learning had occurred to influence the response (white). After 16 training days, S-R learning had become strong enough for the output of the caudate system (dark green) to compete with the hippocampus-based response and take control over the rats' behavior, causing them to make the response acquired during training, leading away from the food. *Middle row:* inactivation of the hippocampus during the test trials. After 8 days, hippocampal inactivation (grey) produced random responding, as predicted by the hypothesis that turning toward the food was the result of hippocampus-based spatial information processing. After 16 days, hippocampal inactivation (grey) did not affect the tendency to turn away from the food, consistent with the hypothesis that the hippocampus was not involved in this S-R type behavior. *Bottom row:* inactivation of the caudate nucleus during the test trials. After 8 days, caudate inactivation (grey) had no effect, as predicted by the idea that this structure was not involved in processing the spatial information that produced the turn toward the food. After 16 days, caudate inactivation (grey) resulted in turning toward the food, reversing the behavior of normal rats, which turned away from the food at this point (top row). This is predicted by the hypothesis that the caudate nucleus mediated the S-R information that produced the turn away from the food in the normal rats. It also shows that the hippocampus-based spatial information was still present and able to influence behavior, but that it was prevented from doing so in normal rats by competition from the output of the caudate system. Eliminating the caudate output allowed the spatial information to resume its influence, allowing the rats to turn toward the food. Data from Packard MG and McGaugh JL (1996) Inactivation of hippocampus or caudate nucleus with lidocaine differentially affects expression of place and response learning. *Neurobiol. Learn. Mem.* 65: 66–72.

Increased release of acetylcholine (ACh) is observed in certain brain structures while learning occurs (Ragozzino et al., 1996). Chang and Gold (2003) measured ACh release in the hippocampus and caudate nucleus while rats were being trained and tested on the cross maze. ACh release in the hippocampus increased early in training and remained high throughout, even after the rats had switched from spatial to S-R behavior. This is consistent with the finding in the inactivation experiment that the hippocampal system continues to process information even when it is no longer reflected in behavior. ACh release in the caudoputamen remained low at first, increasing with repeated trials and reaching its peak in individual rats at the same time as they switched from spatial to S-R behavior. These observations are consistent with those from the inactivation experiment showing that the hippocampal system acquires a coherent spatial representation quickly, but that its influence on behavior is eliminated by competitive behaviors originating from the caudate system that acquires a coherent S-R representation more slowly.

3.5.1.3 Water maze

In this task (Morris, 1981) rats are placed into a large pool of opaque water and allowed to swim in search of a small platform submerged just below the surface so that no local cues, including visual cues, identify its location. The rats can escape from the water by climbing onto the platform. Rats learn to swim directly to the platform location regardless of their starting position in the pool, showing that their behavior does not depend on any specific response or sequence of responses, but on S-S information about its spatial location. If the platform is moved the rats have to relearn its location. This task is usually contrasted with learning to swim to a platform that protrudes just above the surface of the water so that it is visible to the rats. They also learn to swim directly to this platform, but this behavior is not affected when the platform is moved, showing that the rats are responding to a local cue, which could be a result of S-R memory. Morris and coworkers (1982) reported that lesions of the hippocampus impaired learning to swim to a hidden, but not to a visible, platform.

Using a slightly different version of this task Packard and McGaugh (1992) found that learning to discriminate between two identical stimuli on the basis of their spatial locations in a pool was impaired by fimbria-fornix but not by caudate nucleus lesions. Learning to discriminate between two different stimuli that were moved to new locations on each trial was impaired by caudate nucleus but not by fimbria-fornix lesions. This double dissociation between a task requiring spatial information and one that could be performed on the basis of an S-R association is further evidence for the differences in the kinds of information processed in the neural systems that include the hippocampus and the caudate nucleus.

3.5.1.3.(i) Competition in the water maze

McDonald and White (1994) trained rats to find a platform that remained in a constant location in the pool. It was visible on some trials and hidden on others (see **Figure 10**). Normal rats learned to swim to the platform in both conditions. As previously shown, rats with fimbria-fornix lesions swam to the platform normally when it was visible but were severely impaired at finding it when it was hidden because of their inability to process spatial information. Rats with caudate nucleus lesions learned to swim to the hidden platform normally, suggesting normal spatial information processing. Although S-R information processing may have been impaired in these rats, no deficit in their ability to locate the visible platform would be expected because the platform was in the same location on all trials. The spatial information that allowed the caudate-lesioned rats to locate the platform when it was hidden could serve the same purpose when the platform was visible.

To examine the possibility that S-R information processing was impaired in the caudate-lesioned rats, a final test trial was given. The platform was moved to a new location, where it was visible (see **Figure 10**). As shown in **Figure 11**, most of the rats with caudate lesions swam directly to the former location of the platform. When they failed to find it, they swam to the new location, where the platform was visible. This behavior suggests that these rats were impaired at processing S-R information, allowing the competing spatial information to control behavior. In contrast, all of the rats with fimbria-fornix lesions swam directly to the visible platform. This is consistent with an impairment in spatial (S-S) information processing, which allowed acquired S-R information to control behavior. The fact that these shifts in behavior were produced by lesions of fimbria-fornix and caudate nucleus is consistent with the hypothesis that these structures are critical for S-S and S-R information processing, respectively.

Figure 11 also shows that half of the rats in the normal control group swam directly to the visible platform, while the other half swam to its former location first. The behavior of these two subgroups of control rats on the hidden platform trials during training is shown in **Figure 10**. The rats whose behavior was controlled by spatial information on the final trial initially learned the location of the hidden platform much faster than the rats whose behavior was controlled by S-R information

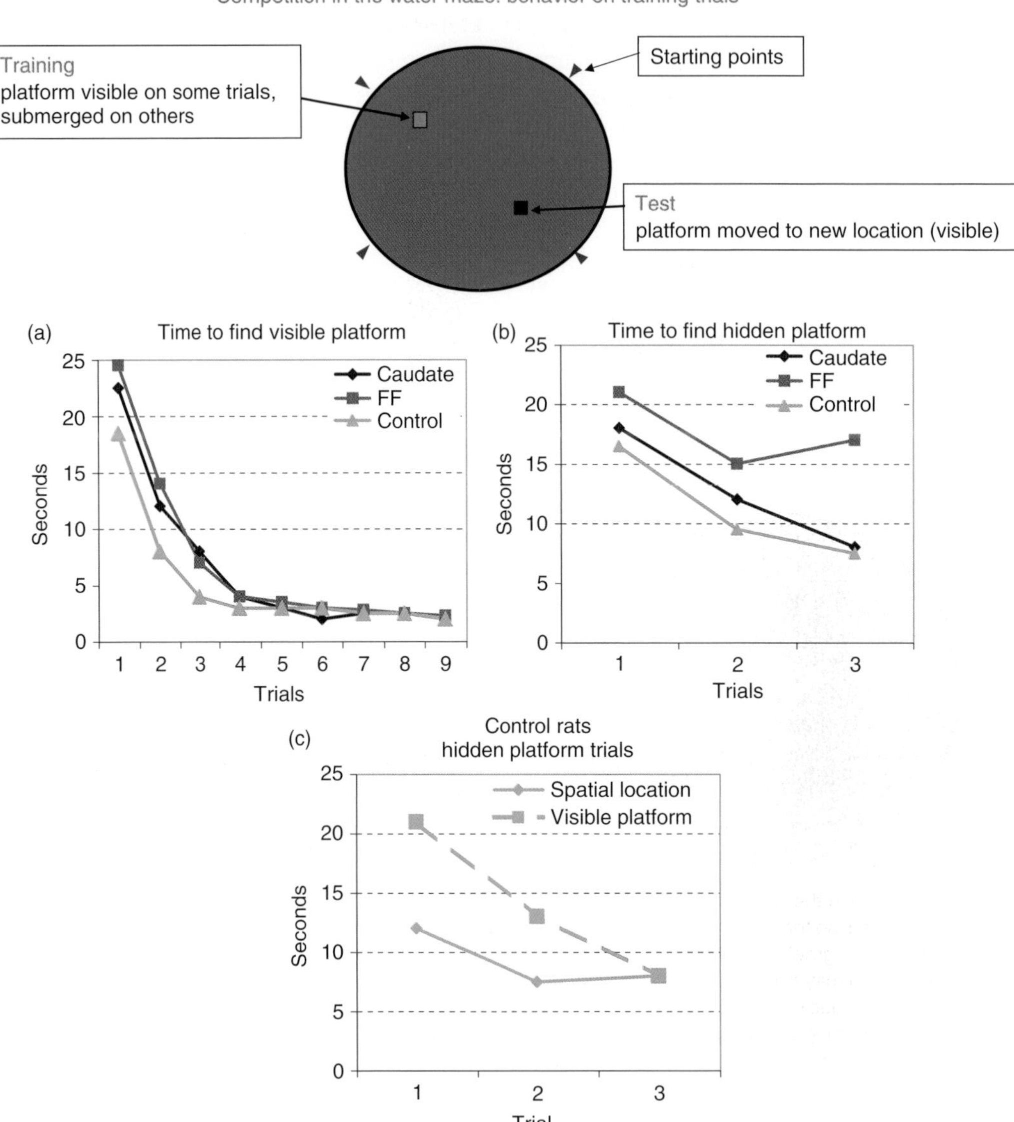

Figure 10 Competition in the water maze: training trials. The blue circle at the top of the figure represents a circular swimming pool about 1.5 m in diameter. Rats were placed into the pool once at each of the four starting points on each training trial. The platform was always in the same location; it was visible on some trials and submerged (invisible) on others. (a) Average time taken to swim to the platform over nine trials when it was visible. (b) Average time to locate the platform during three trials when it was hidden. Hidden platform trials were given after three, five, and nine visible platform trials. Note impairment in fimbria-fornix lesion group on the hidden but not the visible trials. (c) Two subgroups of the control group, which differed in the rate at which they learned to locate the hidden platform. The significance of the difference between these two groups is explained in **Figure 11** and in the text. Data from McDonald RJ and White NM (1994) Parallel information processing in the water maze: Evidence for independent memory systems involving dorsal striatum and hippocampus. *Behav. Neural Biol.* 61: 260–270.

on the final trial. This difference suggests the possibility of constitutional individual differences in the relative learning rates of the hippocampus and caudate systems (see also Colombo and Gallagher, 1998).

3.5.1.3.(ii) Involvement of synaptic functions

Packard and Teather (1997) found that injections of AP5, an *N*-methyl-D-aspartate (NMDA) receptor antagonist (as described elsewhere, NMDA receptors have been implicated in the synaptic events

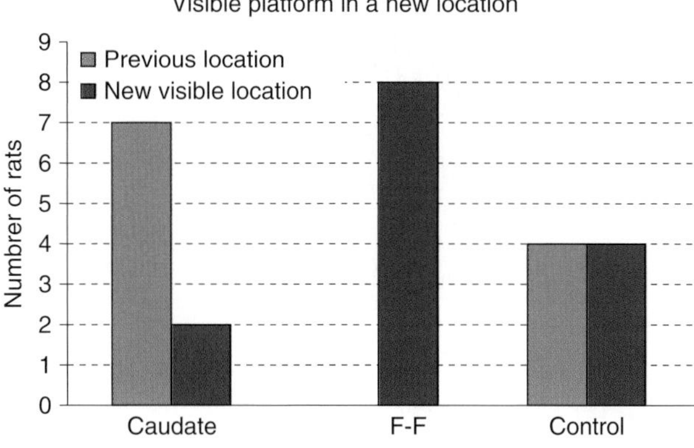

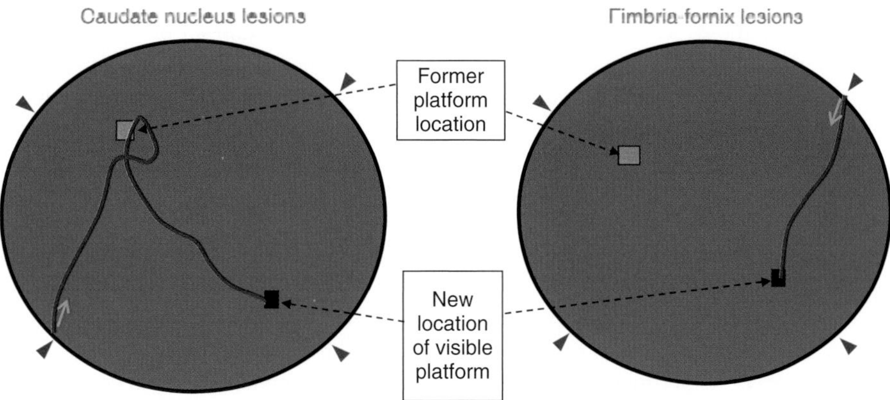

Figure 11 Competition in the water maze: test trial. On the test trial the rats were placed into the pool with the visible platform in a new location, so that spatial learning about the location of the platform competed with the S-R tendency to swim to the visible stimulus. The graph at the top shows that 7/9 rats with caudate nucleus lesions swam to the old spatial location of the platform first; when they failed to find it there, they swam to the visible platform. This is illustrated by the swim path (red line) of a rat with caudate nucleus lesions shown at the bottom left. In the presence of a visible platform, this behavior suggests impaired processing of S-R information, allowing spatial information to control the behavior of most rats in this group. In contrast, as shown in the graph and illustrated on the bottom right, 8/8 rats with fimbria-fornix lesions swam directly to the visible platform. This suggests impaired processing of spatial information, allowing S-R information to control the behavior of these rats. In the control group, four rats swam directly to the visible platform and four swam to its former location first. The behavior of these two subgroups of control rats during the initial hidden platform training trials is shown in **Figure 10**. Data from McDonald RJ and White NM (1994) Parallel information processing in the water maze: Evidence for independent memory systems involving dorsal striatum and hippocampus. *Behav. Neural Biol.* 61: 260–270.

involved in memory storage), into the hippocampus impaired learning to find a hidden but not a visible platform, whereas injections into the caudate nucleus impaired learning to swim to a visible, but not a hidden, platform. These findings suggest the possibility that synaptic changes involved in the storage of S-S and S-R information may occur in the hippocampus and caudate nucleus, respectively.

In another demonstration Teather et al. (2005) counted cells expressing c-Fos and c-Jun (immediate early genes thought to be expressed in the presence of neural activity and synaptic changes involved in memory) after water maze training. In the hippocampus more cells expressing these products were counted following hidden platform training than visible platform training; in the caudate nucleus more expressive cells were found following visible than hidden platform training. These increases were also observed relative to control rats not trained on either task. A similar dissociation has recently been made using cytochrome oxydase as a measure of metabolic activity in the hippocampus and caudate nucleus while rats learned to locate a platform using spatial or local cues (Miranda et al., 2006). Aside from replicating the dissociation between the behavioral tasks and the brain areas with different measures of brain function, these observations again suggest the possibility of synaptic activity related to memory storage in the appropriate brain areas when either S-S or S-R information is being processed.

3.5.1.4 Medial versus lateral caudate nucleus

The caudate nucleus has been described as part of the system that processes S-R information, but evidence shows that in rats, where the structure is often called the caudoputamen, this function is actually confined to its dorsolateral part (White, 1989a; Yin et al., 2004; Featherstone and McDonald, 2004a,b, 2005a,b). This portion of the caudoputamen in the rat may be homologous with the caudate nucleus in primates (Heimer et al., 1985).

There is also evidence that the dorsomedial part of the caudoputamen in the rat processes S-S information (possibly as it interacts with the dorsolateral caudoputamen in the selection of responses – see section 3.3.3). One set of experiments suggesting this possibility shows that fimbria-fornix and dorsomedial caudoputamen lesions have similar effects in the water maze (Devan et al., 1996, 1999). Holahan et al. (2005) found that blocking NMDA receptors in the dorsal hippocampus and dorsomedial caudoputamen had similar effects on the long-term retention of spatial information. Yin and Knowlton (2004) showed that lesions of the posterior dorsomedial caudoputamen, but not of the anterior or dorsolateral parts of the structure, facilitated reinforced S-R responding on the cross maze, an elimination of the competition effect similar to that produced by inactivation or lesions of the hippocampus system. These findings suggest that the dorsomedial caudoputamen in the rat might be considered part of the S-S information processing hippocampal system.

3.5.2 Studies with Humans

Evidence from studies with humans on the dissociation of hippocampus-based declarative (S-S) learning from caudate nucleus-based procedural (or S-R) learning parallel the rat findings quite closely (*See* Chapter 17; Poldrack and Packard, 2003; Hartley and Burgess, 2005). A selection of this evidence is reviewed here.

3.5.2.1 Spatial learning

Iaria et al. (2003) created a virtual eight-arm radial maze on a computer screen and tested normal participants on the win-shift task originally developed for rats. A trial started with the participants at the center of the maze, from where they could look down each of the eight arms and see a virtual landscape of mountains, trees, rocks, and the sun surrounding the maze. They could freely control their movements through the maze with the computer keyboard. Goal objects were not visible from the platform but could be obtained by descending a virtual flight of stairs at the end of each arm. Participants were instructed to obtain all of these objects by entering as few arms as possible. Reentries were scored as errors. Some of the experiments were conducted with the subjects in an fMRI scanner, which is thought to provide indirect information about the relative levels of neural activity in different parts of the brain.

The performance of all participants improved over a series of trials. When asked how they had solved the task, they spontaneously sorted themselves into three groups. One group reported they had used extramaze landmarks, such as proximity to the sun and a tree for one arm and to the sun and a rock for the adjacent arm, to identify and avoid reentering arms. This constitutes a spatial strategy requiring the processing of relational S-S information. Participants using this strategy showed significantly increased activation in the hippocampus. Another group reported using a nonspatial strategy: counting arms in a constant direction from the first arm they saw or from a single landmark. Analysis of this behavior showed that it involved a consistent series of turns to enter each of the correct arms in order around the maze. As the participant returned to the platform from each arm (stimulus), the correct turn (response) was elicited, leading to the retrieval of a goal object (reinforcement). Accordingly, Iaria et al. (2003) concluded that this behavior was produced by processing S-R information. Participants using this strategy showed significantly increased activation in the caudate nucleus.

A third group of participants said they started with the spatial strategy but switched to a nonspatial strategy at some point during the session. Each of these participants started by exhibiting significantly more activation in the hippocampus than in the caudate nucleus, but this relationship was reversed as training progressed and the strategy switch occurred. Throughout the experiment, participants who used the spatial strategy made more errors than those who used a nonspatial strategy. Errors for the group that switched strategies decreased as soon as they switched.

These findings show that two different kinds of information are processed in this task: hippocampus-based spatial (S-S) information and caudate-based nonspatial (S-R) information. This dissociation is similar to the one observed in rats. The findings for the group that switched strategies also corresponds to rat evidence showing that increased training produces a shift from behavior controlled by S-S to behavior controlled by S-R information, processed in the hippocampus and the caudate nucleus, respectively. The basis of the shift may be a difference in the rates at which the two systems acquire coherent representations of the information they process.

Findings similar to those of Iaria et al. (2003) about the relationship between hippocampal and caudate nucleus activation in humans measured in more naturalistic virtual environments have also been reported by Maguire and coworkers (Maguire et al., 1998; Hartley et al., 2003; Hartley and Burgess, 2005).

3.5.2.2 Probabilistic classification

In the probabilistic classification task, also known as the weather forecasting task (Knowlton et al., 1994, 1996), participants are presented with a set of distinct cues selected from a large group and asked whether the set predicts rain or shine. After they respond by pressing one of two keys on a keyboard, they are told that their response was either correct or incorrect (feedback). The feedback provided for a given response to each cue or combination of cues within a set is probabilistic. This means that consistent feedback is given on most trials, but on some trials the opposite feedback is given. Furthermore, the specific mapping between the cues and the feedback is quite complex. Although it is possible to perform the task using declarative information about the feedback given most often, this requires a large number of trials because of the probabilistic feedback and the complexity of the mapping. However, when the probability of consistent feedback for a given response to a set of cues is sufficiently high, and when the stimulus and the reinforced response have been repeated sufficiently often, acquisition of an S-R association that produces the correct response can occur.

Knowlton et al. (1994) found that a group of normal participants and a group of amnesic patients (with impaired hippocampal function) learned this task at the same rate until both groups attained a moderate level of performance (70% correct). This suggests that within this range, performance is not based on information processed by the hippocampal system. However, the amnesic patients did not improve beyond the 70% level, whereas the normal participants continued to improve, possibly because they acquired some declarative knowledge of the mapping between the cues and outcomes (*See* Chapter 2). This finding was subsequently replicated in a study that also reported that Parkinson's patients (with impaired caudate nucleus function) were unable to learn the weather forecasting task at all (Knowlton et al., 1996). When given a series of questions about the conditions of the experiment (declarative memory), the amnesiacs were unable to answer most of the questions, whereas the Parkinson's patients performed normally. These findings constitute a double dissociation between hippocampus and caudate nucleus function with respect to declarative memory for the experimental situation and probabilistic classification (S-R) learning, respectively.

Poldrack and coworkers (1999) studied the brain areas involved in probabilistic classification in normal participants using fMRI. During the early trials, increased activation was seen in the right caudate nucleus (and in the frontal and occipital cortex). Activity in the left hippocampus was suppressed. However, the hippocampus became more active as performance continued to improve and reached levels unattainable by amnesic patients in the Knowlton et al. (1994) study. These findings coincide with the neuropsychological data on the probabilistic classification task (see also Shohamy et al., 2004) and with the general distinction between the processing of procedural or S-R information by a neural system that includes the caudate nucleus, and the processing of declarative, or S-S, information by a hippocampus system.

These findings were replicated and extended by comparing two different versions of the weather forecasting task (Poldrack et al., 2001). One was the standard probabilistic classification task, in which participants are shown the stimulus, make a response, and receive feedback. As already shown, initial acquisition of this task appears to depend on information processed by the caudate system. In a new task the participants were shown the same sets of cues together with the correct response for each set. In this paired associates version of the task, the participants did not make responses or receive feedback. Instead, they acquired information about the relationships among the stimuli and the weather they predicted. This type of task is known to depend on medial temporal lobe function (Warrington and Weiskrantz, 1982; Marchand et al., 2004). By the end of the training trials, the weather prediction performance of both groups was similar.

fMRI scanning showed that the reinforced S-R version of the task activated the caudate nucleus more than the hippocampus, whereas the paired associates version activated the hippocampus more than the caudate nucleus. Accordingly, these findings constitute a double dissociation of caudate-based processing of reinforced S-R information and hippocampus-based processing of S-S information consistent with other animal and human data described.

3.5.3 Summary: Competition and Coherence

As reviewed here and elsewhere (Poldrack and Packard, 2003), data from both animal and human studies strongly suggest that hippocampal function is implicated when the information required to solve a task can be characterized as consisting of S-S associations, and that caudate nucleus function is implicated when the task can be performed using information consisting of S-R associations. The evidence implicating these brain structures includes the effects of impaired function produced by trauma (including lesions made in the laboratory), disease processes, or chemical inactivation, and indices of increased functionality, including activation detected by fMRI, ACh release, and c-Fos expression.

Several instances of competition for control of behavior between the two systems in which these structures reside have been described. These findings are strong evidence for independent, parallel information processing functions in the systems.

The data from studies with normal animals and humans suggest that the kinds of information available in each learning situation – the task demands (Poldrack and Rodriguez, 2004) – determine which neural system controls behavior. This is consistent with the idea that the information processing specialization of each system determines the coherence of the representation it forms of a learning situation (see section 3.4.1.3). The system with the most coherent representation is the one that has the dominant effect on behavior. In the fMRI studies, increased hippocampal activation occurs when S-S information is being processed, and increased activation in the caudate nucleus occurs when S-R information is being processed. These relationships lead to the hypothesis that the level of activation revealed by the fMRI may be a reflection of the coherence of the representations of these information types in the systems.

In some studies an inverse relationship between activation of the hippocampus and caudate nucleus was observed, with depressed activation in the nondominant structure (Poldrack and Rodriguez, 2004). This may be a result of the relationships between the processing capacities of the structures and the information that activates them. Applying Sherry and Shachter's (1987) suggestion that these systems process incompatible information (see section 3.4.1) suggests the possibility that, when one of the two systems develops a coherent representation of a situation, the information available in that situation is incompatible with the specialized representational capacity of the other system. This may lead to an incoherent representation, reflected in decreased activation in the fMRI.

While not ruling out the possible existence of direct or indirect functional interactions, inhibitory or otherwise, between the hippocampus and caudate systems (Poldrack and Rodriguez, 2004), this suggestion shows that it is not necessary to postulate such direct influences to explain the data, which can be understood simply in terms of independent parallel systems that process incompatible information. According to this view, differences in the coherence of the representations formed in the systems determine which one wins the competition to control behavior.

3.6 S-S versus S-Rf Information Processing

The triple dissociation experiment (**Figure 4**) included a double dissociation between performance on the win-shift (impaired by fimbria-fornix lesions) and CCP (impaired by amygala lesions) tasks. This was interpreted as a double dissociation between the neural systems that process S-S and S-Rf information. Other studies with rats and humans support this interpretation.

3.6.1 Studies with Rats

3.6.1.1 CCP with spatial cues

During the CCP training trials in the triple dissociation experiment, the radial maze was surrounded by curtains, and the arms were differentiated by a light in one of them. Similar preferences are learned when the maze is open to the surrounding extramaze cues and the food-paired and no-food arms are on opposite sides of the maze (the separated arms CCP [sCCP]; see **Figure 12**). This preference is eliminated by amygdala but not by fimbria-fornix lesions (White and McDonald, 1993). When the two arms are adjacent to each other (the adjacent arms CCP [aCCP]) the preference is eliminated by hippocampal lesions, but not by amygdala lesions (Chai and White, 2004). This double dissociation is explained by differences in the nature of the extramaze cues visible from separated and adjacent maze arms.

In the sCCP situation, completely different sets of extramaze cues are visible from the ends of the two separated arms (**Figure 12**). The rats acquire a conditioned response to the environmental cues visible from the food-paired arm when they eat while confined on that arm during the training trials. They do not acquire a response to the cues visible from the unpaired arm while confined there, because no food is available. On the test day, the conditioned response causes the rats to approach and spend more time in the presence of the food-paired cues, resulting in a preference for that arm.

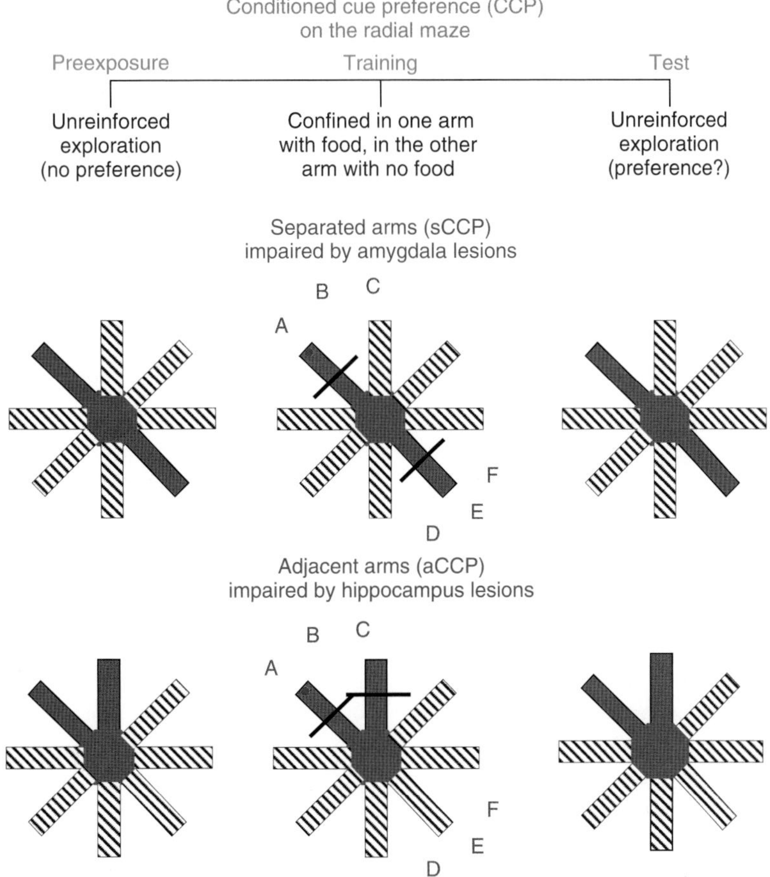

Figure 12 Conditioned cue preference with separate and adjacent radial maze arms. The three phases of the conditioned cue preference (CCP) paradigm (preexposure, training, and test) are shown at the top. The lower part of the figure shows the maze configurations for each phase in the separated and adjacent arms conditions. ABC and DEF are sets of environmental cues visible from the maze arms. In the separated arms CCP situation, completely different sets of cues are visible from the food-paired and no-food arms. During the training trials, a conditioned rewarding response is acquired, with ABC as the conditioned stimulus (CS). No response to DEF is learned. On the test trial, conditioned reward elicited by the CS causes the rat to enter and spend more time in the food-paired than in the unpaired arm. In the adjacent arms CCP situation, the same cues (ABC) are visible from both the food-paired and the unpaired arms. Discrimination between the two arms using these cues requires spatial learning.

This arm discrimination is produced by amygdala-based processing of S-Rf information.

In the aCCP situation, most of the same extramaze cues are visible from the ends of both arms (**Figure 12**). Discriminating between them requires learning about differences in the relationships of their locations to those cues. This is spatial learning, requiring hippocampus-based processing of S-S information. Therefore, the double dissociation between the effects of amygdala and hippocampus system lesions on the aCCP and sCCP tasks constitutes a dissociation between the processing of S-S and S-Rf information, respectively.

3.6.1.2 Cooperation and competition in adjacent arms CCP learning

Although the aCCP and sCCP paradigms differ in the relationship of the arms to be discriminated, all other aspects of the two procedures are identical. If a conditioned response to cues visible from the food-paired arm is acquired in the sCCP procedure, the same response should also be acquired in the aCCP procedure. However, since most of the same cues are visible from both arms in the aCCP procedure, this response should produce an equal tendency to enter both arms. This prediction has been confirmed (Chai and White, 2004).

The parallel occurrence of hippocampus-based spatial learning and amygdala-based S-Rf learning in the aCCP paradigm results in competition between the behavioral outputs of the two systems. Although a conditioned response to the food-paired cues is acquired during the training trials, spatial information about the layout of the maze cannot be acquired during these trials, because spatial learning in rats is severely attenuated when they are prevented from moving around in an environment (Sutherland, 1985; White and Ouellet, 1997; Terrazas et al., 2005). For this reason, rats do not learn the aCCP unless they are preexposed to the maze before the training trials (see **Figure 13**). During these sessions, the rats are allowed to move around freely on the maze with no food present. It has been known for some time that rats acquire spatial information during unreinforced exploration of a novel environment, a phenomenon called latent learning (Blodgett, 1929; Tolman and Honzik, 1930). As shown in **Figure 13**, normal rats require a minimum of three preexposure sessions to express the aCCP.

Interference with expression of this spatial information by the amygdala-based conditioned response is revealed by the finding that rats with amygdala lesions require only one preexposure session to learn the aCCP (**Figure 13**) (Chai and White, 2004). In normal rats, the amygdala-based tendency to enter both arms competes with the hippocampus-based tendency to discriminate between the arms. A minimum of three freely moving preexposures to the maze environment is required for the hippocampus system to acquire a sufficiently coherent representation of the spatial environment for its output to win the competition with the output from the amygdala system for control of behavior. When the competition is eliminated by amygdala lesions, a less coherent hippocampal representation (with, hence, less preexposure) is required to produce output that results in expression of the aCCP.

The competitive interaction between the amygdala and hippocampus systems in the aCCP task has been investigated in more detail (White and Gaskin, 2006). Both amygdala-based S-Rf learning and hippocampus-based S-S learning promote a tendency to enter the food-paired arm, a cooperative interaction. At the same time, the S-Rf learning promotes a tendency to enter the no-food arm, but this tendency is blocked by an interfering tendency resulting from S-S information about the lack of food in the arm, a competitive interaction. These cooperative and competing tendencies are illustrated in **Figure 13**.

3.6.1.3 Path integration versus visual cue conditioning

In addition to using visible spatial cues to navigate in space, rats also use internal cues based on proprioceptive stimuli generated by their movements for this purpose (Etienne et al., 1996; McNaughton et al., 1996). This form of information processing, called path integration, is hippocampus dependent (Smith, 1997; Whishaw et al., 1997, 2001; Whishaw, 1998). Ito et al. (2006) trained rats in an apparatus consisting of a triangular central platform with compartments attached to each of the three sides. Prior to each trial, the rats were exposed to a polarizing cue in the experimental room. The cue was removed before the trial started, so subsequent use of the orienting information it provided was a result of path integration. During the first phase, a flashing light together with a sucrose solution were presented in any of the three compartments, establishing the light as a conditioned cue. The rats acquired a tendency to approach the flashing light; rats with amygdala lesions required more trials than controls, but rats with hippocampal lesions required fewer trials than controls to acquire this behavior. This suggests that the cue preference was a result of amygdala-based processing of S-Rf information and that information processed in the hippocampus of the normal rats interfered with the expression of this behavior. The interference could have been caused by the simultaneous acquisition of information about the location of the sucrose solution based on the polarizing cue. Because this information was irrelevant, its effect on behavior may have interfered with expression of the amygdala-based cue preference in the same way spatial information can interfere with win-stay performance, as described in **Figure 5**.

The rats were then given a series of trials in which flashing lights appeared in any of the three compartments, but sucrose delivery accompanied this cue only when it appeared in one of the compartments. The compartment in which sucrose was available remained constant on all trials. The rats were then given a compartment preference test in the absence of flashing lights and sucrose. The sham-operated rats and the rats with amygdala lesions showed a preference for the compartment in which they had received sucrose, but the rats with hippocampus lesions did not exhibit this preference. Because neither the conditioned cues nor visual spatial cues were available during this test, Ito et al. (2006) attributed the preference to information about the spatial location of the sucrose based on the polarizing cue, processed in the hippocampus system. This information would have been incidentally acquired during the cue-training procedure.

The results of the two tests taken together double dissociate the use of path integration based on the processing of spatial information derived from movement by the hippocampus and the processing of S-Rf information by the amygdala. The demonstration of interference with the expression of the amygdala-based information by hippocampus-based path integration is evidence for independent functioning of the two systems.

3.6.1.4 Fear conditioning

In these experiments, rats are placed into a test cage and given one or more foot shocks as the US. The shock evokes a constellation of URs including an aversive internal state (usually called fear) and skeletal responses, primarily consisting of jumping and running. Neutral stimuli become CSs with the capacity to elicit the internal state of fear without the skeletal responses. This conditioned internal state is thought to be reflected by freezing, a withdrawal response (LeDoux, 1993; Fanselow and Gale, 2003).

Two kinds of stimuli can serve as the CS. In context conditioning, the CS is the test cage itself (as well as the room in which it is located and every other feature of the situation). In cue conditioning, a discrete cue such as a tone or light immediately precedes the shock. The cue becomes a CS, but the context also becomes a CS in this situation (Phillips and LeDoux, 1992). Context conditioning requires a minimum amount of unreinforced preexposure to the context (Fanselow, 1990). This appears to be another instance of latent learning, as in the case of unreinforced preexposure in the appetitive aCCP situation.

Both lesions of the hippocampus (Kim and Fanselow, 1992; Phillips and LeDoux, 1992; Frankland et al., 1998) and lesions of the amygdala (Phillips and LeDoux, 1992; Gale et al., 2004) impair contextual fear conditioning, but only amygdala lesions impair conditioning to a discrete cue CS (Phillips and LeDoux, 1992; Gale et al., 2004). In multiple memory systems terms, the involvement of the amygdala but not the hippocampus when the CS is a discrete cue suggests that this form of fear conditioning is a result of amygdala-based processing of S-Rf information. When the CS is a context requiring preexposure for conditioning to occur, the involvement of the hippocampus suggests that conditioning requires hippocampus-based processing of S-S information. However, context conditioning also requires an intact amygdala, suggesting that S-Rf information is also required for context conditioning. These findings constitute a partial dissociation of S-S and S-Rf information processing by the hippocampus and amygdala in fear conditioning.

This pattern of effects differs from that for the relationship between hippocampus-based spatial learning with appetitive reinforcers and amygdala-based appetitive conditioned responding. However, the fear conditioning studies do not explicitly test multiple memory systems hypotheses, and the numerous differences in the experimental apparatus and procedures used in the two sets of studies make it difficult to conclude that the systems have different functions in appetitive and aversive learning. Examination of this issue requires experiments that directly compare appetitive and aversive learning in the same experimental conditions.

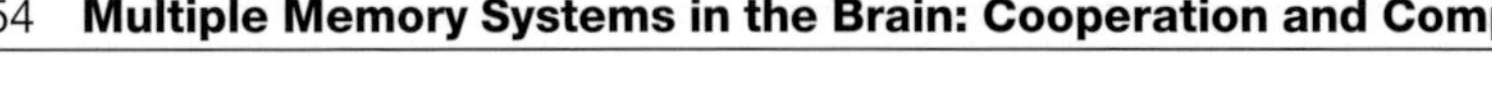

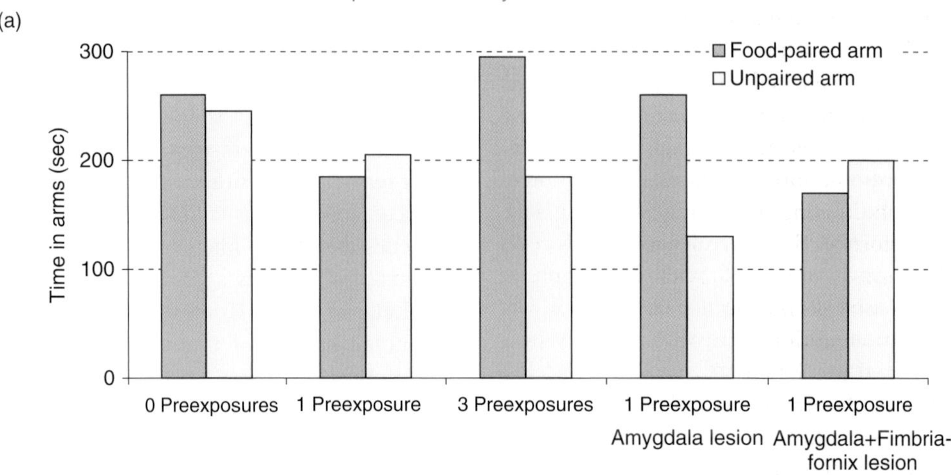

(b)

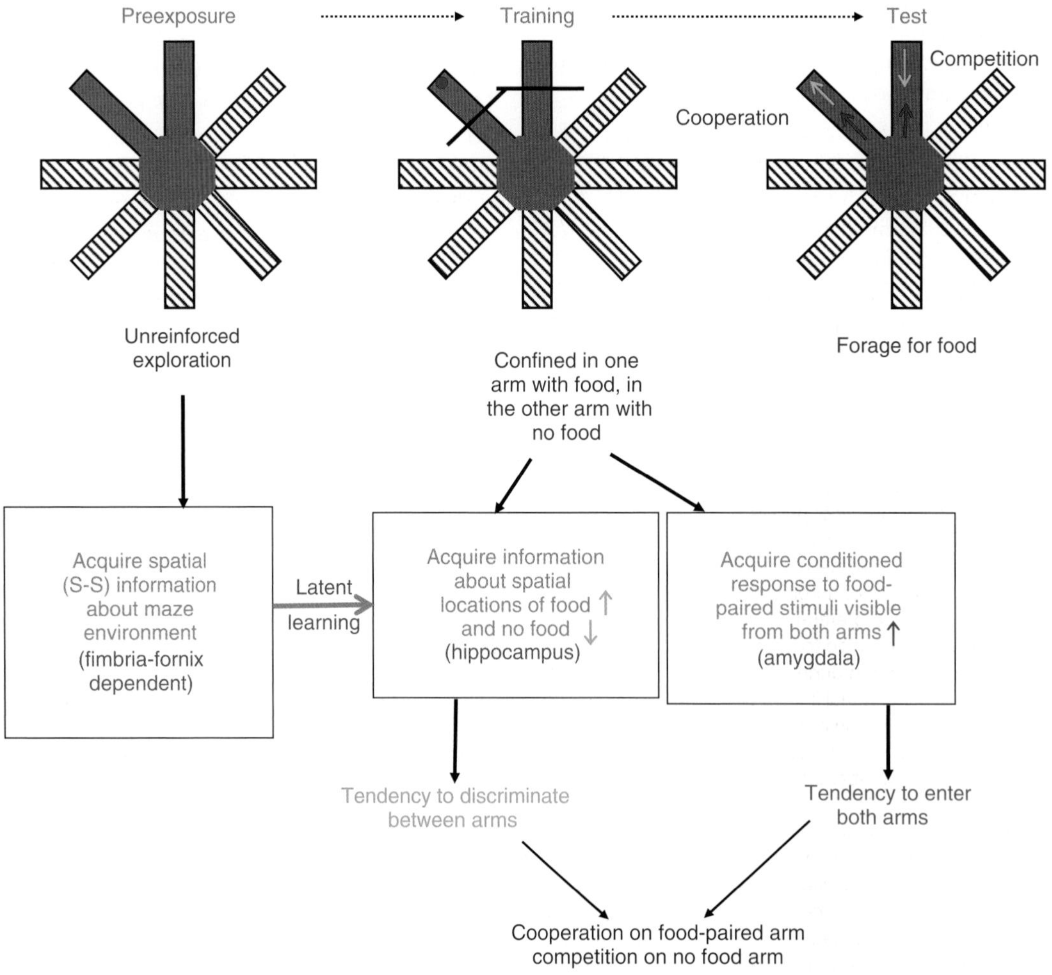

Preexposure → Training → Test

Cooperation

Competition

Unreinforced exploration

Confined in one arm with food, in the other arm with no food

Forage for food

Acquire spatial (S-S) information about maze environment (fimbria-fornix dependent)

Latent learning

Acquire information about spatial locations of food ↑ and no food ↓ (hippocampus)

Acquire conditioned response to food-paired stimuli visible from both arms ↑ (amygdala)

Tendency to discriminate between arms

Tendency to enter both arms

Cooperation on food-paired arm competition on no food arm

3.6.1.5 Skeletal conditioning

The Pavlovian conditioning paradigm has also been used to study at least two overt discrete skeletal responses directly elicited by a US: eye blink (Thompson and Krupa, 1994; Thompson, 2005) and leg flexion (Maschke et al., 2002; Dimitrova et al., 2003, 2004). Only the former will be discussed here. In eye-blink conditioning, a puff of air to the eye or a mild orbital shock (US) elicits a blink (UR). This response is similar to other URs because it is elicited by a reinforcer without previous experience.

In the delay conditioning procedure, the CS is presented first, the US follows after a brief delay, and the two stimuli terminate simultaneously. Using this procedure, eye-blink conditioning in rabbits and cats is impaired by lesions of specific parts of the cerebellum – cortex or nucleus interpositus (Skelton, 1988; Thompson and Krupa, 1994) – but not by lesions of the hippocampus (Christian and Thompson, 2003; Thompson, 2005). These findings suggest that S-Rf information involving a skeletal response (eye blink) is processed in the cerebellum.

In a slightly different procedure, the CS is presented and terminates. After an interval of 0.5–1.0 s, the US is presented. This is called trace conditioning because it is thought that a trace (or representation) of the CS is maintained during the CS-US interval, resulting in the formation of an S-S association between the trace and the US. Trace conditioning is impaired by lesions of the nucleus interpositus of the cerebellum in rabbits (Woodruff-Pak et al., 1985) and by lesions of the hippocampus in rats (Moyer et al., 1990; Thompson and Kim, 1996; Clark et al., 2002). These findings suggest that, in this paradigm, the cerebellum processes S-Rf information only, and the hippocampus processes both S-Rf and S-S information, a partial dissociation. This pattern corresponds to that for aversive fear conditioning with a contextual CS, but not to appetitive CCP learning.

3.6.2 Experiments with Humans

3.6.2.1 Conditioned preference

In an adaptation of the rat CCP task for humans (Johnsrude et al., 1999), normal participants were told that one of three black boxes on a computer screen contained a red ball. Touching a box caused it to open. If the box contained the red ball, the participant received a reward (a raisin or small candy). If the box contained a black ball, a mildly aversive tone sounded. The participants were instructed to count the number of times the red ball appeared in each of the three black boxes. In addition to a ball, each opened box also revealed one of six abstract designs in the background. All designs were presented an equal number of times. Two of them were paired with reward on 90% of the trials on which they appeared, two were paired on 50% of

Figure 13 Competition in the adjacent arms conditioned cue preference (aCCP) task. (a) Learning the aCCP. The top part of the figure shows the effects of preexposure on the separated arms CCP (sCCP) learning. The bars show the mean amounts of time the rats chose to spend in the maze arms during the 20-min test trial with no food present. Rats that received fewer than three sessions of unreinforced preexposure to the maze (see text for explanation) failed to learn the aCCP, but rats that received three sessions of unreinforced preexposure to the maze spent more time in their food-paired than in their unpaired arm, a conditioned cue preference. This suggests that in normal rats, three preexposure sessions permit the acquisition of sufficient spatial information to express an aCCP when combined with information about the locations of food and the absence of food acquired during the training trials. These hippocampus-based behaviors are shown as green arrows on the maze illustrating the test trial in (b). (b) Amygdala-based competition. As shown in (a), rats with amygdala lesions expressed a CCP after only one session of unreinforced preexposure to the maze (compared to a minimum of three for a normal rat), suggesting that amygdala-processed information competed with the hippocampus-based arm discrimination. As explained in the text, an amygdala-based conditioned response to ambiguous cues visible from both arms, acquired during the training trials, results in an equal tendency to enter both arms (red arrows). This results in cooperation between the two systems on the food-paired arm. Amygdala lesions eliminate the amygala-based tendency to enter the food-paired arm, but this does not eliminate the preference, because the hippocampus produces the same tendency. The amygdala-based tendency to enter the no-food arm competes with the hippocampus-based tendency to enter the food-paired arm instead of the no-food arm. Amygdala lesions eliminate the competition, allowing hippocampus-based spatial information to produce the CCP after only a single preexposure session. This is a case of amygdala-based processing of S-Rf information competing with a spatial discrimination resulting from hippocampus-based processing of S-S (spatial) information. Adapted from Chai S-C and White NM (2004) Effects of fimbria-fornix, hippocampus and amygdala lesions on discrimination between proximal locations. *Behav. Neurosci.* 118: 770–784; Gaskin S and White NM (2006) Cooperation and competition between the dorsal hippocampus and lateral amygdala in spatial discrimination learning. *Hippocampus* 16: 577–585.

the trials, and two on 10% of the trials. These designs were not mentioned in the instructions.

After the training trials participants were asked to say how many times the red ball had appeared in each box. All did very well on this task. They were then shown the abstract designs in randomly selected pairs with no balls present and asked to indicate which one they preferred. The 90% patterns were chosen significantly more often than the 10% patterns, a conditioned preference. In the final phase of the experiment the participants were shown their preferred patterns and asked why they preferred them. All participants attributed their preferences to properties of the patterns themselves; none mentioned any relationship between the patterns and reward. This was interpreted to mean that they had acquired a conditioned preference for the reward-paired patterns that did not depend on cognitive or declarative information.

Two groups of surgical patients were tested on this task (Johnsrude et al., 2000). Patients with unilateral resections of the amygdala did not acquire the preference for the reward-paired patterns, but performed accurately on the ball counting task. In contrast, patients with frontal lobe resections acquired normal pattern preferences but were severely impaired on ball counting. This double dissociation between amygdala-based processing of S-Rf information and S-S information requiring an intact frontal cortex corresponds to the dissociations between the processing of these same two kinds of information involving amygdala and the hippocampal systems in the rat.

3.6.2.2 Conditioned fear

Bechara and coworkers (1995) compared three patients, one with bilateral damage restricted to amygdala as a result of Urbach-Weithe disease, one with hippocampal lesions caused by anoxia secondary to cardiac arrests, and one with damage to both structures resulting from herpes simplex encephalitis. The patients were tested on a Pavlovian conditioning task in which the US was a loud horn and the UR was the electrodermal response produced by the startling noise. A series of color slides was shown during conditioning; one color coincided with the presentation of the US, making this discrete cue the CS. Shortly after testing on this task, the subjects were asked a series of questions about the experimental situation as a test of their declarative memory.

The patient with impaired amygdala function failed to acquire a conditioned electrodermal response but had excellent recall of the experimental situation. The patient with impaired hippocampal function acquired the conditioned electrodermal response but had poor memory for details of the experimental situation. The patient with damage to both areas performed poorly on both tasks. These findings dissociate amygdala-mediated processing of S-Rf information from hippocampus-mediated processing of S-S information in humans. This double dissociation corresponds to the dissociation found for appetitive spatial learning in rats and to the data for aversive conditioning in rats with a discrete cue CS.

3.6.2.3 Skeletal responses

As is the case for rats, in humans, eye-blink conditioning with the delay paradigm is impaired by lesions of the cerebellum (Daum et al., 1993), but not by lesions of the hippocampus (Daum et al., 1991; Gabrieli et al., 1995), and trace conditioning is impaired by lesions of the cerebellum (Gerwig et al., 2006) and the hippocampus (Thompson and Kim, 1996; Clark et al., 2002). This partial dissociation coincides with the data from studies of eye-blink conditioning in the rat.

A study measuring the magnetic flux of specific brain areas as an index of neural activity (magnetoencephalography) in humans (Kirsch et al., 2003) found that delay conditioning evoked only activation in the cerebellum, and that trace conditioning evoked only activation in the hippocampus. This suggests a more complete dissociation of processing the information types involved in trace and delay conditioning than the lesion data.

3.6.3 Summary

Several studies, in both rats and humans, consistent with the dissociation of hippocampus-based S-S and amygdala-based S-Rf information processing have been reviewed. These are fewer in number and are usually more difficult to demonstrate than dissociations between S-S and S-R processing. Furthermore, the available data on aversive conditioning in rats are not consistent with the notion of independent parallel processing of the information types required for contextual fear conditioning or for trace conditioning of the eye-blink response. Further experiments are required to determine whether these apparent differences in the relationships among the systems during appetitive and aversive conditioning are real.

3.7 S-Rf versus S-R Information Processing

In the triple dissociation experiment, the CCP task was impaired by lesions of the amygdala but not by lesions of the caudate nucleus; the win-stay task was impaired by lesions of the caudate nucleus but not by lesions of the amygdala. This double dissociation of S-Rf and S-R information processing has been replicated and extended.

Although S-Rf and S-R information both consist of stimulus-response relationships, these differ in important ways. Caudate-mediated S-R information comprises associations between representations of any response an individual can make and representations of contemporaneous stimuli. If the creation of these two representations is temporally contiguous with the occurrence of a reinforcer, the association between them is strengthened, but the reinforcer is not part of the information that constitutes the memory. Amygdala-mediated S-Rf information is limited to associations between responses (URs) that are elicited by reinforcers (USs), which become associated with contemporaneous stimuli (CSs). The responses are unrelated to any spontaneous behavior that may occur in the learning situation and, as already described, are largely unobservable internal changes in autonomic and hormonal function. The behavioral influence of these conditioned responses is often indirect. Observing their existence often requires some form of additional instrumental learning (Dickinson and Dawson, 1989; Dickinson, 1994; Dickinson and Balleine, 1994; Everitt et al., 2001).

In this section, only a single experiment dissociating amygdala-based S-Rf and caudate-based S-R information processing is described. The author is unaware of any other direct dissociations between these two systems with animals or of any parallel experiments with humans.

3.7.1 Win-Stay and CCP Learning

The S-R and S-Rf systems have been dissociated with a simultaneous comparison of the win-stay and CCP radial maze tasks. McDonald and Hong (2004) trained rats with lesions of the dorsolateral caudate nucleus or amygdala on the win-stay task (see **Figure 14**). After reaching a performance criterion, all rats were tested for CCP learning in the same apparatus. The rats were placed on the maze for 20 min with all arms open and no food present. The light used for win-stay training was on in four randomly selected arms; the other four arms were dark. Normal rats spent more time in the lit than in the dark arms, a CCP. Rats with caudate lesions were impaired on win-stay performance but exhibited a preference for the lit arms. Rats with amygdala lesions were normal on win-stay but failed to exhibit a CCP.

These findings dissociate the neural system that processes the S-R information required for win-stay performance (caudate nucleus) from the system that processes the S-Rf information required for the CCP (amygdala). The acquisition of a CCP by rats that were never explicitly trained in that task is a demonstration of the fact that the caudate and amygdala memory systems function simultaneously to acquire different kinds of information in the same learning situation. Since lesions of either structure affected performance of only one of the two tasks and did not improve performance of the other task, there is no evidence of a competitive interaction between the systems in this situation.

3.8 Summary and Some Outstanding Issues

The historical evidence, the triple dissociation on the radial maze, and the double dissociations in both rats and humans all point to the idea that different parts of the brain are involved in learning that requires memory for different kinds of information. The observations of cooperative, and especially competitive, interactions between systems are strong evidence that these parts of the brain, called systems, function independently and in parallel. This is the multiple parallel memory systems hypothesis, as summarized in **Figure 7**. The analysis in this chapter concludes that the hippocampus and related structures process S-S information, the caudate nucleus and connecting structures process S-R information, and a neural system that includes the amygdala processes S-Rf information. These information-processing specializations may result from differences in the internal microstructure of the systems.

The systems are not completely divergent. All of them receive input from the cortex, so the cortex could be considered a shared part of all systems. Points at which the outputs of the systems converge could also be shared parts. However, the evidence shows that there is clearly divergence among the systems, at least at the level of the hippocampus, caudate nucleus, and amygdala.

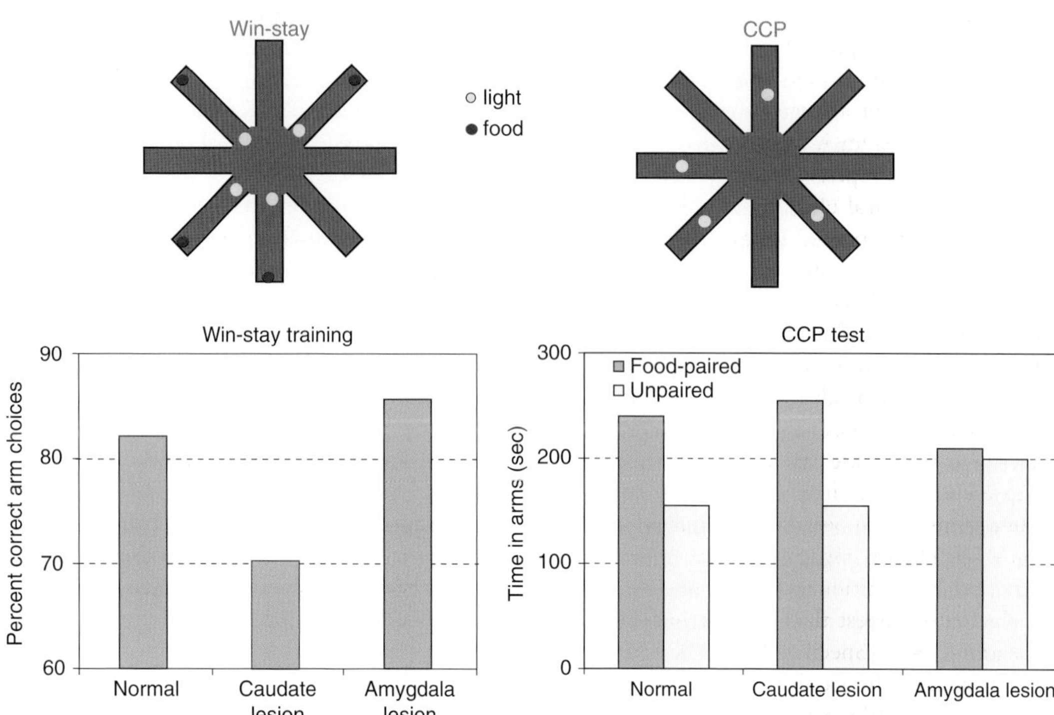

Figure 14 Dissociation of stimulus-response (S-R) and stimulus-reinforcer (S-Rf) information processing in the caudate nucleus and amygdala, respectively. The left side of the figure shows performance of three groups of rats trained on the win-stay radial maze task. Rats with amygdala lesions performed normally, but the performance of rats with caudate nucleus lesions was impaired. The graph shows the mean percent correct responses over the last 3 days of training for each group. In the second part of the experiment, shown on the right, the same rats were given a win-stay test. Four randomly selected arms were lit, and four arms remained dark. The rats were placed on the maze with no food available and allowed to move around freely. The graph shows that the normal rats and the rats with caudate lesions spent more time in the lit arms than in the dark arms, a conditioned cue preference (CCP). The rats with amygdala lesions did not exhibit this preference. This pattern of effects shows that rats can process and store amygdala-based S-Rf information (a conditioned approach response to the light CS) during win-stay training, even if their win-stay performance is very poor because of caudate lesions. The findings dissociate caudate-based processing of S-R information from amygdala-based processing of S-Rf information and are consistent with the hypothesis that the two systems function independently of each other. Adapted from McDonald RJ and Hong NS (2004) A dissociation of dorso-lateral striatum and amygdala function on the same stimulus-response habit task. *Neuroscience* 124: 507–513.

As information flows through the systems (**Figure 7**) it may produce temporary or permanent alterations resulting from the neuroplasticity of their internal structures. These alterations influence the processing of information that flows through the system on future occasions, altering the output of the system and the effect it has on thought and behavior. This is how experience alters behavior. The alterations themselves are memories (note that these neuroplastic changes influence neural activity representing information, but this does not mean the changes actually represent the information). The memories are therefore located in the systems. Although several parts of each system are known to have neuroplastic properties, there is little or no definitive evidence localizing specific memories to specific structures within a system.

Although all information flows through all systems, the specialization of each system means that each can represent only one type of information. For any given situation at any point in time, the representations in each structure will probably differ in coherence. Coherence is a function of two factors. First, the coherence of a representation is determined by the degree to which the information content of a learning situation coincides with the information-processing specialization of a system. When the degree of coincidence is high, most neural elements or microcircuits within the system will be activated in the same way, forming an accurate representation of the situation. This kind of coherent representation produces output with a powerful influence on behavior. When there is a mismatch between the information content of a learning situation and the specialization of a system, it will form a less coherent, or even incoherent, representation of the information. Fewer of its neural elements may be activated, and not all may be activated in the same way. Less coherent representations produce output with weak or no influence on behavior.

The second factor influencing coherence is practice. Increased exposure to a situation (by increasing the number of training trials) increases the coherence of a representation, increasing its influence on behavior. Practice can increase the coherence of even a poor representation sufficiently for the output of the system to influence behavior. This may become apparent when a lesion impairs performance on a task that recovers after additional training.

The data also suggest that the systems have different learning rates. Specifically, the hippocampal system can apparently acquire information about a situation with very little experience (sometimes with a single exposure), but the caudate system requires numerous repeated exposures even to represent situations that correspond to its S-R specialization.

Because all systems receive all information, they all form some kind of coherent or incoherent representation of all situations. A given situation might produce coherent representations in two systems. Even though the representations consist of different information, the outputs of both systems might produce the same behavior. This would be cooperation between the systems. In this case, impairing the function of either system would have no apparent effect. Eliminating the behavior would require impairments of both systems.

The outputs of two systems with coherent representations of a situation might produce different behaviors. This would be a competitive interaction between the systems. Because the outputs may produce different behaviors, they interfere with each other. Impairing the function of either system would eliminate the interference and improve performance of the behavior produced by the intact system.

3.8.1 Some Outstanding Issues

Numerous issues requiring further investigation are suggested by the multiple parallel memory systems theory. This list is necessarily limited to a few of the most general ones.

1. A major question is the degree of genuine functional independence of the proposed systems within which memories are stored. The present summary has emphasized evidence for their independent cooperative or competitive influence on behavior, but possibilities for direct facilitatory or inhibitory actions of one system on another also require further consideration and investigation.

2. The idea that each proposed system is specialized to represent a different type of information, tentatively defined by the triple dissociation experiment, requires further investigation on two levels. First, it should be tested in more different behavioral learning situations that can be parsed into their elements: stimuli, responses, and reinforcers. As more situations are tested, the effects of disabling one or more systems should become increasingly predictable.

3. The idea that systems represent information can also be investigated at the level of the neural microstructure of each system. The theory suggests that experience alters neural systems, which in turn changes how they process the information that flows through them. The implications of this idea for understanding the functional contributions to memory of synaptic and other changes between and within neurons require further examination and definition. Within each system the study of these neuroplastic processes should be done in parallel with an examination of behavioral changes known to be produced by that system. Ultimately, it should be possible to specify how situational information reaches and flows through each system and exactly how this information changes the synaptic relationships in the system so that its processing of similar information on future occasions produces different output.

4. The postulated cooperative and competitive interactions among the outputs of the systems require further investigation on both the anatomical and functional levels of analysis. Specifically, where and how do the outputs of the systems interact?

5. Finally, several criticisms of the multiple memory system concept have been published (Gaffan, 1996, 2001, 2002; Wise, 1996). These complaints largely focus on behavioral evidence from experiments with nonhuman primates and point out that support for the hypothesis is lacking in these species. Experiments directly investigating the multiple memory systems hypothesis in monkeys would either support the theory or reveal its deficiencies.

References

Alzheimer A (1987) About a peculiar disease of the cerebral cortex (Uber eine eingeartige Erkrankung der Hirnrinde, 1907, translated by Jarvik L and Greenson H). *Alzheimer Dis. Assoc. Disord.* 1: 5–8.

Anderson JR and Bower GH (1979) *Human Associative Memory.* Hillsdale, NJ: Lawrence Earlbaum.

Bagshaw M and Benzies S (1968) Multiple measures of the orienting reaction and their dissociation after amygdalectomy in monkeys. *Exp. Neurol.* 20: 175–187.

Beach FH, Hebb DO, Morgan CT, and Nissen HW (1960) *The Neuropsychology of Lashley.* New York: McGraw-Hill.

Bechara A, Tranel D, Damasio H, Adolphs R, Rockland C, and Damasio AR (1995) Double dissociation of conditioning and declarative knowledge relative to the amygdala and hippocampus in humans. *Science* 269: 1115–1118.

Bergmann G and Spence K (1964) Operationism and theory in psychology. *Psychol. Rev.* 48: 1–14.

Blodgett HC (1929) The effect of the introduction of reward upon the maze performance of rats. *Univ. Calif. Publ. Psychol.* 4: 113–134.

Blodgett HC and McCutchan K (1947) Place versus response learning in the simple T-maze. *J. Exp. Psychol.* 37: 412–422.

Burgdorf J and Panksepp J (2006) The neurobiology of positive emotions. *Neurosci. Biobehav. Rev.* 30: 173–187.

Butters N, Martone M, White B, Granholm E, and Wolfe J (1986) Clinical validators: Comparisons of demented and amnesic patients. In: Poon L (ed.) *Handbook of Clinical Assessment of Memory*, pp. 337–352. Washington: American Psychological Association.

Cabanac M (1971) Physiological role of pleasure. *Science* 173: 1103–1107.

Centonze D, Picconi B, Gubellini P, Bernardi G, and Calabresi P (2001) Dopaminergic control of synaptic plasticity in the dorsal striatum. *Eur. J. Neurosci.* 13: 1071–1077.

Chai S-C and White NM (2004) Effects of fimbria-fornix, hippocampus and amygdala lesions on discrimination between proximal locations. *Behav. Neurosci.* 118: 770–784.

Chang Q and Gold PE (2003) Switching memory systems during learning: Changes in patterns of brain acetylcholine release in the hippocampus and striatum in rats. *J. Neurosci.* 23: 3001–3005.

Chozick BS (1983) The behavioral effects of lesions of the corpus striatum: A review. *Int. J. Neurosci.* 19: 143–160.

Christian KM and Thompson RF (2003) Neural substrates of eyeblink conditioning: Acquisition and retention. *Learn. Mem.* 10: 427–455.

Clark RE, Manns JR, and Squire LR (2002) Classical conditioning, awareness, and brain systems. *Trends Cogn. Sci.* 6: 524–531.

Cohen NJ and Eichenbaum H (1991) The theory that wouldn't die: A critical look at the spatial mapping theory of hippocampal function. *Hippocampus* 1: 265–268.

Cohen NJ and Squire LR (1980) Preserved learning and retention of pattern-analyzing skill in amnesia: Dissociation of knowing how and knowing what. *Science* 210: 207–209.

Colombo PJ, Brightwell JJ, and Countryman RA (2003) Cognitive strategy-specific increases in phosphorylated cAMP response element-binding protein and c-Fos in the hippocampus and dorsal striatum. *J. Neurosci.* 23: 3547–3554.

Colombo PJ and Gallagher M (1998) Individual differences in spatial memory and striatal ChAT activity among young and aged rats. *Neurobiol. Learn. Mem.* 70: 314–327.

Cook D and Kesner RP (1988) Caudate nucleus and memory for egocentric localization. *Behav. Neural Biol.* 49: 332–343.

Corkin S (1968) Acqusition of motor skill after bilateral medial temporal lobe excision. *Neuropsychologia* 6: 255–265.

Daum I, Channon S, Polkey CE, and Gray JA (1991) Classical conditioning after temporal lobe lesions in man: Impairment in conditional discrimination. *Behav. Neurosci.* 105: 396–408.

Daum I, Schugens MM, Ackermann H, Lutzenberger W, Dichgans J, and Birbaumer N (1993) Classical conditioning after cerebellar lesions in humans. *Behav. Neurosci.* 107: 748–756.

Davis DM, Jacobson TK, Aliakbari S, and Mizumori SJ (2005) Differential effects of estrogen on hippocampal- and striatal-dependent learning. *Neurobiol. Learn. Mem.* 84: 132–137.

Davis M (1997) Neurobiology of fear responses: The role of the amygdala. *J. Neuropsychiatry Clin. Neurosci.* 9: 382–402.

Devan BD, Goad EH, and Petri HL (1996) Dissociation of hippocampal and striatal contributions to spatial navigation in the water maze. *Neurobiol. Learn. Mem.* 66: 305–323.

Devan BD, McDonald RJ, and White NM (1999) Effects of medial and lateral caudate-putamen lesions on place- and cue-guided behaviors in the water maze: Relation to thigmotaxis. *Behav. Brain Res.* 100: 5–14.

Dickinson A (1994) Instrumental conditioning. In: Mackintosh N (ed.) *Animal Learning and Cognition*, pp. 45–79. New York: Academic Press.

Dickinson A and Balleine BW (1994) Motivational control of goal-directed action. *Animal Learning and Behavior* 22: 1–18.

Dickinson A and Dawson GR (1989) Incentive learning and the motivational control of instrumental performance. *Q. J. Exp. Psychol.* 41: 99–112.

Dickinson A, Nicholas DJ, and Adams CD (1983) The effect of the instrumental training contingency on susceptibility to reinforcer devaluation. *Q. J. Exp. Psychol. B, 35B,* 35–51.

Dimitrova A, Kolb FP, Elles HG, et al. (2003) Cerebellar responses evoked by nociceptive leg withdrawal reflex as revealed by event-related fMRI. *J. Neurophysiol.* 90: 1877–1886.

Dimitrova A, Kolb FP, Elles HG, et al. (2004) Cerebellar activation during leg withdrawal reflex conditioning: An fMRI study. *Clin. Neurophysiol.* 115: 849–857.

Divac I (1968) Functions of the caudate nucleus. *Acta Biol. Exp. (Warsz.)* 28: 107–120.

Divac I, Rosvold HE, and Szwarcbart MK (1967) Behavioral effects of selective ablation of the caudate nucleus. *J. Comp. Physiol. Psychol.* 63: 183–190.

Donahoe JW and Vegas R (2004) Pavlovian conditioning: The CS-UR relation. *J. Exp. Psychol. Anim. Behav. Process.* 30: 17–33.

Douglas RJ and Pribram KH (1966) Learning and limbic lesions. *Neuropsychologia* 4: 197–220.

Ebbinghaus H (1885) *Memory: A Contribution to Experimental Psychology. [Über das gedächtnis. Untersuchungen zur experimentellen psychologie,* translated 1964], Hilgard ER (ed.) (trans.). New York: Dover.

Eichenbaum H and Cohen NJ (2001) *From Conditioning to Conscious Recollection: Memory Systems in the Brain.* Oxford: Oxford University Press.

Eichenbaum H, Otto T, and Cohen NJ (1992) The hippocampus – What does it do? *Behav. Neural Biol.* 57: 2–36.

Etienne AS, Maurer R, and Séguinot V (1996) Path integration in mammals and its interaction with visual landmarks. *J. Exp. Biol.* 199: 201–209.

Everitt BJ, Cador M, and Robbins TW (1989) Interactions between the amygdala and ventral striatum in stimulus-reward associations: Studies using a second-order schedule of sexual reinforcement. *Neuroscience* 30: 63–75.

Everitt BJ, Dickinson A, and Robbins TW (2001) The neuropsychological basis of addictive behaviour. *Brain Res. Brain Res. Rev.* 36: 129–138.

Everitt BJ, Morris KA, O'Brien A, and Robbins TW (1991) The basolateral amygdala-ventral striatal system and conditioned place preference: Further evidence of limbic-striatal interactions underlying reward-related processes. *Neuroscience* 42: 1–18.

Fanselow MS (1990) Factors governing one-trial contextual conditioning. *Anim. Learn. Behav.* 18: 264–270.

Fanselow MS and Gale GD (2003) The amygdala, fear, and memory. *Ann. N. Y. Acad. Sci.* 985: 125–134.

Featherstone RE and McDonald RJ (2004a) Dorsal striatum and stimulus-response learning: Lesions of the dorsolateral, but not dorsomedial, striatum impair acquisition of a simple discrimination task. *Behav. Brain Res.* 150: 15–23.

Featherstone RE and McDonald RJ (2004b) Dorsal striatum and stimulus-response learning: Lesions of the dorsolateral, but not dorsomedial, striatum impair acquisition of a stimulus-response-based instrumental discrimination task, while sparing conditioned place preference learning. *Neuroscience* 124: 23–31.

Featherstone RE and McDonald RJ (2005a) Lesions of the dorsolateral or dorsomedial striatum impair performance of a previously acquired simple discrimination task. *Neurobiol. Learn. Mem.* 84: 159–167.

Featherstone RE and McDonald RJ (2005b) Lesions of the dorsolateral striatum impair the acquisition of a simplified stimulus-response dependent conditional discrimination task. *Neuroscience* 136: 387–395.

Fendt M and Fanselow MS (1999) The neuroanatomical and neurochemical basis of conditioned fear. *Neurosci. Biobehav. Rev.* 23: 743–760.

Ferbinteanu J and Shapiro ML (2003) Prospective and retrospective memory coding in the hippocampus. *Neuron* 40: 1227–1239.

Frankland PW, Cestari V, Filipkowski RK, McDonald RJ, and Silva AJ (1998) The dorsal hippocampus is essential for context discrimination but not for contextual conditioning. *Behav. Neurosci.* 112: 863–874.

Franz SI (1902) On the functions of the cerebrum: I. The frontal lobes in relation to the production and retention of simple sensory-motor habits. *J. Physiol.* 8: 1–22.

Gabrieli JD, Carrillo MC, Cermak LS, McGlinchey-Berroth R, Gluck MA, and Disterhoft JF (1995) Intact delay-eyeblink classical conditioning in amnesia. *Behav. Neurosci.* 109: 819–827.

Gaffan D (1996) Memory, action and the corpus striatum: Current developments in the memory-habit distinction. *Semin. Neurosci.* 8: 33–38.

Gaffan D (2001) What is a memory system? Horel's critique revisited. *Behav. Brain Res.* 127: 5–11.

Gaffan D (2002) Against memory systems. *Philos. Trans. R. Soc. Lond. B Biol. Sci.* 357: 1111–1121.

Gale GD, Anagnostaras SG, Godsil BP, et al. (2004) Role of the basolateral amygdala in the storage of fear memories across the adult lifetime of rats. *J. Neurosci.* 24: 3810–3815.

Gall FJ and Spurzheim J (1819) *Anatomie et Physiologie du Systèm Nerveux en Générale, et du Cerveau en Particulier.* Paris: F. Schoell.

Garcia J and Koelling RA (1966) Relationship of cue to consequence in avoidance learning. *Psychon. Sci.* 7: 439–450.

Gaskin S and White NM (2006) Cooperation and competition between the dorsal hippocampus and lateral amygdala in spatial discrimination learning. *Hippocampus* 16: 577–585.

Gerwig M, Haerter K, Hajjar K, et al. (2006) Trace eyeblink conditioning in human subjects with cerebellar lesions. *Exp. Brain Res.* 170: 7–21.

Gill KM and Mizumori SJ (2006) Context-dependent modulation by D(1) receptors: Differential effects in hippocampus and striatum. *Behav. Neurosci.* 120: 377–392.

Graybiel AM (2001) Neural networks: Neural systems V: Basal ganglia. *Am. J. Psychiatry* 158: 21.

Graybiel AM (2004) Network-level neuroplasticity in cortico-basal ganglia pathways. *Parkinsonism Relat. Disord.* 10: 293–296.

Gross CG, Chorover SL, and Cohen SM (1965) Caudate, cortical, hippocampal, and dorsal thalamic lesions in rats: Alternation and Hebb-Williams maze performance. *Neuropsychologia* 3: 53–68.

Gurney K, Prescott TJ, Wickens JR, and Redgrave P (2004) Computational models of the basal ganglia: From robots to membranes. *Trends Neurosci.* 27: 453–459.

Hartley T and Burgess N (2005) Complementary memory systems: Competition, cooperation and compensation. *Trends Neurosci.* 28: 169–170.

Hartley T, Maguire EA, Spiers HJ, and Burgess N (2003) The well-worn route and the path less traveled: Distinct neural bases of route following and wayfinding in humans. *Neuron* 37: 877–888.

Hatfield T and Gallagher M (1995) Taste-potentiated odor conditioning: Impairment produced by infusion of an *N*-methyl-D-aspartate antagonist into basolateral amygdala. *Behav. Neurosci.* 109: 663–668.

Heimer L, Alheid GF, and Zaborsky L (1985) Basal ganglia. In: Paxinos G (ed.) *The Rat Nervous System, Vol. 1: Forebrain and Midbrain*, pp. 37–86. Sydney: Academic Press.

Heindel WC, Salmon DP, Shults CW, Walicke PA, and Butters N (1989) Neuropsychological evidence for multiple implicit memory systems: A comparison of Alzheimer's, Huntington's, and Parkinson's disease patients. *J. Neurosci.* 9: 582–587.

Hilgard ER and Bower GH (1966) *Theories of Learning,* 3rd edn. New York: Appleton-Century-Crofts.

Hirsh R (1974) The hippocampus and contextual retrieval of information from memory: A theory. *Behav. Biol.* 12: 421–444.

Hirsh R (1980) The hippocampus, conditional operations and cognition. *Physiol. Psychol.* 8: 175–182.

Hirsh R, Holt L, and Mosseri A (1978a) Hippocampal mossy fibers motivation states and contextual retrieval. *Exp. Neurol.* 62: 68–79.

Hirsh R, Leber B, and Gillman R (1978b) Fornix fibers and motivational states as controllers of behavior: A study stimulated by the contextual retrieval theory. *Behav. Biol.* 22: 463–475.

Hirsh R and Segal M (1971) Complete transection of the fornix and reversal of position habit in the rat. *Physiol. Behav.* 8: 1051–1054.

Holahan MR, Rekart JL, Sandoval J, and Routtenberg A (2006) Spatial learning induces presynaptic structural remodeling in the hippocampal mossy fiber system of two rat strains. *Hippocampus* 16: 560–570.

Holahan MR, Taverna FA, Emrich SM, et al. (2005) Impairment in long-term retention but not short-term performance on a water maze reversal task following hippocampal or mediodorsal striatal N-methyl-D-aspartate receptor blockade. *Behav. Neurosci.* 119: 1563–1571.

Hsiao S and Isaacson RL (1971) Learning of food and water positions by hippocampus damaged rats. *Physiol. Behav.* 6: 81–83.

Hull CL (1943) *Principles of Behavior.* New York: Appleton-Century-Crofts.

Humphreys LG (1939) The effect of random alternation of reinforcement on the acquisition and extinction of conditioned eyelid reactions. *J. Exp. Psychol.* 25: 141–158.

Huston JP, Mueller CC, and Mondadori C (1977) Memory facilitation by posttrial hypothalamic stimulation and other reinforcers: A central theory of reinforcement. *Biobehav. Rev.* 1: 143–150.

Iaria G, Petrides M, Dagher A, Pike B, and Bohbot VD (2003) Cognitive strategies dependent on the hippocampus and caudate nucleus in human navigation: Variability and change with practice. *J. Neurosci.* 23: 5945–5952.

Isaacson RL and Kimble DP (1972) Lesions of the limbic system: Their effects upon hypotheses and frustration. *Behav. Biol.* 7: 767–793.

Ito R, Robbins TW, McNaughton BL, and Everitt BJ (2006) Selective excitotoxic lesions of the hippocampus and basolateral amygdala have dissociable effects on appetitive cue and place conditioning based on path integration in a novel Y-maze procedure. *Eur. J. Neurosci.* 23: 3071–3080.

Johnsrude IS, Owen AM, White NM, Zhao WV, and Bohbot VD (2000) Impaired preference conditioning after anterior temporal lobe resection in humans. *J. Neurosci.* 20: 2649–2656.

Johnsrude IS, Owen AM, Zhao WV, and White NM (1999) Conditioned preference in humans: A novel experimental approach. *Learn. Motiv.* 30: 250–264.

Jones B and Mishkin M (1972) Limbic lesions and the problem of stimulus-reinforcement associations. *Exp. Neurol.* 36: 362–377.

Kennedy PJ and Shapiro ML (2004) Retrieving memories via internal context requires the hippocampus. *J. Neurosci.* 24: 6979–6985.

Kentros CG, Agnihotri NT, Hawkins RD, Muller RU, and Kandel ER (2003) Stabilization of the hippocampal representation of space in mice requires attention. *Soc. Neurosci. Abstr.* 24 Abs No 316.15.

Killiany R, Rehbein L, and Mahut H (2005) Developmental study of the hippocampal formation in rhesus monkeys (*Macaca mulatta*): II. Early ablations do not spare the capacity to retrieve conditional object-object associations. *Behav. Neurosci.* 119: 651–661.

Kim JJ and Fanselow MS (1992) Modality-specific retrograde amnesia of fear. *Science* 256: 675–677.

Kim JJ and Jung MW (2006) Neural circuits and mechanisms involved in Pavlovian fear conditioning: A critical review. *Neurosci. Biobehav. Rev.* 30: 188–202.

Kimble DP (1968) Hippocampus and internal inhibition. *Psychol. Bull.* 70: 285–295.

Kimble DP and Kimble RJ (1965) Hippocampectomy and response preservation in the rat. *J. Comp. Physiol. Psychol.* 60: 474–476.

Kirkby RJ (1969) Caudate lesions and perseverative behavior. *Physiol. Behav.* 4: 451–454.

Kirsch P, Achenbach C, Kirsch M, Heinzmann M, Schienle A, and Vaitl D (2003) Cerebellar and hippocampal activation during eyeblink conditioning depends on the experimental paradigm: A MEG study. *Neural Plast.* 10: 291–301.

Knierim JJ, Kudrimoti HS, and McNaughton BL (1998) Interactions between idiothetic cues and external landmarks in the control of place cells and head direction cells. *J. Neurophysiol.* 80: 425–446.

Knowlton BJ, Mangels JA, and Squire LR (1996) A neostriatal habit learning system in humans. *Science* 273: 1399–1402.

Knowlton BJ, Squire LR, and Gluck MA (1994) Probabilistic classification learning in amnesia. *Learn. Mem.* 1: 106–120.

Landauer TK (1969) Reinforcement as consolidation. *Psychol. Rev.* 76: 82–96.

Lashley KS (1950) In search of the engram. *Symp. Soc. Exp. Biol.* 4: 454–482.

LeDoux JE (1993) Emotional memory systems in the brain. *Behav. Brain Res.* 58: 69–79.

Leutgeb S, Leutgeb JK, Barnes CA, Moser EI, McNaughton BL, and Moser MB (2005) Independent codes for spatial and episodic memory in hippocampal neuronal ensembles. *Science* 309: 619–623.

Lever C, Burgess N, Cacucci F, Hartley T, and O'Keefe J (2002) What can the hippocampal representation of environmental geometry tell us about Hebbian learning? *Biol. Cybern.* 87: 356–372.

Ljungberg L (1992) Carl Wernicke and Sergei Korsakoff: Fin de siecle innovators in neuropsychiatry. *J. Hist. Neurosci.* 1: 23–27.

Maguire EA, Burgess N, Donnett JG, Frackowiak RS, Frith CD, and O'Keefe J (1998) Knowing where and getting there: A human navigation network. *Science* 280: 921–924.

Mahut H (1971) Spatial and object reversal learning in monkeys with partial temporal lobe ablations. *Neuropsychologia* 9: 409–424.

Mahut H (1972) A selective spatial deficit in monkeys after transection of the fornix. *Neuropsychologia* 10: 65–74.

Mahut H, Moss M, and Zola-Morgan S (1981) Retention deficits after combined amygdalo-hippocampal and selective hippocampal resections in the monkey. *Neuropsychologia* 19: 201–225.

Maine de Biran P (1804) *Mémoires sur l'influence de l'habitude.* (1987) edn. Paris: Virin.

Marchand AR, Luck D, and Di SG (2004) Trace fear conditioning: A role for context? *Arch. Ital. Biol.* 142: 251–263.

Maren S (2005) Synaptic mechanisms of associative memory in the amygdala. *Neuron* 47: 783–786.

Maren S and Quirk GJ (2004) Neuronal signalling of fear memory. *Nat. Rev. Neurosci.* 5: 844–852.

Martone M, Butters N, Payne M, Becker J, and Sax DS (1984) Dissociations between skill learning and verbal recognition in amnesia and dementia. *Arch. Neurol.* 41: 965–970.

Maschke M, Erichsen M, Drepper J, et al. (2002) Limb flexion reflex-related areas in human cerebellum. *Neuroreport* 13: 2325–2330.

McDonald RJ and Hong NS (2004) A dissociation of dorso-lateral striatum and amygdala function on the same stimulus-response habit task. *Neuroscience* 124: 507–513.

McDonald RJ and White NM (1993) A triple dissociation of memory systems: Hippocampus, amygdala and dorsal striatum. *Behav. Neurosci.* 107: 3–22.

McDonald RJ and White NM (1994) Parallel information processing in the water maze: Evidence for independent memory systems involving dorsal striatum and hippocampus. *Behav. Neural Biol.* 61: 260–270.

McGaugh JL and Herz MJ (1972) *Memory Consolidation.* San Francisco: Albion.

McNaughton BL, Barnes CA, Gerrard JL, et al. (1996) Deciphering the hippocampal polyglot: The hippocampus as a path integration system. *J. Exp. Biol.* 199: 173–185.

Milner B (1958) Psychological defects produced by temporal lobe excision. *Res. Publ. Assoc. Res. Nerv. Ment. Dis.* 36: 244–257.

Milner B (1959) The memory defect in bilateral hippocampal lesions. *Psychiatr. Res. Rep. Am. Psychiatr. Assoc.* 11: 43–58.

Milner B, Corkin S, and Teuber H-L (1968) Further analysis of the hippocampal amnesic syndrome: 14-year follow-up study of H.M. *Neuropsychologia* 6: 215–234.

Milner B and Penfield W (1955) The effect of hippocampal lesions on recent memory. *Trans. Am. Neurol. Assoc.* 42–48.

Miranda R, Blanco E, Begega A, Rubio S, and Arias JL (2006) Hippocampal and caudate metabolic activity associated with different navigational strategies. *Behav. Neurosci.* 120: 641–650.

Mishkin M, Malamut B, and Bachevalier J (1984) Memories and habits: Two neural systems. In: Lynch G, McGaugh JL, and Weinberger NM (eds.) *Neurobiology of Human Memory and Learning*, pp. 65–77. New York: Guilford Press.

Mishkin M, Ungerleider LG, and Macko KA (1983) Object vision and spatial vision: Two cortical pathways. *Trends Neurosci.* 6: 414–417.

Mitchell JA and Hall G (1987) Basal ganglia, instrumental and spatial learning. In: Ellen P and Thinus-Blanc C (eds.) *Cognitive Processes and Spatial Orientation in Animal and Man, Vol. 1: Experimental Animal Psychology and Ethology*, pp. 124–130. Dordrecht, Netherlands: Martinus Nijhoff Publishing.

Mitchell JA and Hall G (1988) Caudate-putamen lesions in the rat may impair or potentiate maze learning depending upon availability of stimulus cues and relevance of response cues. *Q. J. Exp. Psychol. B Comp. Physiol. Psychol.* 40: 243–258.

Mizumori SJ and Leutgeb S (2001) Directing place representation in the hippocampus. *Rev. Neurosci.* 12: 347–363.

Mizumori SJ, Yeshenko O, Gill KM, and Davis DM (2004) Parallel processing across neural systems: Implications for a multiple memory system hypothesis. *Neurobiol. Learn. Mem.* 82: 278–298.

Morris RGM (1981) Spatial localization does not require the presence of local cues. *Learn. Motiv.* 12: 239–261.

Morris RGM, Garrud P, Rawlins JNP, and O'Keefe J (1982) Place navigation impaired in rats with hippocampal lesions. *Nature* 297: 681–683.

Moyer JR Jr., Deyo RA, and Disterhoft JF (1990) Hippocampectomy disrupts trace eye-blink conditioning in rabbits. *Behav. Neurosci.* 104: 243–252.

Muller RU, Stead M, and Pach J (1996) The hippocampus as a cognitive graph. *J. Gen. Physiol.* 107: 663–694.

Nachman M and Ashe JH (1974) Effects of basolateral amygdala lesions on neophobia, learned taste aversions, and sodium appetite in rats. *J. Comp. Physiol. Psychol.* 87: 622–643.

Nadel L (1991) The hippocampus and space revisited. *Hippocampus* 1: 221–229.

Nadel L, O'Keefe J, and Black AH (1975) Slam on the brakes: A critique of Altman, Brunner, and Bayer's response-inhibition model of hippocampal function. *Behav. Biol.* 14: 151–162.

O'Keefe J (1976) Place units in the hippocampus of freely moving rats. *Exp. Neurol.* 51: 78–109.

O'Keefe J and Dostrovsky J (1971) The hippocampus as a spatial map. Preliminary evidence from unit activity in the freely-moving rat. *Brain Res.* 34: 171–175.

O'Keefe J and Nadel L (1978) *The Hippocampus as a Cognitive Map.* Oxford: Oxford University Press.

O'Keefe J, Nadel L, Keightley S, and Kill D (1975) Fornix lesions selectively abolish place learning in the rat. *Exp. Neurol.* 48: 152–166.

Olton DS (1978) Characteristics of spatial memory. In: Hulse SH, Fowler H, and Honig WK (eds.) *Cognitive Processes in Animal Behavior*, pp. 341–373. Hillsdale, NJ: Erlbaum.

Olton DS and Papas BC (1979) Spatial memory and hippocampal function. *Neuropsychologia* 17: 669–682.

Olton DS and Samuelson RJ (1976) Remembrances of places past: Spatial memory in the rat. *J. Exp. Psychol. Anim. Behav. Process.* 2: 97–116.

Olton DS, Walker JA, and Gage FH (1978) Hippocampal connections and spatial discrimination. *Brain Res.* 139: 295–308.

Orbach J, Milner B, and Rasmussen T (1960) Learning and retention in monkeys after amygdala-hippocampus resection. *Arch. Neurol.* 3: 230–251.

Packard MG and Cahill LF (2001) Affective modulation of multiple memory systems. *Curr. Opin. Neurobiol.* 11: 752–756.

Packard MG, Cahill LF, and McGaugh JL (1994) Amygdala modulation of hippocampal-dependent and caudate nucleus- dependent memory processes. *Proc. Natl. Acad. Sci. USA* 91: 8477–8481.

Packard MG, Hirsh R, and White NM (1989) Differential effects of fornix and caudate nucleus lesions on two radial maze tasks: Evidence for multiple memory systems. *J. Neurosci.* 9: 1465–1472.

Packard MG and Knowlton BJ (2002) Learning and memory functions of the Basal Ganglia. *Annu. Rev. Neurosci.* 25: 563–593.

Packard MG and McGaugh JL (1992) Double dissociation of fornix and caudate nucleus lesions on acquisition of two water maze tasks: Further evidence for multiple memory systems. *Behav. Neurosci.* 106: 439–446.

Packard MG and McGaugh JL (1996) Inactivation of hippocampus or caudate nucleus with lidocaine differentially affects expression of place and response learning. *Neurobiol. Learn. Mem.* 65: 66–72.

Packard MG and Teather LA (1997) Double dissociation of hippocampal and dorsal-striatal memory systems by posttraining intracerebral injections of 2-amino-5-phosphonopentanoic acid. *Behav. Neurosci.* 111: 543–551.

Packard MG and Teather LA (1998) Amygdala modulation of multiple memory systems: Hippocampus and caudate-putamen. *Neurobiol. Learn. Mem.* 69: 163–203.

Packard MG and White NM (1991) Dissociation of hippocampal and caudate nucleus memory systems by post-training intracerebral injection of dopamine agonists. *Behav. Neurosci.* 105: 295–306.

Pavlov IP (1927) *Conditioned Reflexes.* Oxford: Oxford University Press.

Peinado-Manzano MA (1988) Effects of biateral lesions of the central and lateral amygdala on free operant successive discrimination. *Behav. Brain Res.* 29: 61–72.

Phillips AG and Carr GD (1987) Cognition and the basal ganglia: A possible substrate for procedural knowledge. *Can. J. Neurol. Sci.* 14: 381–385.

Phillips RG and LeDoux JE (1992) Differential contribution of amygdala and hippocampus to cued and contextual fear conditioning. *Behav. Neurosci.* 106: 274–285.

Pitkänen A, Savander V, and LeDoux JE (1997) Organization of intra-amygdaloid circuitries in the rat: An emerging framework for understanding functions of the amygdala. *Trends Neurosci.* 20: 517–523.

Poldrack RA, Clark J, Pare-Blagoev EJ, et al. (2001) Interactive memory systems in the human brain. *Nature* 414: 546–550.

Poldrack RA and Packard MG (2003) Competition among multiple memory systems: Converging evidence from animal and human brain studies. *Neuropsychologia* 41: 245–251.

Poldrack RA, Prabhakaran V, Seger CA, and Gabrieli JD (1999) Striatal activation during acquisition of a cognitive skill. *Neuropsychology* 13: 564–574.

Poldrack RA and Rodriguez P (2004) How do memory systems interact? Evidence from human classification learning. *Neurobiol. Learn. Mem.* 82: 324–332.

Ragozzino ME, Unick KE, and Gold PE (1996) Hippocampal acetylcholine release during memory testing in rats: Augmentation by glucose. *Proc. Natl. Acad. Sci. USA* 93: 4693–4698.

Restle F (1957) Discrimination of cues in mazes: A resolution of the "place-vs.-response" question. *Psychol. Rev.* 64: 957, 217–228.

Ribot T (1883) *The Diseases of Memory. English translation of Les Maladies de la Mémoire (1881).* New York: Humboldt Library of Popular Science Literature.

Sage JR and Knowlton BJ (2000) Effects of US devaluation on win-stay and win-shift radial maze performance in rats. *Behav. Neurosci.* 114: 295–306.

Sargolini F, Fyhn M, Hafting T, et al. (2006) Conjunctive representation of position, direction, and velocity in entorhinal cortex. *Science* 312: 758–762.

Schafe GE, Doyere V, and LeDoux JE (2005) Tracking the fear engram: The lateral amygdala is an essential locus of fear memory storage. *J. Neurosci.* 25: 10010–10014.

Scoville WB and Milner B (1957) Loss of recent memory after bilateral hippocampal lesions. *J. Neurol. Neurosurg. Psychiatry* 20: 11–21.

Sherry DF and Schacter DL (1987) The evolution of multiple memory systems. *Psychol. Rev.* 94: 439–454.

Shohamy D, Myers CE, Grossman S, Sage J, Gluck MA, and Poldrack RA (2004) Cortico-striatal contributions to feedback-based learning: Converging data from neuroimaging and neuropsychology. *Brain* 127: 851–859.

Skelton RW (1988) Bilateral cerebellar lesions disrupt conditioned eyelid responses in unrestrained rats. *Behav. Neurosci.* 102: 586–590.

Skinner BF (1938) *The Behavior of Organisms.* New York: Appleton-Century-Crofts.

Smith PF (1997) Vestibular-hippocampal interactions. *Hippocampus* 7: 465–471.

Sutherland RJ (1985) The navigating hippocampus: An individual medley of movement, space and memory. In: Buzsaki G and Vanderwolf CH (eds.) *Electrical Activity of the Archicortex*, pp. 255–279. Budapest: Akademiai Kiado.

Sutherland RJ and Dyck RH (1984) Place navigation by rats in a swimming pool. *Can. J. Psychol.* 38: 322–347.

Sutherland RJ and Linggard RC (1982) Being there: A novel demonstration of latent spatial learning in the rat. *Behav. Neural Biol.* 36: 103–107.

Suzuki S, Augerinos G, and Black AH (1980) Stimulus control of spatial behavior on the eight-arm maze in rats. *Learn. Motiv.* 11: 1–18.

Taube JS (1998) Head direction cells and the neurophysiological basis for a sense of direction. *Prog. Neurobiol.* 55: 225–256.

Teather LA, Packard MG, Smith DE, Ellis-Behnke RG, and Bazan NG (2005) Differential induction of c-Jun and Fos-like proteins in rat hippocampus and dorsal striatum after training in two water maze tasks. *Neurobiol. Learn. Mem.* 84: 75–84.

Terrazas A, Krause M, Lipa P, Gothard KM, Barnes CA, and McNaughton BL (2005) Self-motion and the hippocampal spatial metric. *J. Neurosci.* 25: 8085–8096.

Thompson RF (2005) In search of memory traces. *Annu. Rev. Psychol.* 56: 1–23.

Thompson RF and Kim JJ (1996) Memory systems in the brain and localization of a memory. *Proc. Natl. Acad. Sci. USA* 93: 13438–13444.

Thompson RF and Krupa DJ (1994) Organization of memory traces in the mammalian brain. *Annu. Rev. Neurosci.* 17: 519–549.

Thompson WG, Guilford MO, and Hicks LH (1980) Effects of caudate and cortical lesions on place and response learning in rats. *Physiol. Psychol.* 8(4): 473–479.

Thorndike EL (1898) Animal intelligence. An experimental study of the associative processes in animals. *Psychol. Monogr.* 2(4): 1–109.

Thorndike EL (1911) *Animal Intelligence.* New York: Macmillan.

Thorndike EL (1933) A proof of the law of effect. *Science* 77: 173–175.

Tolman EC (1932) *Purposive Behavior in Animals and Men.* New York: Century.

Tolman EC (1948) Cognitive maps in rats and men. *Psychol. Rev.* 56: 144–155.

Tolman EC (1949) There is more than one kind of learning. *Psychol. Rev.* 56: 144–155.

Tolman EC and Honzik CH (1930) Introduction and removal of reward and maze performance in rats. *Univ. Calif. Publ. Psychol.* 4: 257–275.

Tolman EC, Ritchie BF, and Kalish D (1946) Studies in spatial learning II place learning versus response learning. *J. Exp. Psychol. Gen.* 36: 221–229.

Ungerleider LG and Mishkin M (1982) Two cortical visual systems. In: Ingle DJ, Goodale MA, and Masnfield RJW (eds.) *Analysis of Visual Behavior*, pp. 549–586. Cambridge, MA: MIT Press.

Warrington EK and Weiskrantz L (1982) Amnesia: A disconnection syndrome? *Neuropsychologia* 20: 233–248.

Watson JB (1912) Psychology as the behaviorist views it. *Psychol. Rev.* 20: 158–177.

Weiskrantz L (1956) Behavioral changes associated with ablation of the amygdaloid complex in monkeys. *J. Comp. Physiol. Psychol.* 49: 381–391.

Whishaw IQ (1998) Place learning in hippocampal rats and the path integration hypothesis. *Neurosci. Biobehav. Rev.* 22: 209–220.

Whishaw IQ, Hines DJ, and Wallace DG (2001) Dead reckoning (path integration) requires the hippocampal formation: Evidence from spontaneous exploration and spatial learning tasks in light (allothetic) and dark (idiothetic) tests. *Behav. Brain Res.* 127: 49–69.

Whishaw IQ, McKenna JE, and Maaswinkel H (1997) Hippocampal lesions and path integration. *Curr. Opin. Neurobiol.* 7: 228–234.

White NM (1989a) A functional hypothesis concerning the striatal matrix and patches: Mediation of S-R memory and reward. *Life Sci.* 45: 1943–1957.

White NM (1989b) Reward or reinforcement: What's the difference? *Neurosci. Biobehav. Rev.* 13: 181–186.

White NM and Carr GD (1985) The conditioned place preference is affected by two independent reinforcement processes. *Pharmacol. Biochem. Behav.* 23: 37–42.

White NM and Gaskin S (2006) Dorsal hippocampus function in learning and expressing a spatial discrimination. *Learn. Mem.* 13: 119–122.

White NM and McDonald RJ (1993) Acquisition of a spatial conditioned place preference is impaired by amygdala lesions and improved by fornix lesions. *Behav. Brain Res.* 55: 269–281.

White NM and Milner PM (1992) The psychobiology of reinforcers. *Annu. Rev. Psychol.* 43: 443–471.

White NM and Ouellet M-C (1997) Roles of movement and temporal factors in spatial learning. *Hippocampus* 7: 501–510.

Wiener SI, Paul CA, and Eichenbaum H (1989) Spatial and behavioral correlates of hippocampal neuronal activity. *J. Neurosci.* 9: 2737–2763.

Winocur G and Mills JA (1969) Effects of caudate lesions on avoidance behavior in rats. *J. Comp. Physiol. Psychol.* 68: 552–557.

Wise SP (1996) The role of the basal ganglia in procedural memory. *Semin. Neurosci.* 8: 39–46.

Woodruff-Pak DS, Lavond DG, and Thompson RF (1985) Trace conditioning: Abolished by cerebellar nuclear lesions but not lateral cerebellar cortex aspirations. *Brain Res.* 348: 249–260.

Yamamoto T and Fujimoto Y (1991) Brain mechanisms of taste aversion learning in the rat. *Brain Res. Bull.* 27: 403–406.

Yin HH and Knowlton BJ (2002) Reinforcer devaluation abolishes conditioned cue preference: Evidence for stimulus-stimulus associations. *Behav. Neurosci.* 116: 174–177.

Yin HH and Knowlton BJ (2004) Contributions of striatal subregions to place and response learning. *Learn. Mem.* 11: 459–463.

Yin HH, Knowlton BJ, and Balleine BW (2004) Lesions of dorsolateral striatum preserve outcome expectancy but disrupt habit formation in instrumental learning. *Eur. J. Neurosci.* 19: 181–189.

Young PT and Christensen KR (1962) Algebraic summation of hedonic processes. *J. Comp. Physiol. Psychol.* 55: 332–336.

Zola SM and Mahut H (1973) Paradoxical facilitation of object reversal learning after transection of the fornix in monkeys. *Neuropsychologia* 11: 271–284.

4 Implicit Memory and Priming

W. D. Stevens, G. S. Wig, and D. L. Schacter, Harvard University, Cambridge, MA, USA

4.1 Introduction

Priming refers to an improvement or change in the identification, production, or classification of a stimulus as a result of a prior encounter with the same or a related stimulus (Tulving and Schacter, 1990). Cognitive and neuropsychological evidence indicates that priming reflects the operation of implicit or nonconscious processes that can be dissociated from those that support explicit or conscious recollection of past experiences. More recently, neuroimaging studies have revealed that priming is often accompanied by decreased activity in a variety of brain regions (for review, see Schacter and Buckner, 1998; Wiggs and Martin, 1998; Henson, 2003), although conditions exist in which priming-related increases are also observed (e.g., Schacter et al., 1995; Henson et al., 2000; Fiebach et al., 2005). Various terms have been used to describe these neural changes, including adaptation, mnemonic filtering, repetition suppression, and repetition enhancement. These terms often refer to subtly distinct, though related, phenomena, and in some cases belie a theoretical bias as to the nature of such neural changes. Thus, throughout the present review, the term neural priming will be used to refer to changes in neural activity associated with the processing of a stimulus that result from a previous encounter with the same or a related stimulus.

When considering the link between behavioral and neural priming, it is important to acknowledge that functional neuroimaging relies on a number of underlying assumptions. First, changes in information processing result in changes in neural activity within brain regions subserving these processing operations. A second assumption underlying positron emission tomography (PET) and functional magnetic resonance imaging (fMRI) is that these changes in neural activity are accompanied by changes in blood flow, such that the energy expenditure that accompanies increased neuronal processing elicits the delivery of metabolites and removal of by-products to and from active regions, respectively. It is these local vascular changes that are measured: PET measures changes in cerebral blood flow and oxygen or glucose utilization, while fMRI measures the ratio of oxygenated to deoxygenated hemoglobin (i.e., the blood-oxygen-level dependent, or BOLD, signal). Related techniques such as event-related potentials (ERP) and magnetoencephalography (MEG), by contrast, measure the electrophysiological responses of neural populations more directly, although at a cost of decreased spatial resolution. While this chapter will focus on fMRI and to a lesser extent PET studies of priming, ERP and MEG studies will be discussed when they are of special interest to the discussion of a particular topic.

Neuroimaging studies have provided new means of addressing cognitive theories that have traditionally been evaluated through behavioral studies. The primary goal of the present chapter is to examine how neuroimaging evidence has informed, influenced, and reshaped cognitive theories about the nature of priming. We focus on five research areas where such interaction has occurred: influences of explicit versus implicit memory, top-down attentional effects, specificity of priming, the nature of priming-related activation increases, and correlations between brain activity and behavior.

4.2 Influences of Explicit Versus Implicit Memory

Priming is typically defined as a nonconscious or implicit form of memory. This characterization is supported by numerous observations of spared priming in amnesic patients with severe disorders of explicit memory. However, starting with the earliest cognitive studies of priming in healthy volunteers, researchers have been concerned with the possibility that subjects may use some type of explicit retrieval to perform a nominally implicit task. This concern has led to the development of various cognitive procedures for estimating and removing the influences of explicit retrieval (e.g., Schacter et al., 1989; Jacoby, 1991). Two forms of such explicit 'contamination' have received attention in cognitive studies: (1) subjects realize that their memory is being tested, and intentionally retrieve study list words while performing a priming task to augment performance; (2) subjects follow task instructions, and therefore do not engage in intentional retrieval, but nonetheless unintentionally recollect that they had studied target items on the previous study list. With respect to the latter type of contamination, it has been noted that explicit memory often takes the form of unintentional or involuntary recollections of previous experiences in which there is no deliberate, effortful attempt to think back to the past; one is spontaneously 'reminded' of a past event that is accompanied by conscious recollection (e.g., Schacter, 1987; Schacter et al., 1989; Richardson-Klavehn et al., 1994; Richardson-Klavehn and Gardiner, 1998; Bernsten and Hall, 2004). We now consider findings from neuroimaging studies that provide insights into the nature of and relation between implicit and explicit influences on priming.

The explicit contamination issue arose in the first neuroimaging study of priming (Squire et al., 1992). In this experiment, subjects semantically encoded a list of familiar words prior to PET scanning and were then scanned during a stem completion task in which they provided the first word that came to mind in response to visual three-letter word stems. During one scan, subjects could complete stems with study list words (priming), and during another, they could complete stems only with new words that had not been presented on the study list (baseline). In a separate scan, subjects were provided with three-letter stems of study-list words, and were asked to think back to the study list (explicit cued recall).

Priming was associated with decreased activity in the right extrastriate occipital cortex compared with baseline, but there was also increased activity in the right hippocampal formation during priming compared with the baseline condition. In light of previous results from amnesic patients indicating that normal stem-completion priming can occur even when the hippocampal formation is damaged, it seemed likely that the observed activation of the hippocampal region reflects one of the two previously mentioned forms of 'contamination': subjects intentionally retrieved words from the study list or, alternatively, they provided the first word that comes to mind and involuntarily recollected its prior occurrence.

Schacter et al. (1996) attempted to reduce or eliminate explicit influences by using a nonsemantic study task (counting the number of t-junctions in each of target words), which in previous behavioral studies had supported robust stem-completion priming together with poor explicit memory for the target items (e.g., Graf and Mandler, 1984; Bowers and Schacter, 1990). Consistent with the idea that the priming-related hippocampal activation previously observed by Squire et al. reflects contamination from explicit memory that is not essential to observing priming, following the t-junction encoding task there was no evidence of priming-related increases in the vicinity of the hippocampal formation during stem completion performance relative to the baseline task, but there were priming-related decreases in bilateral extrastriate occipital cortex and several other regions.

Using PET, Rugg et al. (1997) found greater left hippocampal activity after deep encoding than after shallow encoding during both intentional (old/new recognition) and unintentional (animate/inanimate decision) retrieval tasks. They also observed greater right anterior prefrontal activity during intentional retrieval than during unintentional retrieval after both deep and shallow encoding. These results suggest that increases in hippocampal activity during explicit retrieval, unaccompanied by corresponding increases in anterior prefrontal activity, reflect the presence of involuntary explicit memory.

A more recent event-related fMRI study by Schott et al. (2005) extends the findings of these early studies. During the study phase, subjects made nonsemantic encoding judgments in which they counted the number of syllables in each word. During the test phase, Schott et al. used a stem completion task and directly compared performance during intentional retrieval (i.e., try to remember a word from the list beginning with these three letters) and incidental retrieval (i.e., complete the stem with the first word that comes to mind). Importantly, they used a behavioral procedure developed by Richardson-Klavehn and Gardiner (1996, 1998) in which participants indicate whether or not they remember that the item they produced on the completion task had appeared earlier during the study task. This procedure could be applied to both the incidental and intentional tests, because on the intentional test subjects were told to complete stems even when they could not recall a study-list item. In the scanner, subjects used a button press to indicate whether they had covertly completed a stem; between these test trials, they provided their completions orally and indicated whether or not they remembered having seen the item during the study task. Stems completed with study-list words that were judged as nonstudied were classified as primed items, whereas stems completed with study-list words judged as studied were classified as remembered items. Both primed and remembered items were compared with baseline items that subjects judged correctly as nonstudied.

Similar to previous studies, Schott et al. (2005) documented activation reductions for primed items compared with baseline items in a number of regions, including extrastriate visual cortex. However, because the primed items in this study were, by definition, ones that subjects did not consciously remember having encountered previously, these data show more convincingly than earlier studies that priming-related activation decreases can reflect strictly nonconscious or implicit memory. Moreover, the authors also reported that their findings concerning priming-related reductions during the incidental tests were largely replicated during the intentional test. Thus, the results support the idea that priming effects can occur during both intentional and unintentional retrieval. Several other regions, including the right prefrontal cortex, showed greater activity during the intentional than the incidental task. In contrast to prior studies, the hippocampus showed greater activity during baseline than during priming, which the authors attributed to novelty encoding. Overall, these neuroimaging results support earlier behavioral distinctions between strategic controlled retrieval (i.e., intentional vs. incidental) and conscious recollection of the occurrence of previously studied items and show clearly that priming-accompanied activation reductions can occur without conscious recollection.

While the foregoing studies attempted to distinguish implicit and explicit aspects of priming by focusing on retrieval, other studies have done so by examining brain activity during encoding. Schott et al. (2006) examined subsequent memory effects, where neural activity during encoding is sorted according to whether items are subsequently remembered or forgotten (e.g., Brewer et al., 1998; Wagner et al., 1998). This study reported fMRI data from the encoding phase of the aforementioned stem completion experiment reported by Schott et al. (2005), where participants counted the number of syllables in each word. Consistent with results from earlier subsequent memory studies that examined explicit retrieval, Schott et al. found greater activation during encoding for subsequently remembered than for forgotten items in left inferior prefrontal cortex and bilateral medial temporal lobe. By contrast, encoding activity in these areas was not associated with subsequently primed items. Instead, subsequent priming was associated with activation decreases during encoding in bilateral extrastriate cortex, left fusiform gyrus, and bilateral inferior frontal gyrus. These regions were distinct from those that showed priming-related decreases during the stem completion test. Schott et al. suggest that their data indicate that priming, in contrast to explicit memory, is associated with sharpening of perceptual representations during encoding, an idea that is consistent with previous theories emphasizing the differential role of a perceptual representation system in priming and explicit memory (Schacter, 1990, 1994; Tulving and Schacter, 1990).

While the combined results from Schott et al.'s (2005, 2006) encoding and retrieval phases highlight clear differences between priming and explicit memory, a related study by Turk-Browne et al. (2006), also using a subsequent memory paradigm, uncovered conditions under which the two forms of memory are associated with one another. Subjects made indoor/outdoor decisions about a series of novel scenes. Each scene was repeated once, at lags ranging from 2 to 11 items. Fifteen minutes after presentation of the final scene, subjects were given a surprise old/new recognition test. Turk-Browne et al. focused on a region of interest in the parahippocampal place area (PPA) that responds maximally to visual scenes (e.g., Epstein and Kanwisher, 1998). The critical outcome was that repeated scenes produced behavioral priming and reduced activation in the PPA, but only for those scenes that were subsequently remembered. Forgotten items did not produce either behavioral or neural priming. A whole-brain analysis revealed similar effects – neural priming for remembered items only – in bilateral PPA as well as in left inferior temporal gyrus and bilateral angular gyrus. However, forgotten items were associated with neural priming in the anterior cingulate.

Given the general trend that behavioral and neural priming both depended on subsequent explicit memory, Turk-Browne et al. suggested that their data reveal a link between implicit and explicit memory that involves some aspect of shared encoding processes – most likely that selective attention during encoding is required for both subsequent priming and explicit memory.

The neuroimaging evidence considered thus far reveals some conditions under which priming can occur independently of explicit memory and others where dependence exists. An experiment by Wagner et al. (2000) showed that priming can sometimes hinder explicit memory. They made use of the well-known spacing or lag effect, where reencoding an item after a short lag following its initial presentation typically produces lower levels of subsequent explicit memory than reencoding an item after a long lag (though in both cases, explicit memory is higher than with no repetition). Using an incidental encoding task (abstract/concrete judgment) and old/new recognition task, Wagner et al. documented greater explicit memory following a long- than a short-lag condition, consistent with previous behavioral findings. By contrast, they showed greater behavioral priming, indexed by reduced reaction time, and greater neural priming, indexed by reduced activity in the left inferior frontal lobe, following a short lag than a long lag. Moreover, there was a negative correlation between the magnitude of neural priming in the left inferior frontal region and the level of subsequent explicit memory. Thus, the short-lag condition that maximized priming also reduced explicit memory. Although the exact mechanism underlying the effect is still not known, Wagner et al. suggested that priming may impair new episodic encoding and later explicit memory by reducing encoding variability, that is, encoding different attributes of repeated items on different trials. To the extent that encoding variability normally enhances subsequent memory by providing multiple retrieval routes to an item (e.g., Martin, 1968), priming might reduce explicit memory because it biases encoding toward sampling the same item features on multiple trials. Whatever the ultimate explanation, these results highlight the role of a previously unsuspected interaction between priming and explicit memory in producing a well-known behavioral effect.

4.3 Top-Down Attentional Effects on Priming

Priming is often considered to be an automatic process (e.g., Jacoby and Dallas, 1981; Tulving and Schacter, 1990; Wiggs and Martin, 1998). However, recent neuroimaging evidence has revealed that, to some extent, behavioral and neural priming may be affected by top-down cognitive processes such as attention or task orientation.

4.3.1 Priming: Automatic/Independent of Attention?

Early evidence supported the notion that perceptual priming effects occur independent of manipulations of attention (for review see Mulligan and Hartman, 1996). However, subsequent findings from behavioral studies began to reveal that some perceptual priming effects do depend to some degree on attention at study (e.g., Mulligan and Hornstein, 2000).

In a seminal review that linked behavioral priming with the phenomenon of repetition suppression, Wiggs and Martin (1998) stated that this process "happens automatically in the cortex" and "is an intrinsic property of cortical neurons," and that "perceptual priming is impervious to . . . attentional manipulations" (Wiggs and Martin, 1998: 231). Indeed, there is some compelling evidence from studies with monkeys to suggest that repetition-related neural priming can occur independent of attention (e.g., Miller et al., 1991; Miller and Desimone, 1993; Vogels et al., 1995), but these findings do not speak directly to neural priming in humans. Some neuroimaging evidence shows that conditions exist under which both behavioral and neural priming are unaffected by manipulations of attention. A PET study by Badgaiyan et al. (2001) investigated the effects of an attentional manipulation during the study phase of a cross-modal priming task. Target words were aurally presented among distracter words at study under either full attention or under a divided-attention task. At test, visual word stems were presented in separate blocks for both target word types. Behavioral priming (faster reaction times) and neural priming (reduced regional cerebral blood flow in superior temporal gyrus) were of similar magnitude for words presented under full and divided attention conditions (see also Voss and Paller, 2006).

An fMRI study that we reviewed earlier (Schott et al., 2005) further demonstrated that changing the nature of the task to be performed during the test phase did not affect the level of behavioral or neural priming. Following shallow encoding of words at study, word stems were presented in separate blocks of either an implicit or an explicit memory task at test. Although the explicit task elicited a higher rate of explicit recollection of previously studied words, there were no differences in behavioral priming effects between the two conditions – i.e., subjects produced an equivalent number of previously studied words when cued with word stems in both test conditions. Moreover, an equivalent degree of neural priming was documented in left fusiform, bilateral frontal, and occipital brain regions in both implicit and explicit conditions. Thus, this experiment demonstrated that changing the task orientation at test had no effect on behavioral or neural priming.

Hasson et al. (2006) demonstrated comparable neural priming in some brain regions despite a change of task orientation across separate sessions (i.e., separate experiments with different tasks). In the first of two experiments, subjects listened to spoken sentences, some grammatically sensible, some nonsensible, and decided whether each sentence was sensible or not. In the second experiment, subjects passively listened to spoken sensible sentences only, making no judgments or responses. A direct contrast between the two tasks indicated that neural priming in temporal regions was equivalent across conditions. However, neural priming was also observed in inferior frontal regions, but only in the active condition in which subjects made sensible/nonsensible judgments. This finding suggests that attentional manipulations have variable effects on different brain regions.

The foregoing studies have demonstrated that behavioral and/or neural priming can occur independent of shifts in attentional demands or task orientation at study (Badgaiyan et al., 2001; Voss and Paller, 2006), at test (Schott et al., 2005), or between different tasks (Hasson et al., 2006). However, consistent with the latter finding by Hasson et al. of concurrent attenuation of priming in prefrontal regions associated with changing task demands, these null results do not rule out the possibility that under different task conditions, and in different brain regions, top-down attentional effects may play an important role in priming. We consider now (and also later in the chapter) recent evidence that supports this claim.

4.3.2 Priming: Modulated by Attention

Henson et al. (2002) reported one of the first neuroimaging studies to demonstrate that neural priming is modulated by top-down cognitive factors. Subjects viewed pictures of famous and nonfamous faces, each presented twice at random intervals within one of two separate, consecutive task sessions. During the implicit task session, subjects performed a continuous famous/nonfamous face discrimination task; during the explicit task session, subjects performed a continuous new/old face recognition task. Neural priming was observed in a face-responsive region in the right fusiform gyrus for repeated famous faces only, consistent with previous findings (Henson et al., 2000), as well as for both famous and nonfamous faces in a left inferior occipital region. Neural priming in these regions occurred only in the implicit task. As stimuli were identical across the different task conditions, the modulation of neural priming was attributed to top-down effects of task orientation.

Although there were effects of attention on neural priming, behavioral priming seemed to be unaffected by top-down factors. Rather, behavioral priming, as indexed by reduced reaction time to respond to repeated presentations of famous faces relative to initial presentations, was equivalent in the implicit and explicit tasks. This result implies a dissociation between behavioral priming and neural priming observed in these brain regions. Further, attentional modulation varied only between sessions, i.e., the same task was performed on each stimulus during the initial and repeated presentations, leaving open the question of whether attentional factors exert an influence at study, at test, or on both occasions.

A subsequent fMRI study tested the hypothesis that attentional factors, specifically at study, have an impact on neural priming (Eger et al., 2004). During fMRI scanning, subjects performed a task at study in which two objects were simultaneously presented, one to the left and one to the right of a central fixation point. Importantly, subjects were cued to attend to either the left or right of center by a visual cue presented onscreen 100 ms prior to presentation of the 'prime' stimuli. A single 'probe' stimulus was subsequently presented in the center of the screen that matched the previously attended stimulus, matched the previously unattended stimulus, was the mirror image of one of these two stimuli, or was novel. Analyses of repetition-related behavioral facilitation (faster reaction times) and neural response reductions (fMRI BOLD signal decreases in fusiform and lateral occipital regions) revealed that behavioral and neural priming occurred only for probes that matched (or mirrored) the attended prime. Conversely, no behavioral or neural priming was documented when the probe stimulus matched (or mirrored) the unattended prime. Thus, this study showed that modulation of spatial attention affects behavioral as well as neural priming in object selective perceptual processing regions, and that these top-down attentional effects exert an influence specifically at the time of study.

In a face-repetition priming study, Ishai et al. (2004) reported that neural priming occurred only for repeated faces that were task relevant. Subjects were presented with a target face and then were shown a series of faces, including three repetitions of the target face, three repetitions of a nontarget face, and seven distracter faces. Participants were required to push a button each time the target face appeared, and thus were required to attend to all faces, although only the target face was task relevant. Significant neural priming (reduced BOLD response for the third relative to the first repetition) was observed in face-responsive regions, including inferior occipital gyri, lateral fusiform gyri, superior temporal sulci, and amygdala, but only for the target face repetitions; no neural priming was associated with repetition of nontarget faces.

Yi and colleagues (Yi and Chun, 2005; Yi et al., 2006) used overlapping scene and face images to also demonstrate that task-relevant attention has an effect even for simultaneously viewed stimuli. In one experiment, participants were presented with overlapping face and scene images and instructed to attend only to the face or the scene on a given trial (Yi et al., 2006). Neural priming in a face-responsive fusiform region was documented only for repeated faces that were attended, and not for scenes or unattended faces. Similarly, neural priming in a scene-responsive parahippocampal region occurred only for repeated scenes that were attended, and not for faces or unattended scenes. Surprisingly, even after sixteen repetitions of a stimulus every 2 s within a block, no trace of neural priming was observed for unattended stimuli in these respective regions (Yi et al., 2006).

Thus, while a number of neuroimaging studies have shown that both behavioral and neural priming can remain constant across study and test manipulations of attention or between different tasks with common stimuli, several studies reviewed here indicate that top-down effects of attention can have an impact on behavioral and/or neural priming, both at the time of study (Henson et al., 2002) and at test (Ishai et al., 2004), and have been shown to involve both spatial attention (Eger et al., 2004) and task-relevant selective attention (Ishai et al., 2004; Yi and Chun, 2005; Yi et al., 2006). To reconcile these ostensibly incongruent conclusions requires a more detailed consideration of the nature of subtle differences in various manipulations of attention, and importantly, of the particular brain regions involved.

Accordingly, recent studies (e.g., Hassan et al., 2006) have begun to dissociate various brain regions that are differentially sensitive to various attentional manipulations. In a study by Vuilleumier et al. (2005), participants viewed overlapping objects drawn in two different colors at study and were instructed to attend only to objects of a specified color. At test, these objects were presented singly among novel real and nonsense objects, and subjects indicated whether each object was a real or nonsense object. Behavioral priming was documented both for previously attended and ignored objects, with a relative boost in performance for objects that were attended. However, different brain regions showed differential sensitivity to the effects of attention on neural priming. A group of regions that comprised right posterior fusiform, lateral occipital, and left inferior frontal regions demonstrated neural priming only for attended objects presented in the original view. By contrast, bilateral anterior fusiform regions were insensitive to changes of viewpoint (original vs.

mirrored), but showed neural priming for unattended objects in addition to more robust neural priming for attended objects. Finally, neural priming in the striate cortex was view specific and more robust for attended than ignored objects.

In keeping with the latter findings, O'Kane et al. (2005) reported a similar dissociation between brain regions differentially sensitive to manipulation of top-down processes. Subjects were presented with words at study and performed a judgment of either size, shape, or composition in separate task blocks. At test, subjects performed a size judgment for all studied words presented among novel words. Behavioral facilitation, as measured by faster reaction times for size judgments at test, was observed for repeated relative to novel words, with an additional benefit when the judgment was the same at study and test (size/size) relative to when the judgment was switched (shape/size or composition/size). Neural priming in left parahippocampal cortex tracked the behavioral trend, showing reduced BOLD responses for repeated relative to novel words, with an additional trend toward increased priming when the task was the same across repetition. In left perirhinal cortex, however, neural priming occurred for repeated words only when the judgment was the same at study and test. The finding that perirhinal cortex is sensitive to semantic but not perceptual repetition provides evidence that this region is involved in conceptual processing.

Considered together, the neuroimaging studies reviewed here suggest that behavioral and neural priming are indeed modulated by top-down cognitive factors of attention or task orientation, but that this modulation exerts differential effects across different brain regions depending on the nature of the task. Neural priming within a given brain region may occur only to the extent that the processing of a stimulus reengages this region in a qualitatively similar manner across repetitions.

4.3.3 Neural Mechanisms of Top-Down Attentional Modulation

Although the effects of attention on priming have now been well documented, little is known about the neural mechanisms that underlie these top-down effects. Efforts to understand these mechanisms have been at the forefront of recently emerging neuroimaging research.

Increased attention at the time of study has been suggested as an important factor in priming. Turk-Browne et al. (2006), as previously reviewed in this chapter, reported that neural priming occurred only for repeated scenes that were later remembered, but not for those scenes that were later forgotten. They found that tonic activation, a general measure of regional neural activity, was elevated for scenes that were later remembered and that also elicited neural priming upon repeated presentation. While previous evidence indicates that increased attention results in increased neural firing rates within process-relevant brain regions, a recent fMRI study suggests that attention may also increase selectivity of the neural population representing an attended stimulus (Murray and Wojciulik, 2004).

Other neuroimaging approaches, including MEG and EEG, have been used to further characterize the nature of attentional modulations of neural priming as well. Evidence supporting the hypothesis that attention serves to increase specificity of perceptual representations was reported by Duzel and colleagues (2005) in a study using MEG. By investigating neural activity at study, they compared words that showed subsequent behavioral priming (faster reaction times) to those that did not show subsequent priming. They reported relatively decreased amplitude, but increased phase alignment, of beta and gamma oscillations for words that showed later priming, indicating increased specificity of the neural response for these words at the time of study. Further, they reported increased coordination of activity between perceptual and higher brain regions for words that showed subsequent priming, as measured by increased interareal phase synchrony of alpha oscillations. Importantly, this increased synchrony between perceptual and higher brain regions was detected immediately prior to the initial presentation of the subsequently primed stimuli, indicating an anticipatory effect. These results suggest that top-down processes, through anticipatory coordination with perceptual brain regions, increase specificity of perceptual representations at study. Such a process may also be necessary at test for successful priming. Gruber et al. (2006) reported that 'sharpening' of the neural response in cell assemblies (as measured by suppression of induced gamma band responses in ERPs) occurred for repeated visual stimuli only when the task was the same at both study and test, but not when the task was switched.

Therefore, through a combination of various neuroimaging techniques, researchers have begun to characterize the neural mechanisms that underlie attentional modulation of priming. These mechanisms may constitute a link between the cognitive functions that are accessible to our conscious awareness and under our volitional control and the unconscious systems that facilitate fluency of mental processing.

4.4 Specificity of Priming

Priming effects vary in their specificity, that is, the degree to which priming is disrupted by changes between the encoding and test phases of an experiment. When study/test changes along a particular dimension produce a reduction in priming, the inference is that the observed priming effect is based to some extent on retention of the specific information that was changed; when level of priming is unaffected by a study/test change, the inference is that priming reflects the influence of an abstract representation, at least with respect to the changed attribute. Questions concerning the specificity of priming have been prominent since the early days of priming research in cognitive psychology, when evidence emerged that some priming effects are reduced when study/test sensory modality is changed (e.g., Jacoby and Dallas, 1981; Clarke and Morton, 1983) and can also exhibit within-modality perceptual specificity, shown by the effects of changing typeface or case for visual words (e.g., Roediger and Blaxton, 1987; Graf and Ryan, 1990), or speaker's voice for auditory words (e.g., Schacter and Church, 1992). Considerable theoretical debate has focused on the key issue raised by studies of specificity effects, namely whether priming reflects the influence of nonspecific, abstract preexisting representations or specific representations that reflect perceptual details of an encoding episode (for review and discussion of cognitive studies, see Roediger, 1990; Schacter, 1990, 1994; Roediger and McDermott, 1993; Tenpenny, 1995; Bowers, 2000).

Considering the early cognitive research together with more recent neuropsychological and neuroimaging studies, Schacter et al. (2004) recently proposed a distinction among three types of specificity effects: stimulus, associative, and response. Stimulus specificity occurs when priming is reduced by changing physical properties of a stimulus between study and test; associative specificity occurs when priming is reduced because associations between target items are changed between study and test; and response specificity occurs when priming is reduced because subjects make different responses to the same stimulus item at study and test. We will review here evidence from neuroimaging studies concerning each of the three types of priming specificity and consider how the imaging data bear on the kinds of theoretical questions that have been of interest to cognitive psychologists.

4.4.1 Stimulus Specificity

Most neuroimaging research has focused on stimulus specificity, which is observed by changing physical features of a stimulus between study and test. As mentioned earlier, cognitive studies have shown that priming effects are sometimes modality specific, that is, reduced when study and test sensory modalities are different compared with when they are the same. Such effects are most commonly observed on tasks such as word or object identification, stem completion, or fragment completion, which require perceptual or data-driven processing (Roediger and Blaxton, 1987). Amnesic patients have shown a normal modality-specific effect in stem completion priming (e.g., Carlesimo, 1994; Graf et al., 1985), suggesting that this effect is not dependent on the medial temporal lobe structures that are typically damaged in amnesics.

Early neuroimaging studies of within-modality visual priming that compared brain activity during primed and unprimed stem completion showed that priming is associated with decreased activity in various posterior and prefrontal cortical regions, but the decreases were observed most consistently in the right occipitotemporal extrastriate cortex (e.g., Squire et al., 1992; Buckner et al., 1995; Schacter et al., 1996). These and related findings raised the possibility that priming-related reductions in extrastriate activity are based on a modality-specific visual representation, perhaps reflecting tuning or sharpening of primed visual word representations (Wiggs and Martin, 1998). Consistent with this possibility, Schacter et al. (1999) directly compared within-modality visual priming to a cross-modality priming condition in which subjects heard words before receiving a visual stem completion task. They found priming-related reductions in extrastriate activity during within- but not cross-modality priming. Surprisingly, however, other neuroimaging studies of within-modality auditory stem completion priming also revealed priming-related activity reductions near the extrastriate region that was previously implicated in visual priming (Badgaiyan et al., 1999; Buckner et al., 2000; Carlesimo et al., 2004). These results remain poorly understood, but it has been suggested that one part of the extrastriate region (V3A, within BA 19) is involved in multimodal functions, perhaps converting perceptual information from one modality to another (Badgaiyan et al., 1999).

Although the results of imaging studies comparing within- and cross-modality priming are not entirely conclusive, studies of within-modality changes in physical properties of target stimuli have provided clear evidence for stimulus-specific neural priming, which in turn implicates perceptual brain mechanisms in the observed priming effects. Studies focusing on early visual areas have provided one source of such evidence. Grill-Spector et al. (1999) found that activation reductions in early visual areas such as posterior lateral occipital complex (LOC) exhibit a high degree of stimulus specificity for changes in viewpoint, illumination, size, and position. By contrast, later and more anterior aspects of LOC exhibit greater invariance across changes in size and position relative to illumination and viewpoint. Evidence from a study by Vuilleumier et al. (2005) considered in the previous section likewise indicates a high degree of stimulus specificity in early visual areas, as indicated by viewpoint-specific neural priming in these regions.

Later visual regions can also show stimulus-specific neural priming, but several studies indicate that this specificity effect is lateralized. In a study by Koutstaal et al. (2001), subjects judged whether pictures of common objects were larger than a 13-inch-square box, and later made the same judgments for identical objects, different exemplars of objects with the same name, and new objects. Behavioral priming, indicated by faster response times, occurred for both identical objects and different exemplars, with significantly greater priming for identical objects. Reductions in activation were also greater for same than for different exemplars in the bilateral middle occipital, parahippocampal, and fusiform cortices. These stimulus-specific activation reductions for object priming were greater in the right than in the left fusiform cortex. Simons et al. (2003) replicated these results and further demonstrated that left fusiform cortex shows more neural priming for different exemplars compared with novel items relative to right fusiform cortex, indicating more nonspecific neural priming in the left fusiform. Also, left but not right fusiform neural priming was influenced by a lexical-semantic manipulation (objects were accompanied by presentation of their names or by nonsense syllables), consistent with a lateralized effect in which right fusiform is modulated by specific physical features of target stimuli and left fusiform is influenced more strongly by semantic features. In a related study by Vuilleumier et al. (2002), subjects decided whether pictorial images depicted real or nonsense objects, and subsequently repeated stimuli were identical, differed in size or viewpoint, or were different exemplars with the same name. Neural priming in the right fusiform cortex was sensitive to changes in both exemplar and viewpoint.

A similar pattern has also been reported for orientation-specific object priming by Vuillemer et al. (2005) in the overlapping shape paradigm described earlier, and Eger et al. (2005) reported a stimulus-specific laterality effect using faces. In the latter experiment, subjects made male/female judgments about famous or unfamiliar faces that were preceded by the identical face, a different view of the same face, or an entirely different face. Behavioral priming, indexed by decreased response times, was greater for same than different viewpoints for both famous and unfamiliar faces. Collapsed across famous and unfamiliar faces, neural priming was more viewpoint dependent in right fusiform gyrus than in left fusiform gyrus. In addition, for famous faces, priming was more nonspecific in anterior than more posterior fusiform cortex. Similarly, Vuillemer et al. (2005) report some evidence for greater stimulus-specific neural priming in posterior compared with anterior fusiform gyrus. Other studies indicate that later perceptual regions can exhibit largely nonspecific priming, both for visual stimuli such as scenes (Blondin and Lepage, 2005) and auditory words (Orfanidou et al., 2006; see also Badgaiyan et al., 2001). However, evidence provided by Bunzeck et al. (2005) suggests that effects in later perceptual regions are characterized by category specificity. In their study, subjects made male/female judgments about faces and indoor/outdoor judgments about scenes. Subjects responded more quickly to repeated faces and scenes compared with initial presentations, thus demonstrating behavioral priming. Face-responsive regions in fusiform and related areas showed selective activation reductions for repeated faces, whereas place-responsive regions in parahippocampal cortex showed decreases for repeated scenes.

By contrast, regions of inferior frontal gyrus and left inferior temporal cortex appear to respond invariantly to an item's perceptual features and are instead sensitive to its abstract or conceptual properties – even when the degree of perceptual overlap between initial and subsequent presentations of a stimulus is minimal to nonexistent. Neural priming has been observed in these regions during reading of mirror-reversed words initially presented in a normal orientation (Ryan and Schnyer, 2006) and also when silently reading semantically related word pairs, but not for pairs that are semantically unrelated (Wheatley et al., 2005). Consistent with this observation, neural priming in these regions is independent of stimulus modality (Buckner et al., 2000) and has even been observed when the modality differs between the first and second presentations of a stimulus (e.g., visual to auditory; Badgaiyan et al., 2001; Carlesimo et al., 2003).

Overall, then, the foregoing studies reveal a fairly consistent pattern in which neural priming in early visual regions exhibits strong stimulus specificity, whereas in later visual regions, right-lateralized stimulus specificity is consistently observed (for a similar pattern in a study of subliminal word priming, see Dehaene et al., 2001). These effects dovetail nicely with previous behavioral studies using divided-visual-field techniques that indicate that visually specific priming effects occur to a greater extent in the left visual field (right hemisphere) than in the right visual field (left hemisphere) (e.g., Marsolek et al., 1992, 1996).

The overall pattern of results from neuroimaging studies of stimulus specificity suggests that, consistent with a number of earlier cognitive theories (e.g., Roediger, 1990; Schacter, 1990, 1994; Tulving and Schacter, 1990), perceptual brain mechanisms do indeed play a role in certain kinds of priming effects.

4.4.2 Associative Specificity

Research concerning the cognitive neuroscience of associative specificity began with studies examining whether amnesic patients can show priming of newly acquired associations between unrelated words. For example, amnesic patients and controls studied pairs of unrelated words (such as window–reason or officer–garden) and then completed stems paired with study list words (window–rea___) or different unrelated words from the study list (officer–rea___). Mildly amnesic patients and control subjects showed more priming when stems were presented with the same words from the study task than with different words, indicating that specific information about the association between the two words had been acquired and influenced priming, but severely amnesic patients failed to show associative priming (Graf and Schacter, 1985; Schacter and Graf, 1986). A number of neuropsychological studies have since examined associative specificity in amnesics with mixed results (for review, see Schacter et al., 2004), and it has been suggested that medial temporal lobe (MTL) structures play a role in such effects. Some relevant evidence has been provided by a PET study that used a blocked design version of the associative stem completion task (Badgaiyan et al., 2002). Badgaiyan et al. found that, as in previous behavioral studies, priming was greater when stems were paired with the same words as during the study task than when they were paired with different words. The same pairing condition produced greater activation in the right MTL than did the different pairing condition, suggesting that associative specificity on the stem completion task may indeed be associated with aspects of explicit memory. Given the paucity of imaging evidence concerning associative specificity, additional studies will be needed before any strong conclusions can be reached.

4.4.3 Response Specificity

While numerous behavioral studies had explored stimulus specificity and associative specificity prior to the advent of neuroimaging studies, the situation is quite different when considering response specificity, where changing the response or decision made by the subject about a particular item influences the magnitude of priming (note that we use the terms 'response specificity' and 'decision specificity' interchangeably, since behavioral data indicate that the effect is likely not occurring at the level of a motor response; see Schnyer et al., in press). Recent interest in response specificity has developed primarily as a result of findings from neuroimaging research. Dobbins et al. (2004) used an object decision priming task that had been used in studies considered earlier (Koutstaal et al., 2001; Simons et al., 2003), but modified the task so that responses either remained the same or changed across repeated trials. In the first scanning phase, pictures of common objects were either shown once or repeated three times, and subjects indicated whether each stimulus was bigger than a shoebox (using a 'yes' or 'no' response). Next, the cue was inverted so that subjects now indicated whether each item was 'smaller than a shoebox'; they made this judgment about new items and a subset of those that had been shown earlier. Finally, the cue was restored to 'bigger than a shoebox,' and subjects were tested on new items and the remaining items from the initial phase.

If priming-related reductions in neural activity that are typically produced by this task represent facilitated size processing, attributable to 'tuning' of relevant aspects of neural representations, then cue reversal should have little effect on priming (though it could disrupt overall task performance by affecting both new and primed items). According to the neural tuning account, the same representations of object size should be accessed whether the question focuses on 'bigger' or 'smaller' than a shoebox. By contrast, if subjects perform this task by rapidly recovering prior responses, and this response learning mechanism bypasses the need to recover size representations, then the cue reversal should disrupt priming-related reductions. When the cue is changed, subjects would have to abandon the learned responses and instead reengage the target objects in a controlled manner in order to recover size information.

During the first scanning phase, standard priming-related activation reductions were observed in both anterior and posterior regions previously linked with priming: left prefrontal, fusiform, and extrastriate regions. But when the cue was reversed, these reductions were eliminated in the left fusiform cortex and disrupted in prefrontal cortex; there was a parallel effect on behavioral response times. When the cue was restored to the original format, priming-related reductions returned (again there was a parallel effect on behavioral response times), suggesting that the reductions depended on the ability of subjects to use prior responses during trials. Accordingly, the effect was seen most clearly for items repeated three times before cue reversal.

Although this evidence establishes the existence of response-specific neural and behavioral priming, there must be limitations on the effect, since a variety of priming effects occur when participants make different responses during study and test. For instance, priming effects on the stem completion task, where subjects respond with the first word that comes to mind when cued with a three-letter word beginning, are typically observed after semantic or perceptual encoding tasks that require a different response (see earlier discussion on top-down attentional influences). Nonetheless, the existence of response specificity challenges the view that all activation reductions during priming are attributable to tuning or sharpening of perceptual representations, since such effects should survive a response change. Moreover, these findings also appear to pose problems for theories that explain behavioral priming effects on object decision and related tasks in terms of changes in perceptual representation systems that are thought to underlie object representation (e.g., Schacter, 1990, 1994; Tulving and Schacter, 1990), since these views make no provisions for response specificity effects. By contrast, the transfer appropriate processing view (e.g., Roediger et al., 1989, 1999) inherently accommodates such effects. According to this perspective, priming effects are maximized when the same processing operations are performed at study and at test. Although this view has emphasized the role of overlapping perceptual operations at study and at test to explain priming effects on tasks such as object decision, to the extent that the subject's decision or response is an integral part of encoding operations, it makes sense that reinstating such operations at test would maximize priming effects.

However, there is one further feature of the experimental paradigm that Dobbins et al. (2004) used to produce response specificity that complicates any simple interpretation. Priming in cognitive studies is usually based on a single study exposure to a target item, but neuroimaging studies of priming have typically used several study exposures in order to maximize the signal strength. As noted earlier, Dobbins et al. found that response specificity effects were most robust for items presented three times during the initial phase of the experiment (high-primed items), compared with items presented just once (low-primed items).

A more recent neuropsychological investigation of response specificity in amnesic patients highlights the potential theoretical importance of this issue (Schnyer et al., 2006). Schnyer et al. compared amnesics and controls on a variant of the object decision task used by Dobbins et al. (2004). Objects were presented either once (low primed) or thrice (high primed), and then responses either remained the same ('bigger than a shoebox?') or were switched ('smaller than a shoebox?'). Consistent with Dobbins et al. (2004), controls showed greater response specificity for high-primed objects compared with low-primed objects. Amnesic patients showed no evidence of response specificity, demonstrating normal priming for low-primed items and impaired priming for high-primed items. That is, healthy controls showed greater priming for high- than for low-primed objects in the same response condition, but amnesics failed to show this additional decrease in response latencies.

These results raise the possibility that different mechanisms are involved in priming for objects presented once versus those presented multiple times. Perhaps single-exposure priming effects on the object decision task depend primarily on perceptual systems that operate independently of the MTL and thus are preserved in amnesic patients. In neuroimaging experiments, such effects might reflect tuning or sharpening of perceptual systems, independent of the specific responses or decisions that subjects make regarding the object. But for items presented several times, subjects may learn to associate the object with a particular response, perhaps requiring participation of medial temporal and prefrontal regions. These considerations also suggest that response or decision specificity in the object decision paradigm used by Dobbins et al. (2004) is better described in terms of stimulus-response or stimulus-decision specificity – that is, the formation of a new link between a particular stimulus and the response or decision. This idea is supported by recent behavioral data showing that response-specific priming occurs only for the exact object that was studied, and not for a different exemplar with the same name (Schnyer et al., in press). In any event, the overall pattern of results suggests that a single-process model is unlikely to explain all aspects of these neural or behavioral priming effects, a point to which we return later in the chapter.

4.5 Priming-Related Increases in Neural Activation

Our review so far has focused on behavioral facilitation and corresponding repetition-related reductions of neural activity associated with priming. However, under some conditions, priming has been associated with decrements in stimulus processing, such as slower responses to previously ignored stimuli relative to novel stimuli (i.e., the 'negative priming' effect – a term coined by Tipper, 1985) and poorer episodic encoding for highly primed items (Wagner et al., 2000). Further, while repetition-related increases in neural activity have long been associated with explicit memory processes, neural increases associated with priming have also been documented, although less frequently. Neuroimaging studies have begun to investigate the nature of such neural increases and the conditions that elicit them. This research suggests a link between performance decrements and increased neural responses associated with priming and provides new evidence that speaks to competing cognitive theories of implicit memory.

4.5.1 Negative Priming

Negative priming (NP) occurs when a stimulus is initially ignored, and subsequent processing of the stimulus is impaired relative to that of novel stimuli. An early example of identity NP was demonstrated by Tipper (1985); overlapping drawings of objects drawn in two different colors were presented, and subjects were instructed to attend to and identify objects of only one specified color. At test, identification of previously presented objects that were ignored was significantly slower than identification of novel objects. The NP effect has since been documented across a diverse range of experimental tasks and stimuli (for review, see Fox, 1995; May et al., 1995). Efforts to characterize the nature of this processing have sparked a number of theoretical debates within the cognitive psychology literature. One of these debates has centered on the cause of NP (e.g., whether it relies on processes during encoding or later retrieval), while another has focused on determining the level of processing that ignored items undergo in order to elicit NP (e.g., perceptual vs. semantic processing).

Competing accounts of the cause of NP are offered by two theories. The selective inhibition model (Houghton and Tipper, 1994) proposes that representations of ignored stimuli are initially activated but are immediately inhibited thereafter by selective attention. Thus, upon subsequent presentation of a previously ignored stimulus, this inhibition must be overcome, resulting in slowed processing relative to novel stimuli. The episodic retrieval model (Neill and Valdes, 1992; Neill et al., 1992) proposes that ignored stimuli are fully encoded into an episodic representation, as are attended stimuli. Upon repeated presentation of a stimulus, episodic information from the initial presentation can provide a 'shortcut' to the previous response associated with that stimulus. Whereas this would facilitate processing of previously attended stimuli that were associated with a particular response, it is detrimental to processing of ignored stimuli with which no response was associated at study. Behavioral experiments have failed to produce unambiguous support for either of these models (Fox, 1995; May et al., 1995; Egner and Hirsch, 2005).

Neuroimaging can provide a useful way to test these theories, because they predict the involvement of different brain regions supporting either inhibitory or episodic processes. Egner and Hirsch (2005) reported data from an fMRI experiment using a color-naming Stroop task that provide support for the episodic retrieval model. A region in the right dorsolateral prefrontal cortex (DLPFC) demonstrated increased activation for probe trials that were subject to NP relative to probe trials that had not been primed. The authors noted that this right DLPFC region has been associated with processes related to episodic retrieval (for review, see Stevens and Grady, 2007). Importantly, across individual subjects, activity in right DLPFC was positively correlated with response times during NP trials, but not nonprimed trials. These data support the theory that ignored stimuli, rather than being actively inhibited, are fully encoded at study, and that episodic retrieval at test contributes to the NP effect.

Another recent fMRI study investigated the level at which ignored stimuli are processed (i.e., perceptual vs. semantic/abstract) (Zubicaray et al., 2006). The authors reasoned that, if ignored stimuli elicit automatic activation of semantic representations at study, then brain regions that have been implicated in the storage and/or processing of these representations, such as the anterior temporal cortex (for review, see McClelland and Rogers, 2003) should be active during study of ignored stimuli. Overlapping drawings of different-colored objects elicited NP (slower reaction time for object identification at test) for previously ignored objects relative to novel objects. Analysis of fMRI data from the study session revealed a positive relationship between the magnitude of BOLD activity in the left anterolateral temporal cortex, including the temporal pole, and the magnitude of the subsequent NP effect. In agreement with Egner and Hirsch (2005), these data suggest that ignored stimuli are actively processed at study, and further indicate that this processing occurs at the level of abstract/semantic representations in higher conceptual brain regions.

4.5.2 Familiar Versus Unfamiliar Stimuli

There has been a long-standing debate in the cognitive psychology literature concerning priming of familiar versus unfamiliar stimuli (for review, see Tenpenny, 1995). According to modification/abstractionist theories (Morton, 1969; Bruce and Valentine, 1985), preexisting representations are required in order for priming to occur; these abstract representations are modified in some way upon presentation of familiar stimuli. According to acquisition/episodic theories (Jacoby, 1983; Roediger and Blaxton, 1987; Schacter et al., 1990), priming does not rely on a preexisting representation; rather, both familiar and unfamiliar stimuli can leave some form of a trace that can facilitate subsequent priming (although there may be limits; see Schacter et al., 1990; Schacter and Cooper, 1995). Neuroimaging studies have produced data relevant to this debate.

In a PET study, Schacter et al. (1995) reported behavioral priming for repeated unfamiliar objects, as shown by increased accuracy of possible/impossible judgments for structurally possible three-dimensional objects. However, in contrast to the more common finding of concomitant reduction in neural activity associated with behavioral priming reviewed earlier in the chapter, the authors reported increased activation in a left inferior fusiform region that was associated with priming of the possible objects.

In a more recent event-related fMRI study, Henson et al. (2000) reported data from four experiments using familiar and unfamiliar faces and symbols that directly tested the hypothesis that repetition-related neural priming entails reduced neural activity for familiar stimuli, but increased neural activity for unfamiliar stimuli. Behavioral priming (faster reaction times for familiarity judgments) was documented for repetition of both familiar and unfamiliar faces and symbols (although priming was greater for familiar than for unfamiliar stimuli). However, in a right fusiform region, repetition resulted in decreased activation for familiar faces and symbols, but increased activation for unfamiliar faces and symbols.

Henson et al. (2000) offered an account of their findings in terms of both modification and acquisition: while priming of familiar stimuli involves modification of preexisting representations, resulting in repetition suppression, priming also occurs for unfamiliar stimuli as a new representation is formed, resulting in repetition enhancement (for a generalized theory, see Henson, 2003). This suggestion is supported by evidence from a study by Fiebach et al. (2005), who concluded that neural decreases accompanying repeated words, in contrast to neural increases accompanying repeated pseudowords, reflect the sharpening of familiar object representations and the formation of novel representations for unfamiliar objects, respectively. Further, data from a previously reviewed study by Ishai et al. (2004) support this hypothesis as well; for unfamiliar faces, neural activation increased for the first repetition, but decreased in a linear trend thereafter, possibly reflecting the initial acquisition of an unfamiliar face representation, followed by subsequent modification of this newly formed representation. Henson et al. (2000) further hypothesized that the repetition enhancement effect for unfamiliar stimuli would only occur in "higher visual areas, such as the fusiform cortex, where the additional processes such as recognition occur" (Henson et al., 2000: 1272). However, in a recent study using event-related fMRI, Slotnick and Schacter (2004) reported increased activation in early visual processing regions (BA 17/18) for repeated, relative to novel, unfamiliar abstract shapes. This finding suggests that earlier perceptual regions may also demonstrate activation attributable to processes involved in acquisition of new representations of unfamiliar stimuli.

4.5.3 Sensitivity Versus Bias

In number of studies by Schacter and colleagues (Schacter et al., 1990, 1991a; Cooper et al., 1992; Schacter and Cooper, 1993) participants studied line drawings of structurally possible and impossible objects and then made possible/impossible judgments at test to repeated presentations of the objects. Behavioral priming is measured as increased accuracy (and/or faster reaction time) for identifying an object as possible or impossible upon repeated presentations; significant priming is consistently observed for possible, but not impossible, objects. As mentioned earlier, a PET study of priming on the possible/impossible decision task revealed that increased activation in a left inferior/fusiform region was associated with priming of possible objects only (Schacter et al., 1995).

Schacter and Cooper proposed that such priming depends on the structural description system (SDS), a subsystem of the more general perceptual representation system (Tulving and Schacter, 1990). The proposal of an SDS was based on evidence of dissociations between priming (for possible, but not impossible, objects) and explicit tests of memory, across study-to-test object transformations (Cooper, et al., 1992; Schacter et al., 1993b), manipulations at encoding (Schacter and Cooper, 1993; Schacter et al., 1990), and in studies with elderly populations and amnesic patients (Schacter et al., 1991b, 1992, 1993b; and for review, see Soldan et al., 2006). In this view, priming of repeated objects reflects increased sensitivity (i.e., accuracy) on the part of the SDS, which is only capable of representing structurally possible objects.

An alternative theory is the bias account of priming in the possible/impossible object-decision task proposed by Ratcliff and McKoon (McKoon and Ratcliff, 1995, 2001; Ratcliff and McKoon, 1995, 1996, 1997, 2000). In this view, an encounter with an object, regardless of whether it is structurally possible or impossible, results in a subsequent bias to classify that object as 'possible,' leading to increased accuracy (i.e., positive priming) for repeated possible objects but decreased accuracy (i.e., negative priming) for impossible objects. However, this account also posits that explicit processes play a role in object-decisions, such that explicit memory of the study episode cues subjects as to whether the object is possible or impossible. It is argued, then, that this combination of bias and episodic information leads to robust positive priming for possible objects. By contrast, for impossible objects, the two factors cancel each other out, resulting in zero priming. Ratcliff and McKoon (1995) reported data from seven experiments that supported their hypothesis (for criticism of their conclusions, see Schacter and Cooper, 1995; for response, see McKoon and Ratcliff, 1995). Other bias accounts of object-decision priming have been proposed as well, such as the structure-extraction bias (Williams and Tarr, 1997).

Behavioral studies relevant to this debate continue to emerge, supporting either the sensitivity account of priming (e.g., Zeelenberg et al., 2002) or the bias account (e.g., Thapar and Rouder, 2001), but behavioral investigations alone have been inconclusive (Soldan et al., 2006). However, neuroimaging studies have recently produced evidence that speaks to the ongoing debate.

In a recent event-related fMRI study (Habeck et al., 2006), subjects performed a continuous possible/impossible object-decision task on structurally possible and impossible objects repeated four times each. Although the behavioral results did not correspond to sensitivity or bias models, or to previous findings (priming, as measured by faster reactions times, was documented for both possible and impossible objects), neural priming was documented for possible objects only. A multivariate analysis of the fMRI data revealed a pattern of brain regions in which activation covaried in a linear fashion (areas showing both repetition suppression and repetition enhancement) with repetition of possible objects only. No such pattern was observed for repetition of impossible objects. Further, there was a correlation between behavioral (faster reaction times) and neural priming for possible objects only.

Similarly, a recent ERP study by Soldan et al. (2006) reported data from two possible/impossible object-decision priming experiments using unfamiliar objects that provide compelling evidence that the visual system differentially encodes globally possible versus globally impossible structures. In the first experiment, subjects made structural decisions (right/left orientation-decision task) about possible and impossible objects at study. In the second experiment, a functional decision (tool/support function-decision task) was performed at study. The behavioral results of the experiments were inconclusive with respect to sensitivity versus bias theories. However, the ERP data clearly failed to support bias theories, which hold that possible and impossible objects are processed similarly in the visual processing system. Rather, two early ERP components (the N1 and N2 responses) showed repetition enhancement for possible objects, but no neural effect for repetition of impossible objects, in both the structural and functional encoding experiments. Moreover, the magnitude of repetition enhancement in the N1 ERP component was correlated with behavioral priming for possible objects. These data support the theory that priming is supported by an SDS that encodes structurally possible objects only.

4.6 Correlations between Behavioral and Neural Priming

While neuroimaging studies have provided considerable evidence bearing on the neural correlates of priming, caution is warranted when interpreting the causal nature of such effects. Although a number of studies have documented the close overlap between neuronal activity and BOLD activity in the primate (Logothetis et al., 2001; Shmuel et al., 2006; for a human analogue see Mukamel et al., 2005), it is critical to determine whether functional neuroimaging data reflect the neural underpinnings of cognitive processes or index spurious activations that are epiphenomenal to the process of interest.

Initial studies used methodologies where blocks during which participants viewed repeated items were contrasted with blocks during which participants viewed novel items (e.g., Squire et al., 1992; Raichle et al., 1994; Buckner et al., 1995; Schacter et al., 1996; Wagner et al., 1997). The introduction of event-related fMRI (Dale and Buckner, 1997) later allowed researchers to intermix old and new items and delineate activity associated with individual trial-types, providing evidence that the neural priming that accompanies repeated items is not simply due to a blunting of attention or vigilance that may permeate extended periods of cognitive processing (e.g., Buckner et al., 1998). Together, studies of this sort have consistently documented the co-occurrence of behavioral priming and neural priming in a subset of the brain regions that are engaged during task performance with novel material (see **Figure 1**).

In order to establish a link between neural priming and behavioral priming, neuroimaging studies have attempted to demonstrate a relationship between the magnitude of both effects. That is, if neural priming is indeed related to behavioral priming, then the two should not only co-occur but should be directly correlated. A number of studies have reported a positive correlation between the magnitudes of behavioral priming and neural priming in frontal regions during tasks of a semantic or conceptual nature. Maccotta and Buckner (2004) showed that behavioral priming for repeated words in a living/nonliving classification task was significantly correlated with the magnitude of neural priming in regions of the left inferior frontal gyrus and pre-supplementary motor areas. Using the same task, Lustig and Buckner (2004) documented significant correlations between behavioral and neural priming in the left inferior frontal gyrus for young adults, healthy older adults, and patients with Alzheimer's disease (also see Golby et al., 2005). A similar pattern has been documented in the auditory domain: Orfanidou et al. (2006) found that the degree of auditory word priming on a lexical decision task was predicted by the extent of neural priming in left inferior frontal gyrus and supplementary motor areas. Others have found that the correlation between behavioral priming and prefrontal neural priming can be category specific. Using a classification task, Bunzeck et al. (2006) provided evidence that the correlations between neural and behavioral priming were specific for scenes in left inferior prefrontal cortex, but for faces in left middle frontal gyrus.

Consistent with the foregoing findings, in the aforementioned study by Dobbins et al. (2004), multiple regression analysis revealed that left prefrontal activity predicted the disruptive effects of response switching on behavioral priming for individual subjects: greater initial reductions in prefrontal activity were associated with greater subsequent disruptions of behavioral response times when the response was changed. To the extent that activation reductions in prefrontal cortex indicate less reliance on controlled processing and greater reliance on automatic processing, these data suggest that performance disruptions attributable to response switching reflect a need to

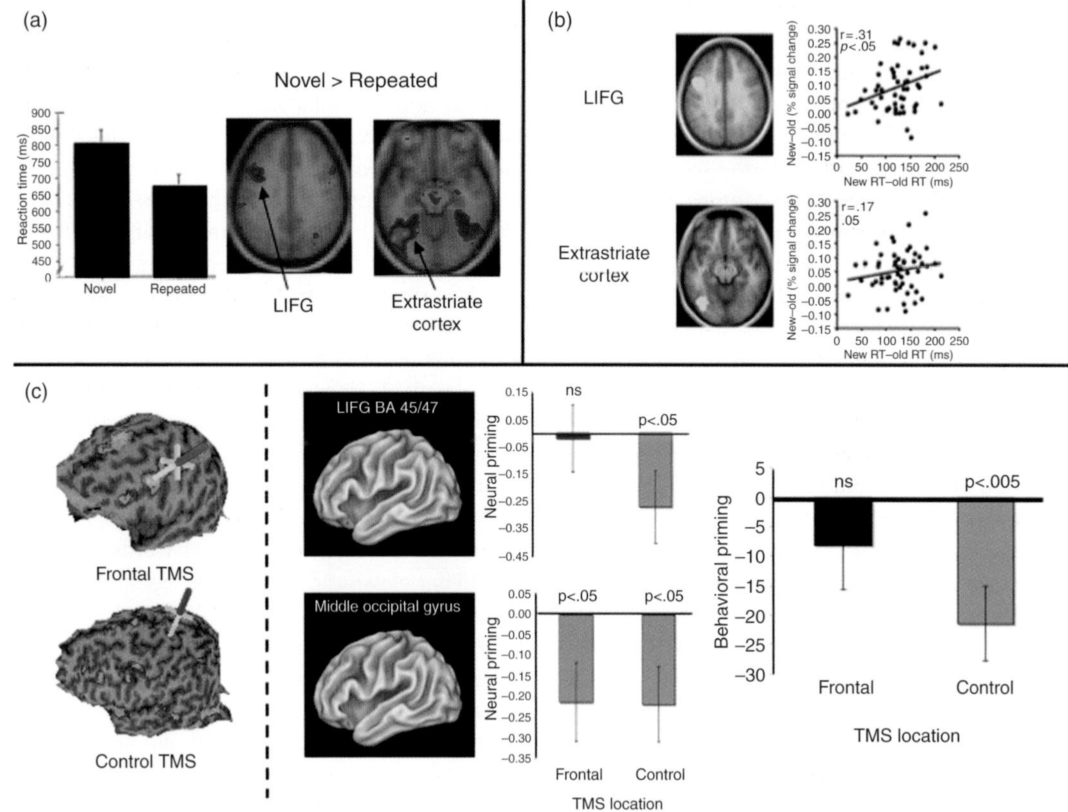

Figure 1 Correlations between behavioral and neural priming. (a) Semantic classification of visual objects using event-related fMRI reveals that the decrease in response time (behavioral priming) that accompanies classification of repeated items co-occurs with decreased activity (neural priming) in regions of the left inferior frontal gyrus (LIFG) and extrastriate cortex. (b) During semantic classification of words, the magnitude of behavioral priming is directly correlated with the magnitude of neural priming in the LIFG, but not the extrastriate cortex. (c) Transcranial magnetic stimulation (TMS) applied to a region of the LIFG (but not of a control location) during semantic classification of visual objects disrupts subsequent behavioral priming and the neural priming in LIFG during fMRI scanning. Neural priming in the middle occipital gyrus is unaffected by frontal or control TMS. Adapted from (a) Buckner RL, Goodman J, Burock M, et al. (1998) Functional-anatomic correlates of object priming in humans revealed by rapid presentation event-related fMRI. *Neuron* 20: 285–296, with permission from Elsevier; (b) Maccotta L and Buckner RL (2004) Evidence for neural effects of repetition that directly correlate with behavioral priming. *J. Cogn. Neurosci.* 16: 1625–1632, with permission from MIT Press; (c) Wig GS, Grafton ST, Demos KE, and Kelley WM (2005) Reductions in neural activity underlie behavioral components of repetition priming. *Nat. Neurosci.* 8: 1228–1233, with permission from the authors.

reengage slower controlled processes in order to make object decisions. This idea is consistent with the further finding that reductions in fusiform activity did not predict behavioral costs of switching cues, suggesting that these reductions may be incidental to behavioral priming during conceptual tasks.

Other evidence indicates that behavioral priming can correlate with neural priming in regions outside the prefrontal cortex as well. Bergerbest et al. (2004) found that behavioral priming for environmental sound stimuli correlated with neural priming in right inferior prefrontal cortex and also in two secondary auditory regions: bilateral superior temporal sulci and right superior temporal gyrus. Using a stem completion task, Carlesimo et al. (2003) found that the magnitude of behavioral cross-modality priming (auditory-to-visual) was correlated with the extent of activation reduction at the junction of the left fusiform and inferior temporal gyrus.

Turk-Browne et al.'s (2006) study of the relation between priming and subsequent memory effects, (where, as discussed earlier, neural activity during encoding is sorted according to whether items are subsequently remembered or forgotten) provided a different perspective on the correlation issue. Repeated scenes produced behavioral and neural priming, but only for those scenes that were subsequently remembered. For these scenes only, there was also a correlation between the magnitude of behavioral and neural priming in the fusiform gyrus; this relationship approached significance in right inferior prefrontal cortex. As discussed earlier, the finding that the degree of behavioral and neural priming depended on subsequent memory points toward a link between implicit and explicit memory, perhaps involving shared attentional processes.

Together, these studies provide evidence for a relationship between behavioral priming and neural priming (also see Zago et al., 2005; Habeck et al., 2006). Correlations between the two variables generalize across paradigms (e.g., semantic classification, stem completion) and are restricted to regions thought to mediate the cognitive operations engaged during the task. Although these correlations have been consistently reported with respect to neural priming in frontal cortices and to a lesser extent temporal cortex, few studies thus far have provided evidence for a correlation between behavioral priming and neural priming in earlier perceptual cortices – even though neural priming in the latter regions frequently accompanies item repetition.

The relationship between behavioral priming and neural priming in early visual regions was explicitly explored by Sayres and Grill-Spector (2006). Participants were scanned using fMRI in an adaptation paradigm during a semantic classification task on objects. Repetition of objects was accompanied by reductions in activity in regions of the LOC and posterior fusiform gyrus. However, in contrast to the correlations that have been observed between neural and behavioral priming in frontal and temporal regions, neural priming in earlier visual regions was unrelated to the facilitation in response time that accompanied repeated classification, thus providing more evidence that these two phenomena may be less tightly associated in these regions.

Although these correlations suggest that neural priming effects in prefrontal and temporal regions may support behavioral priming on a number of tasks, they do not allow conclusions regarding a causal role. It is possible that neural priming in these regions is necessary for behavioral priming. Alternatively, neural priming in other areas of the brain (e.g., regions of perceptual cortex) may subserve behavioral priming, and the neural priming observed in prefrontal and temporal cortex may simply reflect a feedforward propagation of the changes occurring in these other regions. In order to establish a causal relationship between behavioral priming and neural priming in frontal and temporal cortex, one would have to provide evidence of a disruption of behavioral and neural priming in these regions, accompanied by intact neural priming in perceptual cortices.

Wig et al. (2005) provided such evidence by combining fMRI with transcranial magnetic stimulation (TMS). TMS allows for noninvasive disruption of underlying cortical activity to a circumscribed region, thus inducing a reversible temporary virtual lesion (Pascual-Leone et al., 2000). In the study by Wig and colleagues, for each participant, regions of the left prefrontal cortex (along the inferior frontal gyrus) that demonstrated neural priming were first identified during semantic classification (living/nonliving) of repeated objects using fMRI. Each participant was then brought back for a TMS session where they classified a new set of objects using the same task. Short trains of TMS were applied to the previously identified prefrontal region during classification of half of these objects; classification of the remaining half of objects was accompanied by TMS applied to a control region (left motor cortex). Immediately following the TMS session, subjects were rescanned with fMRI while performing the semantic classification task on objects that were previously accompanied by prefrontal stimulation, objects previously accompanied by control-site stimulation, and novel objects. Results revealed that classification of objects that had been previously accompanied by left frontal TMS failed to demonstrate subsequent behavioral priming and neural priming in the left inferior frontal gyrus and lateral temporal cortex. By contrast, neural priming in early visual regions remained intact. Critically, these effects were not due to generalized cortical disruption that accompanied TMS; control-site stimulation had no disruptive effects on either behavioral or neural markers of priming. Consistent with this finding, Thiel et al. (2005) provided evidence for a disruptive effect of left-frontal TMS on behavioral priming during a lexical decision task. Together, these results provide evidence that behavioral and neural markers of priming in frontal and temporal regions are causally related, not just correlated.

In summary, correlations between behavioral and neural priming are observed consistently in prefrontal, and to some extent temporal, regions on priming tasks that include a conceptual component, such as semantic classification and stem completion. Although studies using such tasks have failed to demonstrate a relationship between behavioral priming and neural priming in perceptual regions, behavioral demonstrations of perceptual priming are well documented (e.g., Tulving and Schacter, 1990; Schacter et al., 1993a). A key hypothesis to be evaluated in future investigations is that neural priming in perceptual cortices subserves perceptual priming. Establishing a causal relationship between the two necessitates careful consideration of the behavioral tasks used to demonstrate such effects. Further, it is likely that the behavioral advantage for repeated processing of an item is mediated by multiple processes and components of priming – both conceptual and perceptual – that contribute in an aggregate fashion to facilitate task performance (e.g., Roediger et al., 1999). Neuroimaging research can be helpful in attempting to tease apart the components of such effects and link them with the activity of specific brain regions.

4.7 Summary and Conclusions

Our review demonstrates that neuroimaging research has shed new light on cognitive theories of priming that were originally formulated and investigated through behavioral approaches within the field of cognitive psychology. The contributions of this research include advances with respect to long-standing theoretical debates about the nature of priming, as well as new lines of investigation not previously addressed by cognitive studies.

As alluded to earlier, evidence across several domains of neuroimaging research on priming is inconsistent with a single process account of the phenomenon, and instead supports the idea that multiple processes are involved in different types of behavioral priming and corresponding neural priming. Schacter et al. (2007) recently proposed a multiple-component view of priming, as depicted in **Figure 2**.

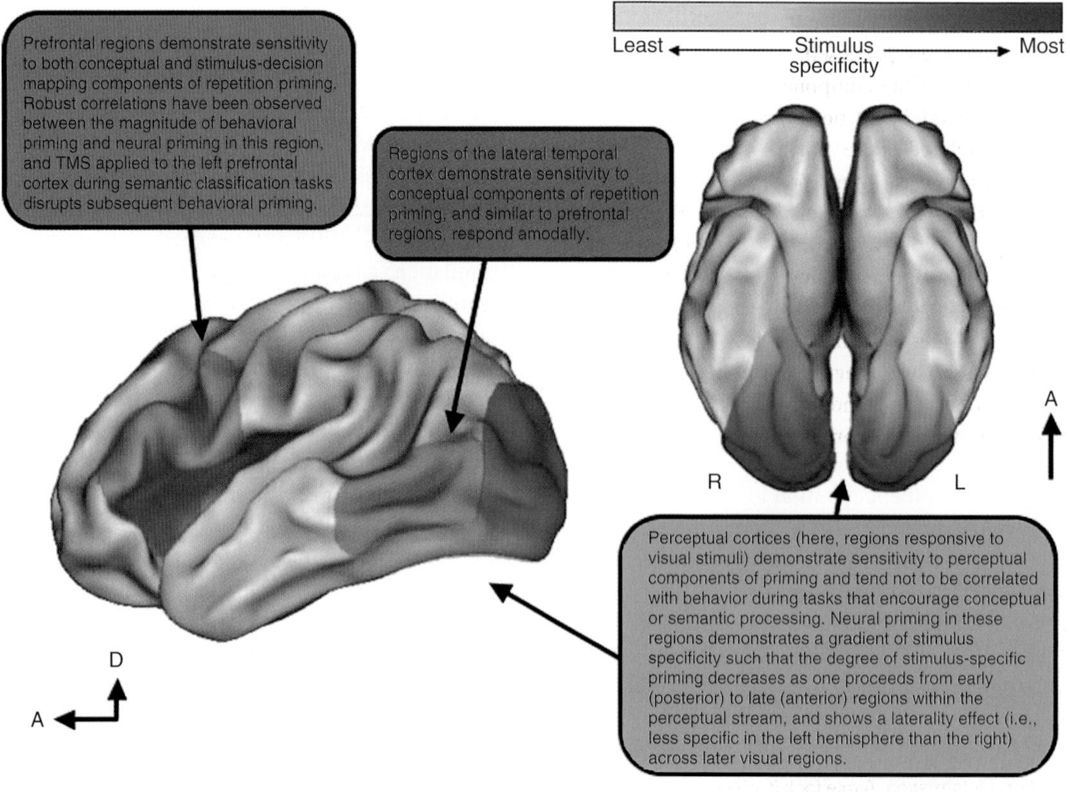

Figure 2 Schematic of proposed components of priming. Figure depicts partially inflated lateral view of the left hemisphere and ventral view of the left and right hemispheres. Lateral view is tilted in the dorsal-ventral plane to expose the ventral surface ('A' denotes anterior direction, 'D' denotes dorsal direction, 'L' and 'R' denote left and right hemispheres, respectively). Color-coding of anatomical regions is meant to serve as a heuristic for the proposed components. The color gradient within the ventral visual stream (blue) is meant to represent approximately the gradient of stimulus specificity that has been observed within these regions. TMS, transcranial magnetic stimulation. Adapted from Schacter DL, Wig GS, and Stevens WD (2007) Reductions in cortical activity during priming. *Curr. Opin. Neurobiol.* 17: 171–176, with permission from Elsevier.

This view suggests that there are at least two distinct mechanisms involved in neural priming. One corresponds roughly to what Wiggs and Martin (1998) called *sharpening* or *tuning*, which occurs when exposure to a stimulus results in a sharper, more precise neural representation of that stimulus (*See* Grill-Spector et al. (2006) for more detailed consideration of sharpening and related ideas). Such tuning effects are likely to predominate in posterior regions that code for the perceptual representations of items, and perhaps in anterior regions that underlie conceptual properties of these items. Tuning effects, however, are unable to account for response-specific priming effects (e.g., Dobbins et al., 2004) and appear to be less correlated with behavioral priming observed during tasks that are semantic or conceptual in nature. The second proposed mechanism primarily reflects changes in prefrontal cortex that drive behavioral priming effects in a top-down manner, as initially controlled processes become more automatic (Logan, 1990; Dobbins et al., 2004).

While the view proposed by Schacter et al. (2007) suggests two possible components of priming, this is a preliminary model that needs to be extended, elaborated, and related more fully to distinctions among types of priming (e.g., perceptual, conceptual, associative) that have been long discussed in the cognitive literature. Traditional theories of priming laid the groundwork for understanding these components, and neuroimaging research will likely play a crucial role in resolving the questions that remain, in suggesting new lines of inquiry not previously conceived of, and in expanding our understanding of the nature of priming and implicit memory more generally.

References

Badgaiyan RD, Schacter DL, and Alpert NM (1999) Auditory priming within and across modalities: Evidence from positron emission tomography. *J. Cogn. Neurosci.* 11: 337–348.

Badgaiyan RD, Schacter DL, and Alpert NM (2001) Priming within and across modalities: Exploring the nature of rCBF increases and decreases. *Neuroimage* 13: 272–282.

Badgaiyan RD, Schacter DL, and Alpert NM (2002) Retrieval of relational information: A role for left inferior prefrontal cortex. *Neuroimage* 17: 393–400.

Bergerbest D, Ghahremani DG, and Gabrieli JD (2004) Neural correlates of auditory repetition priming: Reduced fMRI activation in the auditory cortex. *J. Cogn. Neurosci.* 16: 966–977.

Berntsen D and Hall NM (2004) The episodic nature of involuntary autobiographical memories. *Mem. Cognit.* 32: 789–803.

Blondin F and Lepage M (2005) Decrease and increase in brain activity during visual perceptual priming: An fMRI study on similar but perceptually different complex visual scenes. *Neuropsychologia* 43: 1887–1900.

Bowers BJ (2000) The modality-specific and -nonspecific components of long-term priming are frequency sensitive. *Mem. Cognit.* 28: 406–414.

Bowers JS and Schacter DL (1990) Implicit memory and test awareness. *J. Exp. Psychol. Learn. Mem. Cogn.* 16: 404–416.

Brewer JB, Zhao Z, Glover GH, and Gabrieli JD (1998) Making memories: Brain activity that predicts whether visual experiences will be remembered or forgotten. *Science* 281: 1185–1187.

Bruce V and Valentine T (1985) Identity priming in the recognition of familiar faces. *Br. J. Psychol.* 76: 373–383.

Buckner RL, Goodman J, Burock M, et al. (1998) Functional-anatomic correlates of object priming in humans revealed by rapid presentation event-related fMRI. *Neuron* 20: 285–296.

Buckner RL, Koutstaal W, Schacter DL, and Rosen BR (2000) Functional MRI evidence for a role of frontal and inferior temporal cortex in amodal components of priming. *Brain* 123: 620–640.

Buckner RL, Petersen SE, Ojemann JG, Miezin FM, Squire LR, and Raichle ME (1995) Functional anatomical studies of explicit and implicit memory retrieval tasks. *J. Neurosci.* 15: 12–29.

Bunzeck N, Schutze H, and Duzel E (2006) Category-specific organization of prefrontal response-facilitation during priming. *Neuropsychologia* 44: 1765–1776.

Bunzeck N, Wuestenberg T, Lutz K, Heinze HJ, and Jancke L (2005) Scanning silence: Mental imagery of complex sounds. *Neuroimage* 26: 1119–1127.

Carlesimo GA (1994) Perceptual and conceptual priming in amnesic and alcoholic patients. *Neuropsychologia* 32: 903–921.

Carlesimo GA, Bonanni R, and Caltagirone C (2003) Memory for the perceptual and semantic attributes of information in pure amnesic and severe closed-head injured patients. *J. Clin. Exp. Neuropsychol.* 25: 391–406.

Carlesimo GA, Turriziani P, Paulesu E, et al. (2004) Brain activity during intra- and cross-modal priming: New empirical data and review of the literature. *Neuropsychologia* 42: 14–24.

Clarke R and Morton J (1983) Cross modality facilitation in tachistoscopic word recognition. *Q. J. Exp. Psychol.* 35A: 79–96.

Cooper LA, Schacter DL, Ballesteros S, and Moore C (1992) Priming and recognition of transformed three-dimensional objects: Effects of size and reflection. *J. Exp. Psychol. Learn. Mem. Cogn.* 18: 43–57.

Dale AM and Buckner RL (1997) Selective averaging of rapidly presented individual trials using fMRI. *Hum. Brain Mapp.* 5: 329–340.

Dehaene S, Naccache L, Cohen L, et al. (2001) Cerebral mechanisms of word masking and unconscious repetition priming. *Nat. Neurosc.* 4: 752–758.

Dobbins IG, Schnyer DM, Verfaellie M, and Schacter DL (2004) Cortical activity reductions during repetition priming can result from rapid response learning. *Nature* 428: 316–319.

Duzel E, Richardson-Klavehn A, Neufang M, Schott BH, Scholz M, and Heinze HJ (2005) Early, partly anticipatory, neural oscillations during identification set the stage for priming. *Neuroimage* 25: 690–700.

Eger E, Henson RN, Driver J, and Dolan RJ (2004) Bold repetition decreases in object-responsive ventral visual areas depend on spatial attention. *J. Neurophysiol.* 92: 1241–1247.

Eger E, Schweinberger SR, Dolan RJ, and Henson RN (2005) Familiarity enhances invariance of face representations in human ventral visual cortex: fMRI evidence. *Neuroimage* 26: 1128–1139.

Egner T and Hirsch J (2005) Where memory meets attention: Neural substrates of negative priming. *J. Cogn. Neurosci.* 17: 1774–1784.

Epstein R and Kanwisher N (1998) A cortical representation of the local visual environment. *Nature* 392: 598–601.

Fiebach CJ, Gruber T, and Supp GG (2005) Neuronal mechanisms of repetition priming in occipitotemporal cortex: Spatiotemporal evidence from functional magnetic resonance imaging and electroencephalography. *J. Neurosci.* 25: 3414–3422.

Fox E (1995) Negative priming from ignored distractors in visual selection: A review. *Psychon. Bull. Rev.* 2: 145–173.

Golby A, Silverberg G, Race E, et al. (2005) Memory encoding in Alzheimer's disease: An fMRI study of explicit and implicit memory. *Brain* 128: 773–787.

Graf P and Mandler G (1984) Activation makes words more accessible, but not necessarily more retrievable. *J. Verbal Learn. Verbal Behav.* 23: 553–568.

Graf P and Ryan L (1990) Transfer-appropriate processing for implicit and explicit memory. *J. Exp. Psychol. Learn. Mem. Cogn.* 16: 978–992.

Graf P and Schacter DL (1985) Implicit and explicit memory for new associations in normal subjects and amnesic patients. *J. Exp. Psychol. Learn. Mem. Cogn.* 11: 501–518.

Graf P, Shimamura AP, and Squire LR (1985) Priming across modalities and priming across category levels: Extending the domain of preserved functioning in amnesia. *J. Exp. Psychol. Learn. Mem. Cogn.* 11: 385–395.

Grill-Spector K, Henson R, and Martin A (2006) Repetition and the brain: Neural models of stimulus-specific effects. *Trends Cogn. Sci.* 10: 14–23.

Grill-Spector K, Kushnir T, Edelman S, Avidan G, Itzchak Y, and Malach R (1999) Differential processing of objects under various viewing conditions in the human lateral occipital complex. *Neuron* 24: 187–203.

Gruber T, Giabbiconi CM, Trujillo-Barreto NJ, and Muller MM (2006) Repetition suppression of induced gamma band responses is eliminated by task switching. *Eur. J. Neurosci.* 24: 2654–2660.

Habeck C, Hilton HJ, Zarahn E, Brown T, and Stern Y (2006) An event-related fMRI study of the neural networks underlying repetition suppression and reaction time priming in implicit visual memory. *Brain Res.* 1075: 133–141.

Hasson U, Nusbaum HC, and Small SL (2006) Repetition suppression for spoken sentences and the effect of task demands. *J. Cogn. Neurosci.* 18: 2013–2029.

Henson RN (2003) Neuroimaging studies of priming. *Prog. Neurobiol.* 70: 53–81.

Henson RN, Shallice T, and Dolan R (2000) Neuroimaging evidence for dissociable forms of repetition priming. *Science* 287: 1269–1272.

Henson RN, Shallice T, Gorno-Tempini ML, and Dolan RJ (2002) Face repetition effects in implicit and explicit memory tests as measured by fMRI. *Cereb. Cortex* 12: 178–186.

Houghton G and Tipper SP (1994) A model of inhibitory mechanisms in selective attention. In: Dagenbach D and Carr T (eds.) *Inhibitory Mechanisms in Attention, Memory, and Language*, pp. 53–112. San Diego, CA: Academic Press.

Ishai A, Pessoa L, Bikle PC, and Ungerleider LG (2004) Repetition suppression of faces is modulated by emotion. *Proc. Natl. Acad. Sci. USA* 101: 9827–9832.

Jacoby LL (1983) Perceptual enhancement: Persistent effects of an experience. *J. Exp. Psychol. Learn. Mem. Cogn.* 9: 21–38.

Jacoby LL (1991) A process dissociation framework: Separating automatic from intentional uses of memory. *J. Mem. Lang.* 30: 513–541.

Jacoby LL and Dallas M (1981) On the relationship between autobiographical memory and perceptual learning. *J. Exp. Psychol. Gen.* 110: 306–340.

Koutstaal W, Verfaellie M, and Schacter DL (2001) Recognizing identical vs. similar categorically related common objects: Further evidence for degraded gist representations in amnesia. *Neuropsychology* 15: 268–289.

Logan GD (1990) Repetition priming and automaticity: Common underlying mechanisms? *Cognit. Psychol.* 22: 1–35.

Logothetis NK, Pauls J, Augath M, Trinath T, and Oeltermann A (2001) Neurophysiological investigation of the basis of the fMRI signal. *Nature* 412: 150–157.

Lustig C and Buckner RL (2004) Preserved neural correlates of priming in old age and dementia. *Neuron* 42: 865–875.

Maccotta L and Buckner RL (2004) Evidence for neural effects of repetition that directly correlate with behavioral priming. *J. Cogn. Neurosci.* 16: 1625–1632.

Marsolek CJ, Kosslyn SM, and Squire LR (1992) Form specific visual priming in the right cerebral hemisphere. *J. Exp. Psychol. Learn. Mem. Cogn.* 18: 492–508.

Marsolek CJ, Schacter DL, and Nicholas CD (1996) Form-specific visual priming for new associations in the right cerebral hemisphere. *Mem. Cognit.* 24: 539–556.

Martin E (1968) Stimulus meaningfulness and paired-associate transfer: An encoding variability hypothesis. *Psychol. Rev.* 75: 421–441.

May CP, Kane MJ, and Hasher L (1995) Determinants of negative priming. *Psychol. Bull.* 118: 35–54.

McClelland JL and Rogers TT (2003) The parallel distributed processing approach to semantic cognition. *Nat. Rev. Neurosci.* 4: 310–322.

McKoon G and Ratcliff R (1995) How should implicit memory phenomena be modeled? *J. Exp. Psychol. Learn. Mem. Cogn.* 21: 777–784.

McKoon G and Ratcliff R (2001) Counter model for word identification: Reply to Bowers (1999). *Psychol. Rev.* 108: 674–681.

Miller EK and Desimone R (1993) Scopolamine affects short-term memory but not inferior temporal neurons. *Neuroreport* 4: 81–84.

Miller EK, Gochin PM, and Gross CG (1991) Habituation-like decrease in the responses of neurons in inferior temporal cortex of the macaque. *Vis. Neurosci.* 7: 357–362.

Morton J (1969) Interaction of information in word recognition. *Psychol. Rev.* 76: 165–178.

Mukamel R, Gelbard H, Arieli A, Hasson U, Fried I, and Malach R (2005) Coupling between neuronal firing, field potentials, and fMRI in human auditory cortex. *Science* 309: 951–954.

Mulligan NW and Hartman M (1996) Divided attention and indirect memory tests. *Mem. Cognit.* 24: 453–465.

Mulligan NW and Hornstein SL (2000) Attention and perceptual priming in the perceptual identification task. *J. Exp. Psychol. Learn. Mem. Cogn.* 26: 626–637.

Murray SO and Wojciulik E (2004) Attention increases neural selectivity in the human lateral occipital complex. *Nat. Neurosci.* 7: 70–74.

Neill WT and Valdes LA (1992) Persistence of negative priming: Steady state of decay? *J. Exp. Psychol. Learn. Mem. Cogn.* 18: 565–576.

Neill WT, Valdes LA, Terry KM, and Gorfein DS (1992) Persistence of negative priming: II. Evidence for episodic trace retrieval. *J. Exp. Psychol. Learn. Mem. Cogn.* 18: 993–1000.

O'Kane G, Insler RZ, and Wagner AD (2005) Conceptual and perceptual novelty effects in human medial temporal cortex. *Hippocampus* 15: 326–332.

Orfanidou E, Marslen-Wilson WD, and Davis MH (2006) Neural response suppression predicts repetition priming of spoken words and pseudowords. *J. Cogn. Neurosci.* 18: 1237–1252.

Pascual-Leone A, Walsh V, and Rothwell J (2000) Transcranial magnetic stimulation in cognitive neuroscience – virtual lesion, chronometry, and functional connectivity. *Curr. Opin. Neurobiol.* 10: 232–237.

Raichle ME, Fiez JA, Videen TO, et al. (1994) Practice-related changes in human brain functional anatomy during nonmotor learning. *Cereb. Cortex* 4: 8–26.

Ratcliff R and McKoon G (1995) Bias in the priming of object decisions. *J. Exp. Psychol. Learn. Mem. Cogn.* 21: 754–767.

Ratcliff R and McKoon G (1996) Bias effects in implicit memory tasks. *J. Exp. Psychol. Gen.* 125: 403–421.

Ratcliff R and McKoon G (1997) A counter model for implicit priming in perceptual word identification. *Psychol. Rev.* 104: 319–343.

Ratcliff R and McKoon G (2000) Modeling the effects of repetition and word frequency in perceptual identification. *Psychon. Bull. Rev.* 7: 713–717.

Richardson-Klavehn A and Gardiner JM (1996) Cross-modality priming in stem completion reflects conscious memory, but not voluntary memory. *Psychon. Bull. Rev.* 3: 238–244.

Richardson-Klavehn A and Gardiner JM (1998) Depth-of-processing effects on priming in stem completion: Tests of the voluntary-contamination, conceptual-processing, and lexical-processing hypotheses. *J. Exp. Psychol. Learn. Mem. Cogn.* 24: 593–609.

Richardson-Klavehn A, Gardiner JM, and Java RI (1994) Involuntary conscious memory and the method of opposition. *Memory* 2: 1–29.

Roediger HL III (1990) Implicit memory: A commentary. *Bull. Psychon. Soc.* 28: 373–380.

Roediger HL III and Blaxton TA (1987) Effects of varying modality, surface features, and retention interval on priming in word fragment completion. *Mem. Cognit.* 15: 379–388.

Roediger HL, Buckner RL III, and McDermott KB (1999) Components of processing. In: Foster JK and Jelicic M (eds.) *Memory: Systems, Process, or Function?* pp. 31–65. Oxford: Oxford University Press.

Roediger HL III and McDermott KB (1993) Implicit memory in normal human subjects. In: Spinnler H and Boller F (eds.) *Handbook of Neuropsychology*, pp. 63–131. Amsterdam: Elsevier.

Roediger HL III, Weldon MS, and Challis BH (1989) Explaining dissociations between implicit and explicit measures of retention: A processing account. In: Roediger HLI and Craik FIM (eds.) *Varieties of Memory and Consciousness: Essays in Honor of Endel Tulving*, pp. 3–41. Hillsdale, NJ: Erlbaum.

Rugg MD, Fletcher PC, Frith CD, Frackowiak RSJ, and Dolan RJ (1997) Brain regions supporting intentional and incidental memory: A PET study. *Neuroreport* 8: 1283–1287.

Ryan L and Schnyer D (2006) Regional specificity of format-specific priming effects in mirror word reading using functional magnetic resonance imaging. *Cereb. Cortex* 17: 982–992.

Sayres R and Grill-Spector K (2006) Object-selective cortex exhibits performance-independent repetition suppression. *J. Neurophysiol.* 95: 995–1007.

Schacter DL (1987) Implicit memory: History and current status. *J. Exp. Psychol. Learn. Mem. Cogn.* 13: 501–518.

Schacter DL (1990) Perceptual representation systems and implicit memory: Toward a resolution of the multiple memory systems debate. *Ann. N.Y. Acad. Sci.* 608: 543–571.

Schacter DL (1994) Priming and multiple memory systems: Perceptual mechanisms of implict memory. In: Schacter DL and Tulving E (eds.) *Memory Systems*, pp. 233–268. Cambridge: MIT Press.

Schacter DL, Badgaiyan RD, and Alpert NM (1999) Visual word stem completion priming within and across modalities: A PET study. *Neuroreport* 10: 2061–2065.

Schacter DL, Bowers J, and Booker J (1989) Intention, awareness, and implicit memory: The retrieval intentionality criterion. In: Lewandowsky S, Dunn JC, and Kirsner K (eds.) *Implicit Memory: Theoretical Issues*, pp. 47–69. Hillsdale, NJ: Erlbaum.

Schacter DL and Buckner RL (1998) Priming and the brain. *Neuron* 20: 185–95.

Schacter DL, Chiu CYP, and Ochsner KN (1993a) Implicit memory: A selective review. *Annu. Rev. Neurosci.* 16: 159–182.

Schacter DL and Church B (1992) Auditory priming: Implicit and explicit memory for words and voices. *J. Exp. Psychol. Learn. Mem. Cogn.* 18: 915–930.

Schacter DL and Cooper LA (1993) Implicit and explicit memory for novel visual objects: Structure and function. *J. Exp. Psychol. Learn. Mem. Cogn.* 19: 995–1009.

Schacter DL and Cooper LA (1995) Bias in the priming of object decisions: Logic, assumption, and data. *J. Exp. Psychol. Learn. Mem. Cogn.* 21: 768–776.

Schacter DL, Cooper LA, and Delaney SM (1990) Implicit memory for unfamiliar objects depends on access to structural descriptions. *J. Exp. Psychol. Gen.* 119: 5–31.

Schacter DL, Cooper LA, Delaney SM, Peterson MA, and Tharan M (1991a) Implicit memory for possible and impossible objects: Constraints on the construction of structural descriptions. *J. Exp. Psychol. Learn. Mem. Cogn.* 17: 3–19.

Schacter DL, Cooper LA, Tharan M, and Rubens AB (1991b) Preserved priming of novel objects in patients with memory disorders. *J. Cogn. Neurosci.* 3: 117–130.

Schacter DL, Cooper LA, and Treadwell J (1993b) Preserved priming of novel objects across size transformation in amnesic patients. *Psych. Sci.* 4: 331–335.

Schacter DL, Cooper LA, and Valdiserri M (1992) Implicit and explicit memory for novel visual objects in older and younger adults. *Psychol. Aging* 7: 299–308.

Schacter DL, Dobbins IG, and Schnyer DM (2004) Specificity of priming: A cognitive neuroscience perspective. *Nat. Rev. Neurosci.* 5: 853–862.

Schacter DL and Graf P (1986) Preserved learning in amnesic patients: Perspectives on research from direct priming. *J. Clin. Exp. Neuropsychol.* 8: 727–743.

Schacter DL, Reiman E, Uecker A, Polster MR, Yun LS, and Cooper LA (1995) Brain regions associated with retrieval of structurally coherent visual information. *Nature* 376: 587–590.

Schacter DL, Savage CR, Alpert NM, Rauch SL, and Albert MS (1996) The role of hippocampus and frontal cortex in age-related memory changes: A PET study. *Neuroreport* 7: 1165–1169.

Schacter DL, Wig GS, and Stevens WD (2007) Reductions in cortical activity during priming. *Curr. Opin. Neurobiol.* 17: 171–176.

Schnyer DM, Dobbins IG, Nicholls L, Davis S, Verfaellie M, and Schacter DL (in press) Item to decision mapping in rapid response learning. *Mem Cognit.*

Schnyer DM, Dobbins IG, Nicholls L, Schacter DL, and Verfaellie M (2006) Rapid response learning in amnesia: Delineating associative learning components in repetition priming. *Neuropsychologia* 44: 140–149.

Schott BJ, Henson RN, Richardson-Klavehn A, et al. (2005) Redefining implicit and explicit memory: The functional neuroanatomy of priming, remembering, and control of retrieval. *Proc. Natl. Acad. Sci. USA* 102: 1257–1262.

Schott BJ, Richardson-Klavehn A, Henson RN, Becker C, Heinze HJ, and Duzel E (2006) Neuroanatomical dissociation of encoding processes related to priming and explicit memory. *J. Neurosci.* 26: 792–800.

Shmuel A, Augath M, Oeltermann A, and Logothetis NK (2006) Negative functional MRI response correlates with decreases in neuronal activity in monkey visual area V1. *Nat. Neurosci.* 9: 569–577.

Simons JS, Koutstaal W, Prince S, Wagner AD, and Schacter DL (2003) Neural mechanisms of visual object priming: Evidence for perceptual and semantic distinctions in fusiform cortex. *Neuroimage* 19: 613–626.

Slotnick SD and Schacter DL (2004) A sensory signature that distinguishes true from false memories. *Nat. Neurosci.* 7: 664–672.

Squire LR, Ojemann JG, Miezin FM, Petersen SE, Videen TO, and Raichle ME (1992) Activation of the hippocampus in normal humans: A functional anatomical study of memory. *Proc. Natl. Acad. Sci. USA* 89: 1837–1841.

Soldan A, Mangels JA, and Cooper LA (2006) Evaluating models of object-decision priming: Evidence from event-related potential repetition effects. *J. Exp. Psychol. Learn. Mem. Cogn.* 32: 230–248.

Stevens WD and Grady CL (2007) Insight into frontal lobe function from functional neuroimaging studies of episodic memory. In: Miller BL and Cummings JL (eds.) *The Human Frontal Lobes: Functions and Disorders,* 2nd edn., pp. 207–226. New York: Guildford.

Tenpenny PL (1995) Abstractionist versus episodic theories of repetition priming and word identification. *Psychon. Bull. Rev.* 2: 339–363.

Thapar A and Rouder JN (2001) Bias in conceptual priming. *Psychon. Bull. Rev.* 8: 791–797.

Thiel A, Haupt WF, Habedank B, et al. (2005) Neuroimaging-guided rTMS of the left inferior frontal gyrus interferes with repetition priming. *Neuroimage* 25: 815–823.

Tipper SP (1985) The negative priming effect: Inhibitory priming by ignored objects. *Q. J. Exp. Psychol. A* 37: 571–590.

Tulving E and Schacter DL (1990) Priming and human memory systems. *Science* 247: 301–306.

Turk-Browne NB, Yi DJ, and Chun MM (2006) Linking implicit and explicit memory: Common encoding factors and shared representations. *Neuron* 49: 917–927.

Vogels R, Sary G, and Orban GA (1995) How task-related are the responses of inferior temporal neurons? *Vis. Neurosci.* 12: 207–214.

Voss JL and Paller KA (2006) Fluent conceptual processing and explicit memory for faces are electrophysiologically distinct. *J. Neurosci.* 26: 926–933.

Vuilleumier P, Henson RN, Driver J, and Dolan RJ (2002) Multiple levels of visual object constancy revealed by event-related fMRI of repetition priming. *Nat. Neurosci.* 5: 491–499.

Vuilleumier P, Schwartz S, Duhoux S, Dolan RJ, and Driver J (2005) Selective attention modulates neural substrates of repetition priming and "implicit" visual memory: Suppressions and enhancements revealed by fMRI. *J. Cogn. Neurosci.* 17: 1245–1260.

Wagner AD, Desmond JE, Demb JB, Glover GH, and Gabrieli JDE (1997) Semantic repetition priming for verbal and pictorial knowledge: A functional MRI study of left inferior prefrontal cortex. *J. Cogn. Neurosci.* 9: 714–726.

Wagner AD, Maril A, and Schacter DL (2000) Interactions between forms of memory: When priming hinders new learning. *J. Cogn. Neurosci.* 12: 52–60.

Wagner AD, Schacter DL, Rotte M, et al. (1998) Building memories: Remembering and forgetting of verbal experiences as predicted by brain activity. *Science* 281: 1188–1191.

Wheatley T, Weisberg J, Beauchamp MS, and Martin A (2005) Automatic priming of semantically related words reduces activity in the fusiform gyrus. *J. Cogn. Neurosci.* 17: 1871–1885.

Williams P and Tarr MJ (1997) Structural processing and implicit memory for possible and impossible figures. *J. Exp. Psychol. Learn. Mem. Cogn.* 23: 1344–1361.

Wig GS, Grafton ST, Demos KE, and Kelley WM (2005) Reductions in neural activity underlie behavioral components of repetition priming. *Nat. Neurosci.* 8: 1228–1233.

Wiggs CL and Martin A (1998) Properties and mechanisms of perceptual priming. *Curr. Opin. Neurobiol.* 8: 227–233.

Yi DJ and Chun MM (2005) Attentional modulation of learning-related repetition attenuation effects in human parahippocampal cortex. *J. Neurosci.* 25: 3593–3600.

Yi DJ, Kelley TA, Marois R, and Chun MM (2006) Attentional modulation of repetition attenuation is anatomically dissociable for scenes and faces. *Brain Res.* 1080: 53–62.

Zago L, Fenske MJ, Aminoff E, and Bar M (2005) The rise and fall of priming: How visual exposure shapes cortical representations of objects. *Cereb. Cortex* 15: 1655–1665.

Zeelenberg R, Wagenmakers EJ, and Raaijmakers JG (2002) Priming in implicit memory tasks: Prior study causes enhanced discriminability, not only bias. *J. Exp. Psychol. Gen.* 131: 38–47.

Zubicaray G, McMahon K, Eastburn M, Pringle A, and Lorenz L (2006) Classic identity negative priming involves accessing semantic representations in the left anterior temporal cortex. *Neuroimage* 33: 383–390.

5 Semantic Memory

D. A. Balota and J. H. Coane, Washington University, St. Louis, MO, USA

Semantic memory entails the enormous storehouse of knowledge that all humans have available. To begin with, simply consider the information stored about the words of one's native language. Each of us has approximately 50 000 words stored in our mental dictionary. With each entry, we also have many different dimensions available. For example, with the word 'dog' we have stored information about how to spell it, how to pronounce it, its grammatical category, and the fact that the object the word refers to typically has four legs, is furry, is a common pet, and likes to chase cats (sometimes cars, squirrels, and other rodents), along with additional sensory information about how it feels when petted, the sound produced when it barks, the visual appearance of different types of dogs, emotional responses from past experiences, and much, much more. Of course, our knowledge about words is only the tip of the iceberg of the knowledge we have available. For example, people (both private and public) are a particularly rich source of knowledge. Consider how easy it is to quickly and efficiently retrieve detailed characteristics about John F. Kennedy, Marilyn Monroe, Bill Clinton, a sibling, parent, child, and so on. Indeed, our semantic, encyclopedic knowledge about the world appears limitless.

One concern reflected by the examples above is that semantic memory seems to be all inclusive. In this light, it is useful to contrast it with other forms of memory, and this is precisely what Tulving (1972) did in his classic paper distinguishing semantic and episodic memory. According to Tulving, semantic memory "is a mental thesaurus, organized knowledge a person possesses about words and other verbal symbols, their meaning and referents, about relations among them, and about rules, formulas, and algorithms for the manipulation of these symbols, concepts and relations" (1972, p. 386). In contrast, episodic memory refers to a person's memory for specific events that were personally experienced and remembered. So, the memory for the experience of having breakfast yesterday (e.g., where one was seated, how one felt, the taste of the food, who one was with) would fall under the umbrella of episodic memory, but the fact that eggs, cereal, and toast are typical breakfast foods reflects semantic knowledge. However, as we shall see, there is some controversy regarding where episodic memory ends and semantic memory begins. Indeed, we would argue that semantic memory penetrates all forms of memory, even sensory and working memory (Sperling, 1960; Tulving and Pearlstone, 1966; Baddeley, 2000), because tasks that are assumed to tap into these other types of memory often are influenced by semantic memory.

So, what is indeed unique about semantic memory, and how has this area of research contributed to our understanding of learning and memory in general? One issue that researchers in this area have seriously tackled is the nature of representation, which touches on issues that have long plagued the philosophy of knowledge or epistemology. Specifically, what does it mean to know something? What does it mean to represent the meaning of a word, such as DOG? Is it simply some central tendency of past experiences with DOGS that one has been exposed to (i.e., a prototype DOG), or is there a limited list of primitive semantic features that humans use to capture the meaning of DOG, along with many other concepts and objects? Is the knowledge stored in an abstracted, amodal form that is accessible via different routes or systems, or is all knowledge grounded in specific modalities? For example, the meaning of DOG might be represented by traces laid down by the perceptual motor systems that were engaged when we have interacted with DOGs in the past.

In this chapter, we attempt to provide an overview of the major areas of research addressing the nature of semantic memory, emphasizing the major themes that have historically been at the center of research. Clearly, given the space limitations, the goal here is to introduce the reader to these issues and provide references to more detailed reviews. The vast majority of this work emphasizes behavioral approaches to the study of semantics, but we also touch upon contributions from neuropsychology, neuroimaging, and computational linguistics that have been quite informative recently. We focus on the following major historical developments: (1) the nature of the representation, (2) conceptual development and learning, (3) insights from and limitations of semantic priming studies, (4) interplay between semantic and episodic memory tasks, and (5) cognitive neuroscience constraints afforded by comparisons of different patient populations and recent evidence from neuroimaging studies.

5.1 Nature of the Representation

Although the question of how one represents knowledge has been around since the time of Aristotle, it is clear that cognitive scientists are still actively pursuing this issue. One approach to representation is that we abstract from experience a prototypical meaning of a concept, and these ideal representations are interconnected to other related representations within a rich network of semantic knowledge. This is the network approach. Another approach is that there is a set of primitive features that we use to define the meaning of words. The meanings of different words and concepts reflect different combinations of these primitive features. This is a feature-based approach. Historically, the distinction between these two approaches has been central to research addressing the nature of semantic memory.

5.2 Network Approaches

One of the first landmark studies of knowledge representation came from computer science and was based on the important dissertation of A. M. Quillian. Quillian (1968) developed a model of knowledge representation called the Teachable Language Comprehender. A goal of this model was to formulate a working program that allowed efficient access to an enormous amount of information while minimizing redundancy of information in the network. Quillian adopted a hierarchically organized network, a portion of which is displayed in **Figure 1**. As shown, there are two important aspects to the network: nodes and pathways. The nodes in this network are intended to directly represent a concept in semantic memory, so for example, the word BIRD has a node that represents BIRDNESS. These nodes are interconnected in this network via labeled pathways, which are either 'isa' directional pathways or property pathways. Specifically, one can verify that BIRDS are indeed ANIMALS by finding an isa pathway between BIRDS and ANIMALS. Likewise, one could verify that 'A ROBIN BREATHES' by finding the isa pathway between robin and bird, and between bird and animal, and then accessing the property pathway leading to BREATHES from ANIMALS. In this sense, the model was quite economical, because most properties were stored only at the highest level in the network in which most of the lower exemplars included that property. For example, BREATHES would only be stored at the ANIMAL level, and not at the BIRD or CANARY level, thereby minimizing redundancy (and memory storage) in the network. Quillian also recognized that some features may not apply to all exemplars below that level in the network (e.g., ostriches are birds, and birds fly), so in these cases, one needed to include a

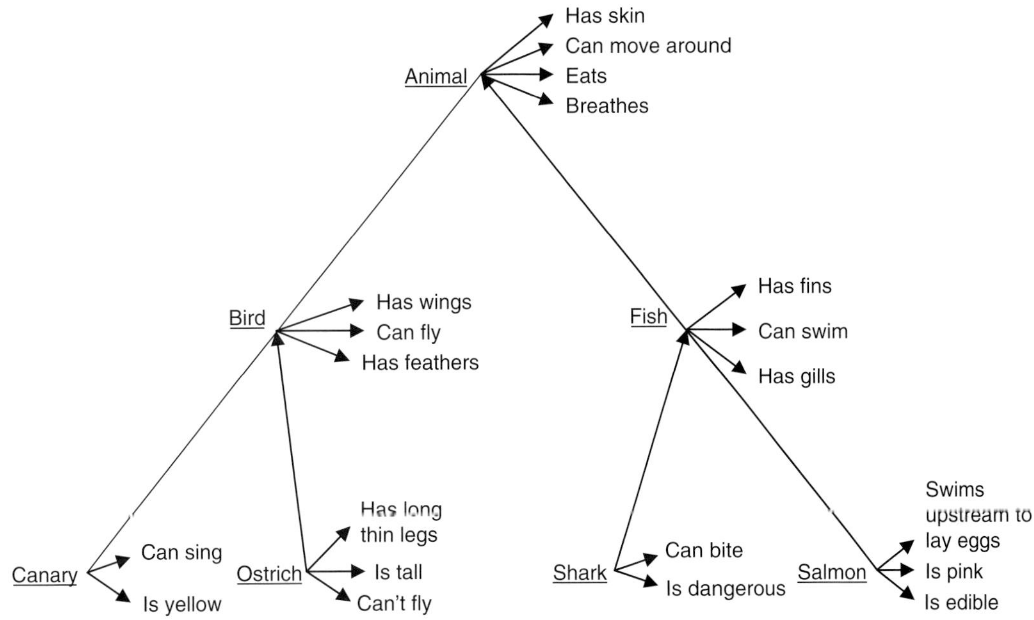

Figure 1 Hierarchically arranged network. Taken from Collins A and Quillian MR (1969) Retrieval time from semantic memory. *J. Verb. Learn. Verb. Behav.* 8: 240–247.

special property for these concepts (such as CAN'T FLY attached to OSTRICHES).

The economy of the network displayed in **Figure 1** does not come without some cost. Specifically, why would one search so deeply in a network to verify a property of a given concept, that is, why would one have to go all the way to the ANIMAL concept to verify that 'CANARIES BREATHE'? It seems more plausible that we would have the property BREATHES directly stored with the CANARY node. Of course, Quillian was not initially interested in how well his network might capture performance in humans, because his goal was to develop a computer model that would be able to verify a multitude of questions about natural categories, within the constraints of precious computer memory available at the time.

Fortunately for cognitive psychologists, Quillian began a collaborative effort with A. Collins to test whether the network model developed by Quillian could indeed predict human performance on a sentence verification task, that is, the speed to verify such sentences as 'A CANARY IS A BIRD'. Remarkably, the Collins and Quillian (1969) study provided evidence that appeared to be highly supportive of the hierarchically organized network structure that Quillian independently developed in artificial intelligence. Specifically, human performance was nicely predicted by how many 'isa' and 'property' pathways one needed to traverse to verify a sentence. The notion is that there was a spreading activation retrieval mechanism that spread across links within the network, and the more links traversed the slower the retrieval time. So, the original evidence appeared to support the counterintuitive prediction that subjects indeed needed to go through the 'CANARY IS A BIRD' link and then the 'BIRD IS AN ANIMAL' link to verify that 'CANARIES BREATHE', because this is where BREATHES is located in the network.

The power of network theory to economically represent the relations among a large amount of information and the confirmation of the counterintuitive predictions via the sentence verification studies by Collins and Quillian (1969) clearly encouraged researchers to investigate the potential of these networks. However, it soon became clear that the initial hierarchically arranged network structure had some limitations. For example, the model encountered some difficulties handling the systematic differences in false reaction times, that is, the finding that correct 'false' responses to 'BUTTERFLIES ARE BIRDS' are slower than responses to 'SPIDERS ARE BIRDS.' Importantly, there was also clear evidence of typicality effects within categories. Specifically, categories have graded structure, that is, some examples of BIRD, such as ROBINS, appear to be better examples than other BIRDS, such as OSTRICHES.

There were numerous attempts to preserve the basic network structure of Collins and Quillian (1969), and indeed, some general models of cognitive performance still include aspects of such network structure. Collins and Loftus (1975) took a major step forward when they developed a network that was not forced into a hierarchical framework. This is displayed in **Figure 2**. As shown, these networks are basically unstructured, with pathways between concepts that are related and the strength of the relationship being reflected by the length of the pathways. Collins and Loftus further proposed that the links between nodes could be dependent on semantic similarity (e.g., items from the same category, such as DOG and CAT, would be linked), or the links could emerge from lexical level factors, such as cooccurrence in the language. Thus, DOG and CAT would be linked because these two items often occur in similar contexts. Because the strength of spreading activation is a function of the distance the activation traversed, typicality effects can be nicely captured in this framework by the length of the pathways. Of course, one might be concerned that such networks are not sufficiently constrained by independent evidence (i.e., if one is slow the pathway must be long). Nevertheless, such networks have been implemented to capture knowledge representation in both semantic and episodic domains (see Anderson, 2000).

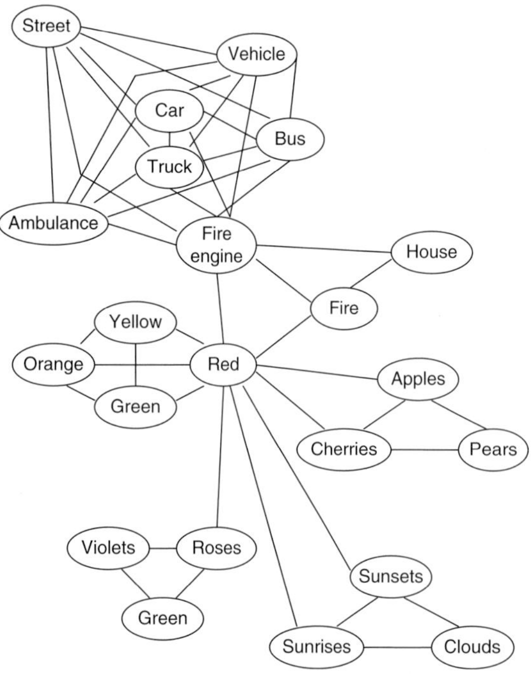

Figure 2 Semantic network. From Collins AM and Loftus EF (1975) A spreading-activation theory of semantic processing. *Psychol. Rev.* 82: 407–428.

More recently, there has been a resurgent interest in a type of network theory. Interestingly, these developments are again driven from fields outside of psychology such as physics (see Albert and Barabasi, 2002) and biology (Jeong et al., 2000). This approach is very principled in nature in that it uses large existing databases to establish the connections across nodes within a network and then uses graph analytic approaches to provide quantitative estimates that capture the nature of the networks. In this light, researchers are not arbitrarily constructing the networks but are allowing the known relations among items within the network to specify the structure of the network. This approach has been used to quantify such diverse networks as the power grid of the Western United States and the neural network of the worm, *C. elegans* (Watts and Strogatz, 1998). Once one has the network established for a given domain (i.e., providing connections between nodes), one can then quantify various characteristics of the network, such as the number of nodes, the number of pathways, the average number of pathways from a node, and the average distance between two nodes. Moreover, there are more sophisticated measures available such as the clustering coefficient, which reflects the probability that two neighbors of a randomly selected node will be neighbors of each other. In this sense, these parameters quantify the characteristics of the targeted network. For example, when looking at such parameters, Watts and Strogatz (1998) found that naturally occurring networks have a substantially higher clustering coefficient and relatively short average distances between nodes compared with randomly generated networks that have the same number of nodes and average connectivity between nodes. This general characteristic of networks is called 'small world' structure. These high clustering coefficients may reflect 'hubs' of connectivity and allow one to access vast amounts of information by retrieving information along the hubs. In popular parlance, such hubs may allow one to capture the six degrees of separation between any two individuals that Milgram (1967) proposed and that has been popularized by the game "six degrees of separation with Kevin Bacon."

What do worms, power grids, and parlor games have to do with semantic memory? Steyvers and Tenenbaum (2005) used three large databases reflecting the meaning of words to construct networks of semantic memory. These included free-association norms (Nelson et al., 1998), WordNet (Miller, 1990), and Roget's Thesaurus (1911). For example, if subjects are likely to produce a word in response to another word in the Nelson et al. free-association norms, then a connection between the two nodes was established in the network. Interestingly, Steyvers and Tenenbaum found that these semantic networks exhibited the same small world structure as other naturally occurring networks; specifically, high-clustering coefficients and a relatively small average path distance between two nodes. As shown in **Figure 3**, if one moves along the hub of highly interconnected nodes, an enormous amount of information becomes readily available via traversing a small number of links.

Of course, it is not a coincidence that naturally occurring networks have small world structure. The seductive conclusion here is that knowledge representation has some systematic similarities across domains. Indeed, Steyvers and Tenenbaum (2005) and others have suggested that such structure reflects central principles in development and representation of knowledge. Specifically, Steyvers and Tenenbaum argue that as the network grows, new nodes are predisposed to attach to existing nodes in a probabilistic manner. It is indeed quite rare that a new meaning of a word is acquired without it being some variation of a preexisting meaning (see Carey, 1978). Hence, across time, nodes that are added to the network will be preferentially attached to existing nodes. This will give rise to a high degree of local clustering, which is a signature of small world network structure. We return to the issue of how concepts develop in a later section.

It is noteworthy that Steyvers and Tenenbaum (2005) have also provided empirical support from their network analyses. For example, they have found that word frequency, or the degree to which a word is encountered in language, and age of acquisition, defined as the average age at which a child learns a given word, effects in naming and lexical decision performance naturally fall from this perspective. Naming and lexical decision are two of the most commonly used word recognition tasks used in research investigating the nature and structure of semantic memory. In naming (or speeded pronunciation), a participant is asked to read a presented stimulus aloud as quickly as possible, whereas in lexical decision, he or she is asked to indicate whether a letter string is a real word or a pseudoword (i.e., a string of letters that does not correspond to the spelling of a real word). In both tasks, the primary dependent measure is response latency. The general assumption is that the speed required to access the pronunciation of a word or to recognize a string of letters reflects processes involved in accessing stored

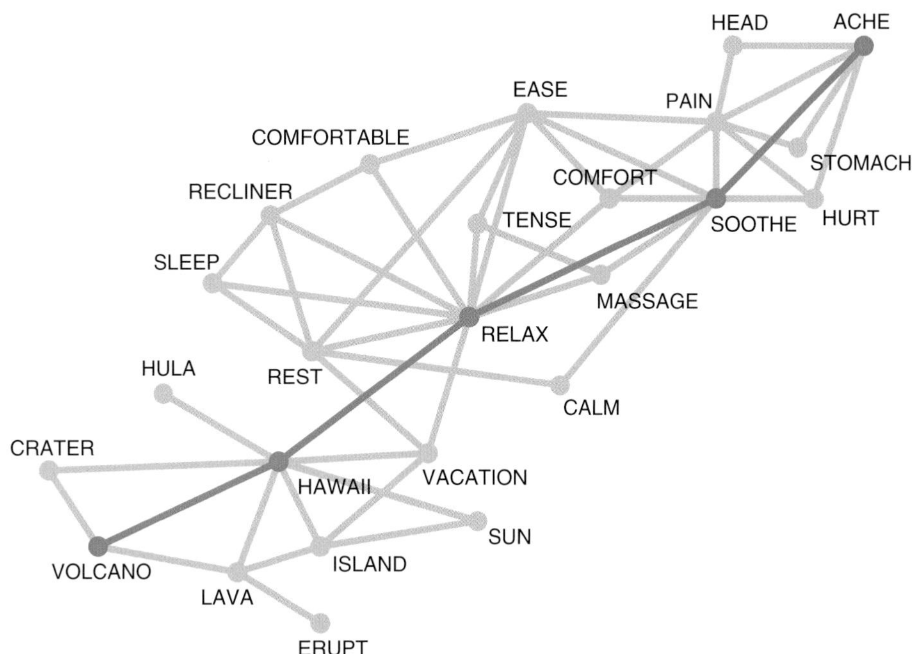

Figure 3 Segment of small world semantic network. Courtesy of Marc Steyvers.

knowledge about that word. Interestingly, Steyvers and Tenenbaum found a reliable negative correlation between number of connections to a node (semantic centrality) in these networks and response latency, precisely as one might predict, after correlated variables such as word frequency and age of acquisition have been partialed out (also see Balota et al., 2004). Clearly, further work is needed to empirically confirm the utility of these descriptions of semantic structure and the mechanisms by which such networks develop over time. However, the recent graph analytic procedures have taken a significant step toward capturing semantic memory within an empirically verified network.

5.3 Feature Analytic Approaches

An alternative to concepts being embedded within a rich network structure is an approach wherein meaning is represented as a set of primitive features that are used in various combinations to represent different concepts. Of course, this issue (distributed representation of knowledge, by way of features, vs. a localist representation, via a node to concept relationship) is central to attempts to represent and quantify learning and memory in general. We now turn to a review of the feature-based approaches in semantic memory.

The original Collins and Quillian (1969) research generated a great deal of attention, and soon researchers realized that categories reflected more graded structures than was originally assumed. Specifically, some members of categories are good members (ROBIN for BIRD), whereas other members appear to be relatively poor members (VULTURE for BIRD) but are still definitely members of the category (see Battig and Montague, 1969; Rosch, 1973). In addition, there was a clear influence of goodness of an exemplar on response latencies in the sentence verification task described above. Specifically, good exemplars were faster to verify than poor exemplars, referred to as the typicality effect. The Collins and Quillian hierarchical network model did not have any obvious way of accommodating such degrees of category membership.

Smith et al. (1974) took a quite different approach to accommodate the results from the sentence verification task. They rejected the strong assumptions of network theory and proposed a model that emphasized the notion of critical semantic features in representing the meaning of a word. So, for example, the word BIRD might be represented as animal, two legged, has wings, sings, is small, flies, and so on. There is no hierarchical organization within this model, but concepts reflect lists of critical features. They also distinguished between two classes of features, defining features and characteristic features. Defining features are the necessary features that an exemplar must have to be a member of a category. So, for example, all birds must eat, move, lay eggs, and so forth. On the other hand, characteristic features are features that most, but not all, exemplars have, such as small, flies, sings.

The second important aspect of the Smith et al. (1974) perspective is the emphasis on the decision processes engaged in the classic sentence verification task (see Atkinson and Juola, 1974; Balota and Chumbley, 1984, for similar decision models applied to short-term memory search and lexical decision, respectively). In verifying a sentence such as 'A ROBIN IS A BIRD,' subjects first access all (both defining and characteristic) features associated with ROBIN and all features associated with BIRD. If there is a high degree of overlap in the features, that is, above some criterion, the subject can make a fast 'yes' response. This would be the case in 'A ROBIN IS A BIRD,' since both defining and characteristic features provide a high degree of overlap. On the other hand, some exemplars of a given category may overlap less in characteristic features such as in 'AN OSTRICH IS A BIRD'. Although ostriches are clearly birds, they are not small and do not fly, which are characteristic features of birds. Hence, in such cases, the subject needs to engage in an additional analytic checking process in which only the defining features are compared. This additional check process takes time and so slows response latencies. Hence, the model can naturally capture the typicality effects mentioned above, that is, robins are better exemplars of birds than ostriches, because robins can be verified based on global overlap in features, whereas ostriches must engage the second, more analytic comparison of only the defining features, thereby slowing response latency.

In addition to accounting for typicality effects, the feature analytic model also captured interesting differences in latencies to respond 'no' in the sentence verification task. Specifically, subjects are relatively fast to reject 'A CARP IS A BIRD' compared with 'A BUTTERFLY IS A BIRD.' Carps do not have many overlapping features with birds, and so the subject can quickly reject this item, that is, there is virtually no overlap in features. However, both butterflies and birds typically have wings, are small, and fly. Hence, the subject must engage the additional check of the defining features for 'BUTTERFLY IS A BIRD,' which ultimately leads to slower response latencies, compared with the sentence 'A CARP IS A BIRD.'

Although there were clear successes of the Smith et al. (1974) feature analytic approach, there were also some problems. For example, the model was criticized for the strong distinction between characteristic and defining features. In fact, McCloskey and Glucksberg (1979) provided a single process random walk model that accommodated many of the same results of the original Smith et al. model without postulating a distinction between characteristic and defining features. According to the random walk framework, individuals sample information across time that supports either a yes or no decision. If the features from the subject and predicate match, then movement toward the yes criterion takes place; if the features do not match, then movement toward the no criterion takes place. This model simply assumed that the likelihood of sampling matching feature information for the subject and predicate is greater for typical members than nontypical members, and therefore the response criterion is reached more quickly for typical than nontypical members, thus producing the influence on response latencies. The distinction between single- and dual-process models is a central issue that pervades much of cognitive science.

A second concern about the Smith et al. (1974) model is that they did not directly measure features but, rather, inferred overlap in features based on multidimensional scaling techniques, in which an independent group of subjects simply rated the similarity of words used in the sentence verification experiment. In this way, one could look at the similarity of the words along an N-dimensional space. Interestingly, Osgood et al. (1957) used a similar procedure to tackle the meaning of words in their classic work on the semantic differential. Osgood et al. found that when subjects rated the similarity across words, and these similarity ratings were submitted to multidimensional scaling procedures, there were three major factors that emerged: Evaluative (good–bad), potency (strong–weak), and activity (active–passive). Although clearly this work is provocative, such similarity ratings do not provide a direct measure of the features available for a concept. So, if there are indeed primitive features, it seems necessary to attempt to more directly quantify these features.

McRae and colleagues have been recently attempting to provide such constraints on feature analytic models (McRae et al., 1997; Cree et al., 1999; Cree and McRae, 2003; McRae, 2004; McRae et al., 2005). The goal here is to develop a feature-based computational model implemented in an attractor network capable of capturing the statistical regularities present in semantic domains. The general notion underlying attractor network models is that knowledge is distributed across units (which might be thought of as features) and that the network settles into a steady pattern of activity that reflects the representation of a concept. The conceptual representations that form the basis of semantic knowledge in the model are derived from feature norming data. To collect norms, groups of participants are asked to list features for a number of concepts (e.g., for DOG, participants might list BARKS, FURRY, CHASES CATS, etc.). McRae and colleagues propose that when participants are asked to list features of various basic-level category exemplars (e.g., DOG and APPLE are basic-level concepts from the superordinate category of MAMMALS and FRUIT, respectively), the resulting lists of features reflect the explicit knowledge people have of these concepts. Importantly, McRae does not claim that the nature of the representation consists of a feature list; rather, he argues, the features are derived from repeated multisensory interactions with exemplars of the concept, and in a feature listing task, subjects temporarily create an abstraction for the purpose of listing features that can be verbally described. Currently, feature norming data are available for 541 concrete objects, representing a wide variety of basic-level concepts. Importantly, the model can account for many empirical observations in semantic tasks, as discussed below.

The major assumption implemented by McRae and colleagues' model is that semantic knowledge, as represented by feature lists, involves the statistical averaging of feature correlations among members of similar categories. Features are correlated if they co-occur in basic-level concepts. For example, HAS FUR is highly correlated with HAS FOUR LEGS, as these two features cooccur in numerous exemplars of the mammal category. However, HAS FUR and HAS WINGS have a low (almost nonexistent) correlation, as these two features do not co-occur frequently. The argument is that individuals are highly sensitive to the regularity of the correlations, which are tapped by semantic tasks. As demonstrated by McRae et al. (1999), the strength of the feature correlations predicted feature verification latencies in both human subjects and model simulations, with stronger correlations yielding faster response latencies than weaker correlations when the concept name was presented before the feature name (e.g., DOG-FUR). In addition, the correlation strength interacted with stimulus onset asynchrony (the time between the onset of the concept name and the onset of the feature name, SOA). Specifically, the effect of feature correlations was larger at shorter SOAs, with only high correlations predicting response latencies. However, at longer SOAs, even weakly correlated features influenced response times, indicating that, as more time was allowed for the effects of correlated features to emerge, even the more weakly correlated feature-concept pairs benefited from the shared representation. In another series of studies, McRae et al. (1997) reported that the strength of feature correlations predicted priming for exemplars from the living things domain but not for exemplars from nonliving things domains, for which priming was instead predicted by individual features. This finding is consistent with evidence that, compared to living things, nonliving things tend to have a lower degree of correlated features (also see section 5.8.1).

Several interesting extensions of McRae and colleagues' work on the role of features in organizing semantic knowledge have been recently reported. Pexman et al. (2002) examined the role of the number of features associated with a concept and found that items with more features were responded to faster in both naming and lexical decision tasks after a number of other variables known to influence visual word recognition latencies had been factored out. Pexman et al. (2003) reported similar results in a semantic categorization task and in a reading task. These findings were interpreted as supporting the distributed nature of semantic representations in which features are assumed to reflect access to conceptual knowledge, and this information quickly comes on line in isolated word recognition tasks.

In a related vein, there is recent evidence from the categorization literature that categories with richer dimensionalities (i.e., more features and more correlations among features) are easier to learn than categories with fewer dimensions (Hoffman and Murphy, 2006). Thus, rather than resulting in combinatorial explosions that make learning impossible, rich categories with many features lend themselves well to learning – a finding that is nicely mirrored in how people, even very young children, quickly and reliably learn to recognize and classify objects in the world. Indeed, it seems that learning to categorize complex objects, which might be quite similar in terms of features, is something most individuals can do reliably and easily. One concern that arises when one examines the richness of the stimuli in the environment, is the potentially infinite number of features that are available to identify a given concept. In fact, critics of feature-based models have argued that the number of possible feature combinations would result in combinatorial explosion, as knowing even a few features of a category could easily result in an enormous number of ways in which the features could be correlated and integrated (see Murphy, 2002, for a discussion). However, as McRae (2004) notes, two points are relevant in addressing this issue. The first is that the feature correlations tend to influence performance largely in implicit tasks – thus reducing the necessity of explaining how an individual can explicitly use the vast amount of information available. The second point is that the feature vectors that underlie semantic representations are generally sparse. In other words, the absence of a specific feature is uninformative, so, for example, knowing that a dog does not have feathers is relatively uninformative. Thus, although feature-based models might not fully capture the richness of the knowledge that individuals have about concepts, they have been useful in advancing research in the field of semantics.

5.4 Concept Learning and Categorization

Since semantic memory deals with the nature of representation of meaning, and categories are central to meaning, it is important to at least touch on the area of categorization and how concepts develop. In their classic book, Bruner et al. (1956) emphasized the importance of categorization in organizing what appears to be a limitless database that drives complex human learning and thought. Categorization has been viewed as a fundamental aspect of learning and indeed has been observed early in childhood (Gelman and Markman, 1986) and in other species such as pigeons (Herrnstein et al., 1976).

One intriguing question that arises when one considers the content of semantic memory concerns the grain size and structure of the representations. In other words, is there a level at which objects in the real world are more or less easy to learn and categorize? One possibility is that the world is initially perceived as a continuum in which there are not separate 'things.' Through repeated interactions with verbal labels or other forms of learning, an individual learns how to discriminate separate objects (e.g., Leach, 1964). This approach places the burden on an extensive and demanding learning process. An alternative approach is that the human cognitive system is ideally suited to detect and recognize objects at a specific grain or level. The assumption that the system is biased toward recognizing specific patterns implies that the process of learning the appropriate verbal labels that refer to specific items in the environment is significantly easier. This problem – how very young children learn that when their mother points to a dog and says 'dog' the referent of the phonological pattern in question refers to an entire object, and not to furry things, things of a certain color, or loosely attached dog parts – has been extensively discussed by Quine (1960).

In an elegant series of experiments, Rosch and colleagues (e.g., Rosch et al., 1976) provided empirical evidence that there is indeed a specific level at which categories of objects are represented that contains the most useful amount of information. For example, identifying a given object as a DOG implies that one recognizes that the specific exemplar is a dog, although it may differ from other dogs one has encountered. Simply knowing something is a dog allows one to draw upon a pool of stored knowledge and experiences to infer appropriate behaviors and interactions with the categorized object. However, knowing the object is an animal is not as informative, given the wide variability among animals. For example, interactions with an elephant are likely to be quite different from those one might have with a spider. Conversely, classifying the exemplar as a Collie or as a German Shepherd does not add a significant amount of inferential power for most purposes.

Rosch et al. (1976) argued that at the basic level, categories are highly informative and can be reliably and easily discriminated from other categories. Exemplars of basic-level categories (e.g., DOGS, BIRDS, CARS, etc.) have many attributes in common, tend to be similar in shape and in how one interacts with them, and allow easy extraction of a prototype or summary representation. The prototype can be accessed and serves as a benchmark against which novel exemplars can be compared: Those that are highly similar to the prototype will be quickly and easily classified as members of the category. Exemplars that differ from the prototype will be recognized as less typical members of a category (e.g., penguins are quite different from many other birds). Hence, typicality effects fall quite nicely from this perspective.

Historically, there has again been some tension between abstract prototype representation and more feature-based approaches. Consider the classic work by Posner and Keele (1968). Although cautious in their interpretation, these researchers reported evidence suggesting that prototypes (in this case a central tendency of dot patterns) were naturally abstracted from stored distortions of that prototype, even though the prototype was never presented for study. They also found that variability across a sufficient number of distortions was critical for abstracting the prototype. These results would appear to support the notion that there is a natural tendency to abstract some representation that is a central tendency of exemplars that share some common elements. So, 'dogness' may be abstracted from the examples of dogs that one encounters. This could suggest that there is indeed a unified representation for dogness.

An alternative approach is that there is nothing unique about these central tendencies but, rather, such representations reflect the similarity of the episodically stored representations in memory. This is a particularly important observation because it suggests that there is a blending of different types of memories, that is, categorical information is simply decontextualized episodic memories. Consider, for example, the classic MINERVA model developed by Hintzman (1986, 1988). In this computational model, each episodic experience lays down a unique trace in memory, which is reflected by a vector of theoretical features. There is no special status of category representations or hierarchical structure. Rather, categorization occurs during retrieval when a probe (the test item) is presented to the system, and the feature vector in the probe stimulus is correlated with all the episodically stored traces. The familiarity of a test probe is a reflection of the strength of the correlations among elements in memory. Because the schema overlaps more with multiple stored representations, that is, it is the central tendency, it will produce a relatively high familiarity signal or strength in a cued recall situation. The importance of the Hintzman approach is that there is no need to directly store central tendencies, as they naturally arise out of the correlation among similar stored traces in the feature vectors. Moreover, as Hintzman argues, there is no need to propose a qualitative distinction between episodic and semantic memories, because both rely on the same memory system, that is, a vast storehouse of individual feature-based episodic traces.

The notion that categories are a reflection of similarity structure across memory traces and can be generated during retrieval clearly has some appeal. Indeed, Barsalou (1985) demonstrated the importance of ad hoc categories that seem to be easily generated from traces that do not inherently have natural category structure; for example, what do photographs, money, children, and pets have in common? On the surface, these items do not appear to be similar – they do not belong to the same taxonomic category, nor do they share many features. However, when given the category label "things to take out of the house in the case of a fire," these items seem to fit quite naturally together because our knowledge base can be easily searched for items that are in the house and are important to us. As Medin (1989) has argued, similarity depends on the theoretical frame that a participant uses to guide a search of memory structures. There appears to be an unlimited number of ways in which similarity can be defined, and hence similarity discovered. For example, lichen and squirrels are similar if one is interested in specifying things in a forest. This brings us to the remarkable context dependency of meaning, and the possibility that meaning is not defined by the stimulus *per se* but is a larger unit involving both the stimulus and the surrounding context. The word DOG in the context of thinking about house pets compared with the word DOG in the context of guard dogs or drug-sniffing dogs probably access quite different interpretations, one in which the focus is on companionship, furriness, and wagging tails, the other in which the more threatening aspects of dogness, such as sharp teeth, are accessed. One might argue that the context activates the relevant set of features, but even this is difficult until one has sufficient constraint on what those features actually are.

5.5 Grounding Semantics

In part because of the difficulties in defining the critical features used to represent meaning and potential problems with the tractability of prototypes of meaning, several researchers attempted to take novel approaches to the nature of the representations. There are two general approaches that we review in this section. First, because of the increase in computational power, there has been an increased reliance on analyses of large-scale databases to extract similarities across the contexts of words used in various situations. This perspective has some similarity to the exemplar-based approach proposed by Hintzman (1986, 1988) and others described earlier. In this sense, meaning is grounded in the context in which words and objects appear. The second approach is to consider the perceptual motor constraints afforded by humans to help ground semantics, that is, the embodied cognition approach. We review each of these in turn.

5.5.1 Grounding Semantics in Analyses of Large-Scale Databases

This approach attempts to directly tackle the poverty of the stimulus problem when considering the knowledge that humans have acquired. Indeed, since the days of Plato, philosophers (and more recently psychologists and linguists) have attempted to resolve the paradox of how humans can acquire so much information based on so little input. Specifically, how is it that children learn so much about the referents of words, when to use them, what their syntactic class is, what the relations among referents are, and so on, without explicit instruction? Some have argued (e.g., Pinker, 1994) that the poverty of the stimulus is indeed the reason one needs to build in genetically predisposed language acquisition devices. However, recent approaches to this issue (e.g., Latent Semantic Analysis, or LSA, Landauer and Dumais, 1997; Hyperspace Analogue to Language, or HAL, Burgess and Lund, 1997) have suggested that the stimulus input is not so impoverished as originally assumed. One simply needs more powerful statistical tools to uncover the underlying meaning and the appropriate database.

In an attempt to better understand how rich the stimulus is when embedded in context, Landauer and Dumais (1997) analyzed large corpora of text that included over 4.6 million words taken from an English encyclopedia, a work intended for young students. This encyclopedia included about 30 000 paragraphs reflecting distinct topics. From this, the authors constructed a data matrix that basically included the 60 000 words across the 30 000 paragraphs. Each cell within the matrix reflected the frequency that a given word appeared in a given paragraph. The data matrix was then submitted to a singular value decomposition, which has strong similarities to factor analysis to reduce the data matrix to a limited set of dimensions. Essentially, singular value decomposition extracts a parsimonious representation of the intercorrelations of variables, but, unlike factor analysis, it can be used with matrices of arbitrary shape in which rows and columns represent the words and the contexts in which the words appear. In this case, the authors reduced the matrix to 300 dimensions. These dimensions reflect the intercorrelations that arise across the words from the different texts. So, in some sense the 300 dimensions of a given word will provide information about the similarity to all other words along these 300 dimensions, that is, the degree to which words co-occur in different contexts. The exciting aspect from this data reduction technique is that by using similarity estimates, the model actually performs quite well in capturing the performance of children acquiring language and adults' performance on tests based on introductory textbooks. In this way, the meaning of a word is being captured by all the past experiences with the word, the contexts with which that word (neighbors) occurs, the contexts that the neighbors occur in, and so on.

The remarkable success of LSA, and other similar approaches such as HAL (Burgess and Lund, 1997), provides a possible answer to the poverty of the stimulus problem, that is, when considering the context, the stimulus is indeed very rich. In the past, we simply have not been able to analyze it appropriately. Moreover, the model nicely captures the apparent contextual specificity of meaning in that meaning is defined by all the contexts that words have appeared in and hence will also be constantly changing ever so slightly across subsequent encounters. Finally, the model is indeed quite important because it does not rely on a strong distinction between semantic and episodic memory since it simply reflects past accumulated exposure to language. In this sense, it has some similarity to the Hintzman (1986) model described above.

5.5.2 Grounding Semantics in Perceptual Motor Systems

An alternative approach that has been receiving considerable recent attention is that meaning can be grounded in perceptual-motor systems (e.g., Barsalou, 1999). Briefly, this perspective is part of the embodied cognition approach that posits that the cognitive system of any organism is constrained by the body in which it is embedded (Wilson, 2002). Thus, cognition (in this case meaning) is not viewed as being separable from perceptual, motor, and proprioceptive systems; rather, it is through the interactions of these systems with the environment that cognition emerges. Furthermore, the type of representations that an organism will develop depends on the structure of the organism itself and how it exists in the world. This approach has its roots in Gibson's (1979) ecological psychology, as it is assumed that structures in the environment afford different interactions to different organisms. It is through repeated interactions with the world that concepts and knowledge emerge. Importantly, the very nature of this knowledge retains its connections to the manner in which it was acquired: Rather than assuming that semantic memory consists of amodal, abstract representations, proponents of embodied approaches argue that representations are grounded in the same systems that permitted their acquisition in the first place (Barsalou et al., 2003).

According to the modality-specific approaches to knowledge, a given concept is stored in adjacent memory systems rather than being abstracted. For example, in Barsolou's (1999) account, knowledge is stored in perceptual symbol systems that emerge through repeated experience interacting with an object or an event. Briefly, Barsalou assumed that when a percept is encountered, selective attention focuses on context-relevant aspects of the percept and allows modal representations to be stored in memory. Repeated interactions with similar events or members of the same category result in the formation of a complex, multimodal representation, and a simulator emerges from these common representations. Simulators are the basic unit of the conceptual system and consist of a frame (which is somewhat similar to a schema), the purpose of which is to integrate the perceptual representations. Simulators provide continuity in the system. Importantly, the representations that are stored include not only modal, perceptual information (e.g., sounds, images, physical characteristics) but also emotional responses, introspective states, and proprioceptive information. Retrieving an exemplar or remembering an event is accomplished by engaging in top-down processing and activating the targeted simulator. Importantly, a given simulator can yield multiple simulations, depending on the organism's goal, the context, and the relevant task demands. For example, different simulations for DOG are possible, such that a different pattern of activity will occur if the warm and furry aspect of dog is relevant or whether the aspect of being a guard or police dog is relevant. Of course, this nicely captures the context sensitivity of meaning. Barsalou (1999) argues that perceptual symbol systems are as powerful and flexible as amodal models, as they are able to implement a complete conceptual system (see also Glenberg and Robertson, 2000).

Evidence in support of modal approaches to semantics can be found in both behavioral and cognitive neuroscience studies. We briefly review some of this evidence here, although a full review of the neuroscience literature is beyond the scope of this chapter (*See* Chapter 6 for further discussion of this area). For example, there is evidence from lesion studies that damage to the pathways supporting a specific modality results in impaired performance in categorization and conceptual tasks that rely on that same modality. Specifically, damage to visual pathways generally results in greater impairment in the domain of living things, which tend to rely heavily on visual processes for recognition. Conversely, damage to motor pathways tends to impair knowledge of artifacts and tools, as the primary mode of interaction with these items is through manipulation (see Martin, 2005). Consistent with the lesion data, neuroimaging studies indicate that different regions of the cortex become active when people process different categories. Regions adjacent to primary visual areas become active when categories such as animals are processed (even if the presentation of the stimulus itself is not in the visual modality), whereas regions close to motor areas become active when categories such as tools are processed. These findings have been interpreted as consistent with the hypothesis that people run perceptual-motor simulations when processing conceptual information (Barsalou, 2003).

Pecher et al. (2003) reported evidence from a property verification task indicating that participants were faster in verifying properties in a given modality (e.g., BLENDER-loud) after verifying a different property for a different concept in the same modality (e.g., LEAVES-rustling) than when a modality switch was required (e.g., CRANBERRIES-tart). Pecher et al. argued that the switch cost observed was consistent with the hypothesis that participants ran perceptual simulations to verify the properties (in this case sounds) rather than accessing an amodal semantic system. In a subsequent study, Pecher et al. (2004) observed that when the same concept in a property verification task was paired with two properties from different modalities, errors and latencies increased when verifying the second property. Pecher et al. interpreted this finding as indicating that recent experiences with a concept influence the simulation of the concept. Importantly, researchers have argued that such results are not simply a result of associative strength (i.e., priming) nor of participants engaging in intentional imagery instructions (Barsalou, 2003; Solomon and Barsalou, 2004).

Although the results summarized above are compelling and are supportive of the hypothesis that sensory-motor simulations underlie many semantic tasks, the majority of these studies have examined tasks such as property verification and property generation. The question thus arises of whether the results are somehow an artifact of the task demands, and specifically whether these results reflect the structure of the semantic memory system or whether subjects are explicitly retrieving information as they notice the relations embedded within the experimental context. Glenberg and Kaschak (2002) extended the evidence for embodiment effects to a novel series of tasks that do not appear as susceptible to task demand effects. In these experiments, participants read a brief sentence and judged whether the sentence made sense or not. The critical sentences contained statements that implied motion either toward the participant (e.g., "Nancy gave you the book") or away from the participant (e.g., "You gave the book to Nancy"). Participants responded by moving their hand toward themselves or away from themselves. Glenberg and Kaschak found what they called the action-sentence compatibility effect: When the required response was consistent with the movement implied in the sentence, participants were faster than when the implied motion and the actual physical response were inconsistent. These data appear most consistent with the view that when processing language, people relate the meaning of the linguistic stimulus to action patterns.

5.6 Measuring Semantic Representations and Processes: Insights from Semantic Priming Studies

As described above, there have been many empirical tools that have been used to provide insights into the nature of semantic memory. For example, as noted earlier, some of the early work by Osgood et al. (1957) attempted to provide leverage on fundamental aspects of meaning via untimed ratings of large sets of words and multidimensional scaling techniques. With the advent of interest in response latencies, researchers turned to sentence verification tasks that dominated much of the early work in the 1970s and 1980s. Although this work has clearly been influential, the explicit demands of such tasks (e.g., explicitly asking subjects to verify the meaningfulness of subject-predicate relations) led some researchers in search of alternative ways to measure both structure and retrieval processes from semantic memory. There was accumulating interest in automatic processes (LaBerge and Samuels, 1974; Posner and Snyder, 1975) that presumably captured the modular architecture of the human processing system (Fodor, 1983), and there was an emphasis on indirect measures of structure and process. Hence, researchers turned to semantic priming paradigms.

Meyer and Schvaneveldt (1971) are typically regarded as reporting the first semantic priming study. In this study, subjects were asked to make lexical decisions (word-nonword decisions) to pairs of stimuli. The subjects' task was to respond yes only if both strings were words. The interesting finding here was that subjects were faster to respond yes when the words were semantically related (DOCTOR NURSE), compared with when they were unrelated (BREAD NURSE). This pattern was quite intriguing because subjects did not need to access the semantic relation between the two words to make the word/nonword decisions. Hence, this may reflect a relatively pure measure of the underlying structure and retrieval processes, uncontaminated by explicit task demands. Moreover, the development of this paradigm was quite important because researchers thought it may tap the spreading activation processes that was so central to theoretical developments at the time.

The research on semantic priming took a significant leap forward with the dissertation work of Neely (1977), who used a framework developed by Posner and Snyder (1975) to decouple the attentional strategic use of the prime-target relations from a more automatic component. In this study, subjects only made lexical decisions to the target, and subjects were given explicit instructions of how to use the prime information. For example, in one condition, subjects were told that when they received the prime BODY, they should think of building parts (Shift condition), whereas in a different condition, subjects were told that when they received the category prime BIRD, they should think of birds (Nonshift condition). Neely varied the time available to process the prime before the target was presented by using SOAs ranging from 250 to 2000 ms. The important finding here is that the instructions of what to expect had no influence on the priming effects at the short SOA (i.e., priming occurred if the prime and target had a semantic relationship, independent of expectancies), but they did have a large effect at the long SOA, when subjects had time to engage an attentional mechanism (i.e., the priming effects were totally dependent on what subjects were told to expect, independent of the preexisting relationship). Hence, Neely argued that the short SOA data reflected pure automatic measures of the semantic structure and retrieval processes and could be used as a paradigm to exploit the nature of such semantic representations.

A full review of the rich semantic priming literature is clearly beyond the scope of the present chapter (see Neely, 1991; Lucas, 2000; Hutchison, 2003, for excellent discussions of the methodological and theoretical frameworks). However, it is useful to highlight a few issues that have been particularly relevant to the current discussion. First, there is some controversy regarding the types of prime-target relations that produce priming effects. For example, returning to the initial observation by Meyer and Schvaneveldt (1971), one might ask if DOCTOR and NURSE are related because they share some primitive semantic features or are simply related because they are likely to co-occur in the same contexts in the language. Of course, this distinction reflects back on core assumptions regarding the nature of semantic information, since models like LSA might capture priming between DOCTOR and NURSE, simply because the two words are likely to cooccur in common contexts. Researchers have attempted to address this by selecting items that vary on only one dimension (see, e.g., Fischler, 1977; Lupker, 1984; Thompson-Schill et al., 1998). Here, semantics is most typically defined by category membership (e.g., DOG and CAT are both semantically related and associatively related, whereas MOUSE and CHEESE are only associatively related). Hines et al. (1986), De Mornay Davies (1998), and Thompson-Schill et al. (1998) have all argued that priming is caused by semantic feature overlap because of results indicating priming only for words that shared semantic overlap versus those did not, when associative strength was controlled. However, Hutchison (2003) has recently argued that the studies that have provided evidence for pure semantic effects (i.e., while equating for associative strength), actually have not adequately controlled for associative strength based on the Nelson et al. (1998) free-association norms. Clearly, equating items on one dimension (associative strength or semantic overlap) while manipulating the other dimension is more difficult than initially assumed. In this light, it is interesting to note that two recent review papers have come to different conclusions regarding the role of semantics in semantic priming based on such item selection studies. Lucas (2000) argued that there was clear evidence of pure semantic effects, as opposed to associative effects, whereas Hutchison (2003) was relatively more skeptical about the conclusions from the available literature.

Balota and Paul (1996) took a different approach to the meaning versus associative influence in priming via a study of multiple primes, instantiating the conditions displayed in **Table 1**. As one can see, the primes were either both related, first related, second related, or both unrelated to the targets, and the targets could either be homographic words with distinct meanings (e.g., ORGAN) or a nonhomographic words (e.g., STRIPES). As one can see, the primes were related to the targets at both the semantic and associative level for the nonhomographs (e.g., LION and STRIPES are both related to TIGER at the associative and semantic level), but for the homographs the primes were related to the targets at only the associative level (e.g., PIANO and KIDNEY are only related to ORGAN at the associative level, since KIDNEY and PIANO are different meanings of ORGAN). Thus, one could compare priming effects in conditions in which primes converged on the same meaning of the target (nonhomographs) and priming effects where the primes diverged on different meanings (homographs). The results from four experiments indicated that the primes produced clear additive effects, that is, priming effects from the single related prime conditions nicely summated to predict the priming effects from the double related prime conditions for both homographs and nonhomographs, suggesting that the effects were most likely a result of associative level information. Only when subjects directed attention to the meaning of the word, via speeded semantic decisions, was there any evidence of the predicted difference between the two conditions. Hence, these results seem to be supportive of the notion that standard semantic priming effects are likely to be the result of associative-level connections instead of meaning-based semantic information. Of course, the interesting theoretical question is how much of our semantic knowledge typically used is caused by overlap in the contexts in which items are stored as opposed to abstracted rich semantic representations.

Table 1 Prime-target conditions from the Balota and Paul (1996) multiprime study

Nonhomographs			
Condition	*Prime 1*	*Prime 2*	*Target*
Related–related	LION	TIGER	STRIPES
Unrelated–related	FUEL	TIGER	STRIPES
Related–unrelated	LION	SHUTTER	STRIPES
Unrelated–unrelated	FUEL	SHUTTER	STRIPES

Homographs			
Condition	*Prime 1*	*Prime 2*	*Target*
Related–related	KIDNEY	PIANO	ORGAN
Unrelated–related	WAGON	PIANO	ORGAN
Related–unrelated	KIDNEY	SODA	ORGAN
Unrelated–unrelated	WAGON	SODA	ORGAN

Balota DA and Paul ST (1996) Summation of activation: Evidence from multiple primes that converge and diverge within semantic memory. *J. Exp. Psychol. Learn. Mem. Cogn.* 22: 827–845.

Hutchison (2003) notes two further findings that would appear to be supportive of associative influences underlying semantic priming effects. First, one can find evidence of episodic priming in lexical decision and speeded word naming tasks. In these studies, subjects study unrelated words such as (CITY-GRASS) and are later presented prime-target pairs in a standard lexical decision study. The interesting finding here is that one can obtain priming effects in such studies, compared to an unrelated/unstudied pair of words (see McKoon and Ratcliff, 1979). Thus, the semantic priming effects obtained in word recognition tasks can also be produced via purely associative information that develops within a single study exposure. However, it should be noted here that there is some question regarding the locus of such priming effects and that one needs to be especially cautious in making inferences from the episodic priming paradigm and the role of task-specific strategic operations (see, e.g., Neely and Durgunoglu, 1985; Durgunoglu and Neely, 1987; Spieler and Balota, 1996; Pecher and Raajmakers, 1999; Faust et al., 2001).

The second pattern of results that Hutchison (2003) notes as being critical to the associative account of semantic priming effects is mediated priming. In these situations, the prime (LION) is related to the target (STRIPES) only through a nonpresented mediator (TIGER). So, the question is whether one can obtain priming from LION to STRIPES, even though these two words appear to be semantically unrelated. Although de Groot (1983) failed to obtain mediated priming effects in the lexical decision task, Balota and Lorch (1986) argued that this may have resulted from the task-specific characteristics of this task. Hence, Balota and Lorch used a speeded pronunciation task and found clear evidence of mediated priming. Evidence for mediated priming has also now been found in versions of the lexical decision task designed to minimize task-specific operations (e.g., McNamara and Altarriba, 1988; McKoon and Ratcliff, 1992; Sayette et al., 1996; Livesay and Burgess, 1998). Of course, it is unclear what semantic features overlap between LION and STRIPES, and so these results would appear to be more consistent with an associative network model, in which there is a relationship between LION and TIGER and between TIGER and STRIPES, along with a spreading activation retrieval mechanism (see McKoon and Ratcliff, 1992; Chwilla and Kolk, 2002, for alternative accounts of the retrieval mechanism).

In sum, although the semantic priming paradigm has been critical in measuring retrieval mechanisms from memory, the argument that these effects reflect amodal semantic representations that are distinct from associative information has some difficulty accommodating the results from multiprime studies, episodic priming studies, and mediated priming studies. As noted earlier, there are available models of semantic memory (e.g., Burgess and Lund, 1997, HAL; Landauer and Dumais, 1997, LSA) and categorization (e.g., Hintzman, 1996, MINERVA) that would strongly support the associative contributions to performance in such tasks and, indeed, question the strong distinction between semantic and episodic memory systems. Hence, this perspective predicts a strong interplay between the systems. We now turn to a brief discussion of the evidence that directly addresses such an interplay.

5.7 The Interplay Between Semantics and Episodic Memory

Memory researchers have long understood the influence of preexisting meaning on learning and memory performance (see Crowder, 1976, for a review). Indeed, in his original memory manifesto, Ebbinghaus (1885) was quite worried about this influence and so purposefully stripped away meaning from the to-be-learned materials by presenting meaningless trigrams (KOL) for acquisition. Of course, semantics has penetrated episodic memory research in measures of category clustering (see Bousfield, 1953; Cofer et al., 1966; Bruce and Fagan, 1970), retrieval-induced inhibition (see Anderson et al., 1994), and release from proactive interference (see Wickens, 1973), among many other paradigms. Indeed, the interplay between preexisting knowledge and recall performance was the centerpiece of the classic work by Bartlett (1932). Researchers realized that even consonant–vowel–consonant trigrams were not meaningless (see Hoffman et al., 1987). At this level, one might even question what it would mean to episodically store in memory totally meaningless information.

One place where researchers have attempted to look at the interplay between semantic and episodic structures is within the episodic priming paradigm described earlier. In these studies, participants receive pairs of unrelated words for study and then are later given prime-target pairs that have either been paired together or not during the earlier acquisition phase. For example, Neely and Durgunoglu (1985) investigated the influence of studying previous pairs of words and word–nonword combinations on both lexical decision performance and episodic recognition performance (also see Durgunoglu and Neely, 1987). Although there were clear differences between the tasks in the pattern of priming effects (suggesting dissociable effects across the two systems), there were also some intriguing similarities. For example, there was evidence of inhibition at a short prime-target SOA (150 ms) in both the episodic recognition task and the lexical decision task from semantically related primes that were in the initial studied list but were not paired with the target. It appeared as if this additional semantic association had to be suppressed in order for subjects to make both the episodic recognition decision and the lexical decision. The finding that this effect occurred at the short SOA also suggests that it may have been outside the attentional control of the participant.

The power of preexisting semantic representations on episodic tasks has recently taken a substantial leap forward with the publication of an important paper by Roediger and McDermott (1995), which revisited an earlier paper published by Deese (1959). This has now become know as the DRM (after Deese, Roediger, and McDermott) paradigm. The procedure typically used in such studies involves presenting a list of 10–15 words for study (REST, AWAKE, DREAM, PILLOW, BED, etc.) that are highly related to a critical nonpresented item (SLEEP). The powerful memory illusion here is that subjects are just as likely to recall (or recognize) the critical nonpresented item (SLEEP) as items that were actually presented. Moreover, when given remember/know judgments (Tulving, 1985), participants often give the critical nonpresented item remember judgments that presumably tapped detailed episodic recollective experience. It is as if the strong preexisting semantic memory structure is so powerful that it overwhelms the episodic study experience.

It should not be surprising that many of the same issues that have played out in the semantic memory research have also played out in the false memory research. Indeed, one model in this area is the activation monitoring (AM) framework (e.g., Roediger et al., 2001a), which suggests that subjects sometimes confuse the activation that is produced by spreading activation that converges on the critical nonpresented item (much akin to the Collins and Loftus, 1975) with the activation resulting from the study event. This framework attempts to keep separate the episodic and semantic systems but also shows how such systems can interact. In contrast, Arndt and Hirshman (1998) have used the Hintzman (1986) MINERVA framework to accommodate the DRM effect by relying on the similarity of the vectors of the individually stored words and the critical nonpresented items. As noted above, the MINERVA framework does not make a strong distinction between episodic and semantic systems. Moreover, the MINERVA model is more a feature-based model, whereas the AM framework *a priori* would appear more akin to a prototype model, but no strong claims have been made along this dimension. A further distinction between the AM framework and the MINERVA approach concerns the relative contributions of backward associative strength (BAS, or the probability that a list item will elicit the target, or critical lure, on a free-association task) and forward associative strength (FAS, or the probability the critical lure will elicit a list item in such a task). According to AM accounts, the critical variable is expected to be BAS, as the activation flows from the list items to the critical lure. However, according to MINERVA, FAS should be more important, as the similarity between the probe (i.e., the critical lure) and the stored episodes (i.e., the list items) should be a more powerful determinant of memory performance. Results from a multiple regression analysis reported by Roediger et al. (2001b) indicated that, in the DRM paradigm, BAS was the better predictor, thus supporting the AM framework. (We thank Roddy Roediger for pointing this out.)

The question of the nature of the representation (i.e., associative vs semantic) underlying these powerful memory illusions has also been studied. For example, Hutchison and Balota (2005) recently utilized the summation paradigm developed by Balota and Paul (1996), described earlier, to examine whether the DRM effect reflects meaning-based semantic information or could also be accommodated by primarily assuming an associative level information. Hence, in this study, subjects studied lists of words that were related to one meaning or related to two different meanings of a critical nonpresented homograph (e.g., the season meaning of FALL or the accident meaning of FALL). In addition, there were standard DRM lists that only included words that were related to the same meaning of a critical nonpresented word (e.g., such as SLEEP). Consistent with the Balota and Paul results, the results from both recall and recognition tests indicated that there was no difference in the pattern of false memory for study lists that converged on the same meaning (standard DRM lists) of the critical nonpresented items and lists that diverged on different meanings (homograph lists) of the critical nonpresented items. However, when subjects were required to explicitly make gist-based responses and directly access the meaning of the list, that is, is this word related to the studied list, there was clear (and expected) difference between homograph and nonhomograph lists. Hutchison and Balota argued that although rich networks develop through strategic use of meaning during encoding and retrieval, the activation processes resulting from the studied information seem to primarily reflect implicit associative information and do not demand rich meaning-based analysis.

There is little doubt that what we store in memory is a reflection of the knowledge base that we already have in memory, which molds the engram. Hence, as noted earlier, semantic memories may be episodic memories that have lost the contextual information across time because of repeated exposures. It is unlikely that a 50-year-old remembers the details of hearing the Rolling Stones' "Satisfaction" for the first time, but it is likely that, soon after that original experience, one would indeed have vivid episodic details, such as where one was, who one was with, and so on. Although this unitary memory system approach clearly has some value (e.g., McKoon et al., 1986), it is also the case that there is some powerful evidence from cognitive neuroscience that supports a stronger distinction.

5.8 Representation and Distinctions: Evidence from Neuropsychology

Evidence for the distinction of multiple memory systems has come from studies of patients with localized lesions that produce strong dissociations in behavior. For example, the classic case of HM (see Scoville and Milner, 1957) indicated that damage to the hippocampus resulted in impairment of the storage of new episodic memories, whereas semantic knowledge appeared to be relatively intact (but see MacKay et al., 1998). Hence, one might be overly concerned about the controversy from the behavioral studies regarding the distinct nature of semantic and episodic memory systems. However, there are additional neuropsychological cases that are indeed quite informative about the actual nature of semantic representations.

5.8.1 Category-Specific Deficits

There have now been numerous cases of individuals who have a specific lesion to the brain and appear to have localized category-specific deficits. For example, there have been individuals who have difficulty identifying items from natural categories (e.g., animals, birds, fruits, etc.) but have a relatively preserved ability to identify items from artificial categories (e.g., clothing, tools, furniture). At first glance, such results would appear to suggest that certain categories are represented in distinct neural tissue that have or have not been disrupted by the lesion. Such a pattern may also be consistent with a localized representation of meaning instead of a distributed feature-based representation in which all concepts share vectors of the same set of primitive features.

Unfortunately, however, the interpretation of impaired performance on natural categories and intact performance on artificial categories has been controversial. For example, such deficits could occur at various stages in the information flow from discriminating visually similar items (e.g., Riddoch and Humphreys, 1987) to problems retrieving the appropriate name of an object (e.g., Hart et al., 1985). Such accounts do not rely on the meaning of the categories but suggest that such deficits may reflect correlated dimensions (e.g., difficulty of the visual discrimination) that differ between natural and artificial categories. In this light, it is particularly important that there have been cases that have shown the opposite pattern. For example, Sacchett and Humphreys (1992) reported an intriguing case that shows disruption of the performance on artificial categories and body parts but relatively preserved performance on natural categories. They argued that one possible reason for this pattern is that this individual had a deficit in representing functional features, which are more relevant to artifactual representations and body parts than natural categories such as fruits and vegetables. Whatever the ultimate explanation of these category-specific deficits, this work has been informative in providing a better understanding of how members within categories may differ on distinct dimensions.

In a similar vein, one hypothesis that has been suggested to explain domain differences in category-specific deficits is the sensory/functional hypothesis (Warrington and McCarthy, 1987; Farah and McClelland, 1991; Caramazza and Shelton, 1998). According to this proposal, natural categories such as animals depend heavily on perceptual information (especially on visual discriminations) for identification and discrimination. Conversely, functional information is more important for recognition of artifacts, such as tools. Thus, damage to regions of sensory cortex is expected to result in selective impairment of natural kinds, whereas damage to regions in or adjacent to motor cortex would result in impairment in artifacts. Although compelling, this view is not endorsed by all researchers. Caramazza and colleagues, in particular, have argued that the sensory/functional hypothesis fails to account for some of the patterns of deficits observed and some of the finer-grain distinctions. In particular, it is difficult for this model to account for the selective sparing or impairment of fruits and vegetables, body parts, and musical instruments that have been reported (see Capitani et al., 2003, for a recent review). Thus, the question of whether and how the type of knowledge that is most critical for supporting the representation of a particular domain is involved in category-specific deficits remains open.

To address this controversy, Cree and McRae (2003) extended the sensory/functional hypothesis to include a broader range of types of knowledge. They developed a brain region taxonomy that included nine different forms of knowledge, including sensory/perceptual in all modalities (vision, taste, audition, etc.), functional, and encyclopedic. Encyclopedic features included information about items such as LIVES IN AFRICA for ELEPHANT – in other words, information that likely was learned and not experienced directly. Cree and McRae then developed a nine-dimensional representation for the 541 concepts for which they had norming data and estimated the salience of each type of knowledge for each object and each category. In a series of cluster analyses, Cree and McRae found that the knowledge types nicely predicted the tripartite distinction between living things, artifacts, and fruits and vegetables reported in several neuropsychological case studies. In addition, Cree and McRae examined several distributional statistics, including the number of distinguishing and distinctive features and similarity to obtain a measure of confusability (i.e., the extent to which a given concept might be confused with another concept from the same category). The categories they examined did appear to be differentially sensitive to these measures, and the implemented model reflected patterns of impairment observed in patients. They concluded that knowledge type does underlie the organization of conceptual representations and that selective impairment in a particular brain region involved in maintaining such knowledge can result in the observed patterns of impairment in patients with category-specific deficits. Although many questions remain, it is clear that evidence from individuals with category-specific deficits has provided considerable insight into both the nature of category representation and the underlying neural representations.

5.8.2 Semantic Dementia

The most common form of dementing illness is dementia of the Alzheimer type (DAT). However, there is also a relatively rare and distinct dementia, referred to as semantic dementia (SD), which overlaps with DAT in features such as insidious onset and gradual deterioration of comprehension and word-finding ability. SD is a variant of frontal temporal dementia and typically involves one or both of the anterior portions of the temporal lobes. The consensus criteria for SD (Hodges et al., 1992) include impairment in semantic memory causing anomia, deficits in both spoken and written word comprehension, a reading pattern consistent with surface dyslexia (i.e., impairment in reading exception words such as PINT but preserved reading of regular words and nonwords that follow standard spelling to sound rules, such as NUST), impoverished knowledge about objects and/or people with relative sparing of phonological and syntactic components of speech output, and perceptual and nonverbal problem solving skills. These individuals are often quite fluent, but their speech is relatively limited in conveying meaning. They are particularly poor at picture naming and understanding the relations among objects. For example, the Pyramids and Palm Trees test developed by Howard and Patterson (1992) involves selecting which of two items (e.g., a palm tree or a fir tree) is most similar to a third item (e.g., a pyramid). Individuals with SD are particularly poor at this task and so would appear to have a breakdown in the representations of the knowledge structures.

An interesting dissociation has been made between SD individuals and DAT individuals. In particular, Simons et al. (2002) recently found a double dissociation, wherein individuals with SD produced poorer picture naming than individuals with DAT; however, individuals with SD produced better performance than individuals with DAT on a later episodic recognition test of these very same pictures (also see Gold et al., 2005). Clearly, the selective impairment across these two groups of participants is consistent with distinct types of information driving these tasks. Of course, one must be cautious about the implications even from this study, because it is unlikely that either task is a process-pure measure of episodic and semantic memory (see Jacoby, 1991), but clearly these results are very intriguing.

Recently, Rogers et al. (2004) proposed a model of semantic memory that maintains strong connections to modality-specific systems in terms of both inputs and outputs and has been particularly useful in accommodating the deficits observed in SD. This model has some interesting parallels to Barsalou's (1999) proposal, in that it assumes that semantic memory is grounded in perception and action networks. In addition, like the model proposed by McRae et al. (1997), Rogers et al. suggest that the system is sensitive to statistical regularities, and these regularities are what underlie the development of semantics. The particular contribution of Rogers et al.'s model, however, is that although semantic representations are grounded in perception–action modality-specific systems, the statistical learning mechanism allows the emergence of abstract semantic representations. Importantly, inputs to semantics are mediated by perceptual representations that are modality specific, and as a result, the content of semantic memory relies on the same neural tissue that supports encoding. However, different from Barsalou and colleagues' account, Rogers et al. do suggest that there is a domain-general, abstracted representation that emerges from cross-modal mappings. Thus, although the system relies on perceptual inputs, the abstract representations can capture cross-modality similarities and structures to give rise to semantic memory.

Rogers et al. (2004) implemented a simple version of their model using a parallel distributed-processing approach in which visual features provided the perceptual input and are allowed to interact in training with verbal descriptors through a mediating semantic level. Importantly, the semantic representations emerge through the course of training as the network learns the mappings between units at the visual and verbal levels. The units the model was trained on consisted of verbal and visual features generated in separate norming sessions. Once training was complete, several simulations were reported in which the model was progressively damaged in a way that was thought to mimic varying levels of impairment observed in individuals with SD. Overall, the model nicely captured the patterns of performance of the patients. Specifically, one pattern often observed in SD is a tendency to overregularize conceptual knowledge. For example, individuals might refer to all exemplars of a category using the superordinate label or a single label that is high in frequency (e.g., calling a DOG an ANIMAL or a ZEBRA a HORSE). This is possibly a result of the progressive failure in retrieving idiosyncratic information that serves to distinguish exemplars, such that only the central tendency (e.g., a prototype or most typical exemplar) remains accessible. Thus, less common items might take on the attributes of higher-frequency exemplars. The model displayed similar patterns of generalization as the SD individuals, a finding explained in terms of changes in attractor dynamics that resulted in the relative sparing of features and attributes shared by many exemplars but a loss of more distinctive features. This model provides an interesting account of semantic memory and the deficits observed in individuals with SD, one in which both perceptually based information and abstracted representations interact to give rise to knowledge of the world.

5.9 Neuroimaging

Investigations into the nature of semantic memory have benefited from recent advances in technology that allow investigators to examine online processing of information in the human brain. For example, positron emission technology (PET) and functional magnetic resonance imaging (fMRI) allow one to measure correlates of neural activity *in vivo* as individuals are engaged in semantic tasks (see Logothetis and Wandell, 2004). Although a full review of the substantial contributions of neuroimaging data to the questions pertaining to semantics is beyond the scope of this chapter (*See* Chapter 6 for a review), we briefly examine some of the major findings that have helped constrain recent theorizing about the nature and locus of semantic representations. Two major brain regions have been identified through neuroimaging studies: left prefrontal cortex (LPC) and areas within the temporal lobes, particularly in the left hemisphere.

The first study to report neuroimaging data relevant to semantic memory was conducted by Petersen et al. (1988), who used PET techniques to localize activation patterns specific to semantic tasks. Subjects were asked to generate action verbs upon presentation of a concrete object noun, and activity during this task was compared with the activity occurring during silent reading of the words. Petersen et al. reported significant patterns of activity in LPC, a finding that has since been replicated and extended to other types of attributes. Martin et al. (1995) extended this work to show that the specific attribute to be retrieved yielded different patterns of activation. Specifically, the locus of activation involved in attribute retrieval tends to be in close proximity to the neural regions that are involved in perception of the specific attributes. Thus, retrieval of visual information, such as color, tends to activate regions adjacent to the regions involved in color perception, whereas retrieval of functional information results in activation of areas adjacent to motor cortex. These findings mesh nicely with the perceptual/motor notions of representation in semantic memory reviewed above (e.g., Barsalou, 1999; Rogers et al., 2004). In addition, Roskies et al. (2001) reported that not only were regions in lateral inferior prefrontal cortex (LIPC) preferentially active during tasks that required semantic processing, but specific regions were also sensitive to task difficulty. Thus, it appears that frontal regions are involved both in the active retrieval from semantic memory and in processing specific semantic information.

Many researchers have suggested, however, that although frontal regions are involved in semantic retrieval, the storage of semantic information is primarily in the temporal regions (see Hodges et al., 1992). Indeed, another area that has been implicated in semantic processing is in the ventral region of the temporal lobes, centered on the fusiform gyrus, and especially in the left hemisphere. This area shows significant activation during word reading and object naming tasks, indicating it is not sensitive to the stimulus form but to the semantic content therein (see Martin, 2005, for a review). Furthermore, within this area, different subregions become more or less activated when subjects view faces, houses, and chairs (e.g., Chao et al., 1999), suggesting that different domains rely on different regions of neural tissue. This, of course, could be viewed as consistent with the category-specific deficits reviewed above. However, as noted by Martin and Chao (2001), although peak activation levels in response to objects from different domains reflect a certain degree of localization, the predominant finding is a pattern of broadly distributed activation throughout the ventral temporal and occipital regions, which is consistent with the idea that representations are distributed over large cortical regions.

Recently, Wheatley et al. (2005) reported data from a semantic priming study using fMRI that also converges on the notion of perceptual motor representations of meaning. Subjects silently read related, unrelated, or identical word pairs at a 250-ms SOA while being scanned. The related pairs consisted of category members that were not strongly associatively related (e.g., DOG-GOAT, but see the discussion above regarding the difficulty of selecting such items). Given the relatively fast SOA and that no overt response was required, Wheatley et al. argued that any evidence for priming should be a reflection of automatic processes. Consistent with other evidence that indicates there are reliable neural correlates of behavioral priming that were evidenced by reduced hemodynamic activity (Wiggs and Martin, 1998; Mummery et al., 1999; Rissman et al., 2003; Maccotta and Buckner, 2004), Wheatley et al. found decreased activity for identity pairs and a slightly smaller, but still significant, decrease for related pairs relative to the unrelated pairs condition. Importantly, Wheatley et al. were able to compare patterns of activation as a function of domain. Consistent with proposals by Barsalou (1999), they found that objects from animate objects yielded more activity in regions adjacent to sensory cortex, whereas manipulable artifacts resulted in greater activity in regions adjacent to motor cortex. These findings were taken as evidence that conceptual information about objects is stored, at least in part, in neural regions that are involved in perception and action.

Although the Wheatley et al. (2005) study used a task that was likely to minimize strategic processing, one question that remains to be addressed is whether the automatic and strategic processes involved in semantic priming tasks (see earlier discussion) can also be dissociated in neural tissue. In a recent study, Gold et al. (2006) reported that several of the brain regions previously implicated in processing during semantic tasks are differentially sensitive to the automatic and strategic processes involved in lexical decision tasks. In three experiments, Gold et al. manipulated prime target relatedness, SOA, and whether primes and targets were orthographically or semantically related. Long and short SOAs were intermixed in scanning runs to assess the relative contributions of strategic and automatic processes (see Neely, 1991). A comparison of orthographic and semantic priming conditions was included to determine whether any areas were particularly sensitive to the two sources of priming or whether priming effects are more general mechanisms. The results clearly indicated that different regions responded selectively to different conditions. Specifically, midfusiform gyrus was more sensitive to automatic than strategic priming, but only for semantically related primes, as this region did not show reduced activity for orthographic primes. Four regions were more sensitive to strategic than automatic priming, two in left anterior prefrontal cortex and bilateral anterior cingulate. Even more intriguing, the two regions in LIPC were further dissociated: The anterior region showed strategic semantic facilitation, as evidenced by decreased activity, relative to a neutral baseline, whereas the posterior region showed strategic semantic inhibition, or increased activity, relative to the neutral baseline. In addition, the medial temporal gyrus showed decreased activation concurrently with the anterior LIPC, supporting previous claims that these regions show greater activation in tasks that are more demanding of strategic processes but reduced activation when the strategic processes are less demanding (Wagner et al., 2000; Gold et al., 2005). In sum, it appears that the behavioral dissociations between automatic and strategic processes in priming tasks are also found in the neuroimaging data. The complexity of the patterns of activation involved in semantic tasks appears to indicate that the retrieval and storage of semantic information is indeed a distributed phenomenon that requires the coordination of a wide array of neural tissue.

5.10 Development and Bilingualism

Although we have attempted to provide a review of the major issues addressed in semantic memory research, there are clearly other important areas that we have not considered in detail because of length limitations. For example, there is a very rich area of developmental research addressing the acquisition of meaning in children (see Bloom, 2000, for a comprehensive review), along with work that attempts to capture the nature of semantic memory in older adulthood (see, e.g., Balota and Duchek, 1989). Of course, we touched upon these issues earlier when discussing how the small world networks of Steyvers and Tenenbaum (2005) develop over time, along with the work by Rosch (1975) on the development of categorization. Given that meaning is extracted from interactions with the environment, the developmental literature is particularly important to understand how additional years of experience mold the semantic system, especially in very early life. There are many interesting connections of this work to topics covered earlier in this chapter. For example, regarding the influence of preexisting structures on false memory, it is noteworthy that young children (5-year-olds) are more likely to produce phonological than semantic false memories, whereas older children (around 11 years and older) are more likely to produce the opposite pattern (see Dewhurst and Robinson, 2004). Possibly, this is a natural consequence of the development of a rich semantic network in early childhood that lags behind a more restricted phonological system.

Another very active area of research involves the nature of semantic representations in bilinguals (see Francis, 1999, 2005, for excellent reviews). For example, researchers have attempted to determine whether there is a common semantic substrate that is amodal, with each language having specific lexical level representations (e.g., phonology, orthography, syntax, etc.) that map onto this system. This contrasts with the view that each language engages distinct semantic level representations. Although there is still some controversy, the experimental results seem more consistent with the assumption that the semantic level is shared across languages, at least for skilled bilinguals. Evidence in support of this claim comes from a diverse range of tasks. For example, in a mixed language list, memory for the language of input is generally worse than memory for the concepts (e.g., Dalrymple-Alford and Aamiry, 1969). In addition, one finds robust semantic priming effects by translation equivalents (words in different languages with the same meaning, e.g., DOG in English and HUND in German), which is consistent with at least a partially shared semantic representation (e.g., de Groot and Nas, 1991; Gollan et al., 1997).

5.11 Closing Comments

The nature of how humans develop, represent, and efficiently retrieve information from their vast repository of knowledge has for centuries perplexed investigators of the mind. Although there is clearly considerable work to be done, recent advances in analyses of large-scale databases, new theoretical perspectives from embodied cognition and small world networks, and new technological developments allowing researchers to measure, *in vivo*, brain activity, are making considerable progress toward understanding this fundamental aspect of cognition.

References

Albert R and Barabasi AL (2000) Topology of evolving networks: Local events and universality. *Phys. Rev. Lett.* 85: 5234–5237.

Anderson JR (2000) *Learning and Memory: An Integrated Approach*, 2nd edn. Pittsburgh: Carnegie Mellon.

Anderson JR and Bower GH (1973) *Human Associative Memory*. Washington DC: Hemisphere Press.

Anderson MC, Bjork RA, and Bjork EL (1994) Remembering can cause forgetting: Retrieval dynamics in long-term memory. *J. Exp. Psychol. Learn. Mem. Cogn.* 20: 1063–1087.

Arndt J and Hirshman E (1998) True and false recognition in MINERVA2: Explanations of a global matching perspective. *J. Mem. Lang.* 39: 371–391.

Atkinson RC and Juola JF (1974) Search and decision processes in recognition memory. In: Krantz DH, Atkinson RC, et al. (eds.) *Contemporary Developments in Mathematical Psychology: I Learning, Memory, and Thinking*, pp. 243–293. San Francisco: Freeman.

Baddeley A (2000) Short-term and working memory. In: Tulving E and Craik FIM (eds.) *The Oxford Handbook of Memory*, pp. 77–92. Oxford: Oxford University Press.

Balota DA and Chumbley JI (1984) Are lexical decisions a good measure of lexical access? The role of word frequency in the neglected decision stage. *J Exp. Psychol. Hum. Percept. Perform.* 10: 340–357.

Balota DA and Duchek JM (1989) Spreading activation in episodic memory: Further evidence for age-independence. *Q. J. Exp. Psychol.* 41A: 849–876.

Balota DA and Lorch RF (1986) Depth of automatic spreading activation: Mediated priming effects in pronunciation but not in lexical decision. *J. Exp. Psychol. Learn. Mem. Cogn.* 12: 336–345.

Balota DA and Paul ST (1996) Summation of activation: Evidence from multiple primes that converge and diverge within semantic memory. *J. Exp. Psychol. Learn. Mem. Cogn.* 22: 827–845.

Balota DA, Cortese MJ, Sergent-Marshall S, Spieler DH, and Yap MJ (2004) Visual word recognition of single syllable words. *J. Exp. Psychol. Gen.* 133: 336–345.

Barsalou LW (1985) Ideals, central tendency, and frequency of instantiation as determinants of graded structure in categories. *J. Exp. Psychol. Learn. Mem. Cogn.* 11: 629–654.

Barsalou LW (1999) Perceptual symbol systems. *Behav. Brain Sci.* 22: 577–609.

Barsalou LW (2003) Abstraction in perceptual symbol systems. *Philos. Trans. R. Soc. Lond. Biol. Sci.* 358: 1177–1187.

Barsalou LW, Simmons WK, Barbey A, and Wilson CD (2003) Grounding conceptual knowledge in modality-specific systems. *Trends Cogn. Sci.* 7: 84–91.

Bartlett FC (1932) *Remembering*. Cambridge: Cambridge University Press.

Battig WF and Montague WE (1969) Category norms for verbal items in 56 categories: A replication and extension of the Connecticut category norms. *J. Exp. Psychol. Monogr.* 80: 1–46.

Bloom P (2000) *How Children Learn the Meanings of Words*. Cambridge MA: MIT Press.

Bousfield WA (1953) The occurrence of clustering in the recall of randomly arranged associates. *J. Gen. Psychol.* 49: 229–240.

Bruce D and Fagan RL (1970) More on the recognition and free recall of organized lists. *J. Exp. Psychol.* 85: 153–154.

Bruner JS, Goodnow JJ, and Austin GA (1956) *A Study of Thinking*. New York: Wiley.

Burgess C and Lund K (1997) Modeling parsing constraints with high-dimensional context space. *Lang. Cogn. Process.* 12: 177–210.

Capitani E, Laiacona M, Mahon B, and Caramazza A (2003) What are the facts of semantic category-specific deficits? A critical review of the clinical evidence. *Cogn. Neuropsychol.* 20: 213–261.

Caramazza A and Shelton JR (1998) Domain-specific knowledge systems in the brain: The animate-inanimate distinction. *J. Cogn. Neurosci.* 10: 1–34.

Carey S (1978) The child as a word learner. In: Halle M, Bresnan J, and Miller GA (eds.) *Linguistic Theory and Psychological Reality*, pp. 264–293. Cambridge MA: MIT Press.

Chao LL, Haxby JV, and Martin A (1999) Attribute-based neural substrates in temporal cortex for perceiving and knowing about objects. *Nat. Neurosci.* 2: 913–919.

Chwilla DJ and Kolk HHJ (2002) Three-step priming in lexical decision. *Mem. Cognit.* 30: 217–225.

Cofer CN, Bruce DR, and Reicher GM (1966) Clustering in free recall as a function of certain methodological variations. *J. Exp. Psychol.* 71: 858–866.

Collins AM and Loftus EF (1975) A spreading-activation theory of semantic processing. *Psychol. Rev.* 82: 407–428.

Collins A and Quillian MR (1969) Retrieval time from semantic memory. *J. Verb. Learn. Verb. Behav.* 8: 240–247.

Cree GS and McRae K (2003) Analyzing the factors underlying the structure and computation of the meaning of chipmunk, cherry, chisel, cheese and cello (and many other such concrete nouns). *J. Exp. Psychol. Gen.* 132: 163–201.

Cree GS, McRae K, and McNorgan C (1999) An attractor model of lexical conceptual processing: Simulating semantic priming. *Cogn. Sci.* 23: 371–414.

Crowder RG (1976) *Principles of Learning and Memory*. Hillsdale, NJ: Erlbaum.

Dalrymple-Alford EC and Aamiry A (1969) Word associations of bilinguals. *Psychon. Sci.* 21: 319–320.

Deese J (1959) On the prediction of occurrence of particular verbal intrusions in immediate free recall. *J. Exp. Psychol.* 58: 17–22.

de Groot AMB (1983) The range of automatic spreading activation in word priming. *J. Verb. Learn. Verb. Behav.* 22: 417–436.

de Groot AMB and Nas GLJ (1991) Lexical representation of cognates and non-cognates in compound bilinguals. *J. Mem. Lang.* 30: 90–123.

de Mornay Davies P (1998) Automatic semantic priming: The contribution of lexical- and semantic-level processes. *Eur. J. Cogn. Psychol.* 10: 398–412.

Dewhurst SA and Robinson CA (2004) False memories in children: Evidence for a shift from phonological to semantic associations. *Psychol. Sci.* 15: 782–786.

Durgunoglu AY and Neely JH (1987) On obtaining episodic priming in a lexical decision task following paired-associate learning. *J. Exp. Psychol. Learn. Mem. Cogn.* 13: 206–222.

Ebbinghaus H (1885) *On Memory*. Ruger HA and Bussenius CE (trans.) New York: Teacher' College, 1913.

Faust ME, Balota DA, and Spieler DH (2001) Building episodic connections: Changes in episodic priming with age and dementia. *Neuropsychology* 15: 626–637.

Farah M and McClelland JL (1991) A computational model of semantic memory impairment: Modality-specificity and emergent category specificity. *J. Exp. Psychol. Gen.* 122: 339–357.

Fischler I (1977) Semantic facilitation without association in a lexical decision task. *Mem. Cognit.* 5: 335–339.

Fodor J (1983) *The Modularity of Mind*. Cambridge MA: MIT Press.

Francis WS (1999) Cognitive integration of language and memory in bilinguals: Semantic representation. *Psychol. Bull.* 125: 193–222.

Francis WS (2005) Bilingual semantic and conceptual representation. In: Kroll JF and de Groot AMB (eds.) *Handbook of Bilingualism: Psycholinguistic Approaches*, pp. 251–267. Oxford: Oxford University Press.

Gelman SA and Markman EM (1986) Categories and induction in young children. *Cognition* 23: 183–208.

Gibson JJ (1979) *The Ecological Approach to Visual Perception*. Hillsdale, NJ: Erlbaum.

Glenberg AM and Kaschak MP (2002) Grounding language in action. *Psychon. Bull. Rev.* 9: 558–565.

Glenberg AM and Robertson DA (2000) Symbol grounding and meaning: A comparison of high-dimensional and embodied theories of meaning. *J. Mem. Lang.* 43: 379–401.

Gold BT, Balota DA, Cortese MJ, et al. (2005) Differing neuropsychological and neuroanatomical correlates of abnormal reading in early-stage semantic dementia and dementia of the Alzheimer type. *Neuropsychologia* 43: 833–846.

Gold BT, Balota DA, Jones SJ, Powell DK, Smith CD, and Andersen AH (2006) Dissociation of automatic and strategic lexical-semantics: fMRI evidence for differing roles of multiple frontotemporal regions. *J. Neurosci.* 26: 6523–6532.

Gollan TH, Forster KI, and Frost R (1997) Translation priming with different scripts: Masked priming with cognates and noncognates in Hebrew-English bilinguals. *J. Exp. Psychol. Learn. Mem. Cogn.* 23: 1122–1139.

Hart J, Berndt RS, and Caramazza A (1985) Category-specific naming deficit following cerebral infarction. *Nature* 316: 439–440.

Herrnstein RJ, Loveland DH, and Cable C (1976) Natural concepts in pigeons. *J. Exp. Psychol. Anim. Behav. Process.* 2: 285–302.

Hines D, Czerwinski M, Sawyer PK, and Dwyer M (1986) Automatic semantic priming: Effect of category exemplar level and word association level. *J. Exp. Psychol. Hum. Percept. Perform.* 12: 370–379.

Hintzman DL (1986) "Schema abstraction" in a multiple trace memory model. *Psychol. Rev.* 93: 411–428.

Hintzman DL (1988) Judgements of frequency and recognition memory in a multiple-trace memory model. *Psychol. Rev.* 95: 528–551.

Hodges JR, Patterson K, Oxbury S, and Funnell E (1992) Semantic dementia: Progressive fluent aphasia with temporal lobe atrophy. *Brain* 115: 1793–1806.

Hoffman AB and Murphy GL (2006) Category dimensionality and feature knowledge: When more features are learned as easily as fewer. *J. Exp. Psychol. Learn. Mem. Cogn.* 32: 301–315.

Hoffman RR, Bringmann W, Bamberg M, and Klein R (1987) Some historical observations on Ebbinghaus. In: Gorfein D and Hoffman R (eds.) *Memory and Learning: The Ebbinghaus Centennial Conference*, pp. 57–76. Hillsdale, NJ: Erlbaum.

Howard D and Patterson K (1992) *The Pyramids and Palm Trees Test*. Bury St. Edmunds: Thames Valley Test Company.

Hutchison KA (2003) Is semantic priming due to association strength or feature overlap? A micro-analytic review. *Psychon. Bull. Rev.* 10: 785–813.

Hutchison KA and Balota DA (2005) Decoupling semantic and associative information in false memories: Explorations with semantically ambiguous and unambiguous critical lures. *J. Mem. Lang.* 52: 1–28.

Jacoby LL (1991) A process dissociation framework: Separating automatic from intentional uses of memory. *J. Mem. Lang.* 30: 513–541.

Jeong H, Kahng B, Lee S, Kwak CY, Barabasi AL, and Furdyna JK (2000) Monte Carlo simulation of sinusoidally modulated superlattice growth. *Phys. Rev. E Stat. Nonlin. Soft Matter Phys.* 65: 031602–031605.

LaBerge D and Samuels SJ (1974) Toward a theory of automatic information processing in reading. *Cogn. Psychol.* 6: 293–323.

Landauer TK and Dumais ST (1997) A solution to Plato's problem: The latent semantic analysis theory of acquisition, induction, and representation of knowledge. *Psychol. Rev.* 104: 211–240.

Leach E (1964) Anthropological aspects of language: Animal categories and verbal abuse. In: Lenneberg EH (ed.) *New Directions in the Study of Language.* Cambridge, MA: MIT Press.

Livesay K and Burgess C (1998) Mediated priming in high-dimensional semantic space: No effect of direct semantic relationships or co-occurrence. *Brain Cogn.* 37: 102–105.

Logothetis NK and Wandell BA (2004) Interpreting the BOLD signal. *Annu. Rev. Physiol.* 66: 735–769.

Lucas M (2000) Semantic priming without association: A meta-analytic review. *Psychon. Bull. Rev.* 7: 618–630.

Lupker SJ (1984) Semantic priming without association: A second look. *J. Verb. Learn. Verb. Behav.* 23: 709–733.

Maccotta L and Buckner RL (2004) Evidence for neural effects of repetition that directly correlate with behavioral priming. *J. Cogn. Neurosci.* 16: 1625–1632.

MacKay DG, Burke DM, and Stewart R (1998) HM's language production deficits: Implications for relationships between memory, semantic binding, and the hippocampal system. *J. Mem. Lang.* 38: 28–69.

Martin A (2005) Functional neuroimaging of semantic memory. In: Cabeza R and Kingstone A (eds.) *Handbook of Functional Neuroimaging of Cognition*, pp. 153–186. Cambridge, MA: MIT Press.

Martin A and Chao LL (2001) Semantic memory and the brain: Structure and processes. *Curr. Opin. Neurobiol. Cogn. Neurosci.* 11: 194–201.

Martin A, Haxby JV, Lalonde FM, Wiggs CL, and Ungerleider LG (1995) Discrete cortical regions associated with knowledge of color and knowledge of action. *Science* 270: 102–105.

McCloskey M and Glucksberg S (1979) Decision processes in verifying category membership statements: Implications for models of semantic memory. *Cogn. Psychol.* 11: 1–37.

McKoon G and Ratcliff R (1979) Priming in episodic and semantic memory. *J. Verb. Learn. Verb. Behav.* 18: 463–480.

McKoon G and Ratcliff R (1992) Spreading activation versus compound cue accounts of priming: Mediated priming revisited. *J. Exp. Psychol. Learn. Mem. Cogn.* 18: 1155–1172.

McKoon G, Ratcliff R, and Dell GS (1986) A critical evaluation of the semantic episodic distinction. *J. Exp. Psychol. Learn. Memo. Cogn.* 12: 295–306.

McNamara TP and Altarriba J (1988) Depth of spreading activation revisited: Semantic mediated priming occurs in lexical decisions. *J. Mem. Lang.* 27: 545–559.

McRae K (2004) Semantic memory: Some insights from feature-based connectionist attractor networks. In: Ross BH (ed.) *Psychology of Learning and Motivation*, vol. 45, pp. 41–86. San Diego: Elsevier.

McRae K, De Sa VR, and Seidenberg MS (1997) On the nature and scope of featural representations of word meaning. *J. Exp. Psychol. Gen.* 126: 99–130.

McRae K, Cree GS, Westmacott R, and de Sa VR (1999) Further evidence for feature correlations in semantic memory. *Can. J. Exp. Psychol.* (Special issue on models of word recognition) 53: 360–373.

McRae K, Cree GS, Seidenberg MS, and McNorgan C (2005) Semantic feature production norms for a large set of living and nonliving things. *Behav. Res. Methods Instr. Comput.* 37: 547–559.

Medin DL (1989) Concepts and conceptual structure. *Am. Psychol.* 44: 1469–1481.

Meyer DE and Schvaneveldt RW (1971) Facilitation in recognizing words: Evidence of a dependence upon retrieval operations. *J. Exp. Psychol.* 90: 227–234.

Milgram S (1967) The small world problem. *Psychol. Today* 2: 60–67.

Miller GA (1990) WordNet: An on-line lexical database. *Int. J. Lexiogr.* 3: 235–312.

Mummery CJ, Shallice T, and Price CJ (1999) Dual-process model in semantic priming: A functional neuroimaging perspective. *Neuroimage* 9: 516–525.

Murphy G (2002) *The Big Book of Concepts*. Cambridge, MA: MIT Press.

Neely JH (1977) Semantic priming and retrieval from lexical memory: Roles of inhibitionless spreading activation and limited-capacity attention. *J. Exp. Psychol. Gen.* 106: 226–254.

Neely JH (1991) Semantic priming effects in visual word recognition: A selective review of current findings and theories. In: Besner D and Humphreys G (eds.) *Basic Processes in Reading: Visual Word Recognition*, pp. 236–264. Hillsdale, NJ: Erlbaum.

Neely JH and Durgunoglu AY (1985) Dissociative episodic and semantic priming effects in episodic recognition and lexical decision tasks. *J. Mem. Lang.* 24: 466–489.

Nelson DL, McEvoy CL, and Schreiber TA (1998) The University of South Florida word association, rhyme, and word fragment norms. http://www.usf.edu/FreeAssociation/.

Osgood CE, Suci GJ, and Tanenbaum PH (1957) *The Measurement of Meaning*. Urbana: University of Illinois Press.

Pecher D and Raaijmakers JGW (1999) Automatic priming effects for new associations in lexical decision and perceptual identification. *Q. J. Exp. Psychol.* 52A: 593–614.

Pecher D, Zeelenberg R, and Barsalou LW (2003) Verifying properties from different modalities for concepts produces switching costs. *Psychol. Sci.* 14: 119–124.

Pecher D, Zeelenberg R, and Barsalou LW (2004) Sensorimotor simulations underlie conceptual representations: Modality-specific effects of prior activation. *Psychon. Bull. Rev.* 11: 164–167.

Petersen SE, Fox PT, Posner M, Mintun M, and Raichle M (1988) Positron emission topographic studies of the cortical anatomy of single word processing. *Nature* 331: 585–589.

Pexman PM, Lupker SJ, and Hino Y (2002) The impact of feedback semantics in visual word recognition: Number of features effects in lexical decision and naming tasks. *Psychon. Bull. Rev.* 9: 542–549.

Pexman PM, Holyk GG, and Monfils M-H (2003) Number of features effects and semantic processing. *Mem. Cognit.* 31: 842–855.

Pinker S (1994) *The Language Instinct*. New York: Harper Collins.

Posner MI and Keele SW (1968) On the genesis of abstract ideas. *J. Exp. Psychol.* 77: 353–363.

Posner MI and Snyder CRR (1975) Attention and cognitive control. In: Solso R (ed.) *Information Processing and Cognition: The Loyola Symposium*, pp. 55–85. Hillsdale, NJ: Erlbaum.

Quillian M (1968) Semantic memory. In: Minsky M (ed.) *Semantic Information Processing*, pp. 227–270. Cambridge, MA: MIT Press.

Quine WVO (1960) *Word and Object*. Cambridge, MA: MIT Press.

Riddoch MJ and Humphreys GW (1987) Visual object processing in optic aphasia: A case of semantic access agnosia. *Cogn. Neuropsychol.* 4: 131–185.

Rissman J, Eliassen JC, and Blumstein SE (2003) An event-related fMRI investigation of implicit semantic priming. *J. Cogn. Neurosci.* 15: 1160–1175.

Roediger HL III and McDermott KB (1995) Creating false memories: Remembering words not presented in lists. *J. Exp. Psychol. Learn. Mem. Cogn.* 21: 803–814.

Roediger HL III, Balota DA, and Watson JM (2001a) Spreading activation and arousal of false memories. In: Roediger HL and Nairne JS (eds) *The Nature of Remembering: Essays in Honor of Robert G. Crowder*, pp. 95–115. Washington DC: American Psychological Association.

Roediger HL III, Watson JM, McDermott KB, and Gallo DA (2001b) Factors that determine false recall: A multiple regression analysis. *Psychon. Bull. Rev.* 8: 385–407.

Rogers TT, Lambon RMA, Garrard P, et al. (2004) Structure and deterioration of semantic memory: A neuropsychological and computational investigation. *Psychol. Rev.* 111: 205–235.

Roget PM (1911) *Roget's Thesaurus of English Words and Phrases*. Available from Project Gutenberg Illinois Benedictine College, Lisle, IL.

Rosch E (1973) On the internal structure of perceptual and semantic categories. In: Moore TE (ed.) *Cognitive Development and the Acquisition of Language*, pp. 111–144. New York: Academic Press.

Rosch E (1975) Cognitive representations of semantic categories. *J. Exp. Psychol. Gen.* 104: 192–233.

Rosch E, Mervis CB, Gray WD, Johnson DM, and Boyes-Braem P (1976) Basic objects in natural categories. *Cogn. Psychol.* 8: 382–440.

Roskies AL, Fiez JA, Balota DA, and Petersen SE (2001) Task-dependent modulation of regions in left inferior frontal cortex during semantic processing. *J. Cogn. Neurosci.* 13: 1–16.

Sachett C and Humphreys GW (1992) Calling a squirrel a squirrel but a canoe a wigwam: A category-specific deficit for artefactual objects and body parts. *Cogn. Neuropsychol.* 9: 73–86.

Sayette MA, Hufford MR, and Thorson GM (1996) Developing a brief measure of semantic priming. *J. Clin. Exp. Neuropsychol.* 8: 678–684.

Scoville WB and Milner B (1957) Loss of recent memory after bilateral hippocampal lesions. *J. Neurol. Neurosurg. Neuropsychiatry* 20: 11–21.

Simons JS, Graham KS, and Hodges JR (2002) Perceptual and semantic contributions to episodic memory: Evidence from semantic dementia and Alzheimer's disease. *J. Mem. Lang.* 47: 197–213.

Smith EE, Shoben EJ, and Rips LJ (1974) Structure and process in semantic memory: A featural model for semantic decisions. *Psychol. Rev.* 81: 214–241.

Solomon KO and Barsalou LW (2004) Perceptual simulation in property verification. *Mem. Cognit.* 32: 244–259.

Sperling G (1960) The information available in brief visual presentation. *Psychol. Monogr.* 74(11) (Whole No. 498).

Spieler DH and Balota DA (1996) Characteristics of associative learning in younger and older adults: Evidence from an episodic priming paradigm. *Psychol. Aging* 11: 607–620.

Steyvers M and Tenenbaum JB (2005) The large-scale structure of semantic networks: Statistical analyses and a model of semantic growth. *Cogn. Sci.* 29: 41–78.

Thompson-Schill SL, Kurtz KJ, and Gabrieli JDE (1998) Effects of semantic and associative relatedness on automatic priming. *J. Mem. Lang.* 38: 440–458.

Tulving E (1972) Episodic and semantic memory. In: Tulving E and Donaldson W (eds.) *Organization of Memory*, pp. 381–403. New York: Academic Press.

Tulving E (1985) Memory and consciousness. *Can. Psychol.* 26: 1–12.

Tulving E and Pearlstone Z (1966) Availability versus accessibility of information in memory for words. *J. Verb. Learn. Verb. Behav.* 5: 381–391.

Wagner AD, Koutstaal W, Maril A, Schacter DL, and Buckner RL (2000) Task-specific repetition priming in left inferior prefrontal cortex. *Cereb. Cortex* 10: 1176–1184.

Warrington EK and McCarthy R (1987) Categories of knowledge: Further fractionations and an attempted integration. *Brain* 110: 1273–1296.

Watts DJ and Strogatz SH (1998) Collective dynamics of "small-world" networks. *Nature* 393: 440–442.

Wheatley T, Weisberg J, Beauchamp MS, and Martin A (2005) Automatic priming of semantically related words reduces activity in the fusiform gyrus. *J. Cogn. Neurosci.* 17: 1871–1885.

Wickens DD (1973) Some characteristics of word encoding. *Mem. Cogn.* 1: 485–490.

Wiggs CL and Martin A (1998) Properties and mechanisms of perceptual priming. *Curr. Opin. Neurobiol.* 8: 227–233.

Wilson M (2002) Six views of embodied cognition. *Psychon. Bull. Rev.* 9: 625–636.

6 Structural Basis of Semantic Memory

A. Martin and W. K. Simmons, National Institute of Mental Health, Bethesda, MD, USA

Published by Elsevier Ltd.

6.1 Introduction

Semantic memory refers to a major division of long-term memory that includes knowledge of facts, events, ideas, and concepts. Thus, semantic memory covers a vast cognitive terrain, ranging from information about historical and scientific facts, to details of public events and mathematical equations, to the information that allows us to identify objects and understand the meaning of words. This chapter focuses on our current understanding of how semantic memories, especially object concepts, are represented in the brain. As we discuss later, ideas about the neural systems underpinning conceptual knowledge have a long history in behavioral neurology and neuropsychology dating back at least to the late nineteenth century. In recent times, however, the idea of semantic memory as a distinct memory system began in 1972 with Endel Tulving's distinction between semantic and episodic memory (Tulving, 1972). Although the notion of episodic memory has undergone considerable evolution since that original formulation (for a brief history see Tulving, 2002), it remains helpful to describe the properties of semantic memory in relation to episodic memory. In current formulations, episodic memory can be thought of as synonymous with autobiographical memory. Episodic memory is the system that allows us to remember (consciously recollect) past experiences (Tulving, 2002) and perhaps may also be critical for imagining and/or simulating future events (Hassabis et al., 2007; Schacter and Addis, 2007). Semantic memories, in contrast, are devoid of information about personal experience. Unlike episodic memories, semantic memories lack information about the context of learning, including situational properties like time and place, and personal dimensions like how we felt at the time the event was experienced. Remembering that you had cereal and toast for breakfast, that you read the newspaper, and that you had a slight headache is dependent on episodic memory. Knowing and, indeed, being able to visually recognize objects like cereal, toast, and newspaper, as well as understanding the words you are now reading, is dependent on semantic memory. In relation to episodic memory, semantic memory is considered to be both a phylogenically and an ontologically older system. In fact, rather than arising as an independent evolutionary development, it is commonly assumed that episodic memory emerged as an add-on or embellishment to semantic memory (Tulving, 2002). Although many animals, especially mammals and birds, acquire information about the world, they are assumed to lack the neural machinery to consciously recollect detailed episodes of their past. Finally, although retrieval of semantic memory often requires explicit, conscious mediation, the organization of semantic memory can also be revealed via implicit tasks such as semantic priming (e.g., Neely, 1991).

The idea that our semantic and episodic memories were dependent on a distinct neural substrate was perhaps first proposed by the American neurologist J.M. Nielsen (1958). As Nielsen noted, amnesia came in two types. One type, which he termed temporal amnesia, was defined by a loss of memory for personal experiences. The other type, which he termed categorical amnesia, was defined by a loss of acquired facts. Nielsen further noted that there were different varieties of categorical amnesias, including amnesias for animate objects and amnesias for inanimate objects (Nielsen, 1946, 1958), presaging a distinction that is prominently highlighted later in this chapter. Nielsen also maintained that the temporal (episodic) and categorical (semantic) amnesias could occur in isolation, thereby noting that their respective neural substrates might be at least partially independent (Nielsen, 1958). Indeed, studies of patients with conceptual deficits have provided some support for Nielsen's claim (Hodges and Graham, 2001; Simons et al., 2002). However, before discussing those patients, we first discuss studies of semantic memory in patients with profound amnesias resulting from damage to the medial temporal lobes. These studies have provided evidence that medial temporal lobe structures play a critical role in acquiring and retrieving both semantic and episodic memories.

6.2 Semantic Memory and the Medial Temporal Lobe Memory System

Studies of patients with impaired episodic memory resulting from damage to the medial temporal lobes have established three broadly agreed-on facts about the functional neuroanatomy of semantic memory. First, like episodic memory, acquisition of semantic memories is dependent on medial temporal lobe structures, including the hippocampal region (CA fields, dentate gyrus, and subiculum) and surrounding neocortex (parahippocampal, entorhinal, and perirhinal cortices). Damage to these structures results in deficient acquisition of new information about vocabulary and famous individuals (e.g., Gabrieli et al., 1988; Hamann and Squire, 1995; Verfaellie et al., 2000, patient SS) and public events (Manns et al., 2003), and the extent of this deficit is roughly equivalent to the deficit for acquiring personal information about day-to-day occurrences.

However, despite broad agreement that acquiring semantic memories requires medial temporal lobe structures, there is disagreement concerning the role of the hippocampal region. One position holds that the hippocampus is necessary for acquiring semantic information (for discussion, see Squire and Zola, 1998). In contrast, others have argued that acquisition of semantic memories can be accomplished by the surrounding neocortical structures alone; participation of the hippocampus is not necessary (for discussion, see Mishkin et al., 1998). Recent studies seem to favor the hippocampal position by showing that carefully selected patients with damage limited to the hippocampus are impaired in learning semantic information about public events (Manns et al., 2003). One potentially important caveat to this claim comes from studies of individuals who have sustained damage to the hippocampus at birth or during early childhood (Vargha-Khadem et al., 1997). These cases of developmental amnesia have disproportionately better semantic than episodic memories, suggesting that the hippocampus may not be necessary for acquiring semantic information. For example, cases of developmental delay resulting from hippocampal damage, although failing to provide accurate descriptions of their daily activities (episodic memory), were able to acquire normal language and social skills, keep up with their schoolwork, and perform in the average range on standard measures of vocabulary and general knowledge (Vargha-Khadem et al., 1997). These findings pose a clear challenge to the standard hippocampal model of declarative memory. Although discussion of this important issue is outside the purview of this chapter, it is certain that a reconciliation of this issue will depend on detailed and direct comparison of adult onset and developmental amnesias with regard to the extent of medial temporal lobe damage and its behavioral consequences.

The second major finding established by studies of amnesic patients is that the medial temporal lobe structures have a time-limited role in the retrieval of semantic memories, which is, in turn, presumably related to a prolonged consolidation process (Squire and Alvarez,1995; but see Moscovitch et al., 2005, for a critique of prolonged consolidation and a reappraisal of the role of the hippocampus in memory retrieval). Evidence in favor of the claim of a time-limited role for the hippocampal region in retrieving semantic memories comes from studies assessing the status of information acquired prior versus after the amnesia onset. Such studies have revealed that, for example, public event knowledge is temporally graded, with increasing accuracy for events further in time from the onset of the amnesia (Kapur and Brooks, 1999; Manns et al., 2003). The length of this temporally graded amnesia, however, can be surprisingly long and probably varies as a function of type of information tested and testing method. For example, in the Manns et al. study, the temporal gradient for news events lasted from 10 to 15 years when evaluated by a test of recall but less than 5 years when evaluated by a recognition test (Manns et al., 2003).

Studies of object and word knowledge are also consistent with the claim that the hippocampus has a time-limited role in retrieving semantic memories. Conceptual information about the meaning of objects and words known to be acquired decades prior to amnesia onset remains intact as assessed by both explicit and implicit tasks. Patients with damage to the hippocampal region are unimpaired on tests of object naming, object property verification, and object category sorting (e.g., Schmolck et al., 2002) and show normal semantic priming (Cave and Squire, 1992).

The third major finding established by studies of amnesic patients is that semantic memories of all types are stored in the cerebral cortex. Most importantly for our present concerns, impaired knowledge about objects and their associated properties acquired prior to amnesia onset is not related to medial temporal lobe damage but rather to the extent of damage to cortex outside this region (e.g., Levy et al., 2004).

6.3 Cortical Lesions and the Breakdown of Semantic Memory

Studies of semantic memory in amnesia have concentrated largely on measures of public event knowledge. The reason for this is that these tasks allow memory performance to be assessed for events known to have occurred either prior to or after amnesia onset. These measures also allow performance to be evaluated for events that occurred at different times prior to amnesia onset to determine whether the memory impairment shows a temporal gradient – a critical issue for evaluating theories of memory consolidation (Moscovitch et al., 2005). However, because these patients have either no or, more commonly, limited damage to regions outside the medial temporal lobes, they are not informative about how semantic information is organized in the cerebral cortex. To address this issue, investigators have turned to patients with relatively focal lesions compromising different cortical areas. In contrast to the studies of amnesic patients, these studies have focused predominantly on measures designed to probe knowledge of object concepts.

6.3.1 Object Concepts

An object concept refers to the representation (i.e., information stored in memory) of an object category (a class of objects in the external world) (Murphy, 2002). The primary function of a concept is to allow us to quickly draw inferences about an object's properties. That is, identifying an object as, for example, a 'hammer' means that we know that this is an object that is used to pound nails, so we do not have to rediscover this property each time the object is encountered (see Murphy, 2002, for an extensive review of cognitive studies of concepts).

A major feature of object concepts is that they are hierarchically organized, with the broadest knowledge represented at the superordinate level, more specific knowledge at an intermediary level commonly referred to as the 'basic level,' and the most specific information at the subordinate level (Rosch, 1978). For example, 'dog' is a basic-level category that belongs to the superordinate categories 'animal' and 'living things' and has subordinate categories such as 'poodle' and 'collie.' As established by Eleanor Rosch and colleagues in the 1970s, the basic level has a privileged status (Rosch et al., 1976; Rosch, 1978). It is the level used nearly exclusively to name objects (e.g., 'dog' rather than 'poodle'). It is also the level at which we are fastest to verify category membership (i.e., we are faster to verify that a picture is a dog than that it is an animal or a poodle). It is also the level at which subordinate category members share the most properties (e.g., collies and poodles have similar shapes and patterns of movement). Finally, the basic level is the easiest level at which to form a mental image (you can easily imagine an elephant but not an animal). As discussed next, studies of patients with cortical damage have documented the neurobiological reality of this hierarchical scheme and the central role of the basic level for representing objects in the human brain.

6.3.2 Semantic Dementia and the General Disorders of Semantic Memory

Several neurological conditions can result in a relatively global or general disorder of conceptual knowledge. These disorders are considered general in the sense that they cut across multiple category boundaries; they are not category specific. Many of these patients suffer from a progressive neurological disorder of unknown etiology referred to as semantic dementia (SD) (Snowden et al., 1989; Hodges et al., 1992). General disorders of semantic memory are also prominent in patients with Alzheimer's disease (who typically have a greater episodic memory impairment than SD patients) (Martin and Fedio, 1983) and can also occur following left hemisphere stroke, prominently involving the left temporal lobe (e.g., Hart and Gordon, 1990).

The defining characteristics of semantic dementia, initially described by Elizabeth Warrington in the mid-1970s, are relatively isolated deficits on measures designed to probe knowledge of objects and their associated properties (Warrington, 1975). These deficits include impaired object naming (with errors typically consisting of semantic errors – retrieving the name of another basic level object from the same category, or retrieving a superordinate category name), impaired generation of the names of objects within a superordinate category (i.e., semantic category fluency), and an inability to retrieve information about object properties – including sensory-based information (shape, color) and functional information (motor-based properties related to the object's customary use – but may include other kinds of information not directly related to sensory or motor properties) (Warrington, 1975; Martin and Fedio, 1983; Patterson and Hodges, 1995). In contrast to modality-specific agnosias, the impairment is not limited to stimuli presented in a single modality like vision but, rather, extends to all tasks probing object knowledge regardless of stimulus presentation modality (visual, auditory, tactile) or format (words, pictures). In agreement with studies of the psychological nature of concepts, the semantic deficit reveals a hierarchical structure. Broad levels of knowledge are often preserved, whereas specific information is impaired. Thus, these patients can sort objects into superordinate categories, having, for example, no difficulty indicating which are animals, which are tools, which are foods, and the like (Warrington, 1975; Martin and Fedio, 1983). Their primary difficulty manifests as a problem distinguishing among the basic level objects as revealed by impaired performance on measures of naming and object property knowledge. For example, when confronted with a picture of a specific basic level object like 'camel,' these patients often produce the name of another object from the same conceptual category (e.g., 'goat') or a superordinate term ('animal') (Warrington, 1975; Martin and Fedio, 1983).

Recent studies have expanded our understanding of SD in two important ways: one related to location of neuropathology, the other to functional characteristics of the disorder. The initial neuropathological and imaging studies of SD indicated prominent atrophy of the temporal lobes, especially to the anterolateral sector of the left temporal lobe, including the temporal polar cortex, the inferior and middle temporal gyri, and the most anterior extent of the fusiform gyrus (Hodges and Patterson, 1996). However, recent advances in neuroimaging that allow for direct and detailed comparison of brain morphology in SD patients relative to healthy control subjects have shown that the atrophy extends more posteriorally along the temporal lobe than previously appreciated (Mummery et al., 2000; Gorno-Tempini et al., 2004; Williams et al., 2005). In fact, the amount of atrophy in ventral occipitotemporal cortex, including the posterior portion of the fusiform gyrus, has been reported to be as strongly related to the semantic impairment in SD as is atrophy in the most anterior regions of the temporal lobes (Williams et al., 2005).

The other major advance in our understanding of SD is that it is not as global a conceptual disorder as initially thought. Rather, certain domains of knowledge may be preserved, and the pattern of impaired and preserved knowledge appears to be related to the locus of pathology. Specifically, left-sided atrophy seems to impair information about all object categories except person-specific knowledge (i.e., information about famous people), which in turn is associated with involvement of the right anterior temporal lobes (Thompson et al., 2004). Also relatively spared is knowledge of number and mathematical concepts (Cappelletti et al., 2005), a domain strongly associated with left posterior parietal cortex (Dehaene et al., 2003).

6.3.3 Category-Specific Disorders of Semantic Memory

Although case reports of relatively circumscribed knowledge disorders date back over 100 years, the modern era of the study of category-specific disorders began in the early 1980s with the seminal reports of Warrington and colleagues (Warrington and Shallice, 1984; Warrington and McCarthy, 1987). Category-specific disorders have the same functional characteristics as SD, except that the impairment is largely limited to members of a single superordinate object category. For example, a patient with a category-specific disorder for 'animals' will have greater difficulty naming and retrieving information about members of this superordinate category relative to members of other superordinate categories (e.g., tools, furniture, flowers). Similar to patients with SD, patients with category-specific disorders have difficulty distinguishing among basic level objects (e.g., between dog, cat, horse), thereby suggesting a loss or degradation of information that uniquely distinguishes members of the superordinate category (e.g., four-legged animals) (for recent collection of papers on these patients see Martin and Caramazza, 2003).

A variety of category-specific disorders have been reported such as relatively circumscribed deficits for knowing about fruits and vegetables (Hart et al., 1985; Crutch and Warrington, 2003). However, consistent with Nielsen's clinical observations (Nielsen 1946, 1958), most common have been reports of patients with relatively greater knowledge deficits for animate entities – especially animals, than for a variety of inanimate object categories. Although less common, other patients show the opposite dissociation: a greater impairment for inanimate manmade objects – including common tools – than for animals and other living things (for extensive review of the clinical literature, see Capitani et al., 2003).

6.3.3.1 Models of category-specific disorders

Two major theoretical positions have been advanced to explain these disorders. Following the explanation posited by Warrington for her initial cases, most current investigators assume that category-specific deficits are a direct consequence of an object property-based organization of conceptual knowledge, an idea that was prominent in the writings of Karl Wernicke, Sigmund Freud, and other behavioral neurologists during the late nineteenth and early twentieth centuries. The central idea is that object knowledge is organized in the brain by sensory (e.g., form, motion, color, smell, taste) and motor properties associated with the object's use (Martin et al., 2000), and in some models other functional/verbally mediated properties such as where an object is typically found (for discussion of sensory/functional models, see Forde and Humphreys, 1999). In this property-based view, category-specific semantic disorders occur when a lesion disrupts information about a particular property or set of properties critical for defining and for distinguishing among category members. Thus, damage to regions that store information about object form, and form-related properties like color and texture, will produce a disorder for animals. This is because visual appearance is assumed to be a critical property for defining animals and because the distinction between different animals is assumed to be heavily dependent on knowing about subtle differences in their visual forms. A critical prediction of sensory-/motor-based models is that the lesion should affect knowledge of all object categories with this characteristic, not only animals. In a similar fashion, damage to regions that store information about how an object is used should produce a category-specific disorder for tools and all other categories of objects defined by how they are manipulated. Cognitive studies with normal individuals on the relationship between and among object features and attributes show broad consistency with the known patterns of category-specific disorders, thus providing additional evidence in support of property-based models (Cree and McRae, 2003).

The alternative to these property-based theories is the domain-specific view championed most recently by Alfonso Caramazza and colleagues (Caramazza and Shelton, 1998; Caramazza and Mahon, 2003). On this account, our evolutionary history provides the major constraint on the organization of conceptual knowledge in the brain. Specifically, the theory proposes that selection pressures have resulted in dedicated neural machinery for solving, quickly and efficiently, computationally complex survival problems. Likely candidate domains offered are animals, conspecifics, plant life, and possibly tools (for a detailed discussion of these models, see Caramazza, 1998). Property-based and category-based accounts are not mutually exclusive. For example, it is certainly possible that concepts are organized by domains of knowledge, implemented in the brain by large-scale property-based systems (Mahon and Caramazza, 2003). Much of the functional neuroimaging evidence to be discussed later is consistent with this view.

6.3.3.2 Functional neuroanatomy of category-specific disorders

There is considerable variability in the location of lesions associated with category-specific disorders for animate and inanimate entities. Nevertheless, some general tendencies can be observed. In particular, category-specific knowledge disorders for animals are disproportionately associated with damage to the temporal lobes (Gainotti, 2000). The most common etiology is herpes simplex encephalitis, a viral condition with a predilection for attacking anteromedial and inferior (ventral) temporal cortices (Adams et al., 1997). Category-specific knowledge disorders for animals also have been reported following focal, ischemic lesions to the more posterior regions of ventral temporal cortex, including the fusiform gyrus (Vandenbulcke et al., 2006). In contrast, category-specific knowledge disorders for tools and their associated actions have been most commonly associated with focal damage to lateral frontal and parietal cortices of the left hemisphere (Tranel et al., 1997; Gainotti, 2000). However, it is important to stress that the lesions in patients presenting with category-specific knowledge disorders are often large and show considerable variability in their location from one patient to another (Capitani et al., 2003). As a result, these cases have been relatively uninformative for questions concerning the organization of object memories in cerebral cortex. In contrast, recent functional neuroimaging studies of the intact human brain have begun to shed some light on this thorny issue.

6.4 The Organization of Conceptual Knowledge: Neuroimaging Evidence

6.4.1 Neuroimaging of Semantic Memory

For nearly two decades cognitive neuroscientists have used positron emission tomography (PET) and functional magnetic resonance imaging (fMRI) to explore the functional neuroanatomy of semantic memory. Although the particular methods, experimental paradigms, and stimuli vary widely, the general tack taken in most studies has been to compare brain activity when subjects engage in tasks requiring the encoding or retrieval of conceptual information (e.g., Is this object a man-made artifact?) versus the activity associated with equally difficult nonconceptual processing (e.g., Does this object's name contain the letter b?), using the same stimuli. The neuroanatomical claims made by these studies are further strengthened when subsequent research observes activity in the same brain regions using stimuli that are conceptually related (e.g., judging whether objects are artifacts) but physically different (e.g., seeing photographs vs. hearing sounds vs. reading names of artifacts). Such findings demonstrate that the regions are responding to the stimuli's conceptual content rather than their physical characteristics. As we will see, however, this does not mean that objects' physical properties are unimportant to their neural representations. On the contrary, using a variety of concepts and object categories, it has been well documented that object concepts are represented in the brain as distributed property circuits, whereby the information most relevant to real-world interactions with an object is stored in the same sensorimotor regions active when that information was acquired.

Studies comparing conceptual to nonconceptual processing consistently identify three brain regions – the left ventrolateral prefrontal cortex (VLPFC) and the ventral and lateral regions of the temporal lobes. A large functional neuroimaging literature demonstrates that the VLPFC serves as a control center for semantic memory, guiding retrieval and postretrieval selection of concept property information stored in other brain regions (Bookheimer, 2002; Martin, 2001; Thompson-Schill, 2003). These functional neuroimaging findings are consistent with neuropsychological findings with patients who, subsequent to left inferior frontal lesions, exhibit word retrieval difficulties while retaining conceptual knowledge for those same words (Baldo and Shimamura, 1998; Thompson-Schill et al., 1998). Information about this region's role in semantic memory has been augmented by recent functional neuroimaging studies that find distinct mechanisms within the VLPFC for information retrieval and selection among competing alternatives (Badre et al., 2005). Although claims for dissociable retrieval and selection subregions in VLPFC remain controversial, there is wide agreement that this region's primary role is to control and manipulate information stored elsewhere (Gold et al., 2005, 2006).

6.4.2 Object Concepts as Sensorimotor Property Circuits

In addition to the VLPFC, a significant body of research demonstrates that various property regions located in or near perceptual cortex store information about object concepts. In particular, these studies find that the posterior ventral and lateral temporal lobes are particularly important for storing information about object concepts (Martin and Chao, 2001; Thompson-Schill, 2003; Martin, 2007). We will see that important clues about how knowledge is represented in the human brain come from how information is organized within these regions.

As described earlier, cases of category-specific deficits point toward a central role for property information in the organization of semantic memory. Early functional neuroimaging research using PET imaging supported these lesion study findings. Using a property production task in which subjects were required to generate a word describing a specific property of a visually presented object, Martin and colleagues (Martin et al., 1995; also see Chao and Martin, 1999; Wiggs et al., 1999) demonstrated that producing color-associate words (e.g., saying 'yellow' in response to an achromatic picture of a pencil or to its written name) elicited activity in the fusiform gyrus just anterior to regions activated when subjects passively viewed color stimuli. In contrast, producing action word associates (e.g., saying 'write' in response to a pencil) elicited activity in premotor cortex as well as a region of the left posterior middle temporal gyrus (pMTG) just anterior to primary visual motion-selective cortex MT/V5. Similar effects have now been observed for other property modalities as well, with sound, touch, and taste properties activating the corresponding auditory, somatosensory, and gustatory cortical regions (Kellenbach et al., 2001; Goldberg et al., 2006).

Functional neuroimaging findings demonstrating that retrieving object property information activated regions near perceptual and motor cortex are highly suggestive of the sensorimotor hypotheses generated in the literature on category-specific disorders. More recently, however, strong evidence for these accounts has come from fMRI studies demonstrating direct overlaps in the neural bases of knowledge, perception, and action. For example, Simmons et al. (in press) demonstrated a direct overlap in the neural bases of color perception and color knowledge retrieval. Using an attention-demanding task requiring fine-grain discriminations among color hues, they first mapped the brain regions underlying color perception. Next, in separate scanning runs, they presented subjects with a verbal property verification task in which they indicated whether color or motor property words could be true of a concept word. Using the color perception task as a functional localizer, they observed that the most color-responsive region in the perception task, located in the left fusiform gyrus, was also activated for color knowledge retrieval relative to retrieving motor knowledge (**Figure 1**). Evidence for direct overlaps between knowledge retrieval and sensorimotor

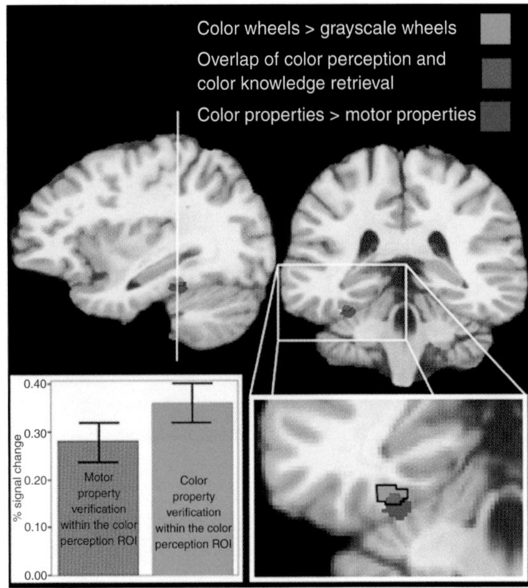

Figure 1 Overlap in perceptual and conceptual color processing. On top, the figure depicts sagittal and coronal sections from the N27 template brain warped to Talairach space (template available in AFNI). The functional overlays represent Talairach-normalized group data from the random effects analysis. Green patches indicate regions where activity was greater for processing color than grayscale wheels in the color perception task ($p < 0.0001$). Blue patches indicate regions where activity was greater for verifying color properties than motor properties in the knowledge retrieval task ($p < 0.01$ with a cluster size of at least 108 mm^3). The red patch in the left fusiform gyrus indicates the region of overlap between the two tasks. The inset bar graph demonstrates that within the left fusiform ROI, where color perception produced a greater response than grayscale perception (in other words, within the combined green and red patches), the average BOLD response to color property words in the property verification task was greater than the response for motor property words ($p = 0.006$). The y-axis indicates percent signal change relative to signal baseline, with error bars representing $\pm$ 1 standard error of the subject means. Adapted from Simmons WK, Ramjee V, Beauchamp MS, McRae K, Martin K, Martin A, and Barsalou LW (in press) A common neural substrate for perceiving and knowing about color. *Neuropsycholgia*.

property systems are not limited to color properties. For example, Pulvermuller and colleagues have demonstrated that simply reading words referring to actions performed with a particular body part (e.g., lick, kick, pick) activated the corresponding motor cortex (e.g., face, foot, and hand representations, respectively) (Hauk et al., 2004).

Together, these findings support claims that knowledge about a particular object property, such as its color or the actions associated with it, resides in the same sensorimotor regions that are active when that information is experienced in the external world. If this is correct, then object categories should have predictable neural representations based on their multimodal property profiles. This appears to be the case. For example, the most salient properties of appetizing foods are how they look, how they taste, and how rewarding they are to eat. Using fMRI, Simmons et al. (2005) demonstrated that viewing images of appetizing foods (e.g., cookies, pizza) while performing a low-level picture repetition detection task was enough to elicit bilateral activity in ventral occipito-temporal regions tuned to represent object form information (e.g., how objects look). Consistent with the sensorimotor account of knowledge representation, the researchers also observed activity in regions of the right insula/operculum (primary gustatory cortex) and left orbitofrontal cortex (OFC) (secondary gustatory cortex) activated in prior fMRI studies when subjects received tastants orally in the scanner (**Figure 2**).

(a)

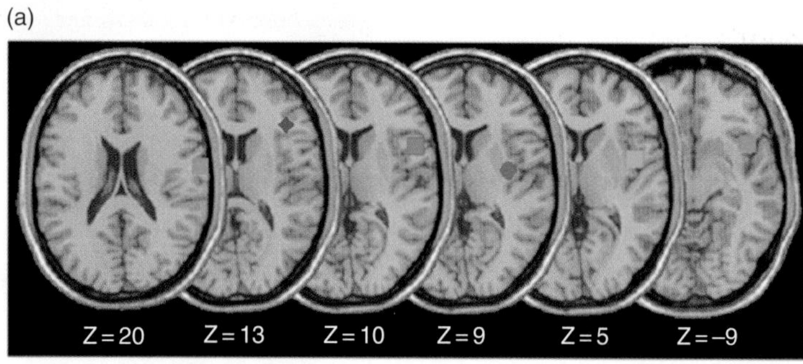

(b)

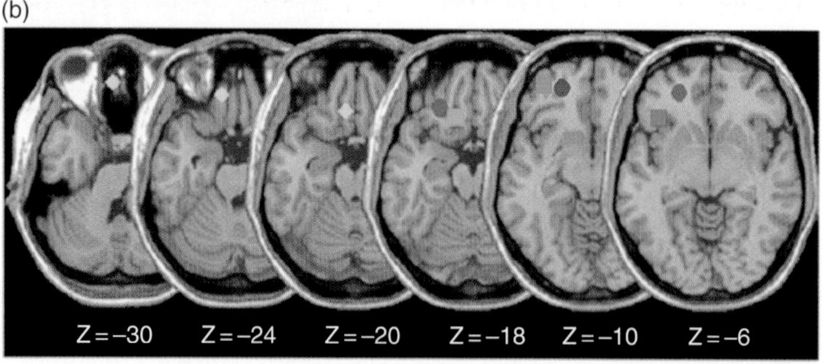

Figure 2 (a) Locations of peak right hemisphere insula/operculum activations reported in taste perception studies. (b) Locations of peak left orbitofrontal cortex (OFC) activations across various tasks. The green squares in the insula/operculum at $Z=20$ and $Z=-9$ represent peak activations observed when participants taste sucrose, whereas the green square in the lateral OFC at $Z=-10$ is the peak activation in the area observed to respond to the combination of gustatory and olfactory stimuli, and thus it is a likely candidate for being the center of flavor representation (de Araujo et al., 2003b). The blue diamond in the insula/operculum at $Z=13$ indicates an area of common activation when participants tasted either glucose or salt (O'Doherty et al., 2001b). The pink squares in the insula/operculum at $Z=10$ and in the OFC at $Z=-6$ indicate the peak activations observed when participants taste umami (de Araujo et al., 2003a). The aqua squares in the insula/operculum at $Z=5$ and in the OFC at $Z=-18$ represent peak activations when participants tasted glucose (Francis et al., 1999). Yellow diamonds in the inferior medial OFC represent peak activations observed when participants receive abstract rewards (O'Doherty et al., 2001a). The blue circle in the OFC at $Z=-10$ represents peak activation observed when participants verify the taste properties of concepts using strictly linguistic stimuli (Simmons, Pecher, Hamann, Zeelenberg, and Barsalou, Poster presented at the Annual Meeting of the Cognitive Neuroscience Society, New York, NY, April 2003). Finally, the red circles in the insula/operculum at $Z=9$ and in the OFC at $Z=-18$ and $Z=-6$ indicate the activation peaks observed in the present study when participants viewed food pictures. When necessary, coordinates reported in other studies were converted from Talairach to MNI space. Adapted from Simmons WK, Martin A, and Barsalou LW (2005) Pictures of appetizing foods activate gustatory cortices for taste and reward. *Cereb. Cortex* 15: 1602–1608.

These findings demonstrate that information about object-associated properties is stored and represented across numerous property regions in the brain, rather than in a single unitary semantic memory storehouse. In addition, the property regions that compose a concept's neural representation overlap with the brain regions mediating that property's perception. Findings to this effect provide strong evidence that at least some aspect of object knowledge is maintained in a modality-specific, perceptual format (Barsalou, 1999). This stands in stark contrast to accounts describing human knowledge solely in terms of amodal, propositional, and linguistic formats that bear arbitrary relationships to the perceptual experiences through which the information was acquired (Fodor, 1975; Pylyshyn, 1984; Kintsch, 1998).

6.4.3 Object Categories in the Brain

The vast majority of studies examining the neural bases of object concept knowledge have presented subjects with photographs of exemplars from various object classes. Given that a large body of monkey neurophysiology and human neuroimaging evidence indicates that the occipitotemporal cortex plays a central role in object perception (Grill-Spector, 2003; Grill-Spector and Malach, 2004), it is unsurprising that in these studies the different object categories invariably activate this region. This does not imply, however, that the ventral occipitotemporal cortex is an undifferentiated object-processing system. Rather, comparisons between classes of objects demonstrate that local regions within the ventral occipitotemporal cortex are particularly responsive to some categories relative to others. Perhaps the most well-known category-responsive brain region is the fusiform face area (FFA), which responds reliably and selectively to face stimuli (Kanwisher et al., 1997; see Kanwisher and Yovel, 2006, for review). Other frequently studied object categories include environmental scenes (places), which reliably activate a region in parahippocampal cortex (Aguirre et al., 1998; Epstein and Kanwisher, 1998), as well as animals and tools, each activating lateral and medial fusiform cortex, respectively (Chao et al., 1999; see Martin and Chao, 2001, and Martin, 2007 for reviews).

The topographic relations among these category-responsive ventral temporal regions are a topic of much research interest. Clearly, distinct categories are associated with activation peaks in particular regions. fMRI pattern analysis techniques, however, have demonstrated that they are also associated with distinct neural signatures across large swaths of ventral occipitotemporal cortex (Haxby et al., 2001; Spiridon and Kanwisher, 2002; Cox and Savoy, 2003). For now, it remains an open question as to how central these nonpeak areas are in the cognitive representation of concepts from any particular category (Haxby et al., 2001; Spiridon and Kanwisher, 2002; Reddy and Kanwisher, 2006). In contrast, however, to this debate about the distributedness of concept representation within a single brain region, human functional neuroimaging evidence leaves little room for debate as to whether conceptual information is distributed across brain regions. Conceptual knowledge is unequivocally distributed throughout the brain, and some of the best evidence to this effect comes from the study of two broad classes of knowledge: animate entities and tools.

6.4.4 Two Case Studies in Category Representation: Animate Entities and Tools

Motivated by category-specific deficits for animals and tools reported in the neuropsychological literature, many functional neuroimaging studies have focused on defining the neural substrate underlying knowledge of animate entities and small, manipulable artifacts such as tools. As we will see, these studies have shown that tasks involving animate objects (i.e., people and animals) are associated with activity in the distributed neural circuit engaged while perceiving animate entities' most salient properties, namely, what they look like and how they move. For example, Chao et al. (1999) demonstrated that naming pictures or reading words denoting animal concepts activated lateral regions in the fusiform gyrus (located along the ventral surface of the temporal lobes and including the FFA), as well as the posterior extent of the superior temporal sulcus (pSTS), located laterally along the temporal lobe (**Figure 3**). In contrast, these authors demonstrated that performing these tasks with manipulable artifacts (e.g., tools) activates a distributed neural circuit underlying not only what these objects look like and how they move but also their function-associated motor properties, including medial regions in the fusiform gyrus, the pMTG, and in a later study, posterior parietal and ventral premotor regions (Chao and Martin, 2000).

The fusiform region activated by animal and tool stimuli is part of a larger object-form processing stream stretching along the ventral surfaces of the

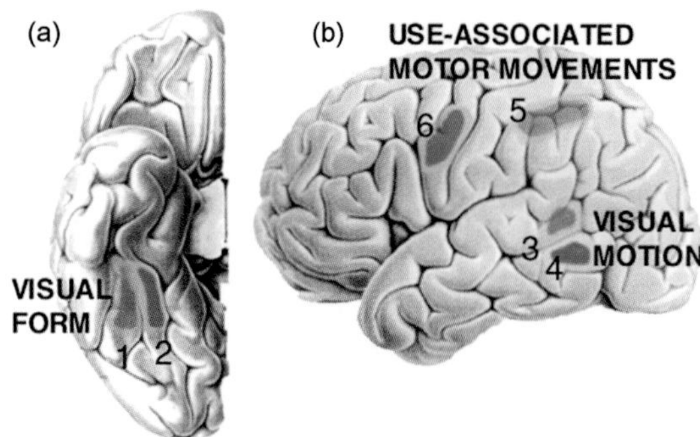

Figure 3 Schematic illustration of regions exhibiting category-related activity for animate entities such as animals and people (red) and manipulable artifacts such as tools (blue). (a) Ventral view of the right hemisphere showing relative location of regions assumed to represent visual form and form-related properties like color and texture of animate entities (1. lateral region of the fusiform gyrus, including, but not limited to, the fusiform face area) and tools; (2. medial region of the fusiform gyrus). (b) Lateral view of the left hemisphere showing relative location of regions assumed to represent biological motion typical of animate entities (3. pSTS) and rigid motion vectors typical of tools (4. pMTG). Also shown are the relative locations of the posterior parietal (5. typically centered on the intraparietal sulcus) and ventral premotor (6.) regions of the left hemisphere assumed to represent information about the motor movements associated with using tools.

occipital and temporal lobes (Ungerleider and Mishkin, 1982). Within this so-called ventral visual stream the form features of visual inputs are processed in a hierarchically organized manner, with more anterior regions representing higher-order information about what objects look like (Riesenhuber and Poggio, 1999; Grill-Spector and Malach, 2004). In contrast, the lateral temporal regions activated by animal and tool stimuli are located immediately anterior to the much-studied visual motion area V5/MT (Watson et al., 1993).

Although the location of these category-responsive regions relative to form and motion processing areas was suggestive as to their functional significance, the clearest evidence for the specific functions played by these two regions in conceptual processing *per se* comes from the work of Beauchamp and colleagues. In a series of studies, subjects were shown static and moving stimuli of humans (photographs and video clips of people performing actions such as jumping, walking, and sitting) and manipulable objects (e.g., photographs and video clips of tools such as hammers, saws, and scissors, moving in characteristic ways) (Beauchamp et al., 2002, 2003). As expected, the two classes of stimuli activated distinct regions in the ventral and lateral temporal lobes (**Figure 4**). Beauchamp et al. (2002) observed that in the fusiform gyrus, lateral regions responded more strongly to depictions of humans, and medial regions responded more to manipulable objects. Importantly, however, both regions responded equally to their preferred stimuli, regardless of whether those stimuli were static or dynamic. In a subsequent study, Beauchamp et al. (2003) observed that the lateral and medial fusiform responded much more to videos of humans and tools, respectively, than they did to point-light displays of humans and tools that lacked the form and color features of the video stimuli, but which maintained their motion vectors. Taking these two sets of findings together, we can infer that the lateral and medial fusiform regions are not modulated by motion but, rather, respond to the form features characterizing object concepts from their preferred categories – form features that are present in both static and dynamic depictions of an object.

Unlike the ventral temporal cortex, lateral temporal regions were more responsive to dynamic than static stimuli, with the pSTS and pMTG exhibiting strong category selectivity. The pSTS responded more strongly to dynamic depictions of human actions than to tool motion. This finding is consistent with monkey neurophysiology and human fMRI studies demonstrating that this region is particularly tuned to flexible, fully articulated motion vectors that characterize biological motion (Oram and Perrett, 1994; Puce et al., 1998; Grossman and Blake, 2001; Pelphrey et al., 2005). In contrast, relative to human actions, the pMTG responded more strongly to the rigid, unarticulated motion vectors characterizing dynamic depictions of tool motions. Thus, in the same way that activity in ventral temporal cortex differentiates along category boundaries, presumably due to different visual form characteristics for animate objects and manipulable artifacts, so activity in lateral temporal cortex similarly differentiates the distinctive motion properties of the two categories.

As reviewed earlier, behavioral (Cree and McRae, 2003) and imaging (see Martin, 2007) evidence demonstrate that an object concept's property profile (e.g., its form, motion, taste, sound) predicts the conglomeration of sensorimotor regions underlying that object concept's storage and representation in the brain. In light of this, it should come as no surprise that in addition to the temporal regions representing their form and motion properties, tasks involving manipulable artifacts also recruit posterior parietal and ventral premotor regions supporting the representation of

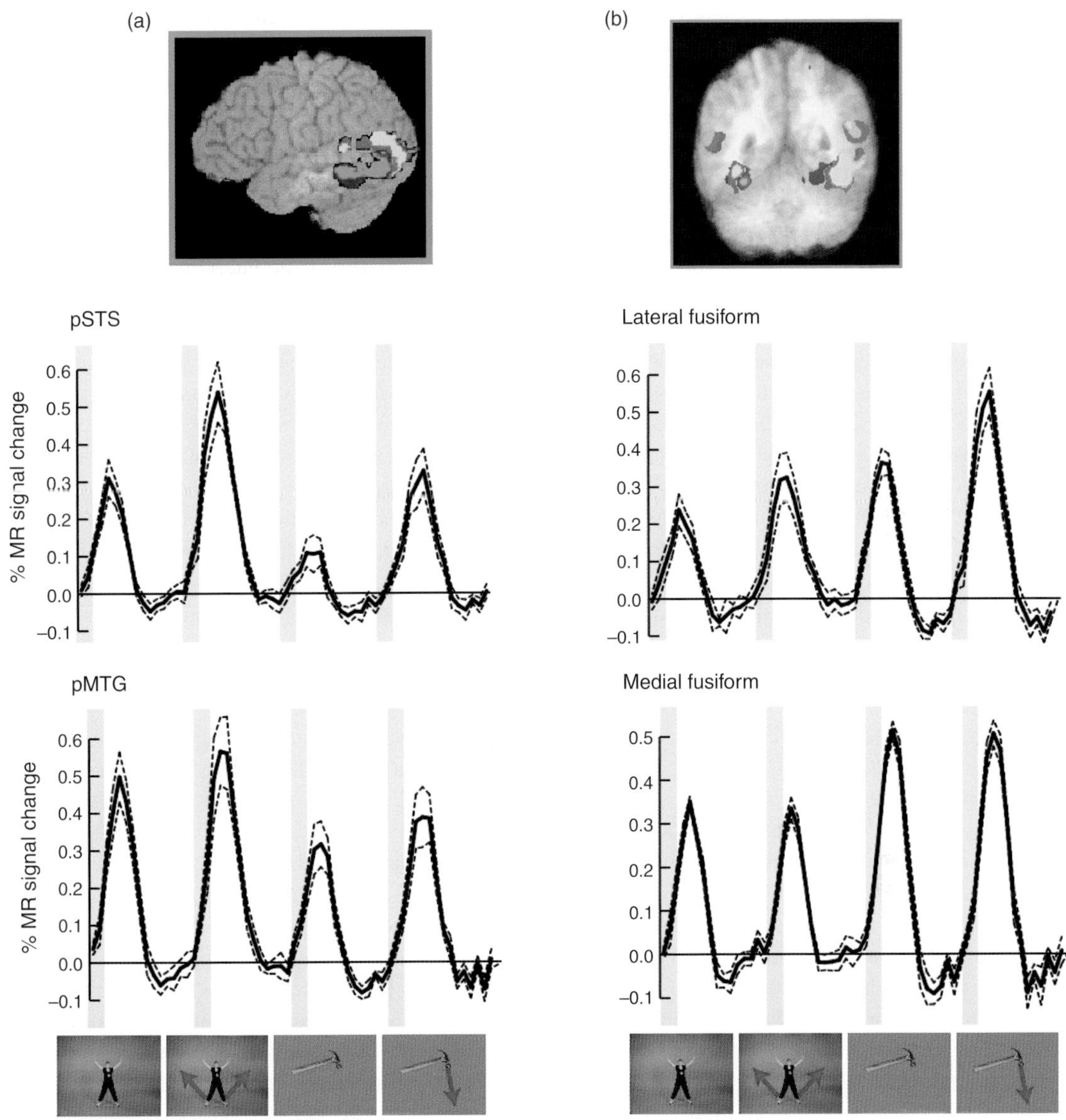

Figure 4 (a) Lateral view of the left hemisphere showing MTG regions that are more responsive when subjects identify static and moving images of tools than people (blue), and pSTS regions that are more responsive for identifying people than tools (yellow). (b) Coronal section illustrating medial fusiform regions that are more responsive when subjects identify static and moving images of tools than people (blue), and the lateral fusiform region that is more active for identifying people (yellow). Below each brain are group-averaged bold response functions depicting activity for static and moving images in each region shown in (a) and (b). The lateral cortical areas in (a) exhibit category and motion effects, where as ventral areas depicted in (b) exhibit only category effects. Vertical gray bars indicate stimulus presentation periods. Dashed lines indicate ±1 SEM. Adapted from Beauchamp MS, Lee KE, Haxby JV, and Martin A (2002) Parallel visual motion processing streams for manipulable objects and human movements. *Neuron* 34: 149–159.

object-associated actions (Chao and Martin, 2000). This finding is consistent with monkey neurophysiology evidence demonstrating that neurons in the ventral premotor and parietal cortices respond when monkeys grasp objects, as well as when they merely see objects they have previously manipulated (Jeannerod et al., 1995; Rizzolatti and Fadiga, 1998).

6.4.5 Category-Related Activations in Property Regions Are the Bases of Conceptual Representations of Objects

Processing various object categories elicits activity in sensorimotor property regions. But how do we know that the activity in property regions represents conceptual information? Three findings in particular from the literature on animate and manipulable artifact object concepts strengthen the case that property regions are involved in conceptual-level processing.

6.4.5.1 Reason #1 to think that property regions are involved in conceptual-level processing: Activity in category regions transcends stimulus features

For both animate and manipulable artifact categories, substantial evidence demonstrates that activity in the categories' property regions is not stimulus specific. For example, differential responses are observed in the lateral fusiform to animate entities in response to pictures and written names of animals (Chao et al., 1999; Okada et al., 2000; Price et al., 2003; Devlin et al., 2005; Rogers et al., 2005; Wheatley et al., 2005; Mechelli et al., 2006), human voices (von Kriegstein et al., 2005), and when simply imagining faces (O'Craven and Kanwisher, 2000). In addition, lateral fusiform activity is also observed in response to stimuli depicting point-light displays of human bodies in motion (Grossman and Blake, 2001, 2002; Beauchamp et al., 2003; Peelen et al., 2006) and degraded and abstract visual stimuli such as human-like stick figures (Peelen and Downing, 2005). These findings are important because they demonstrate that this region is responsive to representations of animate entities, even after most form and color information has been stripped from the stimuli.

Perhaps most significantly, lateral fusiform activity has even been observed when participants view abstract representations of social situations depicted in interactions among simple geometric shapes (Heider and Simmel, 1944). For example, the lateral fusiform gyrus responds to animations suggesting social interactions such as hide-and-seek (Schultz et al., 2003), mocking and bluffing (Castelli et al., 2000, 2002), and sharing (Martin and Weisberg, 2003).

Similarly, differential responses in the medial fusiform to manipulable objects are observed in response to both pictures and written names of tools (Chao et al., 1999, 2002; Whatmough et al., 2002; Devlin et al., 2005; Mechelli et al., 2006), the spoken names of tools (Noppeney et al., 2006), and point-light displays depicting tools in motion (Beauchamp et al., 2003). Medial fusiform activity has even been observed when participants view simple geometric shapes that move and interact in ways that suggest mechanical interactions such as a bowling ball knocking down pins or billiards (Martin and Weisberg, 2003). Clearly, activation in these category-related property areas is not due to particular stimulus features but, rather, appears to be related to high-level conceptual representations.

6.4.5.2 Reason #2 to think that property regions are involved in conceptual-level processing: Activations in property areas occur as property inferences

Further evidence that property regions for animate and manipulable objects are involved in conceptual processing comes from studies in which property inferences manifest as activations in property areas; in other words, when a response occurs within a property area even though that particular property is not, in fact, present in the stimulus. For example, perceiving pictures of animals or people or reading animal names activates the region of the pSTS sensitive to biological motion, even when the stimuli presented are static photographs (Chao and Martin, 1999; Beauchamp et al., 2002). Similarly, perceiving static pictures of tools or reading tool names activates the region of the pMTG known to represent nonbiological motion (Chao and Martin, 1999; Beauchamp et al., 2002; Chao et al., 2002; Phillips et al., 2002; Kellenbach et al., 2003; Creem-Regehr and Lee, 2005; Devlin et al., 2005; Kable et al., 2005; Tranel et al., 2005a, b; Mechelli et al., 2006; Noppeney et al., 2006). In addition to the motion property inferences, however, motor property inferences are also observed in response to tool photographs, with subjects exhibiting activations in premotor cortex, even though they are not physically manipulating the tools (Chao and Martin, 2000; Chao et al., 2002; Creem-Regehr and Lee, 2005; Kan et al., 2006).

These findings are in the same vein as the observations described earlier when subjects viewed appetizing foods. Upon viewing pictures of appetizing foods, activations were observed in insula/operculum and OFC regions known to represent the tastes and taste rewards of foods, even though subjects were not receiving any gustatory stimulation (Simmons et al., 2005).

The ability to make inferences about an entity's properties is at the very core of what most cognitive scientists call conceptual knowledge. Across various categories, human subjects frequently exhibit activations in property regions that correspond to salient object concept information, often when that information is not present in the immediate stimulus. Given its great utility, and likely survival value, we might expect that the ability to infer properties would be preserved across primate species, and recent evidence demonstrates that it is.

In a study demonstrating evolutionary continuity in the neural mechanisms for representing conceptual information, Gil-da-Costa et al. (2004) presented both species-specific calls and nonbiological sounds to awake rhesus macaques undergoing PET imaging. Although both the species-specific calls and nonbiological sounds were attended by activity in auditory cortex, the conspecific calls also elicited activation in area TE/TEO, the presumed monkey homologue of human fusiform gyrus, and in the STS (**Figure 5**). Note that these ventral and lateral temporal activations in visual form and motion property regions occurred to auditory stimuli. As with humans, when monkeys process information about animate entities, in this case other monkeys, activation occurs across a distributed network of property regions to represent those entities' salient features, namely, what they look like and how they move, even when those properties are not immediately present in the stimulus.

6.4.5.3 Reason #3 to think that property regions are involved in conceptual-level processing: Retrieving information from memory depends on reactivating property regions engaged while learning that information

A recent finding using fMRI brain state classification provides yet more evidence that property regions are involved in conceptual processing *per se*, rather than simply responding to features present in experimental stimuli. Polyn et al. (2005) demonstrated that

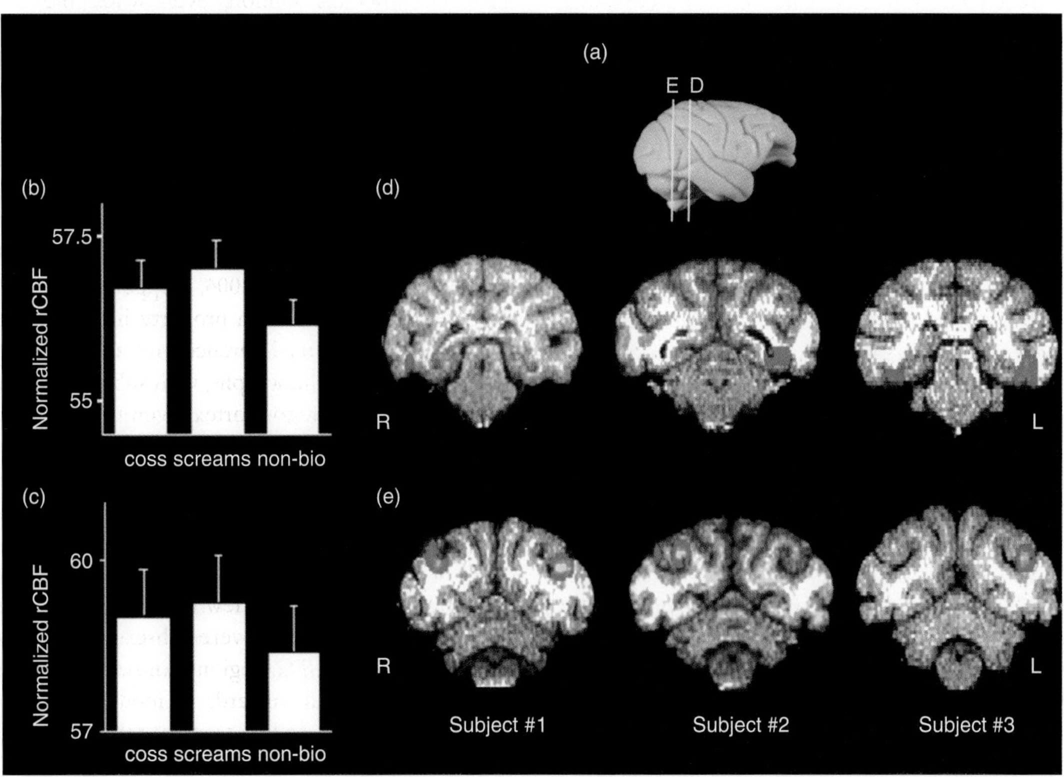

Figure 5 Activation of visual cortical areas in response to species-specific vocalizations in the rhesus macaque. (a) Lateral view of a rhesus monkey brain demonstrating the approximate locations of the coronal sections in (d) and (e). Both (b) and (c) show the mean (± SEM) normalized rCBF for the activations in TE/TEO and MT/MST/STS, respectively. In both regions, coos and screams exhibited reliably greater activation than nonbiological sounds. The coronal slices in (d) and (e) illustrate regions in each monkey that were more responsive to conspecific vocalizations (coos and screams) than to nonbiological sounds. Adapted from Gil-da-Costa R, Braun A, Lopes M, et al. (2004) Toward an evolutionary perspective on conceptual representation: Species-specific calls activate visual and affective processing systems in the macaque. *Proc. Natl. Acad. Sci. USA* 101: 17516–17521.

machine-learning algorithms are capable of detecting activity across the property regions underlying faces, places, and manipulable objects immediately prior to the free recall of information about each of these categories. During the classifier training phase of the study, subjects learned associations between labels and photographs of famous people, places, and common manipulable objects while undergoing fMRI. Later, while still undergoing fMRI, subjects were instructed to recall the items they had learned during the training phase. Brain state classifiers that were trained on data collected during encoding were able to detect distinct patterns of category-related activity that occurred several seconds prior to recall. Importantly, lateral fusiform activity served as the best predictor of famous face recall, left pMTG and parietal cortex activity best predicted manipulable object recall, and parahippocampal activity best predicted recall of places. By demonstrating that retrieving an item from memory depends on reactivating the pattern of activity in property regions that occurred during learning, this finding further establishes the centrality of property-specific information systems in the memory encoding, storage, and retrieval of conceptual information.

6.4.6 Learning about Objects by Building Property Circuits

The close correspondence between brain regions underlying perception and action with an object, and its representation in memory, suggests that conceptual property circuits develop out of experience with objects. A small but growing body of literature demonstrates that this is indeed the case. For example, Weisberg et al. (2007) asked subjects to perform a simple visual matching task on photographs of novel objects while undergoing fMRI. After scanning, the subjects were then given extensive training interacting with the objects, each of which was designed to perform a specific tool-like function. After training, the subjects were once again scanned while performing the visual matching task. Comparing the data from the two imaging sessions revealed that physical experience using the objects in a tool-like manner led to significant changes in the objects' neural representation. Whereas the novel objects elicited only diffuse ventral temporal activation in the first scan session, ventral temporal activity after training was largely restricted to the medial aspect of the fusiform gyrus, the same region previously implicated in representing the visual shape or form of tools. Similarly, new activations emerged after training in other regions observed in studies of tool knowledge, namely, the left pMTG (nonbiological motion) and left intraparietal sulcus and premotor cortex (physical manipulation).

Learning effects have also been observed for animate entities. As described earlier, viewing point-light displays of human forms in motion elicits activity in lateral fusiform and pSTS. Grossman et al. (2004) trained subjects to perceive human forms in point-light displays embedded within visual noise. After training, the subjects were not only better at indicating when a human form was present in a noisy visual display, but they also exhibited greater fusiform and pSTS activity in response to detecting those forms. Interestingly, the amount of activity in both regions was positively correlated with a subject's behavioral performance.

Yet further evidence for the development of property circuits with learning comes from James and Gauthier (2003), who demonstrated that property circuits can develop even through verbal learning. Prior to scanning, subjects learned verbally presented facts about families of novel animate-like entities called greebles. For example, subjects were trained that a particular family of greebles were associated with an auditory property (e.g., roars or squeaks), whereas other types of greebles had action properties (e.g., hops or jumps). After training, subjects underwent fMRI while performing a visual matching task that did not require retrieval of the learned associations. James and Gauthier found that viewing greebles associated with auditory properties produced activity in auditory cortex (as defined by an auditory functional localizer) and viewing greebles associated with action properties produced activity in the biological motion-sensitive region of the pSTS (as localized by moving point-light displays).

James and Gauthier's findings are important for at least two reasons. First, along with the findings of Weisberg et al. (2007), they illustrate how experience with category exemplars leads to the development of property circuits, which can later activate as property inferences. In both studies, simply seeing a particular object from the training set elicited activation in either premotor (for tools) or auditory and motion-sensitive cortex (for greebles), even though that information was unnecessary for successfully performing the task and not present in the stimuli. Second, it illustrates that this process can occur even when experience is verbally mediated. This finding is important precisely because so much of our knowledge is acquired verbally, rather than through direct sensorimotor experience with objects and their properties.

6.5 Summary

The neuropsychological and functional neuroimaging findings presented here tell us much about the organization of conceptual knowledge in the brain. Surveying these studies, it appears that information about any particular object concept is distributed across a discrete network of cortical regions, rather than being represented in a single brain region. In addition, the particular neural circuit for a given object concept includes property regions that are most commonly engaged during perceptual experience with, or functional use of, the object, as demonstrated by training studies that documented the development of property circuits as subjects gained experience with an object.

One reason for suspecting that these property regions are not strictly perceptual but, rather, support conceptual representations is that some property regions activate automatically when an object is identified, regardless of whether their respective properties are immediately present in the stimulus. As such, these activations constitute property inferences about the object. At present, the extant findings suggest that for any given object, properties such as form, motion, and function-associated motor actions are particularly likely to be retrieved automatically. As such, these three property types may form a core set of information that is necessary and sufficient for representing object concepts in memory. There is good reason to believe, however, that future research using a wider array of object categories will reveal important roles for other property types as well (e.g., taste properties may be particularly important for food concepts). Finally, a close physical proximity exists between the neural systems underlying perception and knowledge representation for objects. Indeed, for color and motor properties, the neural bases underlying perceptual and conceptual property representation may partially overlap. Taken together, these findings strongly support so-called embodied cognition accounts of knowledge representation, which claim that conceptual property information is stored in the perceptual and motor systems active when that property information is learned.

References

Adams RD, Victor M, and Ropper AH (1997) *Principles of Neurology*, 6th edn. New York: McGraw-Hill.

Aguirre GK, Zarahan E, and D'Esposito M (1998) An area within human ventral cortex sensitive to "building" stimuli: Evidence and implications. *Neuron* 21: 373–383.

Badre D, Poldrack RA, Pare-Blagoev EJ, Insler RZ, and Wagner AD (2005) Dissociable controlled retrieval and generalized selection mechanisms in ventrolateral prefrontal cortex. *Neuron* 47: 907–918.

Baldo JV and Shimamura AP (1998) Letter and category fluency in patients with frontal lobe lesions. *Neuropsychology* 12: 259–268.

Barsalou LW (1999) Perceptions of perceptual symbols. *Behav. Brain Sci.* 22: 637–660.

Beauchamp MS, Lee KE, Haxby JV, and Martin A (2002) Parallel visual motion processing streams for manipulable objects and human movements. *Neuron* 34: 149–159.

Beauchamp MS, Lee KE, Haxby JV, and Martin A (2003) fMRI responses to video and point light displays of moving humans and manipulable objects. *J. Cogn. Neurosci.* 15: 991–1001.

Bookheimer S (2002) Functional MRI of language: New approaches to understanding the cortical organization of semantic processing. *Annu. Rev. Neurosci.* 25: 151–188.

Caramazza A (1998) The interpretation of semantic category-specific deficits: What do they reveal about the organization of conceptual knowledge in the brain? Introduction. *Neurocase* 4: 265–272.

Caramazza A and Mahon BZ (2003) The organization of conceptual knowledge: The evidence from category-specific semantic deficits. *Trends Cogn. Sci.* 7: 354–361.

Caramazza A and Shelton JR (1998) Domain-specific knowledge systems in the brain: The animate-inanimate distinction. *J. Cogn. Neurosci.* 10: 1–34.

Capitani E, Laiacona M, Mahon B, and Caramazza A (2003) What are the facts of semantic category-specific deficits? A critical review of the clinical evidence. *Cogn. Neuropsychol.* 20: 213–261.

Cappelletti M, Kopelman MD, Morton J, and Butterworth B (2005) Dissociations in numerical abilities revealed by progressive cognitive decline in a patient with semantic dementia. *Cogn. Neuropsychol.* 22: 771–793.

Castelli F, Frith C, Happe F, and Frith U (2002) Autism, Asperger syndrome and brain mechanisms for the attribution of mental stats to animated shapes. *Brain* 125: 1839–1849.

Castelli F, Happe F, Frith U, and Frith C (2000) Movement and mind: A functional imaging study of perception and interpretation of complex intentional movement patterns. *Neuroimage* 12: 314–325.

Cave CB and Squire LR (1992) Intact and long-lasting repetition priming in amnesia. *J. Exp. Psychol. Learn. Mem. Cogn.* 18: 509–520.

Chao LL, Haxby JV, and Martin A (1999) Attribute-based neural substrates in temporal cortex for perceiving and knowing about objects. *Nat. Neurosci.* 2: 913–919.

Chao LL and Martin A (1999) Cortical representation of perception, naming, and knowledge of color. *J. Cogn. Neurosci.* 11: 25–35.

Chao LL and Martin A (2000) Representation of manipulable man-made objects in the dorsal stream. *Neuroimage* 12: 478–484.

Chao LL, Weisberg J, and Martin A (2002) Experience-dependent modulation of category-related cortical activity. *Cereb. Cortex* 12: 545–551.

Cox DD and Savoy RL (2003) Functional magnetic resonance imaging (fMRI) "brain reading": Detecting and classifying distributed patterns of fMRI activity in human visual cortex. *Neuroimage* 19: 261–270.

Cree GS and McRae K (2003) Analyzing the factors underlying the structure and computation of the meaning of chipmunk, cherry, chisel, cheese, and cello (and many other such concrete nouns). *J. Exp. Psychol. Gen.* 132: 153–201.

Creem-Regehr SH and Lee JN (2005) Neural representations of graspable objects: Are tools special? *Cogn. Brain Res.* 22: 457–469.

Crutch SJ and Warrington EK (2003) The selective impairment of fruit and vegetable knowledge: A multiple processing channels account of fine-grain category specificity. *Cogn. Neuropsychol.* 20: 355–372.

de Araujo IET, Kringelbach ML, Rolls ET, and Hobden P (2003a) Representation of umami taste in the human brain. *J. Neurophysiol.* 90: 313–319.

de Araujo IET, Rolls ET, Kringelbach ML, McGlone F, and Phillips N (2003b) Taste-olfactory convergence, and the representation of the pleasantness of flavor, in the human brain. *Eur. J. Neurosci.* 18: 2059–2068.

Dehaene S, Piazza M, Pinel P, and Cohen L (2003) Three parietal circuits for number processing. *Cogn. Neuropsychol.* 20: 487–506.

Devlin JT, Rushworth MFS, and Matthews PM (2005) Category-related activation for written words in the posterior fusiform is task specific. *Neuropsychologia* 43: 69–74.

Epstein R and Kanwisher N (1998) A cortical representation of the local visual environment. *Nature* 392: 598–601.

Fodor JA (1975) *The Language of Thought*. Cambridge, MA: MIT Press.

Forde EME and Humphreys GW (1999) Category-specific recognition impairments: A review of important case studies and influential theories. *Aphasiology* 13: 169–193.

Francis S, Rolls ET, Bowtell R, et al. (1999) The representation of pleasant touch in the brain and its relationship with taste and olfactory areas. *Neuroreport* 10: 453–459.

Gabrieli JD, Cohen NJ, and Corkin S (1988) The impaired learning of semantic knowledge following bilateral medial temporal-lobe resection. *Brain Cogn.* 7: 157–177.

Gainotti G (2000) What the locus of brain lesion tells us about the nature of the cognitive defect underlying category-specific disorders: A review. *Cortex* 36: 539–559.

Gil-da-Costa R, Braun A, Lopes M, et al. (2004) Toward an evolutionary perspective on conceptual representation: Species-specific calls activate visual and affective processing systems in the macaque. *Proc. Natl. Acad. Sci. USA* 101: 17516–17521.

Gold BT, Balota DA, Jones SJ, Powell DK, Smith CD, and Andersen AH (2006) Dissociation of automatic and strategic lexical-semantics: Functional magnetic resonance imaging evidence for differing roles of multiple frontotemporal regions. *J. Neurosci.* 26: 6523–6532.

Gold BT, Balota DA, Kirchhoff BA, and Buckner RL (2005) Common and dissociable activation patterns associated with controlled semantic and phonological processing: Evidence from fMRI adaptation. *Cereb. Cortex* 15: 1438–1450.

Goldberg RF, Perfetti CA, and Schneider W (2006) Perceptual knowledge retrieval activates sensory brain regions. *J. Neurosci.* 26: 4917–4921.

Gorno-Tempini ML, Dronkers NF, Rankin KP, et al. (2004) Cognition and anatomy in three variants of primary progressive aphasia. *Ann. Neurol.* 55: 335–346.

Grill-Spector K (2003) The neural basis of object perception. *Curr. Opin. Neurobiol.* 13: 159–166.

Grill-Spector K and Malach R (2004) The human visual cortex. *Annu. Rev. Neurosci.* 27: 649–677.

Grossman ED and Blake R (2001) Brain activity evoked by inverted and imagined biological motion. *Vision Res.* 41: 1475–1482.

Grossman ED and Blake R (2002) Brain areas active during visual perception of biological motion. *Neuron* 35: 1167–1175.

Grossman ED, Blake R, and Kim CY (2004) Learning to see biological motion: Brain activity parallels behavior. *J. Cogn. Neurosci.* 16: 1669–1679.

Hamann SB and Squire LR (1995) On the acquisition of new declarative knowledge in amnesia. *Behav. Neurosci.* 109: 1027–1044.

Hart J, Brendt RS, and Caramazza A (1985) Category-specific naming deficit following cerebral infarction. *Nature* 316: 439–440.

Hart J and Gordon B (1990) Delineation of single-word semantic comprehension deficits in aphasia, with anatomical correlation. *Ann. Neurol.* 27: 226–231.

Hassabis D, Kumaran D, Vann SD, and Maguire EA (2007) Patients with hippocampal amnesia cannot imagine new experiences. *Proc. Natl. Acad. Sci. USA* 104: 1726–1731.

Hauk O, Johnsrude I, and Pulvermuller F (2004) Somatotopic representation of action words in human motor and premotor cortex. *Neuron* 41: 301–307.

Haxby JV, Gobbini MI, Furey ML, Ishai A, Schouten JL, and Pietrini P (2001) Distributed and overlapping representations of faces and objects in ventral temporal cortex. *Science* 293: 2425–2430.

Heider F and Simmel M (1944) An experimental study of apparent behavior. *Am. J. Psychol.* 57: 243–249.

Hodges JR and Patterson K (1996) Nonfluent progressive aphasia and semantic dementia. *J. Int. Neuropsychol. Soc.* 2: 511–524.

Hodges JR, Patterson K, Oxbury S, and Funnell E (1992) Semantic dementia. Progressive fluent aphasia with temporal lobe atrophy. *Brain* 115: 1783–1806.

Hodges JR and Graham KS (2001) Episodic memory: Insights from semantic dementia. *Philos. Trans. R. Soc. Lond. B Biol. Sci.* 356: 1423–1434.

James TW and Gauthier I (2003) Auditory and action semantic features activate sensory-specific perceptual brain regions. *Curr. Biol.* 13: 1792–1796.

Jeannerod M, Arbib MA, Rizzolatti G, and Sakata H (1995) Grasping objects: The cortical mechanisms of visuomotor transformation. *Trends Neurosci.* 18: 314–320.

Kable JW, Kan IP, Wilson A, Thompson-Schill SL, and Chatterjee A (2005) Conceptual representations of action in the lateral temporal cortex. *J. Cogn. Neurosci.* 17: 1855–1870.

Kan IP, Kable JW, Van Scoyoc A, Chatterjee A, and Thompson-Schill SL (2006) Fractionating the left frontal response to tools: Dissociable effects of motor experience and lexical competition. *J. Cogn. Neurosci.* 18: 267–277.

Kanwisher N, McDermott J, and Chun MM (1997) The fusiform face area: A module in human extrastriate cortex specialized for face perception. *J. Neurosci.* 17: 4302–4311.

Kanwisher N and Yovel G (2006) The fusiform face area: A cortical region specialized for the perception of faces. *Philos. Trans. R. Soc. Lond. B Biol. Sci.* 361: 2109–2128.

Kapur N and Brooks DJ (1999) Temporally-specific retrograde amnesia in two cases of discrete hippocampal pathology. *Hippocampus* 9: 247–254.

Kellenbach ML, Brett M, and Patterson K (2001) Large, colourful or noisy? Attribute- and modality-specific activations during retrieval of perceptual attribute knowledge. *Cogn. Affect. Behav. Neurosci.* 1: 207–221.

Kellenbach ML, Brett M, and Patterson K (2003) Actions speak louder than functions: The importance of manipulability and action in tool representation. *J. Cogn. Neurosci.* 15: 20–46.

Kintsch W. (1998) *Comprehension: A Paradigm for Cognition*. Cambridge, UK: Cambridge University Press.

Levy DA, Bayley PJ, and Squire LR (2004) The anatomy of semantic knowledge: Medial vs. lateral temporal lobe. *Proc. Natl. Acad. Sci. USA* 101: 6710–6715.

Mahon BZ and Caramazza A (2003) Constraining questions about the organization and representation of conceptual knowledge. *Cogn. Neuropsychol.* 2: 433–450.

Manns JR, Hopkins RO, and Squire LR (2003) Semantic memory and the human hippocampus. *Neuron* 38: 127–133.

Martin A (2001) Functional neuroimaging of semantic memory. In: Cabeza R and Kingstone A (eds.) *Handbook of Functional NeuroImaging of Cognition*, pp. 153–186. Cambridge, MA: MIT Press.

Martin A (2007) The representation of object concepts in the brain. *Annu. Rev. Psychol.* 58: 25–45.

Martin A and Caramazza A (eds.) (2003) *The Organization of Conceptual Knowledge in the Brain: Neuropsychological and Neuroimaging Perspectives.* New York: Psychology Press.

Martin A and Chao LL (2001) Semantic memory and the brain: Structure and processes. *Curr. Opin. Neurobiol.* 11: 194–201.

Martin A and Fedio P (1983) Word production and comprehension in Alzheimer's disease: The breakdown of semantic knowledge. *Brain Lang.* 19: 124–141.

Martin A, Haxby JV, Lalonde FM, Wiggs CL, and Ungerleider LG (1995) Discrete cortical regions associated with knowledge of color and knowledge of action. *Science* 270: 102–105.

Martin A, Ungerleider LG, and Haxby JV (2000) Category-specificity and the brain: The sensory-motor model of semantic representations of objects. In: Gazzaniga MS (ed.) *The New Cognitive Neurosciences,* 2nd ed., pp. 1023–1036. Cambridge, MA: MIT Press.

Martin A and Weisberg J (2003) Neural foundations for understanding social and mechanical concepts. *Cogn. Neuropsychol.* 20: 575–587.

Mechelli A, Sartori G, Orlandi P, and Price CJ (2006) Semantic relevance explains category effects in medial fusiform gyri. *Neuroimage* 30: 992–1002.

Mishkin M, Vargha-Khadem F, and Gadian DG (1998) Amnesia and the organization of the hippocampal system. *Hippocampus* 8: 212–216.

Moscovitch M, Rosenbaum RS, Gilboa A, et al. (2005) Functional neuroanatomy of remote episodic, semantic and spatial memory: A unified account based on multiple trace theory. *J. Anat.* 207: 35–66.

Mummery CJ, Patterson K, Price CJ, Ashburner J, Frackowiak RSJ, and Hodges JR (2000) A voxel-based morphometry study of semantic dementia: Relationship between temporal lobe atrophy and semantic memory. *Ann. Neurol.* 47: 36–45.

Murphy GL (2002) *The Big Book of Concepts*. Cambridge, MA: MIT Press.

Neely JH (1991) Semantic priming effects in visual word recognition: A selective review of current findings and theories. In: Besner D and Humphreys GW (eds.) *Basic Processes in Reading: Visual Word Recognition*, pp. 264–336. Hillsdale, NJ: Erlbaum.

Nielsen JM (1946) *Agnosia, Apraxia, Aphasia: Their value in cerebral localization*. New York: Hafner Publishing Company.

Nielsen JM (1958) *Memory and Amnesia.* Los Angeles, CA: San Lucas Press.

Noppeney U, Price CJ, Penny WD, and Friston KJ (2006) Two distinct neural mechanisms for category-selective responses. *Cereb. Cortex* 16: 437–445.

O'Craven KM and Kanwisher N (2000) Mental imagery of faces and places activates corresponding stimulus-specific brain regions. *J. Cogn. Neurosci.* 12: 1013–1023.

O'Doherty J, Kringelbach ML, Rolls ET, Hornak J, and Andrews C (2001a) Abstract reward and punishment representations in the human orbitofrontal cortex. *Nat. Neurosci.* 4: 95–102.

O'Doherty J, Rolls ET, Francis S, Bowtell R, and McGlone F (2001b) Representation of pleasant and aversive taste in the human brain. *J. Neurophysiol.* 85: 1315–1321.

Okada T, Tanaka S, Nakai T, et al. (2000) Naming of animals and tools: A functional magnetic resonance imaging study of categorical differences in the human brain areas commonly used for naming visually presented objects. *Neurosci. Lett.* 296: 33–36.

Oram MW and Perrett DI (1994) Responses of anterior superior temporal polysensory (STPa) neurons to "biological motion" stimuli. *J. Cogn. Neurosci.* 6: 99–116.

Patterson K and Hodges JR (1995) Disorders of semantic memory. In: Baddeley AD, Wilson BA, and Watts FN (eds.) *Handbook of Memory Disorders*, pp. 167–186. New York: John Wiley and Sons.

Peelen MV and Downing PE (2005) Selectivity for the human body in the fusiform gyrus. *J. Neurophysiol.* 93: 603–608.

Peelen MV, Wiggett AJ, and Downing PE (2006) Patterns of fMRI activity dissociate overlapping functional brain areas that respond to biological motion. *Neuron* 49: 815–822.

Pelphrey KA, Morris JP, Michelich CR., Allison T, and McCarthy G (2005) Functional anatomy of biological motion perception in posterior temporal cortex: An fMRI study of eye, mouth and hand movements. *Cereb. Cortex* 15: 1866–1876.

Phillips JA, Noppeny U, Humphreys GW, and Price CJ (2002) Can segregation within the semantic system account for category-specific deficits? *Brain* 125: 2067–2080.

Polyn SM, Natu VS, Cohen JD, and Norman KA (2005) Category-specific cortical activity precedes retrieval during memory search. *Science* 310: 1963–1966.

Price CJ, Noppeney U, Phillips J, and Devlin JT (2003) How is the fusiform gyrus related to category-specificity? *Cogn. Neuropsychol.* 20: 561–574.

Puce A, Allison T, Bentin S, Gore JC, and McCarthy G (1998) Temporal cortex activation in humans viewing eye and mouth movements. *J. Neurosci.* 18: 2188–2199.

Pylyshyn Z (1984) *Computation and Cognition.* Cambridge, MA: MIT Press.

Reddy L and Kanwisher N (2006) Coding of visual objects in the ventral visual stream. *Curr. Opin. Neurobiol.* 16: 408–414.

Riesenhuber M and Poggio T (1999) Hierarchical models of object recognition in cortex. *Nat. Neurosci.* 2: 1019–1025.

Rizzolatti G and Fadiga L (1998) Grasping objects and grasping action meanings: The dual role of monkey rostroventral premotor cortex (area F5). *Novartis Found. Symp.* 218: 81–95.

Rogers TT, Hocking J, Mechelli A, Patterson K, and Price C (2005) Fusiform activation to animals is driven by the process, not the stimulus. *J. Cogn. Neurosci.* 17: 434–445.

Rosch E (1978) Principles of categorization. In: Rosch E and Lloyd BB (eds.) *Cognition and Categorization*, pp. 27–48. Hillsdale, NJ: Erlbaum.

Rosch E, Mervis CB, Gray WD, Johnson DM, and Boyes-Braem P (1976) Basic objects in natural categories. *Cognit. Psychol.* 8: 382–339.

Schacter DL and Addis DR (2007) Constructive memory: The ghosts of past and future. *Nature* 445: 7123–7127.

Schultz RT, Grelotti DJ, Klin A, et al. (2003) The role of the fusiform face area in social cognition: Implications for the pathobiology of autism. *Philos. Trans. R. Soc. Lond. B Biol. Sci.* 358: 415–427.

Schmolck H, Kensinger EA, Corkin S, and Squire LR (2002) Semantic knowledge in patient H. M. and other patients with bilateral medial and lateral temporal lobe lesions. *Hippocampus* 12: 520–533.

Simmons WK, Martin A, and Barsalou LW (2005) Pictures of appetizing foods activate gustatory cortices for taste and reward. *Cereb. Cortex* 15: 1602–1608.

Simmons WK, Ramjee V, Beauchamp MS, McRae K, Martin A, and Barsalou W (in press) A common neural substrate for perceiving and knowing about color. *Neuropsychologia*.

Simons JS, Verfaellie M, Galton CJ, Miller BL, Hodges JR, and Graham KS (2002) Recollection-based memory in frontotemporal dementia: Implications for theories of long-term memory. *Brain* 125: 2523–2536.

Snowden JS, Goulding PJ, and Neary D (1989) Semantic dementia: A form of circumscribed cerebral atrophy. *Behav. Neurol.* 2: 167–182.

Spiridon M and Kanwisher N (2002) How distributed is visual category information in human occipito-temporal cortex? An fMRI study. *Neuron* 35: 1157–1165.

Squire LR and Alvarez P (1995) Retrograde amnesia and memory consolidation: A neurobiological perspective. *Curr. Opin. Neurobiol.* 5: 169–177.

Squire LR and Zola SM (1998) Episodic memory, semantic memory, and amnesia. *Hippocampus* 8: 205–211.

Thompson SA, Graham KS, Williams G, Patterson K, Kapur N, and Hodges JR (2004) Dissociating person-specific from general semantic knowledge: Roles of the left and right temporal lobes. *Neuropsychologia* 42: 359–370.

Thompson-Schill SL (2003) Neuroimaging studies of semantic memory: Inferring "how" from "where." *Neuropsychologia* 41: 280–292.

Thompson-Schill SL, Swick D, Farah MJ, D'Esposito M, Kan IP, and Knight RT (1998) Verb generation in patients with focal frontal lesions: A neuropsychological test of neuroimaging findings. *Proc. Natl. Acad. Sci. USA* 95: 15855–15860.

Tranel D, Damasio H, and Damasio AR (1997) A neural basis for the retrieval of conceptual knowledge. *Neuropsychologia* 35: 1319–1327.

Tranel D, Grabowski TJ, Lyon J, and Damasio H (2005a) Naming the same entities from visual or from auditory stimulation engages similar regions of left inferotemporal cortices. *J. Cogn. Neurosci.* 17: 1293–1305.

Tranel D, Martin C, Damasio H, Grabowski TJ, and Hichwa R (2005b) Effects of noun-verb homonymy on the neural correlates of naming concrete entities and actions. *Brain Lang.* 92: 288–299.

Tulving E (1972) Episodic and semantic memory. In: Tulving E and Donaldson W (eds.) *Organization of Memory*, pp. 381–403. London: Academic Press.

Tulving E (2002) Episodic memory: From mind to brain. *Annu. Rev. Psychol.* 53: 1–25.

Ungerleider LG and Mishkin M (1982) Two cortical visual systems. In: Ingle DJ, Goodale MA, and Mansfield RJW (eds.) *Analysis of Visual Behavior*, pp. 549–586. Cambridge, MA: MIT Press.

Vandenbulcke M, Peeters R, Fannes K, and Vandenberghe R (2006) Knowledge of visual attributes in the right hemisphere. *Nat. Neurosci.* 9: 964–970.

Vargha-Khadem F, Gadian DG, Watkins KE, Connelly A, Van Paesschen W, and Mishkin M (1997) Differential effects of early hippocampal pathology on episodic and semantic memory. *Science* 277: 376–380.

Verfaellie M, Koseff P, and Alexander MP (2000) Acquisition of novel semantic information in amnesia: Effects of lesion location. *Neurpsychologia* 38: 484–492.

von Kriegstein K, Kleinschmidt A, Sterzer P, and Giraud AL (2005) Interaction of face and voice areas during speaker recognition. *J. Cogn. Neurosci.* 17: 367–376.

Warrington EK (1975) The selective impairment of semantic memory. *Q. J. Exp. Psychol.* 27: 635–657.

Warrington EK and McCarthy RA (1987) Categories of knowledge – Further fractionations and an attempted integration. *Brain* 110: 1273–1296.

Warrington EK and Shallice T (1984) Category specific semantic impairments. *Brain* 107: 829–854.

Watson JDG, Myers R, Frackowiak RSJ, et al. (1993) Area V5 of the human brain: evidence from a combined study using positron emission tomography and magnetic resonance imaging. *Cereb. Cortex* 3: 79–94.

Weisberg J, van Turrennout M, and Martin A (2007) A neural system for learning about object function. *Cereb. Cortex* 17: 513–521.

Whatmough C, Chertkow H, Murtha S, and Hanratty K (2002) Dissociable brain regions process object meaning and object structure during picture naming. *Neuropsychologia* 40: 174–186.

Wheatley T, Weisberg J, Beauchamp MS, and Martin A (2005) Automatic priming of semantically related words reduces activity in the fusiform gyrus. *J. Cogn. Neurosci.* 17: 1871–1885.

Wiggs CL, Weisberg J, and Martin A (1999) Neural correlates of semantic and episodic memory retrieval. *Neuropsychologia* 37: 103–118.

Williams GB, Nestor PJ, and Hodges JR (2005) Neural correlates of semantic and behavioural deficits in frontotemporal dementia. *Neuroimage* 24: 1042–1051.

7 Episodic Memory: An Evolving Concept

K. K. Szpunar and K. B. McDermott, Washington University, St. Louis, MO, USA

7.1 Introduction

Although the term episodic memory did not exist until about 35 years ago, it captures much of what philosophers, psychologists, and lay people have meant by memory or remembering. Episodic memory – or the recollection of events from one's personal past – is therefore one of the most fundamentally important concepts in the study of human memory. It is the capacity for episodic memory that enables one to recollect the multitude of details surrounding one's most cherished moments.

A challenge inherent in writing a review chapter on episodic memory is that it is not a static term; the essence of the term episodic memory has morphed and broadened considerably over the short time of the term's existence. It should be no surprise, then, that different empirical evidence has been brought to bear on the different meanings. A further twist is that a single person, Endel Tulving, both introduced the term (in 1972) and has modified its meaning many times in the years since. As a result, his theorizing and adaptation of the concept has spawned much of the relevant literature, and this chapter draws very heavily upon his work and emergent ideas.

We have chosen the following approach in organizing this chapter. We begin by attempting to identify a few of the historical landmarks or prominent features proposed in the conceptual development of episodic memory. We then choose two topics to consider in some depth. Specifically, we consider evidence supporting the proposition that episodic memory is a distinct memory system, different from other types of memory. We then consider research bearing on the suggestion that episodic memory may represent only one facet of a more general cognitive capacity that enables mental time travel into both the subjective past and future.

7.2 Historical Landmarks

7.2.1 A Taxonomic Distinction: Episodic and Semantic Memory

The concept of episodic memory was formally introduced in a seminal chapter by Tulving (1972), who drew a distinction between memory for specific events (episodic memory) and memory for general knowledge and facts (semantic memory). For example, remembering that the word elephant had been present in a list of previously studied words, recounting the events surrounding the day of one's college graduation, or reminiscing about the most recent Christmas dinner with a family member would be considered instances of episodic memory. Knowing that elephants live in Africa, the name of the college one attended, and that a family gathering typically implies a special occasion would be classified as examples of semantic memory (*See* Chapter 5).

In 1972, Tulving explained that laboratory studies of human memory had long been concerned with episodic memory. That is, most experiments were of the same general design: Present events for study and then measure how well they are remembered at a later time. At this time, episodic memory was associated with a certain type of task: Those that required recall or recognition of a prior episode.

Although episodic and semantic memory are both declarative (i.e., may be articulated) and can be differentiated from memory that cannot be expressed in terms of representational information (i.e., procedural memory, or memory of how to perform a skill, see Squire, 1987), there exists a fundamental and straightforward distinction between episodic and semantic memory: Episodic memory involves remembering an episode from one's past that is specific to time and place, whereas semantic memory involves general knowledge that is not associated with specific episodes.

Tulving summarized his seminal 1972 chapter as having made "a case for the possible heuristic usefulness of a taxonomic distinction between episodic and semantic memory and two parallel and partially overlapping information processing systems" (Tulving, 1972: p. 401). At the time, the episodic/semantic distinction was offered as a proposal that the two types of memory may be separable. As will be seen, the concept of episodic memory quickly grew to denote more than its originally intended meaning. The taxonomic distinction between episodic and semantic memory, however, is a central feature of the original conceptualization that has stood the test of time. Indeed, this distinction has been adopted by the field and is in widespread use.

Before proceeding further, it is worth considering the similarities and differences between the term episodic memory and a few other, related terms. Autobiographical memory refers to personal memories of one's own life. These can be of two types: episodic or semantic. Consider the following examples: Remembering the first day of grammar school would rely upon episodic memory, whereas knowing the name of one's grammar school relies upon semantic memory. Both examples, however, represent autobiographical (self-related) memory. We should acknowledge, though, that researchers define autobiographical memory in different ways, so not all would agree with this classification scheme. Explicit memory is another term related to episodic memory. Explicit memory is a term often used as a heuristic for the type of memory used on an explicit test of memory; an explicit test is one in which a person is asked to willfully attempt to retrieve the past. Explicit memory can be contrasted with implicit memory, which is the unintentional manifestation of memory (e.g., if you were to read this chapter a second time, it would likely be read faster).

7.2.2 Subjective Awareness

The role of subjective awareness in memory has long been a topic of interest for the field (e.g., feeling-of-knowing judgments, tip-of-the-tongue states; for a historical review see Metcalfe, 2000). In 1983, Tulving published *Elements of Episodic Memory*, in which he explicitly applied such ideas to his own work. In that volume, Tulving proposed that memories for personal episodes are characterized by a strong feeling of re-experiencing the past. In contrast, Tulving argued that retrieval of general knowledge from semantic memory lacked this phenomenological quality. That is, although someone may know a fact (e.g., that St. Louis is the site of a famous arch) and is aware that he or she acquired knowledge of this fact in the past, one does so in a way that does not necessitate re-experiencing the instance in which the fact had been learned.

Tulving further argued that the feeling of re-experiencing a previously encountered event is the *sine qua non* of episodic memory. He outlined a general framework (General Abstract Processing System, or GAPS; **Figure 1**) by which to understand the act of remembering from episodic memory (Tulving, 1983). The GAPS framework was intended to highlight many issues associated with retrieval from episodic memory. We focus here on how this framework predicts the emergence of subjective awareness (or recollective experience, as it was referred to in 1983). As can be seen in **Figure 1**, an encoded event is converted into a latent memory trace (or engram;

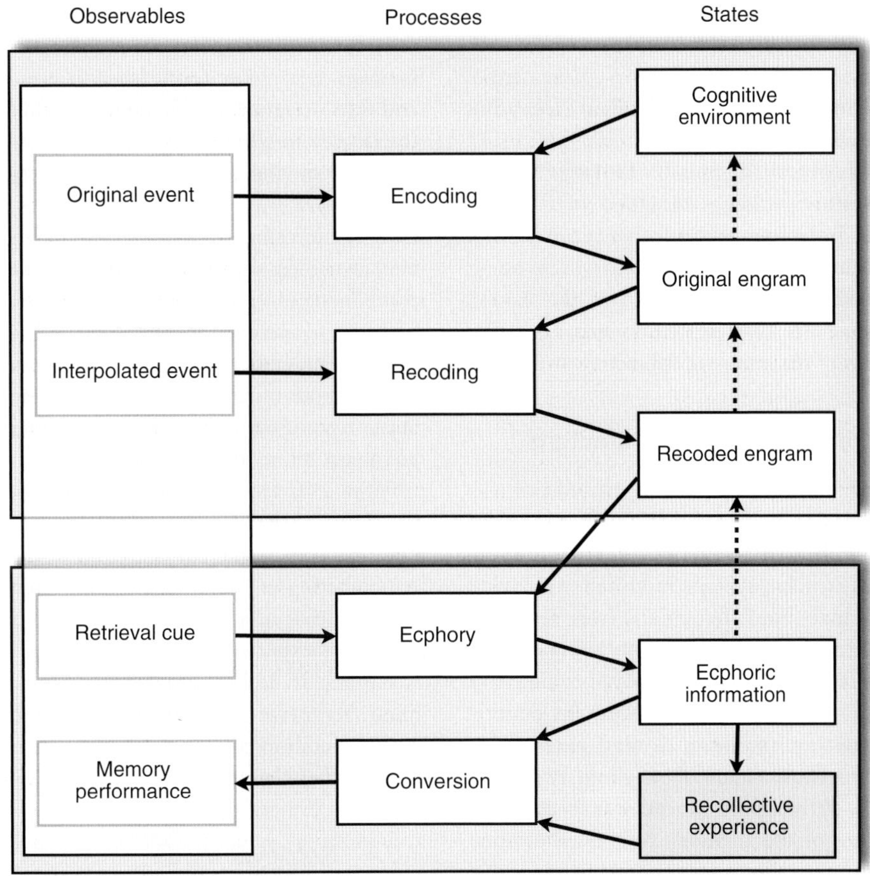

Figure 1 General Abstract Processing System: A conceptual framework for understanding retrieval from episodic memory. Adapted from Tulving E (1983) *Elements of Episodic Memory.* New York: Oxford University Press.

Semon, 1904). However, it is unlikely that the event will be remembered exactly as it had originally occurred. For instance, the latent engram related to that event is subject to recoding (e.g., by virtue of related interpolated events). The recoded engram then interacts with a retrieval cue to produce ecphory: The evocation of information from a latent engram into an active state (Semon, 1904; Tulving and Madigan, 1970; Tulving, 1976; Schacter et al., 1978). That is, the synergistic product of the memory trace and the retrieval cue determine the nature of what is remembered (ecphoric information; Tulving, 1982), which in turn determines recollective experience. Accordingly, the rememberer will become aware of the encoded event to the extent that ecphoric information is representative of the original episode. At this time, no data were presented that directly assessed a participant's recollective experience for the contents of his or her memory.

On the basis of the notable absence of phenomenological data from the majority of verbal learning experiments (but see Metcalfe, 2000, who discusses various exceptions), Tulving (1983) suggested that students of psychology had not yet begun the study of episodic memory. Of course, this claim directly contradicts his previous (Tulving, 1972) assertion, which he declared in 1983 to have been "not very well thought out" (Tulving, 1983: p. 9). Prior research had assumed a correlation between a learner's behavioral response and subjective awareness. That is, if a learner was able to recall or recognize having previously encountered a given stimulus item (e.g., a word from a previously presented list) it was assumed that he or she mentally re-experienced the original event. It is now well-established that there is no direct correlation between behavior on a memory test and the cognitive processes underlying that behavior (Schacter, 1987; Tulving, 1989a; Jacoby, 1991; Roediger and McDermott, 1993; Toth, 2000; *See*

Chapter 4). Tulving (2002b) reflected on this issue by pointing out that episodic memory is concerned with what happened where and when. Typical verbal learning experiments assessed the what aspect but left when and where unqueried.

With this problem in mind, Tulving (1985b) devised a research paradigm designed to illustrate that a learner in a memory experiment does not necessarily remember the instance in which he or she experienced an event that he or she knows occurred in the past. This procedure was a starting point for exploring the nature of subjective awareness.

7.2.3 The Remember/Know Paradigm

The remember/know paradigm was introduced as a tool for investigating a learner's subjective awareness of a prior study episode (Tulving, 1985b), although current procedures have been modified somewhat from the original implementation (see Rajaram, 1993). For the most part, a remember/know experiment takes the form of the typical laboratory memory experiment. Learners study a set of stimulus materials at time one (e.g., a list of words) and take a memory test on those materials at time two. The innovation that Tulving introduced was to ask learners at the time of the memory test whether they actually remembered the exact prior occurrence of a given study item (e.g., the word ocean), or whether they just knew that the item had been presented, but could not remember the precise instance of its original presentation (Tulving, 1985b; Gardiner, 1988; Rajaram, 1993; Gardiner and Richardson-Klavehn, 2000).

Tulving (1985b) showed that learners could easily make these mental distinctions and that both remember and know responses were present during tasks that previously had been thought to tap episodic memory (i.e., recognition, cued recall, and even free recall). This important finding suggested that learners had two routes by which to recover the contents of a past study episode. Remembering was identified as the hallmark of episodic memory and was further associated with a unique mental state called autonoetic (self-knowing) awareness, implying a feeling of personally re-experiencing the past. Knowing was associated with semantic memory and noetic (knowing) awareness, a mental state lacking the feeling of personally re-experiencing the past. Further, memory tasks were found to vary in the degree to which they relied upon remembering, with free recall demonstrating the greatest level of remember responses (i.e., the greatest reliance on episodic memory). Hence, an important conclusion here is that no memory test is a pure measure of episodic memory, and tests designed to assess episodic memory differ in the degree to which they rely on the construct, with none achieving a pure assessment of episodic memory.

It is interesting to note that the subjective (autonoetic) awareness that Tulving had identified as a central component of episodic memory was similar to what pioneers of memory research had in mind when discussing remembering. For instance, William James (1890) wrote of remembering as, "a direct feeling; its object is suffused with a warmth and intimacy to which no object of mere conception ever attains" (James, 1890: p. 239). Hermann Ebbinghaus, (1885) adopted a generally understood conceptualization of memory that had been put forth by John Locke, defining remembering as the emergence of a sought after mental image that is "immediately recognized as something formerly experienced" (Ebbinghaus, 1885: p. 1). According to Locke, memory was the power of the mind "to revive perceptions, which it has once had, with this additional perception annexed to them, that it has had them before" (Locke, 1975: p. 150).

7.2.4 Retrieval Mode

Aside from the subjective awareness (or lack thereof) thought to accompany memory retrieval, Tulving (1983) outlined various other features by which he distinguished episodic from semantic memory (see also Tulving, 2005). At the time, the listing of differences was meant as a starting point for discussion, rather then any acknowledgment of hard-set facts. Importantly, the features on which episodic and semantic memory were hypothesized to differ were divided into three categories, each separately focusing on the information handled by episodic and semantic memory, their operations, and their applications. The main point of these subcategories was to emphasize that the distinction between episodic and semantic memory was more than just a difference in the type of information under consideration.

For instance, Tulving (1983) made a distinction regarding the manner in which access is gained to episodic and semantic knowledge. According to Tulving, access to information from episodic memory is deliberate and requires conscious effort. Conversely, semantic knowledge may be accessed in a relatively automatic fashion. For instance, stimuli in the environment are immediately interpreted on the basis of semantic knowledge. When reading a novel, the meanings of words come to mind with relative ease. However, it is only when one is in a particular state of mind that is focused on their personal past that the same stimulus may remind one of a particular episode. For example, single words have been shown to act as effective cues for the retrieval of personal autobiographical memories (Crovitz and Schiffman, 1974; Robinson, 1976); this is only the case, however, when participants are specifically instructed to use those words as retrieval cues. This state in which one focuses attention on their past and uses incoming information as cues for past experiences is referred to as retrieval mode (Tulving, 1983; Lepage et al., 2000). A potential exception to this rule involves spontaneous conscious recollection, wherein personal memories suddenly come to mind. One common example is the evocation of an emotional memory (e.g., one's first kiss) by a particular piece of music (see Berntsen, 1996, 1998). Similar examples have been offered in the prospective memory literature (McDaniel and Einstein, 2000; Einstein et al., 2005).

Tulving (1983) argued that retrieval mode constituted a necessary condition for retrieval from episodic memory but admitted, "we know next to nothing" about it (Tulving, 1983: p. 169). In terms of the behavioral literature on the topic, the same statement holds true today. Although subsequent research on the topic has illuminated the nature in which the presence/absence of retrieval mode may be manipulated in the context of a memory experiment (e.g., retrieval intentionality criterion, Schacter et al., 1989), we have not learned much more about the state itself.

Recent advances in neuroimaging techniques (see section titled "Functional neuroimaging") have revived interest in the study of retrieval mode. For example, Lepage et al. (2000) suggested that brain regions showing similar patterns of brain activity during either successful or failed attempts of episodic retrieval (relative to a control task that does not engage episodic retrieval processes) can be taken as neuroanatomical correlates of retrieval mode. Reviewing the relevant literature, Lepage et al. identified six frontal lobe regions (mostly right lateralized) that appear to become active whenever participants attempt to retrieve past information, regardless of whether they are successful or not. Thus, the underlying nature of retrieval mode has not yet been delineated, but neuroimaging techniques may prove useful in approaching this issue.

7.2.5 Subjective Awareness, Self, and Time

As we have mentioned, the concept of episodic memory has been considerably refined over the years. According to Tulving's most recent conceptualization, episodic memory is a recently evolved, late-developing, and early-deteriorating past-oriented memory system, more vulnerable than other memory systems to neuronal dysfunction, and probably unique to humans. It makes possible mental time travel through subjective time, from the present to the past, thus allowing one to re-experience, through autonoetic awareness, one's own previous experiences (Tulving, 2002b: p. 5).

Thus far we have highlighted subjective (autonoetic) awareness as the defining feature of retrieval from episodic memory. Equally important are concepts of self and subjective time (Tulving, 2002a,b). That is, episodic memory requires the capacity to represent a psychologically coherent self that persists through subjective time, whose past experiences are recognized as belonging to the present self (self-contiguity; Klein, 2001). Klein (2001; see also Klein et al., 2004) argues that a breakdown of self-contiguity disrupts the ability to represent past and present mental states as being aspects of the same personal identity, thus leaving an individual incapable of identifying a current mental state as one that was previously experienced. Klein (2001) reviews compelling evidence to support this claim. For example, individuals with schizophrenia – a population characterized by impairments in self-contiguity – have profound deficits in episodic memory (McKenna et al., 1994).

7.2.6 The Episodic Memory System

As can be seen by the 2002 definition (quoted in the previous section), episodic memory grew to encompass much more than the type of memory that allowed one to recall or recognize prior events. It became a hypothetical neurocognitive memory system that is characterized, relative to other memory systems, by its unique function and properties (Tulving, 1984, 1985a; Sherry and Schacter, 1987; Schacter and Tulving, 1994). Of course, this basic idea was foreshadowed somewhat by the earlier description (even in the 1972 description regarding partially overlapping processing systems), but the earlier emphasis had been on the basic taxonomic distinction and not on the much more bold claim that it is a memory system.

What exactly is a memory system, and what might the criteria be for establishing one? These questions have spurred a great deal of controversy, much of which appeared in the context of the emerging literature on implicit memory in the late 1980s and early 1990s (Tulving, 1985a; Sherry and Schacter, 1987; Roediger et al., 1990, 1999; Schacter and Tulving, 1994; Buckner, 2007). Some theorists were concerned that the lack of stringent criteria would lead to a proliferation of putative memory systems, many of which were probably not well justified. We wish to sidestep that general debate here; our view is that although the criteria for establishing a memory system are not well-specified (and are often not met even when specified), there is nonetheless strong evidence that episodic memory represents a fundamentally different kind of memory than semantic memory and that the hypothesis that it is indeed a distinct memory system is certainly viable. Here we choose to focus on what was meant by this claim that episodic memory should be considered a memory system and review some of the evidence bearing on the claim.

First, the episodic memory system enables its owner to process (i.e., encode, store, and retrieve) personally experienced episodes. In this way, it allows one to accomplish a feat not possible without the system. Secondly, episodic memory can be differentiated from semantic memory on a variety of dimensions (Tulving, 1972, 1983). We have already addressed one of these dimensions at length, namely the conscious awareness that characterizes episodic (autonoetic awareness) relative to semantic (noetic awareness) memory. Hence, episodic memory has a set of properties that differentiate it from other systems.

It is important to note that the episodic memory system is hypothesized to be related to and have evolved from phylogenetically earlier systems, including semantic memory (Tulving, 1985b, 1995). That is, the ability to consciously re-experience a specific event from the past may have grown out of a more general ability to use the past in an informative fashion, albeit one lacking a sense of subjectively reliving the event (see **Figure 2**). The episodic memory system "depends upon but goes beyond the capabilities of the semantic system. It could not operate in the absence of the semantic system" (Tulving, 1989b: p. 362). Of course, the evolutionary relation between episodic memory and semantic memory is not subject to laboratory investigation. As will be seen, a similar relation appears to exist in the course of ontogenetic development, though, whereby episodic memory emerges in the presence of fully functioning semantic memory.

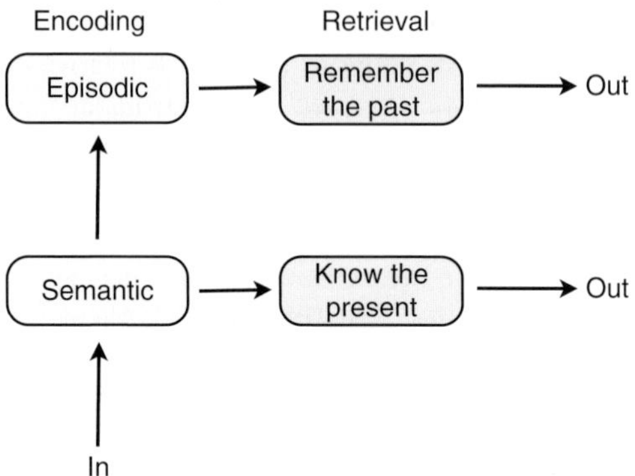

Figure 2 Sketch of the relations between semantic and episodic memory. Information can be encoded into semantic memory independent of episodic memory but must be encoded into episodic memory through semantic memory. Encoded and stored information is potentially available for retrieval from one of the two systems or from both of them. Adapted from Tulving and Markowitsch (1998).

In the following section, we present evidence from neuropsychology, functional brain imaging, and developmental psychology consistent with the idea that episodic memory may in fact represent a viable neurocognitive system or is at least functionally dissociable from semantic memory.

7.3 Converging Evidence for the Episodic Memory System

The idea that episodic memory might represent a distinct memory system emerged largely out of the behavioral psychological literature, where it was shown that a particular independent variable might affect performance on one measure or set of measures (e.g., measures thought to draw largely upon episodic memory) but not affect performance (or affect performance in the opposite direction) on different measures, thought to draw largely on semantic memory. For example, level of processing during encoding affects the likelihood of later remembering but not knowing (when the remember/know paradigm is used; see Yonelinas, 2002, for review). Perhaps the most compelling evidence for the idea comes from brain-based studies, particularly neuropsychological studies. Here it can be shown that some patients lose the ability to use episodic memory while retaining other classes of memory, including semantic memory. Following, we review some of this evidence.

7.3.1 Neuropsychology

Neuropsychological observations of brain-damaged individuals have contributed a great deal to our understanding of the organization of human memory in the brain. Perhaps the most famous contribution is that of Scoville and Milner (1957), who reported the case of patient HM. HM incurred dense amnesia following a bilateral resection of the medial temporal lobes. Since then, a great deal of converging evidence from neuropsychological observations of human patients, neurological experimentation using animal subjects, and more recent advances in functional brain imaging techniques has corroborated Scoville and Milner's original observation: The medial temporal lobes play an important role for memory (for an early reference, see Bekhterev, 1900).

Of particular interest, Scoville and Milner (1957) classified the impairment observed in patient HM as one of declarative memory. That is, no distinction was made between episodic and semantic memory. Of course, this is not surprising given that the distinction was not introduced to the neuropsychological community for another 30 years (Tulving, 1985b; although see Nielsen, 1958, for a foreshadowing of the distinction). Another potential reason the distinction was not made is because it was not readily apparent. HM's surgical resection encompassed large portions of the medial temporal lobes, including, but not limited to, the hippocampal formation. It has recently been considered that hippocampal damage is particularly associated with deficits of episodic memory, whereas semantic memory problems arise as a result of adjacent cortical damage (Mishkin et al., 1997; Aggleton and Brown, 1999). Accordingly, both episodic and semantic memory may have been damaged in patient HM.

Vargha-Khadem and her colleagues have recently reported on a set of three amnesic patients, each of whom sustained bilateral pathology restricted to the hippocampus following an anoxic episode in early life (ranging from birth to 9 years; Vargha-Khadem et al., 1997). Unlike most amnesic patients, their ability to acquire knowledge remains intact. As a result, all three patients have been able to progress through the educational system with little trouble. However, all three are severely impaired in their ability to recall events, even those that occurred minutes previously. These cases represent a clear dissociation between episodic and semantic memory function in the presence of brain damage restricted to the hippocampus.

Although dissociations between episodic and semantic memory are rarely clear-cut, there do exist many case reports in which one is relatively more impaired than the other. Most such cases have reported greater deficits of episodic memory relative to semantic memory (e.g., Cermak and O'Connor, 1983; Calabrese et al., 1996; Kitchener et al., 1998; Levine et al., 1998; Viskontas et al., 2000), although the reverse pattern also occurs (e.g., Grossi et al., 1988; De Renzi et al., 1997; Yasuda et al., 1997; Markowitsch et al., 1999). The reversed pattern (i.e., greater impairment of semantic than episodic memory) is not well accommodated by the idea that episodic memory requires semantic memory to operate.

It is important to note that these case studies are characterized by various etiological factors and resulting patterns of brain impairment that are not restricted to the medial temporal lobes. In general, there is good reason to believe that the operations of various memory systems (including episodic and semantic) depend upon highly distributed and interacting regions of the brain (Mesulam, 1990; Nyberg et al., 2000). For instance, although the role of hippocampus is well established, deficits of episodic memory are also highly correlated with frontal lobe pathology (e.g., Ackerley and Benton, 1947; Freeman and Watts, 1950; Stuss and Benson, 1986; Wheeler et al., 1997).

As an example of relative impairment of episodic memory, consider patient ML (Levine et al., 1998). Following a severe closed-head injury, patient ML became amnesic for pretraumatic events. Although ML retained the capacity to recount many autobiographical facts, he was unable to re-experience any specific event associated with them. For instance, ML could recount the name of a high school teacher perfectly well but was unable to recollect any experience associated with that individual. In brief, the episodic component of patient ML's autobiographical memory was missing. His pathology was restricted to right ventral frontal lobe, including the unicinate fasciculus, a band of fibers connecting frontal and temporal cortices. Patient ML is one of many brain-damaged patients who have lost much of their episodic and semantic memory, with no accompanying anterograde (posttrauma) amnesia.

That is, these patients are able to learn new information. With respect to these patients' retrograde (pretrauma) memory problems, semantic memory typically recovers, while episodic memory remains largely impaired.

As an example of disproportionate impairment of semantic memory, consider the report by Grossi et al. (1988) of a student who lost her ability to reproduce factual knowledge that she had learned prior to her injury. For instance, she was unable to recount various facts learned in school, although she could remember specific meetings with instructors. Summarizing over many such observations, Kapur (1999) concluded that, "loss of factual, semantic memories is readily dissociable from loss of memory for personally experienced events" (p. 819).

Perhaps the most well-documented example of a dissociation between episodic and semantic memory is a patient known as KC, who has been investigated by Tulving (1985b) and his colleagues at the University of Toronto. At the age of 30, patient KC sustained damage to several regions of his brain (including the medial temporal lobes) following a closed-head injury from a motorcycle accident (Rosenbaum et al., 2000, 2005). As with many amnesic patients, neuropsychological testing revealed that KC had retained many of his cognitive capacities. For instance, his intelligence and language faculties remain largely unaffected; he can read and write; he is able to focus and pay close attention to a conversation; he is capable of performing a wide variety of mental tasks, including visual imagery; and his short-term memory is normal.

KC also knows many details about his personal past. Among other things, he knows the names of many of the schools that he attended, the address of his childhood home, the make and color of his former car, and the location of his family's summer home. That is, KC's semantic knowledge of information acquired prior to the brain trauma remains largely intact. Nonetheless, KC cannot remember a single personal episode associated with this knowledge. For instance, although he can readily describe the process of changing a flat tire, he cannot remember ever having performed this task. In fact, KC cannot remember a single episode from his lifetime. This lack of episodic memory extends to highly emotional events; KC has no recollection regarding the untimely death of his brother or a bar fight that left him with a broken arm.

Given the diffuse nature of KC's brain pathology, it remains unclear what the precise cause of the clear dissociation between episodic and semantic memory might be, although strong arguments can be made regarding damage to regions of KC's medial temporal lobes (e.g., Vargha-Khadem et al., 1997; Klein et al., 2002) and frontal cortex (see Wheeler et al., 1997). Regardless, the story of patient KC is a remarkable one and suggests that there may emerge a biological dissociation between episodic and semantic memory.

As a whole, these studies show that various forms of deficits can be found with respect to episodic and semantic memory. Note, however, that there has not yet been successful resolution of how the current concept of episodic memory could accommodate finding a properly functioning episodic memory system occurring in a person with semantic memory deficits. Nonetheless, the more general finding that episodic and semantic memory can be dissociated not just as a function of independent variables but also in neuropsychological patients is consistent with the idea that episodic memory should be considered a memory system.

7.3.2 Functional Neuroimaging

There now exist seemingly countless neuroimaging studies of episodic memory. Here we identify a few general patterns that indicate a brain-based dissociation between episodic and semantic memory. We have found it necessary to be brief, and we suggest that the interested reader seek some of the in-depth reviews that detail the wealth of studies that have shaped our understanding of episodic memory and how it is represented in the brain.

Traditional psychological studies and (especially) lesion studies do not allow the easy separation of retrieval from storage. In neuroimaging studies, however, retrieval effects can arguably be better isolated. Here we focus primarily on retrieval from episodic memory for a couple reasons. First, the encoding of information into episodic memory seems to rely largely upon retrieval of information from semantic memory (Tulving et al., 1994; see also Prince et al., 2007). Storage is a phase not well studied with the methods under consideration here. Finally, retrieval has been argued to be the foundation for understanding memory; indeed, Roediger (2000) entitled a chapter "Why retrieval is the key process in understanding human memory."

Functional neuroimaging techniques, such as positron emission tomography (PET) and functional magnetic resonance imaging (fMRI), allow neuroscientists to examine the healthy human brain at work.

When participants engage in a given cognitive task, PET or fMRI provide information about the level of cerebral blood flow (PET) or blood oxygenation level (fMRI) localized in the brain regions recruited for the task. Such metabolic changes correlate highly with underlying neuronal activity and thus provide important insights into the brain structures that might underlie specific cognitive tasks.

One challenge in conducting brain-imaging research lies in experimental design. In the typical design, metabolic changes associated with two cognitive tasks are contrasted with one another in hopes of isolating the neural correlates of the cognitive process of interest. Researchers attempt to contrast a pair (or in some cases a set) of tasks that are highly similar to one another but that vary on one key dimension. Note that such a contrast highlights differences between tasks but (in the absence of a third, low-level baseline task) is unable to address areas of common activation.

For instance, in order to identify the neural correlates associated with retrieval from episodic memory, studies have contrasted a task that draws upon episodic memory with a second retrieval task that does not involve the reinstatement of specific spatial-temporal details (e.g., retrieval of general knowledge, which draws upon semantic memory). Although one may be certain that one task reasonably depends more on episodic memory and the other more on semantic memory, neither task is a direct window into the type of memory it is designed to reflect; confidence is gained, however, when results replicate across studies and tasks. This approach makes testable the assumption made by Tulving that retrieval from episodic memory relies upon semantic memory but adds to it certain other processes or brain regions. It is therefore possible to see whether episodic memory seems to rely upon the same brain regions as semantic memory with the addition of others.

With the neuropsychological studies just reviewed in mind, one could make some predictions with respect to how episodic and semantic memory might differ. Relative to some lower-level baseline task, semantic and episodic memory would be expected to reveal very similar activity. To the extent that episodic memory indeed builds upon semantic memory, any differences seen would be expected to be in the direction of greater activity for episodic than semantic memory. Specifically, retrieval from episodic memory would be expected to rely more upon hippocampus (and potentially surrounding structures) than would semantic memory.

In general, neuroimaging studies of episodic memory do not line up perfectly with the neuropsychological studies, and the precise reasons behind this situation are still unclear (Buckner and Tulving, 1995). One way in which the data are consistent with the theory is that in general, activation for retrieval from semantic and episodic memory tasks is very similar, with many (but certainly not all) differences tending to go in the direction of episodic retrieval. One puzzling finding is that the hippocampus is not reliably seen as particularly active during retrieval from episodic memory, especially as typically studied, with verbal materials (Fletcher et al., 1997; Schacter and Wagner, 1999). However, neuroimaging studies of episodic memory using autobiographical memories as the content of retrieval, rather than word lists learned in the laboratory, do overlap nicely with lesion studies (e.g., hippocampal activity is commonly reported in neuroimaging studies of autobiographical memory retrieval). Thus, questions regarding the differences obtained using differing methodologies may ultimately need to focus on the tasks being used in conjunction with the method of inquiry.

Direct comparisons of tasks designed to rely on episodic and semantic memory have not been reported as often as one might think (but for some examples see Shallice et al., 1994; Fletcher et al., 1995; Nyberg et al., 1996; McDermott et al., 1999a,b). Those who have done so show that regions within frontal cortex are more active for episodic than semantic memory. In the early 1990s (when the literature was based largely on PET methodology), retrieval-related activation in frontal cortex was almost always right-lateralized in or near Brodmann Area (BA) 10 (for a review see Buckner, 1996); more recent studies using fMRI tend to show bilateral or left-lateralized activity here. Following this relatively unanticipated finding, much work has been devoted to attempting to identify the processing underlying these prefrontal regions involved in episodic retrieval. Some hypotheses regarding the processes include retrieval mode (the mental set of attempting to retrieve the past, LePage et al., 2000), retrieval success (McDermott et al., 2000), postretrieval processing (a set of processes following the initial recovery of information in the retrieval phase; see Rugg and Wilding, 2000), or the amount of retrieval effort extended (Schacter et al., 1996). Different regions certainly contribute to different processes, but it is not yet clear which regions are contributing which processes (or even if the correct processes have been identified). A precise understanding of the situation awaits further work.

Another somewhat surprising finding is the role parietal cortex appears to play in episodic memory. Contrasts of episodic memory tasks with semantic memory tasks tend to activate regions within bilateral inferior parietal cortex (within BA 40) and within medial parietal cortex (precuneus and posterior cingulate/retrosplenial cortex, e.g., McDermott et al., 1999b), and contrasts of episodic retrieval with other comparison tasks have elicited similar findings, which have led to recent attempts to identify the role of parietal cortex in memory (Shannon and Buckner, 2004; Wagner et al., 2005). Although the possible importance of parietal cortex in episodic retrieval was at the time unanticipated from the lesion literature, a closer look at the lesion literature shows that lesions on medial parietal structures can indeed produce what has been called retrosplenial amnesia (Valenstein et al., 1987).

Of historical importance is an early generalization in functional imaging studies of human memory, which suggested an apparent asymmetry between episodic encoding and retrieval processes: Hemispheric Encoding/Retrieval Asymmetry (HERA; Tulving et al., 1994). In general, episodic encoding was thought to be more strongly associated with left frontal lobe activity (than right), whereas episodic retrieval was more strongly associated with right frontal lobe activity (than left). Because episodic encoding is believed to involve a high degree of semantic elaboration of incoming information, semantic retrieval has also been associated with left frontal lobe activity. As reviewed above, most researchers would probably argue that the more profitable approach is to attempt the ascription of processes to specific cortical regions (rather than making broad generalizations to larger regions of cortex, e.g., the role of the right frontal lobe). Nonetheless, the HERA idea was influential in the late 1990s and served as a guiding framework for a number of studies.

In this short review, we have necessarily omitted many relevant issues from consideration. Among those are fMRI studies of remembering and knowing (e.g., Henson et al., 1999; Eldridge et al., 2000; Wheeler and Buckner, 2004) and studies from the tradition of autobiographical memory (see Maguire, 2001 for review). Further, event-related potential (ERP) studies anticipated the importance of parietal cortex in retrieval (Rugg and Allan, 2000) and some of the differences seen in remembering and knowing.

To summarize, initial contrasts of episodic and semantic memory were expected to elucidate the role of the hippocampus in episodic memory. Although some studies showed such activation, many did not. Attention then turned to the role of frontal cortex in remembering (with an accompanying new look at the neuropsychological literature). Most recently, the role of parietal cortex has become of great interest. The questions being asked are essentially of the flavor of which regions contribute which processes. In our view, this approach is the best one to take at this point (see, too, Roediger et al., 1999). Neuroimaging studies have not well adjudicated the question of whether episodic memory is a memory system but have clarified thinking with respect to how (in process terms) episodic and semantic memory differ and what the neural substrates of those different processes might be. Note that this review has focused on studies that are somewhat relevant to the question of whether episodic memory can be thought of as a memory system dissociable from semantic memory; other related issues (e.g., a comparison between remembering and knowing or between successful and unsuccessful retrieval attempts) have not been addressed, as we see them as less critical to the question under consideration here (although they address fundamentally important issues in the topic of remembering).

7.3.3 Development of Episodic Memory: The Magic Number 4 ± 1

Episodic memory is a late-developing memory system that emerges in the context of an already existing ability to draw upon the past in an informative fashion. Beginning at an early age, children are able to acquire vast amounts of knowledge from their surroundings. For instance, within the first few years of life, a child will have learned and retained the meanings of thousands of words and detailed knowledge pertaining to the identities of various objects in their environment. This early accumulation and utilization of knowledge is best characterized in terms of semantic memory. That is, although children know about many things that they have learned in the past, the capacity to reliably remember specific events does not emerge until approximately 4 years of age.

As with various other developmental milestones, episodic memory emerges in a gradual manner. Specifically, although most 3 year olds have great difficulty with tasks that are believed to require episodic memory, there do appear glimpses that this capacity is beginning to manifest itself. For instance, by the age of

3 years, many children are capable of reporting the content of an event that they had previously witnessed in the laboratory (Howe and Courage, 1993; Bauer et al., 1995; Bauer and Werenka, 1995). However, the descriptions are typically vague, and it is difficult to know whether these children remember the precise episodes they describe, or whether they just know about them.

Johnson and Wellman (1980) have presented data suggesting that the ability to discriminate between the mental states of remembering and knowing does not emerge until the age of 5 years. In their study, few 4 year olds, some 5 year olds, and most first-grade children demonstrated an understanding of the distinction. This finding is consistent with the claim that children under the age of 4 years are likely relying upon semantic memory when reporting on events from their past.

A great deal has been learned about the emergence of episodic memory through the use of source memory tests (Johnson and Raye, 1981; Johnson et al., 1993). Not only do such tests require the participant to remember the content of a prior study episode, but the participant must also remember the context (e.g., when, where, etc.) in which that content was learned. Source memory tasks are believed to be good tests of episodic memory in that a correct response requires the reinstatement of specific spatial–temporal aspects of the originally encoded event. Studies that have adapted the source memory paradigm for use with children are consistent in their findings: The capacity for episodic memory appears to emerge around the age of 4 years.

In a particularly clear demonstration, Gopnik and Graf (1988) had 3-, 4-, and 5-year-old children learn the contents of a drawer under one of three conditions. The children were told about the contents of the drawer, were allowed to see the contents of the drawer for themselves, or were given hints so they could infer the contents of the drawer. During a later test, the researchers were interested in the children's ability to answer two questions: What was in the drawer, and how do you know? With regard to the first question, retention of the contents of the drawer was comparable across all age groups. All children knew what they had seen. This was not the case when the children were required to discriminate the source of their knowledge. Although the 5-year-old children made few mistakes in describing the manner in which they had learned about the contents of the drawer, the 3 year olds performed at chance levels (see also Wimmer et al., 1988; O'Neill and Gopnik, 1991). That is, only the 5-year-old children remembered the circumstances under which they had seen the contents.

This basic finding has been replicated many times (e.g., Lindsay et al., 1991; Taylor et al., 1994; see Wheeler, 2000b; Drummery and Newcombe, 2002, for a review). In general, 3 year olds show initial signs of a developing episodic memory system, but for the most part they have great difficulty when they are required to report specific details of past occurrences. By the age of 5 years, most children appear to possess fully functioning episodic memory, although this capacity is likely to continue to develop thereafter (for related discussion, see Nelson, 1984; Gopnik and Slaughter, 1991; Flavell, 1993; Howe et al., 1994; Perner and Ruffman, 1995; Wheeler et al., 1997; Wheeler, 2000a,b; Tulving, 2005; Piolino et al., 2007). With respect to the purposes of our present discussion, children of all ages (except those younger than 8 months; Wheeler, 2000b) possess intact semantic memory, the context in which episodic memory develops.

7.4 Episodic Memory and Mental Time Travel

Finally, we consider the most recent conceptual development regarding episodic memory, namely, its relation to mental time travel. The idea, initially delineated by Tulving (1985a), is roughly that humans (and perhaps only humans) possess the ability to mentally represent their personal past and future (see also Suddendorf and Corballis, 1997; Tulving, 2002a). That is, just as we can vividly recollect our personal past, we can also, with a seemingly equal level of vividness and efficacy, mentally represent personal future scenarios (episodic future thought).

Beginning with the pioneering work of Hermann Ebbinghaus (see also Nipher, 1876), students of psychology and neuroscience have expended more than 100 years of thought and careful experimentation toward an understanding of human memory. However, there has been surprisingly little inquiry into episodic future thought. According to Tulving and his colleagues, both capacities represent an important component of autonoetic consciousness, which is the ability to "both mentally represent and become aware of subjective experiences in the past, present, and future" (Wheeler et al., 1997: p. 331).

Next, we review evidence suggesting that the capacity for episodic future thought (Atance and

O'Neill, 2001) is intricately related to the ability to vividly recollect one's past. Specifically, it has been argued that impairments to both capacities co-occur following brain damage (Tulving, 1985; Klein et al., 2002), that both share similar neural networks (Okuda et al., 2003; Addis et al., 2007; Szpunar et al., 2007), and that both appear rather late in ontogenetic development (Busby and Suddendorf, 2005).

7.4.1 Neuropsychology

For an example of selective damage, consider again patient KC. Along with a selective deficit of episodic memory, KC is unable to project himself mentally into the future. When asked to do either, he states that his mind is "blank"; when asked to compare the kinds of blankness in the two situations, he says it is the "same kind of blankness" (Tulving, 1985: p. 4).

A similar profile is exhibited by patient DB, studied by Klein and colleagues (Klein et al., 2002); DB experienced an anoxic episode following cardiac arrest and can no longer recollect his past, nor can he project himself into the future. Interestingly, Klein et al. revealed that DB was able to think about the past and future in a nonpersonal (semantic) manner. That is, while DB could not report any of what he had personally experienced in the past or any of what he might experience in the future, he could report general facts related to the past, along with what might generally occur in the future (e.g., concerns about global warming).

Hassabis et al. (2007) replicated and extended these findings in a more systematic fashion. In that study, the authors presented a set of five amnesic patients with brain damage localized to the hippocampal formation. Each of these patients is densely amnesic for personal episodes but retains intact semantic memory. To test whether the profound deficit of episodic memory was accompanied by a deficit in episodic future thought, the authors tested the patients' ability to form mental images of novel future experiences. Specifically, the patients were presented with a series of 10 cues and asked to imagine themselves in the context of either novel (e.g., castle) or familiar (e.g., possible event over next weekend) settings. Relative to those of control subjects, the patients' images were "fragmentary and lacking in coherence" (Hassabis et al., 2007: p. 1728).

The aforementioned case studies represent only a few of many reports about amnesic patients. Most other investigations into the phenomenon of amnesia have, for the most part, focused on the memory problems inherent in such patients. For instance, many others have been interested in investigating the relative effects of brain damage on episodic versus semantic memory (Kapur, 1999; Wheeler and McMillan, 2001). Thus, it remains uncertain whether comparable impairments in backward- and forward-going aspects of mental time travel are common in all such patients.

Nevertheless, there do exist prior reports describing amnesic patients as living in the permanent present (Barbizet, 1970; see also Lidz, 1942), and cases similar to the ones mentioned above have been reported (Stuss, 1991; Dalla Barba et al., 1997; Levine et al., 1998). In addition, there exist extensive reviews of case study reports on patients with frontal lobe damage (e.g., Luria and Homskya, 1964; Luria, 1969). One common characterization of these patients is that they seem to be detached from the past and unconcerned about matters related to their personal future (Ackerley and Benton, 1947; see also Freeman and Watts, 1950; Ingvar, 1985; Fuster, 1989; Wheeler et al., 1997; Wheeler, 2000a).

7.4.2 Functional Neuroimaging

The psychological study of episodic future thought has been attempted only sporadically (D'Argembeau and Van der Linden, 2004, 2006; Szpunar and McDermott, in press), and the search for its neural substrates has begun only very recently. Note that we draw an important distinction between episodic future thought and more general thoughts of the future, such as planning, which has received extensive attention in the literature and is thought to rely heavily on regions within frontal cortex (Stuss and Benson, 1986; Shallice, 1988; Fuster, 1989). The set of procedures under examination here – comprising episodic future thought – are arguably a necessary precursor to planning; without the ability to envision oneself spending a weekend with friends on the ski slopes, for example, it is unlikely that one would plan the weekend.

Consider a recent PET study by Okuda et al. (2003). Participants were asked to speak aloud for 1 min about their near future (the next few days), far future (next few years), near past (recent few days), and far past (last few years). Activity during these states was compared to each other and to a fifth, baseline state, which involved talking about the meaning of various words. Two regions in anteromedial frontal cortex and medial temporal cortex were more active for the future conditions than the past conditions; other regions (in nearby medial frontal and medial temporal cortex) exhibited the opposite effects (more activity for past conditions relative to future). The authors suggested that remembering the past and planning for the future likely share common neural correlates and that it may be necessary for past experiences to be reactivated in order to facilitate an effective plan for future events (see too Burgess et al., 2000). Their data suggest that specific regions within frontal and medial temporal cortex might be suited for these functions. Although quite interesting, these data are of questionable relevance to the topic under consideration because in speaking about the future, the participants in this study tended not to focus upon specific future episodes but instead spoke about intentions, conjectures, and schedules. In contrast, these aspects were not much present when speaking about the past (i.e., the past tended to focus on specific episodes). In the other two studies to be considered, participants were asked to focus on specific episodes (either episodes that might take place in the future or ones that indeed took place in the past).

Szpunar et al. (2007) used fMRI to identify brain regions that might be important for representing oneself in time and then to examine those regions to see whether or not they are similarly engaged by past and future thought. In order to accomplish this goal, participants were asked to perform a set of three tasks. In all of these tasks, participants viewed a series of event cues (e.g., birthday party) and were asked to envision a specific scenario in response to the cues. In one task, the instructions were to recollect a personal memory of that kind of event (e.g., a specific previous birthday party). The second task instructed subjects to use the cue to think of a specific future scenario involving the cue. Activity common to both tasks (i.e., a conjunction of the past and future tasks) was contrasted with a third task that involved many of the processes common to past and future thought (e.g., mental construction of lifelike scenarios) but that lacked a sense of representing oneself in time. Specifically, the control task required participants to use the cue as a starting point for imagining former U.S. President Bill Clinton in a specific scenario. Bill Clinton was chosen because pretesting showed that he is easy to visualize in a variety of situations.

As can be seen in **Figure 3**, several regions in the brain's posterior cortex were similarly engaged during personal past and future thought, but not during the control task. These regions were located in the occipital cortex, the posterior cingulate cortex, and the medial temporal lobes. Previous research had shown that these regions are consistently engaged during tasks such as autobiographical memory (Svoboda et al., 2006) and mental navigation of familiar routes (Ghaem et al., 1997; Mellet et al., 2000;

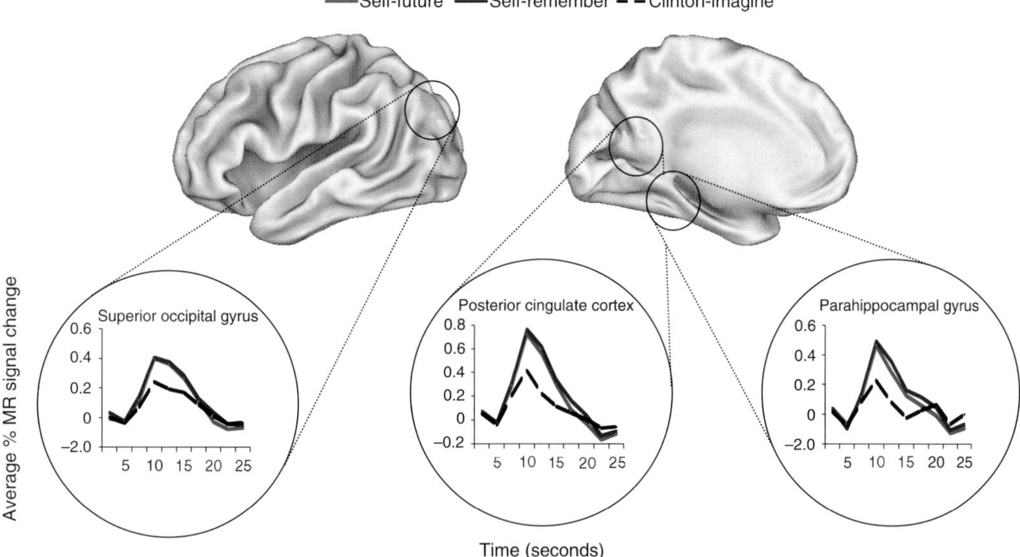

Figure 3 Percent signal change for brain regions exhibiting indistinguishable patterns of activity across time while participants envisioned their personal future and recollected the past. Imagining a familiar individual in similar scenarios resulted in a pattern of activity different from both the past and future tasks. Regions appear within superior occipital gyrus, posterior cingulate cortex, and parahippocampal gyrus. Data from Szpunar, Watson, and McDermott (2007).

Rosenbaum et al., 2004), which encourage participants to recount previously experienced settings (Aminoff et al., 2007). Szpunar et al. hypothesized that asking participants to envision a personal future scenario likely required similar processes. That is, in order to effectively generate a plausible image of the future, participants reactivate contextual associations from posterior cortical regions (cf., Bar and Aminoff, 2003; Okuda et al., 2003; Bar, 2004). Postexperiment questionnaires indicated that participants did tend to imagine future scenarios in the context of familiar settings and people.

A similar pattern of fMRI data has been presented by Addis et al. (2007), who parsed episodic future thought and remembering into two separate phases: construction and elaboration. That is, subjects were given cues (e.g., car) and asked to envision themselves in the future or to remember a past event. Once the event was in mind, they were to press a button and to then keep thinking about the event for the remaining time of the 20 s. They then rated the level of detail, the emotional intensity, and the perspective (first person or third person) before moving to the next trial. Of most interest to the present discussion is the construction phase (in part because the activity during the elaboration phase could not be separated from the activity during the three subsequent rating phases). Relative to baseline tasks that involved sentence generation and imagery, constructing the past and future episodes led to equivalent activity in a set of posterior cortical regions similar to those reported by Szpunar et al. (2007).

In light of such findings, Schacter and Addis (2007a) have proposed what they call the constructive episodic simulation hypothesis. They argue that one important function of retaining personal memories is the ability to sample their contents in mentally constructing (predicting) novel future scenarios (see also Szpunar and McDermott, in press). That past and future thought are so closely related provides insight into why certain populations who lack access to specific personal details of their past (e.g., brain damaged amnesic patients) are also unable to imagine specific personal future scenarios.

Finally, it should be noted that although this is a very recently emerging topic of interest, we anticipate that the above-mentioned studies will act as a catalyst for future research. Several early concept papers and reviews on the topic have also been put forth (Buckner and Carroll, 2007; Miller, 2007; Schacter and Addis, 2007a; Szpunar and McDermott, 2007). There is a recent but clear trend in thinking about episodic memory to include episodic future thought.

7.4.3 Development of Episodic Future Thought

A small but growing line of research suggests that the ability to project oneself into the future emerges in concert with the ability to vividly recollect the past. For instance, Busby and Suddendorf (2005) have shown that it is not until about the age of 5 years that children are able to accurately report what they will or will not do in the future (i.e., tomorrow), as well as what they have or have not done in the past (i.e., yesterday). Many of these studies have focused on requiring children to predict future states (e.g., Suddendorf and Busby, 2005) and have revealed both that the emergence of this capacity is not based simply on semantic knowledge related to the future event (Atance and Meltzoff, 2005) and that it is not dependent on language (Atance and O'Neill, 2005).

7.5 Is Episodic Memory Uniquely Human?

Perhaps the most intensely debated topic regarding episodic memory is whether this capacity, and mental time travel more generally, is uniquely human. There is no dispute that nonhuman animals possess memory. For example, consider a dog that buries a bone in the backyard and retrieves it the following day. How does the dog accomplish this task? Perhaps the animal mentally travels back in time, as we might. Alternatively, the animal may simply know that the backyard is somewhere where things are buried and may be able to make use of salient cues to locate the object it desires. Or the animal may know exactly where the bone is without remembering the episode in which it was placed there. We suspect most dog owners would suggest that the animal surely remembers where it had buried the bone and would likely be willing to offer many other examples to support the claim. But is this what happens?

As it turns out, this is a very difficult question to answer. If we assume that subjective (autonoetic) awareness is the central component of episodic memory, then we are not able to get very far. Much of the evidence for the concept of autonoetic awareness comes by way of verbal reports regarding the subjective state experienced during the act of remembering the past (e.g., remembering vs. knowing). Because we cannot directly ask a nonhuman animal to describe its mental state, the prospect of identifying autonoetic awareness in other species is dim (Clayton et al., 2005). This state of affairs has led some to argue that there should be other means by which to investigate episodic memory in nonhuman animals.

Clayton et al. (2003) suggest that one alternative is to characterize episodic memory in terms of the spatial–temporal information that is encoded about an earlier event (what, where, and when) and the nature by which this information is represented (i.e., as an integrated whole) and utilized. The authors argue that animal studies must consider these behavioral criteria if they are to demonstrate convincing evidence of episodic memory in nonhuman animals. Clayton et al. further review prior attempts using primates, rats, and other animals that fall short of meeting these criteria.

Clayton, Dickinson, and their colleagues have presented several impressive demonstrations of an integrative memory capacity in the western scrub jay (e.g., Clayton and Dickinson, 1998, 1999). In their studies, the scrub jays are given the opportunity to cache both preferable but perishable (e.g., wax worms) and nonpreferable but less perishable (e.g., nuts) foodstuffs (see **Figure 4**). Given that the scrub jays' preferred snack will perish sooner, the birds must remember not only what they stored and where they stored it, but also when the foodstuff had been stored. Although the scrub jays will prefer to search for their favored treat, there is little point if that snack is no longer edible. It appears that the scrub jays are able to integrate these aspects of the original caching episode and search accordingly. That is, the scrub jays are able to appropriately adjust recovery attempts of the differentially perishable caches depending on how long ago they had stored the food items.

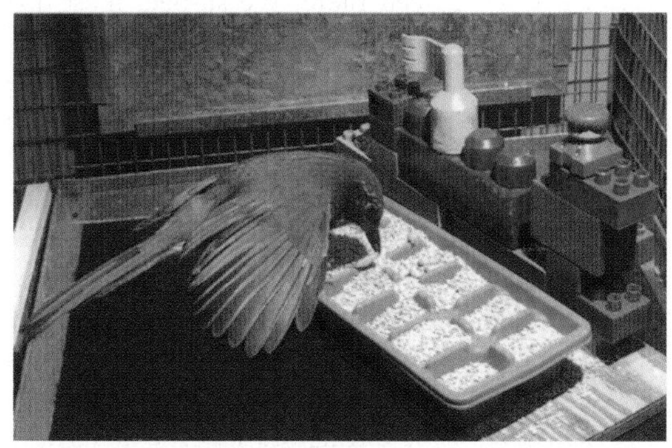

Figure 4 A western scrub-jay caching wax worms.

Even such convincing evidence of an integrated spatial–temporal memory of the past leaves open questions regarding the mental life of this species of bird. As a result, Clayton et al. (2003; Clayton and Dickinson, 1998) refer to this capacity as episodic-like memory, while others question whether this feat represents episodic memory or some other mechanism that may be driven by specific learning algorithms (Suddendorf and Busby, 2003; Suddendorf, 2006; see also Tulving, 2005).

Tulving (2005) has suggested that although mental states cannot be reported by other species, they may in fact be inferred, particularly in the context of mental time travel into the future (e.g., Emery and Clayton, 2001; Dally et al., 2006). Specifically, Tulving argues that comparative studies of episodic memory per se may be futile, in that demonstrations of episodic-like memory in other species may be explained away by simpler mechanisms that need not evoke episodic memory in its true sense (involving autonoetic consciousness). However, it may be possible to construct a situation in which an animal's future-directed behavior may not be attributed to other, simpler means.

Achieving such a situation, however, is no simple matter. A great deal of evidence suggests that even our nearest primitive relatives are incapable of truly future-oriented behavior (for reviews see Roberts, 2002; Suddendorf and Busby, 2003). According to the Bishof-Kohler hypothesis, an animal's foresight is necessarily restricted because it cannot anticipate future needs (for a more in-depth discussion see Suddendorf and Corballis, 1997). For instance, although chimpanzees display preparatory behaviors for future food consumption, it is unclear whether such behaviors indicate foresight beyond the near future (e.g., Boesch and Boesch, 1984; Byrne, 1995). Based on a review of the relevant literature, Roberts (2002) also concluded that higher-order primates appear to be "stuck in time."

Future studies will require clever experimental designs that will allow researchers to examine whether a particular species is able to plan for the future in a manner that is not instigated or maintained by its present motivational state, and in the absence of any immediate benefits associated with a future-directed action (see Mulcahy and Call, 2006; Raby et al., 2007). As it stands, the capacity to mentally represent the personal past and future has only been convincingly demonstrated with human beings (usually over the age of 4 years). Although future research will provide us with a better understanding as to how unique this capacity is to humans, it will likely remain that this capacity holds a special status for humankind (Suddendorf and Corballis, 1997; Tulving, 2002a).

7.6 Concluding Remarks

As with all concepts of scientific inquiry, episodic memory is an evolving one that is largely shaped through the intricate relationship between data, theory, and available methods of inquiry. The concept of episodic memory started out as a taxonomic distinction that might possess some heuristic usefulness for future research. It has now expanded to encompass a dissociable system of the human brain that enables its owner to accomplish a feat (i.e., becoming autonoetically aware of episodes from one's past) that could not otherwise be possible. Currently, episodic memory represents a concept of great interest to many fields (e.g., clinical psychology, comparative psychology, developmental psychology, experimental psychology, functional brain imaging, neuropsychology, and psychopharmacology). There is little doubt that the continuing accumulation of data from these various areas of research, together with their unique methods of inquiry and furthering technological advancements, will ensure that researchers on the topic will continue to ask new and exciting questions.

Acknowledgements

This chapter benefited greatly from comments provided by Endel Tulving and Roddy Roediger.

References

Ackerley SS and Benton AL (1947) Report of a case of bilateral frontal lobe defect. *Res. Publ. Assoc. Res. Nerv. Ment. Dis.* 27: 479–504.

Addis DR, Wong AT, and Schacter DL (2007) Remembering the past and imagining the future: Common and distinct neural substrates during event construction and elaboration. *Neuropsychologia* 45: 1363–1377.

Aggleton JP and Brown MW (1999) Episodic memory, amnesia, and the hippocampal-anterior thalamic axis. *Behav. Brain Sci.* 22: 425–444.

Aminoff E, Gronau N, and Bar M (2007) The parahippocampal cortex mediates spatial and nonspatial associations. *Cereb. Cortex* 17: 1497–1503.

Atance CM and Meltzoff AN (2005) My future self: Young children's ability to anticipate and explain future states. *Cogn. Dev.* 20: 341–361.

Atance CM and O'Neill CM (2001) Episodic future thinking. *Trends Cogn Sci 5*(12): 533–539.

Atance CM and O'Neill DK (2005) The emergence of episodic future thinking in humans. *Learn. Motiv.* 36: 126–144.

Bar M (2004) Visual objects in context. *Nat. Rev. Neurosci.* 5: 617–629.

Bar M and Aminoff E (2003) Cortical analysis of context. *Neuron* 38: 347–358.

Barbizet J (1970) *Human Memory and Its Pathology*. San Francisco: Freeman.

Bauer PJ, Hertsgaard LA, and Werenka SS (1995) Effects of experience and reminding on long-term recall in infancy: Remembering not to forget. *J. Exp. Child Psychol.* 59: 260–298.

Bauer PJ and Werenka SS (1995) One- to two-year olds' recall of events: The more expressed, the more impressed. *J. Exp. Child Psychol.* 59: 475–496.

Bekhterev VM (1900) Demonstration eines Gehirns mit Zerstorung der vorderen und inneren Theile der Hirnrinde beider Schlafenlappen. *Neurol. Zbl.* 19: 990–991.

Berntsen D (1996) Involuntary autobiographical memories. *Appl. Cogn. Psychol.* 10: 435–454.

Berntsen D (1998) Voluntary and involuntary access to autobiographical memory. *Memory* 6: 113–141.

Boesch C and Boesch H (1984) Mental map in wild chimpanzees: An analysis of hammer transport for nut cracking. *Primates* 25: 160–170.

Buckner RL (1996) Beyond HERA: Contributions of specific prefrontal brain areas to long-term memory retrieval. *Psychon. Bull. Rev.* 3: 149–158.

Buckner RL (2007) Memory systems: An incentive, not an endpoint. In: Roediger HL III, Dudai Y, and Fitzpatrick SM (eds.) *Science of Memory: Concepts*, pp. 359–366. Oxford: Oxford University Press.

Buckner RL and Carroll DC (2007) Self-projection and the brain. *Trends Cognitive Sci.* 11: 49–57.

Buckner RL and Tulving E (1995) Neuroimaging studies of memory: Theory and recent PET results. In: Boller F and Grafman J (eds.) *Handbook of Neuropsychology*, pp. 439–466. Amsterdam: Elsevier.

Burgess PW, Veitch E, Costello AL, and Shallice T (2000) The cognitive and neuroanatomical correlates of multitasking. *Neuropsychologia* 38: 848–863.

Busby J and Suddendorf T (2005) Recalling yesterday and predicting tomorrow. *Cogn. Dev.* 20: 362–372.

Byrne R (1995) *The Thinking Ape: Evolutionary Origins of Intelligence*. Oxford: Oxford University Press.

Calabrese P, Markowitsch HJ, Durwen HF, et al. (1996) Right temporofrontal cortex as critical locus for ecphory of old episodic memories. *J. Neurol. Neurosurg. Psychiatry* 61: 304–310.

Cermak L and O'Connor M (1983) The anterograde and retrograde retrieval ability of a patient with amnesia due to encephalitis. *Neuropsychologia* 21: 213–234.

Clayton NS and Dickinson A (1998) Episodic-like memory during cache recovery by scrub jays. *Nature* 395: 272–278.

Clayton NS and Dickinson A (1999) Scrub jays (*Aphelocoma coerulescens*) remember when as well as where and what food item they cached. *J. Comp. Psychol.* 113: 403–416.

Clayton NS, Bussey TJ, and Dickinson A (2003) Can animals recall the past and plan for the future? *Nat. Rev. Neurosci.* 4: 685–691.

Crovitz HF and Schiffman H (1974) Frequency of episodic memories as a function of their age. *Bull. Psychon. Soc.* 4(5B): 517–518.

D'Argembeau A and Van der Linden M (2004) Phenomenal characteristics associated with projecting oneself back into the past and forward into the future: Influence of valence and temporal distance. *Conscious. Cogn.* 13: 844–858.

D'Argembeau A and Van der Linden M (2006) Individual differences in the phenomenology of mental time travel: The effect of vivid visual imagery and emotion regulation strategies. *Conscious. Cogn.* 15: 342–350.

Dalla Barba G, Cappelletti JY, Signorini M, and Denes G (1997) Confabulation: Remembering "another" past, planning "another" future. *Neurocase* 3: 425–436.

Dally JM, Emery NJ, and Clayton NS (2006) Food-caching western scrub-jays keep track of who was watching when. *Science* 312: 1662–1665.

De Renzi E, Lucchelli F, Muggia S, and Spinnler H (1997) Is memory loss without anatomical damage tantamount to a psychogenic deficit? The case of pure retrograde amnesia. *Neuropsychologia* 35: 781–794.

Drummery AB and Newcombe NS (2002) Developmental changes in source memory. *Dev. Sci.* 5: 502–513.

Ebbinghaus H (1885) *Memory: A Contribution to Experimental Psychology*. New York: Dover.

Einstein GO, McDaniel MA, Thomas R, et al. (2005) Multiple processes in prospective memory retrieval: Factors determining monitoring versus spontaneous retrieval. *J. Exp. Psychol. Gen.* 134: 327–342.

Eldridge LL, Knowlton BJ, Furmanski CS, Bookheimer SY, and Engel SA (2000) Remembering episodes: A selective role for the hippocampus during retrieval. *Nat. Neurosci.* 3(11): 1149–1152.

Emery NJ and Clayton NS (2001) Effects of experience and social context on prospective caching strategies by scrub jays. *Nature* 414: 443–446.

Flavell JH (1993) Young children's understanding of thinking and consciousness. *Curr. Dir. Psychol. Sci.* 2: 40–43.

Fletcher PC, Frith CD, Baker SC, Shallice T, Frackowiak R, and Dolan R (1995) The mind's eye-precuneus activation in memory-related imagery. *Neuroimage* 2: 195–200.

Fletcher P, Frith CD, and Rugg MD (1997) Functional neuroanatomy of episodic memory. *Trends Neurosci.* 20: 213–218.

Freeman W and Watts JW (1950) *Pscyhosurgery*, 2nd edn. Springfield, IL: Charles S Thomas.

Fuster JM (1989) *The Prefrontal Cortex. Anatomy, Physiology, and Neuropsychology of the Frontal Lobe*, 2nd edn. New York: Raven.

Gardiner JM (1988) Functional aspects of recollective experience. *Mem. Cognit.* 16: 309–313.

Gardiner JM and Richardson-Klavehn A (2000) Remembering and knowing. In: Tulving E and Craik FIM (eds.) *Oxford Handbook of Memory*, pp. 229–244. Oxford: Oxford University Press.

Ghaem O, Mellet E, Crivello F, et al. (1997) Mental navigation along memorized routes activates the hippocampus, precuneus, and insula. *NeuroReport* 8: 739–744.

Gopnik A and Graf P (1988) Knowing how you know: Young children's ability to identify and remember the sources of their beliefs. *Child Dev.* 59: 1366–1371.

Gopnik A and Slaughter V (1991) Young children's understanding of changes in their mental states. *Child Dev.* 62: 98–110.

Grossi D, Trojano L, Grasso A, and Orsini A (1988) Selective "semantic amnesia" after closed-head injury: A case report. *Cortex* 24: 457–464.

Hampton RR (2005) Can rhesus monkeys discriminate between remembering and forgetting? In: Metcalfe HSTJ (ed.) *The Missing Link in Cognition: Origins of Self-Reflective Consciousness*, pp. 272–295. New York: Oxford University Press.

Hassabis D, Kumaran D, Vann SD, and Maguire EA (2007) Patients with hippocampal amnesia cannot imagine new experiences. *Proc. Natl. Acad. Sci. USA* 104: 1726–1731.

Henson RN, Rugg MD, Shallice T, Josephs O, and Dolan RJ (1999) Recollection and familiarity in recognition memory: An event-related functional magnetic resonance imaging study. *J. Neurosci.* 19(10): 3962–3972.

Howe ML and Courage ML (1993) On resolving the enigma of infantile amnesia. *Psychol. Bull.* 113: 305–326.

Howe ML, Courage ML, and Peterson C (1994) how can I remember when "I" wasn't there: Long-term retention of traumatic experiences and emergence of the cognitive self. *Conscious. Cogn.* 3: 327–355.

Ingvar DH (1985) "Memory of the future": An essay on temporal organization of conscious awareness. *Hum. Neurobiol.* 4(3): 127–136.

Jacoby LL (1991) A process dissociation framework: Separating automatic and intentional uses of memory. *J. Mem. Lang.* 30: 513–541.

James WJ (1890) Memory. In: *The Principles of Psychology*, pp. 643–689. New York: Henry Holt.

Johnson CN and Wellman HM (1980) Children's developing understanding of mental verbs: Remember, know, and guess. *Child Dev.* 51: 1095–1102.

Johnson MK, Hashtroudi S, and Lindsay DS (1993) Source monitoring. *Psychol. Bull.* 114: 3–28.

Johnson MK and Raye CL (1981) Reality monitoring. *Psychol. Rev.* 88: 67–85.

Kapur N (1999) Syndromes of retrograde amnesia: A conceptual and empirical analysis. *Psychol. Bull.* 125: 800–825.

Kitchener EG, Hodges J, and McCarthy R (1998) Acquisition of post-morbid vocabulary and semantic facts in the absence of episodic memory. *Brain* 121: 1313–1327.

Klein SB (2001) A self to remember: A cognitive neuropsychological perspective on how self creates memory and memory creates self. In: Sedikides C and Brewer MB (eds.) *Individual Self, Relational Self, Collective Self*, pp. 25–46. Philadelphia: Psychology Press.

Klein SB, Loftus J, and Kihlstrom JF (2002) Memory and temporal experience: The effects of episodic memory loss on an amnesic patient's ability to remember the past and imagine the future. *Soc. Cogn.* 20(5): 353–379.

Klein SB, German TP, Cosmides L, and Gabriel R (2004) A theory of autobiographical memory: Necessary components and disorders resulting from their loss. *Soc. Cogn.* 22(5): 460–490.

Lepage M, Ghaffar O, Nyberg L, and Tulving E (2000) Prefrontal cortex and episodic memory retrieval mode. *Proc. Natl. Acad. Sci. USA* 97(1): 506–511.

Levine B, Black SE, Cabeza R, et al. (1998) Episodic memory and the self in a case of isolated retrograde amnesia. *Brain* 121: 1951–1973.

Lidz T (1942) The amnesic syndrome. *Arch. Neurol. Psychiatry* 47: 588–605.

Lindsay DS, Johnson MK, and Kwon P (1991) Developmental changes in memory source monitoring. *J. Exp. Child Psychol.* 52: 297–318.

Locke J (1690/1975) *An Essay Concerning Human Understanding*. Nidditch PH (ed.) Oxford: Clarendon Press.

Luria AR (1969) Frontal lobe syndromes. In: Bruyn GW and Vinken PJ (eds.) *Handbook of Clinical Neurology,* vol. 2, pp. 725–757. Amsterdam: North Holland.

Luria AR and Homskya ED (1964) Disturbance in the regulative role of speech with frontal lobe lesions. In: Warren JN and Akert K (ed.) *The Frontal Granular Cortex and Behavior*, pp. 353–371. New York: McGraw-Hill.

Maguire EA (2001) Neuroimaging studies of autobiographical memory. *Philos. Trans. R. Soc. Lond. B* 356: 1441–1451.

Markowitsch HJ, Calabrese P, Neufeld H, Gehlen W, and Durwen HF (1999) Retrograde amnesia for world knowledge

and preserved memory for autobiographical events: A case report. *Cortex* 35: 243–252.
McDaniel MA and Einstein GO (2000) Strategic and automatic processes in prospective memory retrieval: A multiprocess framework. *Appl. Cogn. Psychol.* 14: S127–S144.
McDermott KB, Buckner RL, Petersen SE, Kelley WM, and Sanders AL (1999a) Set- and code-specific activation in frontal cortex: An fMRI study of encoding and retrieval of faces and words. *J. Cogn. Neurosci.* 11(6): 631–640.
McDermott KB, Ojemann JG, Petersen SE, et al. (1999b) Direct comparison of episodic encoding and retrieval of words: An event-related fMRI study. *Memory* 7(5–6): 661–678.
McDermott KB, Jones TC, Petersen SE, Lageman SK, and Roediger HL (2000) Retrieval success is accompanied by enhanced activation in anterior prefrontal cortex during recognition memory: An event-related fMRI study. *J. Cogn. Neurosci.* 12: 965–976.
McKenna PJ, Mortimer AM, and Hodges JR (1994) Semantic memory and schizophrenia. In: David AS and Cutting C (eds.) *The Neuropsychology of Schizophrenia*, pp. 163–178. Hove, UK: Erlbaum.
Mellet E, Bricogne S, Tzourio-Mazoyer N, et al. (2000) Neural correlates of topographic mental exploration: The impact of route versus survey perspective learning. *Neuroimage* 12: 588–600.
Mesulam MM (1990) Large-scale neurocognitive networks and distributed processing for attention, language, and memory. *Annu. Rev. Neurol.* 28: 597–613.
Metcalfe J (2000) Metamemory: Theory and data. In: Tulving E and Craik FIM (eds.) *Oxford Handbook of Memory*, pp. 197–211. New York: Oxford University Press.
Miller G (2007) A surprising conection between memory and imagination. *Science* 315: 312.
Mishkin M, Suzuki WA, Gadian DG, and Vargha-Khadem F (1997) Hierarchical organization of cognitive memory. *Philos. Trans. R. Soci. Lond. B* 352: 1461–1467.
Mulcahy NJ and Call J (2006) Apes save tools for future use. *Science* 312: 1038–1040.
Nelson K (1984) The transition from infant to child memory. In: Moscovitch M (ed.) *Infant Memory: Its Relation to Normal and Pathological Memory in Humans and Other Animals,* vol. 26, pp. 1–24. Hillsdale, NJ: Erlbaum.
Nielsen JM (1958) *Memory and Amnesia*. Los Angeles: San Lucas Press.
Nipher FE (1876) Probability of error in writing a series of numbers. *Am. J. Sci. Arts* 12: 79–80.
Nyberg L, Cabeza R, and Tulving E (1996) PET studies of encoding and retrieval: The HERA model. *Psychon. Bull. Rev.* 3: 135–148.
Nyberg L, Persson J, Habib R, et al. (2000) Large scale neurocognitive networks underlying episodic memory. *J. Cogn. Neurosci.* 12: 163–173.
O'Neill DK and Gopnik A (1991) Young children's ability to identify the sources of their beliefs. *Dev. Psychol.* 27: 134–147.
Okuda J, Fujii T, Ohtake H, et al. (2003) Thinking of the future and past: The roles of the frontal pole and the medial temporal lobes. *Neuroimage* 19: 1369–1380.
Perner J and Ruffman T (1995) Episodic memory and autonoetic consciousness: Developmental evidence and a theory of childhood amnesia. *J. Exp. Child Psychol.* 59: 516–548.
Piolino P, Hisland M, Ruffeveille I, Matuszewski V, Jamaque I, and Eustache F (2007) Do school-age children remember or know the personal past? *Conscious. Cogn.* 16: 84–101.
Prince SE, Tsukiura T, Daselaar SM, and Cabeza R (2007) Distinguishing the neural correlates of episodic memory encoding and semantic memory retrieval. *Psychol. Sci.* 18: 144–151.
Raby CR, Alexis DM, Dickinson A, and Clayton NS (2007) Planning for the future by western scrub-jays. *Nature* 445: 919–921.
Rajaram S (1993) Remembering and knowing: Two means of access to the personal past. *Mem. Cogn.* 21: 89–102.
Roberts WA (2002) Are animals stuck in time? *Psychol. Bull.* 128: 473–489.
Robinson JA (1976) Sampling autobiographical memory. *Cogn. Psychol.* 8: 578–595.
Roediger HL (2000) Why retrieval is the key process in understanding human memory. In: Tulving E (ed.) *Memory, Consciousness, and the Brain: The Tallinn Conference*, pp. 52–75. Philadelphia: Psychology Press.
Roediger HL and McDermott KB (1993) Implicit memory in normal human subjects. In: Boller F and Grafman J (eds.) *Handbook of Neuropsychology,* vol. 8, pp. 63–131. Amsterdam: Elsevier.
Roediger HL, Rajaram S, and Srinivas K (1990) Specifying criteria for postulating memory systems. *Ann. NY Acad. Sci.* 608: 572–589; discussion 589–595.
Roediger HL, Buckner RL, and McDermott KB (1999) Components of processing. In: Foster JK and Jelicic M (eds.) *Memory: Systems, Processes, of Function?* pp. 31–65. Oxford: Oxford University Press.
Rosenbaum RS, Priselac S, Kohler S, et al. (2000) Remote spatial memory in an amnesic person with extensive bilateral hippocampal lesions. *Nat. Neurosci.* 3: 1044–1048.
Rosenbaum SR, Ziegler M, Winocur G, Grady CL, and Moscovitch M (2004) "I have often walked down this street before": fMRI studies on the hippocampus and other structures during mental navigation of an old environment. *Hippocampus* 14: 826–835.
Rosenbaum RS, Kohler S, Schacter DL, et al. (2005) The case of KC: contributions of a memory-impaired person to memory theory. *Neuropsychologia* 43: 999–1021.
Rugg MD and Allan K (2000) Memory retrieval: An electrophysiological perspective. In: Gazzaniga MS (ed.) *The New Cognitive Neurosciences,* 2nd edn. Cambridge, MA: MIT Press.
Rugg MD and Wilding EL (2000) Retrieval processing and episodic memory. *Trends Cogn. Sci.* 4: 108–115.
Schacter DL (1987) Implicit memory: History and current status. *J. Exp. Psychol. Learn. Mem. Cogn.* 13: 501–518.
Schacter DL and Addis DR (2007a) The cognitive neuroscience of constructive memory: Remembering the past and imagining the future. *Philos. Trans. R. Soc. Lond. B* 362: 773–786.
Schacter DL and Addis DR (2007b) Constructive memory: The ghosts of past and future. *Nature* 445: 27.
Schacter DL, Alpert NM, Savage CR, Rauch SL, and Albert MS (1996) Conscious recollection and the human hippocampal formation: Evidence from positron emission tomography. *Proc. Natl. Acad. Sci. USA* 93: 321–325.
Schacter DL, Bowers J, and Booker J (1989) Intention, awareness, and implicit memory: The retrieval intentionality criterion. In: Lewandowsky S, Dunn JC, and Kirsner K (eds.) *Implicit Memory: Theoretical Issues*, pp. 47–65. Hillsdale, NJ: Lawrence Erlbaum.
Schacter DL, Eich JE, and Tulving E (1978) Richard Semon's theory of memory. *J. Verb. Learn. Verb. Behav.* 17: 721–743.
Schacter DL and Tulving E (1994) What are the memory systems of 1994? In: Schacter DL and Tulving E (eds.) *Memory Systems 1994*, pp. 1–38. Cambridge, MA: MIT Press.
Schacter DL and Wagner AD (1999) Medial temporal lobe activations in fMRI and PET studies of episodic encoding and retrieval. *Hippocampus* 9: 7–24.
Scoville W and Milner B (1957) Loss of recent memory after bilateral hippocampal lesions. *J. Neurol. Neurosurg. Psychiatry* 20: 11–21.
Semon R (1904) *Die Mneme Als Erhaltendes Prinzip im Wechsel des Organishen Geschehens*. Leipzig: Wilhelm Engelmann.

Shallice T (1988) *From Neuropsychology to Mental Structure*. Cambridge: Cambridge University Press.

Shallice T, Fletcher JM, Frith CD, Grasby PM, Frackowiak R, and Dolan R (1994) Brain regions associated with acquisition and retrieval of verbal episodic memory. *Nature* 368: 633–635.

Shannon BJ and Buckner RL (2004) Functional-anatomic correlates of memory retrieval that suggest nontraditional processing roles for multiple distinct regions within posterior parietal cortex. *J. Neurosci.* 24: 10084–10092.

Sherry DF and Schacter DL (1987) The evolution of multiple memory systems. *Psychol. Rev.* 94: 439–454.

Squire LR (1987) *Memory and Brain*. New York: Oxford University Press.

Stuss DT (1991) Disturbance of self-awareness after frontal system damage. In: Prigatano GP and Schacter DL (eds.) *Awareness of Deficit After Brain Injury*, pp. 63–83. Oxford: Oxford University Press.

Stuss DT and Benson DF (1986) *The Frontal Lobes*. New York: Raven Press.

Suddendorf T (2006) Foresight and evolution of the human mind. *Science* 312: 1006–1007.

Suddendorf T and Busby J (2003) Mental time travel in animals? *Trends Cogn. Sci.* 7: 391–396.

Suddendorf T and Busby J (2005) Making decisions with the future in mind: Developmental and comparative identification of mental time travel. *Learn. Motiv.* 36: 110–125.

Suddendorf T and Corballis MC (1997) Mental time travel and the evolution of the human mind. *Genet. Soc. Gen. Psychol. Monogr.* 123: 133–167.

Svoboda E, McKinnon MC, and Levine B (2006) The functional neuroanatomy of autobiographical memory: A meta-analysis. *Neuropsychologia* 44: 2189–2208.

Szpunar KK and McDermott KB (2007) Remembering the past to imagine the future. *Cerebrum* February. http://www.dana.org/news/cerebrum/detail.aspx?id=5526 [online].

Szpunar KK and McDermott KB (in press) Episodic future thought and its relation to remembering: Evidence from ratings of subjective experience. *Conscious. Cogn.*

Szpunar KK, Watson JM, and McDermott KB (2007) Neural substrates of envisioning the future. *Proc. Natl. Acad. Sci. USA* 104: 642–647.

Taylor M, Esbensen BM, and Bennett RT (1994) Children's understanding of knowledge acquisition: The tendency for children to report that they have always known what they just learned. *Child Dev.* 65: 1581–1604.

Toth JP (2000) Nonconscious forms of human memory. In: Tulving E and Craik FIM (eds.) *Oxford Handbook of Memory*, pp. 245–261. New York: Oxford University Press.

Tulving E (1972) Episodic and semantic memory. In: Tulving E and Donaldson W (eds.) *Organization of Memory*, pp. 381–403. New York: Academic Press.

Tulving E (1976) Ecphoric processes in recall and recognition. In Brown JS (ed.) *Recall and Recognition*, pp. 37–73. New York: Wiley.

Tulving E (1982) Synergistic ecphory in recall and recognition. *Can. J. Psychol.* 36: 130–147.

Tulving E (1983) *Elements of Episodic Memory*. New York: Oxford University Press.

Tulving E (1984) Relations among components and processes of memory. *Behav. Brain Sci.* 7: 257–268.

Tulving E (1985a) How many memory systems are there? *Am. Psychol.* 40: 385–398.

Tulving E (1985b) Memory and consciousness. *Can. Psychol.* 26: 1–12.

Tulving E (1989a) Memory: Performance, knowledge, and experience. *Eur. J. Cogn. Psychol.* 1: 3–26.

Tulving E (1989b) Remembering and knowing the past. *Am. Sci.* 77: 361–367.

Tulving E (1995) Organization of memory: Quo vidas? In: Gazzaniga MS (ed.) *The Cognitive Neurosciences*, pp. 839–847. Cambridge, MA: MIT Press.

Tulving E (2002a) Chronesthesia: Awareness of subjective time. In: Stuss DT and Knight RC (eds.) *Principles of Frontal Lobe Function*, pp. 311–325. New York: Oxford University Press.

Tulving E (2002b) Episodic memory: From mind to brain. *Annu. Rev. Psychol.* 53: 1–25.

Tulving E (2005) Episodic memory and autonoesis: Uniquely human? In Terrace HS and Metcalfe J (ed.) *The Missing Link in Cognition: Origins of Self-Reflective Consciousness*, pp. 3–56. New York: Oxford University Press.

Tulving E and Madigan SA (1970) Memory and verbal learning. *Annu. Rev. Psychol.* 21: 437–484.

Tulving E, Kapur S, Craik FIM, Moscovitch M, and Houle S (1994) Hemispheric encoding/retrieval asymmetry in episodic memory: Positron emission tomography findings. *Proc. Natl. Acad. Sci. USA* 91: 2016–2020.

Tulving E and Markowitsch HJ (1998) Episodic and declarative memory: Role of the hippocampus. *Hippocampus* 8: 198–204.

Valenstein E, Bowers D, Verfaellie M, Heilman KM, Day A, and Watson RT (1987) Retrospenial amnesia. *Brain* 110: 1631–1646.

Vargha-Khadem F, Gadian DG, Watkins KE, Connelly A, Van Paesschen W, and Mishkin M (1997) Differential effects of early hippocampal pathology on episodic and semantic memory. *Science* 277: 376–380.

Viskontas IV, McAndrews MP, and Moscovitch M (2000) Remote episodic memory deficits in patients with unilateral temporal lobe epilepsy and excisions. *J. Neurosci.* 20: 5853–5857.

Wagner AD, Shannon BJ, Kahn I, and Buckner RL (2005) Parietal lobe contributions to episodic memory retrieval. *Trends Cogn. Sci.* 9: 445–453.

Wheeler MA (2000a) Episodic memory and autonoetic consciousness. In: Tulving E and Craik FIM (eds.) *Oxford Handbook of Memory*, pp. 597–608. New York: Oxford University Press.

Wheeler MA (2000b) Varieties of consciousness and memory. In: Tulving E (ed.), *Memory, Consciousness, and the Brain: The Tallinn Conference*, pp. 188–199. Philadelphia: Psychology Press.

Wheeler ME and Buckner RL (2004) Functional-anatomic correlates of remembering and knowing. *Neuroimage* 21: 1337–1349.

Wheeler MA and McMillan CT (2001) Focal retrograde amnesia and the episodic-semantic distinction. *Cogn. Affect. Behav. Neurosci.* 1: 22–37.

Wheeler MA, Stuss DT, and Tulving E (1997) Toward a theory of episodic memory: The frontal lobes and autonoetic consciousness. *Psychol. Bull.* 121: 331–354.

Wimmer H, Hogrefe G-J, and Perner J (1988) Children's understanding of information access as a source of knowledge. *Child Dev.* 59: 386–396.

Yasuda K, Watanabe D, and Ono Y (1997) Dissociation between semantic and autobiographical memory: A case report. *Cortex* 33: 623–638.

Yonelinas AP (2002) The nature of recollection and familiarity: A review of 30 years of research. *J. Mem. Lang.* 46: 441–517.

8 Working Memory

S. E. Gathercole, University of York, York, UK

8.1 Introduction

A common feature of our everyday mental life is the need to hold information in mind for brief periods of time. We frequently have to remember a new telephone or vehicle registration number, to write down the spelling of an unusual name that has been dictated to us, or to follow spoken instructions to find our destination in an unfamiliar environment. At other times, we need to engage in mental activities that require both temporary storage and demanding cognitive processing. Mental arithmetic provides a good example of this: successfully multiplying two numbers such as 43 and 27 in our heads involves storing not only the numbers but the products of the intermediate calculations, accessing and applying the stored rules of multiplication and addition, and integrating the various pieces of information to arrive at the correct solution. Our conscious experience of the calculation attempt is of a kind of mental juggling, in which we try to keep all elements of the task – the numbers we are trying to remember as well as the calculations – going at the same time. Often, the juggling attempt will fail, either because the capacity of working memory is exceeded, or because we become distracted and our attention is diverted away from the task in hand.

Working memory – which is the term widely used by psychologists to refer to the set of cognitive processes involved in the temporary storage and manipulation of information – supports all of these activities and many more. A useful informal way of conceptualizing working memory is as a mental jotting pad that we can use to record useful material for brief periods of time, as the need arises in the course of our everyday cognitive activities. Although it a valuable and highly flexible resource, working memory has several limitations: its storage capacity is limited, and it is a fragile system whose contents are easily disrupted. Once lost from working memory, material cannot be recovered.

The basic features of working memory are described in this chapter. Leading theoretical accounts of the cognitive processes involved in working memory are described, and key findings and experimental phenomena are outlined. As it is now also known that working memory is important not only for the temporary retention of information, but also for the acquisition of more permanent knowledge, theories of how different aspects of working memory mediate learning are also considered in this chapter.

8.2 The Working Memory Model

One influential theoretical account of working memory has framed much of the research and thinking in this field for several decades. In 1974, Baddeley and Hitch advanced a model of working memory that has been substantially refined and extended over the intervening period. The influence of the working memory model extends far beyond the detailed structure of its cognitive processes, which are considered in the following sections. The radical claim made by Baddeley and Hitch was that working memory is a flexible multicomponent system that satisfies a wide range of everyday cognitive needs for temporary mental storage – in other words, it does important work for the user. The distinction between short-term memory and working memory is a key element in the philosophy of this approach. The term working memory refers to the whole set of cognitive processes that comprise the model, which as we will see includes higher-level attentional and executive processes as well as storage systems specialized for particular information domains. Activities that tap a broad range of the functions of working memory, including both storage and higher-level control functions, are often described as working memory tasks. The term short-term memory, on the other hand, is largely reserved for memory tasks that principally require the temporary storage of information only. In this respect, short-term memory tasks tap only a subset of working memory processes. Detailed examples of each of these classes of memory task are provided in later sections.

A further key element of the Baddeley and Hitch (1974) approach is its use of dual-task methodology to investigate the modular structure of the working memory system. These researchers have developed a set of laboratory techniques for occupying particular components of the working memory system, which can then be used to investigate the extent to which particular activities engage one or another component. By the logic of dual-task methodology, any two activities that are unimpaired when conducted in combination do not tap common limited capacity systems. In contrast, performance decrements when two tasks are combined indicate that they share a reliance on the same component. This empirical approach has proved invaluable in fractionating working memory into its constituent parts, leading to the most recent version of the working memory model, advanced by Baddeley in 2000 (Baddeley, 2000) (**Figure 1**).

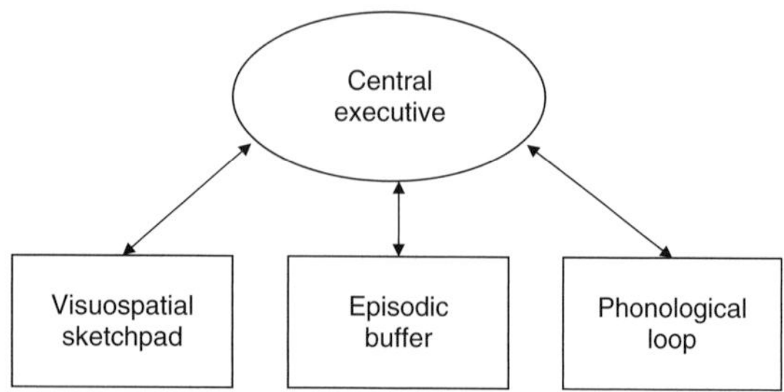

Figure 1 The Baddeley (2000) working memory model.

This model consists of four components. Two of these components, the phonological loop and the visuospatial sketchpad, are slave systems that are specialized for the temporary storage of material in particular domains (verbal and visuospatial, respectively). The central executive is a higher-level regulatory system, and the episodic buffer integrates and binds representations from different parts of the system. The nature of each of these components and associated empirical evidence are described in the following sections. Note also that components of working memory are directly linked with longer-term memory systems in various informational domains. The nature of the interface between working memory and the acquisition of knowledge is considered in later sections of the chapter.

8.2.1 The Phonological Loop

Originally termed the articulatory loop by Baddeley and Hitch (1974), the phonological loop is a slave system dedicated to the temporary storage of material in terms of its constituent sounds, or phonemes. The two-component model of the phonological loop advanced by Baddeley in 1986 is shown in **Figure 2**. Representations in the phonological short-term store are subject to rapid time-based decay. Auditory speech information gains obligatory access to the phonological store.

Subvocal rehearsal reactivates serially the contents of the short-term store, in a process that corresponds closely to overt articulation (speaking), but which does

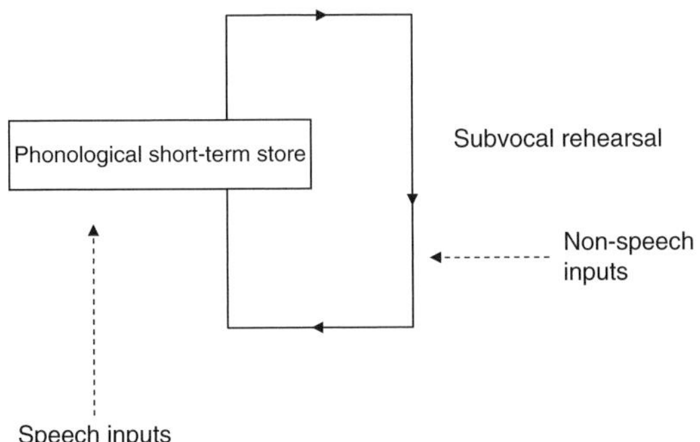

Figure 2 The phonological loop model, based on Baddeley (1986).

not necessarily involve the movement of the speech apparatus or the generation of speech sounds. Representations in the phonological store that are rehearsed before they have time to decay can be maintained in the phonological loop indefinitely, provided that rehearsal continues. Rehearsal consists of the high-level activation of speech-motor planning processes (Bishop and Robson, 1989; Caplan et al., 1992) and is a time-limited process in which lengthier items take longer to activate than short items. Material that is not presented in the form of spoken language but which is nonetheless associated with verbal labels, such as printed words or pictures of familiar objects, can enter the phonological store via rehearsal, which generates the corresponding phonological representations from stored lexical knowledge.

8.2.1.1 Empirical phenomena

This fractionated structure to the phonological loop is consistent with a wide range of experimental phenomena from the serial recall paradigm, in which lists of items are presented serially for immediate recall in the original input sequence. Evidence that verbal material is held in a phonological code is provided by the fact that irrespective of whether the memory lists are presented in auditory form or in the form of print, recall is poorer for sequences in which the items share a high degree of phonological similarity (e.g., C, G, B, V, T) than for those which have little overlap in phonological structure (e.g., X, H, K, W, Q). This effect of phonological similarity, first reported by Conrad (1964) and replicated many times subsequently, indicates that serial recall is mediated by phonological representations. Degradation of these representations, possibly due to decay, will thus cause confusion between representations of items with highly similar phonological structures.

The obligatory access of auditory speech information to the phonological loop is demonstrated by the irrelevant speech effect. Serial recall of visually presented verbal items is impaired if spoken items are presented during list presentation, even though participants are told to ignore these stimuli. Moreover, the recall advantage to phonologically distinct over phonologically similar sequences is eliminated under such conditions of irrelevant speech (Colle and Welsh, 1976; Suprenant et al., 1999). This finding indicates that irrelevant speech operates on the same process that gives rise to the phonological similarity effect, so that the unwanted stimuli generate representations in the phonological store that disrupt those of the list items to be recalled.

Evidence for the existence of a distinct subvocal rehearsal process that operates on the contents of the phonological store is provided by other empirical phenomena. An important finding first reported by Baddeley et al. (1975) is that serial recall accuracy is impaired when memory lists contain lengthy items (e.g., aluminum, hippopotamus, tuberculosis) than otherwise matched short items (e.g., zinc, stoat, mumps). Detailed analyses have established that a linear function related recall accuracy to the rate at which participants can articulate the memory sequence: items that are be spoken more rapidly are recalled more accurately, to a commensurate degree. This phenomenon, known as the word length effect, is present for visually and auditorily presented verbal material and is suggested to reflect the serial rehearsal process, which requires more time to re-activate lengthy than short items. As a consequence, representations in the phonological store of lengthy items are more likely to have decayed between successive rehearsals, leading to decay and loss of information.

Support for this interpretation is provided by findings that the word length effect disappears if participants engage in articulatory suppression by saying something irrelevant such as "hiya, hiya, hiya" during presentation of the memory list, for both visually and auditorily presented lists (Baddeley et al., 1975, 1984). These results can be simply explained. Having to engage in irrelevant articulation during a memory task prevents effective rehearsal of the memory items themselves – it simply is not possible to say one thing and to rehearse subvocally something else. As rehearsal is prevented in this condition, there can be no further impairment of recall with lengthy as opposed to short memory items, as this effect is also tied to the rehearsal process.

It should be noted that because visually presented material requires rehearsal to access the phonological store, preventing rehearsal via articulatory suppression should also eliminate the phonological similarity effect with visual presentation, as the material will not reach the store for the similarity-based interference to occur. This prediction has been supported by findings from many studies (Murray, 1968; Peterson and Johnson, 1971).

The claim that the word length effect arises only from subvocal rehearsal has not gone uncontested. Lengthier items are slower not only to rehearse but also to recall, and there is convincing evidence that the increased delay in recalling longer items is one cause of lower performance, probably due to the increased opportunity for time-based decay of the phonological representations. Cowan et al. (1992) employed mixed lists composed of both short and long words to investigate the effects of recall delay. They found a linear relation between the amount of time elapsing from the beginning of the recall attempt and the accuracy of recall, with recall declining as the delay increased (see also, Cowan et al., 1994). One possibility is that the word length effect is multiply determined, and that the slower rate of rehearsal for long than short items is just one of several mechanisms causing lower levels of recall accuracy for lists composed of lengthy stimuli.

Debate concerning the detailed processes underpinning experimental phenomena such as the effects of word length and irrelevant speech (e.g., Neath et al., 2003; Jones et al., 2006) continues, and will in time result in a fuller understanding of the precise mechanisms of serial recall. More generally, though, the broad distinction between the short-term store and rehearsal subcomponents of the phonological loop has received substantial support from several different empirical traditions. It is entirely consistent with evidence of developmental fractionation of the subcomponents of the phonological loop during the childhood years (see Gathercole and Hitch, 1993; Palmer, 2000, for reviews). The phonological store appears to be in place by the preschool period: by roughly 4 years of age, children show adult-like sensitivity to the phonological similarity of the lists items for auditorily presented material (Hitch and Halliday, 1983; Hulme and Tordoff, 1989). The subvocal rehearsal strategy, in contrast, emerges at a later time, typically after 7 years of age. Flavell et al. (1967) observed many years ago that very young children do not show the overt signs of rehearsal, such as lip movements and overt repetition, that characterize older children. Children below 7 years of age are also not disrupted by recalling memory sequences composed of lengthy rather than short items (Hitch and Halliday, 1983), although word length effects do emerge in children as young as 5 years of age if they are trained in the use of rehearsal strategies (Johnson et al., 1987). Also, there is also no consistent association between the articulatory rate and memory span in 5-year-old children, although strong links are found in adults (Gathercole et al., 1994a). Together, these findings indicate that although the phonological store is present at a very early point in children, the use of subvocal rehearsal as a means of maintaining the rapidly decaying representations in the store emerges only during the middle childhood years.

The phonological store and rehearsal process also appear to be served by distinct neuroanatomical regions of the left hemisphere of the brain. Evidence from patients with acquired brain damage resulting in impairments of verbal short-term memory indicates that short-term phonological storage is associated with the inferior parietal lobule of the left hemisphere, whereas rehearsal is mediated by Broca's area, in the left premotor frontal region (see Vallar and Papagno, 2003; Muller and Knight, 2006, for reviews). Findings from neuroimaging studies using methods such as positron emission tomography and functional magnetic resonance imaging to identify the areas of the brain activated by verbal short-term memory tasks in typical adult participants have further reinforced the neuroanatomical distinction between the phonological store and rehearsal (see Henson, 2005, for review).

8.2.1.2 A computational model of the phonological loop

Despite its simplicity, the Baddeley (1986) model of the phonological loop is capable of explaining much of the evidence outlined in the preceding section and several other experimental phenomena. It does, however, have one notable shortcoming as a model of serial recall. Although this paradigm requires the accurate retention of both the items in the memory list and their precise sequence, the model focuses exclusively on the representation of item information and therefore fails to account for how the serial order of list items is retained in the phonological loop. As a consequence, it cannot accommodate many detailed aspects of serial recall behaviour. One important characteristic of serial recall is the serial position function, the asymmetric bow-shaped curve that arises from high levels of accuracy of recalling initial list items (the primacy effect), relatively poor recall of mid-list items, and a moderate increase in accuracy for items at the end of the sequence (the recency effect). Another key finding is that the most common category of errors in serial recall is order errors, in which items from the original position migrate to nearby but incorrect positions in the output sequence (Bjork and Healy, 1974; Henson et al., 1996). The Baddeley (1986) model of the phonological loop provides no explanation of either of these features of verbal short-term memory.

Burgess and Hitch (1992) addressed this problem by developing and implementing a connectionist network model that incorporated a mechanism for retaining the serial order of items in addition to temporary phonological representations and an analog of rehearsal that corresponds to the phonological loop. The structure of the model is shown in **Figure 3**. It consists of four separate layers of nodes that represent input phonemes, words, output phonemes, and a context signal. Serial order is encoded by associating the activated item representation with a slowly evolving context signal containing a subset of active nodes that change progressively during presentation of the list, and can be conceptualized as a moving window representing time such that successive context states are more similar to one another than temporally distant states. Presentation of an item causes temporary activation of input phoneme nodes, word nodes, and output phoneme nodes via existing interconnections. When one item node succeeds in becoming the most active, a temporary association is formed between the winning item node and currently active context nodes. The item node is then suppressed, allowing the same process to be repeated for the next item in the sequence. In this model, rehearsal consists of feedback from the output phonemes (activated following selection of the winning item node) to the input phonemes.

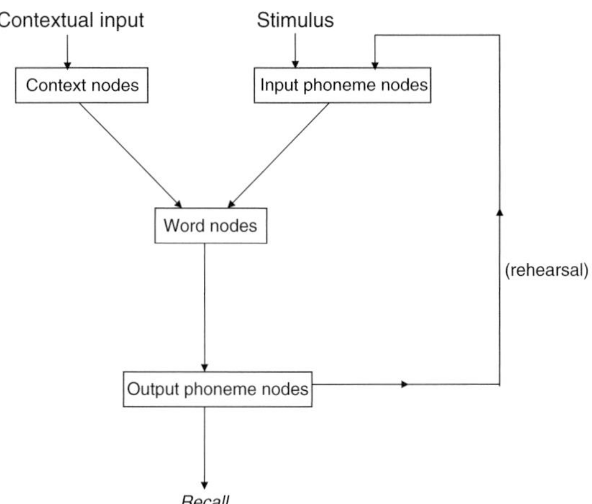

Figure 3 Simplified architecture of the Burgess and Hitch (1992) network model of the phonological loop.

At recall, the original context signal is repeated and evolves over successive items in the same way as at input. For each signal, item nodes receive activation based on their initial pairing with context in the original sequence, and the winning item is selected and activates consistent output phonemes. Noise is added to this final selection process to induce errors. Where serial order errors do occur – that is, incorrect item nodes are selected – they tend to migrate to target-adjacent positions as a consequence of the high degree of overlap in the context nodes active in successive context states.

In addition to generating the classic experimental phenomena associated with the phonological loop such as the phonological similarity, word length, and articulatory suppression effects, this model simulates many of the features of serial order behavior that the phonological loop model on which it was based could not address. Consider first the serial position function. Primacy effects arise largely from the greater number of rehearsals received by early list items, and recall of both initial and final items is enhanced by the reduced degree of order uncertainty at these terminal list positions. A preponderance of order errors is also readily generated because context signals, like item representations, degrade with time. Thus on some occasions, the retrieved item representation will have been associated with an adjacent context signal, yielding recall of a list item at an incorrect output position. When items do migrate in simulations of the model, they show the bell-shaped migration function in which the distances traveled in the sequence are usually small rather than large, which has also been established in the behavioral data.

8.2.1.3 The phonological loop and language

Although the cognitive processes underpinning the phonological loop are well understood, one puzzle for many years was exactly why this system exists. It may have turned out to be useful for remembering telephone numbers, but why do we have the system in the first place? A number of possibilities were considered. One plausible hypothesis was that the phonological loop acts as a buffer for planned speech.

The presence of a phonological output buffer that stores the retrieved phonological specifications of intended lexical items and enables the smooth and rapid production of speech has long been recognized as a logical necessity by speech production theorists (e.g., Bock, 1982; Romani, 1992). There is, however, little evidence that the phonological store fulfills this function (see Gathercole and Baddeley, 1993 for review). It has consistently been found that adult neuropsychological patients with very severe deficits of verbal short-term memory leading to memory spans of only one or two items can nonetheless produce spontaneous speech normally: utterance length rates of hesitations and self-corrections are comparable to those of control adults (Shallice and Butterworth, 1977).

A second hypothesis was that the phonological loop provides an input buffer to incoming language that is consulted in the course of normal comprehension processes (Clark and Clark, 1977). Once again, findings from adult short-term memory patients provided the opportunity to test this hypothesis. The prediction was clear: if short-term memory plays a significant role in comprehension, the very low memory span of short-term memory patients should lead to substantial impairments in processing the meaning of language. Findings from many research groups and many different patients provided little support for this prediction. Despite severe deficits in phonological loop functioning, short-term memory patients typically had few difficulties in processing sentences for meaning, except under conditions in which lengthy, unusual, and ambiguous syntactic structures were used, or the sentences were essentially memory lists (see Vallar and Shallice, 1990; Caplan and Waters, 1990; Gathercole and Baddeley, 1993; for reviews). It therefore appears that although under most circumstances the language processor operates online without recourse to stored representations in the phonological loop, these representations may be consulted in an off-line mode to enable backtracking and possible re-analysis of spoken language under some conditions (McCarthy and Warrington, 1987).

There is, however, one area of language functioning in which the phonological loop appears to play a central role, and that is in learning the sound structure of new words. Evidence from many sources converges on this view. Studies of typically developing children have consistently found close and selective associations between measures of verbal short-term memory and knowledge of both native and foreign language vocabulary (e.g., Gathercole and Baddeley, 1989; Service, 1992; Cheung, 1996; Masoura and Gathercole, 1999). The accuracy of nonword repetition – in which a child hears a spoken nonword such as woogalamic and attempts to repeat it immediately – is particularly highly correlated with vocabulary knowledge, although so too are more conventional measures of verbal short-term memory such as digit span (Gathercole et al., 1994b). A similar link is found between verbal memory skills and the rate of learning nonwords in paired-associate learning paradigms, in which participants learn to associate unfamiliar phonological forms with either novel objects (Gathercole and Baddeley, 1990a, used toy monsters with names such as Pimas), unrelated words (such as fairy-kipser), or semantic attributes (e.g., bleximus is a noisy, dancing fish). Both of the latter examples are from a study reported by Gathercole et al. (1997), in which the phonological memory skills of the participating 5-year-old children were in contrast found to be independent of the ability to learn word–word pairs.

Further evidence that the phonological loop is involved in the long-term learning of phonological structures in particular has been provided by the study of individuals with developmental or acquired deficits in language learning. Specific language impairment (SLI) is a condition in which children fail to develop language at a normal rate despite normal intellectual function. Word learning represents a particular problem for affected children. It has consistently been found that children with SLI have substantial impairments of nonword repetition and of other measures of verbal short-term memory (e.g., Gathercole and Baddeley, 1990b; Bishop et al., 1996; Archibald and Gathercole, 2006). A corresponding neuropsychological patient, PV, had a severe deficit of the phonological loop, and was found to be completely unable to learn word–nonword pairings such as rose–svieti, but performed within the typical range on a word–word learning task (Baddeley et al., 1988). Experimental studies of paired-associate learning with normal adult participants have shown that word–nonword learning is disrupted by variables known to interfere with phonological loop functioning, such as phonological similarity and articulatory suppression (Papagno et al., 1991; Papagno and Vallar, 1992). In contrast, learning of word–word pairs is not influenced by these variables.

On this basis, it has been proposed that the primary function of the phonological loop is to support learning of the sound structures of new words in the course of vocabulary acquisition (Baddeley et al., 1998b). It is suggested that initial encounters with the phonological forms of novel words are represented in the phonological short-term store, and that these representations form the basis for the gradual process of abstracting a stable specification of the sound structure across repeated presentations (Brown and Hulme, 1996). Conditions that compromise the quality of the temporary phonological representation in the phonological loop will reduce the efficiency of the process of abstraction and result in slow rates of learning. In a recent review of this theory and associated evidence, Gathercole (2006) has suggested use of the phonological loop to learn new words is a primitive learning mechanism that dominates at the early stages of learning a language and remains available as a strategy throughout life. However, once a substantial lexicon is established in a language, word learners increasing rely on lexically mediated learning of new words, thereby building on the phonological structures that they have already acquired.

8.2.1.4 Summary

The phonological loop model advanced by Baddeley (1986), consisting of a short-term store and a subvocal rehearsal process, is the most influential current account of verbal short-term memory. Convergent evidence for the model is provided from a range of research traditions including experimental cognitive psychology, developmental psychology, neuropsychology, and neuroimaging. A similar diverse range of findings indicate that the phonological loop plays a key role in vocabulary acquisition (Baddeley et al., 1998; Gathercole, 2006).

The successful implementation of the model in the form of a connectionist network by Burgess and Hitch (1992) is an important development that has stimulated competing computational models of serial recall with distinct architectures. The network model has also been further developed to simulate learning of novel sequences by the phonological loop (Burgess and Hitch, 1999). The availability of detailed models of short-term memory and the reciprocal stimulation of empirical findings and computational simulations is a sign of advanced theoretical development that is in large part due to the guiding influence of the phonological loop concept on this field over many years.

8.2.2 The Visuospatial Sketchpad

8.2.2.1 Theory and empirical phenomena

The second slave system of the working memory model is the visuospatial sketchpad, specialized in the storage and manipulation of information that can be represented in terms of either visual or spatial characteristics. Short-term memory for visuospatial material is associated with increased activity in the right hemisphere regions of the inferior prefrontal cortex, anterior occipital cortex, and posterior parietal cortex, and acquired damage to these regions of the brain leads to selective deficits in remembering these domains of material (see Gathercole, 1999, for review).

Several tasks have been designed to tap the visuospatial sketchpad. These include recognizing the pattern of filled squares in a two-dimensional grid (Phillips and Christie, 1977; Wilson et al., 1987), remembering the order in which a set of blocks are tapped (often known as the Corsi blocks task), using a grid to generate a mental image corresponding to a set of spatial instructions (Brooks, 1967), and recalling the path drawn through a maze (Pickering et al., 2001).

Like its sister slave system the phonological loop, the sketchpad has now been fractionated into two distinct but interrelated components: A visual store or cache that preserves the visual features of perceived or internally generated objects and a spatial or sequential component that may serve a recycling function analogous to subvocal rehearsal (Logie, 1995). The strongest evidence for the separation of the sketchpad into these two components is provided by studies of neuropsychological patients with acquired brain lesions resulting in selective impairments of visual storage but preserved spatial short-term memory (Hanley et al., 1991) and converse deficits in spatial but not visual short-term memory (Della Sala et al., 1999; Della Sala and Logie, 2003).

Dual task studies have played an important role in illuminating the functional organization of the visuospatial sketchpad. One popular method for tapping the capacity for the generation and temporary storage of spatial material is the Brooks (1967) task, in which the participant is presented with a 4 × 4 empty grid in which one particular cell was designated as the starting square. The experimenter then gives a series of verbal instructions which participants are encouraged to remember by mentally filling in the grid, as shown in **Figure 4**. Following the

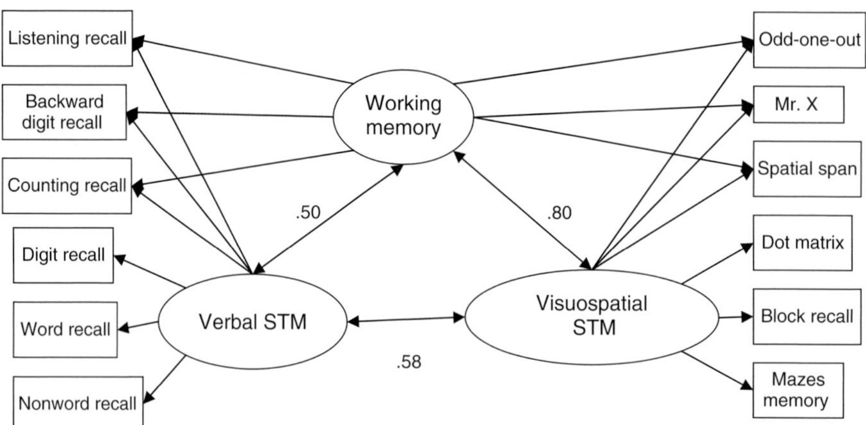

Figure 4 Measurement model of working memory, based on data from children aged 4–11 years. STM, short-term memory. From Alloway TP, Gathercole SE, and Pickering SJ (2006) Verbal and visuo-spatial short-term and working memory in children: Are they separable? *Child Dev.* 77: 1698–1716; used with permission from Blackwell Publishing.

instructions, participants recall the sequence by filling in the grid with the numbers. This condition facilitates the use of spatial imagery and hence the visuospatial sketchpad. In a control condition which does not encourage the use of such spatial imagery, the spatial terms up, down, left, right were replaced by the nonspatial adjectives good, bad, slow, and fast to yield nonsensical sentences. Presumably, recall in this condition was supported by the phonological loop rather than the sketchpad.

Evidence that participants use mental imagery to mediate performance in the spatial but not the nonsense condition is provided by the superior levels of recall accuracy in the former condition (Brooks, 1967). In a systematic study of the effects of concurrent activities on memory performance in the two cases, Baddeley and Lieberman (1980) reported further evidence that distinct components of working memory are employed in the two conditions. Performing a concurrent task – tracking an overhead swinging pendulum – disrupted recall in the spatial but not the nonsense condition. Thus, spatial recall appears to be selectively impaired by the encoding of unrelated spatial content, consistent with the employment of a spatial code to mediate recall performance.

Subsequent investigations indicate that eye movements may play a key role in the maintenance of spatial images in the sketchpad. Postle et al. (2006) reported a series of experiments showing that voluntary eye movements impair memory for spatial locations but not for nonspatial features of visual objects, providing further support for a distinction between visual and spatial components of the sketchpad. Other studies have shown that the engagement of other movement systems such as hands (finger tapping), legs (foot tapping), and arms exerts similar disruptive influences on memory for spatial sequences such as Corsi block recall (e.g., Smyth and Scholey, 1988). It therefore appears that the maintenance of spatial representations in the sketchpad is supported by a central motor plan that is not specific to any particular effector system, by which is recruited the planning and execution of movements in the full range of motor systems.

There is some evidence that the visual storage component of the spatial sketchpad is selectively disrupted by the concurrent perception of irrelevant visual features. In a series of studies reported by Quinn and McDonnell (1996), memory for detailed visual characteristics was selectively impaired by visual noise that corresponded to a randomly flickering display of pixels similar to an untuned television screen that participants were required to view but asked to disregard. This finding is important, as it is directly analogous to the irrelevant speech effect in verbal serial recall (Colle and Welsh, 1976), which has been interpreted as reflecting obligatory access to the short-term store component of the phonological loop for auditory speech material.

One interpretational problem raised by many studies of visuospatial short-term memory is the extent to which these and other similar tasks reflect a genuinely distinct component of working memory, or alternatively draw on the more general resources of the central executive. The central executive, which is described in more detail in the following section, is a limited-capacity domain-general system capable of supporting a wide range of cognitive activities. Several different lines of evidence indicate that the central executive plays a major role in many visuospatial short-term memory tasks. Performance on visual storage tasks has been found to be strongly disrupted by concurrent activities that lack an overt visuospatial component but which are known to tax the central executive, such as mental arithmetic (Phillips and Christie, 1977; Wilson et al., 1987). Also, studies of individual differences have consistently shown that measures of visuospatial short-term memory are much more closely associated with performance on central executive tasks than are phonological loop measures, in both typically developing children (Gathercole et al., 2004a, 2006a; Alloway et al., 2006) and in a clinical study of adults with bipolar mood disorder (Thompson et al., 2006).

8.2.2.2 *Summary*

Although current understanding of the detailed cognitive processes involved in visuospatial short-term memory is less well advanced than that of the phonological loop, two basic facts have now been established. First, the sketchpad functions independently of the phonological loop – it is associated with activity in the right rather than the left hemisphere of the brain and is selectively disrupted by concurrent activities that do not influence the phonological loop. Second, the processes involved in manipulating and storing visual features and spatial patterns appear to be distinct from one another, again showing neuropsychological and experimental dissociations. It is rather less clear to what extent the visuospatial sketchpad represents a distinct component of working memory that is dissociable from the central executive.

8.2.3 The Central Executive

At the heart of the working memory model is the central executive, responsible for the control of the working memory system and its integration with other parts of the cognitive system. The central executive is limited in capacity, and is closely linked with the control of attention and also with the regulation of the flow of information within working memory, and the retrieval of material from more permanent long-term memory systems into working memory. Neuroimaging studies indicate that the frontal lobes of both hemispheres of the brain, and particularly of the prefrontal cortex, are activated by activities known to tax the central executive (See Collette and Van der Linden, 2002; Owen et al., 2005, for reviews).

8.2.3.1 *The supervisory attentional system*

In 1986, Baddeley suggested that central executive may correspond in part at least to the model of the supervisory attentional system (SAS) advanced by Shallice (1982) to explore the control of attention in action. The SAS has two principal components. The contention scheduling system consists of a set of schemas, which are organized structures of behavioral routines that can be activated by either internally or externally generated cues. When a schema reaches a particular level of activation, it is triggered and the appropriate action or set of actions is initiated. Thus, we have schemas that govern all our skilled behaviors: walking and talking, breathing and jumping, opening doors and using a telephone. Schemas can be hierarchically organized. Skilled car drivers, for example, will have a driving schema that is composed of linked subschemas such as steering and braking schemas. Many of our actions are governed by the automatic activation of these schemas in response to environmental cues. So, once we are behind the wheel of a moving car, the sight of a red brake light in the car in front will probably be sufficient to trigger the automatic activation of the braking subschema. Activation levels of all incompatible schemas (such as the accelerating schema, in this case) are inhibited when a schema is triggered.

The second component, the SAS, controls behavior via a very different process. The SAS can directly activate or inhibit schemas, thereby overriding their routine triggering by the contention scheduling system. The intervention of the SAS corresponds to volitional control and prevents us from being endless slaves to environmental cues – it allows us to choose to change the course of our actions at will. However, because the SAS is a limited capacity system, there are finite limits on the amount of attentional control we can apply to our actions.

Baddeley's (1986) suggestion was that the central executive corresponds to the limited-capacity SAS. He also proposed that two types of behavioral disturbance associated with damage to the frontal lobes arise from malfunctioning of the central executive, and coined the term dysexecutive syndrome to describe this disorder. These neuropsychological patients are typically characterized by one of two possible types of behavior. Perseveration is a form of behavioral rigidity in which the individual continually repeats the same action or response. An example would be greeting a newcomer by saying "Hello" and then continuing to make the same response many times to the same individual, increasingly inappropriately. Distractibility consists of unfocused behavior in which the individual fails to engage in meaningful responses but may, for example, continuously walk around a room manipulating objects. Baddeley suggested that such individuals have an impairment in central executive resources that reduces their capacity for volitional control of behavior via the SAS, which is instead dominated by the contention scheduling system. Perseveration results when a schema becomes highly activated and cannot be effectively inhibited by the SAS to allow the triggering of other appropriate behaviors, and distractibility results from the background triggering of behavior by environmental cues with no overriding focus by the SAS.

This conceptualization of the central executive has proved useful in guiding the development of laboratory tasks that engage the central executive. One such task is random generation (Baddeley, 1986). In a typical task, the participant is required to generate in a random manner exemplars from a familiar category, such as digits or letters, paced by a metronome. The importance of generating random sequences rather than stereotyped ones such as 1, 2, 3 or a, b, c is emphasized. In 1998, Baddeley et al. (1998a) conducted a series of experiments to investigate the hypothesis that the central executive is needed to intervene to override the activation of stereotyped response sequences in this task. There were several key findings consistent with this view. First, the degree of randomness of the sequences generated by the participants diminished (i.e., the responses became more stereotyped) when the generation rate was increased. This result indicates that the randomness of the responses was constrained by a limited capacity process. Second, the degree of randomness of the generated sequences was not impaired when the task was combined with other activities requiring stereotyped responses such as counting, but was substantially disrupted by nonstereotyped concurrent activities such as maintaining a digit load or generating exemplars of semantic categories. Applying the logic of dual-task methodology, it appears that both tasks tap a common limited-capacity mechanism, the central executive.

8.2.3.2 Complex memory span

The central executive also plays a key role in complex memory span tasks, which require both processing and storage. The first reported complex span task, reading span, was developed by Daneman and Carpenter in 1980. In this task, participants must read aloud each of a sequence of printed sentences, and at the end of the sequence they must recall the final word of each sentence in the same order as the sentences were presented. The number of sentences read on each trial is then increased until the point at which the participant can no longer reliably recall the sequence of final words. Findings from this task were impressive – complex memory span scores were highly correlated with the performance of the participating college students on their scholastic aptitude tests completed on entry to college. Importantly, the correlations with scholastic aptitude were considerably higher than those found with storage-only measures of verbal short-term memory.

A range of other complex span paradigms have been subsequently developed, all sharing the common feature of requiring both memory storage while participants are engaged in significant concurrent processing activity. A listening span version of the reading span test in which the sentences were heard rather than read by participants was employed by Daneman and Carpenter (1983), and was found to be correspondingly associated with academic abilities. Complex span tasks suitable for use by young children have also been developed. One popular task is counting span, in which the child has to count the number of elements in a series of visual displays, and at the end of the sequence to recall the totals of each array, in the order of presentation (Case et al., 1982). The odd-one-out task (Russell et al., 1996; Alloway et al., 2006) is a complex memory span task that requires visuospatial rather than verbal storage and processing (see also, Shah and Miyake, 1996). Participants view a series of displays each containing three unfamiliar objects, two identical and one different. The task is to point to the location of the odd one out, and then at the end of the sequence to recall the sequence of spatial locations of the different items. In other complex span tasks, the material to be stored is distinct from the contents of the processing activity. An example of one such task is operation span (Turner and Engle, 1989), in which participants attempt to recall digits whose presentation is interpolated with a sequence of simple additions that must be completed.

Despite the large degree of variation in both the processing and storage demands of the different complex memory span tasks, a highly consistent pattern of findings has emerged. Performance on such tasks is strongly related to higher-level cognitive activities such as reasoning and reading comprehension (e.g., Kyllonen and Christal, 1990; Engle et al., 1992), and also to key areas of academic achievement during childhood such as reading and mathematics (e.g., Swanson et al., 1996; Hitch et al., 2001; Jarvis and Gathercole, 2003; Gathercole et al., 2004b, 2006a; Geary et al., 2004; Swanson and Beebe-Frankenberger, 2004). In the majority of these studies, associations with learning were much higher for complex memory span measures than measures such as digit span of verbal short-term memory. Corresponding closer links with measures of intellectual functioning in adulthood such as reading comprehension, scholastic aptitude, and fluid intelligence have also been consistently found in adult populations (for reviews, see Daneman and Merikle, 1996; Engle et al., 1999b).

In order to understand why complex span measures of working memory performance are so strongly associated with learning abilities and other measures of high-level cognition, it is necessary first to consider what cognitive processes these measures tap. It has been suggested that the processing portions of these tasks are supported by the domain-general resources of the central executive, whereas the storage requirements are met by the respective domain-specific slave system (Baddeley and Logie, 1999). By this view, both the central executive and the phonological loop contribute to performance on verbal complex span tasks such as reading span, listening span, and counting span, whereas performance on visuospatial complex span tasks is mediated by the central executive and the visuospatial sketchpad.

There is now substantial evidence to support this proposal. A common processing efficiency factor has been found to underlie both verbal and visuospatial complex memory tasks (Bayliss et al., 2003). Two recent studies have investigated the latent factor structure underlying individuals' performance on both simple (storage-only) and complex span measures in both the verbal and visuospatial domains, in children (Alloway et al., 2006) and in adults (Kane et al., 2004). In both cases, the best-fitting model is a structure consisting of distinct verbal and visuospatial short-term storage components (corresponding to the phonological loop and visuospatial sketchpad, respectively), plus a domain-general factor corresponding to the central executive. A summary of the factor structure of the model from Alloway et al. (2006) is shown in **Figure 4**. It can be seen that the complex span tasks load both on the domain-general factor and the respective domain-specific storage system. These data provide an impressive degree of support for the basic structure of the working memory model.

So why is it the case that slow rates of academic learning therefore characterize children who perform poorly on complex memory measures of working memory (e.g., Pickering and Gathercole, 2004; Gathercole et al., 2006a)? We have suggested that the reason is that working memory acts as a bottleneck for learning (Gathercole, 2004; Gathercole et al., 2006b). The acquisition of knowledge and skill in complex domains such as reading and mathematics requires the gradual accumulation of knowledge over multiple learning episodes, many of which will take place in the structured learning environment of the classroom. Learning is thus an incremental process that builds upon the knowledge structures and understanding that have already been acquired: any factor that disturbs this acquisition process will have deleterious consequences for the rate of learning, as the necessary foundations for progress will not be in place. It is proposed that working memory capacity is one of the factors that constrains learning success in potential learning episodes. Many classroom activities require the child to keep information in mind while engaging in another cognitive activity that might be very demanding for that individual. Mental arithmetic is an example of such a demanding working memory activity for adults. In children, whose working memory capacity is considerably smaller and who do not have the same bedrock of stored knowledge and expertise to support cognitive processing, working memory challenges of a comparable magnitude are present in much simpler activities, such as writing sentences, adding up totals of objects displayed on cards, or detecting rhyming words in a poem read by the teacher. Children with poor working memory capacities will face severe difficulties in meeting the demands of these situations and, as a result of their working memory overload, will fail in part or all of the learning activity. Such situations represent missed learning opportunities and if they occur frequently, will result in a slow rate of learning.

8.2.4 The Episodic Buffer

The episodic buffer is the most recent addition to the working memory model, and was first outlined in a seminal paper by Baddeley in 2000 (Baddeley, 2000).

In this article, Baddeley argued the need for a separate buffer capable of representing and integrating inputs from all subcomponents of working memory and from long-term memory systems in a multidimensional code.

One justification for the episodic buffer is that it solves the binding problem, which refers to the fact that although the separate elements of multimodal experiences such as seeing an object moving and hearing a sound are experienced via separate channels leading to representations in modality-specific codes, our perception is of the event as a coherent unitary whole. At some point, the representations must therefore converge and be chunked together and experienced consciously as a single object or event; Baddeley's suggestion was that the episodic buffer may fulfill this function.

Other evidence also points to a close interface between the subcomponents of working memory and other parts of the cognitive system. It has long been known that meaningful sentences are much better remembered than jumbled sequences of words, with memory spans as high as 16 words compared with the six or seven limit for unrelated words (Baddeley et al., 1987). This indicates that representations in the phonological loop are integrated at some point with conceptual representations arising from the language processing system. Importantly, patients with acquired impairments of verbal short-term memory show reduced memory span for sentences as well as for word lists, but still show the relative advantage of meaningful over the meaningless material. Patient PV, for example, had a sentence span of five and a word span of one (Vallar and Baddeley, 1984). As PV's long-term memory was entirely normal, the reduction in her sentence span must arise from the point of interaction between verbal short-term memory (or the phonological loop). Baddeley (2000) proposed that the episodic buffer may provide the appropriate medium for linking the phonological loop representations with those from long-term memory, and that the central executive may control the allocation of information from different sources into the buffer.

The characteristics of the episodic buffer have been explored in a subsequent experimental programme by Baddeley and collaborators. One line of investigation has looked into whether the episodic buffer plays a role in the binding of different visual features of objects into chunks by comparing memory for arrays of colors or shapes with memory for bound combinations of these features (Allen et al., 2006). In a series of experiments, recognition memory for visually presented objects was tested by presenting an array of objects followed by a probe; the participants' task was to judge whether the probe was present in the original display or not. Across conditions, recognition memory was tested either for shape by presenting a display of different unfilled shapes, for color with a display of squares of different colors, or for both color and shape by presenting objects composed of unique shape/color combinations. In line with previous findings from this paradigm (Wheeler and Treisman, 2002), recognition performance was found to be as accurate in the feature combination as the single feature conditions. Thus, feature binding appears to be a relatively efficient process.

Allen et al. (2006) investigated whether this binding process depends on central executive resources, as might be predicted from the working memory model shown in **Figure 1**, in which information is fed into the episodic buffer from the central executive. To test this possibility, participants also performed demanding concurrent tasks that would be expected to require executive resources – counting backwards and retaining a near-span digit load – while viewing the object arrays. The results were clear: although recognition memory was generally less accurate under dual task conditions, memory for bound features was not selectively disrupted. The only condition that did lead to a greater impairment of recognition for feature combinations than single features was one that involved sequential rather than simultaneous presentation of objects.

On the basis of these findings, Allen et al. concluded that binding the features of simple visual features takes place in the visuospatial sketchpad and does not require executive support. However, it was suggested that storage of such automatically bound information is fragile and may fall apart when further feature combinations need to be encoded and stored in visuospatial memory.

The possible role of the attentional resources of the central executive in integrating linguistic information with representations in the phonological loop in the episodic buffer was investigated by Jefferies et al. (2004). The main focus of this study was the substantial advantage found in the immediate recall of prose compared with unrelated words, which Baddeley (2000) had suggested may be mediated by the integration of linguistic and phonological information in the episodic buffer. Jefferies et al.

conducted a series of experiments in which the relative difficulty of different kinds of lists was equated for individual participants. Thus, an example of an unrelated word list that corresponds to 50% above span for an average participant with a word span of six was the nine items essay, marmalade, is, lots, clowns, wine, spaces, often, a. In the sentence condition of a corresponding level of difficulty, an average participant with a sentence span of 13 would receive the following sequence of unrelated sentences for immediate recall: Railway stations are noisy places. Guns can cause serious injuries. Water is boiled in kettles. Pink roses are pretty flowers. In a further story condition, the sentences were thematically related, as in the following example: A teenage girl loved buying clothes. She went shopping with her mom. They traveled into town by bus.

The possible engagement of attentional processes associated with the central executive was investigated by comparing the impact of a continuous reaction time (CRT) task completed during the presentation of the memory sequence on performance in the different conditions. Following Craik et al. (1996), the CRT task involved pressing one of four keys corresponding to the spatial location of a visual target that appeared on a computer screen; as soon as the key was pressed, the next stimulus was presented. This task is known to place significant demands on controlled attentional processing. If the central executive does play a crucial role in loading phonological and linguistic information into the episodic buffer where it can be integrated into a multidimensional code underpinning sentence span, a selective decrement in the recall of sentences relative to unrelated words would be expected in the concurrent CRT conditions.

Jefferies et al. (2004) found that recall of unrelated words was more or less unaffected by the concurrent task, as was the recall of thematically organized material in the story condition. These findings indicate that the use of the phonological loop places few demands on attentional resources, and also that the activation of preexisting representations relating to the semantic and syntactic content of the stories occurs relatively automatically. In contrast, CRT did markedly impair performance in the condition involving the recall of unrelated sentences. It therefore appears that substantial attentional support from the central executive is required for the retention of unrelated chunks of linguistic information, possibly within the episodic buffer.

Although the study of the episodic buffer is still in its infancy, the concept is being refined in light of new evidence and is proving useful in guiding research on memory for relatively complex forms of material. The simple idea that the central executive is required to feed information through to the episodic buffer for the purposes of feature binding has not received strong support from the research completed so far: there is little evidence for central executive involvement in either the binding of simple visual features (Allen et al., 2006) or in the recall of coherent prose, although attentional support does appear to be crucial for the temporary retention of chunks of unrelated linguistic information (Jefferies et al., 2004). Ongoing and future research designed to delineate the precise conditions under which the central executive and episodic buffer interact seems certain to provide further fruitful insights into the role played by working memory in the storage and manipulation of complex and structured information.

8.2.5 Other Models of Working Memory

The multicomponent model of working memory initially advanced by Baddeley and Hitch (1974) is the most enduring and influential theoretical framework in the field. Its success rests with the breadth of scope of the model – incorporating verbal and visuospatial short-term memory, as well as attentional processes – and also with the capacity of the model to evolve in light of incoming evidence. Although the original tripartite structure of the 1974 model has been largely preserved, each component has been elaborated and differentiated over the intervening years, largely but not exclusively by using the dual task methodology to identify distinct subcomponents of the system. The model has also proved successful in accommodating evidence from a wide range of empirical traditions including cognitive development, neuropsychology, and neuroscience in addition to experimental psychology. It is, however, by no means the only model of working memory, and there are currently several other conceptualizations that are proving to be highly effective in guiding research and thinking in the area. Some of the significant alternative theoretical accounts of working are outlined in the following.

8.2.5.1 Attentional based models

One influential theoretical account of working memory of this type is Cowan's (1995, 2001) embedded process model, summarized in **Figure 5**. According to this model, long-term memory can be partitioned

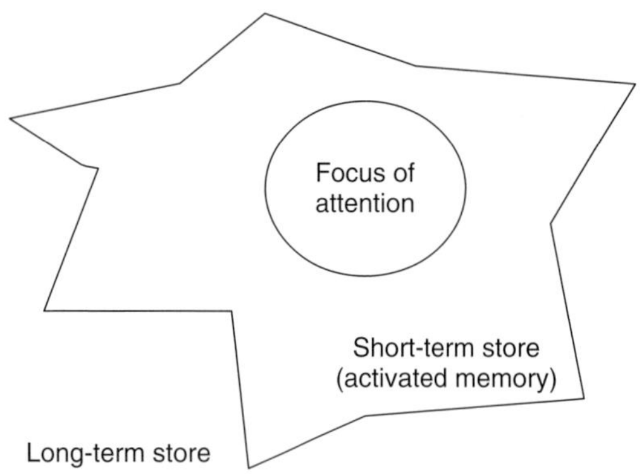

Figure 5 Cowan's (1995) embedded process model of working memory.

in three ways: the larger portion that has relatively low activation at any particular point in time, a subset that is currently activated as a consequence of ongoing cognitive activities and perceptual experience, and a smaller subset of the activated portion that is the focus of attention and conscious awareness. The focus of attention is controlled primarily by the voluntary processes of the executive system that are limited in capacity in chunks. Recent work indicates that typically between three and five chunks of information can be maintained in the focus of attention (Cowan, 2001; see also Chen and Cowan, 2005; Cowan et al., 2005). In contrast, long-term memory activation is time-limited and decays rapidly without further stimulation.

Cowan et al. (2005) have put forward an interpretation of complex memory span performance and its links with scholastic aptitude measures that is markedly divergent from the explanation based on the working memory model considered in the section titled 'The central executive.' By this account, the crucial feature of complex span tasks is that the processing activity prevents the usual deployment of control strategies such as rehearsal and grouping, and thus exposes more directly the scope of the focus of attention, as indexed by the number of chunks that can be maintained simultaneously. Learning ability will be constrained by having a relatively poor scope of attention, laid bare by complex memory span tasks.

An attentional-based account of working memory function has been also advanced by Engle and associates (e.g., Engle et al., 1999b). In some respects, Engle's model shares a similar architecture with the Baddeley and Hitch (1974) framework, combining domain-specific storage of verbal and visuospatial material with controlled attention. The detailed functioning of the components is, however, quite different. Short-term memory consists of traces that have exceeded an activation threshold and represent pointers to specific regions of long-term memory. They therefore do not represent temporary representations in a specialized temporary store, as in the phonological loop. Controlled attention is a domain-general resource that can achieve activation through controlled retrieval, maintain activation, and block interference through the inhibition of distractors.

Unsworth and Engle (2006) have recently put forward a new explanation of why complex memory span tasks correlate more highly with measures of higher-order cognitive function than simple memory span, based upon the distinction between primary and secondary memory. According to this account, memory items that have been recently encountered are held in primary memory, and may also be transferred into the more durable secondary memory system (Waugh and Norman, 1965). The processing activity in complex span tasks displaces items from primary memory, so that recall performance is supported principally by residual activation in secondary memory. Unsworth and Engle suggest that it is the ability to retrieve items from secondary memory that is crucial to more cognitive activities such as reasoning. Note that this interpretation is somewhat similar to that advanced by Cowan et al. (2005); in both cases, the claim is that learning is served most directly by the quality of activation of long-term memory, and not by the capacity of the controlled attention process that generates conscious experience.

8.2.5.2 The resource-sharing model

A contrasting theoretical perspective on working memory was provided by Daneman and Carpenter (1980, 1983; Just and Carpenter, 1992). These researchers conceived working memory as an undifferentiated resource that could be flexibly deployed either to support temporary storage or processing activity. By this account, individuals with relatively low span scores on complex memory span tasks were relatively unskilled at the processing element of the activity (reading, in the case of reading span), thereby reducing the amount of resource available for storage of the memory items. This idea that working memory is a single flexible system fueled by a limited capacity resource that can be flexibly allocated to support processing and storage was applied by Case et al. (1982) to explain developmental increases in working memory performance across the childhood years.

They proposed that the total working memory resource remains constant as the child matures, but that the efficiency of processing increases, releasing additional resource to support temporary storage. Consistent with this view, Case et al. found in a study of 6- to 12-year-old children that counting spans were highly predictable from individual counting speeds. Furthermore, counting spans were reduced to the level typical of 6-year-old children when adults' counting efficiency was reduced by requiring the use of nonsense words rather than digits to count sequences. It was concluded that the decreased memory spans resulted from the greater processing demands imposed by the unfamiliar counting task, leading to a processing/storage trade-off that diminished storage capacity.

8.2.5.3 Time-based theories

The resource-sharing model of working memory has been challenged substantially in recent years. Towse and Hitch (1995) proposed that participants do not process and store material at the same time in complex span tasks as assumed by the resource-sharing approach, but instead strategically switch between the processing and storage elements of the task. Evidence consistent with this task-switching model has been provided in a series of studies that have either varied counting complexity while holding retention interval constant (Towse and Hitch, 1995) or manipulated retention requirements in counting, operation, and reading span tasks, while holding constant the overall processing difficulty (Towse et al., 1998). In each case, the period over which information was stored was a better predictor of complex memory span than the difficulty of the processing activity. This has led to the claim that complex memory span is constrained by a time-based loss of activation of memory items (Hitch et al., 2001).

The consensus view at present is that no single factor constrains complex memory span (Miyake and Shah, 1999; Bayliss et al., 2003; Ransdell and Hecht, 2003). A more complex model recently advanced by Barrouillet and colleagues (Barrouillet and Camos, 2001; Barrouillet et al., 2004) combines concepts of both temporal decay and processing demands in a single metric of cognitive cost that is strongly related to performance on complex span tasks. In this model, the cognitive cost of a processing task is measured as the proportion of time that it requires limited-capacity attentional resources, for example, to support memory retrievals. When attention is diverted from item storage to processing in this way, memory representations cannot be refreshed and therefore decay with time. The heaviest cognitive costs and therefore the lowest levels of complex span performance are therefore expected under conditions in which there is the greatest ratio of number of retrievals to time. Experimental findings reported by Barrouillet et al. (2004) are entirely consistent with this prediction. Using a complex memory span paradigm in which they separately manipulated the rate of presentation of the memory items and the number of intervening items to be processed, complex memory span was found to be a direct linear function of the cognitive cost of the processing activity, computed as a ratio of the number of processing items divided the period over which they were presented. Thus, processing intervals that had relatively high loads (in other words, a relatively large number of items per unit time) were associated with lower span scores than processing intervals with low cognitive loads (low numbers of items per unit time).

8.2.5.4 Summary

In this section, a number of alternative theoretical accounts of working memory have been considered. It can be argued that some of these conceptualizations provide valuable specifications of the nature of central executive processes and are not necessarily incompatible with the Baddeley and Hitch (1974; Baddeley, 2000) model. Certainly, the emphasis on time-based loss of information by Towse and Hitch and the ideas of Barrouillet and colleagues concerning cognitive load could readily be accommodated in an elaborated model of the central executive and its interface with the phonological loop. The majority of these alternative approaches also emphasize the role of attention in working memory, a concept given prominence also by Baddeley (1986). However, other claims that working memory is an activated subset of long-term memory and does not exist as a temporary storage medium distinct from preexisting knowledge are less easy to reconcile.

8.3 Overview

The ability to hold information in mind for brief periods of time, termed working memory by cognitive psychologists, is an essential feature of our everyday mental life. The purpose of this chapter is to provide a contemporary overview of current theoretical understanding of the cognitive processes of working memory. According to the influential model advanced originally by Baddeley and Hitch (1974) and revised and elaborated over the subsequent years (Baddeley, 1986, 2000; Burgess and Hitch, 1992, 1999), working memory consists of an attentional controller, the central executive, supplemented by slave systems specialized in the storage of verbal and nonverbal information (the phonological loop and visuospatial sketchpad, respectively). An additional component is the episodic buffer, capable of integrating information from different parts of working memory and other parts of the cognitive system. Each component of the model is limited in capacity.

This relatively simple model of working memory has proved capable of accommodating a wide range of empirical findings. Its fractionated structure has been informed by findings from experimental studies using dual task methods, by developmental dissociations in studies of children, and by evidence of distinct underlying brain from the fields of neuropsychology and neuroimaging. In the area of the phonological loop in particular, understanding of the underlying cognitive processes is sufficiently well advanced to allow the development of a computational model capable of simulating many detailed aspects of verbal short-term memory behavior.

Two components of the working memory model – the central executive and phonological loop – appear to play key roles not only in the temporary retention of information, but also in supporting longer-term learning, particularly during the childhood years. The phonological loop is important for learning the sound patterns of new words in the course of acquisition of vocabulary in native and foreign languages, whereas the central executive mediates academic learning in areas including reading and mathematics. Detailed theoretical accounts of the possible causal roles of working memory in these elements of learning are considered.

There are also several alternative theoretical accounts of working memory that are currently proving useful in guiding further research and understanding in this field. Some of these theories conceive of working memory as the subset of representations in long-term memory that have been activated either automatically via our interactions with the environment or effortfully, by being the focus of a consciously controlled attentional resource. Whereas the role played by attention is acknowledged in almost all current models of working memory, the distinction between models that assume specialized temporary storage mechanisms and those that see working memory as a property of preexisting knowledge representations is a fundamental one, yet to be resolved by empirical evidence. A further common feature of many theories is that time-based forgetting is a crucial feature of working memory.

Research in the field of working memory continues, stimulated by the availability of detailed theoretical accounts that guide empirical investigations of both typical and atypical working memory functioning. There is also increasing recognition that our current understanding of working memory can be put to more practical use, particularly in the fields of education and remediation (e.g., Gathercole and Alloway, in press). In this respect, working memory represents a strong example of how laboratory investigations of basic cognitive processes have the potential to enhance less esoteric elements of our everyday cognitive experience.

References

Allen RJ, Baddeley AJ, and Hitch GJ (2006) Is the binding of visual features in working memory resource-demanding? *J. Exp. Psychol. Gen.* 135: 298–313.

Alloway TP, Gathercole SE, and Pickering SJ (2006) Verbal and visuo-spatial short-term and working memory in children: Are they separable? *Child Dev.* 77: 1698–1716.

Archibald LMD and Gathercole SE (2006) Short-term and working memory in specific language impairment. *Int. J. Comm. Disord.* 41: 675–693.

Baddeley AD (1996) Exploring the central executive. *Q. J. Exp. Psychol.* 49A: 5–28.

Baddeley AD (2000) The episodic buffer: A new component of working memory? *Trends Cogn. Sci.* 4: 417–422.

Baddeley AD (1986) *Working Memory*. Oxford: Oxford University Press.

Baddeley AD and Hitch G (1974) Working memory. In: Bower G (ed.) *The Psychology of Learning and Motivation*, pp. 47–90. New York: Academic Press.

Baddeley AD and Lieberman K (1980) Spatial working memory. In: Nickerson RS (ed.) *Attention and Performance,* VIII, pp. 521–539. Hillsdale, NJ: Lawrence Erlbaum Associates.

Baddeley AD and Logie RH (1999) The multiple-component model. In: Miyake A and Shah P (eds.) *Models of Working Memory: Mechanisms of Active Maintenance and Executive Control*, pp. 28–61. New York: Cambridge University Press.

Baddeley AD, Thomson N, and Buchanan M (1975) Word length and the structure of short-term memory. *J. Verb. Learn. Verb. Behav.* 14: 575–589.

Baddeley AD, Lewis VJ, and Vallar G (1984) Exploring the articulatory loop. *Q. J. Exp. Psychol.* 36: 233–252.

Baddeley AD, Papagno C, and Vallar G (1988) When long-term learning depends on short-term storage. *J. Mem. Lang.* 27: 5876–5896.

Baddeley AD, Emslie H, Kolodny J, and Duncan J (1998a) Random generation and the executive control of working memory. *Q. J. Exp. Psychol.* 51A: 819–852.

Baddeley AD, Gathercole SE, and Papagno C (1998b) The phonological loop as a language learning device. *Psychol. Rev.* 105: 158–173.

Barrouillet P and Camos V (2001) Developmental increase in working memory span: Resource sharing or temporal decay? *J. Mem. Lang.* 45: 1–20.
Barrouillet P, Bernadin S, and Camos V (2004) Time constraints and resource sharing in adults' working memory spans. *J. Exp. Psychol. Gen.* 133(1): 83–100.
Bayliss DM, Jarrold C, Gunn DM, and Baddeley AD (2003) The complexities of complex span: Explaining individual differences in working memory in children and adults. *J. Exp. Psychol. Gen.* 132: 71–92.
Bishop DVM and Robson J (1989) Unimpaired short-term memory and rhyme judgment in congenitally speechless individuals: Implications for the notion of articulatory coding. *Q. J. Exp. Psychol.* 41A: 123–140.
Bishop DVM, North T, and Donlan C (1996) Nonword repetition as a behavioural marker for inherited language impairment: Evidence from a twin study. *J. Child Psychol. Psychiatry* 37: 391–403.
Bjork EL and Healy AF (1974) Short-term order and item retention. *J. Verb. Learn. Verb. Behav.* 13: 80–97.
Bock JK (1982) Towards a cognitive psychology of syntax: Information processing contributions to sentence formulation. *Psychol. Rev.* 89: 1–49.
Brooks LR (1967) The suppression of visualisation by reading. *Q. J. Exp. Psychol.* 19: 289–299.
Brown GDA and Hulme C (1996) Modeling item length effects in memory span: No rehearsal needed? *J. Mem. Lang.* 34: 594–621.
Brown GDA, Preece T, and Hulme C (2000) Oscillator-based memory for serial order. *Psychol. Rev.* 107: 127–181.
Burgess N and Hitch GJ (1992) Toward a network model of the articulatory loop. *J. Mem. Lang.* 31: 429–460.
Burgess N and Hitch GJ (1999) Memory for serial order: A network model of the phonological loop and its timing. *Psychol. Rev.* 106: 551–581.
Caplan D, Rochon E, and Waters GS (1994) Articulatory length and phonological determinants of word-length effects in span tasks. *Q. J. Exp. Psychol. A* 45: 177–192.
Caplan D and Waters GS (1990) Short-term memory and language comprehension: A critical review of the psychological literature. In: Vallar G and Shallice T (eds.) *Neuropsychological Impairments of Short-Term Memory*, pp. 337–389. Cambridge: Cambridge University Press.
Case R, Kurland DM, and Goldberg J (1982) Working memory capacity as long-term activation: An individual differences approach. *J. Exp. Psychol. Learn. Mem. Cogn.* 19: 1101–1114.
Chen ZJ and Cowan N (2005) Chunk limits and length limits in immediate recall: A reconciliation. *J. Exp. Psychol. Learn. Mem. Cogn.* 31: 1235–1249.
Cheung H (1996) Nonword span as a unique predictor of second-language vocabulary learning. *Dev. Psychol.* 32: 867–873.
Clark HH and Clarke EV (1977) *Psychology and Language*. New York: Harcourt Brace Jovanovitch.
Colle HA and Welsh A (1976) Acoustic masking in primary memory. *J. Verb. Learn. Verb. Behav.* 15: 17–32.
Collette F and Van der Linden M (2002) Brain imaging of the central executive component of working memory. *Neurosci. Biobehav. Rev.* 26: 105–125.
Conrad R (1964) Acoustic confusion in immediate memory. *Br. J. Psychol.* 55: 75–84.
Cowan N (1995) *Attention and Memory: An Integrated Framework*. New York: Oxford University Press.
Cowan N (2001) The magical number 4 in short-term memory: A reconsideration of mental storage capacity. *Behav. Brain Sci.* 24: 87.
Cowan N, Day L, Saults JS, Keller TA, Johnson T, and Flores L (1992) The role of verbal output time in the effects of word length on immediate memory. *J. Mem. Lang.* 31: 1–17.
Cowan N, Keller TA, Hulme C, Roodenrys S, McDougall S, and Rack J (1994) Verbal memory span in children: Speech timing cues to the mechanisms underlying age and word length effects. *J. Mem. Lang.* 33: 234–250.
Cowan N, Johnson TD, and Saults JS (2005) Capacity limits in list item recognition: Evidence from proactive interference. *Memory* 13: 293–299.
Craik FI, Govoni R, Naveh-Benjamin M, and Anderson ND (1996) The effects of divided attention on encoding and retrieval processes in human memory. *J. Exp. Psychol. Gen.* 125: 159–180.
Daneman M and Carpenter PA (1980) Individual differences in working memory and reading. *J. Verbal Learn. Verbal Behav.* 19: 450–466.
Daneman M and Carpenter PA (1983) Individual differences in integrating information between and within sentences. *J. Exp. Psychol. Learn. Mem. Cogn.* 9: 561–584.
Daneman M and Merikle PM (1996) Working memory and language comprehension: A meta-analysis. *Psychon. Bull. Rev.* 3: 422–433.
Della Sala S and Logie RH (2003) Neuropsychological impairments of visual and spatial working memory. In: Baddeley AD, Kopelman MD, and Wilson BA (eds.) *Handbook of Memory Disorders,* 2nd edn., pp. 271–292. New York: Wiley.
Della Sala S, Gray C, Baddeley AD, Allemano N, and Wilson L (1999) Pattern span: A tool for unwelding visuo-spatial memory. *Neuropsychologia* 37: 1189–1199.
Engle RW, Cantor J, and Carullo JJ (1992) Individual differences in working memory and comprehension: A test of four hypotheses. *J. Exp. Psychol. Learn. Mem. Cogn.* 18: 972–992.
Engle RW, Kane MJ, and Tuholski SW (1999a) Individual differences in working memory capacity and what they tell us about controlled attention, general fluid intelligence, and functions of the prefrontal cortex. In: Miyake A and Shah P (eds.) *Models of Working Memory: Mechanisms of Active Maintenance and Executive Control*, pp. 102–134. New York: Cambridge Univ. Press.
Engle RW, Tuholski SW, Laughlin JE, and Conway ARA (1999b) Working memory, short-term memory, and general fluid intelligence: A latent variable approach. *J. Exp. Psychol. Gen.* 125: 309–331.
Flavell JH, Beach DR, and Chinsky JM (1966) Spontaneous verbal rehearsal in a memory task as a function of age. *Child Dev.* 37: 283–299.
Gathercole SE (1999) Cognitive approaches to the development of short-term memory. *Trends Cogn. Sci.* 3: 410–418.
Gathercole SE (2004) Working memory and learning during the school years. *Proc. Br. Acad.* 125: 365–380.
Gathercole SE (2006) Nonword repetition and word learning: The nature of the relationship. *Appl. Psycholing.* 27: 513–543.
Gathercole SE and Alloway TP (in press) *Working Memory and Learning: A Teacher's Guide.* Thousand Oaks, CA: Sage Publications.
Gathercole SE and Baddeley AD (1989) Evaluation of the role of phonological STM in the development of vocabulary in children: A longitudinal study. *J. Mem. Lang.* 28: 200–213.
Gathercole SE and Baddeley AD (1990a) The role of phonological memory in vocabulary acquisition: A study of young children learning new names. *Br. J. Psychol.* 81: 439–454.
Gathercole S and Baddeley A (1990b) Phonological memory deficits in language disordered children: Is there a causal connection? *J. Mem. Lang.* 29: 336–360.
Gathercole SE and Baddeley AD (1993) *Working Memory and Language*. Hove, UK: Lawrence Erlbaum.
Gathercole SE and Hitch G (1993) The development of rehearsal: A revised working memory perspective. In: Collins A,

Gathercole S, Conway M, and Morris P (eds.) *Theories of Memory*. Hove, UK: Lawrence Erlbaum Associates.

Gathercole SE, Adams A-M, and Hitch GJ (1994a) Do young children rehearse? An individual-differences analysis. *Mem. Cogn.* 22: 201–207.

Gathercole SE, Willis C, Emslie H, and Baddeley AD (1994b) The Children's Test of Nonword Repetition: A test of phonological working memory. *Memory* 2: 103–127.

Gathercole SE, Hitch GJ, Service E, and Martin AJ (1997) Short-term memory and new word learning in children. *Dev. Psychol.* 33: 966–979.

Gathercole SE, Pickering SJ, Ambridge B, and Wearing H (2004a) The structure of working memory from 4 to 15 years of age. *Dev. Psychol.* 40: 177–190.

Gathercole SE, Pickering SJ, Knight, and Stedmann (2004b) Working memory skills and educational attainment: Evidence from national curriculum assessments at 7 and 14 years of age. *Appl. Cogn. Psychol.* 18: 1–16.

Gathercole SE, Alloway TP, Willis CS, and Adams AM (2006a) Working memory in children with reading disabilities. *J. Exp. Child Psychol.* 93: 265–281.

Gathercole SE, Lamont E, and Alloway TP (2006b) Working memory in the classroom. In: Pickering S (ed.) *Working Memory and Education*, pp. 219–240. London: Elsevier.

Geary DC, Hoard MK, Byrd-Craven J, and DeSoto MC (2004) Strategy choices in simple and complex addition: Contributions of working memory and counting knowledge for children with mathematical disability. *J. Exp. Child Psychol.* 88: 121–151.

Hanley JR, Young AW, and Pearson NA (1991) Impairment of the visuo-spatial sketchpad. *Q. J. Exp. Psychol.* 43A: 101–125.

Henson R (2005) What can functional neuroimaging tell the experimental psychologist? *Q. J. Exp. Psychol.* 58: 192–233.

Henson RNA, Norris DG, Page MPA, and Baddeley AD (1996) Unchained memory: Error patterns rule out chaining models of immediate serial recall. *Q. J. Exp. Psychol.* 49A: 80–115.

Hitch GJ and Halliday MS (1983) Working memory in children. *Philos. Trans. R. Soc. Lond. B* 302: 324–340.

Hitch GJ, Towse JN, and Hutton U (2001) What limits children's working memory span? Theoretical accounts and applications for scholastic development. *J. Exp. Psychol. Gen.* 130: 184–198.

Hulme C and Tordoff V (1989) Working memory development: The effects of speech rate, word length, and acoustic similarity on serial recall. *J. Exp. Child Psychol.* 47: 72–87.

Jarvis HL and Gathercole SE (2003) Verbal and non-verbal working memory and achievements on national curriculum tests at 11 and 14 years of age. *Educat. Child Psychol.* 20: 123–140.

Jefferies E, Lambon-Ralph MA, and Baddeley AD (2004) Automatic and controlled processing in sentence recall: The role of long-term and working memory. *J. Mem. Lang.* 51: 623–643.

Johnson RA, Johnson C, and Gray C (1987) The emergence of the word length effect in young children: The effects of overt and covert rehearsal. *Br. J. Dev. Psychol.* 5: 243–248.

Jones DM, Hughes RW, and Macken WJ (2006) Perceptual organization masquerading as phonological storage: Further support for a perceptual-gestural view of short-term memory. *J. Mem. Lang.* 54: 265–281.

Just MA and Carpenter PA (1992) A capacity theory of comprehension: Individual differences in working memory. *Psychol. Rev.* 99: 122–149.

Kane MJ, Hambrick DZ, Tuholski SW, Wilhelm O, Payne TW, and Engle RW (2004) The generality of working-memory capacity: A latent-variable approach to verbal and visuo-spatial memory span and reasoning. *J. Exp. Psychol. Gen.* 133: 189–217.

Kyllonen PC and Chrystal RE (1990) Reasoning ability (little more than) working memory capacity. *Intelligence* 14: 389–433.

Logie RH (1995) *Visuo-Spatial Working Memory*. Hove, UK: Erlbaum.

McCarthy RA and Warrington EK (1987) Understanding: A function of short-term memory? *Brain* 110: 1565–1578.

Masoura E and Gathercole SE (1999) Phonological short-term memory and foreign vocabulary learning. *Int. J. Psychol.* 34: 383–388.

Miyake A and Shah P (1999) *Models of Working Memory: Mechanisms of Active Maintenance and Executive Control*. New York: Cambridge University Press.

Muller NG and Knight RT (2006) The functional neuroanatomy of working memory: Contributions of brain lesion studies. *Neuroscience* 139: 51–58.

Murray DJ (1968) Articulation and acoustic similarity in short-term memory. *J. Exp. Psychol.* 78: 679–684.

Neath I, Farley LA, and Surprenant AM (2003) Directly assessing the relationship between irrelevant speech and articulatory suppression. *Q. J. Exp. Psychol.* 56A: 1269–1278.

Owen AM, McMillan KM, Laird AR, et al. (2005) N-back working memory paradigm: A meta-analysis of normative functional neuroimaging. *Hum. Brain Mapp.* 25: 46–59.

Page MPA and Norris D (1998) The Primacy model: A new model of immediate serial recall. *Psychol. Rev.* 105: 761–781.

Palmer S (2000) Working memory: A developmental study of phonological recoding. *Memory* 8: 179–194.

Papagno C and Vallar G (1992) Phonological short-term memory and the learning of novel words: The effects of phonological similarity and item length. *Q. J. Exp. Psychol.* 44A: 47–67.

Papagno C, Valentine T, and Baddeley AD (1991) Phonological short-term memory and foreign-language vocabulary learning. *J. Mem. Lang.* 30: 331–347.

Peterson LR and Johnson ST (1971) Some effects of minimizing articulation on short-term retention. *J. Verb. Learn. Verb. Behav.* 10: 346–354.

Phillips WA and Christie DFM (1977) Interference with visualisation. *Q. J. Exp. Psychol.* 29: 637–650.

Pickering SJ and Gathercole SE (2004) Distinctive working memory profiles in children with special educational needs. *Educat. Psychol.* 24: 393–408.

Pickering SJ, Gathercole SE, and Peaker SM (1998) Verbal and visuo-spatial short-term memory in children: Evidence for common and distinct mechanisms. *Mem. Cogn.* 26: 1117–1130.

Pickering SJ, Gathercole SE, Hall M, and Lloyd SA (2001) Development of memory for pattern and path: Further evidence for the fractionation of visuo-spatial memory. *Q. J. Exp. Psychol.* 54A: 397–420.

Postle BR, Idzikowski C, Della Sala S, and Baddeley AD (2006) The selective disruption of spatial working memory by eye movements. *Q. J. Exp. Psychol.* 59: 100–120.

Quinn JG and McConnell J (1996) Irrelevant pictures in visual working memory. *Q. J. Exp. Psychol.* 49A: 200–215.

Ransdell S and Hecht S (2003) Time and resource limits on working memory: Cross-age consistency in counting span performance. *J. Exp. Child Psychol.* 86: 303–313.

Romani C (1992) Are there distinct input and output buffers – evidence from an aphasic patient with an impaired output buffer? *Lang. Cogn. Process.* 7: 131–162.

Russell J, Jarrold C, and Henry L (1996) Working memory in children with autism and with moderate learning difficulties. *J. Child Psychol. Psychiatry* 37: 673–686.

Service E (1992) Phonology, working memory, and foreign-language learning. *Q. J. Exp. Psychol.* 45A: 21–50.

Shah P and Miyake A (1996) The separability of working memory resources for spatial thinking and language processing: An individual differences approach. *J. Exp. Psychol. Gen.* 125: 4–27.
Shallice T (1982) Specific impairments of planning. *Philos. Trans. R. Soc. Lond. B* 298: 199–209.
Shallice T and Butterworth B (1977) Short-term memory impairment and spontaneous speech. *Neuropsychologia* 15: 729–735.
Smyth MM and Scholey KA (1996) Serial order in spatial immediate memory. *Q. J. Exp. Psychol. A.* 49: 159–177.
Surprenant AM, Neath I, and LeCompte DC (1999) Irrelevant speech, phonological similarity, and presentation modality. *Memory* 7: 405–420.
Swanson HL and Beebe-Frankenberger M (2004) The relationship between working memory and mathematical problem solving in children at risk and not at risk for math disabilities. *J. Educat. Psychol.* 96: 471–491.
Swanson HL, Ashbaker MH, and Lee C (1996) Learning-disabled readers' working memory as a function of processing demands. *J. Exp. Child Psychol.* 61: 242–275.
Thompson JM, Hamilton CJ, Gray JM, et al. (2006) Executive and visuospatial sketchpad resources in euthymic bipolar disorder: Implications for visuospatial working memory architecture. *Memory* 14: 437–451.
Towse JN and Hitch GJ (1995) Is there a relationship between task demand and storage space in tests of working memory capacity? *Q. J. Exp. Psychol.* 48: 108–124.
Towse JN, Hitch GJ, and Hutton U (1998) A reevaluation of working memory capacity in children. *J. Mem. Lang.* 39: 195–217.
Towse JN, Hitch GJ, and Hutton U (2002) On the nature of the relationship between processing activity and item retention in children. *J. Exp. Child Psychol.* 82: 156–184.
Turner MLM and Engle RW (1989) Is working memory capacity task dependent? *J. Mem. Lang.* 28: 127–154.
Unsworth N and Engle RW (2006) Simple and complex memory spans and their relation to fluid abilities: Evidence from list-length effects. *J. Mem. Lang.* 54: 68–80.
Vallar G and Baddeley AD (1984) Fractionation of working memory: Neuropsychological evidence for a short-term store. *J. Verb. Learn. Verb. Behav.* 23: 151–161.
Vallar G and Baddeley AD (1987) Phonological short-term store and sentence processing. *Cogn. Neuropsychol.* 6: 465–473.
Vallar G and Papagno C (2003) Neuropsychological impairments of short-term memory. In: Baddeley AD, Kopelman MD, and Wilson BA (eds.) *Handbook of Memory Disorders*, pp. 249–270. Chichester, UK: John Wiley.
Vallar G and Shallice T (1990) *Neuropsychological Impairments of Short-Term Memory*. Cambridge: Cambridge University Press.
Waugh NC and Norman DA (1965) Primary memory. *Psychol. Rev.* 72: 89–104.
Wheeler ME and Treisman AM (2002) Binding in short-term visual memory. *J. Exp. Psychol. Gen.* 131: 48–64.
Wilson JTL, Scott JH, and Power KG (1987) Developmental differences in the span of visual memory for pattern. *Br. J. Dev. Psychol.* 5: 249–255.

9 Prefrontal Cortex and Memory

C. Ranganath and R. S. Blumenfeld, University of California at Davis, Davis, CA, USA

9.1 Introduction

Dating back at least to the work of Jacobsen (1935), researchers have been interested in characterizing the functional role of the lateral prefrontal cortex (PFC) in memory. In recent years, a wealth of evidence from neuropsychological, neurophysiological, and neuroimaging studies has accumulated, implicating the PFC in a wide variety of memory functions. Here, we will review this evidence and present a general framework for understanding the roles of different prefrontal regions in memory processing.

9.2 Anatomical Organization of the PFC

In order to understand how the PFC contributes to memory, it is useful to start by considering its anatomical characteristics. The PFC is situated in the frontal lobes, rostral to the premotor and motor cortices and, in humans, occupies approximately one third of the cortical mantle (Fuster, 1997). The lateral PFC consists of several highly interconnected subregions that can be distinguished based on cytoarchitectonic characteristics and anatomical connectivity. Many researchers (e.g., Goldman-Rakic, 1987; Petrides, 1994; Fuster, 1997) have proposed functional distinctions between mid-dorsolateral (DLPFC; Brodmann's areas [BA] 9 and 46) and ventrolateral (VLPFC; BA 44, 45, and 47) PFC. VLPFC is situated in the inferior convexity in the monkey brain and in the inferior frontal gyrus in humans. This region is highly connected to ventral posterior sensory areas, and especially to regions of the inferior and superior temporal lobe. DLPFC is situated in the cortex dorsal to the sulcus principalis in the monkey and in the middle frontal gyrus in the human brain. In contrast to VLPFC, DLPFC is more highly interconnected with dorsal stream regions (especially the posterior parietal cortex) and paralimbic cortical regions, including the retrosplenial and parahippocampal cortices.

Although little is known about more anterior regions of lateral PFC (APFC; BA 10), recent research suggests that these regions may be particularly critical for human cognition (Petrides, 1994; Fuster, 1997; Christoff and Gabrieli, 2000; D'Esposito et al., 2000; Koechlin et al., 2003; Ramnani and Owen, 2004). For example, recent comparative neuroanatomical work suggests a twofold increase in the size of APFC in humans relative to chimpanzees (Semendeferi et al., 2001), despite the fact that the relative size of the entire frontal lobe is similar between the two species (Semendeferi et al., 2002). As described in the following, VLPFC, DLPFC, and APFC have been implicated in human memory processes, and there is some evidence that these regions may exhibit different functional characteristics (Wagner, 1999; Buckner and Wheeler, 2001; Fletcher and Henson, 2001; Rainer and Ranganath, 2002; Ranganath and Knight, 2003).

9.3 PFC and Working Memory

9.3.1 PFC Involvement in Working Memory: Short-Term Retention and Cognitive Control

Since the 1980s, a great deal of research has focused on the role of PFC in 'working memory' (WM) processes that support temporary retention and on-line processing of information. Much of this work has characterized the PFC as a global level, but more recent research has been devoted to specifying the different processes implemented by different subregions of PFC (Goldman-Rakic, 1987; Fuster, 1997; D'Esposito et al., 2000; Petrides, 2005). Psychological theories of WM generally distinguish between processes that support temporary retention of information across short delays (or what is now termed 'WM maintenance') and those that support attentional and cognitive control (Baddeley, 1986). The degree to which regions of PFC are necessary for maintenance versus control has been a topic of extensive debate in cognitive neuroscience.

The idea that PFC supports temporary retention of information has largely emerged from single-unit recording studies of monkeys performing the delayed response task, in which the monkey is shown a reward in one of two locations but must wait until after a delay before it can obtain the reward. The task is thought to require the monkey to maintain an internal representation of the remembered location or upcoming movement across the delay period. Critically, lateral prefrontal neurons exhibit persistent activity during the memory delay that is selective for the remembered location (Fuster and Alexander, 1971). This work was extended by Funahashi et al. (1989, 1990), who investigated prefrontal activity during an oculomotor delayed response task, in which a monkey is cued to make an eye movement to a spatial location, but it must wait until after a brief delay before making the saccade. Consistent with other studies of the delayed response task, lateral prefrontal neurons exhibited persistent activity during the memory delay that was specific to the spatial location that was to be remembered. Further research showed that PFC lesions in one hemisphere impaired memory performance specifically for locations in the contralateral hemifield (Funahashi et al., 1993). Based on these findings, it has often been assumed that lateral prefrontal neurons temporarily store information that is to be maintained across a delay (Goldman-Rakic, 1987).

Results from studies by Miller and Desimone seemed to further substantiate this idea by contrasting the activity of neurons in inferior temporal cortex (a region that is involved in visual object processing; cf. Miyashita and Hayashi, 2000) and PFC during a visual WM task. Their findings showed that both inferior temporal and prefrontal neurons showed persistent, stimulus-specific activity during memory delays (Miller et al., 1993, 1996). However, persistent delay period activity in inferior temporal neurons was abolished by the presentation of a distracting stimulus (Miller et al., 1993), whereas activity in PFC remained robust in the face of interference.

Many have interpreted Miller and Desimone's data to support the idea that short-term retention of information is supported by the PFC, rather than by posterior cortical areas that represent the information to be maintained. However, this interpretation rests on the assumption that persistent activity is the sole neural correlate of WM maintenance. This assumption was invalidated in a recent study, in which single-unit activity and local field potentials (LFPs) were recorded in occipital area V4 during a visual WM task (Lee et al., 2005). Unlike neurons in inferior temporal cortex, recordings from V4 did not reveal evidence of persistent, stimulus-specific activity during even an unfilled memory delay. However, results did reveal single-unit activity during the memory delay that was phase-locked to theta oscillations in the electroencephalogram. Critically, the phase-locking of single-unit activity and theta oscillations was selective to the remembered stimulus. These findings strongly suggest that posterior cortical regions can play important roles in WM maintenance even in the absence of overall changes in mean firing rate across the memory delay. Furthermore, converging lines of evidence now suggest that short-term retention of specific kinds of information is supported by activation of the posterior cortical areas that represent that information (Fuster, 1995; Miyashita and Hayashi, 2000; Lee et al., 2005; Ranganath and Blumenfeld, 2005; Ranganath and D'Esposito, 2005; Postle, 2006; Ranganath, 2006).

Results from lesion studies have additionally demonstrated that the PFC contributes to WM by virtue of its role in cognitive control, rather than short-term retention (see D'Esposito and Postle, 1999; Curtis and D'Esposito, 2004; Postle, 2006, for detailed reviews of this topic). Jacobsen (1935) demonstrated that lateral prefrontal lesions caused impairments in the delayed response task, leading him to conclude that the PFC is critical for retaining information across short delays. However, this interpretation was later questioned by Malmo (1942), who demonstrated that prefrontal lesions only impaired monkeys' performance on the task if there was interference present between the instruction and the response. If the lights were turned off between the instruction and response (thus minimizing interference), performance was intact. Subsequent research in the 1960s substantiated the idea that monkeys with PFC lesions performed poorly because they were unable to suppress previously rewarded responses or because they could not maintain the appropriate task set (Mishkin, 1964; Pribram et al., 1964; Pribram and Tubbs, 1967; Nauta, 1971). For instance, Nauta (1971) noted that

> the initial impression that the 'frontal animal' suffers from a memory loss . . . has been effectively refuted, and it now seems certain that frontal-lobe ablation affects a response-guidance other than memory in the customary sense.

This impression has been supported by more recent lesion studies (Mishkin and Manning, 1978; Kowalska et al., 1991; Meunier et al., 1997; Rushworth et al., 1997; Petrides, 2000), as well as single-unit recording (Asaad et al., 2000; Lebedev et al., 2004) studies of monkeys and neuropsychological (Chao and Knight, 1995; D'Esposito and Postle, 1999; D'Esposito et al., 2006) and neuroimaging (Postle et al., 1999; Smith and Jonides, 1999) studies of humans. Indeed, consistent with the monkey literature, humans with prefrontal lesions do not exhibit significant impairments in short-term retention of information, but their performance is impaired on more complex tasks that involve inhibiting distraction and manipulating information (Chao and Knight, 1995, 1998; D'Esposito and Postle, 1999; Ranganath and Blumenfeld, 2005; D'Esposito et al., 2006).

How, then, does one explain the fact that prefrontal regions show persistent activity during WM maintenance? The most likely explanation is that prefrontal neurons do not temporarily store information that is to be maintained, but rather that they represent and maintain context-dependent rules or associations that dictate the kind of information that is currently goal relevant (Fuster, 1997; Miller, 2000). Indeed, this idea can explain not only why PFC neurons exhibit delay period activity, but also why they exhibit activity associated with virtually every relevant aspect of delayed-response tasks (Fuster, 1997). By representing context-dependent stimulus–response associations, PFC networks can use higher-order knowledge to guide behavior in novel situations and override prepotent responses. Because of its connections with posterior cortex, activation of prefrontal representations can increase or decrease the activation of posterior cortical representations, based on what is relevant for current or future goals. This view accords well with most theories of prefrontal function, which generally suggest a role for the PFC in the selection and maintenance of task-relevant information and the inhibition of irrelevant, distracting information (Pribram et al., 1964; Brutkowski, 1965; Luria, 1966a; Nauta, 1971; Stuss and Benson, 1986; Goldman-Rakic, 1987; Cohen and Servan-Schreiber, 1992; Cohen et al., 1996; Fuster, 1997; Knight et al., 1999; Miller, 2000; Shimamura, 2000; Miller and Cohen, 2001; Miller and D'Esposito, 2005).

9.3.2 Functional Imaging of Working Memory: Evidence for Functional Differentiation within PFC

Results from human neuroimaging studies of WM converge with the view described above, and these studies have also provided evidence for functional differentiations within PFC. Based on ideas outlined by Fuster (1997, 2004) and consideration of the available evidence, we suggest one such view, outlining a hierarchy of 'selection' processes implemented by different PFC subregions along the rostro–caudal and dorso–ventral axes (see **Figure 1**).

Anatomically, VLPFC subregions are well positioned to modulate activity in high-level auditory, visual, and multimodal association areas (Petrides and Pandya, 2002). Thus, the VLPFC may be a source of top-down signals that select (i.e., enhance or reduce the activation of) item representations in posterior cortical areas based on current task demands. Consistent with this idea, VLPFC activation is observed when a task requires inhibition of irrelevant or potentially distracting items (Konishi et al., 1999; Aron et al., 2004; Zhang et al., 2004), resolution of proactive interference (Jonides and Nee, 2006), resolution of competition among competing linguistic representations (Thompson-Schill

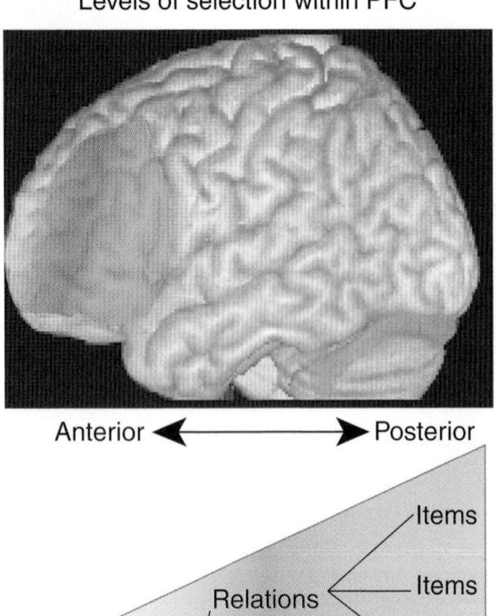

Figure 1 At top, a lateral view of the brain, with a gradient illustrating functional differentiation within the PFC along the rostro–caudal and dorso–ventral axes. At bottom, a hypothesized functional organization is depicted, such that regions in VLPFC (blue) may be involved in selecting relevant items, DLPFC (pink) may be involved in selecting relationships between items that are currently active, and APFC (yellow) may be involved in selecting cognitive sets that determine which items and relations are appropriate targets for selection.

et al., 1997; Wagner et al., 2001a), or activation of an item representation (i.e., WM maintenance; Curtis and D'Esposito, 2003). Furthermore, the topography of VLPFC activation in these studies is material dependent, such that tasks requiring selection, encoding, or maintenance of different kinds of items recruit different subregions of VLPFC (Schumacher et al., 1996; Kelley et al., 1998; Wagner et al., 1998; Poldrack et al., 1999; Wagner, 1999; Braver et al., 2001). In contrast, DLPFC and APFC activation is not material dependent, suggesting that these regions may act at a more abstract level (D'Esposito et al., 1998; Smith and Jonides, 1999; Wagner, 1999; Rainer and Ranganath, 2002; Ranganath and Knight, 2003; Ramnani and Owen, 2004).

Unlike VLPFC, DLPFC is not robustly recruited during tasks that solely require selection of task-relevant information. Instead, evidence from neuroimaging studies suggests that DLPFC is involved in using rules to activate, inhibit, or transform relationships among items that are active in WM. For example, DLPFC activation is reported in 'manipulation' tasks that involve sequencing of information that is being maintained in WM (D'Esposito et al., 1999; Postle et al., 1999; Wagner et al., 2001b; Barde and Thompson-Schill, 2002; Blumenfeld and Ranganath, 2006; Crone et al., 2006; Mohr et al., 2006) or monitoring of previous responses when selecting a future response (Owen, 1997; Owen et al., 1999). DLPFC activation has also been reported in 'chunking' studies which involve processing of relationships to build higher-level groupings among items that are active in memory (Bor et al., 2003, 2004; Bor and Owen, 2006). One parsimonious explanation for this diverse array of findings is that DLPFC may implement selection processes that accentuate or inhibit the activation of relationships among items that are active in memory.

Although APFC is not nearly as well characterized as DLPFC and VLPFC, available evidence is consistent with the idea that APFC is at the apex of the hierarchy of selection processes implemented by PFC. One way of conceptualizing this role is that APFC implements the selection of appropriate cognitive sets – that is, sets of goal-directed rules that determine which types of relations and items are appropriate for selection by DLPFC and VLPFC, respectively. Although virtually every type of task involves some kind of cognitive set, APFC recruitment specifically occurs during tasks that place demands on the *selection* of an appropriate cognitive set (Rogers and Monsell, 1995; Mayr and Kliegl, 2000; Rogers et al., 2000; Mayr, 2002). Consistent with this prediction, several functional magnetic resonance imaging (fMRI) studies have reported APFC activation using paradigms in which subjects must actively maintain a task set (Braver et al., 2003; Bunge et al., 2003; Sakai and Passingham, 2003) or hold a primary task set in mind while processing secondary subgoals (Koechlin et al., 1999; Braver and Bongiolatti, 2002; Koechlin et al., 2003; Kubler et al., 2003; Badre and Wagner, 2004). As we describe later, the role of APFC in selection and maintenance of cognitive sets might explain why APFC activation is routinely observed during long-term memory (LTM) retrieval tasks.

To summarize, it is clear that the PFC is involved in WM processes, but that role has been misinterpreted in recent years. Available evidence indicates that PFC is not necessary for short-term retention per se, and that it is more specifically critical for WM control processes that guide behavior under a range of circumstances. These processes may emerge through prefrontal representations that use context information to select relevant information and inhibit irrelevant information. We suggest that this selection mechanism is common across prefrontal regions, and that different prefrontal regions act to select information at different levels (**Figure 1**). Specifically, VLPFC acts to activate or inhibit item representations, whereas DLPFC acts to activate or inhibit relationships between items that are actively selected or maintained through VLPFC operations. Finally, APFC may play a role in activating or inhibiting representations of cognitive sets that determine which types of items and relations are appropriate for selection (Bunge et al., 2003; Sakai and Passingham, 2003). As we will describe, this hypothesized division of labor corresponds well to the imaging literature on PFC and LTM processes (see also Fletcher and Henson, 2001, for a similar perspective).

9.4 Effects of Prefrontal Lesions on LTM Encoding and Retrieval

9.4.1 Neuropsychological Studies of Patients with Prefrontal Lesions

Clinicians have long noted that focal prefrontal lesions in humans produce subtle but noticeable memory deficits, and this impression accords well with results from neuropsychological studies (Stuss and Benson, 1986; Shimamura, 1995; Ranganath and Knight, 2003). In general, patients with PFC lesions show impairments on a wide range of memory tasks that tax executive control during encoding and/or retrieval (Stuss and Benson, 1986; Moscovitch, 1992; Shimamura, 1995; Ranganath and Knight, 2003). For instance, PFC patients exhibit impaired performance on unconstrained memory tests such as free-recall (Jetter et al., 1986; Janowsky et al., 1989a; Eslinger and Grattan, 1994; Gershberg and Shimamura, 1995; Wheeler et al., 1995; Dimitrov et al., 1999). In contrast to healthy control participants, PFC patients tend not to spontaneously cluster or group recall output according to semantic relationships within a categorized word list (Hirst and Volpe, 1988; Incisa della Rochetta and Milner, 1993; Stuss et al., 1994; Gershberg and Shimamura, 1995). Furthermore, when presented with several study-test trials with the same word list, healthy participants tend to recall items in the same order across recall trials, a phenomenon termed 'subjective organization.' Patients with prefrontal lesions, however, show less trial-to-trial consistency of recall output order compared to controls (Stuss et al., 1994; Gershberg and Shimamura, 1995; Alexander et al., 2003).

Patients with prefrontal lesions also exhibit impaired performance on tests of source memory (Janowsky et al., 1989c; Duarte et al., 2005), memory for temporal order (Shimamura et al., 1990; McAndrews and Milner, 1991; Butters et al., 1994; Kesner et al., 1994; Mangels, 1997), and judgments of frequency (Stanhope et al., 1998). Furthermore, PFC patients often fail to spontaneously use common memory strategies and lack insight into their own memory problems (Hirst and Volpe, 1988; Janowsky et al., 1989b; Moscovitch and Melo, 1997; Vilkki et al., 1998).

In contrast to these deficits, patients with prefrontal lesions can often perform at near-normal levels when given structured encoding tasks or tests that do not tax strategic retrieval processes. For instance, PFC patients perform better at cued recall compared to free recall and have only a mild impairment in item recognition (Wheeler et al., 1995). Moreover, patients can show marked improvements on a variety of recall measures if given sufficient practice or environmental support at encoding or retrieval (Hirst and Volpe, 1988; Incisa della Rochetta and Milner, 1993; Gershberg and Shimamura, 1994; Stuss et al., 1994).

9.4.2 Recollection and Familiarity in Patients with Prefrontal Lesions

As noted above, patients with prefrontal lesions tend to show only mild deficits in recognition memory performance. Behavioral research has supported the idea that item recognition can be supported either by the assessment of familiarity, or by the recollection of specific details associated with the item (Yonelinas, 2002). Some researchers have speculated that prefrontal damage may selectively affect the recollection process (Knowlton and Squire, 1995; Davidson and Glisky, 2002; Gold et al., 2006), based on reports of recollection deficits among the healthy elderly (Davidson and Glisky, 2002) and among amnesic patients with Korsakoff's syndrome (Knowlton and Squire, 1995) that may be correlated with performance on the Wisconsin card sorting task and other tasks thought to be dependent on PFC function. However, it is highly unlikely that performance on such tests uniquely indexes the functioning of the PFC and no other brain region.

To directly test the role of PFC in recognition memory, it is necessary to directly assess recollection and familiarity in patients with focal prefrontal lesions. One methodological challenge in addressing this question is that prefrontal lesions are typically unilateral (due to stroke or tumor excision), and therefore patients might rely on the intact hemisphere to support performance. A recent study dealt with this issue by using a divided-field presentation method to specifically assess memory performance for information that was encoded in the visual field contralateral to the lesioned hemisphere ('contralesional') and the field ipsilateral to the lesioned hemisphere ('ipsilesional'). Thus, if PFC regions contribute to familiarity or recollection, one would expect deficits in these processes to be most substantial when objects were encoded in the contralesional visual field. Patients and controls were tested using the remember-know method, in which they decided whether each test object was shown during the study phase, and if so, whether they could recollect specific details about the study episode. These data were then used to create quantitative indices of familiarity and recollection for objects encoded in the contralesional and ipsilesional hemifields in each patient, and similar indices were created for each visual field in the corresponding age- and education-matched control participant. As shown in **Figure 2**, patients showed impaired familiarity for objects that were presented in the contralesional field at the time of encoding. Furthermore, although PFC patients did not exhibit deficits in subjective recollection, patients with left frontal lesions exhibited impairments in memory for the context in which each word was encountered (i.e., source memory).

Findings from this study demonstrate that, contrary to previous assertions, the PFC is necessary for normal familiarity-based recognition. Additionally, although patients with PFC lesions may have a subjective experience of recollection, they may still exhibit impairments in the ability to use recollected information to make source attributions (particularly following left frontal lesions – see the section titled 'Laterality of PFC activation during LTM encoding and retrieval' for more on this topic). This finding makes sense if one assumes that PFC damage affects control processes, rather than memory storage. That is, engagement of PFC-dependent control processes most likely impacts encoding of overall familiarity strength as well as encoding of distinctive contextual information that would support recollection (Ranganath et al., 2003b, 2005a; Blumenfeld and Ranganath, 2006). Furthermore, engagement of PFC-dependent control processes at retrieval most likely affect strategic search and decision processes that influence the retrieval and use of familiarity and recollective information (Ranganath et al., 2000, 2003a, 2007).

9.4.3 Theoretical Accounts of Memory Deficits following Prefrontal Lesions

Theoretical accounts of memory deficits in patients with prefrontal lesions generally fall into two categories. Some theories emphasize the role of the PFC in selection processes that direct attention toward goal-relevant information and task-appropriate responses. Thus, memory deficits may arise in patients with prefrontal lesions because they are unable to select goal-relevant information or inhibit distracting or interfering items or responses during encoding or retrieval (Luria, 1966b; Perret, 1974; Shimamura, 1995). One finding consistent with this account comes from a study of paired associate learning in patients with focal PFC lesions and matched controls (Shimamura et al., 1995). In this study, participants learned a list of word pairs ('A–B') and then learned an overlapping list of word pairs ('A–C') across several trials. Recall success on the A–C list required subjects to inhibit the 'A–B' pairing and select the appropriate 'A–C' pairing. Critically, patients with PFC lesions showed a disproportionate decrease in recall performance between the first trial of A–B learning and the first trial of A–C learning (i.e., a measure of proactive interference), as compared to controls. Furthermore, during cued recall of the A–C list, PFC patients recalled significantly more intrusions from the A–B list. These finding suggest that patients with prefrontal lesions were unable to inhibit the influence of previously learned associations during encoding or retrieval of new associations.

The second category of theories to explain memory deficits following prefrontal lesions emphasizes the role of the PFC in guiding spontaneous organization of information (Milner et al., 1985; Hirst and Volpe, 1988; Incisa della Rochetta and Milner, 1993; Gershberg and Shimamura, 1995). In psychology, 'organization' refers to memory strategies that emphasize forming or utilizing relationships among items in a list during encoding and/or retrieval. Some common organizational strategies during encoding include

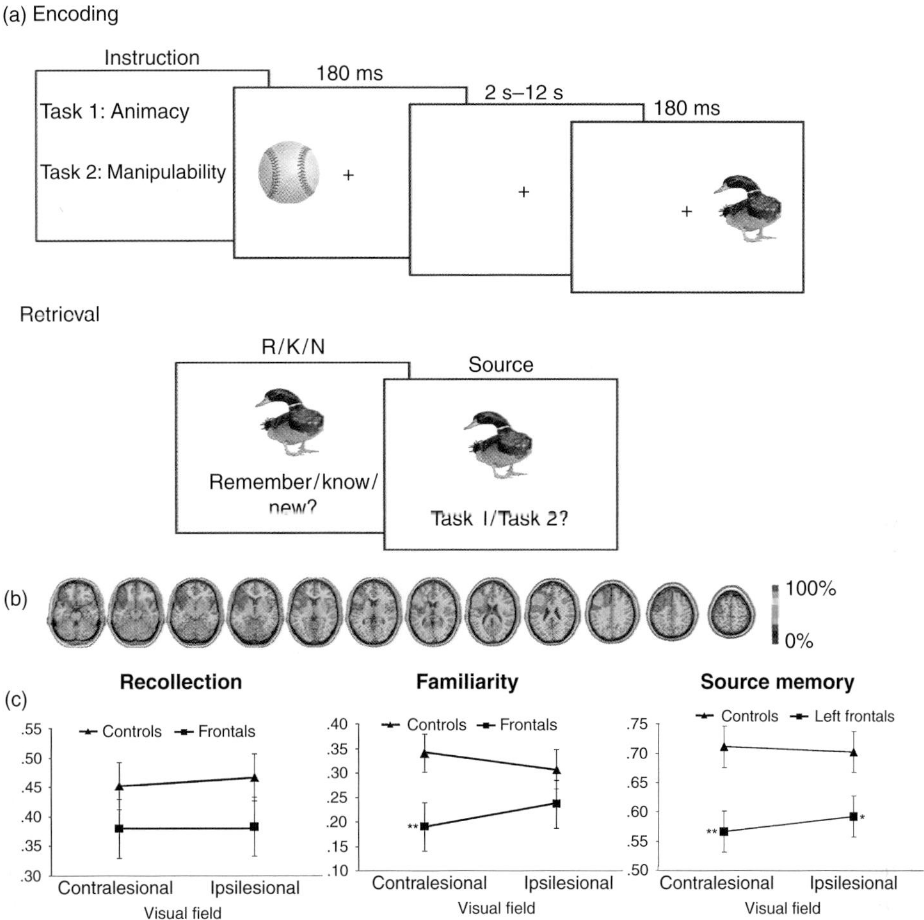

Figure 2 (a) Participants with lateral prefrontal lesions and controls encoded objects that were briefly flashed to the left or right hemifield, and then performed retrieval tests assessing memory for each item and the task that was performed during encoding. (b) Lesion overlap for patients. Right frontal lesions have been transcribed to the left hemisphere to determine the overlap across all patients. The color scale indicates the percentage of patients with lesions in a specific area. (c) Results showed that subjective measures of recollection (left) were relatively spared in the patients, whereas familiarity (middle) was impaired, particularly for objects encoded in the contralesional visual field. Source memory (right) performance was also impaired in patients with left frontal lesions. Experimental design and results from Duarte A, Ranganath C, and Knight RT (2005) Effects of unilateral prefrontal lesions on familiarity, recollection, and source memory. *J. Neurosci.* 25: 8333–8337.

categorizing words in a list according to semantic features, imagining two or more items interacting, or forming a sentence out of two or more words. Organizational processes do not facilitate LTM by enhancing features of specific items in memory, but rather by promoting memory for associations among items.

The organizational account described above can explain free recall deficits seen in patients with PFC lesions, because free recall is thought to rely heavily on organization of information in the study list. One study directly tested this hypothesis by comparing performance of patients with lateral prefrontal lesions and healthy controls on learning of lists of words that were either semantically related or unrelated (Gershberg and Shimamura, 1995). Patients with PFC lesions showed impaired recall of items from both related and unrelated lists. Furthermore, the patients failed to demonstrate normal levels of subjective organization and failed to show semantic clustering following study of semantically related lists, two indices of organizational processing during encoding. Interestingly, recall and clustering performance increased for semantically related word lists when patients were explicitly asked to make a category judgment during encoding, when they were provided with the category names at test, or both. The same was not true for the healthy controls, who performed at similar levels regardless of whether they were given cues or instructions. This pattern of results suggests that patients were capable of using semantic information to guide encoding and retrieval, but that they lacked the ability to spontaneously use semantic organizational strategies. In contrast, controls were spontaneously using organizational strategies during encoding and/or retrieval. These findings, and others (Hirst and Volpe, 1988; Incisa della Rochetta and Milner, 1993; Stuss et al., 1994; Alexander et al., 2003) suggest that LTM deficits following prefrontal lesions may emerge partly from a failure to organize information during encoding and capitalize on organizational structure during retrieval.

Many researchers have suggested that both selection and organizational processes depend on the functioning of the PFC, and there are several studies that have found support for both the interference and organizational accounts in the same study (Hirst and Volpe, 1988; Stuss et al., 1994; Gershberg and Shimamura, 1995; Shimamura et al., 1995; Alexander et al., 2003). One question that cannot be addressed by the neuropsychological evidence is whether selection and organization depend upon the same regions of PFC, because these studies typically use subject groups that have significant heterogeneity in lesion size and location. However, in light of the evidence from imaging studies of WM control processes, it is possible that VLPFC is particularly critical for selection of relevant item information, whereas DLPFC is particularly critical for building of relationships between items in a manner that supports organization. As we will describe below, this hypothesis is consistent with results from neuroimaging studies of LTM encoding and retrieval.

9.5 Functional Neuroimaging of LTM Encoding and Retrieval

9.5.1 Subsequent Memory Effects and the PFC

Event-related fMRI studies have investigated LTM encoding by identifying 'subsequent memory' or 'Dm' (difference due to memory) effects (Paller and Wagner, 2002). In these paradigms, brain activity is monitored during the performance of an incidental encoding task (i.e., semantic processing of a single word). Following scanning, a surprise memory test is administered, and brain activation during encoding is analyzed as a function of later memory success or failure. For example, participants might be given a semantic encoding task in the scanner, and then once out of the scanner, they receive an item-recognition test on the items they studied. The results can then be used to contrast brain activity during successful versus unsuccessful encoding.

Results from studies using the subsequent memory paradigm have demonstrated significant pre-frontal involvement in LTM encoding. Inspection of the spatial distribution of activation peaks (or 'local maxima') from these studies, shown in **Figure 3**, reveals

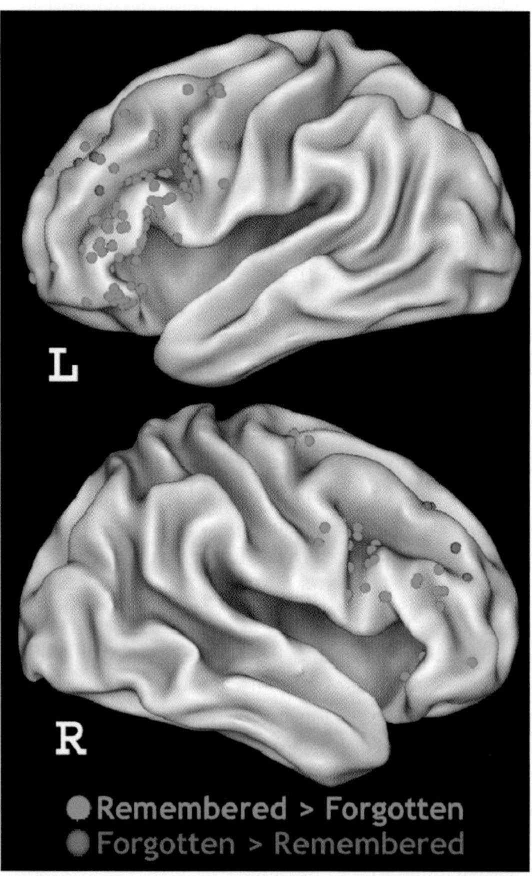

Figure 3 Activation peaks from fMRI studies investigating prefrontal activation during memory encoding. Each green dot represents an activation peak in an analysis that reported increased activation during encoding of items that were subsequently remembered, as compared with items that were subsequently forgotten (i.e., a 'subsequent memory effect'). Each red dot represents an activation peak in an analysis that reported increased activation during encoding of items that were subsequently forgotten, as compared with items that were subsequently remembered (i.e., 'a subsequent forgetting effect').

not only that PFC activation is routinely linked with successful LTM encoding, but also that the degree of involvement seems to differ between different PFC subregions. There is overwhelming support for the idea that VLPFC contributes to LTM formation. Out of 150 local maxima associated with subsequent memory, 132 fall within the VLPFC. Furthermore, 33 of the 35 studies that reported prefrontal subsequent memory effects find local maxima within the VLPFC. Given that the ability to select relevant item information is essential for many forms of goal-directed cognitive processing, including memory encoding, it makes sense that VLPFC should be strongly linked to memory encoding in a wide variety of behavioral contexts.

The imaging literature seems to tell a different story about the DLPFC. Out of 150 local maxima throughout the PFC, only 18 fall within the DLPFC. Furthermore, five studies have found increased DLPFC activation during processing of items that were subsequently forgotten, as compared with items that were subsequently remembered. Thus, based on the numbers alone, there does not appear to be much support for the idea that DLPFC contributes to LTM encoding. This pattern of findings could suggest either that DLPFC implements processes that do not contribute to successful LTM encoding, or that previous studies were insensitive to its role in LTM formation.

Relevant to the latter possibility, it is notable that imaging studies of WM have implicated DLPFC in processing of relationships between items, and that imaging studies of LTM encoding typically do not elicit relational processing. Most imaging studies have examined encoding of single items studied in isolation, using encoding tasks that orient attention toward specific attributes of a study item and away from relationships between items. In these studies, it is unlikely that participants would spontaneously process relationships among items in the study list, and engagement of relational processing might have even been deleterious to later memory performance (i.e., because allocating resources toward processing the relationships among items might take attentional resources away from processing the distinctive features of the items themselves). Accordingly, it is possible that the encoding conditions in many previous imaging studies were not conducive to revealing the contribution of DLPFC to successful LTM encoding. The retrieval tests used in subsequent memory paradigms might also be a relevant factor. Most imaging studies of encoding assess successful LTM formation with tests of item recognition memory. However, processing of relationships between items facilitates memory by enhancing interitem associations, and item recognition memory tests may not be sensitive to detecting these effects (Bower, 1970). Thus, sorting encoding activation by subsequent item recognition performance might mask the role of DLPFC in successful LTM encoding.

If DLPFC contributes to LTM encoding through its role in relational processing, the ability to detect this contribution may depend on the kinds of encoding and retrieval tasks that are used. Indeed, in imaging studies that used encoding tasks that encouraged relational processing or retrieval tests that are sensitive to memory for associations among items, DLPFC activity during encoding predicts subsequent memory (Addis and McAndrews, 2006; Blumenfeld and Ranganath, 2006; Staresina and Davachi, 2006; Summerfield et al., 2006). In one such study, we found evidence that DLPFC activation is related to successful LTM encoding specifically under conditions that emphasize processing of relationships between items (Blumenfeld and Ranganath, 2006). In this study, participants were scanned during the performance of two WM tasks (**Figure 4(a)**). On 'rehearse' trials, participants were presented with a set of three words and required to maintain the set across a 12-s delay period, in anticipation of a question probing memory for the identity and serial position of the items. On 'reorder' trials, participants were required to rearrange a set of three words based on the weight of the object that each word referred to. They maintained this information across a 12-s delay period in anticipation of a question probing memory for serial order of the items in the rearranged set. Although both rehearse and reorder trials required maintenance of the three-item set, reorder trials additionally required participants to compare the items in the set and transform the serial order of the items. Thus, reorder trials forced participants to actively process relationships between the items in the memory set, whereas rehearse trials simply required maintenance of the memory set across a delay. Analyses of subsequent recognition memory performance showed that there were significantly more reorder trials in which all three items were recollected than would be expected based on the overall item hit-rates alone (**Figure 4(b)**). The same was not true for memory for rehearse trials, for which the proportion of trials on which all three items were subsequently recollected was no different than would be expected by

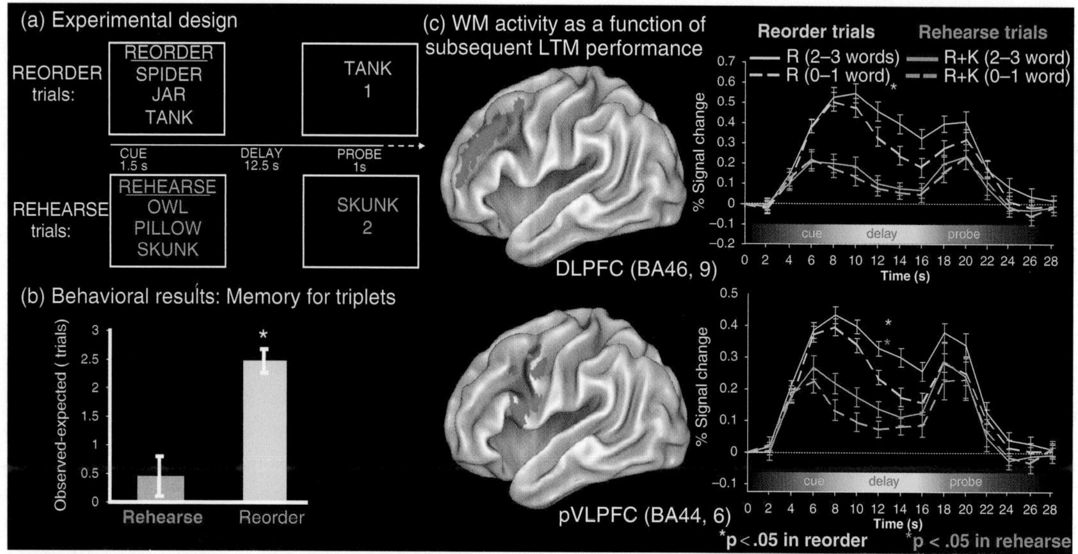

Figure 4 (a) Schematic depiction of the two tasks performed during fMRI scanning. (b) Behavioral results, showing that participants recalled significantly more triplets from each reorder trial (yellow) than would be expected based on the overall hit rate. This finding suggests that, on reorder trials, memory performance was supported by associations among the items in the memory set. (c) fMRI data showing that DLPFC (top) exhibited increased activation during the delay period of reorder trials for which 2–3 items were subsequently remembered (solid yellow), as compared with trials in which 0–1 items were remembered (dashed yellow). No such effect is seen on rehearse trials (gray lines). At bottom, activation in a region of posterior VLPFC (pVLPFC) is plotted, showing that delay period activation in this region during both rehearse and reorder trials was predictive of subsequent memory performance. Experimental design and results from Blumenfeld RS and Ranganath C (2006) Dorsolateral prefrontal cortex promotes long-term memory formation through its role in working memory organization. *J. Neurosci.* 26: 916–925.

the item hit-rates alone. These findings suggest that, on reorder trials, processing of the relationships among the items in each memory set resulted in successful encoding of the associations among these items.

Consistent with the idea that the DLPFC is involved in processing of relationships between items in WM, fMRI data revealed that DLPFC activation was increased during reorder trials, as compared with rehearse trials (**Figure 4(c)**). Furthermore, DLPFC activation during reorder but not rehearse trials was positively correlated with subsequent memory performance. Specifically, DLPFC activation was increased on reorder trials for which 2–3 items were later recollected, as compared with trials for which 1 or 0 items were later recollected. No such relationship was evident during rehearse trials. In contrast, activation in a posterior region of left VLPFC (BA 44/6) was correlated with subsequent memory performance on both rehearse and reorder trials. Thus, results from this study suggest that DLPFC and VLPFC may play dissociable roles in LTM encoding. DLPFC activation may specifically promote successful LTM formation through its role in processing of relationships among items, whereas VLPFC activation seems to promote LTM formation under a broader range of conditions.

Results from another recent study demonstrated the specific nature of DLPFC contributions to memory encoding by comparing the relationship between activation and subsequent performance on free recall and item recognition memory tests (Staresina and Davachi, 2006). As described earlier, item recognition tests are often insensitive to memory for inter-item associations in LTM, whereas recall performance is significantly influenced by encoding of interitem associations (Tulving, 1962). Consistent with a role for DLPFC in encoding inter-item associations, DLPFC activation was specifically enhanced during encoding of items that were recalled compared to those that were not. DLPFC activation was not correlated with subsequent item recognition performance. In contrast, encoding time activation in VLPFC was positively correlated with subsequent memory performance on both the recall and the recognition tests. These results are consistent with the idea that DLPFC activation will contribute to subsequent LTM performance specifically under retrieval conditions that are sensitive to memory for associations among items.

The role of APFC in promoting LTM formation has not been well characterized in prior studies. We suspect that this is because activation in this region, like DLPFC, is not typically reported in studies of LTM encoding. Future work will be necessary to determine whether or how APFC contributes to successful LTM formation.

9.5.2 PFC Activation during LTM Retrieval

Numerous imaging studies have investigated the role of prefrontal regions in memory retrieval, showing that regions in DLPFC, VLPFC, and APFC are routinely activated during performance of such tasks (Fletcher and Henson, 2001; Ranganath et al., 2003a; Ranganath and Knight, 2003; Ranganath, 2004). Unlike studies of encoding, retrieval studies have not shown a consistent relationship between activation in any prefrontal region and successful retrieval. However, this is not surprising if PFC activation reflects control processes that are engaged during retrieval tasks even when retrieval fails (Ranganath et al., 2000, 2007; Dobbins et al., 2002; Simons et al., 2005a). If different prefrontal regions contribute to different control processes, then it may be more fruitful to compare and contrast activation between retrieval conditions that are more or less likely to engage these processes, rather than contrasting activation between successful and unsuccessful retrieval (Fletcher and Henson, 2001). Results from such studies have converged in many respects with results from studies of WM and LTM encoding in implicating VLPFC in item processing and DLPFC in relational processing.

One study conducted by Fletcher and colleagues is particularly relevant, in that they observed a double dissociation between the roles of VLPFC and DLPFC across two LTM retrieval tasks. In this study, positron emission tomography was used to measure prefrontal activation during two different retrieval tests. In one condition, the study lists were structured lists of 16 single words that were organized according to an overall theme and then broken down into four subcategories. For these lists, participants were given a free recall test, with the instruction to use the organizational structure of the list to guide retrieval. In the other condition, the study lists consisted of 16 category–exemplar word pairs (e.g., 'fruit–banana'). For these lists, participants performed a cued recall test, in which they had to recall the appropriate exemplar in response to each category name (e.g., 'fruit–?'). These two retrieval conditions differed in terms of the control processes that should be engaged during retrieval. In the free recall condition, participants were encouraged to use relational processing in order to generate appropriate retrieval cues, whereas in the cued recall condition, the specific cue was already provided. However, in the cued recall condition, presentation of a category name would presumably activate many semantic associations, and therefore, item-based selection processes would be required to resolve this conflict (Thompson-Schill et al., 1997; Wagner et al., 2001a). Critically, the authors found a double dissociation between activation within the PFC, such that DLPFC activation (BA 46) was increased during the free recall condition, whereas VLPFC activation (BA 44) was increased during the cued recall condition. This finding is consistent with findings from WM and LTM encoding studies suggesting that VLPFC regions implement processes that modulate activation of item representations, whereas DLPFC regions implement processes that activate representations of relationships among items.

In addition to more lateral regions of PFC, anterior prefrontal regions (BA 10) are also routinely activated in studies of LTM retrieval, and particularly during source memory tasks that require retrieval of detailed information (Nolde et al., 1998; Fletcher and Henson, 2001; Ranganath and Knight, 2003). An interesting finding to emerge from many of these studies is that APFC activation is often not contingent on successful retrieval, or even on the difficulty of the retrieval decision (Henson et al., 1999; Rugg et al., 1999; Ranganath et al., 2000, 2007; Dobbins et al., 2002, 2003; Simons et al., 2005a,b). As noted earlier, APFC activation during WM tasks tends to be associated with the demand to select or maintain a cognitive set that dictates what information is relevant for selection. Cognitive models of memory retrieval suggest that this may be particularly relevant for accurate performance on source memory tasks (Johnson et al., 1993, 1997a; Mather et al., 1997; Norman and Schacter, 1997; Marsh and Hicks, 1998). This is because episodic memories are complex and consist of multiple characteristics (e.g., records of perceptual information in multiple modalities, cognitive operations, actions, affective reactions; Johnson et al., 1993). In many instances, a potential retrieval cue can activate several potential memories, including information that is irrelevant to a particular source decision (Koriat and Goldsmith, 1996;

Johnson, 1997; Koriat et al., 2000). Source memory decisions therefore demand the selection of an appropriate cognitive set in order to constrain retrieval of information associated with a cue and to narrow down the criteria for subsequent decision processes (Johnson et al., 1993; Mather et al., 1997; Norman and Schacter, 1997; Marsh and Hicks, 1998). This set would be initiated in response to a retrieval cue in order to constrain retrieval of information associated with the cue and narrow down the criteria for subsequent decision processes (Johnson et al., 1993; Johnson and Raye, 1998; Rugg and Wilding, 2000). This process has been described as setting 'decision criteria,' 'feature weights,' or a 'retrieval orientation.' We hypothesize that APFC is critical for selecting cognitive sets, and that source memory decisions constitute an example of when this process must be engaged.

One way of testing this idea is to contrast APFC activation between retrieval tasks that vary in terms of the specificity of the memory decision that is to be made (Ranganath et al., 2000, 2007). In one such study (Ranganath et al., 2000), brain activity was contrasted between a retrieval task that required participants to make a general item recognition decision versus a retrieval task that required participants to make a recognition decision specifically based on the match between the visual features of test items relative to studied items (**Figure 5**). Not surprisingly, participants were slower and less accurate at making responses to previously studied items in the more specific test condition. However, for unstudied items, accuracy and reaction times were comparable across the two test conditions. Results showed that activation in left APFC was increased during the more specific test, as compared with the more general test. What is more remarkable, however, is that activation during specific test trials was also increased for new items that

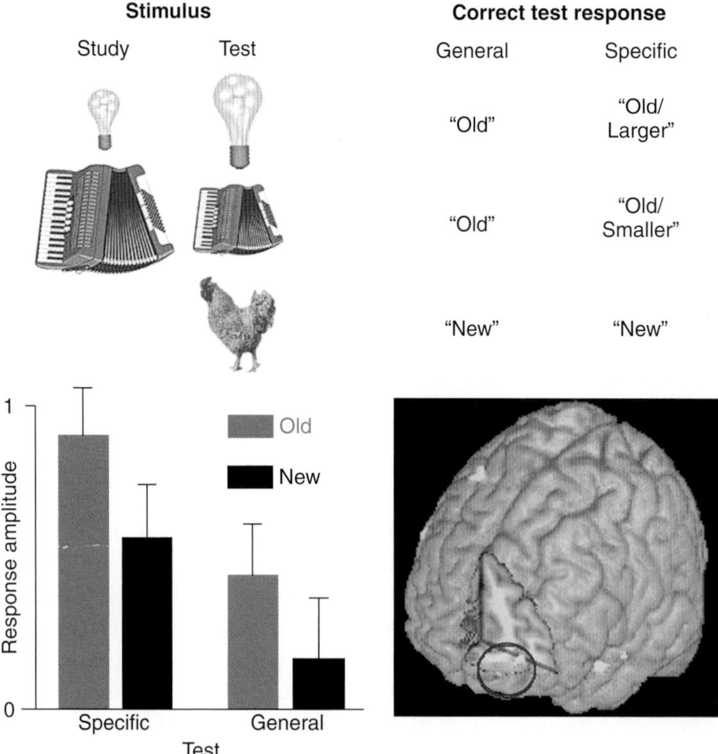

Figure 5 Participants studied objects that were shown in a large or small size, and then at test were shown objects that were either larger or smaller than the studied objects. In the 'General' test condition, participants were instructed to make a decision as to whether each object was studied, whereas on specific test trials, participants were additionally instructed to decide whether each test object was larger or smaller than the studied objects. In a region of left APFC, shown in the lower right panel, activation was increased for both old and new items in the specific test, as compared with the more general test condition (lower left panel). Experimental design and results from Ranganath C, Johnson MK, and D'Esposito M (2000) Left anterior prefrontal activation increases with demands to recall specific perceptual information. *J. Neurosci.* 20: RC108: 1–5.

were not seen during the study phase, despite the fact that behavioral performance was the same across the two test conditions. Thus, APFC activation during specific test trials reflected the need to constrain retrieval of information associated with each test item and to narrow down the criteria for subsequent decision processes. In this sense, APFC activation in source memory tasks might be analogous to activations in WM tasks in which one must select and maintain sets of rules that dictate the items or relationships that are currently relevant (Braver et al., 2003; Bunge et al., 2003; Sakai and Passingham, 2003).

Relevant to this idea, some researchers have suggested that APFC may be involved in maintaining an 'episodic retrieval mode' – a cognitive set which ensures that stimuli will be treated as cues for episodic retrieval (Lepage et al., 2000; Rugg and Wilding, 2000; Buckner, 2003). This view is supported by recent functional imaging studies showing sustained anterior prefrontal activity during episodic retrieval tasks, sometimes extending across multiple retrieval trials (Duzel et al., 1999; Lepage et al., 2000; Velanova et al., 2003). Additionally, retrieval mode-related activation in APFC appears to depend on the degree of control that is required in a given episodic memory test (Velanova et al., 2003). These findings are consistent with the idea that APFC is more generally involved in selection and maintenance of cognitive sets that support accurate episodic retrieval and source monitoring.

9.5.3 Laterality of PFC Activation during LTM Encoding and Retrieval

Another issue of interest that emerged from imaging studies of LTM retrieval concerns hemispheric asymmetries in the PFC. The question emerged from results of positron emission tomography studies of verbal memory that repeatedly observed left prefrontal activation during semantic decision tasks and right-lateralized prefrontal activation during tasks that engaged episodic retrieval processes (Tulving et al., 1994). Reviewing these findings, Tulving and his colleagues proposed the hemispheric encoding retrieval asymmetry (HERA) model, in which the left PFC was proposed to play a disproportionate role in episodic encoding (via its role in semantic processing) and the right PFC was proposed to play a disproportionate role in episodic retrieval (Tulving et al., 1994; Nyberg et al., 1996).

Shortly after its introduction, HERA was criticized, based on findings showing that left and right VLPFC are typically recruited during both encoding and retrieval tasks, and that the relative laterality of these effects is more dependent on the types of material that are being processed than on the type of memory operation (encoding or retrieval) being performed (Kelley et al., 1998; Wagner et al., 1998; McDermott et al., 1999; Golby et al., 2001). In response to this criticism, Habib et al. (2003) have argued that such findings

> . . . have no relevance to HERA. They provide good evidence in support of material-specific hemispheric asymmetry, but, because encoding and retrieval processes were not systematically varied and their interaction with hemispheres was not examined in these studies, the data are neutral with respect to HERA.

Another criticism of HERA is that, in focusing on left–right asymmetries, the model failed to account for perhaps more compelling functional differences along the rostro–caudal and dorsal–ventral axes (Buckner, 1996). Furthermore, laterality effects in DLPFC and APFC remain difficult to characterize. Laterality effects in these regions have typically not varied according to material, but also have not strictly followed predictions of the HERA model (Nolde et al., 1998; Ranganath and Knight, 2003; Ranganath, 2004).

Following up on the HERA model, Cabeza and colleagues (2003) recently proposed that the left PFC is engaged by tasks requiring semantically guided generation of information, whereas the right PFC is engaged by tasks requiring monitoring and checking of retrieved information. Another idea that has been proposed is that that left PFC is more engaged during the monitoring of specific memory characteristics, whereas right PFC is more engaged during the monitoring of undifferentiated information (Mitchell et al., 2004). A related idea is that the left PFC may disproportionately contribute to the use of specific contextual information to make a memory decision, whereas the right PFC may disproportionately contribute to the use of familiarity to make a memory decision (Dobbins et al., 2004). Like the HERA model, these accounts also do not specify whether the proposed hemispheric asymmetries would be expected to be constant across different subregions of PFC (e.g., DLPFC, VLPFC, APFC). At present, it is unclear if any of these models can fully account for patterns of hemispheric asymmetry in PFC activation during LTM retrieval, but this is in part due to the fact that the models have not been directly contrasted in many studies (Ranganath, 2004).

9.6 Conclusions and Future Prospects

Converging evidence from neuropsychology and neuroimaging supports the idea that prefrontal regions play an important role in WM and LTM encoding and retrieval. Research on WM has shown that the PFC is not necessary for short-term retention of information per se, and instead that prefrontal regions contribute to WM performance by using goals and prior knowledge to guide activation of mnemonic representations. For example, regions in VLPFC may be more involved in modulating the activation of relevant items, whereas DLPFC may be more involved in modulating the activation of relationships between items that are currently being processed. Regions in APFC may be involved in selecting sets of rules that determine which items and relations are appropriate for selection.

Studies of LTM converge with the findings described earlier by demonstrating a role for the PFC in control processes that support encoding and retrieval. Neuropsychological research has shown that PFC regions may support LTM encoding by subserving controlled selection of attention toward goal-relevant items and by building or assessing relationships between relevant items. Imaging studies have shown that VLPFC may support LTM encoding by enhancing the strength and distinctiveness of memory for item information, whereas DLPFC may support encoding by building associations among items. During retrieval, VLPFC may support the ability to resolve competition in order to retrieve relevant items from memory, whereas DLPFC may support the ability to use relational information to guide successful retrieval and to inhibit previously learned associations. Additionally, some evidence suggests that APFC may support the selection of rules to determine the dimensions on which a retrieval cue and retrieved information should be processed.

Although our model can explain the extant evidence, future research will be needed to more extensively test it and to specify some important and currently unresolved issues. One important question is the nature of functional interactions within the PFC, and between different prefrontal and posterior cortical regions. Given the functional role for APFC suggested above, it would seem that APFC should modulate activation in corresponding regions of DLPFC and VLPFC, depending on the task set that is to be implemented (Sakai and Passingham, 2003). Furthermore, to the extent that VLPFC implements processes that select features of relevant items, one might expect that VLPFC should show increased connectivity with posterior areas that represent those features (Gazzaley et al., 2004). DLPFC regions, however, might process relational information in a number of ways. For instance, it is possible that DLPFC processes relational information by directly modulating activation in posterior cortical areas (Summerfield et al., 2006), perhaps by modulating the relative timing of neural firing within and across different areas (Shastri, 1996). Another possibility is that the posterior parietal cortex maintains dynamic relational bindings on line (Vogel et al., 2001), and that DLPFC can alter these bindings through its interconnections with parietal regions (Wendelken, 2001). A third possibility is that the DLPFC might modulate activation of relationships between items through its interactions with VLPFC (Blumenfeld and Ranganath, unpublished observations). Of course, none of the three accounts are mutually exclusive, and much more research needs to be done to address this fundamental question.

Another critical question for future research is to understand the role of orbitofrontal cortex (BA 11, on the ventromedial surface of the PFC) in memory processes. Research on orbitofrontal cortex and WM has generally focused on its role in integrating emotional and cognitive influences on behavior. However, given the extensive connectivity between the orbitofrontal cortex and medial temporal regions (perirhinal and entorhinal cortex) that are critical for LTM, it is reasonable think that orbitofrontal cortex should play an important role in LTM (Ranganath et al., 2005b). Evidence from patients with orbitofrontal lesions (due to anterior communicating artery aneurysms) is consistent with this idea (Rapcsak et al., 1996, 1999; Johnson et al., 1997b; Moscovitch and Melo, 1997; Schnider and Ptak, 1999; Schnider, 2000).

In conclusion, human neuropsychology and neuroimaging research has revealed significant insights into the roles of different regions of PFC in different kinds of memory processes. We have presented an integrative framework to characterize these roles, but further research needs to be done to flesh out this framework and to address several important, and as yet unresolved, questions. Given the fact that disturbances in memory and prefrontal functioning are associated with normal aging (Tisserand and Jolles, 2003), cerebrovascular disease (Wu et al., 2002; Nordahl et al., 2005, 2006), and psychiatric (Cohen and Servan-Schreiber, 1992; Glahn et al., 2005) and neurological (Elliott, 2003; Levin and Hanten, 2005; Neary et al., 2005) conditions, addressing these questions will be of fundamental importance.

Acknowledgments

Our research has been supported by National Institute of Mental Health grant 1R01MH68721.

References

Addis DR and McAndrews MP (2006) Prefrontal and hippocampal contributions to the generation and binding of semantic associations during successful encoding. *Neuroimage* 33: 1194–1206.

Alexander MP, Stuss DT, and Fansabedian N (2003) California Verbal Learning Test: Performance by patients with focal frontal and non-frontal lesions. *Brain* 126: 1493–1503.

Aron AR, Robbins TW, and Poldrack RA (2004) Inhibition and the right inferior frontal cortex. *Trends Cogn. Sci.* 8: 170–177.

Asaad WF, Rainer G, and Miller EK (2000) Task-specific neural activity in the primate prefrontal cortex. *J. Neurophysiol.* 84: 451–459.

Baddeley A (1986) *Working Memory*. New York: Oxford University Press.

Badre D and Wagner AD (2004) Selection, integration, and conflict monitoring; assessing the nature and generality of prefrontal cognitive control mechanisms. *Neuron* 41: 473–487.

Barde LH and Thompson-Schill SL (2002) Models of functional organization of the lateral prefrontal cortex in verbal working memory: Evidence in favor of the process model. *J. Cogn. Neurosci.* 14: 1054–1063.

Blumenfeld RS and Ranganath C (2006) Dorsolateral prefrontal cortex promotes long-term memory formation through its role in working memory organization. *J. Neurosci.* 26: 916–925.

Bor D, Duncan J, Wiseman RJ, and Owen AM (2003) Encoding strategies dissociate prefrontal activity from working memory demand. *Neuron* 37: 361–367.

Bor D, Cumming N, Scott CE, and Owen AM (2004) Prefrontal cortical involvement in verbal encoding strategies. *Eur. J. Neurosci.* 19: 3365–3370.

Bor D and Owen AM (2006) A common prefrontal–parietal network for mnemonic and mathematical recoding strategies within working memory. *Cereb. Cortex* 17: 778–786.

Bower GH (1970) Organizational factors in memory. *Cogn. Psychol.* 1: 18–46.

Braver TS, Barch DM, Kelley WM, et al. (2001) Direct comparison of prefrontal cortex regions engaged by working and long-term memory tasks. *Neuroimage* 14: 48–59.

Braver TS and Bongiolatti SR (2002) The role of frontopolar cortex in subgoal processing during working memory. *Neuroimage* 15: 523–536.

Braver TS, Reynolds JR, and Donaldson DI (2003) Neural mechanisms of transient and sustained cognitive control during task switching. *Neuron* 39: 713–726.

Brutkowski S (1965) Functions of prefrontal cortex in animals. *Physiol. Rev.* 45: 721–746.

Buckner RL (1996) Beyond HERA: Contributions of specific prefrontal brain areas to long-term memory retrieval. *Psychonom. Bull. Rev.* 3: 149–158.

Buckner RL (2003) Functional-anatomic correlates of control processes in memory. *J. Neurosci.* 23: 3999–4004.

Buckner RL and Wheeler ME (2001) The cognitive neuroscience of remembering. *Nat. Rev. Neurosci.* 2: 624–634.

Bunge SA, Kahn I, Wallis JD, Miller EK, and Wagner AD (2003) Neural circuits subserving the retrieval and maintenance of abstract rules. *J. Neurophysiol.* 90: 3419–3428.

Butters MA, Kaszniak AW, Glisky EL, and Eslinger PJ (1994) Recency discrimination deficits in frontal lobe patients. *Neuropsychology* 8: 343–354.

Cabeza R, Locantore JK, and Anderson ND (2003) Lateralization of prefrontal activity during episodic memory retrieval: Evidence for the production-monitoring hypothesis. *J. Cogn. Neurosci.* 15: 249–259.

Chao LL and Knight RT (1995) Human prefrontal lesions increase distractibility to irrelevant sensory inputs. *Neuroreport* 6: 1605–1610.

Chao LL and Knight RT (1998) Contribution of human prefrontal cortex to delay performance. *J. Cogn. Neurosci.* 10: 167–177.

Christoff K and Gabrieli JD (2000) The frontopolar cortex and human cognition: Evidence for a rostrocaudal hierarchical organization within the human prefrontal cortex. *Psychobiology* 28: 168–186.

Cohen JD, Braver TS, and O'Reilly RC (1996) A computational approach to prefrontal cortex, cognitive control and schizophrenia: Recent developments and current challenges. *Philos. Trans. R. Soc. Lond. B Biol. Sci.* 351: 1515–1527.

Cohen JD and Servan-Schreiber D (1992) Context, cortex, and dopamine: A connectionist approach to behavior and biology in schizophrenia. *Psychol. Rev.* 99: 45–77.

Crone EA, Wendelken C, Donohue S, van Leijenhorst L, and Bunge SA (2006) Neurocognitive development of the ability to manipulate information in working memory. *Proc. Natl. Acad. Sci. USA* 103: 9315–9320.

Curtis CE and D'Esposito M (2003) Persistent activity in the prefrontal cortex during working memory. *Trends Cogn. Sci.* 7: 415–423.

Curtis CE and D'Esposito M (2004) The effects of prefrontal lesions on working memory performance and theory. *Cogn. Affect. Behav. Neurosci.* 4: 528–539.

D'Esposito, Aguirre GK, Zarahn E, and Ballard D (1998) Functional MRI studies of spatial and non-spatial working memory. *Cogn. Brain Res.* 7: 1–13.

D'Esposito M, Cooney JW, Gazzaley A, Gibbs SE, and Postle BR (2006) Is the prefrontal cortex necessary for delay task performance? Evidence from lesion and FMRI data. *J. Int. Neuropsychol. Soc.* 12: 248–260.

D'Esposito M and Postle BR (1999) The dependence of span and delayed-response performance on prefrontal cortex. *Neuropsychologia* 37: 1303–1315.

D'Esposito M, Postle BR, Ballard D, and Lease J (1999) Maintenance versus manipulation of information held in working memory: An event-related fMRI study. *Brain Cogn.* 41: 66–86.

D'Esposito M, Postle BR, and Rypma B (2000) Prefrontal cortical contributions to working memory: Evidence from event-related fMRI studies. *Exp. Brain Res.* 133: 3–11.

Davidson PS and Glisky EL (2002) Neuropsychological correlates of recollection and familiarity in normal aging. *Cogn. Affect. Behav. Neurosci.* 2: 174–186.

Dimitrov M, Granetz J, Peterson M, Hollnagel C, Alexander G, and Grafman J (1999) Associative learning impairments in patients with frontal lobe damage. *Brain Cogn.* 41: 213–230.

Dobbins IG, Foley H, Schacter DL, and Wagner AD (2002) Executive control during episodic retrieval: Multiple prefrontal processes subserve source memory. *Neuron* 35: 989–996.

Dobbins IG, Rice HJ, Wagner AD, and Schacter DL (2003) Memory orientation and success: Separable neurocognitive components underlying episodic recognition. *Neuropsychologia* 41: 318–333.

Dobbins IG, Simons JS, and Schacter DL (2004) fMRI evidence for separable and lateralized prefrontal memory monitoring processes. *J. Cogn. Neurosci.* 16: 908–920.

Duarte A, Ranganath C, and Knight RT (2005) Effects of unilateral prefrontal lesions on familiarity, recollection, and source memory. *J. Neurosci.* 25: 8333–8337.

Duzel E, Cabeza R, Picton TW, et al. (1999) Task-related and item-related brain processes of memory retrieval. *Proc. Natl. Acad. Sci. USA* 96: 1794–1799.

Elliott R (2003) Executive functions and their disorders. *Br. Med. Bull.* 65: 49–59.

Eslinger PJ and Grattan LM (1994) Altered serial position learning after frontal lobe lesion. *Neuropsychologia* 32: 729–739.

Fletcher PC and Henson RN (2001) Frontal lobes and human memory: Insights from functional neuroimaging. *Brain* 124: 849–881.

Funahashi S, Bruce CJ, and Goldman-Rakic PS (1989) Mnemonic coding of visual space in the monkey's dorsolateral prefrontal cortex. *J. Neurophysiol.* 61: 331–349.

Funahashi S, Bruce CJ, and Goldman-Rakic PS (1990) Visuospatial coding in primate prefrontal neurons revealed by oculomotor paradigms. *J. Neurophysiol.* 63: 814–831.

Funahashi S, Bruce CJ, and Goldman-Rakic PS (1993) Dorsolateral prefrontal lesions and oculomotor delayed-response performance: Evidence for mnemonic "scotomas." *J. Neurosci.* 13: 1479–1497.

Fuster JM (1995) *Memory in the Cerebral Cortex*. Cambridge: MIT Press.

Fuster JM (1997) *The Prefrontal Cortex: Anatomy, Physiology, and Neuropsychology of the Frontal Lobes,* 3rd edn. New York: Raven Press.

Fuster JM (2004) Upper processing stages of the perception–action cycle. *Trends Cogn. Sci.* 8: 143–145.

Fuster JM and Alexander GE (1971) Neuron activity related to short-term memory. *Science* 173: 652–654.

Gazzaley A, Rissman J, and D'Esposito M (2004) Functional connectivity during working memory maintenance. *Cogn. Affect. Behav. Neurosci.* 4: 580–599.

Gershberg FB and Shimamura AP (1994) Serial position effects in implicit and explicit tests of memory. *J. Exp. Psychol. Learn. Mem. Cogn.* 20: 1370–1378.

Gershberg FB and Shimamura AP (1995) Impaired use of organizational strategies in free recall following frontal lobe damage. *Neuropsychologia* 33: 1305–1333.

Glahn DC, Ragland JD, Abramoff A, et al. (2005) Beyond hypofrontality: A quantitative meta-analysis of functional neuroimaging studies of working memory in schizophrenia. *Hum. Brain Mapp.* 25: 60–69.

Golby AJ, Poldrack RA, Brewer JB, Spencer D, Desmond JE, Aron AP, and Gabrieli JD (2001) Material-specific lateralization in the medial temporal lobe and prefrontal cortex during memory encoding. *Brain* 124: 1841–1854.

Gold JJ, Smith CN, Bayley PJ, et al. (2006) Item memory, source memory, and the medial temporal lobe: Concordant findings from fMRI and memory-impaired patients. *Proc. Natl. Acad. Sci. USA* 103: 9351–9356.

Goldman-Rakic PS (1987) Circuitry of the prefrontal cortex and the regulation of behavior by representational memory. In: Plum F and Mountcastle V (eds.) *Handbook of Physiology, Sec 1: The Nervous System*, Vol. 5, pp 373–417. Bethesda: Americal Physiological Society.

Habib R, Nyberg L, and Tulving E (2003) Hemispheric asymmetries of memory: The HERA model revisited. *Trends Cogn. Sci.* 7: 241–245.

Henson RNA, Shallice T, and Dolan RJ (1999) Right prefrontal cortex and episodic memory retrieval: A functional MRI test of the monitoring hypothesis. *Brain* 122: 1367–1381.

Hirst W and Volpe BT (1988) Memory strategies with brain damage. *Brain Cogn.* 8: 379–408.

Incisa della Rochetta A and Milner B (1993) Strategic search and retrieval initiation: The role of the frontal lobes. *Neuropsychologia* 31: 503–524.

Jacobsen CF (1935) Functions of frontal association areas in primates. *Arch. Neurol. Psychiatry* 33: 558–560.

Janowsky JS, Shimamura AP, Kritchevsky M, and Squire LR (1989a) Cognitive impairment following frontal lobe damage and its relevance to human amnesia. *Behav. Neurosci.* 103: 548–560.

Janowsky JS, Shimamura AP, and Squire LR (1989b) Memory and metamemory: Comparisons between patients with frontal lobe lesions and amnesic patients. *Psychobiology* 17: 3–11.

Janowsky JS, Shimamura AP, and Squire LR (1989c) Source memory impairment in patients with frontal lobe lesions. *Neuropsychologia* 27: 1043–1056.

Jetter W, Poser U, Freeman RB, and Markowitsch HJ (1986) A verbal long-term memory deficit in frontal lobe damaged patients. *Cortex* 22: 229–242.

Johnson MK (1997) Source monitoring and memory distortion. *Philos. Trans. R. Soc. Lond. B Biol. Sci.* 352: 1733–1745.

Johnson MK, Hashtroudi S, and Lindsay DS (1993) Source monitoring. *Psychol. Bull.* 114: 3–28.

Johnson MK, Kounios J, and Nolde SF (1997a) Electrophysiological brain activity and memory source monitoring. *Neuroreport* 8: 1317–1320.

Johnson MK, O'Connor M, and Cantor J (1997b) Confabulation, memory deficits, and frontal dysfunction. *Brain Cogn.* 34: 189–206.

Johnson MK and Raye CL (1998) False memories and confabulation. *Trends Cogn. Sci.* 2: 137–145.

Jonides J and Nee DE (2006) Brain mechanisms of proactive interference in working memory. *Neuroscience* 139: 181–193.

Kelley WM, Miezin FM, McDermott KB, et al. (1998) Hemispheric specialization in human dorsal frontal cortex and medial temporal lobe for verbal and nonverbal memory encoding. *Neuron* 20: 927–936.

Kesner RP, Hopkins RO, and Fineman B (1994) Item and order dissociation in humans with prefrontal cortex damage. *Neuropsychologia* 32: 881–891.

Knight RT, Staines WR, Swick D, and Chao LL (1999) Prefrontal cortex regulates inhibition and excitation in distributed neural networks. *Acta Psychol. (Amst.)* 101: 159–178.

Knowlton BJ and Squire LR (1995) Remembering and knowing: Two different expressions of declarative memory. *J. Exp. Psychol. Learn. Mem. Cogn.* 21: 699–710.

Koechlin E, Basso G, Pietrini P, Panzer S, and Grafman J (1999) The role of the anterior prefrontal cortex in human cognition. *Nature* 399: 148–151.

Koechlin E, Ody C, and Kouneiher F (2003) The architecture of cognitive control in the human prefrontal cortex. *Science* 302: 1181–1185.

Konishi S, Nakajima K, Uchida I, Kikyo H, Kameyama M, and Miyashita Y (1999) Common inhibitory mechanism in human inferior prefrontal cortex revealed by event-related functional MRI. *Brain* 122(Pt 5): 981–991.

Koriat A and Goldsmith M (1996) Monitoring and control processes in the strategic regulation of memory accuracy. *Psychol. Rev.* 103: 490–517.

Koriat A, Goldsmith M, and Pansky A (2000) Toward a psychology of memory accuracy. *Annu. Rev. Psychol.* 51: 481–537.

Kowalska DM, Bachevalier J, and Mishkin M (1991) The role of the inferior prefrontal convexity in performance of delayed nonmatching-to-sample. *Neuropsychologia* 29: 583–600.

Kubler A, Murphy K, Kaufman J, Stein EA, and Garavan H (2003) Co-ordination within and between verbal and visuospatial working memory: Network modulation and anterior frontal recruitment. *Neuroimage* 20: 1298–1308.

Lebedev MA, Messinger A, Kralik JD, and Wise SP (2004) Representation of attended versus remembered locations in prefrontal cortex. *PLoS. Biol.* 2: e365.

Lee H, Simpson GV, Logothetis NK, and Rainer G (2005) Phase locking of single neuron activity to theta oscillations during working memory in monkey extrastriate visual cortex. *Neuron* 45: 147–156.

Lepage M, Ghaffar O, Nyberg L, and Tulving E (2000) Prefrontal cortex and episodic memory retrieval mode. *Proc. Natl. Acad. Sci. USA* 97: 506–511.

Levin HS and Hanten G (2005) Executive functions after traumatic brain injury in children. *Pediatr. Neurol.* 33: 79–93.

Luria AR (1966a) *The Working Brain*. New York: Penguin.

Luria AR (1966b) *Higher Cortical Functions in Man*. New York: Basic Books.

Malmo RB (1942) Interference factors in delayed response in monkey after removal of the frontal lobes. *J. Neurophysiol.* 5: 295–308.

Mangels JA (1997) Strategic processing and memory for temporal order in patients with frontal lobe lesions. *Neuropsychology* 11: 207–221.

Marsh RL and Hicks JL (1998) Test formats change source-monitoring decision processes. *J. Exp. Psychol. Learn. Mem. Cogn.* 24: 1137–1151.

Mather M, Henkel LA, and Johnson MK (1997) Evaluating characteristics of false memories: Remember/know judgments and memory characteristics questionnaire compared. *Mem. Cognit.* 25: 826–837.

Mayr U (2002) Inhibition of action rules. *Psychon. Bull. Rev.* 9: 93–99.

Mayr U and Kliegl R (2000) Task-set switching and long-term memory retrieval. *J. Exp. Psychol. Learn. Mem. Cogn.* 26: 1124–1140.

McAndrews MP and Milner B (1991) The frontal cortex and memory for temporal order. *Neuropsychologia* 29: 849–859.

McDermott KB, Buckner RL, Petersen SE, Kelley WM, and Sanders AL (1999) Set- and code-specific activation in frontal cortex: An fMRI study of encoding and retrieval of faces and words. *J. Cogn. Neurosci.* 11: 631–640.

Meunier M, Bachevalier J, and Mishkin M (1997) Effects of orbital frontal and anterior cingulate lesions on object and spatial memory in rhesus monkeys. *Neuropsychologia* 35: 999–1015.

Miller BT and D'Esposito M (2005) Searching for "the top" in top-down control. *Neuron* 48: 535–538.

Miller EK (2000) The prefrontal cortex and cognitive control. *Nat. Rev. Neurosci.* 1: 59–65.

Miller EK and Cohen JD (2001) An integrative theory of prefrontal cortex function. *Annu. Rev. Neurosci.* 24: 167–202.

Miller EK, Erickson CA, and Desimone R (1996) Neural mechanisms of visual working memory in prefrontal cortex of the macaque. *J. Neurosci.* 16: 5154–5167.

Miller EK, Li L, and Desimone R (1993) Activity of neurons in anterior inferior temporal cortex during a short-term memory task. *J. Neurosci.* 13: 1460–1478.

Milner B, Petrides M, and Smith ML (1985) Frontal lobes and the temporal organization of memory. *Hum. Neurobiol.* 4: 137–142.

Mishkin M (1964) Perseveration of central sets after frontal lesions in monkeys. In: Warren JM and Akert K (eds.) *The Frontal Granular Cortex and Behavior*, pp. 219–237. New York: McGraw-Hill.

Mishkin M and Manning FJ (1978) Non-spatial memory after selective prefrontal lesions in monkeys. *Brain Res.* 143: 313–323.

Mitchell KJ, Johnson MK, Raye CL, and Greene EJ (2004) Prefrontal cortex activity associated with source monitoring in a working memory task. *J. Cogn. Neurosci.* 16: 921–934.

Miyashita Y and Hayashi T (2000) Neural representation of visual objects: Encoding and top-down activation. *Curr. Opin. Neurobiol.* 10: 187–194.

Mohr HM, Goebel R, and Linden DE (2006) Content- and task-specific dissociations of frontal activity during maintenance and manipulation in visual working memory. *J. Neurosci.* 26: 4465–4471.

Moscovitch M (1992) Memory and working-with-memory: A component process model based on modules and central systems. *J. Cogn. Neurosci.* 4: 257–267.

Moscovitch M and Melo B (1997) Strategic retrieval and the frontal lobes: Evidence from confabulation and amnesia. *Neuropsychologia* 35: 1017–1034.

Nauta WJH (1971) The problem of the frontal lobe: A reinterpretation. *J. Psychiatr. Res.* 8: 167–187.

Neary D, Snowden J, and Mann D (2005) Frontotemporal dementia. *Lancet Neurol.* 4: 771–780.

Nolde SF, Johnson MK, and Raye CL (1998) The role of prefrontal regions during tests of episodic memory. *Trends Cogn. Sci.* 2: 399–406.

Nordahl CW, Ranganath C, Yonelinas AP, Decarli C, Fletcher E, and Jagust WJ (2006) White matter changes compromise prefrontal cortex function in healthy elderly individuals. *J. Cogn. Neurosci.* 18: 418–429.

Nordahl CW, Ranganath C, Yonelinas AP, DeCarli C, Reed BR, and Jagust WJ (2005) Different mechanisms of episodic memory failure in mild cognitive impairment. *Neuropsychologia* 43: 1688–1697.

Norman KA and Schacter DL (1997) False recognition in younger and older adults: Exploring the characteristics of illusory memories. *Mem. Cognit.* 25: 838–848.

Nyberg L, Cabeza R, and Tulving E (1996) PET studies of encoding and retrieval: The HERA model. *Psychonom. Bull. Rev.* 3: 135–148.

Owen AM (1997) The functional organization of working memory processes within human lateral frontal cortex: The contribution of functional neuroimaging. *Eur. J. Neurosci.* 9: 1329–1339.

Owen AM, Herrod NJ, Menon DK, et al. (1999) Redefining the functional organization of working memory processes within human lateral prefrontal cortex. *Eur. J. Neurosci.* 11: 567–574.

Paller KA and Wagner AD (2002) Observing the transformation of experience into memory. *Trends Cogn. Sci.* 6: 93–102.

Perret E (1974) The left frontal lobe of man and the suppression of habitual responses in verbal categorical behaviour. *Neuropsychologia* 12: 323–330.

Petrides M (1994) Frontal lobes and working memory: Evidence from investigations of the effects of cortical excisions in nonhuman primates. In: Boller F and Grafman J (eds.)

Handbook of Neuropsychology, pp. 59–82. Amsterdam: Elsevier Science B.V.

Petrides M (2000) Dissociable roles of mid-dorsolateral prefrontal and anterior inferotemporal cortex in visual working memory. *J. Neurosci.* 20: 7496–7503.

Petrides M (2005) Lateral prefrontal cortex: Architectonic and functional organization. *Philos. Trans. R. Soc. Lond. B Biol. Sci.* 360: 781–795.

Petrides M and Pandya DN (2002) Association pathways of the prefrontal cortex and functional observations. In: Stuss DT and Knight RT (eds.) *Principles of Frontal Lobe Function*, pp. 31–50. New York: Oxford University Press.

Poldrack RA, Wagner AD, Prull MW, Desmond JE, Glover GH, and Gabrieli JD (1999) Functional specialization for semantic and phonological processing in the left inferior prefrontal cortex. *Neuroimage* 10: 15–35.

Postle BR (2006) Working memory as an emergent property of the mind and brain. *Neuroscience* 139: 23–38.

Postle BR, Berger JS, and D'Esposito M (1999) Functional neuroanatomical double dissociation of mnemonic and executive control processes contributing to working memory performance. *Proc. Natl. Acad. Sci. USA* 96: 12959–12964.

Pribram KH, Ahumada A, Hartog J, and Roos L (1964) A progress report on the neurological processes disturbed by frontal lesions in primates. In: Warren JM and Akert K (eds.) *The Frontal Granular Cortex and Behavior*, pp. 28–55. New York: McGraw-Hill Book Company.

Pribram KH and Tubbs WE (1967) Short-term memory, parsing, and the primate frontal cortex. *Science* 156: 1765–1767.

Rainer G and Ranganath C (2002) Coding of objects in the prefrontal cortex in monkeys and humans. *Neuroscientist* 8: 6–11.

Ramnani N and Owen AM (2004) Anterior prefrontal cortex: Insights into function from anatomy and neuroimaging. *Nat. Rev. Neurosci.* 5: 184–194.

Ranganath C (2004) The 3-D prefrontal cortex: Hemispheric asymmetries in prefrontal activity and their relation to memory retrieval processes. *J. Cogn. Neurosci.* 16: 903–907.

Ranganath C (2006) Working memory for visual objects: Complementary roles of inferior temporal, medial temporal, and prefrontal cortex. *Neuroscience* 139: 277–289.

Ranganath C and Blumenfeld RS (2005) Doubts about double dissociations between short- and long-term memory. *Trends Cogn. Sci.* 9: 374–380.

Ranganath C, Cohen MX, and Brozinsky CJ (2005a) Working memory maintenance contributes to long-term memory formation: Neural and behavioral evidence. *J. Cogn. Neurosci.* 17: 994–1010.

Ranganath C and D'Esposito M (2005) Directing the mind's eye: Prefrontal, inferior and medial temporal mechanisms for visual working memory. *Curr. Opin. Neurobiol.* 15: 175–182.

Ranganath C, Heller A, Cohen MX, Brozinsky CJ, and Rissman J (2005b) Functional connectivity with the hippocampus during successful memory formation. *Hippocampus* 15: 997–1005.

Ranganath C, Heller AS, and Wilding EL (2007) Dissociable correlates of two classes of retrieval processing in prefrontal cortex. *Neuroimage* 35: 1663–1673.

Ranganath C, Johnson MK, and D'Esposito M (2000) Left anterior prefrontal activation increases with demands to recall specific perceptual information. *J. Neurosci.* 20: RC108: 1–5.

Ranganath C, Johnson MK, and D'Esposito M (2003a) Prefrontal activity associated with working memory and episodic long-term memory. *Neuropsychologia* 41: 378–389.

Ranganath C and Knight RT (2003) Prefrontal cortex and episodic memory: Integrating findings from neuropsychology and event-related functional neuroimaging. In: Parker A, Wildng E, and Bussey T (eds.) *The Cognitive Neuroscience of Memory Encoding and Retrieval*, pp. 83–99. Philadelphia: Psychology Press.

Ranganath C, Yonelinas AP, Cohen MX, Dy CJ, Tom SM, and D'Esposito M (2003b) Dissociable correlates of recollection and familiarity within the medial temporal lobes. *Neuropsychologia* 42: 2–13.

Rapcsak SZ, Polster MR, Glisky MR, and Comer JF (1996) False recognition of unfamiliar faces following right hemisphere damage: Neuropsychological and anatomical observations. *Cortex* 32: 593–611.

Rapcsak SZ, Reminger SL, Glisky EL, Kaszniak AW, and Comer JF (1999) Neuropsychological mechanisms of false facial recognition following frontal lobe damage. *Cogn. Neuropsychol.* 16: 267–292.

Rogers RD, Andrews TC, Grasby PM, Brooks DJ, and Robbins TW (2000) Contrasting cortical and subcortical activations produced by attentional-set shifting and reversal learning in humans. *J. Cogn. Neurosci.* 12: 142–162.

Rogers RD and Monsell S (1995) Costs of a predictable switch between simple cognitive tasks. *J. Exp. Psychol. Gen.* 124: 207–231.

Rugg MD, Fletcher PC, Chua PM, and Dolan RJ (1999) The role of the prefrontal cortex in recognition memory and memory for source: An fMRI study. *Neuroimage* 10: 520–529.

Rugg MD and Wilding EL (2000) Retrieval processing and episodic memory. *Trends Cogn. Sci.* 4: 108–115.

Rushworth MF, Nixon PD, Eacott MJ, and Passingham RE (1997) Ventral prefrontal cortex is not essential for working memory. *J. Neurosci.* 17: 4829–4838.

Sakai K and Passingham RE (2003) Prefrontal interactions reflect future task operations. *Nat. Neurosci.* 6: 75–81.

Schnider A (2000) Spontaneous confabulations, disorientation, and the processing of 'now.' *Neuropsychologia* 38: 175–185.

Schnider A and Ptak R (1999) Spontaneous confabulators fail to suppress currently irrelevant memory traces. *Nat. Neurosci.* 2: 677–681.

Schumacher EH, Lauber E, Awh E, Jonides J, Smith EE, and Koeppe RA (1996) PET evidence for an amodal verbal working memory system. *Neuroimage* 3: 79–88.

Semendeferi K, Armstrong E, Schleicher A, Zilles K, and Van Hoesen GW (2001) Prefrontal cortex in humans and apes: A comparative study of area 10. *Am. J. Phys. Anthropol.* 114: 224–241.

Semendeferi K, Lu A, Schenker N, and Damasio H (2002) Humans and great apes share a large frontal cortex. *Nat. Neurosci.* 5: 272–276.

Shastri L (1996) Temporal synchrony, dynamic bindings, and SHRUTI: A representational but nonclassical model of reflexive reasoning. *Behav. Brain Sci.* 19: 331–337.

Shimamura AP (1995) Memory and frontal lobe function. In: Gazzaniga MS (ed.) *The Cognitive Neurosciences*, pp. 803–813. Cambridge, MA: MIT Press.

Shimamura AP (2000) The role of the prefrontal cortex in dynamic filtering. *Psychobiology* 28: 207–218.

Shimamura AP, Janowsky JS, and Squire LR (1990) Memory for the temporal order of events in patients with frontal lobe lesions and amnesic patients. *Neuropsychologia* 28: 803–813.

Shimamura AP, Jurica PJ, Mangels JA, Gershberg FB, and Knight RT (1995) Susceptibility to memory interference effects following frontal lobe damage: Findings from tests of paired-associate learning. *J. Cogn. Neurosci.* 7: 144–152.

Simons JS, Gilbert SJ, Owen AM, Fletcher PC, and Burgess PW (2005a) Distinct roles for lateral and medial anterior

prefrontal cortex in contextual recollection. *J. Neurophysiol.* 94: 813–820.
Simons JS, Owen AM, Fletcher PC, and Burgess PW (2005b) Anterior prefrontal cortex and the recollection of contextual information. *Neuropsychologia* 43: 1774–1783.
Smith EE and Jonides J (1999) Storage and executive processes in the frontal lobes. *Science* 283: 1657–1661.
Stanhope N, Guinan E, and Kopelman MD (1998) Frequency judgements of abstract designs by patients with diencephalic, temporal lobe or frontal lobe lesions. *Neuropsychologia* 36: 1387–1396.
Staresina BP and Davachi L (2006) Differential encoding mechanisms for subsequent associative recognition and free recall. *J. Neurosci.* 26: 9162–9172.
Stuss DT, Alexander MP, Palumbo CL, Buckle L, Sayer L, and Pogue J (1994) Organizational strategies of patients with unilateral or bilateral frontal lobe injury in word list learning tasks. *Neuropsychology* 8: 355–373.
Stuss DT and Benson DF (1986) *The Frontal Lobes*. New York: Raven Press.
Summerfield C, Greene M, Wager T, Egner T, Hirsch J, and Mangels J (2006) Neocortical connectivity during episodic memory formation. *PLoS. Biol.* 4: e128.
Thompson-Schill SL, D'Esposito M, Aguirre GK, and Farah MJ (1997) Role of left inferior prefrontal cortex in retrieval of semantic knowledge: A reevaluation. *Proc. Natl. Acad. Sci. USA* 94: 14792–14797.
Tisserand DJ and Jolles J (2003) On the involvement of prefrontal networks in cognitive ageing. *Cortex* 39: 1107–1128.
Tulving E (1962) Subjective organization in free recall of "unrelated" words. *Psychol. Rev.* 69: 344–354.
Tulving E, Kapur S, Craik FI, Moscovitch M, and Houle S (1994) Hemispheric encoding/retrieval asymmetry in episodic memory: Positron emission tomography findings [see comments]. *Proc. Natl. Acad. Sci. USA* 91: 2016–2020.
Velanova K, Jacoby LL, Wheeler ME, McAvoy MP, Petersen SE, and Buckner RL (2003) Functional-anatomic correlates of sustained and transient processing components engaged during controlled retrieval. *J. Neurosci.* 23: 8460–8470.
Vilkki J, Servo A, and Surma-aho O (1998) Word list learning and prediction of recall after frontal lobe lesions. *Neuropsychology* 12: 268–277.
Vogel EK, Woodman GF, and Luck SJ (2001) Storage of features, conjunctions and objects in visual working memory. *J. Exp. Psychol. Hum. Percept. Perform.* 27: 92–114.
Wagner AD (1999) Working memory contributions to human learning and remembering. *Neuron* 22: 19–22.
Wagner AD, Pare-Blagoev EJ, Clark J, and Poldrack RA (2001a) Recovering meaning: Left prefrontal cortex guides controlled semantic retrieval. *Neuron* 31: 329–338.
Wagner AD, Maril A, Bjork RA, and Schacter DL (2001b) Prefrontal contributions to executive control: fMRI evidence for functional distinctions within lateral Prefrontal cortex. *Neuroimage* 14: 1337–1347.
Wagner AD, Poldrack RA, Eldridge LL, Desmond JE, Glover GH, and Gabrieli JD (1998) Material-specific lateralization of prefrontal activation during episodic encoding and retrieval. *Neuroreport* 9: 3711–3717.
Wendelken C (2001) The role of mid-dorsolateral prefrontal cortex in working memory: A connectionist model. *Neurocomputing* 44–46: 1009–1016.
Wheeler MA, Stuss DT, and Tulving E (1995) Frontal lobe damage produces episodic memory impairment. *J. Int. Neuropsychol. Soc.* 1: 525–536.
Wu CC, Mungas D, Petkov CI, et al. (2002) Brain structure and cognition in a community sample of elderly Latinos. *Neurology* 59: 383–391.
Yonelinas AP (2002) The nature of recollection and familiarity: A review of 30 years of research. *J. Mem. Lang.* 46: 441–517.
Zhang JX, Feng C, Fox PT, Gao J, and Tan L (2004) Is left inferior frontal gyrus a general mechanism for selection? *Neuroimage* 23: 596–603.

10 Anatomy of the Hippocampus and the Declarative Memory System

R. D. Burwell and K. L. Agster, Brown University, Providence, RI, USA

10.1 Introduction

10.1.1 A Short History of the Anatomy of Declarative Memory

A half century ago, Scoville and Milner (1957) described profound memory loss following bilateral medial temporal lobe resection in the landmark patient HM. In the following years, scientists studying memory and the brain narrowed in on the hippocampus as the critical structure for everyday memory for facts and events. In the past two decades, however, we have come full circle: It is now apparent that the cortical areas surrounding the hippocampal formation also play critical roles in memory. Today, it is generally accepted that the hippocampal formation and the nearby parahippocampal region together are necessary for human declarative memory, but many questions remain concerning the functional diversity of structures within the so-called declarative memory system. To what extent can the function of hippocampal and parahippocampal substructures be dissociated? How discrete are such functions? How do these structures interact to permit encoding, storage, consolidation, and retrieval of representations of facts and events? What additional cognitive functions might be supported? Understanding the structure and connectivity of these regions is necessary for generating and testing sound hypotheses about the neurobiology of memory.

10.1.2 Overview of the Hippocampal System

10.1.2.1 Nomenclature

The structures that are the topic of this chapter have variously been termed the medial temporal lobe memory system (Squire and Zola-Morgan, 1991), the hippocampal memory system (Eichenbaum et al., 1994), and the hippocampal region (Witter and Amaral, 2004). The terms hippocampal region or hippocampal system have the advantage that the terminology translates effectively from humans to animal models of human memory, including rodents.

These regions are thought to support a type of memory that has been variously called episodic memory, declarative memory, or autobiographical memory. For research on memory using animal models, the terms episodic or episodic-like memory may be most appropriate.

The hippocampal system comprises the hippocampal formation and the parahippocampal region (**Figure 1**). The hippocampal formation includes the dentate gyrus, the hippocampus proper (fields CA1, CA2, and CA3), and the subiculum (**Figure 2**). The primary criterion for inclusion in the hippocampal formation is the trilaminar character of the structures. In addition, the included structures are connected by largely unilateral pathways beginning with the dentate gyrus granule cell input to the CA3 (**Figure 3**). CA3 pyramidal cells, in turn, provide a unidirectional input to the CA1. Finally, CA1 projects to the subiculum. Because corticocortical connections in the brain are overwhelmingly reciprocal, such a multisynaptic, unidirectional circuit is unique. In contrast, the entorhinal cortex projects to all portions of the hippocampal formation. The connectivity and laminar structure of the entorhinal cortex differentiate it from hippocampal formation structures. The dentate gyrus, hippocampus proper, and subiculum are therefore collectively referred to as the hippocampal formation (**Figure 3**, structures shown in yellow), and the entorhinal cortex is considered part of the parahippocampal region.

The parahippocampal region, also called the retrohippocampal region, includes the perirhinal, postrhinal (or parahippocampal), entorhinal, presubicular, and parasubicular cortices (**Figure 1**). The postrhinal cortex in the rodent brain is considered the

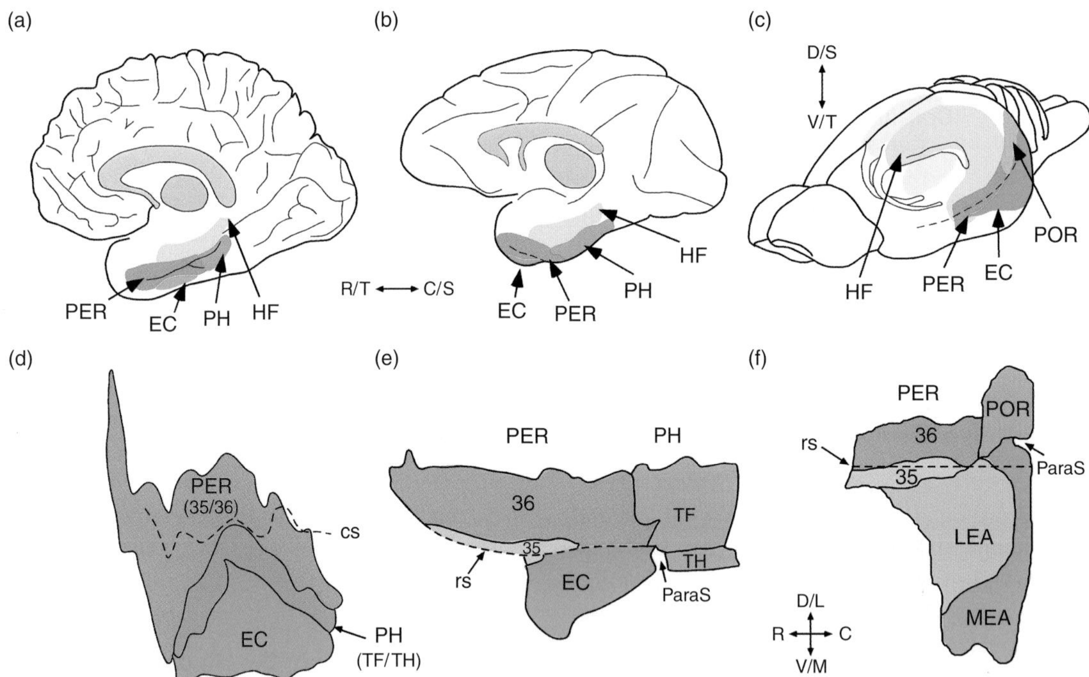

Figure 1 Comparative views of the hippocampal system for the human (left), monkey (middle), and rat (right). The upper panel shows the relevant structures in lateral views of the human brain (a), the monkey brain (b), and the rodent brain (c). The lower panel shows unfolded maps of the relevant cortical structures for the human brain (d), the monkey brain (e), and the rodent brain (f). Shown for the human and monkey brain are unfolded layer IV maps of the perirhinal (PER) areas 35 and 36, parahippocampal (PH) areas TF and TH, and entorhinal cortex (EC). Figures adapted from Burwell RD, Witter MP, and Amaral DG (1995) The perirhinal and postrhinal cortices of the rat: A review of the neuroanatomical literature and comparison with findings from the monkey brain. *Hippocampus* 5: 390–408; Insausti R, Tuñón T, Sobreviela T, Insausti AM, and Gonsalo LM (1995) The human entorhinal cortex: A cytoarchitectonic analysis. *J. Comp. Neurol.* 355: 171–198. Shown for the rodent brain are unfolded surface maps of the PER areas 35 and 36, the postrhinal cortex (POR), and the lateral and medial entorhinal areas (LEA and MEA). The rodent POR is the homolog of the primate PH (see text for details). In the monkey and the rat brain, the parasubiculum (ParaS) is interposed between the entorhinal and POR/PH (arrows). The pre- and parasubiculum, which are components of the parahippocampal region, are not shown (but see Figure 2). Abbreviations: cs, collateral sulcus; rs, rhinal sulcus; DG, dentate gyrus; D, dorsal; L, lateral; M, medial; ParaS, parasubiculum; PreS, presubiculum; S, septal; Sub, subiculum; T, temporal; V, ventral.

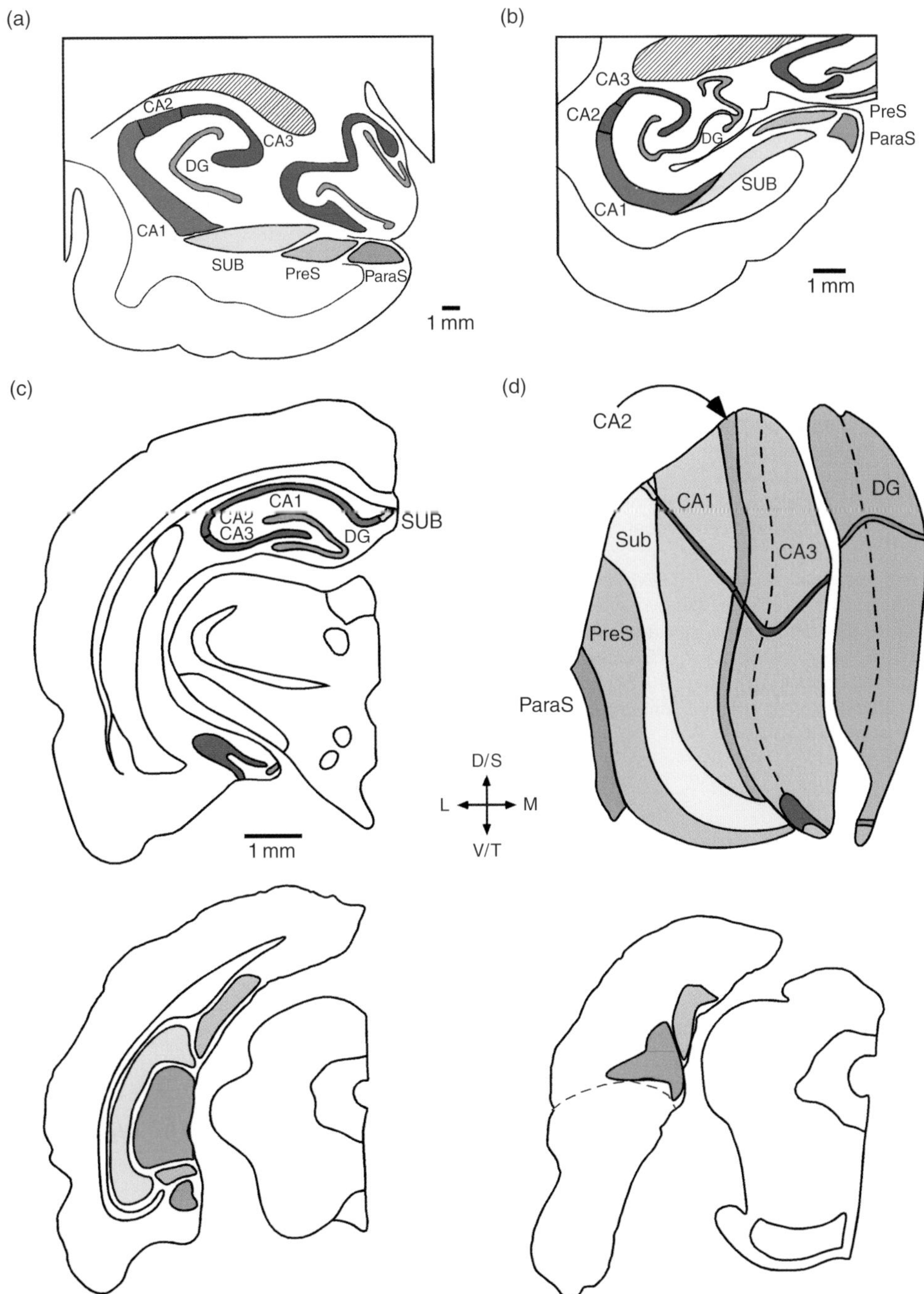

Figure 2 Comparative views of the hippocampal formation with the pre- and parasubiculum. (a) Coronal sections of the human brain (a), monkey brain (b), and rat brain (c) showing the cellular layers of the hippocampal formation structures: the dentate gyrus (green), CA3 (blue), CA2 (purple), CA1 (red), and the subiculum (yellow). (d) An unfolded map of the rodent hippocampal formation. Rodent schematics adapted from Burwell RD and Witter MP (2002) Basic anatomy of the parahippocampal region in monkeys and rats. In: Witter MP and Wouterlood FG (eds.) *The Parahippocampal Region, Organization and Role in Cognitive Functions.* London: Oxford University Press. The presubiculum (light orange) and parasubiculum (dark orange) are also shown at two rostrocaudal levels in panels (e) and (f). Also shown are perirhinal areas 36 and 35 (panels (c) and (e)), the lateral and medial entorhinal areas (LEA and MEA, panels (e) and (f)), and the postrhinal cortex (POR, panel (f)). Abbreviations: DG, dentate gyrus; D, dorsal; L, lateral; M, medial; ParaS, parasubiculum; PreS, presubiculum; S, septal; Sub, subiculum; T, temporal; V, ventral.

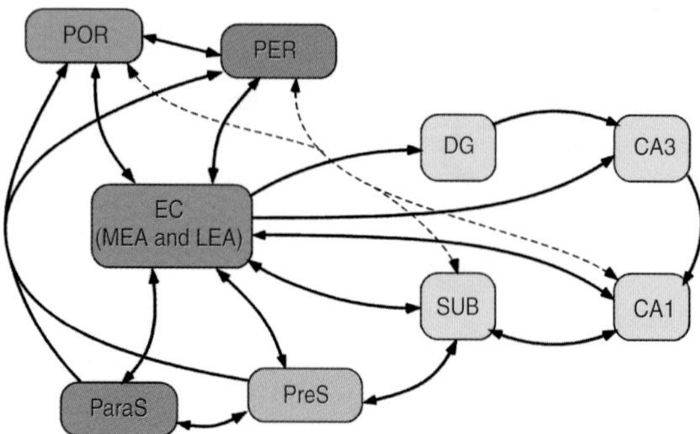

Figure 3 Simplified schematic of the hippocampal system. The schematic includes the hippocampal formation (structures in yellow) and the parahippocampal region (structures in red, blue, green, and orange). The hippocampal formation comprises three-layered structures characterized by largely unidirectional connections, whereas the parahippocampal region comprises six-layered cortices characterized by reciprocal connections. Note that the perirhinal and postrhinal cortices (PER and POR) have reciprocal connections with CA1 and the subiculum. Abbreviations: DG, dentate gyrus; EC, entorhinal cortex; LEA, lateral entorhinal area; MEA, medial entorhinal area; ParaS, parasubiculum; PER, perirhinal cortex; PH, parahippocampal cortex in the primate brain; POR, postrhinal cortex in the rodent brain; PreS, presubiculum; subiculum (SUB).

homolog of the parahippocampal cortex in the primate brain. The perirhinal and postrhinal cortices are the major recipients of cortical afferents, and they project heavily to entorhinal cortex. The entorhinal cortex and the pre- and parasubiculum also receive direct cortical inputs. The entorhinal cortex projects directly to all components of the hippocampal formation and all other components of the parahippocampal region (**Figure 3**). The entorhinal connections with CA1, the subiculum, and all other parahippocampal structures are reciprocal.

One practical problem in the comparative anatomy of these structures is the confusing use of the term parahippocampal. In the rodent brain, the term has only one use (i.e., in the phrase 'parahippocampal region'). In the human and monkey brains, the term is used in two additional ways. First is the parahippocampal cortex, a cortical region in the medial temporal lobe that is a component of the parahippocampal region (and is the homolog of the rodent postrhinal cortex). Second, the parahippocampal gyrus is the fold or gyrus that contains a large portion of the entorhinal, perirhinal, and parahippocampal cortices.

There are also discrepancies in the terminology for the perirhinal cortex. In Brodmann's (1909) nomenclature, which includes verbal and numeric terms, the verbal term for area 35 was perirhinal, and the verbal term for area 36 was ectorhinal. Although Brodmann defined area 36 as a very narrow strip of cortex that did not include the temporal pole, other classic studies, which reported more detailed cytoarchitectonic analyses of these regions, included the temporal pole in area 36 (von Economo, 1929; Von Bonin and Bailey, 1947). There was no designation in Brodmann's nomenclature for the caudally located region we now call the parahippocampal cortex (reviewed in Suzuki and Amaral, 2003b). Using a different nomenclature, von Economo and Koskinsas named the rostral perirhinal/ectorhinal region areas TG and TGa and the caudal (parahippocampal) region areas TF and TH. In modern terminology, the term perirhinal cortex was used to designate the combined areas 35 and 36 (Amaral et al., 1987) or 35a and 35b (Van Hoesen and Pandya, 1975). In the latter nomenclature, area 36 was termed TL.

Currently, the most commonly used nomenclature for memory research in the primate brain is perirhinal cortex comprising areas 35 and 36. Burwell and colleagues (Burwell et al., 1995; Burwell, 2001) adapted that nomenclature for use in the rodent brain. The term ectorhinal is no longer in use except in rodent brain atlases. Thus, within a comparative framework for experimental neuroscience, it seems reasonable to adhere to the nomenclature of perirhinal cortex as designating the combined areas 35 and 36 for both the rodent and primate brains.

10.1.2.2 Location of the hippocampal system structures

The focus of this chapter is the rat hippocampal system about which we have the most detailed anatomical information, but it is worth noting that there are surprising similarities and interesting differences between these structures in the rodent and the primate brains. The upper panel of **Figure 1** shows that the hippocampus is C-shaped and relatively larger in the rodent brain (**Figure 1(c)**). The dorsal or septal portion of the region is associated with the fimbria-fornix and the septal nuclei. The ventral or temporal portion of the structure is associated with the temporal cortices. The hippocampus is relatively smaller in the primate brain (**Figure 1(b)**). The structure is still shaped like a C, though shallower and rotated about 90° clockwise, such that the opening is pointing upward. In the primate brain, the rostral hippocampus is associated with the temporal cortices, and the caudal hippocampus is associated with the septal nuclei. Accordingly, for cross-species comparisons, the best terminology for the long axis of the hippocampus is the term septotemporal.

In the human brain, the rhinal sulcus is relatively small and is associated with only the most rostral portion of the perirhinal cortex. The collateral sulcus forms the lateral border of the parahippocampal gyrus (**Figure 1(d)**). As in the monkey brain, the entorhinal, perirhinal, and parahippocampal cortices occupy the parahippocampal gyrus and the temporal pole. The perirhinal cortex occupies the temporal pole and continues caudally. The entorhinal cortex lies in the medial portion of the anterior parahippocampal gyrus and is bordered rostrally and laterally by the perirhinal cortex. The parahippocampal cortex forms the caudal border of the perirhinal cortex.

In the monkey brain, which is less gyrencephalic (smoother) than the human brain and more gyrencephalic than the rat brain, the rhinal sulcus is associated with the full extent of the perirhinal cortex. Area 35 is a narrow band of agranular cortex that occupies the fundus and the lateral bank of the rhinal sulcus. Area 36 is a larger strip of dysgranular cortex located lateral to area 35 and including the temporal pole (**Figure 1(b)** and **1(e)**). All but the most rostral part of the lateral border of area 36 is shared with area TE of inferotemporal cortex. The rostrolateral border is formed by the superior temporal gyrus. Suzuki and Amaral (2003a) extended the border of area 36 rostrally and septally to include the medial half of the temporal pole on cytoarchitectonic and connectional grounds. The monkey parahippocampal cortex, comprising areas TH and TF, is located caudal to the perirhinal and entorhinal cortices (**Figure 1(b)** and **1(e)**). Area TF is larger than area TH and is laterally adjacent to area TH. Area TH is a thin strip of largely agranular cortex medially adjacent to area TF. The parahippocampal cortex is bordered rostrally by the entorhinal and perirhinal cortices, laterally by TE, medially by the para- and presubiculum, and caudally by visual area V4.

In the rodent brain, the rhinal sulcus, or fissure as it is sometimes called, is the only prominent sulcus (**Figure 1(c)** and **1(f)**). It extends along the entire lateral surface of the brain, though it is quite shallow in its caudal extent. The region is bordered rostrally by the insular cortex. Insular cortex is classically defined as the region overlying the claustrum. The transition from insular cortex to the perirhinal cortex occurs when claustral cells underlying layer VI of the cortex are no longer visible. The perirhinal cortex comprises two cytoarchitectonically distinct strips of cortex, areas 35 and 36. Area 36 lies dorsally adjacent to area 35. The entorhinal cortex provides the ventral border of area 35. The dorsal border of area 36 is formed by secondary somatosensory cortex, rostrally, secondary auditory cortex at midrostrocaudal levels, and ventral temporal association cortex at caudal levels. The postrhinal cortex is located caudal to perirhinal cortex and provides the caudal border. It lies ventral to the ventral temporal area and dorsal to the medial entorhinal cortex (**Figure 2(f)**).

10.1.2.3 Cross-species comparisons: Human, monkey, and rodent

A comparative analysis of the unfolded maps of the human, monkey, and rat brains shows that the spatial relationships of the perirhinal, parahippocampal/postrhinal, and entorhinal cortices are similar (**Figure 1**). Aside from the obvious differences in scale, the relative size differences are also interesting. Studies in rats, monkeys, and humans suggest that the perirhinal cortex accounts for roughly 3% of the cortical surface area, suggesting that the region scales linearly with cortical surface area. Also, in all three species, the surface area of the perirhinal cortex is roughly twice that of the postrhinal/parahippocampal cortex. Therefore, postrhinal/parahippocampal cortex also appears to scale linearly with brain size. The relative size of the entorhinal cortex, however, differs dramatically across species. In the rat brain, its surface area is more than three times that of the perirhinal cortex, but in the primate brain, entorhinal cortex is considerably smaller than the perirhinal cortex.

The homology of the rodent postrhinal cortex with the primate parahippocampal cortex is based on the structural and connectional similarities. In rodents and primates, the region receives substantial input from visual associational, retrosplenial, and posterior parietal cortices. Subcortical connections are also similar. For example, the rat postrhinal cortex is strongly and reciprocally connected with the lateral posterior nucleus of the thalamus (LPO). Likewise, the monkey parahippocampal cortex is connected with the pulvinar, the homolog of the lateral preoptic area (LPO) in the rodent.

In human, monkey, and rat, the entorhinal cortex is a six-layered cortex characterized by a cell sparse layer (lamina dissecans) separating the deep and superficial layers. The medial part of the entorhinal area is, structurally, more highly differentiated as compared to the lateral part, and the lamina dissecans is more evident. It should be noted that in the rat, the medial entorhinal area is more caudal and ventral, whereas the lateral entorhinal area is more rostral and dorsal (**Figure 1(c)** and **1(f)**). In both rat and monkey, the intrinsic connectivity of the entorhinal cortex appears to be organized into intrinsic bands of interconnectivity that form discrete associational networks. In the rat, these bands of intrinsic connectivity project to different levels of the dentate gyrus, suggesting a functional topography. There is evidence that a similar topography exists for the monkey.

All hippocampal formation structures observed in the human brain are also present in the monkey and rat brains (**Figure 2**). The absolute size of the hippocampal formation is largest in the human brain and smallest in the rodent brain, though the structure is relatively larger in the rodent brain. As previously mentioned, the hippocampus is situated differently in different species. In the human and monkey brains, it is as if the hippocampal formation has swung down and forward, such that rostral hippocampus in the primate brain is comparable to ventral hippocampus in the rodent brain. Similarly, caudal hippocampus in the primate brain is comparable to dorsal hippocampus in the rodent brain. For ease of comparative analysis, it is most efficient to use the terms septal and temporal to describe the long axis because these terms can be applied similarly across all species. The septotemporal axis in the rodent hippocampus is equivalent to dorsoventral axis, and the septotemporal axis in the primate hippocampus is equivalent to the caudorostral axis.

10.2 The Parahippocampal Region

10.2.1 The Postrhinal Cortex

The postrhinal cortex is located near the caudal pole of the rat brain, caudal to the perirhinal cortex, dorsal to the rhinal sulcus and to the medial entorhinal area (**Figure 1(c)**). Usually the postrhinal cortex arises at the caudal limit of the angular bundle when subicular cells are no longer present in coronal sections (**Figure 4(a)**). At this level, postrhinal cortex is characterized by the presence of ectopic layer II cells at the perirhinal–postrhinal border near the ventral border with the medial entorhinal cortex (**Figure 4(b)**, arrow). Moving caudally, the postrhinal cortex rises dorsally above the caudal extension of the rhinal fissure and wraps obliquely around the

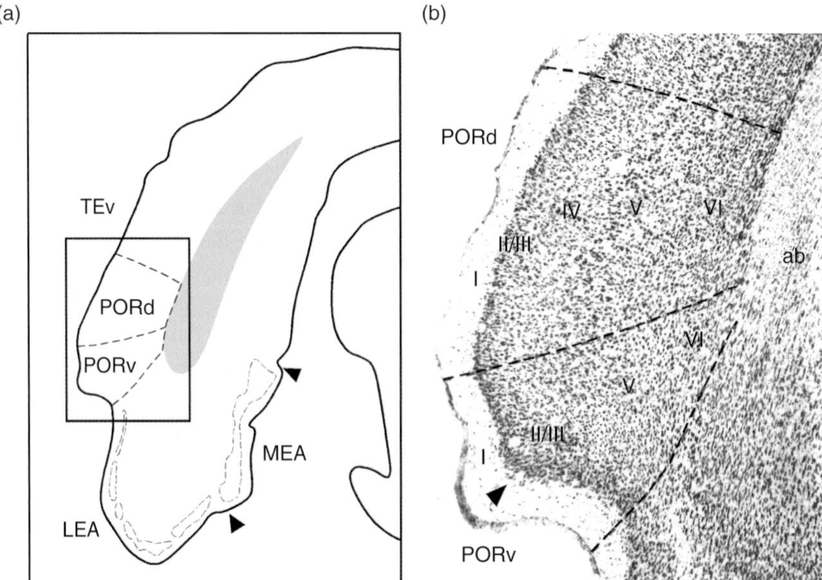

Figure 4 Location and photomicrograph of the postrhinal cortex (POR). (a) Drawing of a coronal section of the rat brain at the level of the rostral limit of the postrhinal cortex. (b) Nissl-stained coronal section showing the septal and temporal subregions of the POR (PORd and PORv, respectively). Layers are labeled I–VI. The septal subregion has a more differentiated laminar pattern. The ventral subregion is characterized by ectopic layer II cells (arrow) that appear near the rostral border with area 36. Abbreviations: ab, angular bundle.

caudal pole of the brain. Visual association cortex, which forms the dorsal border of postrhinal cortex, has a more differentiated laminar pattern and a broader layer IV. The precise location of the dorsal border is difficult to distinguish cytoarchitectonically. A convenient landmark, however, is provided by the parasubiculum. The dorsal border of the postrhinal cortex on the lateral surface tends to be at the same dorsoventral level as the parasubiculum on the medial surface. The medial entorhinal cortex borders the postrhinal cortex ventrally and is easily distinguished by the large layer II cells and distinct laminar look of the cortex.

The cell layers of the postrhinal cortex have a homogeneous look because the packing density of cells is similar across layers (**Figure 4(b)**). In coronal sections, there is a broadening of the deep layers, which is due to the conformation of the region at the caudal pole of the brain (**Figure 4**). In sagittal sections, however, layers II–III, V, and VI each occupy about one-third of the cortical depth. The region can be subdivided into dorsal and ventral subdivisions based on cytoarchitectonic features. In general, the dorsal subregion has a more organized and radial appearance. The primary difference between the two subdivisions is that the dorsal portion has a distinguishable granule cell layer IV. Another difference is that layer V of the dorsal subregion is slightly narrower than in the ventral subdivision.

Retrograde tract tracing studies show that three-quarters of postrhinal afferentation arise in neocortex. The remainder is roughly evenly divided between subcortical and hippocampal afferents. The neocortical connections of the postrhinal cortex distinguish it from the nearby perirhinal cortex, in that cortical input to the postrhinal cortex is strongly dominated by visual and visuospatial inputs. In terms of sensory input, the postrhinal cortex receives almost a third of its total input from visual associational regions. The strongest associational input arises in the posterior parietal cortex. Dorsal retrosplenial cortex also provides a strong projection. The input from frontal associational regions largely arises in ventrolateral orbital frontal cortex. A strong input arises in the caudal and ventral temporal area, which is itself strongly interconnected with visual association cortices. For the most part, all cortical connections are equally reciprocated. The exception is that the postrhinal cortex projects strongly to the perirhinal cortex, but the return projection is substantially weaker.

The subcortical afferents are dominated by the thalamic inputs, which arise predominantly in the lateral posterior nucleus of the thalamus. That projection is reciprocal. There is also input from the anteromedial dorsal thalamic group and the intralaminar nucleus of the thalamus. The input from the amygdala is very small and is mainly from the lateral and basolateral nuclei. The postrhinal cortex also projects back to the lateral and basolateral amygdala nuclei. The inputs from the septum are also relatively small and are dominated by the medial septum.

The postrhinal cortex projects strongly to the medial entorhinal cortex, particularly to the lateral band. The entorhinal projection is weakly reciprocal. Postrhinal cortex has strong reciprocal connections with the septal presubiculum and the parasubiculum. In addition to these parahippocampal connections, there are strong direct connections with the hippocampus. The postrhinal cortex projects directly to the septal CA1 and subiculum, and both projections are returned. Connections with the temporal hippocampus are modest.

10.2.2 The Perirhinal Cortex

The perirhinal cortex arises at the caudal limit of the insular cortex and can be distinguished from insular cortex by the absence of the underlying claustrum. It is bordered dorsally by temporal association regions, ventrally by piriform and entorhinal cortex, and caudally by the postrhinal cortex. For most of its rostrocaudal extent, the perirhinal cortex includes the fundus and both banks of the rhinal sulcus (**Figure 1(f)**). At its caudal limit, the region rises dorsal to the fundus. A signature feature of the perirhinal cortex in the rodent and monkey brains is the presence of large heart-shaped cells in deep layer V that appear in both area 36 and area 35 (**Figure 5**).

Perirhinal area 36 is located dorsal to the rhinal sulcus. Although the region has a more prominent laminar structure dorsally than ventrally, area 36 is generally described as dysgranular cortex. The dorsal border of area 36 is best discerned by characteristics of the granular cell layer, layer IV. Area 36 has a fairly rudimentary layer IV as compared to the discrete granular layer of the dorsally adjacent neocortical areas. Another feature of the region is the patchy layer II in which medium-sized cells are organized in clumps or patches. The organization of layer V cells into lines gives the region a radial look, especially dorsally. Layer VI has a bilaminar appearance in that the cells in the deep portion of the layer

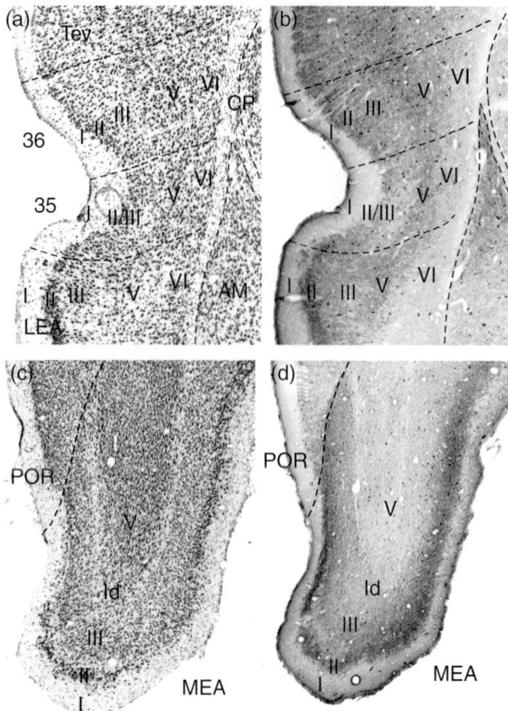

Figure 5 Photomicrographs of the perirhinal (PER), postrhinal (POR) and lateral and medial entorhinal cortices (LEA and MEA). (a) Nissl-stained coronal section showing PER areas 36 and 35 and the LEA. (b) Adjacent section stained for parvalbumin. Heavy staining of layer II in the LEA provides a useful marker for the PER-LEA border. (c) Nissl-stained coronal section showing MEA and POR. (d) Adjacent section stained for parvalbumin. Layers are labeled I–VI. Parvalbumin staining also differentiates the MEA-POR border. Other abbreviations: AM, amygdala; CP, caudate putamen.

are smaller, darker, and more densely packed than the cells in the superficial portion of the layer.

Area 35 is generally characterized by a broad layer I. Layers II and III tend to blend together (**Figure 5**). The region lacks a layer IV and is thus considered agranular cortex. Layer V of area 35 has a disorganized look as compared to the radial appearance in area 36. As in area 36, layer VI has a bilaminate appearance. A general characteristic of area 35 is the organization of its cells into an arcing formation that spans all layers. This feature is most evident below the rhinal sulcus. The entorhinal cortex forms most of the ventral border and can be distinguished from ventral area 35 by the medium to large darkly staining stellate cells of layer II and by the appearance of the lamina dissecans, a cell-sparse area between layers III and V.

The input to the perirhinal cortex is roughly evenly divided between cortical and subcortical structures. The perirhinal cortex receives input from nearly all unimodal and polymodal associational regions of neocortex, but there are subregional differences. For example, area 36 receives roughly equal input from olfactory, auditory, visual and visuospatial, and sensorimotor regions, whereas area 35 is dominated by olfactory input from piriform cortex. There are also subregional similarities and differences in polymodal association input. Area 36 receives the largest cortical input from temporal association regions followed by insular and frontal regions. In contrast, area 35 receives the larger input from insular cortex followed by temporal association and frontal regions. Of course, there is also a heavy intrinsic input from area 36. Areas 36 and 35 each receive only small inputs from posterior associational regions. As would be expected, these associational connections are largely reciprocal.

Perirhinal areas 36 and 35 are also differentiated by subcortical connections. The strongest subcortical connections of area 36 are with the amygdala. The afferent input arises largely in the lateral nucleus, but the basolateral and basomedial nuclei also provide substantial inputs. Substantial thalamic input arises largely in the dorsolateral group and in the reticular thalamic nucleus. In contrast, area 35 receives its strongest subcortical afferents from olfactory structures, primarily from the endopiriform nucleus, but also from the piriform transition area. Other substantial inputs arise in the amygdala, the midline and lateral thalamic groups, and the medial geniculate nucleus of the thalamus.

Like the postrhinal cortex, the perirhinal cortex projects strongly to the lateral entorhinal cortex. The projection arises in area 35 and terminates most heavily in the so-called lateral band of the entorhinal cortex (see following). The entorhinal projection is weakly reciprocated. Area 36 is weakly connected with hippocampal and subicular structures, although these connections may be functionally important. Area 35 receives input back from the septal presubiculum. The strongest projection back to area 35 arises in temporal CA1, but it also receives input from temporal subiculum and presubiculum. Other smaller inputs arise in septal CA1 and the parasubiculum.

10.2.3 Entorhinal Cortex

The entorhinal cortex is of considerable interest in memory research. Not only does it provide the major conduit for sensory information to the hippocampal formation, but a number of recent discoveries also suggest that the region may make unique contributions to the processing of spatial information. The entorhinal cortex is a relatively large and complicated structure, and its connections are topographically organized. Thus, understanding the areal differences in entorhinal structure could provide insight into its role in memory.

In rats and other animals, the entorhinal cortex has been divided into two subdivisions roughly equivalent to modern definitions of the lateral and medial entorhinal areas (LEA and MEA, **Figure 1(f)**) (Brodmann, 1909; Krieg, 1946). The LEA (**Figure 5**, top) is perhaps most easily distinguished from the MEA (**Figure 5**, bottom) by differences in layer II. LEA has a very clumpy layer II as compared to the more homogeneous layer II of the MEA. The sparsely populated layer IV, also called the lamina dissecans, is considered a landmark feature of the entorhinal cortex, but there are subregional differences. In general, the LEA exhibits a less prominent lamina dissecans as compared to the MEA (compare **Figure 5**).

Some time ago, the monkey entorhinal cortex was further subdivided on the basis of structural and connectional criteria (Van Hoesen and Pandya, 1975; Amaral et al., 1987). The rat entorhinal cortex has now been subdivided into six fields according to similar criteria (**Figure 6(a)**) (Insausti et al., 1997). The LEA comprises four fields: the dorsal lateral entorhinal field (DLE), the dorsal intermediate entorhinal field (DIE), the amygdalo-entorhinal transitional field (AE), and the ventral intermediate entorhinal field (VIE). Each field has unique connectional and/or structural characteristics. The medial entorhinal area (MEA) is subdivided into a caudal field (CE) and a medial field (ME). Medially, the MEA is bordered by the parasubiculum. The MEA border with the parasubiculum is marked by a layer II that thickens into a characteristic club-shaped formation.

The intrinsic connections of the entorhinal cortex are organized in a rostrocaudal manner, such that the cells located in each of three bands of the entorhinal area are highly interconnected but do not project outside the band of origin (**Figure 6(b)**) (Dolorfo and Amaral, 1998). Interestingly, each band of intrinsic connectivity spans the MEA and LEA. An important recent discovery about these regions has to do with the relationship of these bands of intrinsic connectivity with the perforant pathway, the entorhinal projection to the dentate gyrus. Briefly, the lateral band projects to the septal half of the dentate gyrus, whereas the intermediate and medial bands project to the third and fourth septotemporal quarters, respectively (**Figure 6(c)**). This connectional topography suggests that functional diversity within the entorhinal cortex may be in register with functional diversity in the hippocampus.

The entorhinal cortex is strongly connected with other parahippocampal region structures. Perirhinal

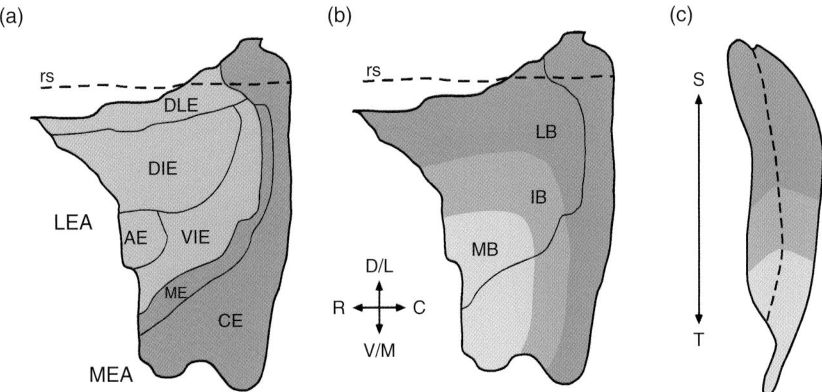

Figure 6 Unfolded maps of the entorhinal cortex and the target of the perforant pathway, the dentate gyrus. (a) Unfolded map of the rodent entorhinal cortex showing the LEA in light green and the MEA in dark green. Further parcellation of each subregion is noted by black lines (Insausti et al., 1997). (b) Unfolded map of the rodent entorhinal cortex showing the lateral (LB) in dark green, the intermediate band (IB) in medium green, and medial band (MB) in pale green. (c) The unfolded dentate gyrus, color coded to denote the terminations of the perforant pathway. The entorhinal LB projects to the septal half of the dentate gyrus, the IB projects to the third quarter, and the MB projects to the temporal quarter. Abbreviations: AE, amygdalo-entorhinal transitional field; CE, caudal entorhinal field; D, dorsal; DLE, dorsal lateral entorhinal field; DIE, dorsal intermediate entorhinal field; L, lateral; M, medial; ME, medial entorhinal field; S, septal; T, temporal; V, ventral.

input arises largely in area 35 and terminates preferentially to the lateral band of the LEA. The postrhinal input arises in all portions of the region and terminates primarily in the lateral band of the MEA. There is a heavy return projection to perirhinal cortex that arises in all layers and all portions of the entorhinal cortex, though the strongest projection arises in the lateral band. Strong inputs originate from the pre- and parasubiculum. The parasubiculum targets the entire entorhinal cortex, septal presubiculum projects more heavily to the MEA, and temporal presubiculum projects more heavily to the LEA. The entorhinal cortex provides modest reciprocal connections with the pre- and parasubiculum (Witter and Amaral, 2004).

The entorhinal cortex has neocortical connections, through weaker than perirhinal and postrhinal cortices. The LEA receives very strong input from the piriform and agranular insular cortices. Medial and orbital frontal regions provide a strong projection. Input from the cingulate, parietal, and occipital cortices is relatively weak. There is little differentiation across the lateral to medial bands. Piriform cortex also projects to the MEA, but the projection terminates in the lateral and intermediate bands. In contrast, the lateral band receives moderate to strong projections from frontal, cingulate, parietal, and occipital cortices. Projections to the medial frontal and olfactory structures tend to arise in the intermediate and medial bands. A very narrow strip of the entorhinal cortex that is positioned closest to the rhinal fissure gives rise to the major projections to other cortical areas, including the lateral frontal, temporal, parietal, cingulate, and occipital cortices.

The entorhinal cortex has widespread connections with subcortical structures, and it is possible that the subcortical afferents are as influential as the cortical afferents. Strong projections arise in claustrum, olfactory structures, the amygdala, and dorsal thalamus. The olfactory input arises in the endopiriform nucleus and the piriform transition area and is stronger to the LEA than the MEA. The dorsal thalamic input arises primarily in the midline thalamic nuclei and is stronger to MEA than to LEA. The LEA and MEA receive input from septal nuclei, though the inputs are relatively small. The amygdala input arises in all nuclei except the central nucleus and amygdalohippocampal area and is stronger to LEA than MEA. In addition, the entorhinal cortex projects to all amygdaloid structures except the nucleus of the lateral olfactory tract and the central nucleus (Pikkarainen and Pitkanen, 1999).

The entorhinal cortex projects to all hippocampal formation structures including the dentate gyrus, fields CA3, CA2, and CA1 of the hippocampus proper, and the subiculum (reviewed in Witter and Amaral, 2004). The entorhinal projections to the dentate gyrus, CA3, and CA2 originate in layer II of the entorhinal cortex. The terminations of the layer II projections exhibit a radial topography in that the LEA terminates in the outer DG molecular layer, whereas the MEA projects to the middle DG molecular layer (**Figure** 7). The projections to CA1 and the subiculum originate in layer III. The terminations of the layer III projections

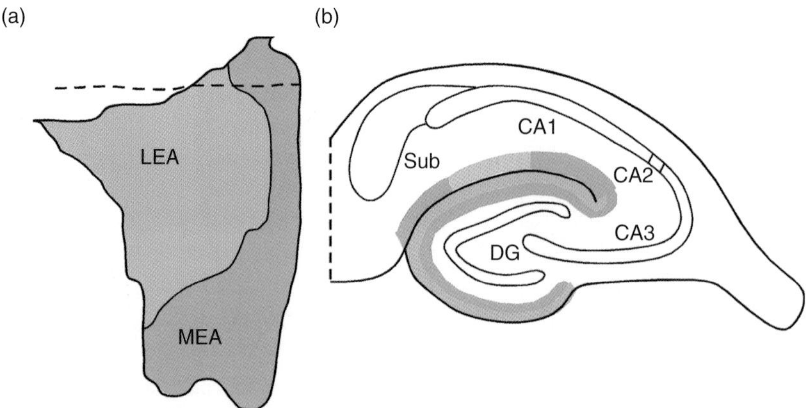

Figure 7 Illustration of the radial and transverse topography of the entorhinal projection to the hippocampal formation. (a) Unfolded map of the entorhinal cortex showing the LEA in light green and the MEA in dark green. (b) Line drawing of a hippocampal section perpendicular to the long axis. Adapted from Witter MP and Amaral DG (2004) Hippocampal Formation. In: Paxinos G (ed.) *The Rat Nervous System,* 3rd ed. San Diego, CA: Academic Press. The terminations of the LEA are in light green, and the terminations of the MEA are in dark green. The projection to the DG exhibits a radial topography, whereas the projection to CA1 and subiculum (sub) exhibits a transverse topography. See text for details.

exhibit a transverse topography such that the LEA projects to distal CA1 and proximal subiculum, and the MEA projects to the proximal CA1 and distal subiculum. The organization of the CA1 and subicular projections back to deep layers of the LEA and MEA roughly reciprocates the forward projections.

10.2.4 Presubiculum

The presubiculum is bordered dorsally by retrosplenial cortex, medially by the subiculum, and ventrolaterally by the parasubiculum (**Figures 2(e)**, **2(f)**, and **8(a)**). Areas 48 and 27 according to Brodmann (1909) are both included in the presubiculum. Area 48, the most dorsal extension of the presubiculum, is sometimes called the postsubiculum. Because the presubiculum and this dorsal component exhibit considerable cytoarchitectonic similarities, it may be more appropriate to designate the area collectively with a single term.

Layer II of the six-layered presubiculum is thick and contains small, densely packed, and darkly staining pyramidal cells (**Figure 8(b)**). Cells in layer III are even smaller, round, and also darkly staining. Whereas cells in layer II tend to form clusters, cells in layer III have a more homogeneous look. Layer III is separated from the deep layers by a narrow, sparsely populated gap that is continuous with the lamina dissecans of the parasubicular cortex. Deep to this cell-sparse gap are two layers. Layer V is very thin and contains pyramidal cells. Layer VI is slightly thicker and contains a mixture of cell types.

As it turns out, acetylcholinesterase (AChE) is an excellent marker for the presubiculum. Layer II stains moderately darkly (**Figure 8(c)**). Deep to layer II is a dark band that contains layers III, the cell-sparse gap, and layer V. Layer VI is moderately to lightly stained in AChE preparations. AChE is also a good marker for the parasubiculum.

The presubiculum has extensive associational, commissural, and hippocampal parahippocampal connections (Witter and Amaral, 2004). The septal and temporal parts of the presubiculum are highly interconnected. Connections with the contralateral presubiculum are also extensive, though commissural connectivity may be stronger ventrally than dorsally. The presubiculum provides a weak input to the dentate gyrus and all fields of the hippocampus proper. It is reciprocally connected with the subiculum. The presubiculum projects to superficial layers of the subiculum. The projection to the septal subiculum is moderately strong, and the temporally directed projection is relatively weak. The input from the subiculum terminates in layer I.

Regarding parahippocampal connectivity, the presubiculum projects to superficial layers of the

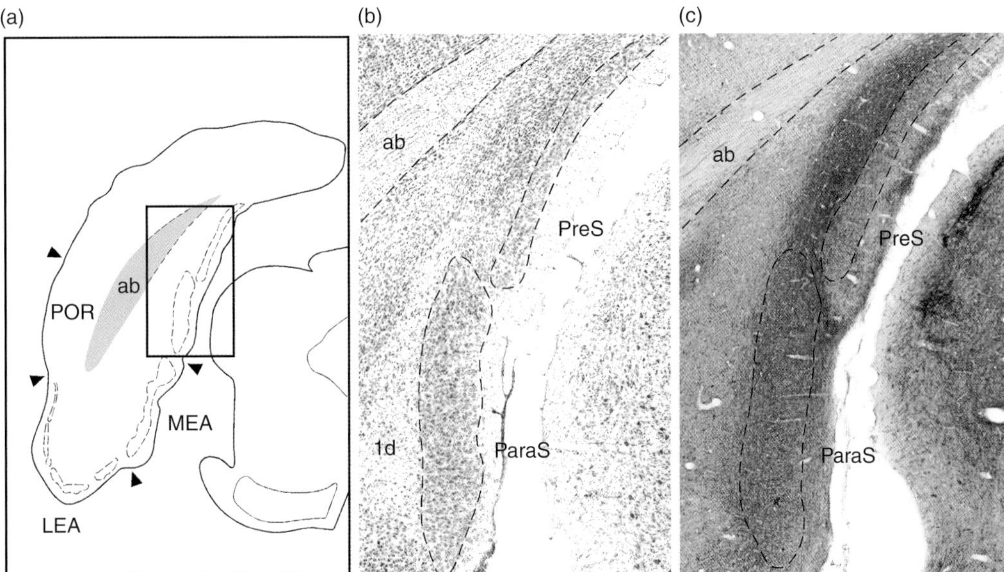

Figure 8 Photomicrographs of the presubiculum (PreS) and parasubiculum (ParaS). (a) Drawing of a coronal section of the rat brain at the level of the angular bundle (ab). The inset designates the areas shown in panels (b) and (c). (b) Nissl-stained coronal section showing the PreS and ParaS. Layer II is outlined for the PreS, and the combined layer II/III is outlined for ParaS. (c) Adjacent section stained for acetylcholinesterase (AChE). AChE provides an excellent marker for these regions.

parasubiculum, but the connections with the entorhinal cortex are by far the strongest. The presubicular–entorhinal projection is bilateral, largely directed to medial entorhinal cortex, and almost exclusively terminates in layer III. Septal presubiculum projects much more heavily to the MEA than the LEA, but temporal presubiculum projects heavily to both entorhinal divisions. Septal presubiculum also provides a moderately heavy input to the postrhinal cortex. The dorsal extension (Brodman's area 48, sometimes termed the postsubiculum) projects massively to postrhinal cortex. Temporal presubiculum projects heavily to the LEA and the MEA and moderately heavily to perirhinal areas 36 and 35. Septal presubiculum receives heavy input from postrhinal cortex and a moderately heavy input from the MEA portion of the lateral band. Temporal presubiculum receives a very heavy input from the MEA portion of the medial band, weak input from the LEA, and virtually nothing from the perirhinal and postrhinal cortices.

The heaviest neocortical input to the presubiculum arises in the granular retrosplenial cortex, but weaker inputs arise in prelimbic cortex, dorsomedial prefrontal areas, and the anterior cingulate cortex (Witter and Amaral, 2004). The primary subcortical inputs are from the dorsal thalamus, specifically, the anteroventral, the anterodorsal, and the laterodorsal nuclei. The presubiculum receives subcortical input from the thalamus, primarily the anterior thalamic nuclei including the anteroventral, anterodorsal, and laterodorsal nuclei. A massive return projection targets the same nuclei. There is also a strong cholinergic input arising from septal nuclei. Finally, the presubiculum has reciprocal connections with the mamillary nuclei of the hypothalamus.

10.2.5 The Parasubiculum

For most of its rostrocaudal extent, the parasubiculum is bordered by presubiculum dorsally and the medial entorhinal area ventrally (**Figure 2(e)** and **2(f)**). At more caudal levels, the parasubiculum is interposed between the postrhinal cortex and the medial entorhinal area. A broad, combined layer II/III contains large, densely packed, moderately darkly staining pyramidal cells. This layer is separated from the deep layers by a broad lamina dissecans. Layers V and VI can be distinguished from one another and tend to run continuously with deep layers of the medial entorhinal area. In AChE preparations, layers I and II/III are darkly stained (**Figure 8(c)**). The lamina dissecans and layer V are lightly stained, and layer V is moderately darkly stained.

The parasubiculum has associational connections that project dorsally and ventrally. The ventral projections are heavier and more extensive than the dorsal ones. Commissural projections terminate in layers I and III of the contralateral homotopic region.

The hippocampal input to the parasubiculum arises mainly in the subiculum and terminates in layer I and superficial layer II. There are also return projections to the hippocampal formation. The structure projects directly to the molecular layer of the dentate gyrus. This is especially interesting given that the parasubiculum receives strong inputs from anterior thalamic nuclei. As has been previously noted, the anterior thalamic projection to the parasubiculum provides a pathway by which the anterior thalamus can affect hippocampal processing of incoming information at very early stages.

Like the presubiculum, the parasubiculum exhibits substantial connections with other parahippocampal structures. The parasubiculum projects selectively to layer II of the entorhinal cortex. The entorhinal projection is much heavier to MEA than to the LEA. Interestingly, the parasubicular projection to POR is even heavier than that to the MEA. Parahippocampal inputs arise mainly from the MEA, with the medial band providing the heaviest return projection. There is also a modest presubicular input.

Extrinsic connections of the parasubiculum are few. The only neocortical afferents arise in retrosplenial cortex and visual cortex, and these inputs are quite weak. Other than the input from the anterior thalamus, the only other subcortical afferents arise in the amygdala from the lateral, basal, and accessory basal nuclei.

10.3 The Hippocampal Formation

The structures of the hippocampal formation are grouped together partly because of the sequential activation pattern that was identified several decades ago. The entorhinal cortex activates the dentate gyrus via the perforant pathway, the mossy fiber pathway from the denate gyrus activates CA3, and the CA3 Schaffer collaterals activate CA1. Some of the earliest and most famous studies of the structure of the nervous system were conducted by Ramón y Cajal, who used a technique developed by Camillo Golgi for darkly staining a small number of neurons in the brain. Cajal's elegant studies and drawings, including the rodent hippocampus (**Figure 9**), provided the basis for the neuron doctrine.

Because of the complex architecture of the hippocampus, it is helpful to describe its structure in terms of three axes, the longitudinal, transverse, and radial axes. As previously discussed, we use the term septotemporal for the longitudinal axis of the hippocampus. Along the transverse axis, which is orthogonal to the long axis of the hippocampus, the dentate gyrus can be considered the proximal limit and transverse locations designated according to position relative to the dentate gyrus. Thus, the part of the CA3 lying in the V of the dentate gyrus is proximal CA3, and the part closest to CA1 is distal (**Figure 10**). Similarly, the part of CA1 closest to CA3 is proximal, and so on. Finally, the laminar structure is perpendicular to the radial axis. In this terminology, the molecular layers are superficial and the layers on the opposite side of the principle cell layers are deep.

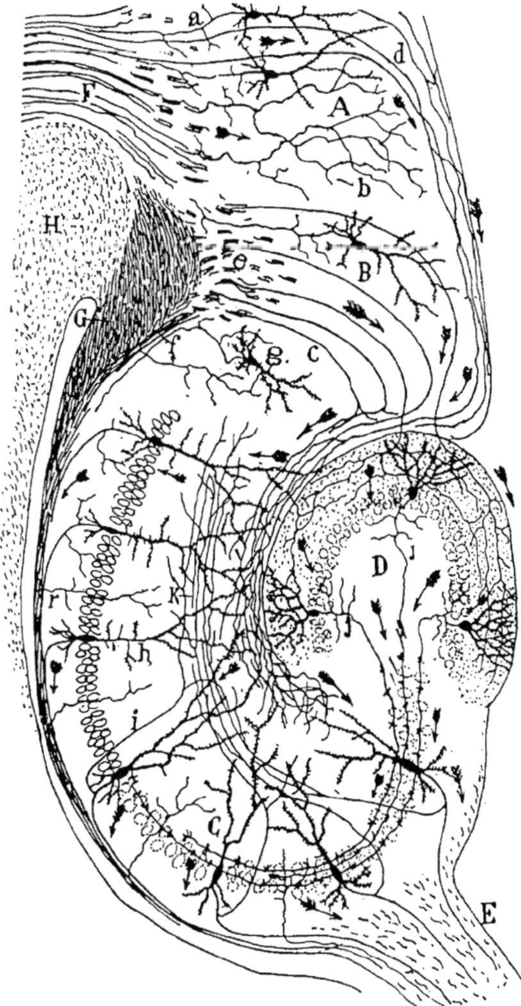

Figure 9 Drawing of the circuitry of the hippocampal formation by Ramón y Cajal (1909). Cajal proposed that the nervous system is made up of countless separate units, or nerve cells composed of dendrites, soma, and axons, each of which is a conductive device. He further proposed that information is received on the cell bodies and dendrites and conducted to distant locations through axons. Abbreviations: A, retrosplenial area; B, subiculum; C, Ammon's horn; D, dentate gyrus; E, fimbria; F, cingulum; G, angular bundle; H, corpus callosum; K, recurrent collaterals; a, axon entering the cingulum; b, cingulum fibers; c-e, perforant path fibers; g, subicular cell; h, CA1 pyramidal cells; i, Schaffer collaterals; collaterals of alvear fibers.

Based primarily on electrophysiological data and mapping of vasculature, Anderson and colleagues (1971) proposed that the hippocampal formation was organized in parallel lamellae stacked along the longitudinal axis. They further proposed that this lamellar organization would permit strips, or slabs, of the hippocampus to function as independent units. Although the lamellar hypothesis shaped research on the hippocampus for years to come and continues to influence modern concepts of hippocampal function, modern neuroanatomical research has revealed that the hippocampal projections are much more divergent than is suggested by the lamellar hypothesis. Indeed, the major hippocampal and dentate associational projections extend along the septotemporal axis as well as the transverse axis.

10.3.1 The Dentate Gyrus

The dentate gyrus is three-layered cortex whose principle cell layer is V shaped (**Figure 10**). The molecular layer lies outside the V, and the polymorphic layer lies inside the V. The beginning of the CA3 principle cell layer protrudes into the polymorphic area of the dentate gyrus. This conformation has generated some confusion over the border between CA3 and the dentate gyrus polymorphic layer, as well as the identity of these cells. In earlier nomenclatures, and occasionally in modern reports, the part of CA3 next to the dentate gyrus was sometimes called CA4. With modern techniques for defining connectional characteristics, however, it is now clear that those pyramidal cells belong to CA3.

The dentate granule cell layer contains small, very densely packed, oval cells that have a dark appearance in cell stains (**Figure 10(a)**). Each granule cell has a small number of primary dendrites (one to four) that are covered with spines. The dendrites

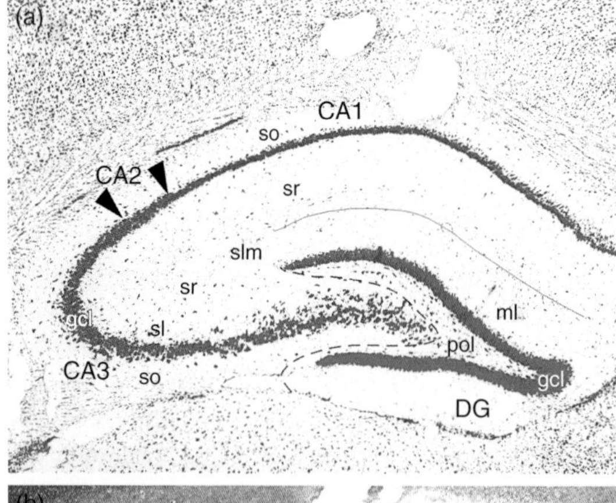

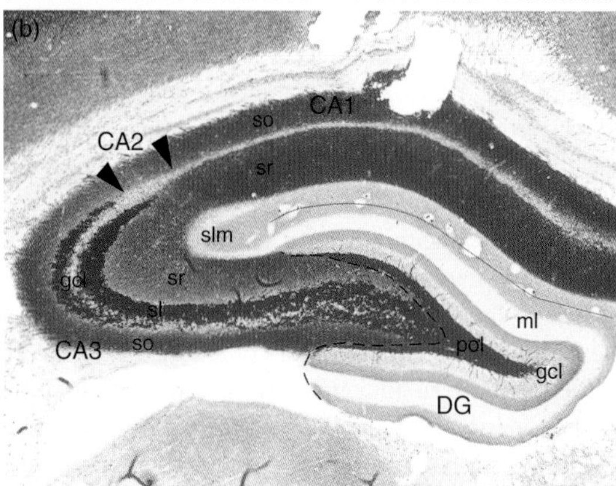

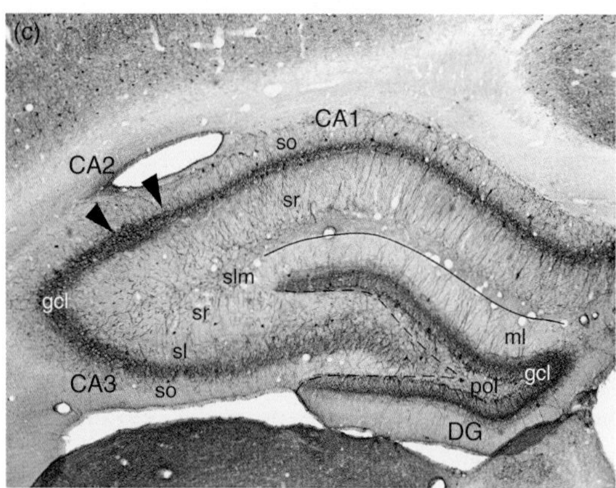

Figure 10 Photomicrographs of the hippocampal formation. (a) Nissl-stained coronal section showing the dentate gyrus (DG) and hippocampus proper, comprising fields CA3, CA2, and CA1. (b) Adjacent section stained for heavy metals using the Timm's method. (c) Parvalbumin-stained section showing the same regions. Layers of the DG are the outer molecular layer (ml), the granule cell layer (gcl), and the polymorphous layer (pol). The CA fields contain the outer stratum lacunosum-moleculare (slm), the stratum radiatum (sr), the gcl, and the stratum oriens (so). CA3 also contains the stratum lucidum (sl). The dashed line demarcates the border between the DG and CA3. The solid line shows the location of the hippocampal fissure and demarcates the border between DG and CA1.

extend into the molecular layer all the way to the hippocampal fissure. In the subgranular region, between the granule cell layer and the polymorphic layer, there are several cell types, most of which are immunoreactive for gamma-aminobutyric acid (GABA). A subset of these cells is also immunoreactive for the calcium-binding protein, parvalbumin (**Figure 10(c)**). The most prominent types are the basket cell and the axo-axonic, or chandelier, cell. The basket cell interneurons are quite large with a single, aspiny apical dendrite extending into the molecular layer and several basal dendrites extending into the polymorphic layer. Axo-axonic cells have a dendritic tree of radial branches extending through the molecular layer. The axon arborizes extensively in the granule cell layer.

The molecular layer contains mostly dendrites from cells of the granule and polymorphic layers. In material stained for heavy metals using the Timm's method, it is possible to visualize the three sublayers of the molecular layer (**Figure 10(b)**). The inner third of the molecular layer, next to the lightly colored granule cell layer, stains a reddish brown. The middle sublayer stains yellow, and the outer sublayer stains orange. Though the molecular layer mostly contains dendrites, there are a few cell types that stain for VIP, GABA, and parvalbumin. One interesting type of GABA-immunoreactive cell, with its soma in the molecular layer, has an axon restricted to the outer two-thirds of the molecular layer. Thus, its terminal field coincides with the perforant path terminations in the dentate molecular layer.

The polymorphic layer contains a number of cell types, but the best characterized is the mossy cell. These large multipolar cells are so named because of their large dendritic spines, the so-called thorny excrescences. The mossy fiber axons from the granule layer terminate on these spines. There are a number of interneurons with somata in the polymorphic layer that make inhibitory connections on the dentate granule cells. One such cell type is the hilar perforant-path (HIPP) associated cell, which has a dendritic tree in the polymorphic layer but extensive axonal arbor in the outer two-thirds of the molecular layer where the perforant path input terminates. Another type is the hilar commissural-associational pathway (HICAP) related cell, which innervates the inner molecular layer, the molecular layer perforant-path (MOPP) associated cell. The dendritic tree and axonal arbor of this cell occupy the outer two-thirds of the molecular layer, where the perforant path input terminates.

The entorhinal cortex provides the only cortical input to the dentate gyrus through the perforant pathway. There is substantial subcortical input from the septal nuclei, the hypothalamus, and the brain stem modulatory systems. The cholinergic input from the septal region originates in the medial septal nucleus and in the nucleus of the diagonal band of Broca. It is topographically organized such that cells in the medial septal areas tend to terminate septally, and cells in lateral septal structures terminate temporally. The projection terminates in the polymorphic layer. The primary hypothalamic input is from the supramamillary area and terminates in a narrow band of the molecular layer just superficial to the granule cell layer. This projection is probably excitatory and appears to target both granule cells and interneurons. The dentate gyrus receives input from each of the modulatory neurotransmitter systems in the brainstem. The noradrenergic input is from the pontine nucleus of the locus coeruleus and terminates in the polymorphic layer. The serotonergic input is from several of the raphe nuclei and also terminates in the polymorphic region. Minor dopaminergic inputs arise in the ventral tegmental area and the substantia nigra.

The only output of the dentate gyrus is the granule cell mossy fiber projection to CA3. Axon collaterals of each cell project to the full extent of the transverse axis. This is the one component of the hippocampal circuitry that does show a lamellar projection pattern. The fibers travel along or within the CA3 pyramidal layer, eventually reaching the stratum lucidum. In addition to the CA3 projection, the mossy fibers give rise to an associational connection consisting of about seven collaterals that terminate in the dentate gyrus polymorphic layer before entering CA3. The mossy fiber axons can be easily identified in Timm's preparations in which they stain very darkly (**Figure 10(b)**).

10.3.2 The Hippocampus Proper

The hippocampus proper consists of three fields. Proximal to distal from the dentate gyrus, they are the Ammon's horn fields CA3, CA2, and CA1 (**Figure 10**). Like the dentate gyrus, these fields are a three-layered cortex consisting of a principle layer located between cell-sparse layers. Deep to the principle cell layer is the stratum oriens. Superficial to the principle cell layer are the stratum radiatum and the stratum lacunosum-moleculare. CA3 has an additional thin layer, the stratum lucidum, which lies just superficial to the principle cell layer and deep to the stratum radiatum.

The principal cell layer consists, primarily, of pyramidal cells. The pyramidal cells in CA3 are larger and the layer thicker compared with CA1. The small and often-overlooked field CA2 contains larger pyramids, similar to CA3, but is similar to CA1 in other ways. For example, it lacks mossy fiber input. Each pyramidal cell has an apical dendritic arbor extending upward through the stratum radiatum and the stratum lacunosum-moleculare and a basal dendritic arbor extending into the stratum oriens. CA3 cells proximal to the dentate gyrus have smaller dendritic trees than the cells distal to the dentate gyrus, but overall, the dendritic arbors of cells in CA3 are larger than those in CA1. The dendritic arbors of pyramidal cells in CA2 are mixed, some with large arbors, similar to CA3, and some with small arbors, similar to CA1.

Interneurons undoubtedly play an important role in the regulation of local circuits in the hippocampus proper. Hippocampal interneurons differ in morphology, immunoreactivity, synaptic properties, laminar location, and connectivity. Hippocampal interneurons are GABAergic, but they may also be immunoreactive for somatostatin, neuropeptide Y, vasopressin, cholecystokinin, parvalbumin, calbindin, and calretinin. Most hippocampal interneurons have short axons, but there are also interneurons with long axons that project outside the hippocampal formation. We mention a few types here, but for a full discussion, see Freund and Buzsaki (1996).

One prominent interneuron type in the pyramidal cell layer is the chandelier or axo-axonic cell. The apical dendrites are radially oriented and span all superficial layers to the hippocampal fissure. The basal dendrites form a thick arbor in the stratum oriens. There is also a heterogeneous group of basket cells whose apical dendrites extend into the stratum moleculare and whose extensive basal dendrites span the entire depth of the stratum oriens. The axo-axonic cells and the basket cells are conveniently positioned to receive excitatory input from all afferents of the hippocampus proper.

Some hippocampal interneuron cell types have cell bodies in stratum oriens and innervate principal cell dendrites, similar to those described for the dentate gyrus. The oriens lacunosum-moleculare (O-LM) cells have a dense axonal arbor restricted to the stratum lacunosum moleculare. The dendritic tree is localized to layers that receive recurrent collaterals. There are many other interneuron types including the bistratisfied, horizontal trilaminar, and radial trilaminar cells.

The CA3 pyramidal cell axons are highly collateralized and project to all CA fields both ipsilaterally and contralaterally. There is also a small collateral projection to the polymorphic layer of the dentate gyrus. CA3 does not, however, project to the subiculum, presubiculum, parasubiculum, or entorhinal cortex. The projection to CA1 is called the Schaffer collateral projection, the projections to CA3/CA2 are called the associational projections, and the projections to contralateral structures are called the commissural projections. The Schaffer collateral projection exhibits a topography such that proximal CA3 cells (closer to the dentate gyrus) tend to project to levels of CA1 that extend farther in the septal than temporal directions. Distal CA3 cells (farther from the dentate gyrus) tend to project farther in the temporal direction. In addition, projections of proximal CA3 cells tend to terminate more superficially in stratum radiatum, whereas distal CA3 cells tend to terminate more deeply in stratum radiatum and in stratum oriens. The associational projections exhibit complex transverse and radial topographies, but in general the CA3-CA3 associational projections terminate extensively along the septotemporal axis (Witter and Amaral, 2004). The pattern of the terminations of the commissural projections mirrors those of the associational projections.

Extrinsic connections of CA3 are not robust except for the substantial projection to the lateral septal nucleus. The major subcortical input to CA3 is cholinergic and arises in the medial septal nucleus and the nucleus of the diagonal band of Broca. There is a GABAergic component of the projection that terminates primarily on the GABAergic interneurons of the stratum oriens. Temporal CA3 receives a minor input from the amygdala basal nucleus, which terminates in the stratum oriens and the stratum radiatum. Inputs from piriform cortex have also been reported. A noradrenergic projection arises in the locus coeruleus, and a serontonergic input arises in the raphe nucleus.

Field CA2 can be differentiated from CA3 by the lack of mossy fiber input and the associated thorny excrescences (**Figure 10(b)**). The pyramidal cell layer also stains more intensely for parvalbumin (**Figure 10(c)**). The intrinsic projections are similar to those of CA3, although the topographies may not be the same. For example, like CA3, CA2 also provides a small collateral projection back to the dentate gyrus. Not much is known specifically about CA2 extrinsic connections, but available evidence suggests that the region is differentiated from CA3 by hypothalamic input from the supramamillary area.

Field CA1 exhibits only a weak associational/commissural connection, a feature that is in striking contrast to the robust associational network present in CA3. This difference has been interpreted as underlying some of the putative functional differences in CA3 and CA1. Other intrahippocampal connections, however, are extensive. CA1 interneurons project to CA3 and to the polymorphic layer of the dentate gyrus. The major projection from CA1, however, is to the subiculum, and that projection exhibits a strict topography. Distal CA1 projects to proximal subiculum, and proximal CA1 projects to distal subiculum. The mid-CA1 projection terminates in midproximodistal subiculum.

Field CA1 receives substantial cortical and subcortical input from extrahippocampal structures. Cortical input arrives from the perirhinal, postrhinal, and entorhinal cortices. Subcortical input to CA1 is grossly similar to the subcortical input to CA3 but differs in the details. The septal input is weaker and terminates in stratum oriens. The input from the amygdala is more substantial, especially to distal CA1. Amygdala input arises in the basal and accessory basal nuclei. There is a prominent input from the nucleus reuniens of the thalamus that terminates in the stratum lacunosum moleculare. Like CA3, CA1 receives weak noradrenergic input from the locus coeruleus and weak serotonergic input from the raphe nucleus. There is also a weak dopaminergic input.

Of the hippocampal CA fields, CA1 has the more robust extrinsic projections. The cortical projections include the perirhinal, postrhinal, entorhinal, retrosplenial cortices, preinfralimbic, and medial prefrontal cortex. In general, the septal half projects more heavily to postrhinal cortex, the medial entorhinal area, and retrosplenial cortex, whereas the temporal half of CA1 projects more heavily to perirhinal cortex, the lateral entorhinal area, and infralimbic cortex. Temporal levels also project to the anterior olfactory nucleus, the hypothalamus, nucleus accumbens, and the basal nucleus of the amygdala.

10.3.3 The Subiculum

The subiculum is widely considered the output structure of the hippocampal formation. In this way, it differs from its parahippocampal neighbors, the pre- and parasubiculum, which are considered to be input structures. Like the CA fields of the hippocampus proper and the dentate gyrus, the subiculum is a three-layered cortex with a deep, polymorphic layer, a pyramidal cell layer containing the principle cells, and a molecular layer, which is continuous with the stratum lacunosum moleculare of field CA1. The subiculum can be distinguished from the proximally situated CA1 and the distally situated presubiculum by a principle cell layer that is more loosely packed. The border with CA1 is further demarcated by the widening of the middle layer of the subiculum.

The principle cell layer contains large pyramidal cells. The basal dendrites terminate in the deep part of the principle layer, and the apical dendrites extend into the molecular layer. The pyramidal cells are large and of uniform shape. Electrophysiological findings suggest that there are two populations of pyramids, though they cannot be distinguished morphologically. So-called regular spiking cells tend to be located superficially, and bursting cells tend to be located deep in the layer. Although both types are projection cells, it is possible that only the bursting cells project to the entorhinal cortex. Among the pyramids are numerous smaller cells, probably representing varied types of interneurons. Perforant pathway fibers contact GABAergic cells that stain for parvalbumin. Not much is known about subicular interneurons, but in general, the population of interneurons appears similar to that observed in field CA1 (Witter and Amaral, 2004).

The associational connections of the subiculum extend temporally from the point of origin and terminate in all layers. There is no commissural projection. There are also local associational connections confined to the pyramidal layer and the deepest part of the molecular layer. The available data suggests that the bursting pyramidal cells form a columnar network that is roughly interconnected.

Connections of the subiculum with other hippocampal structures is limited to input from CA1, which is massive. The projection exhibits a topography such that proximal CA1 projects to distal subiculum, midproximodistal CA1 projects to midsubiculum, and distal CA1 projects to proximal subiculum. The projection is not truly lamellar, however, as any part of CA1 projects to about one-third of the septotemporal extent of the subiculum.

The parahippocampal connections of the subiculum are more diverse, but the best-characterized projection is to deep layers of entorhinal cortex. Septal levels of the subiculum provide substantial input to the lateral and medial entorhinal cortices. Septal subicular input to the postrhinal cortex is equally strong, but input to perirhinal cortex, especially area 35, is modest. Temporal subiculum provides massive input to the entorhinal cortex and moderate input to perirhinal and postrhinal cortices. The subiculum also receives a substantial input from the entorhinal cortex. The entorhinal lateral band projects more strongly to septal subiculum, and the entorhinal intermediate and medial bands project more strongly to temporal subiculum. There is also modest input from the perirhinal and postrhinal cortices. Perirhinal cortex projects relatively more strongly to temporal subiculum, and the postrhinal cortex projects relatively more strongly to septal subiculum. The subiculum also projects heavily to the pre- and parasubicular cortices, though the return projections are modest (O'Mara et al., 2001).

The most prominent neocortical projections are to retrosplenial and prefrontal cortices. The distal and septal part of the subiculum projects to the ventral retrosplenial cortex. The presubiculum projections to frontal areas include the medial orbital, prelimbic, infralimbic, and anterior cingulate cortices. The retrosplenial projection is reciprocated, but available evidence suggests that the frontal projections are not.

The diverse subcortical projections target the septal complex, the amygdala, the nucleus accumbens, the hypothalamus, and the thalamus. All septotemporal levels of the subiculum project to the lateral septum, but the projection arises primarily in the proximal part. Septal input arises mainly in the nucleus of the diagonal band. The amygdala projection arises primarily in the temporal subiculum and targets the posterior and basolateral nuclei. The projection to the nucleus accumbens is topographic such that the proximal part of the septal subiculum projects to rostrolateral nucleus accumbens, and the proximal part of the temporal subiculum projects to the caudomedial nucleus accumbens. The hypothalamic projection also arises primarily in the temporal subiculum. It terminates in the medial preoptic area and the ventromedial, dorsomedial, and ventral premammillary nuclei. Finally, there are documented connections with thalamic nuclei, though the details are not well described. The proximal part of the septal subiculum projects to the anteromedial nucleus of the thalamus, but the distal part projects to the anterior thalamic complex. The latter projection is reciprocated. Temporal subiculum receives input from the nucleus reuniens. Available evidence suggests that the anteroventral nucleus of the thalamus also projects to the subiculum.

10.4 Conclusions

10.4.1 The Flow of Sensory Information through the Hippocampal System

The entorhinal cortex is widely recognized as the primary way station for sensory information on its way from the neocortex to the hippocampus. Much of the neocortical input arrives by way of the perirhinal and postrhinal cortices, but there are also direct neocortical inputs to the entorhinal cortex. The presubiculum and parasubiculum are also considered input structures for the hippocampal memory system. The distinct patterns of cortical afferentation to parahippocampal structures, the intrinsic connections, and the topography of the parahippocampal–hippocampal connections suggest that parahippocampal structures are involved in the preprocessing of sensory information provided to the hippocampus, and that there is functional diversity within the parahippocampal region. The view that parahippocampal structures have different functions is consistent with emerging evidence that there is also substantial functional diversity among hippocampal formation structures.

In **Figure 11**, we have attempted to schematize the flow of sensory information through the hippocampal memory system. Beginning with the input structures, perirhinal area 36 receives sensory input from visual, auditory, and somatosensory regions. Longitudinal intrinsic connections integrate across modalities before transmission to perirhinal area 35. This polymodal input to area 35 is joined by olfactory information and then passed on to entorhinal cortex, primarily the lateral band of the LEA. The postrhinal cortex receives visual and visuospatial input from posterior parietal, retrosplenial, and visual association regions, along with a small input from auditory association cortex. That information is integrated and transmitted to entorhinal cortex, primarily to the lateral band of the MEA. Presubiculum is targeted by the subiculum in a topographical manner such that septotemporal levels of the subiculum map onto septotemporal levels of the presubiculum. Subicular input is integrated with direct visuospatial input to the presubiculum, especially the septal component. That information is forwarded to the parasubiculum, the postrhinal cortex, and the MEA.

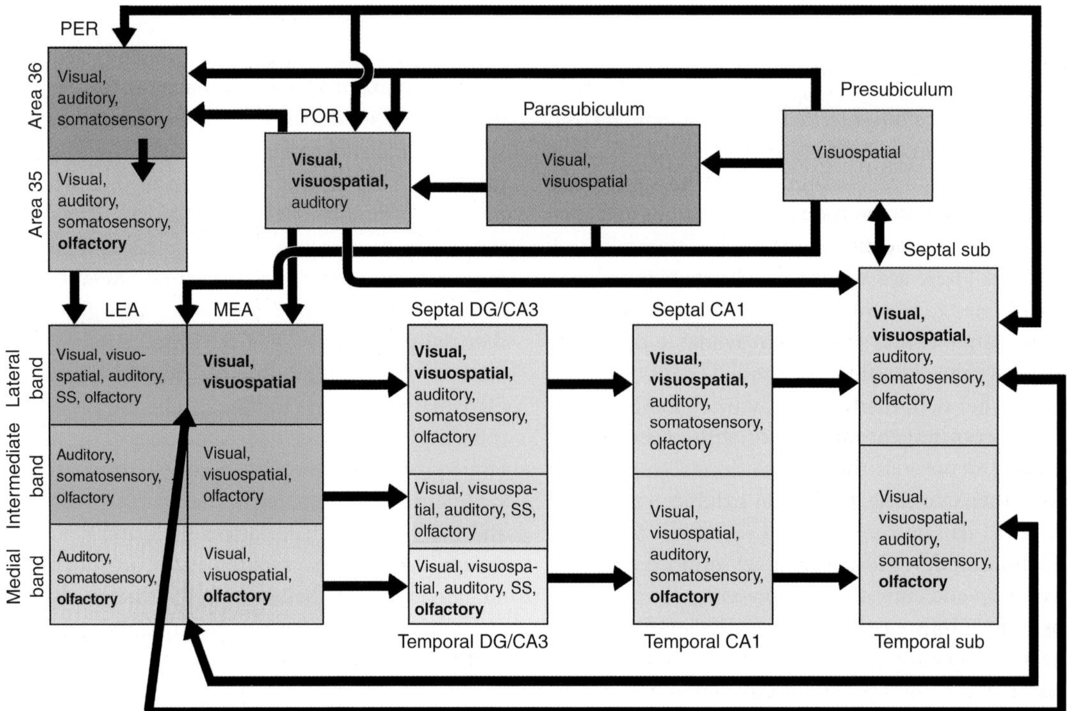

Figure 11 Diagram of the flow of sensory information through the hippocampal memory system. Black arrows indicate the primary pathways by which sensory information traverses the hippocampal memory system. Note that only the stronger connections are indicated and that emphasis is on the feedforward connections as opposed to the feedback connections. Abbreviations: CA, CA field; DG, dentate gyrus; LEA, lateral entorhinal area; MEA, medial entorhinal area; PER, perirhinal cortex; POR, postrhinal cortex; sub, subiculum.

The most septal component of the presubiculum, the area sometimes termed the postsubiculum, projects massively to the postrhinal cortex. Finally, the parasubiculum, which receives direct, but modest, visual and visuospatial input along with its subicular input, projects to postrhinal cortex and the MEA.

To summarize, information from all modalities reaches the full septotemporal extent of the hippocampus, but the degree of processing of different modalities is weighted differently along the septotemporal axis. Visual and visuospatial input is processed and elaborated along a pathway that includes the postrhinal cortex, lateral MEA, the septal hippocampal formation, septal presubiculum, parasubiculum, and then back to postrhinal cortex and lateral MEA. Olfactory information is less segregated but follows a pathway that includes the perirhinal cortex, medial LEA, and temporal hippocampal formation structures. Thus, there appears to be functional diversity in the processing of sensory information that is organized along the septotemporal axis; visual and visuospatial information is predominant in the septal hippocampus, and olfactory information is predominant in the temporal hippocampus.

10.4.2 The Comparative Anatomy of the Hippocampal System

As indicated earlier, all components of the parahippocampal region and the hippocampal formation are represented in both the rodent and the primate brain. Many of the connectional principles are also conserved. Taking into account the differences in brain size and sensory processing needs, cortical afferentation of the parahippocampal structures is similar across species. Additionally, the available evidence suggests that the architecture of the perforant pathway is similar in the primate and rodent brains. In the monkey and the rat, the perforant pathway projections to the dentate gyrus, CA3, and CA2 originate in layer II of the entorhinal cortex. Also in both, the projections to CA1 and the subiculum originate in layer III. In addition, the terminations of the projections originating in entorhinal layer III exhibit a transverse topography. The rostral entorhinal cortex in the monkey and the lateral entorhinal area in the rat project to the border of the CA1 and subiculum; the caudal entorhinal cortex in the monkey and the medial entorhinal area in the rat project to proximal CA1 and distal subiculum (Witter, 1986, 1993, Amaral, 1993). The intrinsic connections of the monkey entorhinal cortex also exhibit patterns similar to the lateral to medial bands of intrinsic connectivity observed in the rodent entorhinal cortex. Taken together, the evidence suggests that both the rat and monkey hippocampal memory systems are excellent models for the medial temporal lobe memory system in the human brain.

References

Amaral DG (1993) Emerging principles of intrinsic hippocampal organization. *Curr. Opin. Neurobiol.* 3: 225–229.

Amaral DG, Insausti R, and Cowan WM (1987) The entorhinal cortex of the monkey: I. Cytoarchitectonic organization. *J. Comp. Neurol.* 264: 326–355.

Anderson P, Bliss TV, and Skrede KK (1971) Lamellar organization of hippocampal pathways. *Exp. Brain Res.* 13: 222–38.

Brodmann K (1909) *Vergleichende Lokalisationslehre der Grosshirnrinde in ihren Prinzipien dargestellt auf Grund des Zellenbaues*. Liepzig: Barth.

Burwell RD (2001) The perirhinal and postrhinal cortices of the rat: Borders and cytoarchitecture. *J. Comp. Neurol.* 437: 17–41.

Burwell RD and Witter MP (2002) Basic anatomy of the parahippocampal region in monkeys and rats. In: Witter MP and Wouterlood FG (eds.) *The Parahippocampal Region, Organization and Role in Cognitive Functions*. London: Oxford University Press.

Burwell RD, Witter MP, and Amaral DG (1995) The perirhinal and postrhinal cortices of the rat: A review of the neuroanatomical literature and comparison with findings from the monkey brain. *Hippocampus* 5: 390–408.

Dolorfo CL and Amaral DG (1998) Entorhinal cortex of the rat: Organization of intrinsic connections. *J. Comp. Neurol.* 398: 49–82.

Eichenbaum H, Otto T, and Cohen NJ (1994) Two functional components of the hippocampal memory system. *Behav. Brain Sci.* 17: 449–518.

Freund TF and Buzsaki G (1996) Interneurons of the hippocampus. *Hippocampus,* 6: 347–470.

Insausti R, Herrero MT, and Witter MP (1997) Entorhinal cortex of the rat: Cytoarchitectonic subdivisions and the origin and distribution of cortical efferents. *Hippocampus* 7: 146–183.

Insausti R, Tuñón T, Sobreviela T, Insausti AM, and Gonsalo LM (1995) The human entorhinal cortex: A cytoarchitectonic analysis. *J. Comp. Neurol.* 355: 171–198.

Krieg WJS (1946) Connections of the cerebral cortex. I. The albino rat. B. Structure of the cortical areas. *J. Comp. Neurol.* 84: 277–323.

O'Mara SM, Commins S, Anderson M, and Gigg J (2001) The subiculum: A review of form, physiology and function. *Prog. Neurobiol.* 64: 129–55.

Pikkarainen M and Pitkanen A (1999) Projections from the lateral, basal, and accessory basal nuclei of the amygdala to the hippocampal formation in rat. *J. Comp. Neurol.* 403: 229–260.

Ramón y Cajal S (1909) *Histologie du systáeme nerveux de l'homme and des vertâebrâes*. Paris: Maloine.

Scoville WB and Milner B (1957) Loss of recent memory after bilateral hippocampal lesions. *J. Neurol. Neurosurg. Psychiatry* 20: 11–21.

Squire LR and Zola-Morgan S (1991) The medial temporal lobe memory system. *Science* 253: 1380–6.

Suzuki WA and Amaral DG (2003a) Perirhinal and parahippocampal cortices of the macaque monkey: Cytoarchitectonic and chemoarchitectonic organization. *J. Comp. Neurol.* 463: 67–91.

Suzuki WA and Amaral DG (2003b) Where are the perirhinal and parahippocampal cortices? A historical overview of the nomenclature and boundaries applied to the primate medial temporal lobe. *Neuroscience* 120: 893–906.

Van Hoesen GW and Pandya DN (1975) Some connections of the entorhinal (area 28) and perirhinal (area 35) cortices of the rhesus monkey. I. Temporal lobe afferents. *Brain Res.* 95: 1–24.

Von Bonin G and Bailey P (1947) *The Neocortex of Macaca Mulatta*. Urbana: University of Illinois Press.

Von Economo C (1929) *The Cytoarchitectonics of the Human Cerebral Cortex*. London: Oxford University Press.

Witter MP (1986) A survey of the anatomy of the hippocampal formation, with emphasis on the septotemporal organization of its intrinsic and extrinsic connections. *Adv. Exp. Med. Biol.* 203: 67–82.

Witter MP (1993) Organization of the entorhinal-hippocampal system: A review of the current anatomical data. *Hippocampus* 3: 33–44.

Witter MP and Amaral DG (2004) Hippocampal Formation. In: Paxinos G (ed.) *The Rat Nervous System,* 3rd edn. San Diego, CA: Academic Press.

11 Long-Term Potentiation: A Candidate Cellular Mechanism for Information Storage in the CNS

J. D. Sweatt, University of Alabama at Birmingham, Birmingham, AL, USA

In a very practical way, this chapter is a transition point for this volume. With this chapter, we transition from analyzing behavior to investigating cellular and molecular mechanisms for altering synaptic strength. We transition to attempting to understand mammalian memory by the reductionist approach of studying a simpler cellular phenomenon at the molecular level. Thus, this chapter will serve to place the many molecular details presented in other chapters into a broader context. In addition, wherever possible this chapter will be used as a launching point for further reading of other chapters in the volume by specifically citing other chapters at appropriate points along the way.

The particular circuits and neuronal connections that underlie most forms of mammalian learning and memory are mysterious at present, especially for hippocampus-dependent forms of learning. There is little understanding of the means by which complex memories are stored and recalled at the neural circuit level – this will be a very important avenue of future research. Thus in many ways the study of long-term potentiation (LTP) serves as a surrogate for studying hippocampus-dependent memory directly. LTP can only be viewed as a surrogate at present because very few studies are available directly implicating LTP (especially hippocampal LTP, which has been most widely studied) in defined memory behaviors. Even considering the vast number of published studies of LTP, we are left with a tentative causal link between LTP and memory *per se*.

Nevertheless, this chapter will focus on LTP. We will focus on it for three main reasons. First, it has been extensively studied and is the form of synaptic plasticity that is best understood at the molecular level. Second, it is a robust form of synaptic plasticity and worthy of investigation in its own right. Finally, it is a specific candidate cellular mechanism for mediating certain forms of associative learning, spatial learning, and adaptive change in the central nervous system (CNS), in particular in the amygdala, hippocampus, and cerebral cortex, respectively.

11.1 Hebb's Postulate

Despite the various caveats concerning the specific role of LTP in hippocampus-dependent memory formation, there is a general hypothesis for memory storage that is available and broadly accepted. This hypothesis is the following:

> Memories are stored as alterations in the strength of synaptic connections between neurons in the CNS.

The significance of this general hypothesis should be emphasized – this is one of the few areas of contemporary cognitive research for which there is a unifying hypothesis.

This general hypothesis has a solid underlying rationale. Learning and memory manifest themselves as a change in an animal's behavior, and scientists capitalize on this to study these phenomena by observing and measuring changes in an animal's behavior in the wild or in experimental situations. However, all the behavior exhibited by an animal is a result of activity in the animal's nervous system. The nervous system comprises many kinds of cells, but the primary functional units of the nervous system are neurons. Because neurons are cells, all of an animal's behavioral repertoire is a manifestation of an underlying cellular phenomenon. By extension, changes in an animal's behavior such as occurs with learning must also be subserved by an underlying cellular change.

In general, the vast majority of the communication between neurons in the nervous system occurs at synapses. As synapses mediate the neuron–neuron communication that underlies an animal's behavior, changes in behavior are ultimately subserved by alterations in the nature, strength, or number of interneuronal synaptic contacts in the animal's nervous system. The capacity for alterations of synaptic connections between neurons is referred to as *synaptic plasticity*, and as described earlier, one of the great unifying theories to emerge from neuroscience research in the last century was that synaptic plasticity subserves learning and memory. LTP (of some sort at least) is the specific form of synaptic plasticity that is the leading candidate as a mechanism subserving behavior-modifying changes in synaptic strength that mediate higher-order learning and memory in mammals.

One of the pioneers in advancing the idea that changes in neuronal connectivity are a mechanism for memory was the Canadian psychologist Donald Hebb, who published his seminal formulation as what is now generally known as Hebb's postulate:

> When an axon of cell A . . . excites cell B and repeatedly or persistently takes part in firing it, some growth process or metabolic change takes place in one or both cells so that A's efficiency as one of the cells firing B is increased. (Hebb, 1949)

Note the important contrast between Hebb's postulate and its popular contemporary formulation – one (Hebb's) specifies cell firing, and the other (the modern formulation) specifies synaptic change. These two phenomena are clearly different, and the current, exclusively synaptic, variant is incomplete. Changes in synapses are certainly important in information storage in the CNS, but we need to consider that the postsynaptic receptors sit in a membrane whose biophysical properties are carefully controlled. Regulation of membrane sodium channels, chloride channels, and potassium channels also contributes significantly to the net effect in the cell that any neurotransmitter-operated process can achieve.

Thus, limitations arise from ignoring potential long-term regulation of membrane biophysical properties. We need to consider that local changes in dendritic membrane excitability may be involved in cellular information processing and also that global changes in cellular excitability that alter the likelihood of the cell firing an action potential may also be a mechanism for information storage. These topics are addressed elsewhere in this volume (*See* Chapter 14). Another potential mechanism involved in memory that involves the entire cell and not specific synapses is adult neurogenesis, the growth and functional integration of new neurons in the adult CNS. Neurogenesis will be addressed in other chapters (*See* Chapter 36). Finally, one can think of inhibition (e.g., GABAergic (GABA: gamma-aminobutyric acid) modulation) as operating above the level of the single synapse because it can control the likelihood of the cell firing an action potential.

The possibility that global or cellwide alterations might be involved in memory is also relevant when considering global genomic (transcriptional) and epigenomic changes, which affect the nucleus and thereby potentially the entire cell as well. These mechanisms are discussed elsewhere (*See* Chapter 36). One solution to the problem of global changes due to altered transcription is specific trafficking of the products of global changes in transcription.

The idea of the involvement of processes such as excitability in memory, processes that encompass the entire cell, has been criticized as too limiting because with global changes in excitability, one loses the computational power of selectively altering the response at a single synaptic input (i.e., synapse specificity). However, we don't know how the neuron or the CNS computes a memory output. The fundamental unit of information storage may not be the synapse but the neuron. Future experiments will be necessary to resolve this issue, but it is nevertheless worthwhile to keep in mind the possibility that regulation of excitability, and regulation of neuronal properties cellwide, as well as the more typically considered alterations in synaptic connections, may play roles in memory storage.

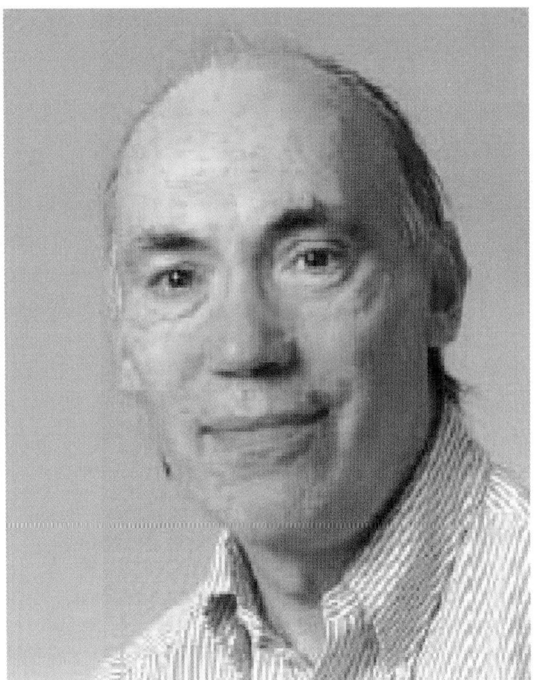

Figure 1 T. V. P. Bliss, *FRS*. Photo courtesy of Tim Bliss.

11.2 A Breakthrough Discovery – LTP in the Hippocampus

As a young postdoctoral researcher, Tim Bliss (**Figure 1**) set out to find a long-lasting form of synaptic plasticity in the hippocampus. By teaming up with Terje Lomo in Per Anderson's laboratory in Oslo, Bliss did just that. The seminal report by Bliss and Lomo in 1973, describing a phenomenon they termed long-term potentiation of synaptic transmission, set the stage for what is now over three decades of progress in understanding the basics of long-term synaptic alteration in the CNS.

In their experiments, Bliss and Lomo recorded synaptic responses in the dentate gyrus, stimulating the perforant path inputs from the entorhinal cortex (Bliss and Lomo, 1973). They used extracellular stimulating and recording electrodes implanted into the animal, and the basic experiment was begun by recording baseline synaptic transmission in this pathway. They discovered that a brief period of high-frequency (100-Hz 'tetanic') stimulation led to a robust increase in the strength of synaptic connections between the perforant path inputs from the entorhinal cortex onto the dentate granule neurons in the dentate gyrus (**Figure 2**). They also observed an increased likelihood of the cells firing action potentials in response to a constant synaptic input, a phenomenon they termed E-S (excitatory postsynaptic potential (EPSP)-to-spike) potentiation. These two phenomena together were termed LTP. LTP lasted many, many hours in this intact rabbit preparation. The appeal of LTP as an analog of memory was immediately apparent – it is a long-lasting change in neuronal function that is produced by a brief period of unique stimulus, exactly the sort of mechanism that had long been postulated to be involved in memory formation. This pioneering work of Bliss and Lomo set in motion a several-decades-long pursuit by numerous investigators geared toward understanding the attributes and mechanisms of LTP.

11.2.1 The Hippocampal Circuit and Measuring Synaptic Transmission in the Hippocampal Slice

Bliss and Lomo did their experiment using the intact rabbit, stimulating and recording in the anesthetized animal using implanted electrodes. In recent times, this preparation has been largely supplanted by the use of recordings from hippocampal slices maintained *in vitro* (**Figure 3**). Because most of the LTP

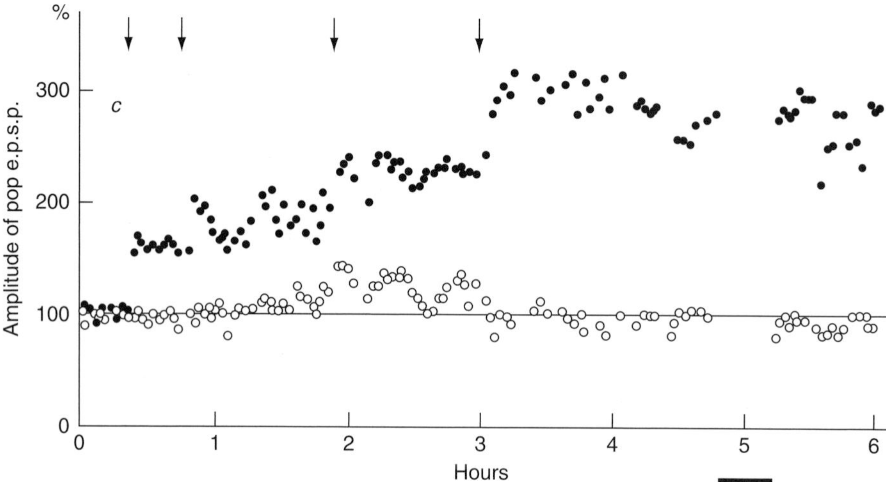

Figure 2 Bliss and Lomo's first published LTP experiment. As described in more detail in the text, in this pioneering work Tim Bliss and Terje Lomo demonstrated LTP of synaptic transmission. This specific experiment investigated synaptic transmission at perforant path inputs into the dentate gyrus (see **Figure 4**). Arrows indicate the delivery of high-frequency synaptic stimulation, resulting in LTP. Filled circles are responses from the tetanized pathways; open circles are a control pathway that did not receive tetanic stimulation. The bar, where no data points are available, indicates a period of time where Tim Bliss fell asleep. Data acquisition in this era involved the investigator directly measuring by hand synaptic responses from an oscilloscope screen. Moreover, it was not unusual for experiments to extend overnight due to the long amount of time involved in preparing the rabbit for the experiment, implanting the electrodes into the brain, and establishing a stable recording configuration. From Bliss TV and Lomo T (1973) Long-lasting potentiation of synaptic transmission in the dentate area of the anaesthetized rabbit following stimulation of the perforant path. *J. Physiol.* 232: 331–356. Used with permission.

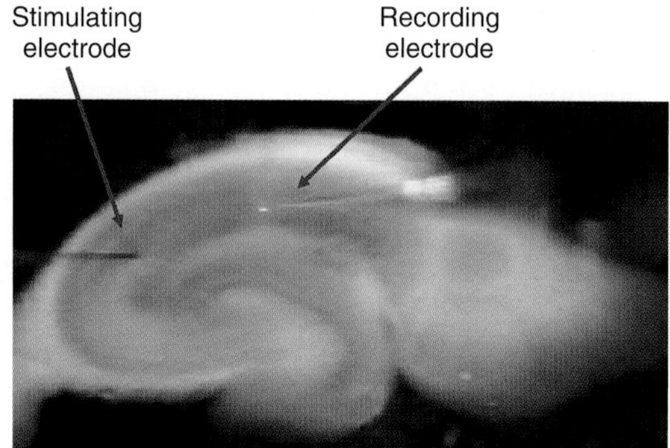

Figure 3 Electrodes in a living hippocampal slice. This photograph illustrates the appearance of a mouse hippocampal slice, maintained in a recording chamber. Responses in area CA1 are recorded using a saline-filled glass micropipette electrode (right) and a bipolar platinum stimulating electrode (left). See text and **Figure 4** for additional details.

experiments that will be described in the rest of the book come from this type of preparation, the next section will describe the hippocampal neuronal and synaptic circuit and give an overview of extracellular recording in a typical LTP experiment.

The main information processing circuit in the hippocampus is the relatively simple trisynaptic pathway, and much of this basic circuit is preserved in transverse slices across the long axis of the hippocampus (**Figure 4**). Various types of LTP can be induced at all three of these synaptic sites, and we will discuss later some mechanistic differences among the various types of LTP that can be induced. Most experiments on the basic attributes and mechanisms of LTP have been studies of the synaptic connections between axons from area CA3 pyramidal neurons that extend into area CA1. These are the synapses onto CA1 pyramidal neurons that are known as the Schaffer collateral inputs.

The main excitatory (i.e., glutamatergic) synaptic circuitry in the hippocampus, in overview, consists of three modules (see **Figure 4**) (van Groen and Wyss, 1990; Johnston and Amaral., 1998; Naber and Witter, 1998). Information enters the dentate gyrus of the hippocampal formation from cortical and subcortical structures via the perforant path inputs from the entorhinal cortex (**Figure 4**). These inputs make synaptic connections with the dentate granule cells of the dentate gyrus. After synapsing in the dentate gyrus, information is moved to area CA3 via the mossy fiber pathway, which consists of the axonal outputs of the dentate granule cells and their connections with pyramidal neurons in area CA3. After

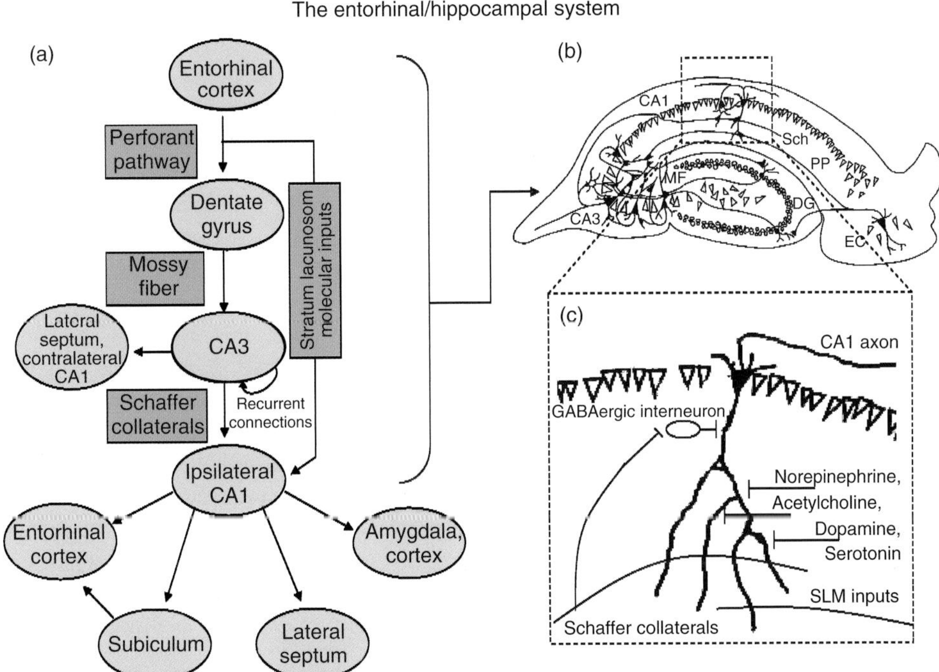

Figure 4 The entorhinal/hippocampal system. (a) This panel diagrams the principal inputs, outputs, and intrinsic connections. (b) In this panel, the central components of the circuit are delineated in a more anatomically correct fashion, illustrating the principal intrinsic connections of the dentate gyrus and hippocampus proper. (c) This is an expansion of area CA1 showing some of the synaptic inputs onto a single pyramidal neuron in area CA1. See text for additional details. Diagram by J. David Sweatt and Sarah E. Brown. Hippocampal diagram from Johnston D and Wu SM (1995) *Foundations of Cellular Neurophysiology*, p. 433. Cambridge, MA: MIT Press. Used with permission.

synapsing in area CA3, information is moved to area CA1 via the Schaffer collateral path, which consists largely of the axons of area CA3 pyramidal neurons along with other projections from area CA3 of the contralateral hippocampus as well. After synapsing in CA1, information exits the hippocampus via projections from CA1 pyramidal neurons and returns to subcortical and cortical structures.

The connections in this synaptic circuit are retained in a fairly impressive manner if one makes transverse slices of the hippocampus, as the inputs, 'trisynaptic circuit,' and outputs are laid out in a generally laminar fashion along the long axis of the hippocampal formation. This is a great advantage for *in vitro* electrophysiological experiments.

It is important to emphasize that the trisynaptic circuit outlined earlier is a great oversimplification, as there are a great many additional synaptic components of the hippocampus. For example, inhibitory GABAergic interneurons make synaptic connections with all of the principal excitatory neurons outlined earlier. These GABAergic inputs serve in both a feedforward and feedback fashion to control excitability. There are many recurrent and collateral excitatory connections between the excitatory pyramidal neurons as well, particularly in the area CA3 region. There is a direct projection from the entorhinal cortex to the distal regions of CA1 pyramidal neuron dendrites, a pathway known as the stratum lacunosum moleculare.

Finally, there are many modulatory projections into the hippocampus that make synaptic connections with the principal neurons (see **Figure 4**). These inputs are via long projection fibers from various anatomical nuclei in the brainstem region, and they are generally not directly excitatory or inhibitory, but rather serve to modulate synaptic connectivity in a fairly subtle way. There are four predominant extrinsic modulatory projections into the hippocampus. First, there are inputs of norepinephrine (NE)-containing fibers that project from the locus ceruleus. Second, there are dopamine (DA)-containing fibers that arise from the substantia nigra. There also are inputs using acetylcholine (ACh) from the medial septal nucleus and 5-hydroxytryptamine (5HT, serotonin) from the raphe nuclei.

11.2.2 LTP of Synaptic Responses

In a popular variation of the basic LTP experiment, extracellular field potential recordings in the dendritic regions of area CA1 are utilized to monitor synaptic transmission at Schaffer collateral synapses (see **Figure 5**). A bipolar stimulating electrode is placed in the *stratum radiatum* subfield of area CA1 and stimuli (typically constant current pulses ranging from 1 to 30 μA) are delivered. Stimuli delivered in this fashion stimulate the output axons of CA3 neurons that pass nearby, causing action potentials to propagate down these axons. Cellular responses to this stimulation are recorded using extracellular or intracellular electrophysiologic recording techniques.

The typical waveform in an extracellular recording consists of a fiber volley, which is an indication of the presynaptic action potential arriving at the recording site and the excitatory postsynaptic potential (EPSP) itself. The EPSP responses are a manifestation of synaptic activation (depolarization) in the CA1 pyramidal neurons. For measuring field (i.e., extracellularly recorded) EPSPs, the parameter typically measured is the initial slope of the EPSP waveform (see **Figure 5**). Absolute peak amplitude of EPSPs can also be measured, but the initial slope is the preferred index. This is because the initial slope is less subject to contamination from other sources of current flow in the slice. For example, currents are generated by feedforward inhibition due to GABAergic neuron activation. Also, if the cells fire action potentials, this also can contaminate later stages of the EPSP, even when one is recording from the dendritic region.

Extracellular field recordings measure responses from a population of neurons, so EPSPs recorded in this fashion are referred to as population EPSPs (pEPSPs). Note that pEPSPs are downward deflecting for stratum radiatum recordings (see **Figure 5**). If one is recording from the cell body layer (stratum pyramidale), the EPSP is an upward deflection, and if

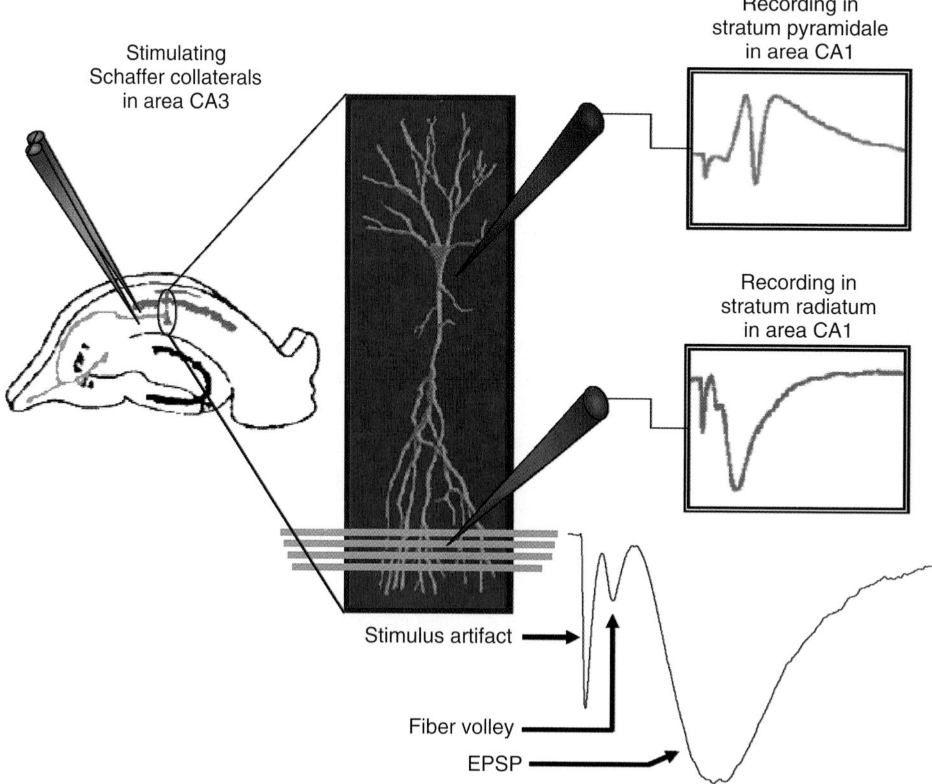

Figure 5 Recording configuration and typical physiologic responses in a hippocampal slice recording experiment. Electrode placements and responses from stratum pyramidale (cell body layer) and stratum radiatum (dendritic regions) are shown. In addition, the typical waveform of a population excitatory postsynaptic potential (EPSP) is illustrated, showing the stimulus artifact, fiber volley, and population EPSP. Figure and data by Joel Selcher.

the cells fire action potentials, the EPSP has superimposed on it a downward deflecting spike, the population spike. As mentioned earlier, for both stratum radiatum and stratum pyramidale recordings the EPSP slope measurements are taken as early as possible after the fiber volley to eliminate contamination by population spikes.

As a prelude to starting an LTP experiment, input-output (I/O) functions for stimulus intensity versus EPSP magnitude are recorded in response to increasing intensities of stimulation (see **Figure 6**). For the remainder of the experiment, the test stimulus intensity is set to elicit an EPSP that is approximately 35–50% of the maximum response

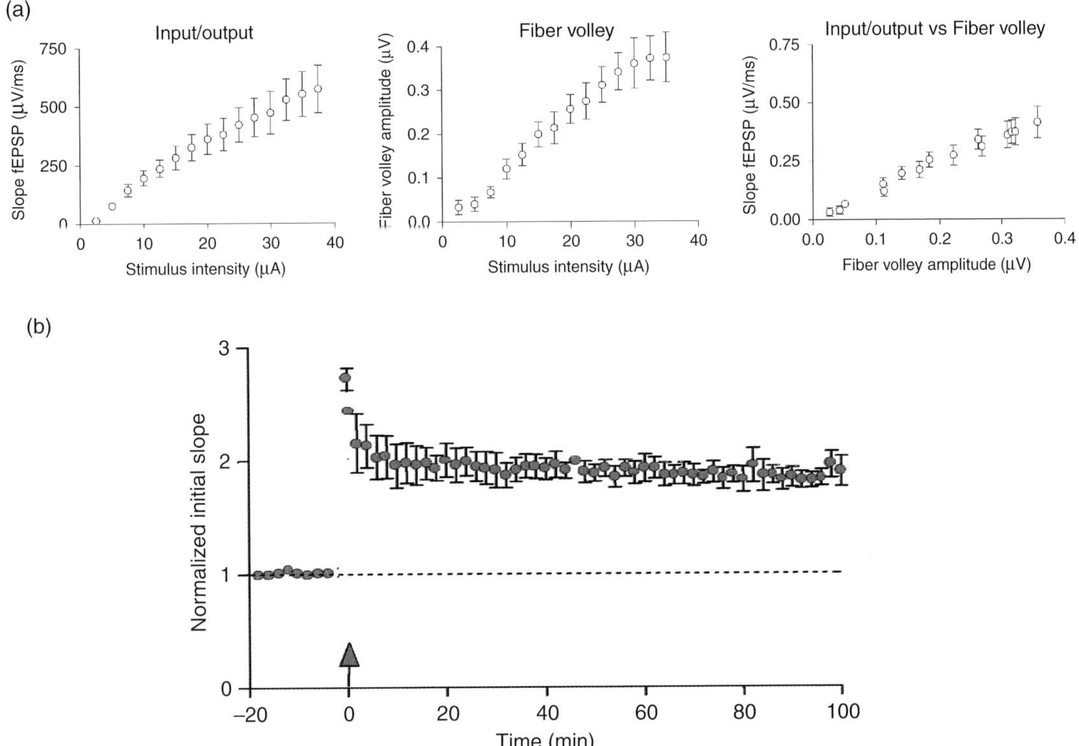

Figure 6 An input-output curve and typical LTP experiment. (a) The relationship of EPSP magnitude (field EPSP, EPSP) versus stimulus intensity (in microamperes), and the same data converted to an input-output relationship for EPSP versus fiber volley magnitude to allow an evaluation of postsynaptic response versus presynaptic response in the same hippocampal slice. (b) A typical high-frequency stimulation-induced potentiation of synaptic transmission in area CA1 of a rat hippocampal slice *in vitro*. The arrow indicates the delivery of 100-Hz (100 pulses/second) synaptic stimulation. Data courtesy of Ed Weeber and Coleen Atkins. In most pharmacologic experiments using physiologic recordings in hippocampal slice preparations, effects of drug application on baseline synaptic transmission can be evaluated by simply monitoring EPSPs before and after drug application, using a constant stimulus intensity. A more elaborate alternative is to produce input-output curves for EPSP initial slope (or magnitude) versus stimulus intensity for the presynaptic stimulus. These types of within-slice experiments are very straightforward, but in some experimental comparisons, this type of within-preparation design is not possible. For example, if one is comparing a wild type with a knockout animal, there of necessity must be a comparison across preparations. How does one evaluate if there is a difference in basal synaptic transmission in this situation? The principal confound is because although one has control over magnitude of the stimulus one delivers to the presynaptic fibers, differences in electrode placement, slice thickness, etc., from preparation to preparation cause variability in the magnitude of the synaptic response elicited by a constant stimulus amplitude. One commonly used approach to compare from one preparation (or animal strain) to the next is to quantitate the EPSP relative to the amplitude of the fiber volley in that same hippocampal slice. The rationale is that the fiber volley, which represents the action potentials firing in the presynaptic fibers, is a presynaptic physiologic response from within the same slice and that one can at least normalize the EPSP to a within-slice parameter. The underlying assumption is that the magnitude of the fiber volley is representative of the number of axons firing an action potential. Although not a perfect control, evaluating input-output relationships for fiber volley magnitude versus EPSP is a great improvement when making comparisons between different types of animals. If differences are observed, an increase in the fiber volley amplitude – EPSP slope relationship suggests an augmentation of synaptic transmission.

recorded during the I/O measurements. Baseline synaptic transmission at this constant test stimulus intensity is usually monitored for a period of 15–20 min to ensure a stable response.

Once the health of the hippocampal slice is confirmed as indicated by a stable baseline synaptic response, LTP can be induced using any one of a wide variety of different LTP induction protocols. Many popular variations include a single or repeated period of 1-s, 100-Hz stimulation (with delivery of the 100-Hz trains separated by 20 s or more) where stimulus intensity is at a level necessary for approximately half-maximal stimulation (see **Figure 6**). A variation is a strong induction protocol where LTP is induced with three pairs of 100-Hz, 1-s stimuli, where stimulus intensity is near that necessary for a maximal EPSP. This latter protocol gives robust LTP that lasts for essentially as long as one can keep the hippocampal slice alive. A final major variation is high-frequency stimulation patterned after the endogenous hippocampal theta rhythm; this will be described in more detail in a later section of this chapter.

11.2.3 Short-Term Plasticity: PTP and PPF

Two types of short-term plasticity are exhibited at hippocampal Schaffer collateral synapses and elsewhere that are activity dependent, just as is LTP. These are paired-pulse facilitation (PPF) and posttetanic potentiation (PTP). PPF is a form of short-term synaptic plasticity that is commonly held to be due to residual calcium augmenting neurotransmitter release presynaptically. When two single-stimulus pulses are applied with interpulse intervals ranging from 20 to 300 ms, the second EPSP produced is larger than the first (see **Figure 7**). This effect is referred to as PPF. The role of this type of synaptic plasticity in the behaving animal is unknown at this time; however, it clearly is a robust form of temporal integration of synaptic transmission and could be used in information processing behaviorally. The second form of short-term plasticity, PTP, is a large enhancement of synaptic efficacy observed after brief periods of high-frequency synaptic activity. For example, in experiments where LTP is induced with one or two 1-s, 100-Hz tetani, a large and transient increase in synaptic efficacy is produced immediately after high-frequency tetanus (see **Figure 7**). This is PTP. The mechanisms for PTP are unknown, but both PTP and PPF are *N*-methyl-D-aspartate (NMDA) receptor-independent phenomena.

11.3 NMDA Receptor Dependence of LTP

In 1983, Graham Collingridge made the breakthrough discovery that induction of these tetanus-induced forms of LTP is blocked by a blockade of a specific subtype of glutamate receptor, the NMDA receptor (Collingridge et al., 1983). Collingridge's fascinating discovery was that the glutamate analog

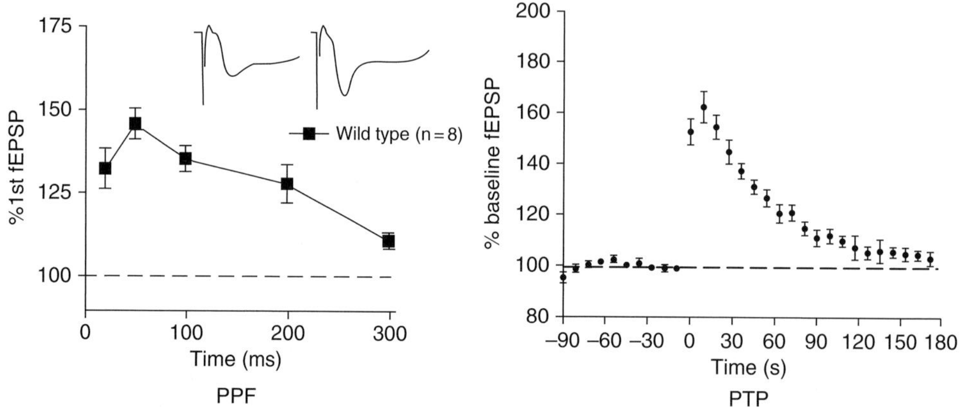

Figure 7 Paired-pulse facilitation (left) and posttetanic potentiation (right). See text for details. Data for both panels courtesy of Michal Levy. fEPSP, field EPSP.

aminophosphonovaleric acid (APV), an agent that selectively blocks the NMDA subtype of glutamate receptor, could block LTP induction while leaving baseline synaptic transmission entirely intact (**Figure 8**).

This was the first experiment to give a specific molecular insight into the mechanisms of LTP induction. The properties of the NMDA receptor that allow it to function in this unique role of triggering LTP are important. For our purposes right now, pharmacologic blockers of NMDA receptor function have allowed the definition of different types of LTP that can be selectively induced with various physiologic stimulation protocols. For example, subsequent work has shown that an NMDA receptor-independent type of LTP can be induced in area CA1 and elsewhere in the hippocampus (mossy fibers to be precise), as well as in other parts of the CNS. We will return to a brief description of these types of LTP at the end of this chapter, but for now, we will continue to focus on NMDA receptor-dependent types of LTP.

Early studies of LTP used mostly high-frequency (100-Hz) stimulation in repeated 1-s-long trains as the LTP-inducing stimulation protocol. Although these protocols are still widely used to good effect, it is clear that such prolonged periods of high-frequency firing do not occur physiologically in the behaving animal. However, LTP can also be induced by stimulation protocols that are much more like naturally occurring neuronal firing patterns in the hippocampus. To date the forms of LTP induced by these types of stimulation have all been found to be NMDA receptor dependent in area CA1. Two popular variations of these protocols are based on the natural occurrence of an increased rate of hippocampal pyramidal neuron firing while a rat or mouse is exploring and learning about a new environment. Under these circumstances hippocampal pyramidal neurons fire bursts of action potentials at about 5 bursts/s (i.e., 5 Hz). This is the hippocampal 'theta' rhythm that has been described in the literature. One variation of LTP-inducing stimulation that mimics this pattern of firing is referred to as theta-frequency stimulation (TFS), which consists of 30 s of single stimuli delivered at 5 Hz. Another variation, theta burst stimulation (TBS) consists of three trains of stimuli delivered at 20-s intervals, each train composed of ten stimulus bursts delivered at 5 Hz, with each burst consisting of four pulses at 100 Hz (see **Figure 9**). It is worth noting that these patterns of stimulation, which are based on naturally occurring firing patterns *in vivo*, lead to LTP in hippocampal slice preparations as well.

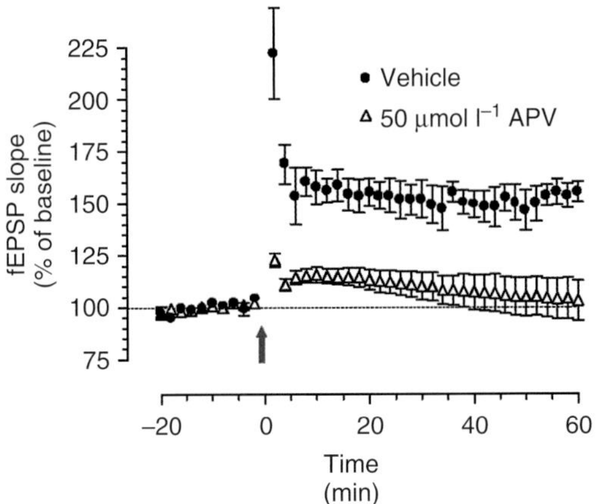

Figure 8 APV block of LTP. These data are from recordings *in vitro* from mouse hippocampal slices, demonstrating the NMDA receptor dependence of tetanus-induced LTP. Identical high-frequency synaptic stimulation was delivered in control (filled circles) and NMDA receptor antagonist (APV, open triangles) treated slices. fEPSP, field EPSP. Data courtesy of Joel Selcher.

11.3.1 Pairing LTP

Of course, much more sophisticated electrophysiologic techniques than extracellular recording can be used to monitor synaptic function. Intracellular recording and patch clamp techniques that measure electrophysiologic responses in single neurons have also been used widely in studies of LTP. These types of recording techniques perturb the cell that is being recorded from and lead to 'run-down' of the postsynaptic response in the cell impaled by the electrode. This limits the duration of the LTP experiment to however long the cell stays alive – somewhere in the range of 60 to 90 min for an accomplished physiologist. Regardless, in these recording configurations one can induce synaptic potentiation using tetanic stimulation or theta-pattern stimulation and measure LTP as an increase in postsynaptic currents through glutamate-gated ion channels or as an increase in postsynaptic depolarization when monitoring the membrane potential.

Control of the postsynaptic neuron's membrane potential with cellular recording techniques also allows for some sophisticated variations of the LTP induction paradigm. In one particularly important

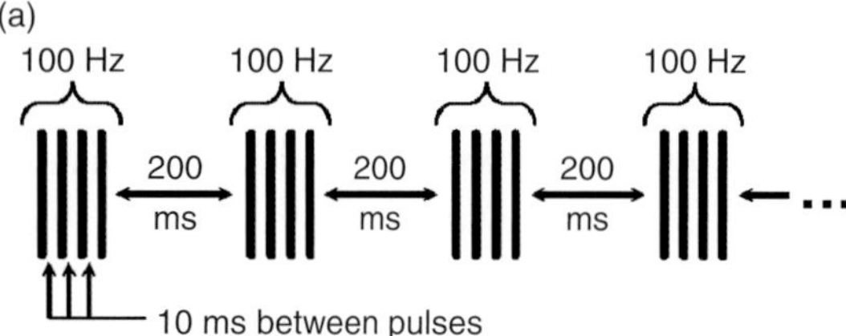

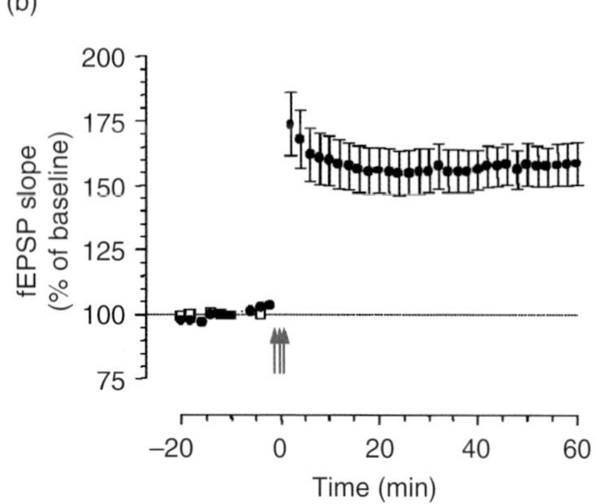

Figure 9 LTP triggered by theta-burst stimulation (TBS) in the mouse hippocampus. (a) Schematic depicting TBS. This LTP induction paradigm consists of three trains of 10 high-frequency bursts delivered at 5 Hz. (b) LTP induced with TBS (TBS-LTP) in hippocampal area CA1. The three red arrows represent the three TBS trains. fEPSP, field EPSP.

series of experiments, it was discovered that LTP can be induced by pairing repeated single presynaptic stimuli with postsynaptic membrane depolarization, so-called pairing LTP (Wigstrom and Gustafsson, 1986) (**Figure 10**).

The basis for pairing LTP comes from one of the fundamental properties of the NMDA receptor (**Figure 11**). The NMDA receptor is both a glutamate-gated channel and a voltage-dependent one. The simultaneous presence of glutamate and a depolarized membrane is necessary and sufficient (when the coagonist glycine is present) to gate the channel. Pairing synaptic stimulation with membrane depolarization provided via the recording electrode (plus the low levels of glycine always normally present) opens the NMDA receptor channel and leads to the induction of LTP.

How does the NMDA receptor trigger LTP? The NMDA receptor is a calcium channel, and its gating leads to elevated intracellular calcium in the postsynaptic neuron. This calcium influx triggers LTP, and indeed other chapters in this volume deal with the various processes this calcium influx triggers. It is important to remember that it is not necessarily the case that every calcium molecule involved in LTP induction actually comes through the NMDA receptor. Calcium influx through membrane calcium channels and calcium released from intracellular stores may also be involved.

The gating of the NMDA receptor/channel involves a voltage-dependent Mg^{++} block of the channel pore. Depolarization of the membrane in which the NMDA receptor resides is necessary to drive the divalent Mg^{++} cation out of the pore, which then allows calcium ions to flow through. Thus, the simultaneous occurrence of both glutamate in the synapse and a depolarized postsynaptic membrane are necessary to open the channel and allow LTP-triggering calcium into the postsynaptic cell.

These properties, glutamate dependence *and* voltage dependence, of the NMDA receptor allow it to function as a coincidence detector. This is a critical aspect of NMDA receptor regulation, and this allows for a unique contribution of the NMDA receptor to information processing at the molecular level. Using the NMDA receptor, the neuron can trigger a unique event, calcium influx, specifically when a particular synapse is both active presynaptically (glutamate is present in the synapse) and postsynaptically (when the membrane is depolarized).

This confers a computational property of associativity on the synapse. This attribute is nicely illustrated by 'pairing' LTP, as described earlier, where low-frequency synaptic activity paired with postsynaptic depolarization can lead to LTP. The associative property of the NMDA receptor allows for many other types of sophisticated information processing as well, however. For example, activation of a weak input to a neuron can induce potentiation, provided a strong input to the same neuron is activated at the same time (Barrionuevo and Brown, 1983). These particular features of LTP induction have stimulated a great deal of interest, as they are reminiscent of classical conditioning, with depolarization and synaptic input roughly corresponding to unconditioned and conditioned stimuli, respectively.

The associative nature of NMDA receptor activation allows for synapse specificity of LTP induction as well, which has been shown to occur experimentally. If one pairs postsynaptic depolarization with activity at one set of synaptic inputs to a cell, while leaving a second input silent or active only during

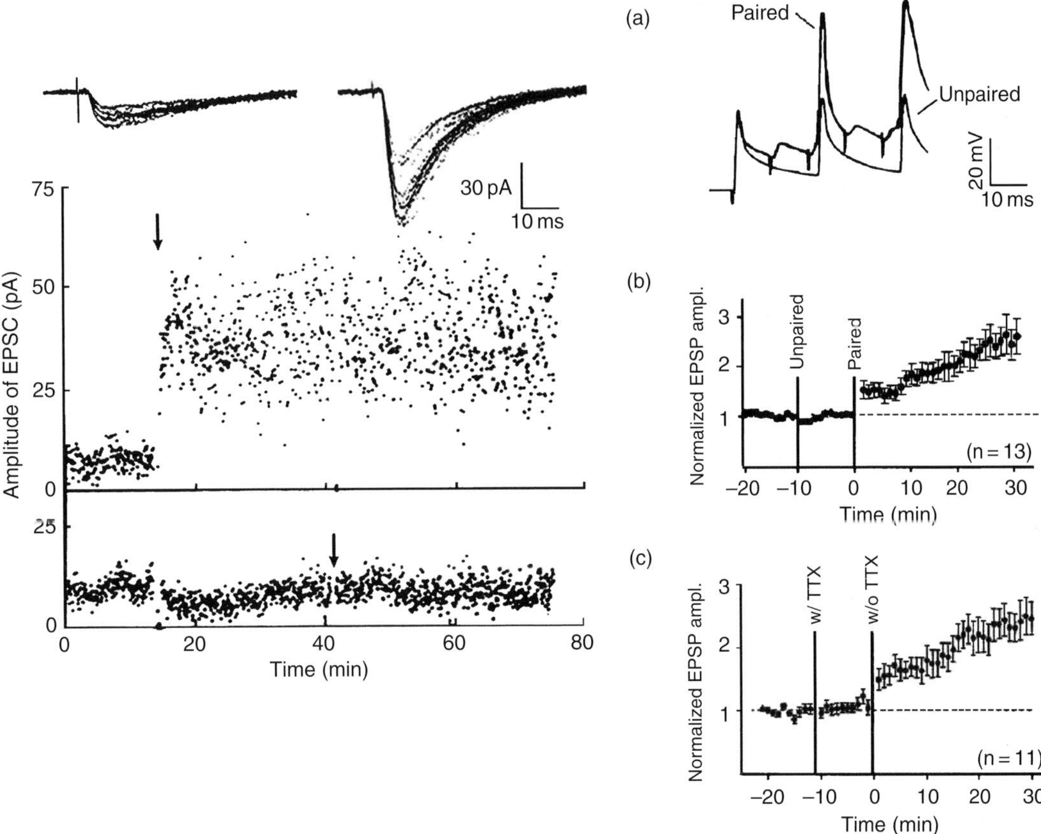

Figure 10 Pairing LTP. (Left panel) LTP of synaptic transmission induced by pairing postsynaptic depolarization with synaptic activity. The upper panels illustrate postsynaptic currents (EPSCs) recorded directly from the postsynaptic neuron using voltage-clamp techniques. The data shown are a pairing LTP experiment (upper) and control, nonpaired pathway (lower). In the pairing LTP experiment, hippocampal CA1 pyramidal neurons were depolarized from −70 mV to 0 mV while the paired pathway was stimulated at 2 Hz 40 times. Control received no stimulation during depolarization. From Malinow R and Tsien RW (1990) Presynaptic enhancement shown by whole-cell recordings of long-term potentiation in hippocampal slices. *Nature* 346: 177–180. (Right panels) Pairing small EPSPs with back-propagating dendritic action potentials induces LTP. Inset (a): Subthreshold EPSPs paired with back-propagating action potentials increase dendritic action potential amplitude. Voltage-clamp recording at approximately 240 μm from soma, that is, in the dendritic tree of the neuron (see **Figure 12**). Action potentials were evoked by 2-ms current injections through a somatic whole-cell electrode at 20-ms intervals. Alone, action potential amplitude was small (unpaired). Paired with EPSPs (5 stimuli at 100 Hz), the action potential amplitude increased greatly (paired). Inset (b): Grouped data showing normalized EPSP amplitude after unpaired and paired stimulation. The pairing protocol shown in (a) was repeated 5 times at 5 Hz at 15-s intervals for a total of 2 times. Inset (c): A similar pairing protocol was given with and without applying the sodium channel blocker tetrodotoxin (TTX, to block action potential propagation) to the proximal apical dendrites to prevent back-propagating action potentials from reaching the synaptic input sites. LTP was induced only when action potentials fully back-propagated into the dendrites. Reproduced with permission from Magee JC and Johnston D (1997) A synaptically controlled, associative signal for Hebbian plasticity in hippocampal neurons. *Science* 275: 209–213.

periods at which the postsynaptic membrane is near the resting potential, then selective potentiation of the paired input pathway occurs.

Similarly, in field stimulation experiments LTP is restricted to tetanized pathways – even inputs convergent on the same dendritic region of the postsynaptic neuron are not potentiated if they receive only baseline synaptic transmission in the absence of synaptic activity sufficient to adequately depolarize the postsynaptic neuron (Anderson et al., 1977). This last point illustrates the basis for LTP cooperativity. LTP induction in extracellular stimulation experiments requires cooperative interaction of afferent fibers, which in essence means there is an intensity threshold for triggering LTP induction. Sufficient total synaptic activation by the input fibers must be

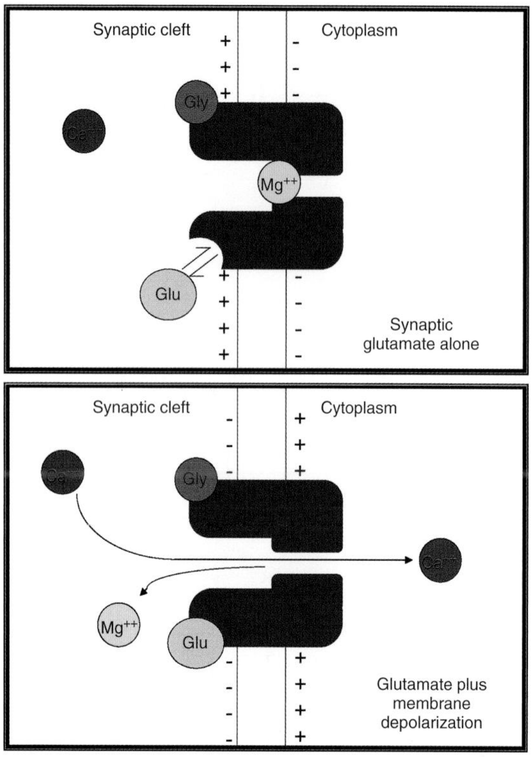

Figure 11 Coincidence detection by the NMDA receptor. The simultaneous presence of glutamate and membrane depolarization is necessary for relieving Mg^{++} blockade and allowing calcium influx. Figure by J. David Sweatt and Sarah E. Brown.

achieved such that the postsynaptic membrane is adequately depolarized to allow opening of the NMDA receptor (McNaughton et al., 1978).

11.3.2 Dendritic Action Potentials

In the context of the functioning hippocampal neuron *in vivo*, the associative nature of NMDA receptor activation means that a given neuron must reach a critical level of depolarization for LTP to occur at any of its synapses. Specifically, in the physiologic context the hippocampal pyramidal neuron generally must reach the threshold for firing an action potential, although there are some interesting alternatives to this that we will discuss later in this chapter. Although action potentials are, of course, triggered in the active zone of the cell body, hippocampal pyramidal neurons along with many other types of CNS neurons can actively propagate action potentials into the dendritic regions: the so-called back-propagating action potential (Magee and Johnston, 1997) (see **Figure 12**). These dendritic action potentials are just like action potentials propagated down axons in that they are carried predominantly by voltage-dependent ion channels such as sodium channels. The penetration of the back-propagating action potential into the dendritic region provides a wave of membrane depolarization that allows for the opening of the voltage-dependent NMDA receptor/ion channels. *Active* propagation of the action potential is necessary because the biophysical properties of the dendritic membrane dampen the passive propagation of membrane depolarization, thus an active process such as action potential propagation is required. As a generalization, in many instances in the intact cell, back-propagating action potentials are what allow sufficient depolarization to reach hippocampal pyramidal neuron synapses to open NMDA receptors. In an ironic twist, this has brought us back to a more literal reading of Hebb's postulate, where, as we discussed at the beginning of this chapter, Hebb actually specified *firing* of the postsynaptic neuron as being necessary for the strengthening of its connections.

In fact, the timing of the arrival of a dendritic action potential with synaptic glutamate input appears to play an important part in precise, timing-dependent triggering of synaptic plasticity in the hippocampus (Magee and Johnston, 1997) (*See* **Figures 10** and **13**). It has been observed that a critical timing window is involved vis-à-vis back-propagating action potentials: glutamate arrival in the synaptic cleft must slightly precede the back-propagating action potential for the NMDA receptor to be effectively opened. This timing dependence arises in part due to the time required for glutamate to bind to and open the NMDA receptor. The duration of an action potential is, of course, quite short, so in essence the glutamate must be there first and already be bound to the receptor for full activation to occur. (Additional factors are also involved; *See* Bi and Poo, 1998; Kamondi et al., 1998; Linden, 1999; and Johnston et al., 2000 for a discussion.)

This order-of-paring specificity allows for a precision of information processing – not only must the membrane be depolarized but also as a practical matter, the cell must fire an action potential. Moreover, the timing of the back-propagating action potential arriving at a synapse must be appropriate. It is easy to imagine how the nervous system could capitalize on these properties to allow for forming precise timing-dependent associations between two events.

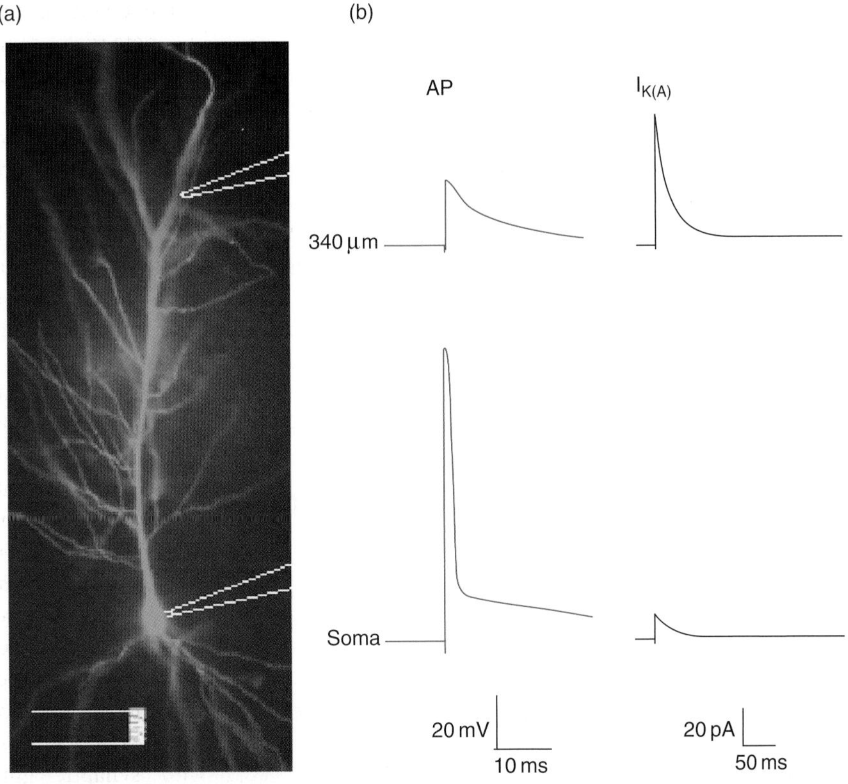

Figure 12 Back-propagating action potentials in dendrites of CA1 pyramidal neurons. (a) Indicates the recording setup, with a bipolar stimulating electrode used to trigger action potentials at the cell body region (lower left), a recording electrode in the cell soma to monitor firing of an action potential, and a recording electrode in the dendrites (upper right) to monitor propagation of the action potential into the distal dendritic region. (b) Traces in (b) indicate the data recorded from the soma (lower) and dendritic (upper) electrodes. The left-hand traces from (b) (labeled AP) indicate the membrane depolarization achieved at the soma and dendrite when an action potential is triggered and propagates into the dendritic region. Note that the dendritic action potential is of lower magnitude and broader due to the effects of dendritic membrane biophysical properties as the action potential propagates down the dendrite. The right half of (b) shows current flow through 'A-type' voltage-dependent potassium currents observed in the soma and dendrites. The density of A-type potassium currents increases dramatically as one progresses outward from the soma into the dendritic regions, as illustrated by the much larger potassium current observed in the distal dendritic electrode. These voltage-dependent potassium channels are key regulators of the likelihood of back-propagating action potentials reaching various parts of the dendritic tree. Data and figure reproduced from Yuan LL, Adams JP, Swank M, Sweatt JD, and Johnston D (2002) Protein kinase modulation of dendritic K+ channels in hippocampus involves a mitogen-activated protein kinase pathway. *J. Neurosci.* 22: 4860–4868, with permission.

One twist to the order-of-pairing specificity is that if the order is reversed and the action potential arrives before the EPSP, then synaptic depression is produced. The mechanisms for this attribute are under investigation at present. One hypothesis is that the backward pairing by various potential mechanisms leads to a lower level of calcium influx, which produces synaptic depression (*See* following discussion and Chapter 12).

Overall it is important to note that the dendritic membrane in which the NMDA receptors reside is not passive, but contains voltage-dependent ion channels. Thus controlling the postsynaptic membrane biophysical properties can be a critical determinant for regulating the triggering of synaptic change.

11.4 NMDA Receptor-Independent LTP

Although the vast majority of studies of LTP and its molecular mechanisms have investigated NMDA receptor-dependent processes, as mentioned earlier there also are several types of NMDA receptor-independent LTP. The next section will briefly

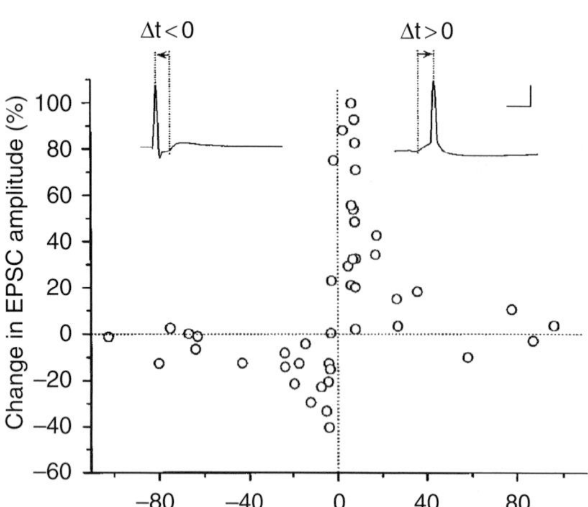

Figure 13 The timing of back-propagating action potentials with synaptic activity determines whether synaptic strength is altered, and in which direction. Precise timing of the arrival of a back-propagating action potential (a 'spike') with synaptic glutamate determines the effect of paired depolarization and synaptic activity. A narrow window when the arrival of the synaptic EPSP immediately precedes or follows the arrival of the back-propagating action potential determines whether synaptic strength is increased, is decreased, or remains the same. See text for additional discussion. EPSC, excitatory postsynaptic current. Figure adapted from Bi GQ and Poo MM (1998) Synaptic modifications in cultured hippocampal neurons: Dependence on spike timing, synaptic strength, and postsynaptic cell type. *J. Neurosci.* 18: 10464–10472, with permission.

describe a few different types of NMDA receptor-independent LTP as background material and to highlight them as important areas of investigation.

11.4.1 200-Hz LTP

NMDA receptor-independent LTP can be induced at the Schaffer collateral synapses in area CA1, the same synapses discussed thus far. This allows for somewhat of a comparison and contrast of two different types of LTP at the same synapse. A protocol that elicits NMDA receptor-independent LTP in area CA1 is the use of four 0.5-s, 200-Hz stimuli separated by 5 s (Grover and Teyler, 1990). LTP induced with this stimulation protocol is insensitive to NMDA receptor-selective antagonists such as APV (see **Figure 14**). It is interesting that simply doubling the rate of tetanic stimulation from 100 Hz to 200 Hz appears to shift activity-dependent mechanisms for synaptic potentiation into NMDA receptor independence. At the simplest level of thinking, this indicates that there is some unique type of temporal integration going on at the higher frequency stimulation that allows for superseding the necessity for NMDA receptor activation. What might the 200-Hz stimulation be uniquely stimulating? One appealing hypothesis arises from the observation that 200-Hz LTP is blocked by blockers of voltage-sensitive calcium channels. Thus, the current working model is that 200-Hz stimulation elicits sufficiently large and sufficiently prolonged membrane depolarization, resulting in the opening of voltage-dependent calcium channels, to trigger elevation of postsynaptic calcium sufficient to trigger LTP synaptic potentiation. One observation consistent with this hypothesis is that injection of postsynaptic calcium chelators blocks 200-Hz stimulation-induced LTP.

11.4.2 TEA LTP

NMDA receptor-independent LTP in area CA1 can also be induced using tetraethylammonium (TEA^+) ion application, a form of LTP that is referred to as LTP_k (Aniksztejn and Ben-Ari, 1991; Powell et al., 1994). TEA^+ is a nonspecific potassium channel blocker, the application of which greatly increases membrane excitability. Like 200-Hz LTP, LTP_k is insensitive to NMDA receptor antagonists and is blocked by a blockade of voltage-sensitive calcium channels. Moreover, LTP_k is also blocked by postsynaptic calcium chelator injection as well. The induction of LTP_k is dependent on synaptic activity, as AMPA receptor antagonists block its induction. Similar to 200-Hz LTP, the current model for TEA LTP is that synaptic depolarization via alpha-amino-3-hydroxy-5-methyl-4 isoxazole propionic acid (AMPA) receptor activation, augmented by the hyperexcitable membrane due to K^+ channel blockade, leads to a relatively large and prolonged membrane depolarization. This leads to the triggering of LTP through postsynaptic calcium influx.

11.4.3 Mossy Fiber LTP in Area CA3

The predominant model system for studying NMDA receptor-independent LTP is not the Schaffer collateral synapses, but rather the mossy fiber inputs into area CA3 pyramidal neurons. Considerable excitement accompanied the discovery of NMDA receptor-independent LTP at these synapses by Harris and Cotman (1986). The mossy fiber synapses are unique, large synapses with unusual presynaptic specializations, and there has been much interest in comparing the attributes and mechanisms of induction of mossy fiber LTP (MF-LTP) with those of NMDA receptor-dependent LTP in area CA1.

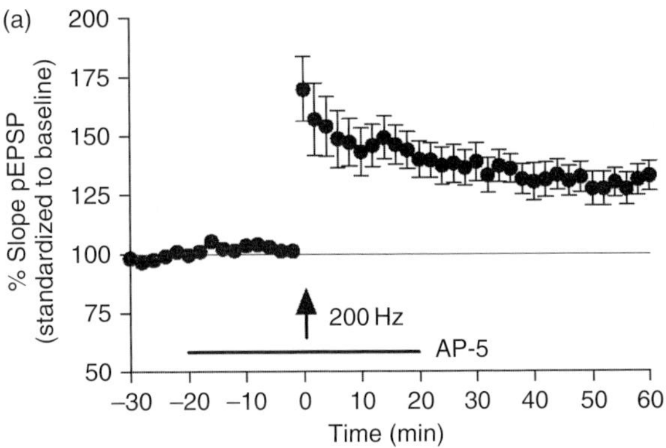

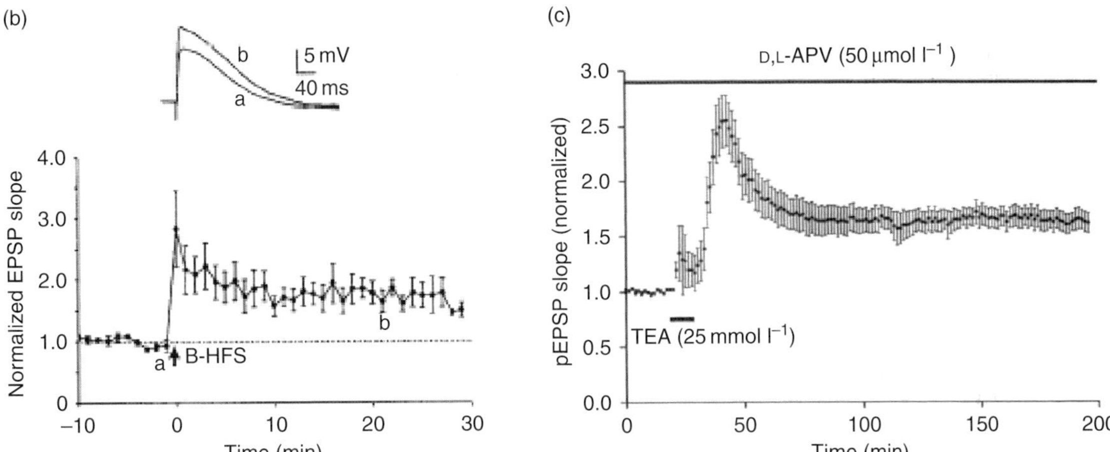

Figure 14 Examples of NMDA receptor-independent LTP. (a) 200-Hz stimulation in area CA1 elicits LTP even in the presence of the NMDA receptor antagonist APV. pEPSP, population EPSP. Data courtesy of Ed Weeber. (b) LTP at mossy fiber inputs into area CA3 is also NMDA receptor independent – the potentiation shown occurred in the presence of blockers of the NMDA receptor. Data courtesy of Rick Gray. From Kapur A, Yeckel MF, Gray R, and Johnston D (1998) L-Type calcium channels are required for one form of hippocampal mossy fiber LTP. *J. Neurophysiol.* 79: 2181–2190; used with permission. (c) Application of the K channel blocker tetra-ethyl ammonium (TEA) also elicits NMDA receptor-independent LTP in area CA1. Data courtesy of Craig Powell (Ph.D. thesis, Baylor College of Medicine, p. 50).

However, subsequent progress in investigating the mechanistic differences between these two types of LTP has been relatively slow for several reasons. First, the experiments are technically difficult physiologically – typically area CA3 is the first part of the hippocampal slice preparation to die *in vitro*. The local circuitry in area CA3 is complex, with many recurrent excitatory connections between neurons there: synapses that also are plastic and exhibit NMDA receptor-dependent LTP. Most problematic has been that there has been an ongoing controversy about the necessity of postsynaptic events, especially elevations of postsynaptic calcium, for the induction of MF-LTP. There are basically two schools of thought on MF-LTP. One line of thinking is that MF-LTP is entirely presynaptic in its induction and expression (Zalutsky and Nicoll, 1990). A second line of thinking is that MF-LTP has a requirement for postsynaptic signal transduction events for its induction (see, e.g., Kapur et al., 1998; Yeckel et al., 1999). Based on the available literature, it is difficult to come up with a definitive answer to the locus and mechanisms of induction of MF-LTP. For the purposes of this chapter, which focuses on NMDA receptor-dependent forms of LTP, I will simply note that this has been an area of controversy.

11.5 A Role for Calcium Influx in NMDA Receptor-Dependent LTP

In contrast to the story with MF-LTP, NMDA receptor-dependent LTP at Schaffer collateral synapses has achieved a broad consensus of a necessity for elevations of postsynaptic calcium for triggering LTP (Lynch et al., 1983). In fact, this is one of the few areas of LTP research in which there is almost universal agreement.

The case for a role for elevated postsynaptic calcium in triggering LTP is quite clear-cut and solid. It is well established and has been reviewed adequately a sufficient number of times (Johnston et al., 1992; Nicoll and Malenka, 1995; Chittajallu et al., 1998), so this material will only be presented in overview here. A principal line of evidence is that injection of calcium chelators postsynaptically blocks the induction of LTP. Also, inhibitors of a variety of calcium-activated enzymes also block LTP induction, including when they are specifically introduced into the postsynaptic neuron. Fluorescent imaging experiments using calcium-sensitive indicators have clearly demonstrated that postsynaptic calcium is elevated with LTP-inducing stimulation. Finally, elevating postsynaptic calcium is sufficient to cause synaptic potentiation (although there has been some controversy on this point). Thus the hypothesis of a role for postsynaptic calcium elevation in triggering LTP has met the three classic criteria (block, measure, mimic) necessary for 'proving' a hypothesis (Sweatt, 2003), and this idea is on a solid experimental footing.

11.6 Presynaptic versus Postsynaptic Mechanisms

One of the most intensely studied and least satisfactorily resolved aspects of LTP concerns the locus of LTP maintenance and expression. One component of LTP is an increase in the EPSP, which could arise from increasing glutamate concentrations in the synapse or by increasing the responsiveness to glutamate by the postsynaptic cell (**Figure 15**). The 'pre' versus 'post' debate is whether the relevant changes reside presynaptically, manifest as an increase in neurotransmitter release or similar phenomenon, or whether they reside postsynaptically as a change in glutamate receptor responsiveness. Over the last 15 years or so there have been numerous experiments performed to try to address this question, and as of yet there is no clear consensus answer. Popularity of the 'pre' hypothesis versus the 'post' hypothesis has waxed and waned, and this oscillation may continue for some time yet. The next few paragraphs will summarize a few representative findings to provide background on these issues. Reading the recent papers by Choi et al. (2000), Bolshakov et al. (1997), and Nicoll and Malenka (1999) will provide a feel for the nature of the ongoing debate.

In some of the earliest studies to begin to get at LTP mechanistically, it became clear that infusing compounds into the postsynaptic cell led to a block of LTP. A few of these studies involving calcium chelators were described in the last section. If compounds that are limited in their distribution to the postsynaptic compartment block LTP, the most parsimonious hypothesis is that LTP resides postsynaptically.

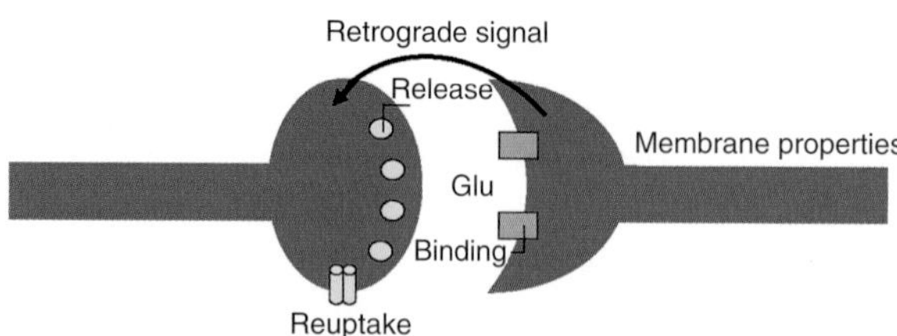

Presynaptic = Altered
- Neurotransmitter amount in vesicles
- Number of vesicles released
- Kinetics of release
- Glutamate reuptake
- Probability of vesicle fusion

Postsynaptic = Altered
- Number of AMPA receptors
- Insertion of AMPA receptors
- Ion flow through AMPA channels
- Membrane electrical properties

Additional possibilities include changes in number of total synaptic connections between two cells

Figure 15 Potential sites of synaptic modification in LTP. Figure by J. David Sweatt and Sarah E. Brown.

However, shortly thereafter, evidence began to accumulate suggesting that presynaptic changes were involved in LTP expression as well. For example, various types of 'quantal' analysis that had been successfully applied at the neuromuscular junction to dissect presynaptic changes from postsynaptic changes suggested that LTP is associated with changes presynaptically. In a series of investigations, several laboratories used whole-cell recordings of synaptic transmission in hippocampal slices and found an increase in the probability of release, a strong indicator of presynaptic changes in classic quantal analysis (Dolphin et al., 1982; Bekkers and Stevens, 1990; Malinow and Tsien, 1990; Malinow, 1991; Malgaroli et al., 1995; Zakharenko et al., 2001). These findings fit nicely with earlier studies from Tim Bliss's laboratory suggesting an increase in glutamate release in LTP as well (Dolphin et al., 1982). Given findings supporting postsynaptic locus on the one hand and presynaptic locus on the other, why not just hypothesize that there are changes both presynaptically and postsynaptically? The rub came in that some of the quantal analysis results seemed to exclude postsynaptic changes as occurring.

These findings in the early 1990s ushered in an exciting phase of LTP research that was important independent of the pre versus post debate *per se.* If there are changes presynaptically but these changes are triggered by events originating in the postsynaptic cell, as the earlier inhibitor-perfusion experiments had indicated, then the existence of a *retrograde messenger* is implied. A retrograde messenger is a compound generated in the postsynaptic compartment that diffuses back to and signals changes in the presynaptic compartment – the opposite (retrograde) direction from normal synaptic transmission. Moreover, if the compound is generated intracellularly in the postsynaptic neuron then the compound must be able to traverse the postsynaptic membrane somehow. The data supporting presynaptic changes in LTP implied the existence of such a signaling system, and this hypothesis launched a number of interesting and important experiments to determine what types of molecules might serve such a role – some of these are highlighted in **Figure 16**.

However, in the mid-1990s the pre/post pendulum began to swing back in the opposite direction, toward the postsynaptic side. Several groups found evidence for postsynaptic changes that could account for the apparently presynaptic changes identified by quantal analysis studies. Specifically, evidence was generated for what are termed *silent synapses* (see **Figure 17**). These are synapses that contain NMDA receptors but no AMPA receptors – they are capable of synaptic plasticity mediated by NMDA receptor activation but are physiologically silent in terms of baseline synaptic transmission. Silent synapses are rendered active by NMDA receptor-triggered activation of latent AMPA receptors postsynaptically. Such uncovering of silent AMPA receptors could involve membrane insertion or posttranslational activation of already-inserted receptors. Activation of silent synapses is a postsynaptic mechanism that could explain the effects (decreased failure rate, for example) in quantal analysis experiments that implied presynaptic changes. Thus, there is now an argument that all of LTP physiology and biochemistry could be postsynaptic.

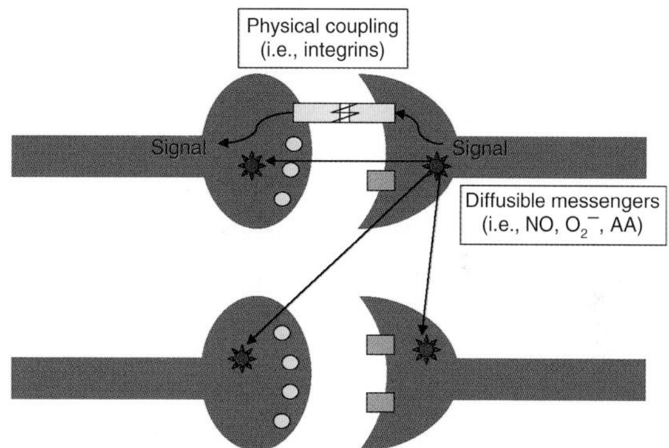

Figure 16 Potential mechanisms for retrograde signaling. Figure by J. David Sweatt and Sarah E. Brown.

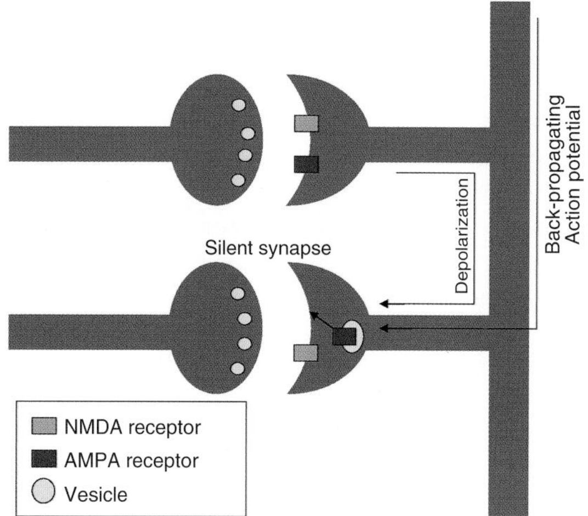

Figure 17 A simplified model of silent synapses. Figure by J. David Sweatt and Sarah E. Brown.

This model for conversion of silent synapses into active synapses by AMPA receptor insertion is an entirely postsynaptic phenomenon. However, there has been a variation of this idea proposed, which has been referred to as a whispering synapse. A whispering synapse has both AMPA and NMDA receptors in it, but because of a number of hypothetical factors such as glutamate affinity differences between NMDA and AMPA receptors, kinetics of glutamate elevation in the synapse, or spatial localization of the receptors, the AMPA receptors are silent. A whispering synapse is converted to being fully active by a presynaptic mechanism. An increase in glutamate release presynaptically, resulting in an elevation of glutamate levels in the synapse, then allows the effective activation of preexisting AMPA receptors with baseline synaptic transmission. By this mechanism, a synapse that was previously silent with respect to baseline synaptic transmission is rendered detectably active. However, this alternative mechanism requires no change in the postsynaptic compartment whatsoever.

Like the retrograde messenger hypothesis, the silent synapses hypothesis has also led to a number of important and interesting experiments that warrant attention aside from the pre versus post debate. Specifically, these experiments have focused new attention on the importance of considering the postsynaptic compartment in a cell-biological context. Mechanisms of receptor insertion, trafficking, and turnover that had been studied in nonneuronal cells are now beginning to get the attention they deserve in neurons as well. Like retrograde signaling, experiments arising from investigating mechanisms for activation of silent synapses have led to important 'spin-off' studies that are important independent of the precipitating issue of pre versus post.

Given the variety of evidence described so far, should one conclude that LTP resides presynaptically, postsynaptically, or both? Although there is not yet an unambiguous consensus in the pre versus post debate, overall the available literature indicates that changes are occurring in both the presynaptic and postsynaptic compartments. Two different types of approaches are briefly mentioned here, but these types of experiments are described in much more detail in another chapter in this volume (*See* Chapter 13). First, a number of experiments using sophisticated imaging techniques have found LTP to be associated with presynaptic changes such as increased vesicle recycling and increased presynaptic membrane turnover (see, for example, Malgaroli et al., 1995; Zakharenko et al., 2001). Also, direct biochemical measurements of the phosphorylation of proteins selectively localized to the presynaptic compartment have shown LTP-associated changes. Conceptually similar experiments looking at phosphorylation of postsynaptic proteins have found the same thing. Thus, imaging and biochemistry studies have fairly clearly illustrated that sustained biochemical changes are happening in both the presynaptic and postsynaptic cell.

This conclusion and indeed all of the pre versus post experiments have a very important caveat to keep in mind. In trying to reach a consensus conclusion, one is making a comparison across a wide spectrum of different types of experiments and different preparations. For example, one is comparing results with cultured cells versus hippocampal slices. One is trying to compare results for different types of LTP, LTP induced using pairing versus tetanic stimulation protocols. One likely is looking at different stages of LTP in comparing results from different experimental time points. Finally, in these experiments the various investigators are using material from different developmental stages in the animal, where the neurons under study are in different stages of their differentiation pathway. These considerations are a good reason to exercise caution in interpreting the experiments at this point, and indeed these issues may be contributing greatly to the apparent incompatibility of the results obtained in different labs.

11.7 LTP Can Include an Increased Action Potential Firing Component

Another caveat to keep in mind is that the preceding discussion deals only with mechanisms contributing to increases in synaptic strength. The increased EPSP is typically measured in field recording experiments as an increase in the initial slope of the EPSP (or EPSP magnitude), and as was discussed earlier, a second component of LTP is referred to as EPSP-spike (E-S) potentiation. As was already mentioned, E-S potentiation was identified by Bliss and Lomo in the first published report of LTP (1973) and is defined as an increase in population spike amplitude that cannot be attributed to an increase in synaptic transmission (i.e., initial EPSP slope in field recordings). Thus, E-S potentiation is a term used to refer to the postsynaptic cell having an increased probability of firing an action potential at a constant strength of synaptic input.

E-S potentiation at Schaffer collateral synapses can be observed using recordings in stratum pyramidale, as is illustrated in **Figure 18**. In this example, Eric Roberson generated I/O curves for the initial slope of the EPSP and the population spike amplitude, using various stimulus intensities, before and after LTP induction. E-S potentiation is manifest as an increase in population spike amplitude, even when responses are normalized to EPSP slope. Roberson's research also found that the probability of induction and magnitude of EPSP-spike (E-S) potentiation in area CA1 is more variable than LTP of synaptic transmission. A similar greater variability in E-S potentiation was observed by Bliss and Lomo in their original report as well.

What is the mechanism for this long-term increase in the likelihood of firing an action potential? One possibility is that there are changes in the intrinsic excitability of the postsynaptic neuron. Particularly appealing is the idea that long-term downregulation of dendritic potassium channel function could cause a persisting increase in cellular excitability and action potential firing. Although investigations of this hypothesis are still at an early stage, some recent work has suggested that E-S potentiation has a component due to intrinsic changes in the postsynaptic neuron. This idea is discussed further in another chapter (*See* Chapter 14).

Progress in testing this hypothesis has been slow due to the technically difficult nature of the experiments. Most patch-clamp physiologic studies of LTP have utilized recordings from the cell body, which are not capable of detecting changes in channels localized to the dendrites due to technical limitations. Thus, testing the idea of changes in dendritic excitability as a mechanism contributing to E-S potentiation requires dendritic patch-clamp recording, which at present only a few laboratories do routinely.

However, a more thoroughly investigated mechanism for E-S potentiation is based on alterations in feed-forward inhibitory connections onto pyramidal neurons in area CA1 (see **Figure 19**). The next few paragraphs present an overview of this area.

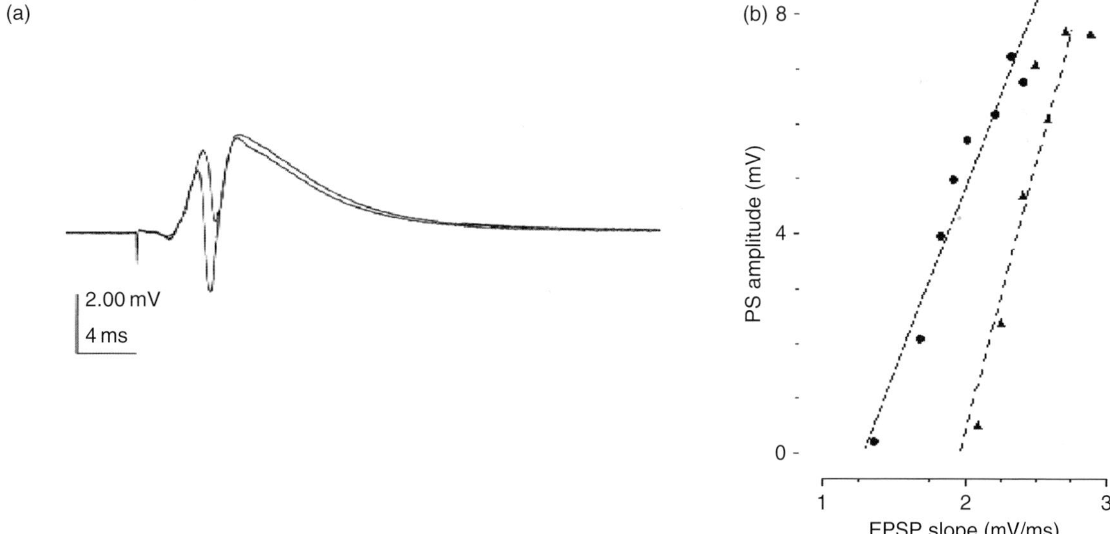

Figure 18 EPSP-spike (E-S) potentiation in area CA1. Extracellular recordings were made in the cell body layer of area CA1 (using stimulation of the Schaffer collateral inputs), and input-output (I/O) curves were performed using a range of 5 to 45 μA constant current stimulation. Initial slopes of the EPSP and population spike (PS) amplitude were then determined from the tracings and the data plotted as PS amplitude versus EPSP slope. (a) Superimposed representative tracings for before and 75 min after tetanic stimulation, showing the increased PS amplitude after tetanic stimulation. (b) Plots are shown for pretetanus (triangles) and 75 min posttetanus (circles). In this experiment five 100-Hz tetani were delivered. E-S coupling was assayed in hippocampal slices by taking a second set of I/O measurements after the induction of LTP. The baseline I/O curve and the poststimulation I/O curve were then compared to assess whether a change in excitability has occurred over the course of the experiment. Although in the illustration both EPSP slope and PS amplitude were measured from the same waveform, recording from the cell body layer, the preferred approach is to record EPSPs in the dendritic region and simultaneously record spikes independently from the cell body layer. This minimizes cross contamination of the PS changes in the EPSP measurements and vice versa. Data and figure courtesy of Erik Roberson.

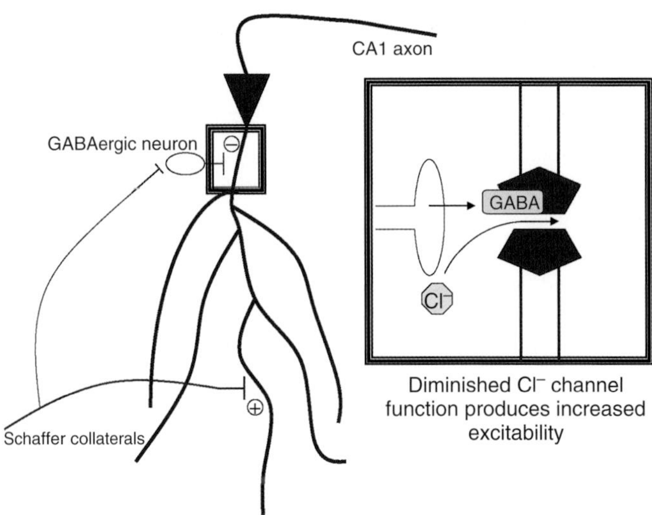

Figure 19 The GABAergic interneuron model of ES potentiation. One potential mechanism for E-S potentiation is diminution of inhibitory feed-forward inhibition through GABAergic interneurons in area CA1. Specific possible sites for this effect include LTD of the Schaffer collateral inputs onto GABAergic neurons, or synaptic depression of the interneuron-CA1 pyramidal neuron synapse. Figure by J. David Sweatt and Sarah E. Brown.

A number of different types of neurons in the hippocampus are called interneurons (or intrinsic neurons) because their inputs and outputs are restricted to local areas of the hippocampus itself. In other words, they only communicate with other neurons nearby in the hippocampus. Most of these neurons in area CA1 use the inhibitory neurotransmitter GABA, and their actions are to inhibit firing of CA1 pyramidal neurons. Different GABAergic interneurons make connections in all the dendritic regions of CA1 pyramidal neurons as well as the initial segment of the axon where the action potential originates. A single GABAergic interneuron may contact a thousand pyramidal neurons; thus, the effects of altered interneuron function are not generally limited to a single follower cell.

Interneurons in area CA1 receive glutamatergic Schaffer collateral projections just as the pyramidal neurons do – in fact, the inputs to the interneurons are branches of the same axons impinging the pyramidal neurons. Glutamate release at these interneuron synapses activates the interneurons and causes downstream release of GABA onto the pyramidal neurons. This inhibitory action is of course slightly delayed at the level of the single cell that receives input from the same Schaffer collateral axon that is activating the GABAergic interneuron, because there is an extra synaptic connection involved.

How does this local circuit contribute to E-S potentiation? Two different groups have shown that the same stimulation that produces LTP at the Schaffer collateral pyramidal neuron synapses simultaneously produces a decreased efficacy of coupling (long-term depression, LTD) of the Schaffer collateral interneuron synapses (McMahon and Kauer, 1997; Lu et al., 2000). Thus, although the excitatory input to the pyramidal neuron is being enhanced, the feed-forward inhibitory GABA input is diminished. This causes a net increase in excitability and increased likelihood of firing an action potential, added on top of the increased EPSP due to the normal LTP mechanisms. This is, of course, the definition of E-S potentiation.

There are a couple of interesting properties for this LTD at the Schaffer collateral interneuron synapse. First, it is NMDA receptor dependent just like LTP. This explains why one does not see E-S potentiation independent of synaptic potentiation in experiments where APV is infused onto the slice. Second, and more interesting, the LTD is not specific to the activated synapse – other Schaffer collateral inputs onto the same interneuron are also depressed (McMahon and Kauer, 1997). Therefore, there is decreased feed-forward inhibition across all the inputs (and outputs of course) for the whole interneuron. The interneuron has a diminished response to all its inputs and, therefore, decreased feedforward inhibition to all its outputs. Thus, the interneuron LTD appears to be serving to modulate the behavior of an entire small local circuit of neuronal connections. The precise role this interesting attribute plays in hippocampal information processing is unclear at present, but it is under study.

11.8 Temporal Integration Is a Key Factor in LTP Induction

At one level, it is a statement of the obvious to say that LTP induction depends on temporal integration. After all, the characteristic that distinguishes LTP induction protocols from baseline stimulation is that during an LTP induction protocol, stimulation is delivered at a higher rate. It obviously is the case that if the only attribute that is different is that the synapse is seeing activity at 100 pulses per second rather than once per 20 seconds, then unique timing-dependent processes are triggering LTP, which is simply a restatement of one definition of temporal integration. But what are the unique events that are happening physiologically with high-frequency stimulation? Stated briefly, the answer to this question is that temporal integration is occurring such that the cell is reaching a threshold of depolarization to fire an action potential (Scharfman and Sarvey, 1985; Johnston et al., 1999; Linden, 1999). This action potential firing then leads to membrane depolarization to allow opening of NMDA receptors. The following paragraphs will describe two different ways in which this can happen.

The first mechanism can be illustrated by considering what happens during the 1-s period of 100-Hz tetanus. Such closely spaced stimulation means that postsynaptic depolarization from the first EPSP carries over into the second stimulation, and so on, and so on, 96 more times. Stated more precisely, the postsynaptic membrane potential does not recover to the original resting potential before an additional depolarizing EPSP is triggered, and temporal summation of postsynaptic depolarization occurs. The summed depolarization eventually reaches threshold for the cell to fire an action potential. This is one of the classic examples of neuronal temporal integration, and of course, such a process is not limited to hippocampal pyramidal neurons. One unique aspect of this in hippocampal neurons, and probably other cortical neurons as well, is that triggering of the action potential is used to generate a back-propagating action potential into the dendrites, which is involved in depolarizing the NMDA receptor and triggering synaptic plasticity.

A second example comes from considering LTP induced by theta-pattern stimulation. With this type of LTP induction protocol, delivered at the slower 5 Hz (once/200 ms) rate, temporal integration is similarly involved but occurs via a different route. After all, 200 ms is long enough for the postsynaptic membrane potential to completely recover before the next wave of depolarization, so temporal integration of the sort described earlier is inadequate as an explanation. Joel Selcher investigated this question by examining the physiologic events occurring during the period of TFS. For illustrative purposes, his results with TFS stimulation will be discussed, although he and others observed similar effects with TBS as well.

These experiments used TFS consisting of 30 s of 5-Hz stimulation. This stimulation paradigm evokes stable LTP as described earlier and illustrated in **Figure 20**. Population spikes were assessed during the TFS period, utilizing a dual-recording electrode technique. The stimulating electrode remained in hippocampal area CA3 and activated Schaffer collateral fibers innervating area CA1. One recording electrode was positioned in stratum radiatum of area CA1 to record synaptic responses, field EPSPs (**Figure 20(b)**). Another electrode was placed in stratum pyramidale, the cell body layer, to record action potential firing in response to the same input. For each single stimulus, the initial slope of the EPSP recorded in stratum radiatum and the amplitude of the population spike recorded in stratum pyramidale were measured throughout the period of 5-Hz stimulation.

TFS resulted in a short-lived increase in action potential firing during the 30 seconds of 5-Hz stimulation (see **Figures 20(c)** and **20(d)**). For roughly the first 20 s of the stimulation, the amplitude of the population spike increased dramatically. Meanwhile, over this same time period, the EPSP slope recorded in stratum radiatum gradually declined. Therefore, the ratio of the population spike amplitude to the EPSP slope increased over time, indicating an increased likelihood of action potential firing over the short time course of the TFS (**Figure 20(d)**). Once again, for TFS as for 100-Hz tetanic stimulation, some temporal integration process is taking place to cause action potential firing during the period of LTP-inducing stimulation.

The mechanism for this temporal integration is not clear at present: clearly temporal summation of the sort operating in 100-Hz stimulation is not sufficient to explain it. However, a variety of previous studies have suggested that for LTP induced by TFS, there is an important role for attenuation of feed-forward GABAergic inhibition onto pyramidal neurons (Davies et al., 1991; Mott and Lewis, 1991; Chapman et al., 1998) (**Figure 21**). One current hypothesis is that short-term synaptic depression in the GABAergic local circuit during TFS, due to stimulation of presynaptic GABA-B

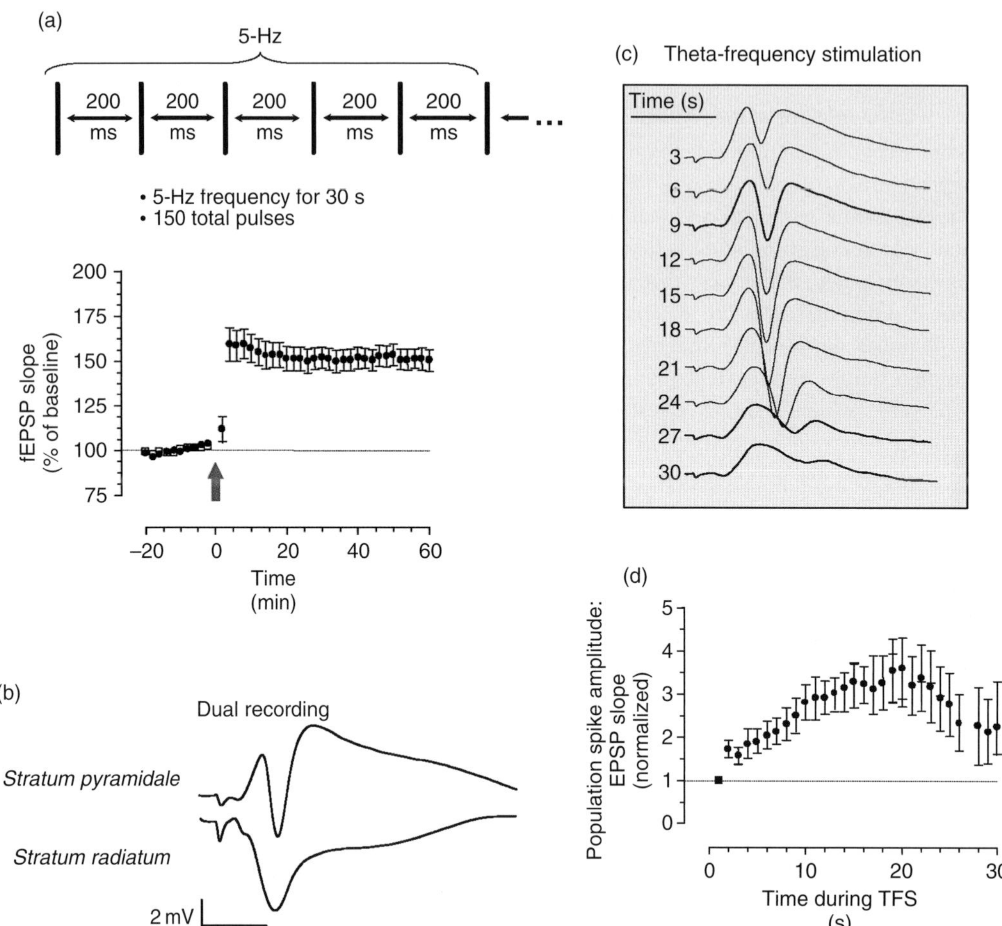

Figure 20 Increased action potential firing over the course of theta-frequency stimulation (TFS). (a) The TFS protocol and TFS-induced LTP in mouse hippocampal slices. (b) Electrode placement configuration for recording EPSP and population spikes simultaneously during TFS. (c) Representative traces in response to TFS from a hippocampal slice. Note the difference in the population spike between the first and 18th stimulation of the stimulation paradigm. (d) Quantitation of increased spike amplitude during TFS. Population spike counts recorded in stratum pyramidale of hippocampal area CA1 during theta-burst stimulation is plotted versus burst number during TFS. Slices showed a progressive increase in spike generation during the first two-thirds of TFS. Data and figures courtesy of Joel Selcher.

autoreceptors, leads to a loss of GABA-mediated inhibition, increased excitability, and increased firing of action potentials during the period of TFS.

11.9 LTP Can Be Divided into Phases

Contemporary models divide very long-lasting LTP (i.e., LTP lasting in the range of 5 to 6 h) into at least three phases. LTP comprising all three phases can be induced with repeated trains of high-frequency stimulation in area CA1 (see **Figure 22**), and the phases are expressed sequentially over time to constitute what we call 'LTP.' Late LTP (L-LTP) is hypothesized to be dependent for its induction on changes in gene expression, and this phase of LTP lasts many hours (see also Winder et al., 1998). Early LTP (E-LTP) is likely subserved by persistently activated protein kinases and starts at around 30 min or less posttetanus and is over in about 2–3 h. The first stage of LTP, generally referred to as short-term potentiation (STP), is independent of protein kinase activity for its induction and lasts about 30 min. I prefer to refer to the first stage of LTP as initial LTP to emphasize that it is a persistent form of NMDA receptor-dependent synaptic plasticity that is induced by LTP-inducing tetanic stimulation and

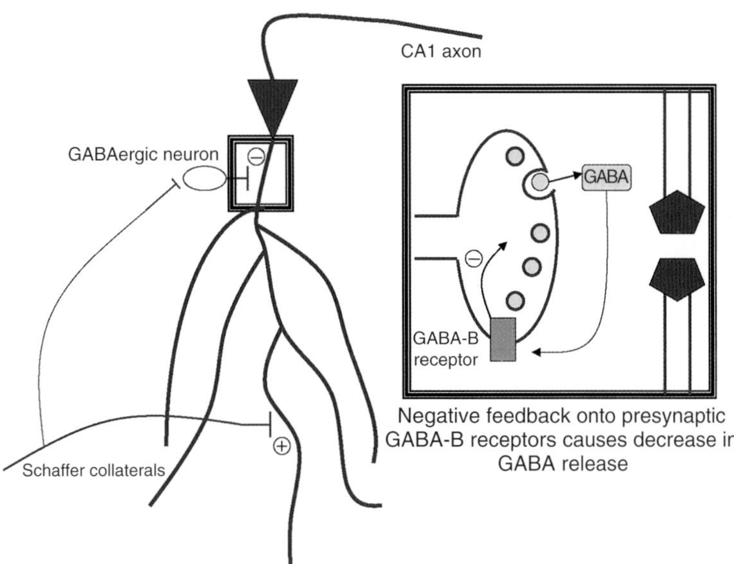

Figure 21 GABA-B receptors in temporal integration with TBS. This figure presents one model for the increased excitability that occurs during TBS, based on autoinhibition at GABAergic inputs onto CA1 pyramidal neurons during the period of stimulation. Figure by J. David Sweatt and Sarah E. Brown.

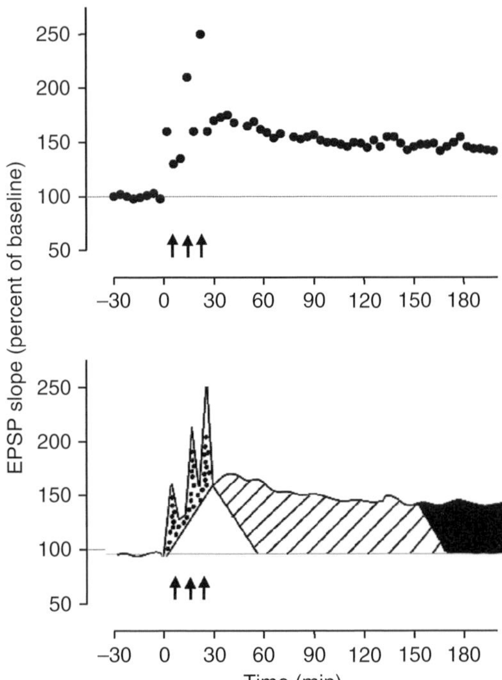

Figure 22 Immediate, early, and late LTP. The upper panel is real data from a late-phase LTP experiment, courtesy of Eric Roberson. The lower panel is a cartoon adaptation of the same data approximating the initial, early, and late stages of LTP. Adapted from Roberson ED, English JD, and Sweatt JD (1996) A biochemist's view of long-term potentiation. *Learn. Mem.* 3: 1–24, with permission.

is a prelude to E-LTP and L-LTP (Roberson et al., 1996). The mechanisms for initial LTP (aka STP) are essentially a complete mystery at present.

Readers may note some degree of ambiguity in the times specified for each phase of LTP. This is in part because the phases are very descriptive, and different labs often use slightly different conditions for their LTP experiments. For example, for technical reasons most L-LTP experiments are performed at room temperature, or 27–28°C, because it is much easier to maintain a healthy slice for many hours at these lower temperatures. Many E-LTP experiments, especially those involving direct biochemical measurements, are performed at 32–35°C. Comparing studies done at different temperatures is complicated by the pronounced temperature dependence of essentially all chemical reactions. A doubling of reaction rate for a change from room temperature to 32°C is fairly common for biochemical reactions. For these many reasons, it is difficult to try to compare experiments done at one temperature to experiments done at another. 'Late' LTP may start at 3 h at room temperature, start at 1.5 h at 32°C, and start at 45 min *in vivo.*

11.9.1 E-LTP and L-LTP – Types versus Phases

E-LTP and L-LTP refer to different *temporal* phases of LTP. These phases are subserved by different *maintenance* mechanisms of different time courses and durations. These two phases of LTP, E-LTP and L-LTP, are not exclusive of each other. In fact, depending on the LTP induction protocol used, E-LTP can be ongoing while L-LTP is developing, and one supplants the other over time. This has certain theoretical implications that are discussed in more detail in Roberson et al. (1996). These definitions are important as we transition to molecular mechanisms in another chapter of this volume (*See* Chapter 13). These definitions contain an underlying assumption about the biochemistry of LTP that is an organizing principle for the rest of this volume, that is, that different phases of LTP are subserved by distinct molecular mechanisms.

However, the terms E-LTP and L-LTP have been used in a slightly different fashion as well, in particular as popularized by the Kandel laboratory (*See* Winder et al., 1998). The Kandel laboratory and others use a terminology that divides the NMDA receptor-dependent form of LTP in area CA1 into E-LTP and L-LTP as well. E-LTP and L-LTP in this terminology refer to what one can characterize as two subtypes of LTP – a transient form (typically lasting 1–2 h) and a long-lasting form (lasting at least 5 h or more). The latter form of LTP is characterized by its dependence on intact protein synthesis, and the induction of this form of LTP requires delivery of multiple tetanic stimuli. E-LTP in this alternative nomenclature is induced by fewer tetanic stimuli and is protein synthesis independent. In this usage, E-LTP and L-LTP are defined as different *types* of LTP, not as temporal phases of LTP. Thus, one must keep in mind that two slightly different variations in the use of the terms E-LTP and L-LTP exist in the literature.

Before turning to a discussion of some implications of LTP having phases, a final set of three terms must be introduced – three terms widely used in the LTP literature. These terms arose from pharmacological inhibitor studies of LTP, and these types of studies will be reviewed in a moment. However, first we will simply introduce the terms.

Induction refers to the transient events serving to trigger the formation of LTP. *Maintenance*, or more specifically a maintenance mechanism, refers to the persisting biochemical signal that lasts in the cell. This persisting biochemical signal acts on an effector, for example, a glutamate receptor or the presynaptic release machinery, resulting in the *expression* of LTP.

It is important to keep in mind that, depending on the design of the experiment, induction, maintenance, and expression could be differentially inhibited (see **Figure 23**). The simplest type of experiment does not do this – for example, imagine if one applies an enzyme inhibitor (or knocks out a gene) before, during, and after the period of LTP-inducing high-frequency stimulation, this manipulation may block LTP. However, this does not distinguish whether the missing activity is required for the induction, the expression, or the maintenance of LTP. To distinguish among these

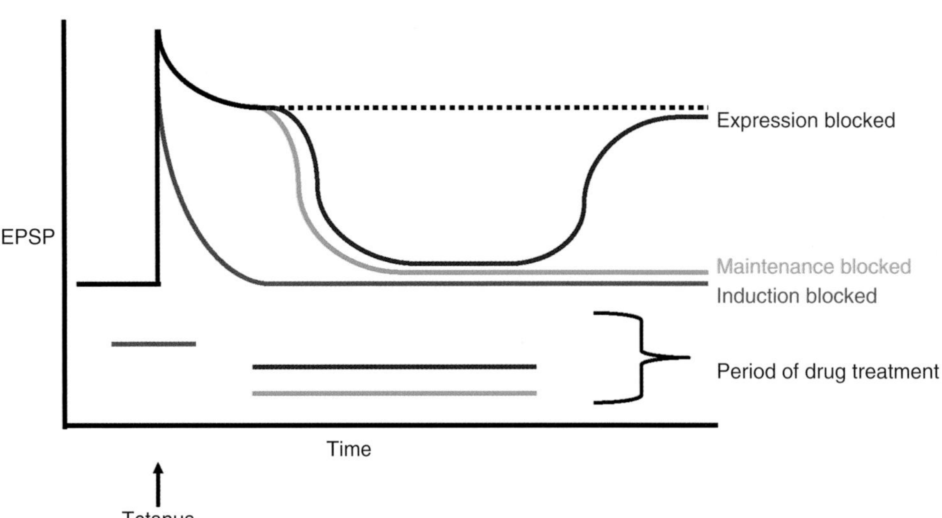

Figure 23 Induction, maintenance, and expression of LTP. This schematic illustrates the different experimental approaches to dissecting effects on the biochemical mechanisms subserving LTP induction, maintenance, or expression. See text for additional details.

possibilities, imagine instead applying the inhibitor selectively at different time points during the experiment. If inhibitor is applied only during the tetanus and then washed out and it blocks the generation of LTP, one can conclude that the enzyme is necessary for LTP induction. If the inhibitor is applied after the tetanus and it reverses the potentiation, it may be blocking either the maintenance or expression of LTP, as was nicely illustrated in an early experiment by Malinow et al. (1988), where they applied a protein kinase inhibitor after LTP induction. In this experiment, transient application of a kinase inhibitor after tetanus blocked synaptic potentiation, but the potentiation recovered after removal of the inhibitor. This is a blockade of LTP *expression*. However, if the kinase inhibitor had caused the potentiation to be lost irreversibly, the inhibitor would then by definition have blocked the *maintenance* of LTP.

Finally, it is important to synthesize the concepts of induction, maintenance, and expression with the concept of phases. Simply stated, three phases of LTP (initial-, E-, and L-LTP) times three distinct underlying mechanisms for each phase (induction, maintenance, and expression) give nine separate categories into which any particular molecular mechanism contributing to LTP may fit (see **Figure 24**). Added to this is the complexity that one phase could be largely presynaptic and another largely postsynaptic. Interesting implications begin to arise from thinking about LTP this way: How is it that the different mechanisms for the different phases interact with each other? Is the maintenance mechanism for one phase the induction mechanism for the next, or do the mechanisms for the phases operate independently? If the maintenance and expression mechanisms for the phases are independent, how does the magnitude of LTP stay constant as the shorter-lasting phase decays? How does the mechanism for L-LTP know where to stop, so that the magnitude of L-LTP is the same as the magnitude that E-LTP had attained? Roberson et al. (1996) discusses some hypothetical answers to these questions. It also is important to keep in mind that in many ways the same considerations apply to memory itself. If memory is encoded as some complex set of molecular changes, how is it that fidelity of memory maintained as short-term memory fades into long-term memory, for example? Although we will not arrive at an answer to these many questions, it is instructive to begin to formulate a hypothetical framework for their discussion.

11.10 Spine Anatomy and Biochemical Compartmentalization

So far we have discussed the synapse in largely abstract terms related mostly to its function. However, the synapse is also a physical entity, and the structural attributes of this entity confer some interesting properties (reviewed in Chapter 13 of this volume). This brief section will describe certain physical aspects of the synapse that will be important to consider. In brief, three points are highlighted in this section. First, most synapses in the CNS and almost all excitatory synapses in the hippocampus are at specialized structures called *dendritic spines*. Second, spines are small, well-circumscribed biochemical compartments that localize proteins and signal molecules to a specific postsynaptic compartment. Third, spines are, of course, contiguous with dendrites and thus continuously sense the local dendritic membrane potential.

A picture of part of the dendritic region of an area CA1 pyramidal neuron is shown in **Figure 25**. The fuzzy appearance of the CA1 dendritic tree in this picture is due to the abundance of small dendritic spines protruding at right angles to the dendritic shaft. Almost all (about 95%) of the Schaffer collateral synapses we have been discussing in the abstract are actually physically present at spines. Most spines have a fairly simple, elongated, mushroomlike (i.e., chicken drumstick) shape, although there is clearly

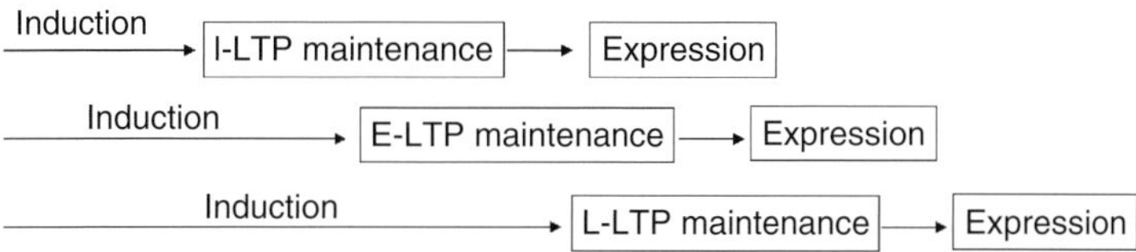

Figure 24 Mechanisms of induction, maintenance, and expression. This diagram highlights the importance of considering that each different phase of LTP may have separate and parallel induction, maintenance, and expression mechanisms. Figure by J. David Sweatt and Sarah E. Brown.

(a)
mCD8
Distal

(b)

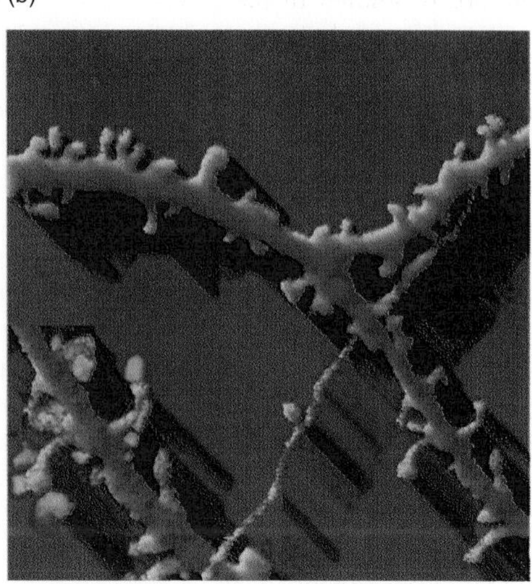

Figure 25 Dendrites with spines in a hippocampal pyramidal neuron. This figure illustrates the presence and shapes of dendritic spines on pyramidal neurons in the hippocampus. The spines are the small mushroom-shaped lateral projections containing synaptic contacts. (a) Courtesy of Liqun Lou, Stanford University. (b) Courtesy of E. Korkotian, The Weizmann Institute.

great diversity of their morphology. For example, a low percentage (about 2%) of CA1 pyramidal neuron spines are bifurcated and actually have two synapses on them. Spines have an actin-based cytoskeleton, and most have both smooth endoplasmic reticulums that can contribute to local calcium release and polyribosomes, where local protein synthesis occurs. In hippocampal pyramidal neurons, microtubules and mitochondria are limited to the dendritic shaft.

A distinguishing feature of the area of synaptic contact at the spine is the postsynaptic density, or PSD. This is a highly compact biochemical structure containing scaffolding proteins, receptors, and signal transduction components. The calcium/calmodulin-sensitive protein kinase CaMKII is particularly enriched at the PSD, as is a structural protein called PSD-95, a name that is based on its molecular weight.

The dendritic spine membrane surrounds the PSD and the area immediately below it and thus circumscribes a discrete biochemical compartment. The spine neck, however, is open to the dendritic shaft so there is still considerable diffusion of soluble spine contents (such as calcium and second messengers) into the local dendritic region. Nevertheless, on short time scales the spine compartment may serve to effectively localize signaling molecules to a specific synapse. Moreover, molecules tethered to the PSD by scaffolding proteins and the like probably have fairly limited diffusion because the spine compartment will make them tend to rebind at the same PSD as they unbind and rebind. Thus, this spine morphology is likely to be an important component for achieving synaptic specificity in LTP and other forms of synaptic plasticity.

The compartmentalization of molecules by the dendritic spine is not generally paralleled by an electrical compartmentalization. At one point, a popular line of thinking was that the shape and properties of the spine neck might regulate the capacity of electrical signals to get to and from the spine head compartment. This idea is no longer considered tenable, and as a first approximation, we can assume that the spine membrane potential reflects the local dendritic shaft membrane potential. However, it is likely that electrical compartmentalization does occur in dendrites, but this is at the level of the various dendritic branches as well as a component contributed by their overall distance from the soma (Johnston and Wu, 1995). This introduces the fascinating possibility that local generation and restricted propagation of action potentials within a specific dendritic subregion might be used as a mechanism for generating dendritic branch-specific plasticity.

11.11 LTP Outside the Hippocampus

The abundance of literature dedicated to studying LTP in the hippocampus might lead a newcomer to the field to suppose that LTP is somehow restricted to these synapses. However, plasticity of synaptic function, including phenomena such as LTP and LTD, is the rule rather than the exception for most forebrain synapses. LTP outside the hippocampus has been mostly studied in the cerebral cortex and the amygdala. The likely functional roles for LTP at these other sites are quite diverse, but two specific examples are worth highlighting. LTP-like processes in the cerebral cortex play a role in activity-dependent development of the visual system and other sensory systems. LTP in the amygdala has received prominent attention as a mechanism contributing to cued fear conditioning. The role of LTP in amygdala-dependent fear conditioning, in fact, is the area for which the strongest case can be made for a direct demonstration of a behavioral role for LTP. This will be discussed in more detail elsewhere (*See* Chapter 21). It is important to keep in mind through the rest of this volume that cortical LTP and amygdalar LTP probably exhibit some mechanistic differences from the NMDA receptor-dependent LTP that we will be focusing on. However, the molecular similarities are likely to greatly outweigh the differences (Schafe et al., 2000).

11.12 Modulation of LTP Induction

In one sense, the hippocampal slice is a denervated preparation. In the intact animal, the hippocampus receives numerous input fibers that provide modulatory inputs of the neurotransmitters DA, NE, 5HT, and ACh. Functionally these inputs are largely lost as a necessity of physically preparing the hippocampal slice for the experiment. However, these lost modulatory inputs can be partially reconstituted by directly applying the neurotransmitters (or more commonly pharmacologic substitutes) to the slice preparation *in vitro*. This approach has been used quite successfully to gain insights into the physiologic mechanisms and functional roles of these inputs in the intact brain.

NE, DA, and ACh-mimicking compounds can all modulate the induction of LTP at Schaffer collateral synapses. Specifically, agents acting at various subtypes of receptors for these compounds can increase the likelihood of LTP induction and the magnitude of LTP that is induced. Several examples of this type of modulation experiment are shown in **Figure 26**. In one example (panel A), 5-Hz stimulation of Schaffer collateral synapses, for 3 min, gives essentially no potentiation. Coapplication of isoproterenol, a beta-adrenergic receptor agonist that mimics endogenous NE, converts a nonpotentiating signal into a potentiating one (Thomas et al., 1996). Under other conditions beta-adrenergic agonists can augment the *magnitude* of LTP induced as well, if different physiologic stimulation protocols are used that evoke modest LTP. Similar types of effects can be observed for activation of various subtypes of receptors for ACh and DA (see Yuan et al., 2002).

One known site of action of neuromodulators is regulation of back-propagating action potentials in pyramidal neuron dendrites. All of these agents, which modulate LTP induction, can modulate the magnitude of back-propagating action potentials (see **Figure 26(b)**). The augmentation of back-propagating action potentials is a means by which these neurotransmitters can enhance membrane depolarization and thereby enhance NMDA receptor opening.

The growth factor BDNF (brain-derived neurotrophic factor) can also modulate the induction of LTP by a number of mechanisms, at least one of which is presynaptic (Gottschalk et al., 1998; Lu and Chow, 1999; Xu et al., 2000; **Figure 26(c)**). BDNF, acting through its cell-surface receptor TrkB, acts on presynaptic terminals to selectively facilitate neurotransmitter release during high-frequency stimulation. This is an interesting example of modulation of LTP induction that is activity dependent but localized to the presynaptic compartment. The mechanisms controlling the levels of BDNF in the adult hippocampus are not entirely clear at this point, but it is fairly well established that hippocampal BDNF levels can be regulated by a variety of neuronal activity-dependent processes and indeed in response to environmental signals impinging on the behaving animal.

11.13 Depotentiation and LTD

If synapses can be potentiated and this potentiation is very long-lasting, over time the synapses will be driven to their maximum synaptic strength. In this condition, there is no longer synaptic plasticity and no further capacity for that synapse to participate in synaptic-plasticity-dependent processes. Worse yet, over the lifetime of an animal, synapses will by random chance experience LTP-inducing conditions (presynaptic activity coincident with a postsynaptic action potential, for example) numerous times. If LTP is irreversible, ultimately every synapse will be maximally potentiated – obviously not a desirable condition vis-à-vis memory storage.

Consideration of this conundrum raises two implications. First, synapses that are involved in lifelong memory storage must be rendered essentially aplastic. In order to have good fidelity of memory storage over the lifetime of an animal, a synapse involved in permanent memory storage must be rendered immutable to a change in synaptic strength due to the random occurrence of what would normally be LTP-inducing stimulation.

But what about synapses like those in the hippocampus that are not sites of memory storage, but rather whose plasticity is part of the active processing of forming new long-term memories? To retain their plasticity and hence their capacity to contribute to memory formation, their potentiation must be reversible. Schaffer collateral synapses can undergo activity-dependent reversal of LTP, a phenomenon termed depotentiation (see **Figure 27**). Another activity-dependent way to decrease synaptic strength is LTD, the mirror image of LTP. LTD is a long-lasting decrease of synaptic strength below baseline. Using a logic similar to that of the first paragraph of this section, the phenomenon of dedepression of synaptic transmission is implied, although this has not been widely studied at this point.

As a practical matter it is often difficult to separate depotentiation from LTD experimentally. For example, a 'baseline' response in hippocampal slices or *in vivo* likely is a mixture of basal synaptic activity and activity at previously potentiated synapses. Moreover, for the most part the stimulation protocols used to induce depotentiation are variations of the protocols used to induce LTD. Nevertheless, mechanistic investigations have made clear that depotentiation and LTD use different mechanisms (Lee et al., 1998, 2000) and thus must be considered as distinct processes.

Physiologic LTD (and depotentiation) induction protocols generally involve variations of repetitive

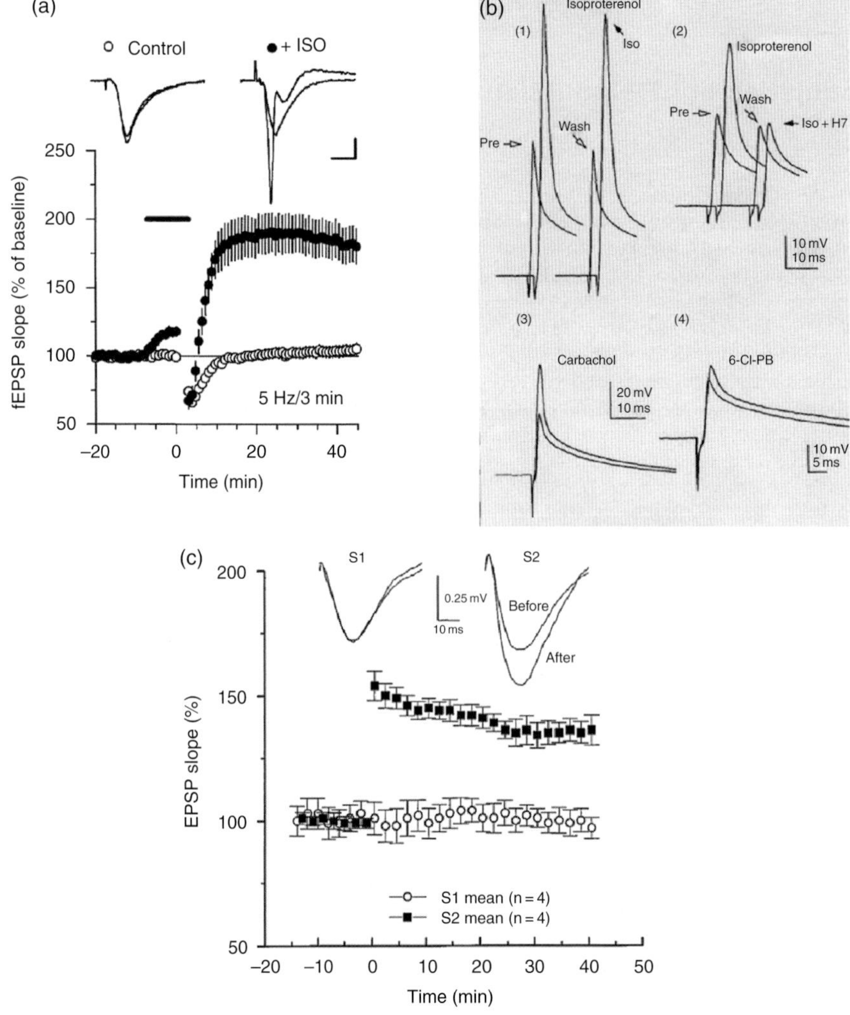

1-Hz stimulation (Lee et al., 1998; Kemp et al., 2000). A common protocol is to deliver 900 stimuli at 1 Hz, but there also are LTD protocols that use random small variations in frequency in the 1-Hz region and variations that use paired-pulse stimuli delivered at 1 Hz. Synaptic depression appears to be fairly robust *in vivo*, but is quite difficult to induce in hippocampal slices from adult animals. LTD *in vitro* is almost always studied using slices from immature animals, or cultured immature neurons, and it is possible that LTD as it is currently studied *in vitro* is largely a manifestation of what is normally a developmental mechanism.

One ironic aspect of the LTP/LTD story is that both phenomena at Schaffer collateral synapses can be blocked by NMDA receptor antagonists. This suggests that calcium influx triggers both processes, and indeed current models of LTD induction hypothesize that LTD is caused by an influx of calcium that achieves a lower level than that needed for LTP induction. This lower level of calcium is hypothesized to selectively activate protein phosphatases and, by this mechanism, to lower synaptic efficacy.

Another very different type of LTD is cerebellar LTD. Cerebellar LTD occurs at synapses onto Purkinje neurons in the cerebellar cortex. Cerebellar LTD is a very interesting phenomenon because its behavioral role is much better understood than the hippocampal plasticity phenomena we are discussing throughout this book. Among other things, cerebellar LTD is involved in associative eye-blink conditioning, a cerebellum-dependent classical conditioning paradigm. Considerable progress has been made in inves-tigating the roles and mechanisms of cerebellar LTD, as will be described in another chapter (*See* Chapter 12).

Figure 26 Neuromodulation of LTP induction. (a) Modulation of LTP induction by the beta-adrenergic agonist isoproterenol (ISO). Activity-dependent β-adrenergic modulation of low-frequency stimulation-induced LTP in the hippocampus CA1 region. In control experiments (no ISO), 3 min of 5-Hz stimulation (delivered at time = 0, open symbols, n = 26) had no lasting effect on synaptic transmission (45 min after 5-Hz stimulation, field EPSPs (fEPSPs) were not significantly different from pre–5-Hz baseline, t(25) = 1.01). However, 3 min of 5-Hz stimulation delivered at the end of a 10-min application of 1.0 mmol l^{-1} ISO (indicated by the bar) induced LTP (closed symbols, $p < 0.01$ compared with baseline). The traces are fEPSPs recorded during baseline and 45 min after 5-Hz stimulation in the presence and absence (control) of ISO. Calibration bars are 2.0 mV and 5.0 ms. Reproduced from Thomas MJ, Moody TD, Makhinson M, and O'Dell TJ (1996) Activity-dependent beta-adrenergic modulation of low frequency stimulation induced LTP in the hippocampal CA1 region. *Neuron* 17: 475–482, with permission. (b) One potential mechanism for neuromodulation is regulation of back-propagating action potentials in CA1 dendrites. The data shown illustrate amplification of dendritic action potentials by isoproterenol (1) and its susceptibility to inhibition by the protein kinase inhibitor H7 (2). The traces shown are from dendritic patch-clamp recordings from hippocampal pyramidal neurons. Muscarinic agonist (carbachol, (3)) and the dopamine receptor agonist 6-Cl-PB also can give various degrees of action-potential modulation as well. (1) Bath application of 1 µmol l^{-1} isoproterenol resulted in a 104% increase in amplitude, from 41 mV ('Pre') to 84 mV, of an antidromically initiated action potential recorded 220 µm from the soma. Wash-out of isoproterenol amplitude (38 mV; 'wash'). With a second application of isoproterenol (dark arrow labeled 'Iso'), the amplitude again increased twofold to 80 mV. (2) In a different recording 300 µmol l^{-1} H-7, a generic kinase inhibitor, was included in the control sine during the wash-out of isoproterenol. The subsequent second application of isoproterenol failed to lead to a second increase in amplitude (dark arrow labeled 'Iso + H7'). (3) In a distal recording (300 µM), 1 µmol l^{-1} carbachol increased the action potential amplitude by 81%, from 27–60 mV. In the carbachol experiments, cells were held hyperpolarized to –80 mV to remove Na+ channel inactivation. (4) One of the 6 out of 10 recordings where 6-Cl-PB led to an increase in amplitude. In a recording 220 µm from the soma, 10 µmol l^{-1} 6-Cl-PB increased dendritic action potential amplitude by 26%, from 21 to 26.5 mV. The cells were held at –70 mV in all 6-Cl-PB experiments. Adapted from Johnston D, Hoffman DA, Colbert CM, and Magee JC (1999) Regulation of back-propagating action potentials in hippocampal neurons. *Curr. Opin. Neurobiol.* 9: 288–292, with permission. (c) BDNF also modulates LTP induction in response to theta-frequency type stimulation. Two stimulating electrodes were positioned on either side of a single recording electrode to stimulate two different groups of afferents converging in the same dendritic field in CA1. Stimulation was applied to Schaffer collaterals alternately at low frequency (1 per min). After a period of baseline recording, LTP was induced with a theta-burst stimulation applied at time 0 only to one pathway (S1, filled squares). Simultaneous recording of an independent pathway (S2, open circles) showed no change in its synaptic strength after the theta burst was delivered to S1. BDNF (closed squares) selectively facilitates the induction of LTP in the tetanized pathway without affecting the synaptic efficacy of the untetanized pathway. EPSPs were recorded in the CA1 area of BDNF-treated slices. Synaptic efficacy (initial slope of field EPSPs) is expressed as a percentage of baseline value recorded during the 20 min before the tetanus. Representative traces of field EPSPs from S1 and S2 pathways were taken 10 min before and 40 min after the theta-burst stimulation. Adapted from Gottschalk W, Pozzo-Miller LD, Figurov A, and Lu B (1998) Presynaptic modulation of synaptic transmission and plasticity by brain-derived neurotrophic factor in the developing hippocampus. *J. Neurosci.* 18: 6830–6839, with permission.

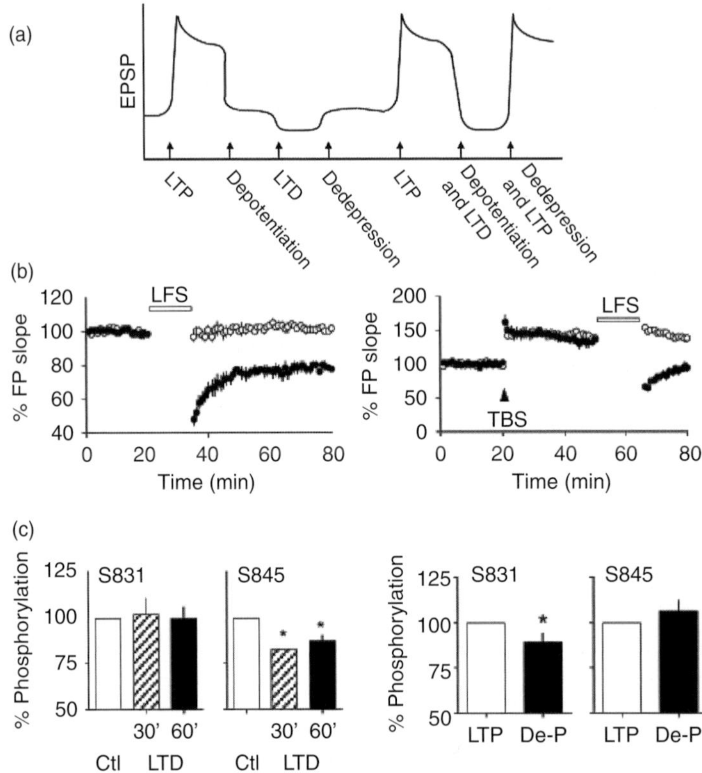

Figure 27 Depotentiation and LTD. (a) Schematic illustrating LTP, depotentiation, LTD, dedepression, and combinations of them. Figure by J. David Sweatt and Sarah E. Brown. (b) LTD and depotentiation in hippocampal neurons. Simultaneous recording of slices receiving baseline stimulation (control, open circles) and 1-Hz stimulation (closed circles). FP, Field potential. Regulation of distinct AMPA receptor phosphorylation sites during bidirectional synaptic plasticity. (c) Homosynaptic LTD in CA1 is associated with dephosphorylation of GluR1 at a PKA site (ser845). Depotentiation gives dephosphorylation at a CaMKII/PKC site (ser831). Adapted from Lee HK, Barbarosie M, Kameyama K, Bear MF, and Huganir RL (2000) Regulation of distinct AMPA receptor phosphorylation sites during bidirectional synaptic plasticity. *Nature* 405: 955–959, with permission from Elsevier.

11.14 Summary

Like learning, LTP can be defined as a long-lasting change in output in response to a transient input. The persistence of this effect has been demonstrated to extend many hours *in vitro* and several weeks *in vivo.* We do not know how LTP relates to memory, and there is evidence for and against the hypothesis that hippocampal LTP is involved in memory. Regardless, it is the best-understood example of long-lasting synaptic plasticity in the mammalian CNS, and it is a model for how long-lasting memory-associated changes are likely to occur in the CNS. One premise of some other chapters of this volume is that understanding LTP will yield valid insights into the mechanisms of plasticity that underlie learning and memory in the brain. The bona fide changes in neuronal connections that occur *in vivo* may or may not be identical to LTP as it is presently studied in the laboratory, but this does not diminish its utility as a cellular model system for studying lasting neuronal change in the mammalian CNS.

Acknowledgments

This chapter is adapted from *Mechanisms of Memory*, J. David Sweatt, Elsevier, 2003.

References

Andersen P, Sundberg SH, Sveen O, and Wigstrom H (1977) Specific long-lasting potentiation of synaptic transmission in hippocampal slices. *Nature* 266: 736–737.

Ankisztejn L and Ben-Ari Y (1991) Novel form of long-term potentiation produced by a K+ channel blocker in the hippocampus. *Nature* 349: 67–69.

Barrionuevo G and Brown TH (1983) Associative long-term potentiation in hippocampal slices. *Proc. Natl. Acad. Sci. USA* 80: 7347–7351.

Bekkers JM and Stevens CF (1990) Presynaptic mechanism for long-term potentiation in the hippocampus. *Nature* 346: 724–729.

Bi GQ and Poo MM (1998) Synaptic modifications in cultured hippocampal neurons: Dependence on spike timing, synaptic strength, and postsynaptic cell type. *J. Neurosci.* 18: 10464–10472.

Bliss TV and Lomo T (1973) Long-lasting potentiation of synaptic transmission in the dentate area of the anaesthetized rabbit following stimulation of the perforant path. *J. Physiol.* 232: 331–356.

Bolshakov VY, Golan H, Kandel ER, and Siegelbaum SA (1997) Recruitment of new sites of synaptic transmission during the cAMP-dependent late phase of LTP at CA3–CA1 synapses in the hippocampus. *Neuron* 19: 635–651.

Chapman CA, Perez Y, and Lacaille JC (1998) Effects of GABA(A) inhibition on the expression of long-term potentiation in CA1 pyramidal cells are dependent on tetanization parameters. *Hippocampus* 8: 289–298.

Chittajallu R, Alford S, and Collingridge GL (1998) Ca2+ and synaptic plasticity. *Cell Calcium* 24: 377–385.

Choi S, Klingauf J, and Tsien RW (2000) Postfusional regulation of cleft glutamate concentration during LTP at 'silent synapses'. *Nat. Neurosci.* 3: 330–336.

Collingridge GL, Kehl SJ, and McLennan H (1983) Excitatory amino acids in synaptic transmission in the Schaffer collateral-commissural pathway of the rat hippocampus. *J. Physiol.* 334: 33–46.

Davies CH, Starkey SJ, Pozza MF, and Collingridge GL (1991) GABA autoreceptors regulate the induction of LTP. *Nature* 349: 609–611.

Dolphin AC, Errington ML, and Bliss TV (1982) Long-term potentiation of the perforant path *in vivo* is associated with increased glutamate release. *Nature* 297: 496–498.

Gottschalk W, Pozzo-Miller LD, Figurov A, and Lu B (1998) Presynaptic modulation of synaptic transmission and plasticity by brain-derived neurotrophic factor in the developing hippocampus. *J. Neurosci.* 18: 6830–6839.

Grover LM and Teyler TJ (1990) Two components of long-term potentiation induced by different patterns of afferent activation. *Nature* 347: 477–479.

Harris EW and Cotman CW (1986) Long-term potentiation of guinea pig mossy fiber responses is not blocked by N-methyl D-aspartate antagonists. *Neurosci. Lett.* 70: 132–137.

Hebb DO (1949) *The Organization of Behavior: A Neuropsychological Theory.* New York: Wiley.

Johnston D and Amaral DG (1998) Hippocampus. In: Shepherd GM (ed.) *The Synaptic Organization of the Brain,* 4th edn., pp. 417–458. New York: Oxford University Press.

Johnston D, Hoffman DA, Colbert CM, and Magee JC (1999) Regulation of back-propagating action potentials in hippocampal neurons. *Curr. Opin. Neurobiol.* 9: 288–292.

Johnston D, Hoffman DA, Magee JC, et al. (2000) Dendritic potassium channels in hippocampal pyramidal neurons. *J. Physiol.* 525(Pt 1): 75–81.

Johnston D, Williams S, Jaffe D, and Gray R (1992) NMDA-receptor-independent long-term potentiation. *Annu. Rev. Physiol.* 54: 489–505.

Johnston D and Wu SM (1995) *Foundations of Cellular Neurophysiology.* Cambridge, MA: MIT Press.

Kamondi A, Acsady L, and Buzsaki G (1998) Dendritic spikes are enhanced by cooperative network activity in the intact hippocampus. *J. Neurosci.* 18: 3919–3928.

Kapur A, Yeckel MF, Gray R, and Johnston D (1998) L-Type calcium channels are required for one form of hippocampal mossy fiber LTP. *J. Neurophysiol.* 79: 2181–2190.

Kemp N, McQueen J, Faulkes S, and Bashir ZI (2000) Different forms of LTD in the CA1 region of the hippocampus: Role of age and stimulus protocol. *Eur. J. Neurosci.* 12: 360–366.

Lee HK, Barbarosie M, Kameyama K, Bear MF, and Huganir RL (2000) Regulation of distinct AMPA receptor phosphorylation sites during bidirectional synaptic plasticity. *Nature* 405: 955–959.

Lee HK, Kameyama K, Huganir RL, and Bear MF (1998) NMDA induces long-term synaptic depression and dephosphorylation of the GluR1 subunit of AMPA receptors in hippocampus. *Neuron* 21: 1151–1162.

Linden DJ (1999) The return of the spike: Postsynaptic action potentials and the induction of LTP and LTD. *Neuron* 22: 661–666.

Lu B and Chow A (1999) Neurotrophins and hippocampal synaptic transmission and plasticity. *J. Neurosci. Res.* 58: 76–87.

Lu YM, Mansuy IM, Kandel ER, and Roder J (2000) Calcineurin-mediated LTD of GABAergic inhibition underlies the increased excitability of CA1 neurons associated with LTP. *Neuron* 26: 197–205.

Lynch G, Larson J, Kelso S, Barrionuevo G, and Schottler F (1983) Intracellular injections of EGTA block induction of hippocampal long-term potentiation. *Nature* 305: 719–721.

Magee JC and Johnston D (1997) A synaptically controlled, associative signal for Hebbian plasticity in hippocampal neurons. *Science* 275: 209–213.

Malgaroli A, Ting AE, Wendland B, et al. (1995) Presynaptic component of long-term potentiation visualized at individual hippocampal synapses. *Science* 268: 1624–1628.

Malinow R, Madison DV, and Tsien RW (1988) Persistent protein kinase activity underlying long-term potentiation. *Nature* 335: 820–824.

Malinow R and Tsien RW (1990) Presynaptic enhancement shown by whole-cell recordings of long-term potentiation in hippocampal slices. *Nature* 346: 177–180.

Malinow R (1991) Transmission between pairs of hippocampal slice neurons: Quantal levels, oscillations, and LTP. *Science* 252: 722–724.

McMahon LL and Kauer JA (1997) Hippocampal interneurons express a novel form of synaptic plasticity. *Neuron* 18: 295–305.

McNaughton BL, Douglas RM, and Goddard GV (1978) Synaptic enhancement in fascia dentata: Cooperativity among coactive afferents. *Brain Res.* 157: 277–293.

Mott DD and Lewis DV (1991) Facilitation of the induction of long-term potentiation by GABAB receptors. *Science* 252: 1718–1720.

Naber PA and Witter MP (1998) Subicular efferents are organized mostly as parallel projections: A double-labeling, retrograde-tracing study in the rat. *J. Comp. Neurol.* 393: 284–297.

Nicoll RA and Malenka RC (1995) Contrasting properties of two forms of long-term potentiation in the hippocampus. *Nature* 377: 115–118.

Nicoll RA and Malenka RC (1999) Expression mechanisms underlying NMDA receptor-dependent long-term potentiation. *Ann. N. Y. Acad. Sci.* 868: 515–525.

Powell CM, Johnston D, and Sweatt JD (1994) Autonomously active protein kinase C in the maintenance phase of N-methyl-D-aspartate receptor-independent long term potentiation. *J. Biol. Chem.* 269: 27958–27963.

Roberson ED, English JD, and Sweatt JD (1996) A biochemist's view of long-term potentiation. *Learn Mem.* 3: 1–24.

Schafe GE, Atkins CM, Swank MW, Bauer EP, Sweatt JD, and LeDoux JE (2000) Activation of ERK/MAP kinase in the amygdala is required for memory consolidation of Pavlovian fear conditioning. *J. Neurosci.* 20: 8177–8187.

Scharfman HE and Sarvey JM (1985) Postsynaptic firing during repetitive stimulation is required for long-term potentiation in hippocampus. *Brain Res.* 331: 267–274.

Sweatt JD (2003) *Mechanisms of Memory.* London: Elsevier.

Thomas MJ, Moody TD, Makhinson M, and O'Dell TJ (1996) Activity-dependent beta-adrenergic modulation of low frequency stimulation induced LTP in the hippocampal CA1 region. *Neuron* 17: 475–482.

van Groen T and Wyss JM (1990) Extrinsic projections from area CA1 of the rat hippocampus: Olfactory, cortical, subcortical, and bilateral hippocampal formation projections. *J. Comp. Neurol.* 302: 515–528.

Wigstrom H and Gustafsson B (1986) Postsynaptic control of hippocampal long-term potentiation. *J. Physiol. (Paris)* 81: 228–236.

Winder DG, Mansuy IM, Osman M, Moallem TM, and Kandel ER (1998) Genetic and pharmacological evidence for a novel, intermediate phase of long-term potentiation suppressed by calcineurin. *Cell* 92: 25–37.

Xu B, Gottschalk W, Chow A, et al. (2000) The role of brain-derived neurotrophic factor receptors in the mature hippocampus: Modulation of long-term potentiation through a presynaptic mechanism involving TrkB. *J. Neurosci.* 20: 6888–6897.

Yeckel MF, Kapur A, and Johnston D (1999) Multiple forms of LTP in hippocampal CA3 neurons use a common postsynaptic mechanism. *Nat. Neurosci.* 2: 625–633.

Yuan LL, Adams JP, Swank M, Sweatt JD, and Johnston D (2002) Protein kinase modulation of dendritic K+ channels in hippocampus involves a mitogen-activated protein kinase pathway. *J. Neurosci.* 22: 4860–4868.

Zakharenko SS, Zablow L, and Siegelbaum SA (2001) Visualization of changes in presynaptic function during long-term synaptic plasticity. *Nat. Neurosci.* 4: 711–717.

Zalutsky RA and Nicoll RA (1990) Comparison of two forms of long-term potentiation in single hippocampal neurons. *Science* 248: 1619–1624.

12 LTD – Synaptic Depression and Memory Storage

C. Hansel, Erasmus University Medical Center, Rotterdam, The Netherlands

M. F. Bear, Massachusetts Institute of Technology, Cambridge, MA, USA

12.1 Introduction

A widely held assumption among neuroscientists is that experience is capable of persistently modifying the properties of synapses, and that this use-dependent modification is central to both neuronal memory storage and the refinement of connections in brain development. This general idea was initially voiced by Sechenov and Cajal and was later formalized by Hebb (1949) in his famous synaptic modification postulate:

> When an axon of cell A is near enough to excite a cell B and repeatedly or persistently takes part in firing it, some growth process or metabolic change takes place in one or both cells such that A's efficiency, as one of the cells firing B, is increased. (Hebb, 1949)

However, it was not until many years later that an electrophysiological model system emerged that appeared to embody this idea of activity-dependent synaptic memories in the mammalian brain. Bliss and Lomo (1973) showed that brief, high-frequency stimulation of a population of axons, the perforant path projection to the hippocampal dentate gyrus, produced an increase in the strength of these synapses which could last for hours. This phenomenon, called long-term potentiation (LTP), has since been seen to last for days to weeks in chronic preparations. The duration of LTP, together with its initial discovery in the hippocampus, a brain region known from behavioral studies to be important for the storage of declarative memory, produced a surge of interest in LTP as a putative cellular model system for memory. This interest was only increased when it became clear that under certain conditions LTP could display some of the formal properties of learning such as specificity (LTP is confined to activated synapses) and associativity (weak stimulation of an input to a postsynaptic cell will only induce LTP when paired with a neighboring strong input to that same cell).

While the first studies of LTP relied upon field potential recording in the intact hippocampus, this phenomenon has subsequently been observed in almost every type of glutamatergic synapse in the brain and has been extensively studied in reduced preparations such as brain slices and cultures of embryonic neurons. At the same time that LTP was gradually 'escaping' from the hippocampus, it was becoming clear that it was not the only form of use-dependent synaptic modification. The converse phenomenon, long-term depression (LTD) was also initially observed in the hippocampus before being found in other brain regions. At present, it appears likely that there are no synapses that express only LTP or LTD. In most synapses, LTP and LTD are typically evoked by brief, strong stimulation and sustained, weak stimulation, respectively. The direction of change in synaptic strength (LTP vs. LTD) is believed to be determined, at most types of synapses, by the amount of postsynaptic activity (as indexed by Ca influx) which occurs during induction: a small amount of postsynaptic Ca influx results in LTD, while a larger amount results in LTP (see Linden, 1999; Zucker, 1999, for review).

If LTP in the mature brain truly functions to underlie memory storage, then what is the function of LTD? One proposal has been that LTD is a "neuronal substrate of forgetting" (Tsumoto, 1993). While there is no definitive evidence to dispute this view, there is no definitive support for it either. A potentially more useful construct is to consider that information is likely to be stored in the brain, at least in part, as an array of synaptic weights. If these synapses are driven to their maximal or minimal strengths, then those elements of the array become limited in their ability to contribute to subsequent plasticity. Thus, neural circuits containing synapses that can actively both increase and decrease their strength are at a distinct computational advantage.

Experience-dependent refinement of connections during brain development can also potentially benefit from having both LTP and LTD mechanisms. Synapses which undergo strong, correlated activity can be strengthened and thereby retained, while synapses which have weak uncorrelated activity can be weakened and ultimately removed. Like memory storage, one could imagine that developmental refinement of connections could proceed using either LTD or LTP alone, but the presence of both allows for faster and more flexible change.

In this article we will not attempt to provide a comprehensive overview of LTD at the many synapses in the brain where it has been studied. Rather, we will focus on the two best-understood forms (LTD at the hippocampal Schaffer collateral/commissural-CA1 pyramidal cell synapse and LTD at the cerebellar parallel fiber–Purkinje cell synapse) as case studies to examine both the cellular processes which underlie LTD and its larger role in behavior and development.

12.2 LTD of the Hippocampal Schaffer Collateral-CA1 Synapse

The Schaffer collateral-CA1 synapse is widely used as a model synapse for the study of LTP and of synaptic plasticity in general. The hippocampus is not necessarily the brain area of choice when it comes to relating synaptic gain changes to their behavioral consequences, because it is many synapses from the sensory periphery. Nevertheless, the hippocampus does store certain types of information, and it is reasonable to expect that synaptic plasticity participates in this process (Riedel et al., 1999). Moreover, available evidence suggests that what has been learned about synaptic plasticity in the hippocampus is also widely applicable to synapses elsewhere in the brain. For example, it seems that synaptic plasticity at glutamatergic synapses onto some (but not all) neocortical pyramidal cells operates using similar rules for induction as its counterpart at CA1 hippocampal synapses.

Although the original discovery of LTP (in the dentate gyrus, by Terje Lømo) was accidental (the unexpected outcome of experiments designed to study synaptic responses during repetitive stimulation), it was quickly embraced as a potential synaptic mechanism for memory (Bliss and Lomo, 1973). Excitement grew in the mid-1980s, when the properties of LTP in CA1 were shown to satisfy the requirements of Hebb's famous postulate that active synapses strengthen when their activity correlates specifically with a strong postsynaptic response (Wigstrom and Gustafsson, 1985; Kelso et al., 1986; Malinow and Miller, 1986; Sastry et al., 1986). However, theoreticians had concluded years before that 'Hebbian' synaptic modifications alone were not likely to be sufficient to account for memory storage; the efficient storage of information by synapses requires bidirectional synaptic modifications; i.e., LTD as well as LTP. Thus, the search for homosynaptic LTD in the hippocampus was theoretically motivated; it was not an accident (the reasons that it was not stumbled on accidentally will become clear in the discussion below). The theoretical suggestion was that synapses should depress when their activity *fails* to correlate with a strong postsynaptic response. To realize this situation experimentally, induction of LTD was attempted in CA1 using prolonged trains of presynaptic stimulation, delivered at frequencies (0.5–10 Hz) that fail to evoke a strong postsynaptic response (Dudek and Bear, 1992). Trains of low-frequency stimulation (LFS) are now the standard protocol for induction of homosynaptic LTD in CA1 and at synapses throughout the forebrain.

When discussing induction and expression mechanisms of LTD, it is important to note that LFS induces at least two, and possibly three (Berretta and Cherubini, 1998), mechanistically distinct forms of LTD in CA1, whose discovery solved previously existing contradictions (see Bear and Abraham, 1996). One form depends on the activation of *N*-methyl-D-aspartate receptors (NMDARs); another depends on the activation of group 1 metabotropic glutamate receptors (mGluRs), which are postsynaptic glutamate receptors coupled to phosphoinositide metabolism. These two forms will be described separately here.

12.3 Theoretical Framework

The bidirectional modification of excitatory synaptic transmission is not just an abstract theoretical construct. We need to understand mechanisms of bidirectional synaptic plasticity because direct experimental observations have shown, repeatedly, that synapses in the cerebral cortex are, in fact, bidirectionally modifiable. The value added by a theoretical structure is that it helps to make sense of what bidirectional synaptic plasticity accomplishes with respect to information storage and provides insight into how it might be implemented.

Neurons throughout the cerebral cortex, including area CA1 of the hippocampus, have stimulus-selective receptive fields. Chronic recording from cortical neurons has shown that as something new is learned, stimulus selectivity changes – some synaptic inputs potentiate and others depress. In CA1, for example, neurons show selectivity for positions in space, and this selectivity shifts rapidly as animals learn a new spatial environment (Breese et al., 1989; Wilson and McNaughton, 1993). What does a stable shift in selectivity tell us about memory? Neural network theory suggests that the selectivity shift reflects the creation of new neural representations. The memory is encoded by changing the pattern of synaptic weights across the network of neurons (Bear, 1996).

Now consider what happens when more new information is learned: stimulus selectivity (i.e., the pattern of synaptic weights) shifts further. An implication of this finding is that previously encoded memories can remain stable, even as the pattern of synaptic strengths is again modified to create new representations. According to this way of thinking, memory requires the episodic (if not continual) bidirectional modification of synaptic transmission to fine-tune the patterns of synaptic weights in the neural network. It is important to emphasize, of course, that in the absence of new learned information, synaptic weights must remain stable. Passive decay of synaptic weight (that is, back to an initial value that might be larger or smaller) leads to a loss of the stored representations.

The bidirectional modification of synaptic transmission obviously requires that individual synapses on neurons be capable of some form of LTP and some form of LTD. However, every theory of memory storage that assumes bidirectional synaptic modification places an important constraint on the mechanisms of LTP and LTD: reversibility. Consider the problem that would arise if the LTP and LTD mechanisms were distinct and irreversible. While it is true that synaptic weights could be fine-tuned initially by simple summation of the two independent processes, eventually saturation would occur as the synapses underwent rounds of bidirectional modification (see **Figure 6**). This problem does not occur if LTP and LTD are inverse processes mechanistically.

Now we come to the question of what distinguishes stimulation conditions that yield synaptic potentiation from those that yield synaptic depression. To specifically encode memory, synaptic modifications must depend on the presynaptic activation of the synapses bringing information into the network. In other words, the modifications must be 'homosynaptic.' The variables that determine the polarity or sign of the modification, in principle, could be the absolute amount of presynaptic activity, the concurrent level and timing of postsynaptic activity, or some combination of these variables. There are many abstract theoretical 'learning rules' based on these variables, but the most useful are those that attempt to account for what has actually been observed experimentally. One very influential proposal was made by Bienenstock, Cooper, and Munro (1982) in what is known as the BCM theory. In order to account for the development and plasticity of neuronal stimulus selectivity, they proposed that active synapses are potentiated when the total postsynaptic response exceeds a critical value, called the 'modification threshold' (qm), and that active synapses are depressed when the total postsynaptic response is greater than zero but less than qm. In addition, it was proposed that the value of qm varies as a function of the average integrated postsynaptic activity.

Once the requirements for LTP induction in CA1 had been elucidated, a specific physiological basis for the BCM theory became apparent. The proposal was made (1) that the term qm corresponds to the critical level of postsynaptic depolarization at which the Ca flux through the NMDAR exceeds the threshold for inducing LTP; (2) that LTD should be a consequence of presynaptic activity that consistently fails to evoke a postsynaptic Ca response large enough to induce LTP; and (3) that the postsynaptic threshold for LTP should vary depending on the stimulation history of the postsynaptic neuron (Bear et al., 1987). These hypotheses have now all been validated experimentally.

The BCM theory motivated the search for LTD using LFS (Dudek and Bear, 1992). The rationale was to provide a high level of presynaptic activity that did not evoke a large postsynaptic response. Critical variables for LTD induction in rat hippocampal slices proved to be the stimulation strength (it could not be so strong as to elicit orthodromic action potentials), healthy inhibition, stimulation frequency (<10 Hz), the number of stimuli (typically hundreds), and the age of the animal (greater magnitude before 35 days of age). LTD was found to be a very reliable phenomenon when the appropriate conditions were met. Even so, there was concern that LTD might be an artifact. First, there was heightened skepticism because several previous reports of LTD induction using different protocols had proven difficult to replicate in the hippocampus; second, the same LFS protocol that was found to induce LTD had previously been reported by others to be ineffective in altering baseline synaptic transmission; and third, synaptic depression could easily be dismissed as a pathological change rather than a form of synaptic plasticity. Most of these concerns faded when it was found that at least one form of LTD depended specifically upon activation of NMDARs and a rise in postsynaptic Ca, that the same synapses that showed LTD could subsequently be potentiated, and that LTD could be elicited *in vivo* (Dudek and Bear, 1992, 1993; Mulkey and Malenka, 1992; Thiels et al., 1994; Heynen et al., 1996; Debanne et al., 1997; Manahan-Vaughan, 1997).

It is now apparent that multiple forms of LTD exist in CA1, possibly at the same synapses. Remarkably, however, all forms of LTD can be elicited using variations of the LFS protocol, specifically under conditions that fail to evoke a large postsynaptic response. Thus, the hypothesis of homosynaptic LTD, inspired by the BCM theory, has been amply confirmed. As we will discuss further, it is also noteworthy that the NMDAR-dependent form of LTD appears to be the functional inverse of LTP, thus satisfying the theoretical requirement that synaptic modifications be both bidirectional and reversible. Thus, at least in theory, the mechanisms of LTD as well as LTP can contribute to the receptive field plasticity underlying memory storage in the hippocampus and elsewhere.

12.4 NMDAR-Dependent LTD

12.4.1 Induction by Calcium

Induction of homosynaptic LTD in CA1 using the standard 1-Hz LFS protocol *in vivo*, and under most experimental conditions *in vitro*, is blocked by NMDAR antagonists (Dudek and Bear, 1992; Mulkey and Malenka, 1992; Heynen et al., 1996; Manahan-Vaughan, 1997). Although this form of LTD shares with LTP a dependence upon NMDA receptor activation and a rise in postsynaptic Ca ion concentration, there is a systematic difference in the type of stimulation that yields the two types of synaptic modification. This difference is easily demonstrated simply by varying the frequency of tetanic stimulation. In rat CA1, for example, 900 pulses at 0.5–3 Hz typically yields LTD, whereas the same amount of stimulation at frequencies greater than 10 Hz yields LTP (**Figure 1(a)**; Dudek and Bear, 1992). The different consequences of stimulation at different frequencies have been attributed to systematic differences in the postsynaptic Ca currents through the postsynaptic NMDA receptors. Indeed, it is now well established that the critical variables are postsynaptic depolarization and Ca entry, not stimulation frequency *per se*. For example, while 1-Hz stimulation normally produces LTD, postsynaptic hyperpolarization during conditioning prevents any change, and depolarization leads to induction of LTP (Mulkey and Malenka, 1992). Likewise, while high-frequency stimulation normally produces LTP, it produces LTD instead if delivered in the presence of subsaturating concentrations of an NMDA receptor antagonist (Cummings et al., 1996; **Figure 1(b)**, **(c)**).

The appropriate activation of postsynaptic NMDARs appears to be sufficient to induce LTD; presynaptic activity is not necessary. This conclusion is supported by the observation that photolysis of caged extracellular glutamate (Kandler et al., 1998; Dodt et al., 1999) and brief bath application of NMDA (Lee et al., 1998; Kamal et al., 1999) induce LTD without concurrent presynaptic stimulation. In agreement with the idea that Ca passing through NMDARs is the trigger for LTD, photolysis of caged Ca in the postsynaptic neuron can also induce synaptic depression (Neveu and Zucker, 1996). This finding is important, as it indicates that LTD can be induced by Ca entry through the NMDAR without the need to invoke any other Ca-independent signaling or triggering process. Curiously, however, a modest, brief elevation in Ca concentration ([Ca]) was found to induce LTP and LTD with equal probability. Subsequent analysis suggests that LTD is most reliably induced (and LTP is never induced) by a modest (~0.7 μmol l^{-1}) but prolonged (~60 s) rise in [Ca]. LTP, in contrast, is most reliably induced by a large (~10 μmol l^{-1}) and brief (~3 s) increase in [Ca] (Yang et al., 1999). Although these findings are all consistent with the proposal that LTD and LTP are triggered by distinct Ca responses during NMDAR activation (Bear et al., 1987; Lisman, 1989; Artola and Singer, 1993; Bear and Malenka, 1994) and with imaging studies that confirmed

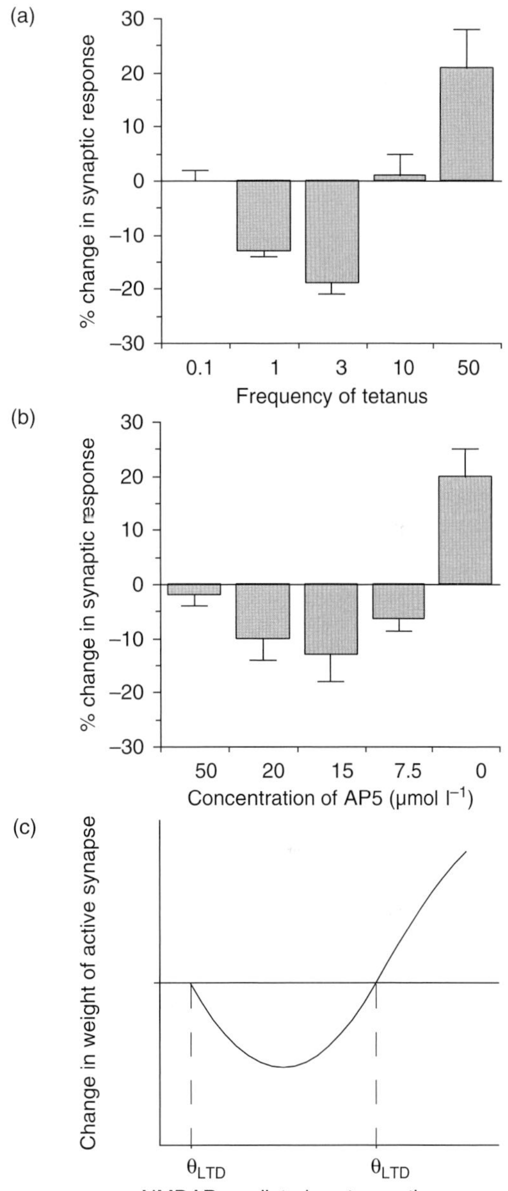

Figure 1 Induction of NMDAR-dependent bidirectional plasticity of the Schaffer collateral synapse in CA1. (a) Summary of the effects of a 900-pulse tetanus delivered at different frequencies (replotted from Dudek SM and Bear MF (1992) Homosynaptic long-term depression in area CA1 of hippocampus and effects of NMDA receptor blockade. *Proc. Natl. Acad. Sci. USA* 89: 4363–4367, with permission from the National Academy of Sciences, USA). (b) Summary of the effects of a 600-pulse, 20-Hz tetanus in different concentrations of the NMDA receptor antagonist AP5 (replotted from Cummings JA, Mulkey RM, Nicoll RA, and Malenka RC (1996) Ca signalling requirements for long-term depression in the hippocampus. *Neuron* 16: 825–833, with permission from Elsevier). (c) A synaptic 'learning rule' based on data such as those given in (a) and (b). This learning rule is formally similar to that proposed in the BCM theory.

that LTP-inducing stimuli elicit larger Ca transients than LTD-inducing stimuli (Hansel et al., 1997; Cormier et al., 2001), they argue against a simple relationship between synaptic modification and Ca level. The dynamics of the Ca response are also important determinants of the polarity of synaptic modification.

Perhaps not surprisingly, under certain circumstances voltage-gated Ca channels may also contribute to the Ca signal that triggers LTD (Christie et al., 1996). However, this role appears to be supplementary, since NMDAR activation is still required to observe homosynaptic LTD under these conditions, and Ca channel activation is not always necessary (Selig et al., 1995b). Nonetheless, the modulation of synaptic plasticity by active dendritic Ca conductances can be striking. Markram et al. (1997) made the remarkable observation that a back-propagating dendritic action potential, precisely timed to occur a few milliseconds before a synaptically evoked excitatory postsynaptic potential (EPSP), could promote induction of LTD in neocortical pyramidal neurons by stimuli that otherwise are ineffective. Similar findings have been reported in hippocampal cultures (Bi and Poo, 1998). The relative timing of coincident pre- and postsynaptic activity determines the amplitude of Ca transients in dendritic spines: Ca transients are larger when an EPSP precedes an action potential (AP) than when it follows it (Koester and Sakmann, 1998). As the former condition favors LTP induction (Markram et al., 1997), these results demonstrate that, under physiological conditions, larger Ca signals are indeed associated with LTP induction, whereas lower Ca signals more likely result in the induction of LTD.

An appealing hypothesis for this observation is that voltage-gated Ca influx inactivates NMDARs, thus causing a relatively lower Ca transient upon subsequent synaptic activation (Linden, 1999; Zucker, 1999). From a computational perspective, the observation that LTP results from EPSPs followed by APs, whereas LTD results from activation in the reverse order, provides a perfect correlate of Hebbian (and anti-Hebbian) concepts. APs following EPSPs suggest that the activated input repetitively and successfully contributed sufficient depolarization so that the spike threshold was reached, which is a Hebbian requirement for strengthening of that synapse. On the other hand, EPSPs following APs can be interpreted as random, uncorrelated presynaptic activity, leading to weakening of those synaptic inputs.

To summarize what has been learned to date, LTD is induced by an elevation of Ca that is constrained, apparently, by three variables: (1) proximity to the postsynaptic membrane, (2) peak concentration, and (3) duration. Synaptic stimulation causes LTD when it yields the appropriate response within the 'box' defined by these parameters. While LFS at 1 Hz is usually effective, under different experimental conditions different protocols may be required (e.g., Thiels et al., 1994; Debanne et al., 1994). Ca entry through the NMDA receptor is sufficient to induce LTD, but this can also be supplemented by other Ca sources (Christie et al., 1996; Reyes and Stanton, 1996).

12.5 The Role of Calcium-Dependent Enzymatic Reactions

A key component in the theory of synaptic memory formation is that synaptic efficacy is controlled by the phosphorylation state of alpha-amino-3-hydroxy-5-methyl-4-isoxazole propionic acid receptors (AMPARs) which can mediate biophysical changes at the individual receptor level and/or can modify the insertion/internalization balance of AMPARs (for review see Song and Huganir, 2002). Induction of LTP requires activation of Ca-dependent serine-threonine protein kinases in the postsynaptic neuron. Key molecules in hippocampal LTP are Ca/calmodulin-dependent protein kinase II (CaMKII; Malenka et al., 1989; Malinow et al., 1989; Silva et al., 1992; Pettit et al., 1994; Lledo et al., 1995) and protein kinase C (PKC), whose ζ isoform is upregulated during LTP maintenance (Hrabetova and Sacktor, 1996). Lisman (1989) proposed that LTD might result from activation of a protein phosphatase cascade, leading to dephosphorylation of the same synaptic proteins that are involved in LTP. Subsequent experiments by Mulkey and coworkers confirmed an essential role for postsynaptic protein phosphatase 1 (PP1) and calcineurin (PP2B) in the induction of LTD with LFS (Mulkey et al., 1993, 1994).

The basic working hypothesis continues to be that LTD results from dephosphorylation of postsynaptic PP1 substrates and that CaMKII and PP1 act as a kinase/phosphatase switch, regulating the phosphorylation state of AMPARs and their auxiliary proteins (Lisman and Zhabotinsky, 2001; Malleret et al., 2001). As will be discussed, there is now direct evidence for dephosphorylation of synaptic proteins following

LTD induction protocols (Lee et al., 1998, 2000, 2003; Ramakers et al., 1999). Moreover, there is evidence that PP1 activity is persistently increased by LTD-inducing stimulation (Thiels et al., 1998) and that peptides that inhibit PP1 binding to target proteins block LTD induction (Morishita et al., 2001). PP1 is regulated by the protein inhibitor-1 (I-1). When I-1 is phosphorylated by protein kinase A (PKA), PP1 is inactive. Dephosphorylation of I-1 by PP2B releases PP1 from inhibition (Cohen, 1989; Nairn and Shenolikar, 1992). PP2B is activated by Ca/calmodulin and, therefore, is believed to be key for translating an increase in [Ca] into LTD (**Figure 2**).

Before moving on to consider expression mechanisms, it should be noted that there are also data suggesting that Ca/calmodulin triggers LTD by activating nitric oxide synthase (Izumi and Zorumski, 1993; Gage et al., 1997). The proposed mechanism of nitric oxide action is the retrograde activation of a second messenger cascade in the presynaptic terminal involving soluble guanylyl cyclase and cyclic guanosine monophosphate (cGMP)-dependent protein kinase (Reyes et al., 1999). This scenario is not universally agreed upon, however, since others report no effect of nitric oxide inhibitors on LTD (Cummings et al., 1994). At the present time, it appears that this mechanism lies in parallel with

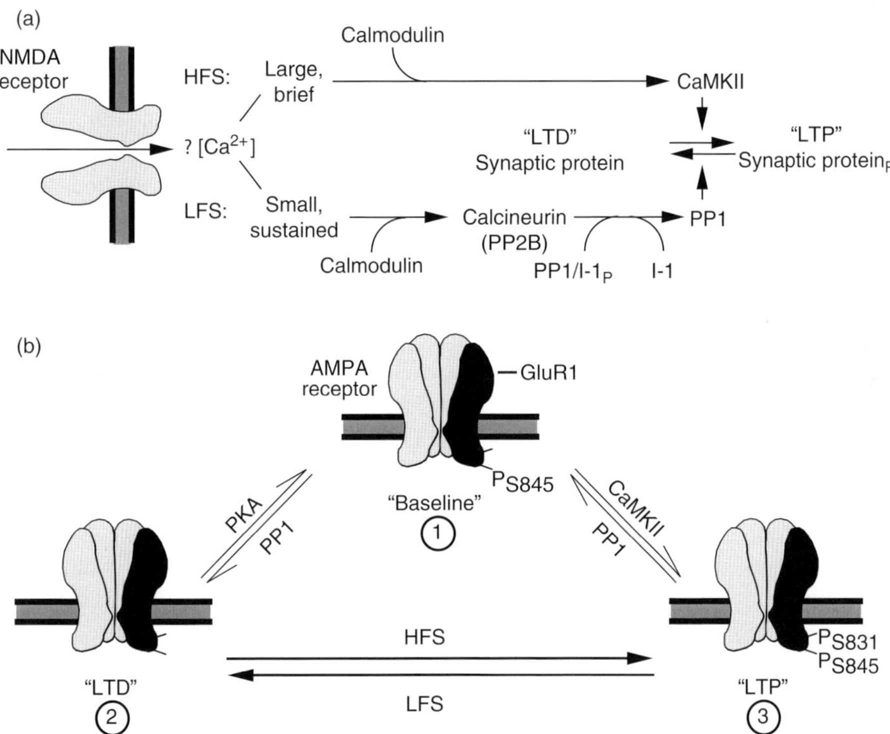

Figure 2 Molecular models for bidirectional plasticity of the Schaffer collateral synapse in CA1. (a) Induction. Strong NMDA receptor activation resulting from high-frequency stimulation (HFS) causes a large, brief rise in intracellular calcium. This calcium signal triggers activation of CaMKII and the induction of LTP by phosphorylation of synaptic proteins. Weak NMDA receptor activation resulting from low-frequency stimulation (LFS) produces a smaller but more sustained rise in intracellular calcium. This calcium signal selectively activates calcineurin which dephosphorylates inhibitor-1 (I-1). Dephosphorylation of I-1 relieves protein phosphatase 1 (PP1) from inhibition. LTD results from dephosphorylation of the same synaptic proteins involved in LTP. (b) Expression. (1) Under baseline conditions, the GluR1 subunit of AMPA receptors is highly phosphorylated at ser-845, a protein kinase A (PKA) substrate. (2) LFS causes dephosphorylation of ser-845 and LTD. (3) From the baseline state, HFS causes phosphorylation of ser-831, a CaMKII substrate, and LTP. According to this model, LTD and LTP result from bidirectional modifications of AMPA receptor phosphorylation, but at different sites. Thus, dedepression and LTP are not formally equivalent, nor are depotentiation and LTD. (4) The fourth possible state, in which ser-831 is phosphorylated and ser-845 is not, has not been observed experimentally. Adapted from Kameyama K, Lee HK, Bear MF, and Huganir RL (1998) Involvement of a postsynaptic protein kinase A substrate in the expression of homosynaptic long-term depression. *Neuron* 21: 1163–1175, with permission from Elsevier.

that involving postsynaptic phosphatase activation. It is plausible that nitric oxide signaling is involved in the mGluR-dependent form of LTD (discussed in the following section), but this remains to be examined explicitly.

12.5.1 Expression Mechanisms

It now seems very clear that a modification of postsynaptic glutamate sensitivity is a major expression mechanism for the NMDAR-dependent form of LTD. As mentioned earlier, liberating caged glutamate in CA1, under conditions where synaptic transmission is blocked, results in LTD of the glutatmate-evoked currents. This LTD is restricted spatially to the site of glutamate release and depends upon NMDAR activation and postsynaptic protein phosphatase activity (Kandler et al., 1998). The possibility remains that this form of LTD is actually expressed at extrasynaptic glutamate receptors and therefore could be mechanistically distinct from LFS-induced LTD. However, very similar findings have recently been obtained in rat neocortex where, in addition, it was shown that synaptically induced LTD results in a decrease in sensitivity to laser-stimulated photolysis of caged glutamate. Moreover, LFS-induced LTD occluded further synaptic depression by glutamate pulses (Dodt et al., 1999). The close similarities between CA1 and neocortical LTD (Kirkwood et al., 1993; Kirkwood and Bear, 1994) suggest that these findings may apply generally to NMDAR-dependent LTD in the cerebral cortex, at least in some layers.

A very interesting picture has emerged recently to account for decreased glutamate sensitivity following LTD. The model of bidirectional synaptic modification through reversible changes in the phosphorylation of postsynaptic substrates (Lisman, 1989; Bear and Malenka, 1994) begged the question of which synaptic phosphoproteins are involved. Now there is direct evidence that LTD is associated with dephosphorylation of AMPAR subunits, the consequence of which is known to be depression of glutamate-evoked currents. In addition, there are converging lines of evidence that LTD is associated with the removal of glutamate receptors from the postsynaptic membrane (for review see Song and Huganir, 2002; Collingridge et al., 2004). We shall discuss each of these mechanisms, in turn.

AMPARs are heteromeric complexes assembled from four homologous subunits (GluR1–4) in various combinations (Seeburg, 1993; Hollmann and Heinemann, 1994). The large majority of AMPARs in the hippocampus contain both GluR1 and GluR2 subunits (Wenthold et al., 1996). Hippocampal LTP largely rests on modifications of the GluR1 subunits, which determine trafficking behavior in GluR1/GluR2 heteromers (Song and Huganir, 2002). The GluR1 subunit is highly regulated by protein phosphorylation and contains identified phosphorylation sites on the intracellular carboxy-terminal domain. Serine-831 is phosphorylated by CaMKII and PKC, while serine-845 is phosphorylated by PKA (Roche et al., 1996; Barria et al., 1997a). Phosphorylation of either of these sites has been shown to potentiate AMPAR function through distinct biophysical mechanisms (Derkach et al., 1999). Phosphorylation site-specific antibodies have been used to measure the phosphorylation state of receptors *in situ* (Mammen et al., 1997). The PKA site shows higher basal phosphorylation than the CaMKII/PKC site (Lee et al., 1998).

To investigate the changes in AMPAR phosphorylation that occur following synaptic plasticity, Lee et al. (1998) devised a method to induce LTD chemically in hippocampus slices. The rationale behind this approach was to increase the probability of detecting biochemical changes by maximizing the number of affected synapses in the slice. They showed that brief bath application of NMDA induces synaptic depression (called chem-LTD) that shares a common expression mechanism with LFS-induced LTD. Biochemical analysis showed a selective dephosphorylation of serine-845 (the PKA site) following induction of chem-LTD. Phosphorylation of serine-831 (the CaMKII/PKC site), in contrast, was not altered by the treatment. This result was unexpected, since serine-831 is the site phosphorylated during LTP (Barria et al., 1997b). Thus, these findings contradict the simple notion that LTD and LTP reflect bidirectional changes in the phosphorylation of the same site. By refining the biochemical detection method, these findings have now been confirmed using synaptically induced LTD and LTP (Lee et al., 2000). LFS delivered to naive synapses causes dephosphorylation of the PKA site and LTD. Conversely, theta-burst stimulation (TBS) delivered to naive synapses causes phosphorylation of the CaMKII/PKC site and LTP. Both types of synaptic change are reversible, however. Thus, LFS delivered after prior induction of LTP causes dephosphorylation of the CaMKII/PKC site and depotentiation of the synaptic response. TBS delivered after prior induction of LTD causes phosphorylation of the

PKA site and de-depression of the synaptic response (**Figure 2**; Kameyama et al., 1998). This PKA-mediated recovery from depression is associated with AMPA receptor reinsertion (Ehlers, 2000).

Despite the progress that has been made in characterizing the phosphorylation events underlyling LTP and LTD induction, some important aspects still remain unsolved. While the CaMKII/PKC phosphorylation site serine-831 is phosphorylated during LTP (Lee et al., 2000) and this phosphorylation event leads to an increase in receptor conductance (Derkach et al., 1999), serine-831 phosphorylation does not affect receptor trafficking (Hayashi et al., 2000). A current hypothesis is that synaptic targeting of GluR1/GluR2 receptors ultimately requires CaMKII-mediated phosphorylation of a family of small transmembrane AMPAR regulatory proteins (TARPs), such as stargazin (for review see Nicoll et al., 2006). Phosphorylation at the PKA site serine-845 seems to act as a 'priming' step for GluR1 membrane insertion (Esteban et al., 2003). As described above, dephosphorylation at serine-845 occurs during LTD (Lee et al., 2000), and indeed promotes internalization of AMPARs (Lee et al., 2003). PKC also plays a role in the delivery of GluR1 subunits to synapses. In a recent study, it was demonstrated that a PKC (all isoforms)-mediated phosphorylation at serine-818 is required for GluR1 insertion and LTP (Boehm et al., 2006). Moreover, it has been shown that the constitutively active PKC isoform PKMζ promotes AMPAR membrane insertion and might be crucial for maintaining increased receptor numbers (Ling et al., 2006). Taken together, the available data suggest that all three GluR1 phosphorylation sites discussed here, namely serine-818, -831, and -845, are involved in the induction of LTP, which likely sets constraints for LTP-inducing stimuli, but also opens up routes to modify the probability for GluR1 insertion and LTP.

While the available evidence for the role of GluR1 insertion in LTP is compelling and the remaining questions mostly focus on the underlying phosphorylation steps, the events underlying hippocampal LTD induction are less clear. As pointed out earlier, it has been shown that dephosphorylation of the GluR1 subunit at serine-845 is involved in LTD and GluR1 endocytosis. In mutant mice, in which phosphorylation at serine-831 and -845 is prevented by mutations to alanine ('phospho-free mice') NMDAR-dependent LTD is blocked (Lee et al., 2003). This finding is consistent with earlier reports demonstrating that inhibition of PP2B blocks GluR1 internalization, which has been interpreted as showing that phosphatase activity is required for GluR1 endocytosis and LTD (Beattie et al., 2000). However, a recently promoted hypothesis gains weight, which states that LTP is mediated by membrane delivery of AMPA receptors with long cytoplasmic termini (i.e., GluR1-, GluR2L-, GluR4-containing AMPARs), whereas LTD is mediated by the endocytosis of AMPA receptors with short cytoplasmic termini (GluR2-containing AMPARs) (for review see Malinow, 2003). The refilling of receptor 'pools' required to maintain plasticity would then occur through a slow exchange of AMPARs (McCormack et al., 2006). Time will tell how these findings can be reconciled. However, there is indeed plenty of evidence showing that GluR2 subunits can cycle in and out of the membrane as well.

The carboxy terminus of GluR2 binds to N-ethylmaleimide-sensitive factor (NSF), a protein previously shown to play an essential role in membrane fusion events (Nishimune et al., 1998; Osten et al., 1998; Song et al., 1998; Lüscher et al., 1999; Noel et al., 1999). NSF-GluR2 binding promotes GluR2 insertion at hippocampal synapses (Lüscher et al., 1999). Under physiological conditions, NSF is activated by NO-mediated S-nitrosylation, which enables NSF to bind to GluR2, thus promoting GluR2 surface expression (Huang et al., 2005). Conversely, GluR2 phosphorylation at serine-880 promotes a clathrin-mediated GluR2 endocytosis (Man et al., 2000), which leads to LTD (Seidenman et al., 2003). GluR2 endocytosis involves unbinding of GluR2 from the glutamate receptor-interacting protein GRIP1 (Dong et al., 1997) and binding to protein interacting with C-kinase 1 (PICK1) (Xia et al., 1999; Chung et al., 2000).

The pool of NSF-regulated AMPARs appears to be required for expression of LTD, because LFS has no effect after these receptors are internalized (Lüscher et al., 1999; Luthi et al., 1999). Three lines of evidence suggest that AMPAR internalization is an expression mechanism for LTD. First, in hippocampal slices, prior saturation of LTD renders the AMPARs at the depressed synapses (but not at other synapses on the same neuron) insensitive to inhibitors of the NSF-GluR2 interaction (Luthi et al., 1999). Second, in hippocampal cell culture, field stimulation at 5 Hz causes an NMDAR-dependent depression of spontaneous miniature excitatory postsynaptic current (EPSC) amplitudes and the loss of surface-expressed GluR1 (Carroll et al., 1999). Third, in the adult hippocampus *in vivo*, there is an NMDAR-dependent loss of GluR1 and GluR2 from the synaptoneurosomal biochemical fraction following induction of LTD (Heynen et al., 2000).

In keeping with the evidence cited, the magnitude of the postsynaptic response to quantal release of glutamate (the quantal size) is decreased after LTD (Oliet et al., 1996). However, in addition, a robust finding is that the number of quantal responses to synaptic stimulation (the quantal content) is also decreased (Stevens and Wang, 1994; Goda and Stevens, 1996; Oliet et al., 1996; Carroll et al., 1999). According to traditional assumptions, decreased quantal content reflects the failure of neurotransmitter release in response to a presynaptic action potential. It is interesting, therefore, that a decrease in quantal content is also a consequence of disrupting the NSF-GluR2 interaction (Luthi et al., 1999). Presumably this results from the total loss of AMPARs from some synapses. Thus, although presynaptic changes may also occur following LFS (Ramakers et al., 1999), there is apparently no need to invoke a presynaptic mechanism to account for the key properties of NMDAR-dependent LTD of AMPAR-mediated responses.

Another robust finding is that responses to activation of NMDARs are also depressed following LTD (Xiao et al., 1994, 1995; Selig et al., 1995a). While these observations are consistent with the parallel loss of AMPA receptors and NMDA receptors from synaptoneurosomes following LTD *in vivo* (Heynen et al., 2000), they could also reflect a component of LTD expression that is presynaptic. The GluR internalization in response to intracellular manipulations of the NSF-GluR2 interaction (Luthi et al., 1999), or of clathrin-mediated endocytosis (Lüscher et al., 1999; Man et al., 2000; Wang and Linden, 2000), has been restricted to AMPARs only. Thus, the mechanism for NMDAR regulation is apparently distinct from that for AMPAR regulation.

12.6 Modulation of LTD

As discussed, induction of LTD depends on postsynaptic phosphatase activation by Ca passing through NMDAR channels. Thus, it comes as no surprise that LTD is subject to modulation by factors that alter the Ca flux in response to synaptic stimulation and by factors that alter the intracellular enzymatic response to a change in Ca concentration.

An example of the first type of modulation is the effect of altered inhibition. Under some experimental conditions, reduced inhibition may be required to allow the NMDAR activation that is necessary to induce LTD (Wagner and Alger, 1995). However, under other conditions, reduced inhibition may suppress LTD in response to LFS at certain frequencies by facilitating induction of LTP instead (Steele and Mauk, 1999). Similarly, the conditions required for LTD induction depend on the properties of postsynaptic NMDARs. For example, overexpression of the NR2B subunit, which leads to a prolongation of NMDAR-mediated synaptic currents, changes the frequency-response function to promote LTP and suppress LTD across a range of stimulation frequencies (Tang et al., 1999). Modulation of inhibition and NMDAR subunit composition are physiologically relevant, as these parameters change during development and are regulated by activity.

The intracellular response to a change in Ca depends on the availability of Ca binding proteins, such as calmodulin, and on the location, concentration, and activity of the kinases and phosphatases that regulate synaptic strength. Mutations that alter these parameters have been shown to enhance (Mayford et al., 1995) or disrupt (Brandon et al., 1995; Qi et al., 1996; Migaud et al., 1998) LTD. PKA seems to play a pivotal role in the intracellular regulation of LTD. According to the current model for LTD induction, activation of PKA would be expected to inhibit LTD by preventing the activation of PP1 (via I-1 phosphorylation) and by maintaining AMPAR phosphorylation at a high level. Regulation of LTD via PKA is also physiologically relevant. For example, there is evidence that PKA activation in response to stimulation of noradrenergic b-receptors shifts the frequency response function to favor LTP over LTD (Blitzer et al., 1995, 1998; Thomas et al., 1996; Katsuki et al., 1997). Conversely, activation of muscarinic acetylcholine receptors facilitates LTD (Kirkwood et al., 1999), possibly by PKC-mediated inhibition of adenylyl cyclase (Stanton, 1995; Nouranifar et al., 1998).

Other variables that impact LTD are postnatal age and the behavioral state of the animal. Although the mechanism remains to be determined, it is well established that the magnitude and reliability of LTD decline with increasing age (Dudek and Bear, 1993; Errington et al., 1995; Wagner and Alger, 1995a; Kamal et al., 1998), supporting the idea that this mechanism plays an important role in the refinement of circuits during critical periods of development (Rittenhouse et al., 1999). However, the existence of LTD in the adult hippocampus has been the subject of some controversy, with some labs reporting success (Thiels et al., 1994; Heynen et al., 1996; Manahan-Vaughan, 1997) and others reporting failure (Errington et al., 1995; Doyle et al., 1997; Staubli and Scafidi, 1997) to observe LTD *in vivo*. Resolution of this controversy may now be at hand. First, it has been established that there are rat strain differences in the expression of LTD (Manahan-Vaughan and Braunewell, 1999). Second, and most importantly, it has been shown that LTD is powerfully modulated by the behavioral state of the animal. When LTD-resistant animals are exposed to mild stress (Kim et al., 1994; Xu et al., 1997), or even simply to a novel environment (Manahan-Vaughan and Braunewell, 1999), there is a striking facilitation of LTD. The stress effect may be mediated by glucocorticoids (Coussens et al., 1997; Xu et al., 1998b); the mechanism for the novelty effect is unknown, although modulation by acetylcholine has been suggested (Bear, 1999). Whatever the mechanism, the results show that brain-state is a crucial variable that must be controlled during studies of LTD in adults.

The effect of novelty exposure on LTD is particularly interesting. When LFS is delivered as animals explore a novel environment, the resulting LTD lasts for weeks regardless of the strain of rat. However, the facilitation of synaptic plasticity is so marked that the usual 1-Hz tetanus is no longer required to induce LTD. The low-frequency electrical stimulation normally used to monitor synaptic transmission (5 pulses given at 0.1 Hz every 5 min for 15 min) is enough to significantly depress synaptic transmission for several hours if it is delivered during novelty exposure. An exciting possibility is that the pattern of electrical stimulation imposed on the brain during the novel experience is incorporated into the memory of that experience, and this memory is stored as LTD of the synapses that were active at that time. Indeed, recordings from neurons in the temporal lobes have consistently revealed that a cellular correlate of recognition memory is a diminished response to the learned stimulus (Xiang and Brown, 1998). Perhaps this reduced response, and the memory trace, is accounted for by the mechanisms of homosynaptic LTD.

A final type of LTD modulation was suggested by the BCM theory. The idea was that the value of qm (the LTD-LTP crossover point) should vary depending on the history of the integrated postsynaptic response (Bear et al., 1987; Bear, 1995). After periods of strong postsynaptic activity, the modification threshold slides to promote LTD over LTP; after periods of postsynaptic inactivity, the threshold adjusts to promote LTP over LTD. In this way, the properties of synaptic plasticity adjust to keep the network of modifiable synapses within a useful dynamic range. There is now compelling evidence from a number of systems that the stimulation requirements for induction of LTD are indeed altered by prior postsynaptic activity (Kirkwood et al., 1996; Holland and Wagner, 1998; Wang and Wagner, 1999). The mechanisms for this plasticity of synaptic plasticity, or 'metaplasticity' (Abraham and Bear, 1996), remain to be determined, but the obvious candidates are clear from this discussion of LTD modulation. Changes in inhibition (Huang et al., 1999b; Steele and Mauk, 1999), NMDAR properties (Quinlan et al., 1999), and the balance of postsynaptic kinases and phosphatases (Mayford et al., 1995; Migaud et al., 1998) have all been proposed as mechanisms for the sliding modification threshold of the BCM theory.

12.7 mGluR-Dependent LTD

12.7.1 Induction

In addition to activating ionotropic receptors, glutamate stimulates G-protein coupled mGluRs. There are three classes of mGluR, defined by their pharmacology and coupling to second messenger pathways (Pin and Bockaert, 1995). Group 1 mGluRs (designated mGluR1 and mGluR5) stimulate phosphoinositide (PI) turnover via activation of phospholipase C (PLC). It is of historical interest to note that, based on theoretical considerations, the proposal was made that PI-coupled mGluRs play a role in triggering synaptic depression in the cerebral cortex (Dudek and Bear, 1989), and that the protocol of using LFS to induce homosynaptic LTD was designed originally with the aim of testing this hypothesis (Dudek and Bear, 1992). Although this early work implicated NMDARs instead, it was not long before a role for mGluRs was suggested for LTD. In particular, Bolshakov and Siegelbaum (1994) found that the mGluR antagonist α-methyl-4-carboxyphenylglycine (MCPG) prevents homosynaptic LTD in response to LFS in slices from very young rats (postnatal day 3–7). LTD in this preparation also required a rise in intracellular [Ca] and activation of voltage-gated Ca channels during LFS, but not activation of NMDARs.

Confusion about mGluR involvement in LTD persisted for a number of years due to some failures to replicate (Selig et al., 1995b), exacerbated by the finding that MCPG is actually a very weak antagonist of the action of glutamate at mGluR5 (Brabet et al., 1995; Huber et al., 1998). Fortunately, the smoke has now cleared. First, it is now clear that the activation of mGluRs necessary to induce LTD is often not achieved using the usual 1- to 5-Hz stimulus trains. Protocols that work reliably are those that enhance glutamate release during conditioning stimulation, such as delivering prolonged trains of paired pulses (Kemp and Bashir, 1997a), or by antagonizing the adenosine inhibition of glutamate release (de Mendonca et al., 1997; Kemp and Bashir, 1997b). These protocols produce LTD of large magnitude with a component that cannot be blocked with NMDAR antagonists. Second, the use of new, potent mGluR antagonists and genetically altered mice has established that the NMDAR-independent LTD requires activation of mGluR5, and, conversely, that induction of NMDAR-dependent LTD does not (Bortolotto et al., 1999; Huber et al., 2001; Sawtell et al., 1999).

It has now been established that activation of group 1 mGluRs induces LTD by a mechanism that is entirely distinct from that engaged by NMDAR activation (Oliet et al., 1997). This mGluR-dependent LTD (mGluR-LTD) can be induced by synaptic stimulation in the presence of NMDAR antagonists, or by simple pharmacological activation of mGluRs using the group 1 mGluR-selective agonist DHPG ((RS)-3,5-dihydroxyphenylglycine) (Fitzjohn et al., 1999; Huber et al., 2001). Remarkably, the specific group 1 mGluRs involved differ for chemically and synaptically induced LTD. Whereas DHPG-induced LTD involves mGluR1 and mGluR5 activation, synaptically induced LTD is only mGluR5-dependent (Volk et al., 2006). The requirement of voltage-gated Ca entry for induction of mGluR-dependent LTD (mGluR-LTD) by synaptic stimulation has been confirmed, although the type of channel (L- or T-type) apparently varies depending on the circumstances (Bolshakov and Siegelbaum, 1994; Oliet et al., 1997; Otani and Connor, 1998). In addition, synaptically induced mGluR-LTD requires activation of postsynaptic PLC (Reyes and Stanton, 1998) and PKC (Bolshakov and Siegelbaum, 1994; Oliet et al., 1997; Otani and Connor, 1998). Unlike the NMDAR-dependent LTD (NMDAR-LTD), mGluR-LTD is not affected by inhibition of postsynaptic PP1 (Oliet et al., 1997).

Biochemical experiments suggest that activation of group 1 mGluRs in synaptoneurosomes stimulates, in a PKC-dependent manner, the aggregation of ribosomes and mRNA, and the synthesis of the fragile X mental retardation protein (Weiler and Greenough, 1993; Weiler et al., 1997). Thus, it is of considerable interest that mGluR-LTD is prevented by manipulations that interfere with protein synthesis. Huber et al. (2001) have shown that induction of mGluR-LTD is prevented by the postsynaptic inhibition of mRNA translation during conditioning stimulation. Because the LTD is homosynaptic and occurs even when the dendrites are isolated from their cell bodies, a requirement for rapid, synapse-specific synthesis of proteins from preexisting mRNA is strongly suggested. These findings are consistent with a number of converging lines of evidence suggesting a major role for mRNA translation in the mechanisms of mGluR5 action (Merlin et al., 1998; Raymond et al., 2000).

The discovery of polyribosomes at the base of dendritic spines has long invited speculation that synaptic activity regulates the protein composition, and therefore function, of synapses in the brain (Steward et al., 1988). Available data now indicate that mGluR5 activation triggers synapse-specific mRNA translation, and that one functional consequence is LTD (**Figure 3**). The obvious questions to be examined next concern the mechanism of translation regulation, the identity of the essential transcripts, and the mechanism that couples new protein synthesis to a change in synaptic function. The mGluR-LTD model should prove extremely valuable for answering these questions.

12.7.2 Expression

At the present time, more is known about how mGluR-LTD is *not* expressed than about how it is expressed. Specifically, mGluR-LTD is not expressed via the same mechanism as NMDAR-LTD. This conclusion is supported by the finding that the two forms of LTD are additive and do not mutually occlude one another. Moreover, while NMDAR-LTD is reversed by induction of LTP (and vice versa), mGluR-LTD is not (Oliet et al., 1997; Fitzjohn et al., 1999; Huber et al., 2001). It has been reported that after mGluR-LTD the quantal content, but not the quantal size, is reduced (Bolshakov and Siegelbaum, 1994; Oliet et al., 1997), consistent with a presynaptic expression side. However, this observation could also be explained by an all-or-none loss of postsynaptic AMPARs at individual synapses (all-or-none because a graded decrease would be reflected in a decrease in quantal size). Studies on the phosphorylation state of AMPARs in mGluR-LTD could not provide a consistent view on the expression side of mGluR-LTD so far. Whereas one study reported that

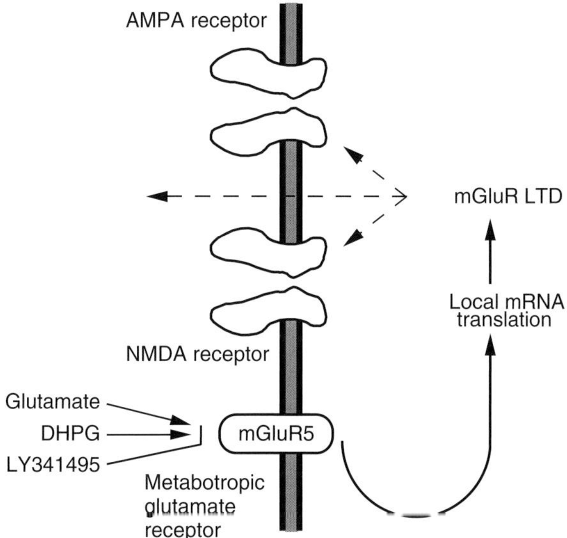

Figure 3 Model for metabotropic glutamate receptor-dependent LTD (mGluR-LTD) in CA1. Activating mGluR5 during synaptic stimulation, or by the selective agonist DHPG, triggers LTD that can be prevented by the selective mGluR antagonist LY341495. Synaptically evoked mGluR-LTD requires local translation of preexisting mRNA.

mGluR-LTD, unlike NMDAR-LTD, is not associated with a dephosphorylation of AMPA receptors (Huber et al., 2001), another found that in DHPG-induced LTD the activation of tyrosine phosphatases leads to a tyrosine dephosphorylation of AMPARs and their subsequent endocytosis (Moult et al., 2006). A possible explanation for this discrepancy might be that a developmental switch occurs between the second and the third postnatal week from a pre- to a postsynaptic expression side of mGluR-LTD (Nosyreva and Huber, 2005).

12.8 Depotentiation

The term 'depotentiation' refers to the reversal of previously established LTP, which can be elicited by variations of the LFS protocol. Confusion has arisen because the same term has been used to describe two phenomena. One type of depotentiation, of course, is homosynaptic LTD of synapses from a potentiated baseline, which can be induced at any time following LTP induction and utilizes the same mechanisms discussed above. The second type of depotentiation refers to the disruption of LTP that occurs when LFS is delivered within a relatively brief time window immediately following LTP induction. This time-sensitive depotentiation apparently is caused by interference with the transient intracellular biochemical reactions that are required to 'fix' LTP in the period that follows strong NMDAR activation.

12.8.1 Time-Sensitive Depotentiation

High-frequency synaptic stimulation (HFS) typically induces LTP in CA1. However, establishment of stable LTP is prevented if the HFS is followed by certain types of synaptic stimulation including, but not restricted to, LFS (Hesse and Teyler, 1976; Barrionuevo et al., 1980; Arai et al., 1990; Staubli and Lynch, 1990; Fujii et al., 1991; Barr et al., 1995; Holscher et al., 1997). This retrograde disruption of LTP is time dependent. LFS within 5 min of HFS can completely prevent LTP; however, the same stimulation may have no effect when delivered 1 h after HFS.

A clear picture of the mechanism for time-sensitive depotentiation (TS-DP) has finally emerged (**Figure 4**). Although the upstream regulation varies depending on the type of stimulation used, the critical downstream requirement for TS-DP is activation of postsynaptic PP1 during the sensitive period (O'Dell and Kandel, 1994; Staubli and Chun, 1996; Huang et al., 1999a). This period coincides with the time when LTP can be disrupted by inhibition of protein kinases (Huber et al., 1995). Thus, the data indicate that stable establishment of LTP requires the active serine-threonine phosphorylation of synaptic substrates for a defined time period. If this phosphorylation is prevented or reversed, so is LTP.

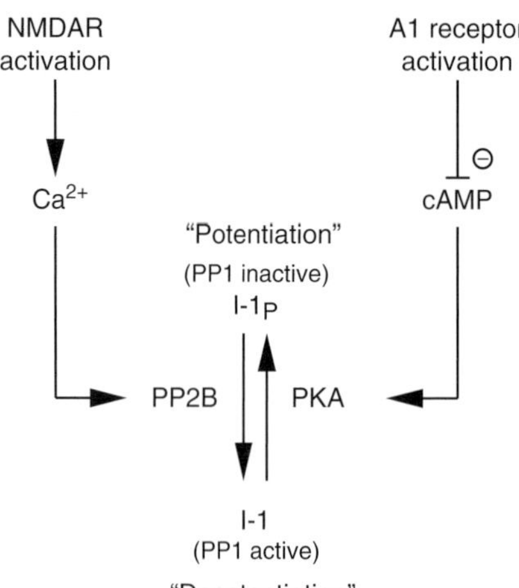

Figure 4 Converging pathways to depotentiation. Depotentiation occurs if synapses are given LFS in a narrow time window immediately following induction of LTP. Available evidence suggests that depotentiations results from dephosphorylation of postsynaptic proteins by protein phosphatase 1 (PP1). PP1 is activated when inhibitor 1 (I-1) is dephosphorylated by calcineurin (PP2B) at a PKA site. Stimuli that cause depotentiation include those that activate PP2B (e.g., NMDAR activation) and those that inhibit PKA (e.g., adenosine A1 receptor activation).

Upstream regulation of TS-DP can occur in different ways. One route for TS-DP induction appears to be the now-familiar pathway involving NMDAR stimulation (Fujii et al., 1991; O'Dell and Kandel, 1994; Barr et al., 1995; Xiao et al., 1996) followed by activation of PP2B and dephosphorylation of I-1 (O'Dell and Kandel, 1994; Zhuo et al., 1999). A second route to TS-DP induction, also leading to dephosphorylation of I-1, is the activation of A1 adenosine receptors (Larson et al., 1993; Staubli and Chun, 1996; Fujii et al., 1997; Huang et al., 1999a). A1 receptor activation inhibits adenylyl cyclase and, as a consequence, PKA (Dunwiddie and Fredholm, 1989). Injection of PKA activators into the postsynaptic neuron can prevent depotentiation caused by A1 receptor activation (Huang et al., 1999a).

Despite the apparent mechanistic similarities of TS-DP and NMDAR-LTD, the two phenomena differ. For example, TS-DP shows much less developmental regulation than LTD, and the patterns of activity that are optimal for induction are different (O'Dell and Kandel, 1994). In addition, TS-DP shows greater sensitivity to PP1 inhibitors and to deletion of the Aα isoform of PP2B than does LTD (O'Dell and Kandel, 1994; Zhuo et al., 1999). Interestingly, however, like LTD, TS-DP *in vivo* is dramatically facilitated by exposure of animals to a novel environment (Xu et al., 1998a).

A simple way to reconcile the findings is if we assume that LTP induction results in the transient exposure of postsynaptic phosphorylation sites to both protein kinases and phosphatases. Normally, the kinase activation that follows strong NMDAR stimulation leads to a net phosphorylation of these sites and LTP. However, the sites are also vulnerable to dephosphorylation if PP1 is activated. Because the phosphorylation sites are exposed, the threshold level of PP1 activation for TS-DP is much lower than that for NMDAR-LTD. Thus, while stimulation that induces LTD also can always produce TS-DP, the converse is not true. However, the common requirement for PP1 activation makes both forms of synaptic modification subject to very similar types of modulation.

12.8.2 Time-Insensitive Depotentiation

Under conditions in which *de novo* LTD is induced by LFS, the same stimulation can also reverse LTP that was induced hours before. The precise mechanism of LTD and LTP reversal may not be identical, however. For example, LTD *de novo* is associated with the dephosphorylation of GluR1 at a PKA site. However, the same induction protocol given 1 h after induction of LTP causes dephosphorylation of the CaMKII/PKC site instead (Lee et al., 2000; see **Figure 2(b)**). On the other hand, both LTD and LTP reversal *in vivo* are associated with a parallel decrease in AMPAR and NMDAR protein in the synaptoneurosomal biochemical fraction (Heynen et al., 2000).

12.9 LTD of the Cerebellar Parallel Fiber–Purkinje Cell Synapse

The second type of synapse that we want to use as an example to discuss LTD mechanisms is the parallel fiber–Purkinje cell synapse in the cerebellum. For comparison, we will also describe a more recently characterized form of LTD at the climbing fiber–Purkinje cell synapse. Why bother to study synaptic plasticity in an obscure and atypical part of the brain like the cerebellum? The answer is that it is one of only two locations where learning and memory can be understood at the level of circuits (the other being the amygdala; for comparison see Medina et al., 2002). In contrast, the hippocampus, for all of its experimental utility, receives information that is so highly processed that its content cannot be easily characterized (what is the nature of the information conveyed by the perforant path?).

12.10 Cerebellar Anatomy and Some Useful Models

The cerebellum functions largely to integrate various forms of sensory information to smooth and fine-tune complex voluntary movements and reflexes (see Ito, 1984, for review). Therefore, cerebellar damage in humans is associated not with outright paralysis, but rather with dysmetric and ataxic syndromes, as well as impairments in motor learning. In addition, some recent work on human cerebellar lesions complemented by functional imaging studies has implicated the cerebellum in certain forms of non-motor procedural learning as well (see Schmahmann, 1997, for review).

The cerebellum comprises ~10% of the total weight of the human brain, but contains >50% of the total number of neurons, packed into the most infolded and convoluted structure in the brain. This degree of specialization suggests that, throughout evolution, fast, accurate, coordinated movements have been highly adaptive. To coordinate many joints and muscles, it is necessary that sensory and proprioceptive signals from any location in the body or sensory world be able to influence motor commands to any muscle in the body. Essentially, this requires a giant switchboard, which is implemented in the following way. The cerebellar circuitry is essentially composed of a relay station in the deep cerebellar nuclei (DCN) and a cortical 'side-loop' (see **Figure 5(a)**). The neurons of the DCN receive their main excitatory drive from glutamatergic mossy fibers which are the axons of a large number of precerebellar nuclei. The main outflow of information from this structure is carried by excitatory axons which originate from the large neurons of the DCN and project to premotor areas including the red nucleus and thalamus. In addition, there are small projection neurons in the DCN which are GABAergic (Kumoi et al., 1988; Batini et al., 1992) and send axons to the inferior olive (Fredette and Mugnaini, 1991).

The sole output of the cortical side-loop is the inhibitory, GABAergic (GABA: gamma-aminobutyric acid) projection from Purkinje cells to the neurons of the DCN (both large and small projection neurons are innervated; see De Zeeuw and Berrebi, 1995; Teune et al., 1998). Purkinje cells receive two major excitatory inputs, which are organized in very different ways. Each Purkinje cell is innervated by a single climbing fiber. This climbing fiber, which originates in the neurons of the inferior olive, will innervate ~10 Purkinje cells. This is potentially the most powerful synaptic contact in the brain, as each Purkinje cell receives ~1400 synapses from a single climbing fiber axon (Strata and Rossi, 1998). Climbing fibers also provide a very weak innervation of the DCN, consisting of a few synapses in the most distal dendrites, the function of which is poorly understood. In contrast, each Purkinje cell receives ~200 000 synapses from parallel fibers, which are the axons of granule cells. Because of the large number of granule cells (~50 billion) and the divergent output of their parallel fibers (each contacts ~1000 Purkinje cells), this synapse is the most abundant of any in the brain. Closing the loop, granule cells receive excitatory synapses from branches of the same mossy fibers which innervate the DCN directly. Because there are ~10 000-fold more granule cells than DCN cells, the innervation of granule cells by mossy fibers is highly convergent.

Putting this circuit together, it appears as if cerebellar output is driven by direct excitatory input from the mossy fibers and is modulated by the inhibitory input from the Purkinje cell axons, the latter of which will reflect computations and interactions in the Purkinje cell. These computations will be performed upon very subtle and informationally rich excitatory parallel fiber input and massive, synchronous excitation produced by the climbing fiber. This striking anatomical organization has inspired some notable models of motor learning. In particular, Marr (1969) proposed that the parallel fiber–Purkinje cell synapses could provide contextual information, that climbing fiber–Purkinje cell synapses could signal an 'error' in motor performance that required alteration of subsequent behavior, and that the conjunction of these two signals could strengthen the parallel fiber–Purkinje cell synapse to create a memory trace for motor learning. This model was modified by Albus (1971), who noted that a decrease in synaptic strength would be more appropriate, given the sign-reversing function of the Purkinje cell inhibitory output. Importantly, Albus also noted that this model is analogous to classical conditioning, with the parallel fibers conveying a conditioned stimulus (CS), the climbing fiber an unconditioned stimulus (US), and a depression of the parallel fiber–Purkinje cell synapse giving rise to a conditioned response (CR) via disinhibition of

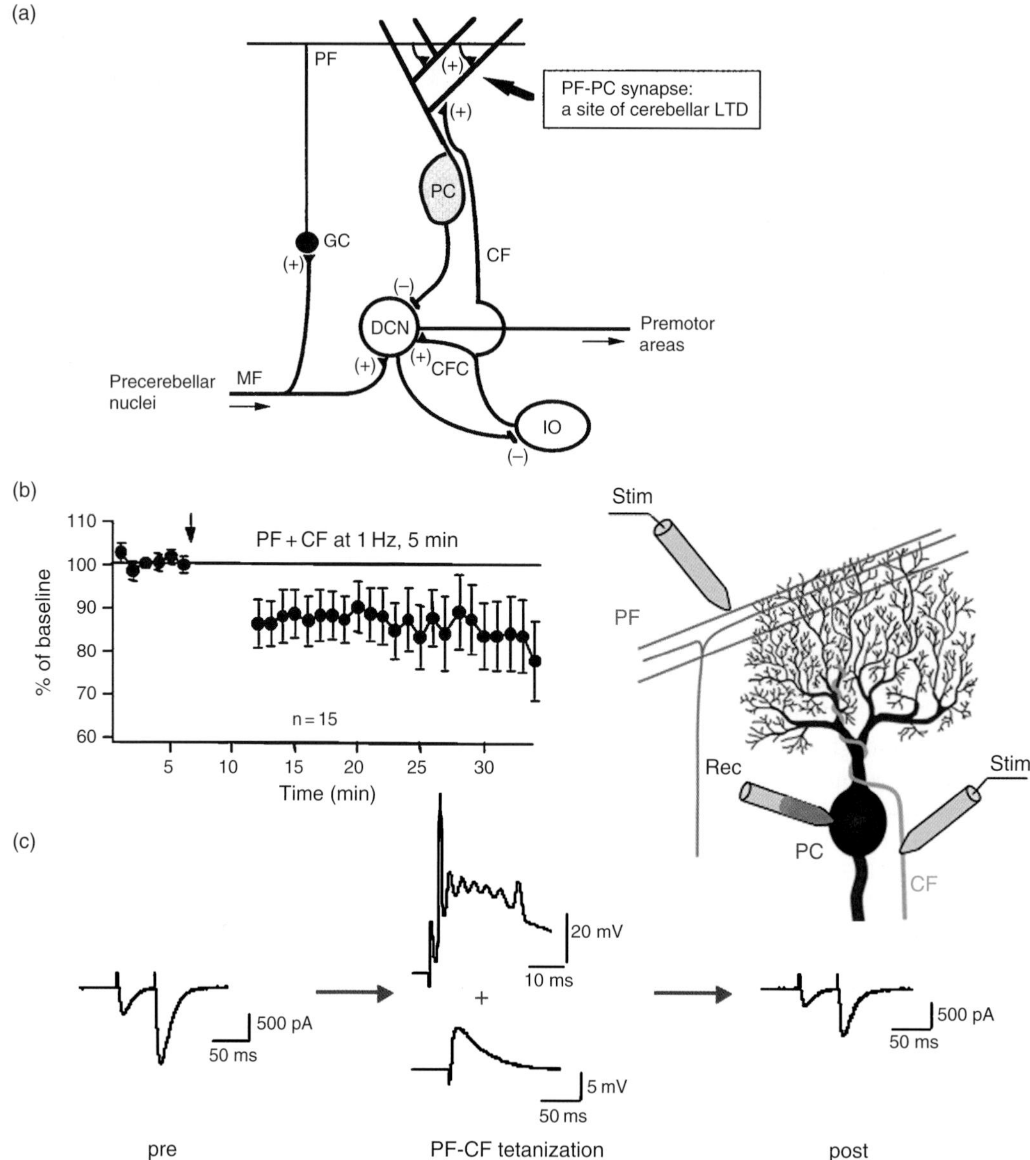

Figure 5 Basic cerebellar functional anatomy and LTD of the parallel fiber–Purkinje cell synapse. (a) A simplified diagram of cerebellar circuitry. Information flow through the main relay pathway consisting of precerebellar nuclei, their axons, the mossy fibers (MF), their targets in the deep cerebellar nuclei (DCN), and DCN excitatory axons projecting to premotor centers, is indicated with arrows. Excitatory synapses are denoted with a (+) and inhibitory synapses with a (–). IO, inferior olive; CF, climbing fiber; CFC, climbing fiber collateral; PC, Purkinje cell; GC, granule cell; PF, parallel fibers. (b) Left: parallel fiber LTD is obtained after paired parallel fiber and climbing fiber tetanization (1 Hz, 5 min; n = 15). Arrow indicates the time point of tetanization. Right: Diagram showing the electrode arrangement used for LTD induction *in vitro*. Whole-cell patch-clamp recording (rec) is used to monitor electrical responses to parallel fiber (PF) and/or climbing fiber (CF) stimulation. For extracellular stimulation, glass pipettes are used (stim) that are filled with ACSF. (c) Test responses to PF stimulation are recorded before and after tetanization in voltage-clamp mode. The paired-pulse facilitation ratio is monitored to screen for presynaptic changes. For tetanization, recordings are switched to current-clamp mode. CF activation results in a typical complex spike (top). The PF-EPSP is shown here in isolation (bottom), but in these recordings is masked by the complex spike. Following tetanization, the PF-EPSC amplitude is reduced.

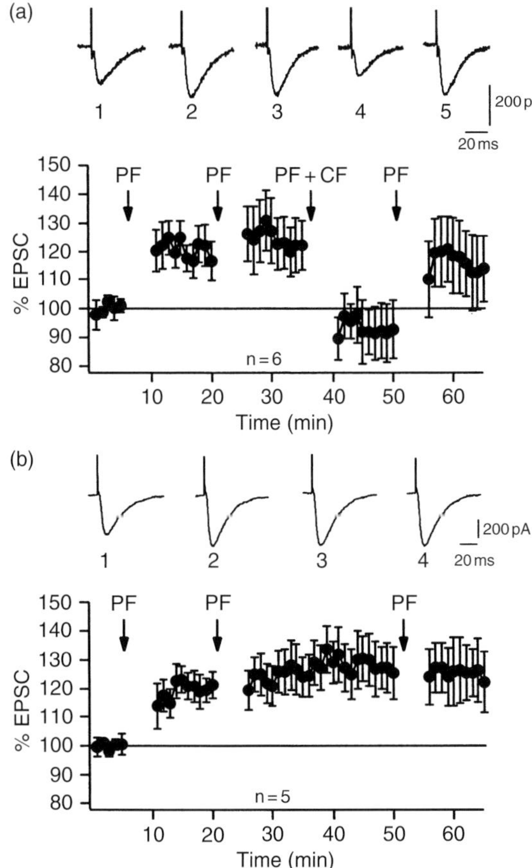

Figure 6 Reversal of parallel fiber LTP by LTD. (a) Saturated LTP is reversed by the application of the LTD protocol. Two LTP protocols were followed by an LTD protocol and, finally, by a third LTP protocol (n = 6). The LTD protocol consists of a paired parallel fiber and climbing fiber stimulation at 1 Hz for 5 min. The LTP protocol consists of the same parallel activation pattern in the absence of climbing fiber activation. Tetanization periods are indicated by the arrows. (b) Omission of the LTD protocol reveals LTP saturation after the application of two LTP protocols (n = 5). In (a) and (b), traces on top show EPSCs from the time points indicated. This figure is taken from Coesmans M, Weber JT, De Zeeuw CI, and Hansel C (2004) Bidirectional parallel fiber plasticity in the cerebellum under climbing fiber control. *Neuron* 44: 691–700, with permission from Elsevier.

the DCN. To place this model in a behavioral context, let us consider a well-characterized form of classical conditioning, associative eyeblink conditioning in the rabbit. Before training, an airpuff to the eye (US) gives rise to an immediate reflexive blink (the unconditioned response, UR). During training, a neutral stimulus such as a tone (CS) is paired with the airpuff stimulation so that the tone onset precedes the airpuff and the two stimuli coterminate. As the rabbit acquires the association, it performs a blink carefully timed to immediately precede the airpuff (CR). This associative learning can also be actively reversed. In well-trained animals which reliably perform CRs, this response can undergo rapid extinction if tone stimuli are repeatedly presented without airpuffs.

12.11 The Role of the Cerebellum in Associative Eyeblink Conditioning

There is extensive evidence to support the involvement of cerebellar circuits in associative eyeblink conditioning (see Kim and Thompson, 1997, for review). Similar evidence implicates the cerebellum in other forms of motor learning such as limb-load adjustment and adaptation of the vestibulo-ocular reflex (VOR; du Lac et al., 1995; De Zeeuw et al., 1998). Extracellular recording showed that populations of cells in the nucleus interpositus (a particular portion of the DCN) discharge during the UR before training and, in well-trained animals, begin to fire during the CS-US interval. This firing is predictive of and correlated with the performance of the CR, suggesting that the CR behavior is expressed in the firing rate and pattern of DCN neurons (McCormick and Thompson, 1984a,b; Berthier and Moore, 1986, 1990). This notion is further supported by the finding that microstimulation in the appropriate region of the nucleus interpositus elicited a strong eyelid response in either trained or untrained animals (McCormick and Thompson, 1984a). Moreover, during training, stimulation of mossy and climbing fibers can substitute for the CS and US, respectively (Mauk et al, 1986; Steinmetz et al., 1986, 1989).

The data obtained using lesions and reversible inactivation have been somewhat more complex (see Mauk, 1997, for review). A Marr/Albus model would predict that lesions of the cerebellar cortex would both delete the memory trace in previously trained animals and prevent further learning. Initially, it was observed that lesioning either the whole cerebellum (ipsilateral to the trained eye) or the anterior interpositus nucleus completely abolished the CR but *not* the UR (McCormick et al., 1982; McCormick and Thompson, 1984a,b; Yeo et al., 1985a; Steinmetz et al., 1992; but see Welsh and Harvey, 1989). These experiments suggested that cerebellar lesions abolished the memory trace for eyeblink conditioning, but their irreversibility made it difficult to dissociate this interpretation from a performance deficit. A more convincing case was made when experiments showed that reversible inactivation of the DCN with muscimol (a $GABA_A$ receptor agonist) prevented the acquisition of the eyeblink CR, but not the performance of the UR (Krupa et al., 1993; Hardiman et al., 1996; Krupa and Thompson, 1997; but see Bracha et al., 1994). In contrast, inactivation of the superior cerebellar peduncle or red nucleus, sites through which excitatory DCN output is conveyed, prevented the expression of the CR during training, but not its acquisition, as evidenced by the fact that the CR was present after inactivation (Krupa et al., 1993; Krupa and Thompson, 1995). These studies suggest that the cerebellum and its associated projections are essential for acquisition and expression of the eyeblink CR. More specifically, the memory trace seems to be localized 'upstream' of the red nucleus, in the cerebellar cortex and/or the DCN.

While there is general agreement that lesions or inactivation of the DCN block the acquisition of the eyeblink CR, there has been considerable debate over the specific role of the cerebellar cortex in eyeblink conditioning. Reports using lesions and inactivation of the cerebellar cortex have ranged from those which have found a complete blockade of CR acquisition (Yeo et al., 1985b), to those which have slowed, but not prevented acquisition (Lavond and Steinmetz, 1989; Yeo and Hardiman, 1992), to those which have found no effect at all (McCormick and Thompson, 1984a,b). Some recent reports point to a potential resolution of this problem. Lesions which included the anterior cerebellar cortex (a region previously thought not to be important), or infusion of picrotoxin (a $GABA_A$ receptor antagonist, the opposite of muscimol) into the DCN to block Purkinje cell input, did not abolish the CR entirely but affected its timing (Perrett et al., 1993; Perrett and Mauk, 1995; Garcia and Mauk, 1998). Recently, a model has been proposed to explain these findings. In this model, the memory trace of the eyeblink CR is sequentially stored, initially as a depression of the parallel fiber–Purkinje cell synapse in the cerebellar cortex. This would result in an attenuation of Purkinje cell firing and hence Purkinje cell–DCN synaptic drive, thereby disinhibiting the DCN targets. This disinhibition, when coupled with activation of the mossy fiber–DCN synapse, could then potentiate the latter, resulting in storage of the CR at the mossy fiber–DCN synapse while the timing of the conditioned response is retained in the cerebellar cortex (Raymond et al., 1996; Mauk, 1997; Mauk and Donegan, 1997; Medina and Mauk, 1999).

12.12 Potential Cellular Substrates of Associative Eyeblink Conditioning

LTD of the parallel fiber–Purkinje cell synapse has been proposed as a cellular mechanism which could, at least in part, underlie the acquisition of associative eyeblink conditioning. This phenomenon, which was first described by Ito and colleagues (1982), results when the climbing fiber (corresponding to the US) and parallel fiber (corresponding to the CS) inputs are activated together at low frequencies (1–4 Hz; see **Figure 5(b)**). In addition, stimulation of parallel fibers alone can produce LTP of the parallel fiber–Purkinje cell synapse, thus providing a form of bidirectional control (Lev-Ram et al., 2002; Coesmans et al., 2004). LTD in the parallel fiber–Purkinje cell synapse requires association of parallel fiber (CS) and climbing fiber (US) activation and would result in decreased firing of the Purkinje cell, causing increased firing of DCN neurons and enhanced expression of the CR. Essentially, this is a cellular restatement of the Marr/Albus model. Conversely, repeated activation of the parallel fiber (CS) alone could, through enhanced inhibition resulting from parallel fiber LTP, decrease firing of the DCN and thereby reduce expression of the CR during extinction.

As indicated by the lesion and inactivation studies described above, it is likely that the parallel fiber–Purkinje cell synapse is not the only site of information storage during cerebellar motor learning. At a cellular level, extinction of the CR, as results from repeated application of a tone CS, could be mediated not only by LTP of the parallel fiber–Purkinje cell synapse, but also by LTD of the mossy fiber–DCN synapse. This idea is consistent with reports that both cortical lesions which include the anterior region (Perrett and Mauk, 1995) and reversible inactivation of the DCN with muscimol (Hardiman et al., 1996; Ramnani and Yeo, 1996) block CR extinction.

Recently, both LTD and LTP have been described at the mossy fiber–DCN synapse. Whereas LTD can be observed after high-frequency mossy fiber burst stimulation, either alone or paired with postsynaptic depolarization (Zhang and Linden, 2006), LTP can be elicited when high-frequency mossy fiber stimulation is paired with postsynaptic hyperpolarization followed by a rebound current (Pugh and Raman, 2006). The existence of mossy fiber LTP has been suggested by a model of Mauk and coworkers, in which disinhibition of the DCN from reduced Purkinje cell input, when coupled with activation of the mossy fiber–DCN synapses, results in LTP of mossy fiber–DCN synapses, constituting a portion of the memory trace of the CR (Raymond et al., 1996; Mauk, 1997; Mauk and Donegan, 1997). A recent computational analysis has suggested that an LTP induction rule for the mossy fiber–DCN synapse that depends upon specific patterns of Purkinje cell input (plus ongoing mossy fiber activity) could constitute a memory trace that is unusually resistant to degradation by ongoing 'background' activity in the cerebellar circuit (Medina and Mauk, 1999). The dependence of mossy fiber LTP on paired hyperpolarization and subsequent rebound currents (Pugh and Raman, 2006), mimicking the response to Purkinje cell activity and the transient interruption of inhibition (e.g., related to a complex spike pause), fits this theoretical framework and underlines the importance of a specific timing of mossy fiber and Purkinje cell activity for LTP induction. A missing piece that remains in the puzzle, however, is whether previous parallel fiber–LTD induction (resulting in a reduction of the inhibitory tone imposed by Purkinje cells) not only leads to increased activity levels in DCN cells, but also facilitates the induction of mossy fiber LTP.

12.13 Parallel Fiber LTD Induction

12.13.1 Parametric Requirements

Cerebellar LTD was first described in the intact cerebellum (Ito et al., 1982) and, since that time, has been analyzed in acute slice preparations, primary cultures, acutely dissociated Purkinje cells, and macropatches of Purkinje cell dendrite. In slice or *in situ*, the standard induction protocol consists of stimulating the parallel and climbing fiber inputs together at low frequency (1–4 Hz) for a period of 2–6 min. This results in a selective attenuation of the parallel fiber–Purkinje cell synapse (typically a 20–50% reduction of baseline synaptic strength), which reaches its full extent in ~10 min and persists for the duration of the experiment, typically 1–2 h.

LTD is said to result from coactivation of parallel fibers and climbing fibers, but what are the precise timing constraints on this coactivation? This is an important point, because if parallel fiber LTD underlies associative eyeblink conditioning, then the temporal constraints on CS/US association should be reflected in the temporal constraints on LTD induction. One study, using intracellular recording in rabbit cerebellar slice, has indicated that LTD is optimally induced when climbing fiber stimulation precedes parallel fiber stimulation by 125–250 ms (Ekerot and Kano, 1989). Another study using a similar preparation has shown that LTD may be induced by climbing fiber–parallel fiber stimulation with an interval of 50 ms, but claims that LTD induced by climbing fiber–parallel fiber pairing will not occur unless disynaptic inhibition is blocked by addition of a $GABA_A$ antagonist (Schreurs and Alkon, 1993). Neither of these intervals (in which the US precedes CS) will support robust eyeblink conditioning. However, with slightly different stimulation protocols (small trains of parallel fiber stimulation instead of single pulses in one case) parallel fiber before climbing fiber pairing, at intervals which support eyeblink conditioning, may also be effective in inducing LTD in the absence of $GABA_A$ receptor blockade (Chen and Thompson, 1995; Schreurs et al., 1996). In a more recent study, which combined whole-cell patch-clamp recordings with two-photon Ca imaging, it was shown that LTD is optimally induced when parallel fiber activation precedes climbing fiber activation by 50–200 ms and that coincident parallel fiber and climbing fiber activation results in supralinear Ca signals (Wang et al., 2000). Thus, the timing requirements found in cerebellar motor learning paradigms can indeed be matched by timing requirements characterized in cerebellar slice preparations. Moreover, the optimal timing conditions for LTD induction also yielded the largest spine Ca signals, providing an explanation why this particular activation sequence was beneficial for LTD induction.

12.13.2 Climbing Fiber Signals

The climbing fiber contributes to LTD induction by causing sufficient postsynaptic depolarization (through activation of AMPARs) to strongly activate voltage-sensitive Ca channels in the dendrites, thereby causing a complex spike and a large Ca influx (see **Figure 7**; for review see Schmolesky et al., 2002). In fact, climbing fiber activation may be replaced in the LTD induction protocol by direct depolarization of the Purkinje cell (Crepel and Krupa, 1988; Hirano, 1990; Linden et al., 1991). Furthermore, LTD induction is blocked by postsynaptic application of a Ca chelator (Sakurai, 1990; Linden and Connor, 1991; Konnerth et al., 1992), electrical inhibition of Purkinje cells during parallel

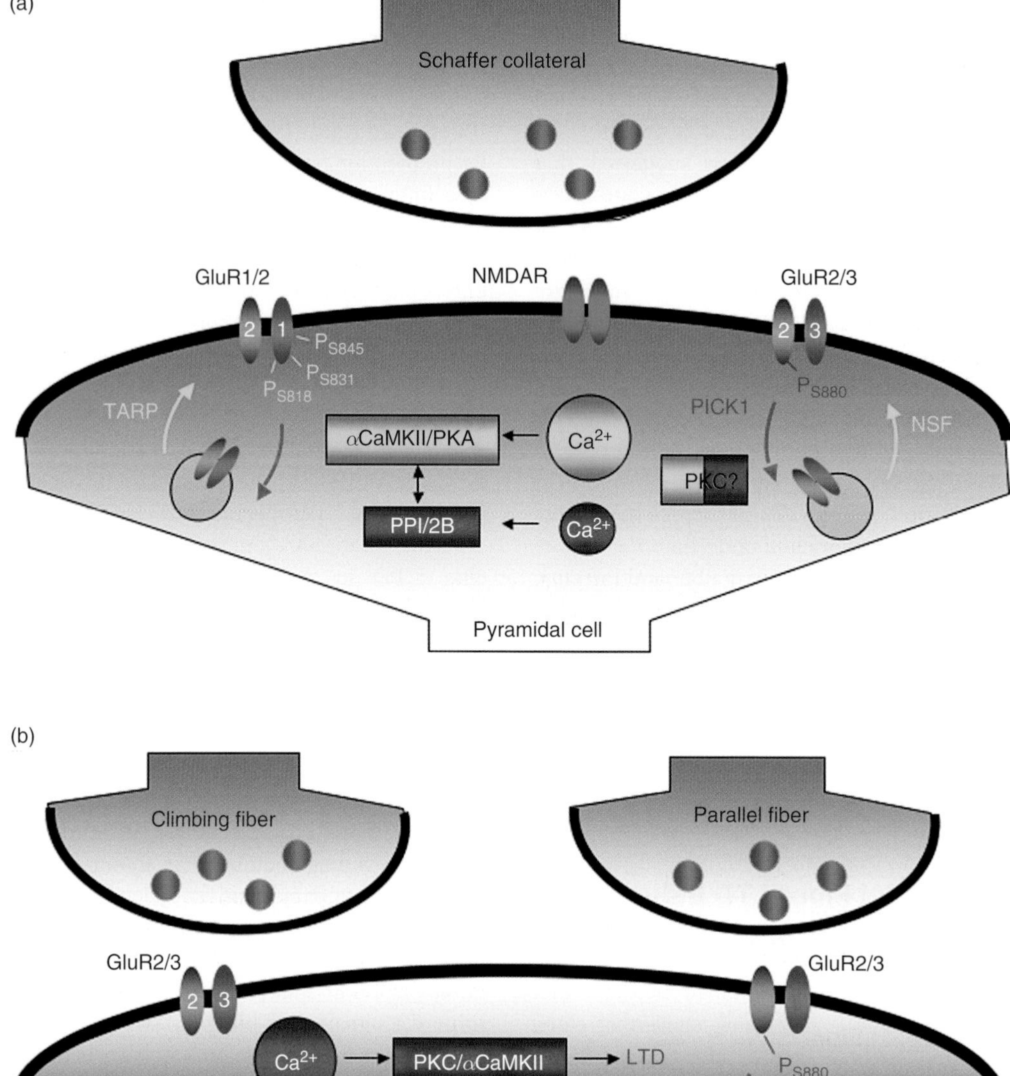

Figure 7 Comparison of LTP and LTD induction cascades at CA1 hippocampal (a) and cerebellar synapses (b). LTP induction cascades are shown in yellow, and LTD induction cascades in red. (a) LTP and LTD induction at Schaffer collateral synapses onto CA1 hippocampal pyramidal cells. Functional NMDARs are present in pyramidal cells, but not in Purkinje cells. Other calcium sources present in both types are neurons are not displayed. Note that PKA and protein phosphatase 1 (PP1) are not directly calcium activated. PKC has been implicated in hippocampal LTP, but also in the endocytosis of GluR2 subunits. Abbreviations are used as explained in the text. (b) LTP and LTD induction at cerebellar parallel fiber–Purkinje cell synapses. For simplicity, climbing fiber and parallel fiber terminals are shown to contact the same postsynaptic compartment; (b) is modified from Hansel C (2005) When the B-team runs plasticity: GluR2 receptor trafficking in cerebellar long-term potentiation. *Proc. Natl. Acad. Sci. USA* 102: 18245–18246, with permission from the National Academy of Sciences, USA.

fiber/climbing fiber conjunctive stimulation (Ekerot and Kano, 1985, 1989; Hirano, 1990; Crepel and Jaillard, 1991), or removal of external Ca (Linden and Connor, 1991). In addition, studies using optical indicators have shown large Ca accumulations in Purkinje cell dendrites following climbing fiber stimulation (Ross and Werman, 1987; Knöpfel et al., 1990; Konnerth et al., 1992). These Ca transients reach supralinear levels when the climbing fiber stimulation is paired with parallel fiber activation (see above; Wang et al., 2000). While these studies have suggested that Ca influx is the sole mediator of climbing fiber action, another view has come from studies which have examined a peptide released from climbing fiber terminals, corticotropin releasing factor. Miyata et al. (1999) have found that LTD induced by either parallel fiber/climbing fiber conjunction or parallel fiber/depolarization conjunction can be blocked by antagonists of the corticotropin releasing factor receptor in a slice preparation. Furthermore, parallel fiber/depolarization conjunction fails to induce LTD in slices prepared from rats in which climbing fibers were chemically prelesioned, but this may be restored with exogenous corticotropin releasing factor. These observations have led to the suggestion that corticotropin releasing factor plays a permissive role in LTD of parallel fiber synapses. A similar facilitatory role of corticotropin releasing factor can be found for LTD induction at climbing fiber–Purkinje cell synapses (see following; Schmolesky et al., 2007).

12.13.3 Parallel Fiber Signals

Parallel fiber activation results in glutamate release, which activates glutamate receptors in the Purkinje cell dendrite. While mature Purkinje cells do not express functional NMDARs, they are found on both cultured embryonic Purkinje cells and acutely dissociated Purkinje cells in early postnatal life (Linden and Connor, 1991; Rosenmund et al., 1992). Purkinje cells also express AMPARs of the GluR2-containing, Ca-impermeable variety (Linden et al., 1993; Tempia et al., 1996) as well as a particular metabotropic receptor, mGluR1, at high levels in the dendritic spines where parallel fiber synapses are received (Martin et al., 1992).

The first evidence indicating that activation of metabotropic receptors was required for parallel fiber LTD induction came from experiments using cerebellar cultures, which showed that agonists that activated both AMPA and metabotropic receptors (such as glutamate and quisqualate) could substitute for parallel fiber activation during LTD induction, but that agonists that failed to activate metabotropic receptors (such as AMPA or aspartate) could not (Kano and Kato, 1987; Linden et al, 1991). Complementary evidence was found in which metabotropic receptor antagonists blocked LTD induction (Linden et al., 1991; Hartell, 1994; Narasimhan and Linden, 1996; Lev-Ram et al., 1997a). These results, while they indicated that metabotropic receptor activation was required, did not specify which metabotropic receptor(s) were important for LTD induction. The first findings to address this issue were those of Shigemoto et al. (1994), who demonstrated that specific inactivating antibodies directed against mGluR1 could block LTD induction in cell culture. This result was confirmed and extended by two different groups using mGluR1 knockout mice (Aiba et al., 1994; Conquet et al., 1994).

Activation of mGluR1 results in the activation of phospholipase C and the consequent production of two initial products, inositol-1,4,5-trisphosphate (IP_3) and 1,2-diacylglycerol. The former binds to specific intracellular IP_3 receptors, resulting in the liberation of Ca from internal stores, while the latter results in activation of PKC. Are both of these products required for parallel fiber LTD induction? Purkinje cells express IP_3 receptors, particularly the type I isoform, at unusually high levels (Nakanishi et al., 1991), and it has been shown through photolysis of caged IP_3 that these receptors are functionally coupled to intracellular Ca release in situ (Khodakhah and Ogden, 1993; Wang and Augustine, 1995). Several lines of evidence have supported a role for IP_3 receptor activation in the induction of parallel fiber LTD. First, compounds which interfere with IP_3 receptor function have been shown to block LTD. Application of heparin, a nonspecific (Herbert and Maffrand, 1991; Bezprozvanny et al., 1993) inhibitor of the IP_3 receptor, blocked LTD induced by glutamate/depolarization conjunction in cultured Purkinje cells (Kasono and Hirano, 1995) or by parallel fiber/depolarization conjunction in Purkinje cells in a cerebellar slice (Khodakhah and Armstrong, 1997). A specific inactivating antibody directed against the IP_3 receptor was similarly effective (Inoue et al., 1998). Application of thapsigargin, a drug which depletes internal Ca stores through inhibition of the endoplasmic reticulum Ca-ATPase, also blocked LTD induction (Kohda et al., 1995). Thapsigargin would be expected to deplete Ca stores gated by both the IP_3 receptor and the ryanodine receptor, the latter of which mediates Ca-induced Ca release. Second, photolysis of IP_3 in cultured Purkinje cells can induce LTD when combined with depolarization plus AMPAR activation (Kasano and Hirano, 1995). Similarly, IP_3 photolysis combined with depolarization can induce LTD in slices derived from either wild-type (Khodakhah and Armstrong, 1997) or mGluR1 knockout mice (Daniel et al., 1999). Finally, parallel fiber LTD is blocked in slices derived from a mutant mouse which lacks the type I IP_3 receptor (Inoue et al., 1998).

While these experiments would appear to provide a strong case for the involvement of IP_3 receptors in cerebellar LTD induction, it is worth noting that not all evidence has been consistent with this view. For example, thapsigargin application in slices was found to block LTD induced by bath application of the mGluR agonist trans-DL-1-amino-1,3-cyclopentanedicarboxylic acid (ACPD) together with depolarization, but not parallel fiber/depolarization conjunction (Hemart et al., 1995). Furthermore, Narasimhan et al. (1998) performed ratiometric imaging of free cytosolic Ca on both acutely dissociated and cultured Purkinje cells. It was determined that the threshold for glutamate pulses to contribute to LTD induction was below the threshold for producing a Ca transient. Furthermore, the Ca transients produced by depolarization alone and glutamate plus depolarization were not significantly different. In addition, the potent and selective IP_3 receptor channel blocker xestospongin C (an improvement over heparin) was not found to affect the induction of LTD in either acutely dissociated or cultured Purkinje cells at a concentration which was sufficient to block mGluR1-evoked Ca mobilization. Finally, replacement of mGluR1 activation by exogenous synthetic diacylglycerol in an LTD induction protocol was successful. At present it is not clear why an IP_3 signaling cascade is not required for induction of cerebellar LTD in these experiments using reduced preparations, while other experiments using both slice and culture preparations have suggested otherwise.

12.13.4 Second Messengers

Two major postsynaptic signals resulting from cerebellar LTD induction are 1,2-diacylglycerol and Ca. These signals are known to synergistically activate the enzyme PKC. The involvement of PKC in LTD induction was suggested by experiments in which PKC inhibitors blocked induction when applied during glutamate/depolarization conjunction in cultured Purkinje cells (Linden and Connor, 1991). Application of these compounds after LTD had been induced had no effect, suggesting that continued PKC activation is not required for LTD to persist. Blockade of LTD induction by PKC inhibitors has since been confirmed using several preparations including cerebellar slices (Hartell, 1994; Freeman et al., 1998), acutely dissociated Purkinje cells and Purkinje cell dendritic macropatches (Narasimhan and Linden, 1996), as well as cultured Purkinje cells derived from a transgenic mouse which expresses a PKC inhibitor peptide (De Zeeuw et al., 1998). These observations are complemented by the finding that bath application of PKC-activating phorbol esters induces an LTD-like attenuation of Purkinje cell responses to exogenous glutamate or AMPA (Crepel and Krupa, 1988; Linden and Connor, 1991) which occludes pairing-induced LTD. In a recent study using αCaMKII knockout mice, it was shown that αCaMKII is involved in cerebellar LTD induction as well (Hansel et al., 2006). Moreover, LTD was blocked when the CaMKII inhibitor KN-93 was bath applied, but not when its inactive analogue, KN-92, was used. These observations show that, similar to hippocampal LTP (but operating in an 'inverse' manner), multiple kinases are involved in the induction process.

In addition to PKC and αCaMKII activation, a number of studies have indicated that release of the gaseous second messenger, nitric oxide (NO) by the action of the Ca/calmodulin-sensitive enzyme NO synthase (NOS), is necessary for parallel fiber LTD induction. They have shown that an LTD-like phenomenon could be induced when climbing fiber stimulation was replaced by bath application of NO via donor molecules such as sodium nitroprusside (Crepel and Jaillard, 1990; Shibuki and Okada, 1991; Daniel et al., 1993; but see Glaum et al., 1992). Likewise, induction of LTD by more conventional means could be blocked by inhibitors of NOS (such as N^G-nitro-L-arginine), agents that bind NO in the extracellular fluid (such as hemoglobin), or genetic deletion of the neuronal isoform of NOS (Lev-Ram et al., 1997b). Application of NO donors, cGMP analogs, or cGMP phosphodiesterase inhibitors directly to the Purkinje cell (via a patch pipette) also resulted in depression of parallel fiber responses (Daniel et al., 1993; Hartell, 1994, 1996), while postsynaptic application of a NOS inhibitor did not block LTD induction (Daniel et al., 1993). In contrast, postsynaptic application of a specific guanylyl cyclase inhibitor was effective in blocking LTD induction (Boxall and Garthwaite, 1996;

Lev-Ram et al., 1997a). These findings suggested a model in which climbing fiber activation resulted in NO production, which then diffused to the Purkinje cell to activate soluble guanylyl cyclase. However, this model was complicated by the fact that both climbing fibers (Bredt et al., 1990; Vincent and Kimura, 1992; Ikeda et al., 1993) and Purkinje cells (Bredt et al., 1990; Vincent and Kimura, 1992; Crepel et al., 1994) lack NOS.

A proposal which addresses this complication has been that climbing fiber–evoked Ca influx into Purkinje cell dendrites causes K-efflux, which depolarizes adjacent parallel fiber terminals, resulting in Ca influx and the consequent activation of NOS in these compartments (Daniel et al., 1998). Another approach has been taken by Lev-Ram et al. (1995), who found that photolysis of caged NO loaded into Purkinje cells could substitute for parallel fiber activation in LTD induction. When NO photolysis was followed by direct Purkinje cell depolarization within a 50-ms window, LTD of parallel fiber EPSCs was produced. LTD induced in this manner could be blocked by a postsynaptic application of a Ca chelator or NO scavenger, but not external application of a NOS inhibitor or an NO scavenger. In contrast, LTD produced by parallel fiber/depolarization conjunction could be blocked by either an internally or externally applied NO scavenger, or an externally applied NOS inhibitor, but not an internally applied NOS inhibitor. This pattern of results suggests a model in which activation of parallel fibers causes an anterograde NO signal which acts inside the Purkinje cell. A subsequent investigation by this group showed that, when photolysis of caged Ca was used in place of Purkinje cell depolarization, the coincidence requirement for NO and Ca pairing was <10 ms, and the resultant LTD could be blocked by an inhibitor of soluble guanylyl cyclase (Lev-Ram et al., 1997a). However, when caged Ca and cGMP were used, the inhibition of guanylyl cyclase could be overcome, and the coincidence requirement was lengthened to $\sim$200 ms.

The production of cGMP by this cascade is likely to be exerting its effect through activation of cGMP-dependent protein kinase (PKG). LTD induced by parallel fiber/depolarization conjunctive stimulation (Hartell, 1994) or photolytic NO/depolarization stimulation (Lev-Ram et al, 1997a) may be blocked with PKG inhibitors. While the mechanisms by which PKG might contribute to LTD induction are not known, one suggestion has been that phosphorylation of G-substrate by PKG could result in inhibition of protein phosphatases (Ito, 1990), which in turn promote LTP induction (Belmeguenai and Hansel, 2005).

In contrast to the extensive evidence indicating a requirement for a NO/cGMP/PKG cascade in slice preparations, LTD of glutamate currents produced without synaptic stimulation in cultured Purkinje cells is unaffected by reagents that stimulate (sodium nitroprusside) or inhibit (hemoglobin, N^G-nitro-L-arginine) NO signaling (Linden and Connor, 1992). Furthermore, in cerebellar cultures made from neuronal NOS knockout mice, LTD was indistinguishable from that in cultures from wild-type mice (Linden et al., 1995). In wild-type cultures, neither an activator of soluble guanylate cyclase, nor an inhibitor of type V cGMP-phosphodiesterase, nor inclusion of cGMP analogs in the patch pipette produced an LTD like effect. Induction of LTD was not blocked by inclusion in the patch pipette of three different PKG inhibitors. These results suggest that a NO/cGMP/PKG cascade is not required for cerebellar LTD induction in culture.

A recent study suggests that in slices NO might indeed be required for LTD induction, but that NO is not released from parallel fiber terminals, but instead from interneurons (Shin and Linden, 2005). Using combined patch-clamp recordings and presynaptic confocal Ca imaging, the authors demonstrated that there are no NMDAR-mediated Ca transients in parallel fiber terminals, which had previously been suggested to promote NOS activation and subsequent NO production (Casado et al., 2002). Rather, functional NMDAR and NMDAR-mediated Ca signaling were found in the somata, dendrites, and presynaptic terminals of stellate cells (Shin and Linden, 2005). Thus, it is likely that under certain activation conditions NO diffuses from interneurons to Purkinje cells and facilitates LTD induction by promoting phosphatase inhibition.

12.14 Parallel Fiber LTD Expression

While considerable attention has been paid to the molecular mechanisms of cerebellar LTD induction, significant effort has only recently been focused upon its expression. A widely accepted notion has been that LTD is expressed, at least in part, as a down-regulation of the postsynaptic sensitivity to AMPA, as LTD may be detected using AMPA or glutamate test pulses in intact (Ito et al., 1982), slice (Crepel and Krupa, 1988), and culture (Linden et al., 1991) preparations. These experiments have been extended with ultrareduced preparations that completely lack functional presynaptic terminals (Linden, 1994) including outside-out dendritic macropatches and acutely dissociated Purkinje cells (Narasimhan and Linden, 1996, Narasimhan et al., 1998) which provide definitive evidence for a postsynaptic locus of expression. This idea has received further support from a study showing that the coefficient of variation of parallel fiber EPSCs was altered by manipulations known to act presynaptically (such as transient synaptic attenuation produced by addition of adenosine), but was not altered by induction of LTD (Blond et al., 1997).

In CA1 pyramidal cells, synaptic plasticity is implemented by changes both in the properties of postsynaptic AMPA receptors and in the insertion/internalization balance of AMPA receptor subunits (see above). In contrast, parallel fiber LTD is not associated with changes in AMPA receptor properties, such as glutamate affinity, conductance, or kinetics (Linden, 2001; for review see Ito, 2001). Rather, synaptic plasticity at parallel fiber synapses seems to rely entirely on changes in AMPA receptor trafficking. In Purkinje cells, GluR1 expression is low (Baude et al., 1994), and GluR2/GluR3 heteromers constitute the majority of AMPA receptors. PF-LTD results from a clathrin-mediated endocytosis of GluR2 (Wang and Linden, 2000), which requires PKCα-dependent phosphorylation of GluR2 at serine-880 (Chung et al., 2003; Leitges et al., 2004). The internalization of GluR2 involves unbinding from GRIP (Dong et al., 1997) and binding to PICK1 (Xia et al., 1999, 2000; Chung et al., 2000; Steinberg et al., 2006), thus using the same molecular machinery as described for GluR2 endocytosis in CA1 pyramidal cells (**Figure 7**). The role of αCaMKII activation, which is needed for LTD induction (Hansel et al., 2006), in GluR2 subunit trafficking remains to be examined.

12.15 Another Type of Cerebellar LTD: Climbing Fiber LTD

In the classic Marr-Albus-Ito models of cerebellar function and learning, paired parallel fiber and climbing fiber stimulation leads to LTD at the parallel fiber synapses, but the climbing fiber input was considered invariant (Marr, 1969; Albus, 1971; Ito, 1984). This reputation is a result of early studies by Eccles and colleagues demonstrating a high degree of reliability of complex spike occurrence upon tetanization at frequencies exceeding 100 Hz (e.g., Eccles et al., 1966). However, a different perspective of the 'invariance' of the complex spike emerges when it comes to modifications of the complex spike waveform. The search for plasticity at climbing fiber synapses was actually started using recordings of climbing fiber–mediated EPSCs in voltage-clamp mode, enabling an electrophysiological isolation of synaptic events underlying the complex spike. Climbing fiber activation at 5 Hz for 30 s resulted in a lasting reduction of EPSC amplitudes (Hansel and Linden, 2000; Carta et al., 2006). This form of LTD at the climbing fiber input was not accompanied by changes in parallel fiber responses, but it turned out that climbing fiber LTD shares induction requirements with parallel fiber LTD, namely a dependence on postsynaptic Ca transients, mGluR1, and PKC activation (Hansel and Linden, 2000). Climbing fiber LTD is not accompanied by changes in the paired-pulse depression ratio (Hansel and Linden, 2000) and also does not alter the degree of AMPA receptor blockade by a low-affinity competitive antagonist, γ-D-glutamylglycine, which unbinds rapidly from AMPA receptors and can be used as a reporter for changes in glutamate release (Shen et al., 2002). These results suggest that climbing fiber LTD, just like parallel fiber LTD, is postsynaptically expressed. When discussing plasticity at the climbing fiber synapse, it has to be kept in mind that this is a very unusual type of synapse, as climbing fiber activity under physiological conditions results in an all-or-none complex spike. The waveform of complex spikes is composed of an initial Na action potential in the soma, followed by smaller spikelets on top of a plateau. These spikelets likely reflect calcium spike activity in the dendrite, although at the somatic level (where typically the recordings are performed) resurgent Na conductances might be involved as well (for review see Schmolesky et al., 2002). As complex spikes are the physiological responses to climbing fiber stimulation, climbing fiber plasticity was also characterized when complex spikes were recorded in current-clamp mode. Under these conditions, 5-Hz climbing fiber activation for 30 s resulted in a selective reduction of slow complex spike components (most reliably the first spikelet) (Hansel and Linden, 2000; see also Hansel et al., 2001). This effect could be mimicked by partial AMPA receptor blockade using NBQX (1,2,3,4-tetrahydro-6-nitro-2,3-dioxo-benzo-[f]quinoxaline-7-sulfonamide) (Weber et al., 2003), suggesting that climbing fiber LTD is primarily caused by a reduction in AMPAR-mediated transmission, which subsequently affects dendritic Ca spike activity. This interpretation is supported by experiments in which whole-cell patch-clamp recordings and microfluorometric Ca measurements were simultaneously performed. These recordings showed that climbing fiber LTD is accompanied by a long-term depression of dendritic Ca transients (Weber et al., 2003). Finally, it was shown that climbing fiber LTD is associated with a reduction in the afterhyperpolarization (AHP) following complex spikes (Schmolesky et al., 2005), which might result from the depression of Ca transients. These observations show that LTD at the climbing fiber synapse affects all components of a climbing fiber response, namely the underlying synaptic transmission and subsequently the complex spike, the complex spike-evoked Ca transient, as well as the complex spike AHP. As will be discussed, these alterations (particularly the 'Ca-LTD') have a large effect on the function of Purkinje cells and on parallel fiber plasticity.

12.16 Interactions Between LTP and LTD at Parallel Fiber Synapses

Parallel fiber LTD is postsynaptically induced and expressed (for review see Hansel et al., 2001; Ito, 2001, 2002). A mechanism allowing for activity-dependent reversibility of LTD therefore needs to operate postsynaptically as well. Recently, a postsynaptic form of parallel fiber LTP has indeed been described (Lev-Ram et al., 2002; Coesmans et al., 2004). LTP had been reported in earlier studies under conditions when LTD was blocked (e.g., Sakurai, 1990; Shibuki and Okada, 1992), but in these studies the expression side of LTP was not specifically addressed. The first type of parallel fiber LTP that was actually examined in detail turned out to be a presynaptic phenomenon (Salin et al., 1996).

This presynaptic form of LTP is typically induced by brief (4–8 Hz) parallel fiber tetanization and requires presynaptic Ca influx (Salin et al., 1996; Linden, 1997) and activation of Ca-sensitive adenylyl cyclase I (Storm et al., 1998), an enzyme which is concentrated in granule cell presynaptic terminals. The resulting cyclic adenosine monophosphate elevation then activates PKA (Salin et al., 1996) in this same compartment (Linden and Ahn, 1999). A PKA substrate involved in the induction of presynaptic parallel fiber LTP is the active zone protein RIM1α (Lonart et al., 2003).

The postsynaptic form of parallel fiber LTP can be obtained with the same parallel fiber tetanization protocol used for the induction of parallel fiber LTD (1 Hz; 5 min), but in the absence of climbing fiber activity (Lev-Ram et al., 2002; Coesmans et al., 2004). Therefore, the polarity of synaptic gain changes at the parallel fiber input depends on the activity level of the heterosynaptic climbing fiber input. Climbing fiber activity can exert such function as a polarity switch, because LTD induction requires a larger Ca transient than LTP induction (Coesmans et al., 2004). This is a remarkable observation, as it indicates that bidirectional parallel fiber plasticity is governed by a Ca-threshold mechanism that operates inverse to its hippocampal counterpart (**Figure 7**). The additional Ca needed for parallel fiber LTD induction is contributed by climbing fiber–evoked complex spike activity (Konnerth et al., 1992; Wang et al., 2000). In fact, previous induction of climbing fiber LTD (and the associated reduction in dendritic Ca transients) reduces the probability for subsequent induction of parallel fiber LTD (Coesmans et al., 2004). Postsynaptic parallel fiber LTP depends on the activation of protein phosphatases 1, 2A, and 2B, but neither requires PKC activity (Belmeguenai and Hansel, 2005) or αCaMKII activity (Hansel et al., 2006). The postsynaptic expression side of this form of parallel fiber LTP suggests that it might provide a reversal mechanism for LTD. The postsynaptic expression of LTP was confirmed by the absence of changes in the paired-pulse facilitation ratio (Lev-Ram et al., 2002; Coesmans et al., 2004) and by the absence of changes in the degree of AMPA receptor blockade by the low-affinity competitive AMPA receptor antagonist γ-DGG (Coesmans et al., 2004). Postsynaptic LTD and LTP can indeed reverse each other: when LTP was saturated first by applying the LTP-inducing protocol twice, application of the LTD protocol resulted in a depotentiation (**Figure 6**). Subsequent application of the LTP protocol for the third time again potentiated the parallel fiber EPSCs, indicating that the previous LTD protocol had reversed LTP and that the LTP mechanism was not saturated any longer (Coesmans et al., 2004). The mutual reversibility of postsynaptic parallel fiber LTD and LTP is also suggested by the observation that LTP induction involves an NSF-dependent membrane delivery of GluR2 subunits (Kakegawa and Yuzaki, 2005), which are internalized during LTD (**Figure 7**).

12.17 Comparison of Bidirectional Plasticity at Hippocampal and Cerebellar Synapses

While this article largely focuses on the description of LTD mechanisms and the function of LTD, we have also discussed how at both hippocampal and cerebellar synapses LTD relates to LTP. This relation is crucial for an understanding of brain plasticity when it comes to the cellular machinery involved in synaptic memory storage, but also when it comes to the functions of LTP and LTD, respectively. A postsynaptic form of parallel fiber LTP was only recently discovered (Lev-Ram et al., 2002), but its arrival on the scene finally establishes bidirectional plasticity at parallel fiber synapses and allows us to directly compare the cellular mechanisms involved in LTP and LTD induction at hippocampal synapses to their cerebellar counterparts. To start with, at both types of synapses different 'tools' are available for plasticity: in contrast to pyramidal neurons, mature Purkinje cells lack functional NMDARs (Crepel et al., 1982) and only weakly express the AMPAR subunit GluR1 (Baude et al., 1994). Purkinje cells, in turn, express the orphan glutamate receptor $\delta 2$ (GluR$\delta 2$), which plays a not well-understood role in parallel fiber LTD (for review see Yuzaki, 2004), but is not expressed in pyramidal cells. Moreover, Purkinje cells lack back-propagating action potentials in the dendrites (Stuart and Häusser, 1994), but fire complex spikes in response to climbing fiber activation (for review see Schmolesky et al., 2002).

Our current understanding of plasticity mechanisms is not yet advanced enough to pinpoint, for example, what consequences the absence of functional NMDARs has for Purkinje cells, or the absence of GluR$\delta 2$ receptors for pyramidal cells. However, we can describe an emerging picture of remarkable differences between hippocampal and cerebellar plasticity, but also of astonishing similarities (see also Hansel, 2005). In several aspects, cerebellar plasticity provides a mirror image of hippocampal plasticity. As described in detail earlier, hippocampal LTP induction requires large Ca transients and the activation of protein kinases (e.g., CaMKII, PKA, PKC), whereas LTD relies on lower Ca transients and the activation of protein phosphatases. In cerebellar plasticity, the Ca and kinase/phosphatase dependencies are inverse to the hippocampal ones (**Figure 7**): LTD induction (by paired parallel fiber and climbing fiber activity) requires larger Ca transients than LTP induction (by parallel fiber activity alone) (Coesmans et al., 2004). Moreover, LTD is PKC dependent (Linden and Connor, 1991; De Zeeuw et al., 1998) and αCaMKII dependent (Hansel et al. 2006), whereas LTP induction requires the activation of protein phosphatases 1, 2A, and 2B (Belmeguenai and Hansel, 2005).

At the level of AMPAR trafficking, the mirror image–like arrangement of induction events is partially confirmed and partially breaks down. Kinase activity promotes the membrane insertion of GluR1 subunits, which dominate trafficking behavior in GluR1/GluR2 heteromers (Song and Huganir, 2002). Three GluR1 phosphorylation sites are discussed in the context of hippocampal LTP induction, namely serine-831 (CaMKII, but for conductance changes), serine-845 (PKA), and most recently, serine-818 (PKC). In GluR1 'phospho-free' mice, NMDAR-dependent LTD is blocked, which has been interpreted as further evidence for the hypothesis that a dephosphorylation at GluR1 promotes GluR1 endocytosis and LTD (Lee et al., 2003). This scenario would indeed provide a mirror image to the phosphorylation events involved in parallel fiber plasticity, which, however, is mediated by GluR2 subunit trafficking. PKCα-mediated phosphorylation at serine-880 causes GluR2 endocytosis and LTD (Leitges et al., 2004), while LTP is phosphatase dependent (PP1/2A/2B; Belmeguenai and Hansel, 2005) and is associated with a membrane insertion of GluR2 subunits (Kakegawa and Yuzaki, 2005).

However, the phosphorylation/AMPAR trafficking events involved in LTP and LTD, particularly at hippocampal synapses, are still not sufficiently well understood to reach such a comprehensive and simplifying view. At the moment it seems safe to say that the cellular events underlying LTP induction indeed differ significantly, simply because there is compelling evidence that hippocampal LTP is mediated in part by a membrane insertion of GluR1 subunits, which are only weakly expressed in Purkinje cells. However, GluR2 subunit trafficking, which clearly mediates parallel fiber plasticity, works similarly in pyramidal cells. GluR2 phosphorylation at serine-880 triggers a clathrin-mediated GluR2 endocytosis at both hippocampal (Man et al., 2000; Seidenman et al., 2003) and cerebellar synapses (Wang and Linden, 2000; Chung et al., 2003). On the other hand, NSF-GluR2 binding promotes GluR2 insertion at both types of synapses (Lüscher et al., 1999; Kakegawa and Yuzaki, 2005). Moreover, recent evidence suggests that GluR2 rather than GluR1 endocytosis mediates LTD in CA1 pyramidal cells (for review see Malinow, 2003), which would suggest that both types of synapses use the same mechanism for LTD expression. How this scenario fits together with the obviously different Ca signaling requirements and kinase/phosphatase dependences of LTD induction at hippocampal and cerebellar synapses remains to be seen.

12.18 Is LTD of the Parallel Fiber–Purkinje Cell Synapse Involved in Motor Learning?

A fruitful approach to testing the hypothesized LTD/motor learning connection has been provided by the generation of mutant mice that lack proteins thought to be required for cerebellar LTD (see Chen and Tonegawa, 1997, for review). Several forms of knockout mice have been reported which have shown impairments in both parallel fiber LTD and motor learning. Mutant mice which lack mGluR1 have severely impaired cerebellar LTD (Aiba et al., 1994; Conquet et al., 1994; Ichise et al., 2000), consistent with previous studies using mGluR1 antagonists or inactivating antibodies. These mice had normal postsynaptic voltage-gated Ca currents and normal paired-pulse facilitation and depression of parallel and climbing fiber synapses, respectively. mGluR1 mutant mice were severely ataxic and showed impairments in several motor coordination tasks. When associative eyeblink conditioning was performed, these animals showed a partial deficit in CR acquisition (Aiba et al, 1994), which may not reflect an inability to produce a CR, but rather an inability to produce the optimal timing of the eyelid closure.

Other knockout mice also have LTD and motor learning deficits. Unfortunately, in some of these cases it is not understood how the missing protein functions in LTD induction. GluRδ2 is a protein which is expressed almost exclusively in Purkinje cell dendritic spines. While a point mutation in this receptor gives rise to a constitutive cation conductance and the *lurcher* phenotype (Zuo et al., 1997), the function of wild-type GluRδ2 is not clear. A GluRδ2 null mouse has impaired cerebellar LTD (Kashiwabuchi et al., 1995), consistent with reports that have used application of antisense oligonucleotides to suppress expression of this protein in culture preparations (Hirano et al., 1995; Jeromin et al., 1996). While the cerebellar cortex appears normal by light microscopy, electron microscopic analysis revealed an ~50% reduction in the number of parallel fiber–Purkinje cell synapses. This mouse is severely ataxic and is retarded in its ability to achieve a form of vestibular compensation: the righting response under a rotation load following unilateral middle ear destruction (Funabiki et al., 1995). These results are supported by more recent observations that injection of an anti-GluRδ2 antibody into the subarachnoidal supracerebellar space caused ataxic gait and poor rotorod test performance (Hirai et al., 2003).

A puzzling LTD defect is found in a mutant mouse which lacks glial fibrillary acidic protein (GFAP), which is, of course, not expressed in neurons. Since at least the early phase of cerebellar LTD may be expressed in reduced preparations that lack glia (Narasimhan and Linden, 1996, Narasimhan et al., 1998), it is likely that this knockout is exerting its effect indirectly. These mice show normal motor coordination, but are severely impaired in parallel fiber LTD and partially impaired in acquisition of associative eyeblink conditioning (Shibuki et al., 1996). Interestingly, these mice show clear improvement with training in a motor coordination task (the rotating rod), indicating that there are forms of motor learning that do not require cerebellar LTD.

There have been several major problems which have complicated the analysis of knockout mice. First, knockout mice have the gene of interest deleted from the earliest stages of development. As a result, these mice often have a complex developmental phenotype. For example, PKCγ, mGluR1 and GluRδ2 (but not GFAP) knockout mice all have cerebellar Purkinje cells that fail to undergo the normal developmental conversion from multiple to mono climbing fiber innervation in early postnatal life (Chen et al., 1995; Kano et al., 1995, 1997; Kurihara et al., 1997). Second, knockout of one gene sometimes produces compensatory upregulation in the expression of other related genes during development. In the CREBa-d (CREB: cAMP response element binding protein) knockout mouse, there is compensatory upregulation of the related transcription factor cAMP response element modulator (Hummler et al., 1994; Blendy et al., 1996). A third complicating factor is that knockout mice have the gene of interest deleted in every cell of the body, not just the cells of interest, making it more difficult to ascribe the knockout's behavioral effects to dysfunction in any one particular structure or cell type. This could be a potential problem for the analysis of behaviors such as associative eyeblink conditioning and VOR adaptation, which are likely to require use-dependent plasticity at multiple sites, synapses received by both cerebellar Purkinje cells and their targets in the DCN or vestibular nuclei.

To address the latter two complications, an alternative approach has been used (De Zeeuw et al., 1998). Using the promoter of the Purkinje cell-specific gene *pcp-2* (also known as L7; Oberdick et al., 1990), transgenic mice have been created in which a selective inhibitor to a broad range of PKC isoforms (House and Kemp, 1987; Linden and Connor, 1991) is chronically overexpressed. This strategy ensures that, in L7-PKCI mice, PKC inhibition will be restricted to Purkinje cells, and that compensation via upregulation of different PKC isoforms will not succeed in blunting the biochemical effect of the transgene. This transgenic strategy resulted in nearly complete suppression of both cerebellar LTD as assessed in culture and adaptation of the VOR in the intact, behaving animal. In addition, L7-PKCI mice show impaired learning-dependent timing of conditioned eyeblink responses (Koekkoek et al., 2003). The phenotype of these animals was remarkably delimited. They showed normal motor coordination as measured by their ability to display the normal eye movement reflexes, optokinetic reflex, and VOR, as well as by several tests of gross motor coordination (rotorod, thin rod). Basal electrophysiological and morphological features of Purkinje cells were unaltered (with the exception that the Purkinje cells remained multiply innervated by climbing fibers). Similarly, conditional knockout mice lacking cGMP-dependent protein kinase type I (cGKI) selectively in Purkinje cells show impaired LTD and VOR gain adaptation (Feil et al., 2003).

While these mice with Purkinje cell–specific deficits represent a refinement in testing the relationship between parallel fiber LTD and motor learning, there are still caveats and complications which remain. First, the one basal physiological abnormality found in L7-PKCI mice is that about 50% of the Purkinje cells show a persistent multiple climbing fiber innervation, raising the possibility that this could be a cause of their failure to demonstrate VOR adaptation. However, this is unlikely because a PKCγ knockout mouse shows multiple climbing fiber innervation with normal cerebellar LTD and no motor learning deficit (Chen et al., 1995; Kano et al., 1995). Moreover, it has been shown more recently that the elimination of surplus climbing fibers is not entirely blocked in L7-PKCI mice, but only delayed, and that the elimination process is completed in 3- to 6-month-old mice (Goossens et al., 2001) A strategy to alleviate this kind of problem in the future will be to make the L7-PKCI transgene inducible in adult mice. Second, it has recently been reported that the climbing fiber–Purkinje cell synapse undergoes LTD, which, like parallel fiber LTD, requires activation of PKC (Hansel and Linden, 2000). Thus, even inhibition of PKC that is restricted to Purkinje cells cannot have its behavioral effects solely ascribed to parallel fiber LTD. Third, it is clear that PKC does not function in Purkinje cells only to produce LTD of various synapses. For example, it is known that voltage-gated K channels are modulated by PKC in Purkinje cells. Could this or some other function of PKC that is unrelated to LTD underlie the VOR adaptation deficit? While this is not an easy problem to address, future studies will benefit from *in vivo* recording during the appropriate behavioral tasks to distinguish among these possibilities.

While the mutant mouse studies cited here provide strong support for the widely accepted notion that LTD mediates forms of cerebellar motor learning (for review see De Zeeuw and Yeo, 2005), there are also examples of failures to establish such relationship: it has been shown that T-588, a drug that affects Ca release from internal stores, blocks parallel fiber LTD *in vitro* (Kimura et al., 2005), but does not impair associative eyelid conditioning (Welsh et al., 2005). Studies are on the way to examine the effects of disrupting PF-LTP on motor learning. These studies may provide additional insight into how synaptic plasticity contributes to learning and memory. In VOR gain conditioning, LTD is assumed to provide the cellular basis for increasing the VOR gain. When examining properties of reversibility, it has been found that complete reversal can be reached by gain-down training after gain-up training. In contrast, gain-up training after gain-down training led to an incomplete reversal (Boyden and Raymond, 2003; Boyden et al., 2004). It was suggested that this asymmetric reversibility was caused by an involvement of both pre- and postsynaptic LTP in the downregulation of the VOR gain, with only the postsynaptic form of LTP providing a true reversal mechanism. It will also be interesting to study the role of (postsynaptic) LTP in associative eyeblink conditioning. LTP can be observed after parallel fiber stimulation alone, which makes it an ideal candidate mechanism to mediate extinction of conditioned eyeblink responses, as extinction can be obtained by application of the conditioned stimulus alone (for review see Hansel et al., 2001).

12.19 Conclusion

In this article, we have provided a portrait of LTD by describing the phenomenon *per se* and by summarizing and explaining the cellular signaling cascades that are involved in LTD induction and expression. At the end of this article, we would like to address a question (once more) that appears particularly crucial for plasticity at large: if LTP provides a cellular correlate of information storage and learning (synaptic memory), why is there a need for LTD?

We would like to discuss this question using again the hippocampal area CA1 (and with it, glutamatergic synapses onto cortical pyramidal cells in general) and the cerebellum as examples.

We hasten to add, however, that the list of possible LTD mechanisms is not exhausted by the study of the two synapses we have highlighted in this article. Inhibitory synapses have also been shown to exhibit LTD (Marty and Llano, 1995; Aizenman et al., 1998). Other forms of LTD have been described in excitatory synapses at other locations, such as the striatum (Lovinger et al., 1993; Calabresi et al., 1999), amygdala (Li et al., 1998; Wang and Gean, 1999), neocortex (Artola et al., 1996; Egger et al., 1999), other parts of the hippocampal formation (Kobayashi et al., 1996; Manahan-Vaughan, 1998), and the olfactory bulb (Mutoh et al., 2005). Time will tell whether these forms of LTD use expression mechanisms which overlap with those we have described here.

By intuition, most researchers in the plasticity field would likely associate LTP with learning and LTD with forgetting. This might be due to the fact that a strengthening of synaptic transmission is easily perceived as information storage, and a weakening of synaptic strength as erasing previously stored information. Moreover, LTP and LTD, as characterized in the adult, have strong overlap with cellular mechanisms involved in strengthening (establishing) and weakening (disconnecting) synapses in the developing brain (e.g., Rittenhouse et al., 1999; for review see Singer, 1995), and synapse elimination certainly qualifies as a form of deleting previously present 'information.' Over the last years, experimental evidence from the hippocampus supports this view; agents that block signaling factors for LTP induction (e.g., NMDARs), or corresponding genetic manipulations, impair hippocampus-dependent learning, for example, in spatial learning tasks (for review see Silva, 2003). Along these lines, mutations that enhance LTP enhance learning. This effect was observed in transgenic mice overexpressing NR2B receptors (Tang et al., 1999), but also in transgenic mice expressing a constitutively active form of H-ras, which facilitates glutamate release through increased extracellular signal-regulated protein kinase (ERK)-dependent phosphorylation of synapsin I (Kushner et al., 2005). Similarly, the protein phosphatases PP1 and PP2B (calcineurin), which are involved in LTD induction, have been shown to constrain LTP and learning (Malleret et al., 2001; Genoux et al., 2002), suggesting that LTD itself constrains learning and promotes forgetting. On the other hand, a forebrain-specific calcineurin knockout resulted in a blockade of LTD, but selectively impaired hippocampus-dependent working and episodic-like memory tasks (Zeng et al., 2001), which suggests that LTD inhibition does not automatically facilitate learning. Moreover, LTD is involved in novelty acquisition (Manahan-Vaughan and Braunewell, 1999; Etkin et al., 2006). It might, therefore, be impossible to generally state that LTP equals learning and LTD equals forgetting. Rather, it will be necessary to look in detail at the type of synapse involved and the particular learning task. At cortical synapses, where the correlation to behavioral outputs is far more difficult to establish, the concept of LTD and LTP as extremes along an array of graded synaptic weights might be more useful. At this synaptic level, the need for reversal mechanisms (e.g., LTD for potentiated synapses) is more obvious, as reversibility prevents saturation and, consequently, the subsequent loss of plasticity. It has to be kept in mind, though, that LTP can act as much as a reversal mechanism for LTD as LTD can be a reversal mechanism for LTP.

In the cerebellum, it is easier to assign a role in motor learning to parallel fiber LTD, although even in the cerebellum this link is not established beyond any doubt (see earlier). A final question then is why the cerebellum uses LTD for learning. A possible answer can be found in the range of spontaneous action potential discharge rates observed in pyramidal cells and Purkinje cells. Recent *in vivo* whole-cell patch-clamp recordings in awake animals show that the spontaneous spike rates in cortical neurons are extremely low; e.g., in the somatosensory cortex they are well below 0.1 Hz (Margrie et al., 2002). In contrast, Purkinje cells have spontaneous discharge rates of 30 Hz, and simple spike rates can transiently exceed 200 Hz upon sensory activation (see Monsivais et al., 2005). These high discharge rates provide a strong, tonic inhibition to the target cells in the

DCN. Parallel fiber LTD leads to a disinhibition of DCN cells, facilitating transmission and/or LTP induction at mossy fiber–DCN synapses (Medina et al., 2002). Thus, it seems that Purkinje cells use different plasticity rules than pyramidal cells, because they are GABAergic projection neurons and because they belong to the few types of neurons with a high spontaneous discharge rate. These features assign different roles to Purkinje cells in the local cerebellar network than those assigned to pyramidal cells in their local networks and projection areas.

Ten years ago, the LTD club was very small, and LTD seemed like an obscure synaptic phenomenon. Indeed, it is probably safe to say that at the end of the 1980s there was little general interest in LTD, or even any strong conviction that homosynaptic depression existed at all outside the cerebellum. This situation has clearly changed. The major challenge for the next 10 years will be to see if the role of LTD in the brain lives up to its lofty theoretical promise.

Acknowledgments

This chapter builds on a previous book chapter by Mark F. Bear and David J. Linden (2000), as well as on a recent commentary by Christian Hansel (2005). We would like to thank David Linden for his previous contribution, which made work on this chapter significantly easier.

References

Abraham W and Bear M (1996) Metaplasticity: The plasticity of synaptic plasticity. *TINS* 19: 126–130.

Aiba A, Kano M, Chen C, et al. (1994) Deficient cerebellar long-term depression and impaired motor learning in mGluR1 mutant mice. *Cell* 79: 377–388.

Aizenman C, Manis PB, and Linden DJ (1998) Polarity of long-term synaptic gain change is related to postsynaptic spike firing at a cerebellar inhibitory synapse. *Neuron* 21: 827–835.

Albus JS (1971) A theory of cerebellar function. *Math. Biosci.* 10: 25–61.

Arai A, Larson J, and Lynch G (1990) Anoxia reveals a vulnerable period in the development of long-term potentiation. *Brain Res.* 511: 353–357.

Artola A, Hensch T, and Singer W (1996) Calcium-induced long-term depression in the visual cortex of the rat. *J. Neurophysiol.* 76: 984–994.

Artola A and Singer W (1993) Long-term depression of excitatory synaptic transmission and its relationship to long-term potentiation. *Trends Neurosci.* 16: 480–487.

Barr DS, Lambert NA, Hoyt KL, Moore SD, and Wilson WA (1995) Induction and reversal of long-term potentiation by low- and high- intensity theta pattern stimulation. *J. Neurosci.* 15: 5402–5410.

Barria A, Derkach V, and Soderling T (1997a) Identification of the Ca/calmodulin-dependent protein kinase II regulatory phosphorylation site in the alpha-amino-3-hydroxyl-5-methyl-4-isoxazole-propionate-type glutamate receptor. *J. Biol. Chem.* 272: 32727–32730.

Barria A, Muller D, Derkach V, Griffith LC, and Soderling TR (1997b) Regulatory phosphorylation of AMPA-type glutamate receptors by CaM-KII during long-term potentiation. *Science* 276: 2042–2045.

Barrionuevo G, Schottler F, and Lynch G (1980) The effects of low frequency stimulation on control and "potentiated" synaptic responses in the hippocampus. *Life Sci.* 27: 2385–2391.

Batini C, Compoint C, Buissert-Delmas C, Daniel H, and Guegan M (1992) Cerebellar nuclei and the nucleocortical projections in the rat: Retrograde tracing coupled to GABA and glutamate immunohistochemistry. *J. Comp. Neurol.* 315: 74–84.

Baude A, Molnar E, Latawiec D, McIlhinney RAJ, and Somogyi P (1994) Synaptic and nonsynaptic localization of the GluR1 subunit of the AMPA-type excitatory amino acid receptor in the rat cerebellum. *J. Neurosci.* 14: 2830–2843.

Bear M (1995) Mechanism for a sliding synaptic modification threshold. *Neuron* 15: 1–4.

Bear MF (1996) A synaptic basis for memory storage in the cerebral cortex. *Proc. Natl. Acad. Sci. USA* 93: 13453–13459.

Bear MF (1999) Homosynaptic long-term depression: A mechanism for memory? *Proc. Natl. Acad. Sci. USA* 96: 9457–9458.

Bear MF and Abraham WC (1996) Long-term depression in hippocampus. *Annu. Rev. Neurosci.* 19: 437–462.

Bear MF, Cooper LN, and Ebner FF (1987) A physiological basis for a theory of synaptic modification. *Science* 237: 42–48.

Bear MF and Linden DJ (2000) The mechanisms and meaning of long-term synaptic depression in the mammalian brain. In: Cowan WN, Südhof T, and Stevens CF (eds.) *Synapses*, pp. 455–517. Baltimore: Johns Hopkins.

Bear MF and Malenka RC (1994) Synaptic plasticity: LTP and LTD. *Curr. Opin. Neurobiol.* 4: 389–399.

Beattie EC, Carroll RC, Yu X, et al. (2000) Regulation of AMPA receptor endocytosis by a signaling mechanism shared with LTD. *Nat. Neurosci.* 3: 1291–1300.

Belmeguenai A and Hansel C (2005) A role for protein phosphatases 1, 2A, and 2B in cerebellar long-term potentiation. *J. Neurosci.* 25: 10768–10772.

Berretta N and Cherubini E (1998) A novel form of long-term depression in the CA1 area of the adult rat hippocampus independent of glutamate receptors activation. *Eur. J. Neurosci.* 10: 2957–2963.

Berthier NE and Moore JW (1986) Cerebellar Purkinje cell activity related to the classically conditioned nictitating membrane response. *Exp. Brain Res.* 63: 341–350.

Berthier NE and Moore JW (1990) Activity of deep cerebellar nuclear cells during classical conditioning of nictitating membrane extension in rabbits. *Exp. Brain Res.* 83: 44–54.

Bezprozvanny IB, Ondrias K, Kattan E, Stoyanovsky DA, and Erlich BA (1993) Activation of the calcium release channel ryanodine receptor by heparin and other polyanions is calcium dependent. *Mol. Biol. Cell.* 4: 347–352.

Bi GQ and Poo MM (1998) Synaptic modifications in cultured hippocampal neurons: Dependence on spike timing, synaptic strength, and postsynaptic cell type. *J. Neurosci.* 18: 10464–10472.

Bienenstock EL, Cooper LN, and Munro PW (1982) Theory for the development of neuron selectivity: Orientation specificity and binocular interaction in visual cortex. *J. Neurosci.* 2: 32–48.

Blendy JA, Kaestner KH, Schmid W, and Schutz G (1996) Targeting of the CREB gene leads to up-regulation of a novel CREB mRNA isoform. *EMBO J.* 15: 1098–1106.

Bliss TVP and Lomo T (1973) Long-lasting potentiation of synaptic transmission in the dentate area of the anaesthetized rabbit following stimulation of the perforant path. *J. Physiol.* 232: 331–356.

Blitzer RD, Connor JH, Brown GP, et al. (1998) Gating of CaMKII by cAMP-regulated protein phosphatase activity during LTP. *Science* 280: 1940–1942.

Blitzer RD, Wong T, Nouranifar R, Iyengar R, and Landau EM (1995) Postsynaptic cAMP pathway gates early LTP in hippocampal CA1 region. *Neuron* 15: 1403–1414.

Blond O, Daniel H, Otani S, Jaillard D, and Crepel F (1997) Presynaptic and postsynaptic effects of nitric oxide donors at synapses between parallel fibres and Purkinje cells: Involvement in cerebellar long-term depression. *Neuroscience* 77: 945–954.

Boehm J, Kang MG, Johnson RC, Esteban J, Huganir RL, and Malinow R (2006) Synaptic incorporation of AMPA receptors during LTP is controlled by a PKC phosphorylation site on GluR1. *Neuron* 51: 213–225.

Bolshakov VY and Siegelbaum SA (1994) Postsynaptic induction and presynaptic expression of hippocampal long-term depression. *Science* 264: 1148–1152.

Bortolotto ZA, Fitzjohn SM, and Collingridge GL (1999) Roles of metabotropic glutamate receptors in LTP and LTD in the hippocampus. *Curr. Opin. Neurobiol.* 9: 299–304.

Boxall AR and Garthwaite J (1996) Long-term depression in rat cerebellum requires both NO synthase and NO-sensitive guanylyl cyclase. *Eur. J. Neurosci.* 8: 2209–2212.

Boyden ES, Katoh A, and Raymond JL (2004) Cerebellum-dependent learning: The role of multiple plasticity mechanisms. *Ann. Rev. Neurosci.* 27: 581–609.

Boyden ES and Raymond JL (2003) Active reversal of motor memories reveals rules governing memory encoding. *Neuron* 39: 1031–1042.

Brabet I, Mary S, Bockaert J, and Pin J-P (1995) Phenylglycine derivatives discriminate between mGluR1- and mGluR5-mediated responses. *Neuropharmacology* 34: 895–903.

Bracha V, Webster ML, Winters NK, Irwin KB, and Bloedel JR (1994) Effects of muscimol inactivation on the cerebellar interposed-dentate nuclear complex on the performance of the nictitating membrane response of the rabbit. *Exp. Brain Res.* 100: 453–468.

Brandon EP, Zhuo M, Huang YY, et al. (1995) Hippocampal long-term depression and depotentiation are defective in mice carrying a targeted disruption of the gene encoding the RI beta subunit of cAMP-dependent protein kinase. *Proc. Natl. Acad. Sci. USA* 92: 8851–8852.

Bredt DS, Hwang PM, and Snyder SH (1990) Localization of nitric oxide synthase indicating a neural role for nitric oxide. *Nature* 347: 768–770.

Breese C, Hampson R, and Deadwyler S (1989) Hippocampal place cells: Stereotypy and plasticity. *J. Neurosci.* 9: 1097–1111.

Calabresi P, Centonze D, Gubellini P, Marfia GA, and Bernardi G (1999) Glutamate-triggered events inducing corticostriatal long-term depression. *J. Neurosci.* 19: 6102–6110.

Carroll RC, Lissin DV, von Zastrow M, Nicoll RA, and Malenka RC (1999) Rapid redistribution of glutamate receptors contributes to long-term depression in hippocampal cultures. *Nat. Neurosci.* 2: 454–460.

Carta M, Mameli M, and Valenzuela CF (2006) Alcohol potently modulates climbing fiber–Purkinje neuron synapses: Role of metabotropic glutamate receptors. *J. Neurosci.* 26: 1906–1912.

Casado M, Isope P, and Ascher P (2002) Involvement of presynaptic N-methyl-D-aspartate receptors in cerebellar long-term depression. *Neuron* 33: 123–130.

Chen C, Kano M, Abeliovich A, et al. (1995) Impaired motor coordination correlates with persistent multiple climbing fiber innervation in PKC-mutant mice. *Cell* 83: 1233–1242.

Chen C and Thompson RF (1995) Temporal specificity of long-term depression in parallel fiber–Purkinje synapses in rat cerebellar slice. *Learn. Mem.* 2: 185–198.

Chen C and Tonegawa S (1997) Molecular genetic analysis of synaptic plasticity, activity-dependent neural development, learning and memory in the mammalian brain. *Annu. Rev. Neurosci.* 20: 157–184.

Christie BR, Magee JC, and Johnston D (1996) The role of dendritic action potentials and Ca influx in the induction of homosynaptic long-term depression in hippocampal CA1 pyramidal neurons. *Learn. Mem.* 3: 160–169.

Chung HJ, Steinberg JP, Huganir RL, and Linden DJ (2003) Requirement of AMPA receptor GluR2 phosphorylation for cerebellar long-term depression. *Science* 300: 1751–1755.

Chung HJ, Xia J, Scannevin RH, Zhang X, and Huganir RL (2000) Phosphorylation of the AMPA receptor subunit GluR2 differentially regulates its interaction with PDZ domain-containing proteins. *J. Neurosci.* 20: 7258–7267.

Coesmans M, Weber JT, De Zeeuw CI, and Hansel C (2004) Bidirectional parallel fiber plasticity in the cerebellum under climbing fiber control. *Neuron* 44: 691–700.

Cohen P (1989) The structure and regulation of protein phosphatases. *Annu. Rev. Biochem.* 58: 453–508.

Collingridge GL, Isaac JTR, and Wang YT (2004) Receptor trafficking and synaptic plasticity. *Nat. Rev. Neurosci.* 5: 952–962.

Conquet F, Bashir ZI, Davies CH, et al. (1994) Motor deficit and impairment of synaptic plasticity in mice lacking mGluR1. *Nature* 327: 237–243.

Cormier RJ, Greenwood AC, and Connor JA (2001) Bidirectional synaptic plasticity correlated with the magnitude of dendritic calcium transients above a threshold. *J. Neurophysiol.* 85: 399–406.

Coussens CM, Kerr DS, and Abraham WC (1997) Glucocorticoid receptor activation lowers the threshold for NMDA-receptor-dependent homosynaptic long-term depression in the hippocampus through activation of voltage-dependent calcium channels. *J. Neurophysiol.* 78: 1–9.

Crepel F, Audinat E, Daniel H, et al. (1994) Cellular locus of the nitric oxide-synthase involved in cerebellar long-term depression induced by high external potassium concentration. *Neuropharmacology* 33: 1399–1405.

Crepel F, Dhanjal SS, and Sears TA (1982) Effect of glutamate, aspartate and related derivatives on cerebellar Purkinje cell dendrites in the rat: An *in vitro* study. *J. Physiol. (Lond.)* 329: 297–317.

Crepel F and Jaillard D (1990) Protein kinases, nitric oxide and long-term depression of synapses in the cerebellum. *NeuroReport* 1: 133–136.

Crepel F and Jaillard D (1991) Pairing of pre- and postsynaptic activities in cerebellar Purkinje cells induces long-term changes in synaptic efficacy *in vitro*. *J. Physiol.* 432: 123–141.

Crepel F and Krupa M (1988) Activation of protein kinase C induces a long-term depression of glutamate sensitivity of cerebellar Purkinje cells. An *in vitro* study. *Brain Res.* 458: 397–401.

Cummings JA, Mulkey RM, Nicoll RA, and Malenka RC (1996) Ca signalling requirements for long-term depression in the hippocampus. *Neuron* 16: 825–833.

Cummings JA, Nicola SM, and Malenka RC (1994) Induction in the rat hippocampus of long-term potentiation (LTP) and long-term depression (LTD) in the presence of a nitric oxide synthase inhibitor. *Neurosci. Lett.* 176: 110–114.

Daniel H, Hemart N, Jaillard D, and Crepel F (1993) Long-term depression requires nitric oxide and guanosine 3′-5′ cyclic

monophosphate production in cerebellar Purkinje cells. *Eur. J. Neurosci*. 5: 1079–1082.
Daniel H, Levenes C, and Crepel F (1998) Cellular mechanisms of cerebellar LTD. *Trends Neurosci*. 21: 401–407.
Daniel H, Levenes C, Fagni L, Conquet F, Bockaert J, and Crepel F (1999) Inositol-1,4,5-trisphosphate-mediated rescue of cerebellar long-term depression in subtype 1 metabotropic glutamate receptor mutant mouse. *Neuroscience* 92: 1–6.
Debanne D, Gahwiler BH, and Thompson SM (1994) Asynchronous pre- and postsynaptic activity induces associative long-term depression in area CA1 of the rat hippocampus *in vitro*. *Proc. Natl. Acad. Sci. USA* 91: 1148–1152.
Debanne D, Gahwiler BH, and Thompson SM (1997) Bidirectional associative plasticity of unitary CA3-CA1 EPSPs in the rat hippocampus *in vitro*. *J. Neurophysiol*. 77: 2851–2855.
de Mendonca A, Almeida T, Bashir ZI, and Ribeiro JA (1997) Endogenous adenosine attenuates long-term depression and depotentiation in the CA1 region of the rat hippocampus. *Neuropharmacology* 36: 161–167.
Derkach V, Barria A, and Soderling TR (1999) Ca/calmodulin-kinase II enhances channel conductance of alpha-amino-3-hydroxy-5-methyl-4-isoxazolepropionate type glutamate receptors. *Proc. Natl. Acad. Sci. USA* 96: 3269–3274.
De Zeeuw CI and Berrebi AS (1995) Postsynaptic targets of Purkinje cell terminals in the cerebellar and vestibular nuclei of the rat. *Eur. J. Neurosci*. 7: 2322–2333.
De Zeeuw CI, Hansel C, Bian F, et al. (1998) Expression of a protein kinase C inhibitor in Purkinje cells blocks cerebellar long-term depression and adaptation of the vestibulo-ocular reflex. *Neuron* 20: 495–508.
De Zeeuw CI and Yeo CH (2005) Time and tide in cerebellar memory formation. *Curr. Opin. Neurobiol*. 15: 667–674.
Dodt H, Eder M, Frick A, and Zieglgansberger W (1999) Precisely localized LTD in the neocortex revealed by infrared-guided laser stimulation. *Science* 286: 110–113.
Dong H, O'Brien RJ, Fung ET, Lanahan AA, Worley PF, and Huganir RL (1997) GRIP: A synaptic PDZ domain-containing protein that interacts with AMPA receptors. *Nature* 386: 279–284.
Doyle CA, Cullen WK, Rowan MJ, and Anwyl R (1997) Low-frequency stimulation induces homosynaptic depotentiation but not long-term depression of synaptic transmission in the adult anaesthetized and awake rat hippocampus *in vitro*. *Neuroscience* 77: 75–85.
Dudek SM and Bear MF (1989) A biochemical correlate of the critical period for synaptic modification in the visual cortex. *Science* 246: 673–675.
Dudek SM and Bear MF (1992) Homosynaptic long-term depression in area CA1 of hippocampus and effects of N-methyl-D-aspartate receptor blockade. *Proc. Natl. Acad. Sci. USA* 89: 4363–4367.
Dudek SM and Bear MF (1993) Bidirectional long-term modification of synaptic effectiveness in the adult and immature hippocampus. *J. Neurosci*. 13: 2910–2918.
du Lac S, Raymond JL, Sejnowski TJ, and Lisberger SG (1995) Learning and memory in the vestibulo-ocular reflex. *Ann. Rev. Neurosci*. 18: 409–441.
Dunwiddie TV and Fredholm BB (1989) Adenosine A1 receptors inhibit adenylate cyclase activity and neurotransmitter release and hyperpolarize pyramidal neurons in rat hippocampus. *J. Pharmacol. Exp. Ther*. 249: 31–37.
Eccles JC, Llinas R, Sasaki K, and Voorhoeve PE (1966) Interaction experiments on the responses evoked in Purkinje cells by climbing fibres. *J. Physiol*. 182: 297–315.
Egger V, Feldmeyer D, and Sakmann B (1999) Coincidence detection and changes of synaptic efficacy in spiny stellate neurons in rat barrel cortex. *Nat. Neurosci*. 2: 1098–1105.
Ehlers MD (2000) Reinsertion or degradation of AMPA receptors determined by activity-dependent endocytic sorting. *Neuron* 28: 511–525.
Ekerot C-F and Kano M (1985) Long-term depression of parallel fibre synapses following stimulation of climbing fibres. *Brain Res*. 342: 357–360.
Ekerot C-F and Kano M (1989) Stimulation parameters influencing climbing fibre induced long-term depression of parallel fibre synapses. *Neurosci. Res*. 6: 264–268.
Errington ML, Bliss TVP, Richter-Levin G, Yenk K, Doyere V, and Laroche S (1995) Stimulation at 1–5 Hz does not produce long-term depression or depotentiation in the hippocampus of the adult rat *in vivo*. *J. Neurophysiol*. 74: 1793–1799.
Esteban JA, Shi SH, Wilson C, Nuriya M, Huganir RL, and Malinow R (2003) PKA phosphorylation of AMPA receptor subunits controls synaptic trafficking underlying plasticity. *Nat. Neurosci*. 6: 136–143.
Etkin A, Alarcon JM, Weisberg SP, et al. (2006) A role in learning for SRF: Deletion in the adult forebrain disrupts LTD and the formation of an immediate memory of a novel context. *Neuron* 50: 127–143.
Feil R, Hartmann J, Luo C, et al. (2003) Impairment of LTD and cerebellar learning by Purkinje cell-specific ablation of cGMP-dependent protein kinase I. *J. Cell Biol*. 163: 295–302.
Fitzjohn SM, Kingston AE, Lodge D, and Collingridge GL (1999) DHPG-induced LTD in area CA1 of juvenile rat hippocampus; characterisation and sensitivity to novel mGlu receptor antagonists. *Neuropharmacology* 38: 1577–1583.
Fredette BJ and Mugnaini E (1991) The GABAergic cerebello-olivary projection in the rat. *Anat. Embryol*. 184: 225–243.
Freeman JH, Shi T, and Schreurs BG (1998) Pairing-specific long-term depression prevented by blockade of PKC or intracellular Ca. *NeuroReport*. 9: 2237–2241.
Fujii S, Saito K, Miyakawa H, Ito K, and Kato H (1991) Reversal of long-term potentiation (depotentiation) induced by tetanus stimulation of the input to CA1 neurons of guinea pig hippocampal slices. *Brain Res*. 555: 112–122.
Fujii S, Sekino Y, Kuroda Y, Sasaki H, Ito K, and Kato H (1997) 8-cyclopentyltheophylline, an adenosine A1 receptor antagonist, inhibits the reversal of long-term potentiation in hippocampal CA1 neurons. *Eur. J. Pharmacol*. 331: 9–14.
Funabiki K, Mishina M, and Hirano T (1995) Retarded vestibular compensation in mutant mice deficient in $\delta 2$ glutamate receptor subunit. *Neuroreport* 7: 189–192.
Gage AT, Reyes M, and Stanton PK (1997) Nitric-oxide-guanylyl-cyclase-dependent and -independent components of multiple forms of long-term synaptic depression. *Hippocampus* 7: 286–295.
Garcia KS and Mauk MD (1998) Pharmacological analysis of cerebellar contributions to the timing and expression of conditioned eyelid responses. *Neuropharmacology* 37: 471–480.
Genoux D, Haditsch U, Knobloch M, Michalon A, Storm D, and Mansuy IM (2002) Protein phosphatase 1 is a molecular constraint on learning and memory. *Nature* 418: 970–975.
Glaum SR, Slater NT, Rossi DJ, and Miller RJ (1992) The role of metabotropic glutamate receptors at the parallel fiber–Purkinje cell synapse. *J. Neurophysiol*. 68: 1453–1462.
Goda Y and Stevens CF (1996) Long-term depression properties in a simple system. *Neuron* 16: 103–111.
Goossens J, Daniel H, Rancillac A, et al. (2001) Expression of protein kinase C inhibitor blocks cerebellar long-term depression without affecting Purkinje cell excitability in alert mice. *J. Neurosci*. 21: 5813–5823.
Hansel C (2005) When the B-team runs plasticity: GluR2 receptor trafficking in cerebellar long-term potentiation. *Proc. Natl. Acad. Sci. USA* 102: 18245–18246.

Hansel C, Artola A, and Singer W (1997) Relation between dendritic Ca2+ levels and the polarity of synaptic long-term modifications in rat visual cortex neurons. *Eur. J. Neurosci.* 9: 2309–2322.

Hansel C, de Jeu M, Belmeguenai A, et al. (2006) αCaMKII is essential for cerebellar LTD and motor learning. *Neuron* 51: 835–843.

Hansel C and Linden DJ (2000) Long-term depression of the cerebellar climbing fiber–Purkinje neuron synapse. *Neuron* 26: 473–482.

Hansel C, Linden DJ, and D'Angelo E (2001) Beyond parallel fiber LTD: The diversity of synaptic and non-synaptic plasticity in the cerebellum. *Nat. Neurosci.* 4: 467–475.

Hardiman MJ, Ramnani N, and Yeo CH (1996) Reversible inactivations of the cerebellum with muscimol prevent the acquisition and extinction of conditioned nictitating membrane responses in the rabbit. *Exp. Brain Res.* 110: 235–247.

Hartell NA (1994) cGMP acts within cerebellar Purkinje cells to produce long-term depression via mechanisms involving PKC and PKG. *NeuroReport* 5: 833–836.

Hartell NA (1996) Strong activation of parallel fibers produces localized calcium transients and a form of LTD which spreads to distant synapses. *Neuron* 16: 601–610.

Hayashi Y, Shi SH, Esteban JA, Piccini A, Poncer JC, and Malinow R (2000) Driving AMPA receptors into synapses by LTP and CaMKII: Requirement for GluR1 and PDZ domain interaction. *Science* 287: 2262–2267.

Hebb DO (1949) *The Organization of Behavior*. New York: Wiley.

Hemart N, Daniel H, Jaillard D, and Crepel F (1995) Receptors and second messengers involved in long-term depression in rat cerebellar slices *in vitro*: A reappraisal. *Eur. J. Neurosci.* 7: 45–53.

Herbert J-M and Maffrand J-P (1991) Effect of pentosan polysulphate, standard heparin and related compounds on protein kinase C activity. *Biochim. Biophys. Acta.* 1091: 432–441.

Hesse GW and Teyler TJ (1976) Reversible loss of hippocampal long term potentiation following electronconvulsive seizures. *Nature* 264: 562–564.

Heynen AJ, Abraham WC, and Bear MF (1996) Bidirectional modification of CA1 synapses in the adult hippocampus *in vivo*. *Nature*. 381: 163–166.

Heynen A, Quinlan EM, Bae D, and Bear MF (2000) Bidirectional, activity-dependent regulation of glutamate receptors in the adult hippocampus *in vivo*. *Nat. Neurosci.* 28: 527–536.

Hirai H, Launey T, Mikawa S, et al. (2003) New role of δ2-glutamate receptors in AMPA receptor trafficking and cerebellar function. *Nat. Neurosci.* 6: 869–876.

Hirano T (1990) Effects of postsynaptic depolarization in the induction of synaptic depression between a granule cell and a Purkinje cell in rat cerebellar culture. *Neurosci. Lett.* 119: 145–147.

Hirano T, Kasono K, Araki K, and Mishina M (1995) Suppression of LTD in cultured Purkinje cells deficient in the glutamate receptor-2 subunit. *NeuroReport* 6: 524–526.

Holland LL and Wagner JJ (1998) Primed facilitation of homosynaptic long-term depression and depotentiation in rat hippocampus. *J. Neurosci.* 18: 887–894.

Hollmann M and Heinemann S (1994) Cloned glutamate receptors. *Annu. Rev. Neurosci.* 17: 31–108.

Holscher C, Anwyl R, and Rowan MJ (1997) Stimulation on the positive phase of hippocampal theta rhythm induces long-term potentiation that can be depotentiated by stimulation on the negative phase in area CA1 *in vivo*. *J. Neurosci.* 17: 6470–6477.

House C and Kemp BE (1987) Protein kinase C contains a pseudosubstrate prototype in its regulatory domain. *Science* 238: 1726–1728.

Hrabetova S and Sacktor TC (1996) Bidirectional regulation of protein kinase ζ in the maintenance of long-term potentiation and long-term depression. *J. Neurosci.* 16: 5324–5333.

Huang CC, Liang YC, and Hsu KS (1999a) A role for extracellular adenosine in time-dependent reversal of long-term potentiation by low-frequency stimulation at hippocampal CA1 synapses. *J. Neurosci.* 19: 9728–9738.

Huang JZ, Kirkwood A, Pizzorusso T, et al. (1999b) BDNF regulates the maturation of inhibition and the critical period of plasticity in mouse visual cortex. *Cell* 98: 739–755.

Huang Y, Man HY, Sekine-Aizawa Y, et al. (2005) S-nitrosylation of N-ethylmaleimide sensitive factor mediates surface expression of AMPA receptors. *Neuron* 46: 533–540.

Huber KM, Mauk MD, Thompson C, and Kelly PT (1995) A critical period of protein kinase activity after tetanic stimulation is required for the induction of long-term potentiation. *Learn. Mem.* 2: 81–100.

Huber KM, Roder JC, and Bear MF (2001) Chemical induction of mGluR5- and protein synthesis-dependent long-term depression in hippocampal area CA1. *J. Neurophysiol.* 86: 321–325.

Huber KM, Sawtell NB, and Bear MF (1998) Effects of the metabotropic glutamate receptor antagonist MCPG on phosphoinositide turnover and synaptic plasticity in visual cortex. *J. Neurosci.* 18: 1–9.

Hummler E, Cole TJ, Blendy JA, et al. (1994) Targeted mutation of the CREB gene: Compensation within the CREB/ATF family of transcription factors. *Proc. Natl. Acad. Sci. USA* 91: 5647–5651.

Ichise T, Kano M, Hashimoto K, et al. (2000) mGluR1 in cerebellar Purkinje cells essential for long-term depression, synapse elimination, and motor coordination. *Science*. 288: 1832–1835.

Ikeda M, Morita I, Murota S, Sekiguchi F, Yuasa T, and Miyatake T (1993) Cerebellar nitric oxide synthase activity is reduced in nervous and Purkinje cell degeneration mutants but not in climbing fiber–lesioned mice. *Neurosci. Lett.* 155: 148–150.

Inoue T, Kato K, Kohda K, and Mikoshiba K (1998) Type 1 inositol 1,4,5-trisphosphate receptor is required for induction of long-term depression in cerebellar Purkinje neurons. *J. Neurosci.* 15: 5366–5373.

Ito M (1984) *The Cerebellum and Neural Control*. New York: Raven Press.

Ito M (1990) Long-term depression in the cerebellum. *Semin. Neurosci.* 2: 381–390.

Ito M (2001) Cerebellar long-term depression: Characterization, signal transduction, and functional roles. *Physiol. Rev.* 81: 1143–1194.

Ito M (2002) The molecular organization of cerebellar long-term depression. *Nat. Rev. Neurosci.* 3: 896–902.

Ito M, Sakurai M, and Tongroach P (1982) Climbing fibre induced depression of both mossy fiber responsiveness and glutamate sensitivity of cerebellar Purkinje cells. *J. Physiol.* 324: 113–134.

Izumi Y and Zorumski CF (1993) Nitric oxide and long-term synaptic depression in the rat hippocampus. *NeuroReport* 4: 1131–1134.

Jeromin A, Huganir R, and Linden DJ (1996) Suppression of the glutamate receptor δ2 subunit produces a specific impairment in cerebellar long-term depression. *J. Neurophysiol.* 76: 3578–3583.

Kakegawa W and Yuzaki M (2005) Novel mechanism underlying AMPA receptor trafficking during cerebellar long-term potentiation. *Proc. Natl. Acad. Sci. USA* 102: 17846–17851.

Kamal A, Biessels GJ, Gispen WH, and Urban IJ (1998) Increasing age reduces expression of long-term depression and dynamic range of transmission plasticity in CA1 field of the rat hippocampus. *Neuroscience* 83: 707–715.

Kamal A, Ramakers GM, Urban IJ, De Graan P, and Gispen WH (1999) Chemical LTD in the CA1 field of the hippocampus from young and mature rats. *Eur. J. Neurosci.* 11: 3512–3516.

Kameyama K, Lee HK, Bear MF, and Huganir RL (1998) Involvement of a postsynaptic protein kinase A substrate in the expression of homosynaptic long-term depression. *Neuron* 21: 1163–1175.

Kandler K, Katz LC, and Kauer JA (1998) Focal photolysis of caged glutamate produces long-term depression of hippocampal glutamate receptors. *Nature Neurosci.* 1: 119–123.

Kano M, Hashimoto K, Chen C, et al. (1995) Impaired synapse elimination during cerebellar development in PKC-mutant mice. *Cell* 83: 1223–1231.

Kano M, Hashimoto K, Kurihara H, et al. (1997) Persistent multiple climbing fiber innervation of cerebellar Purkinje cells in mice lacking mGluR1. *Neuron* 18: 71–79.

Kano M and Kato M (1987) Quisqualate receptors are specifically involved in cerebellar synaptic plasticity. *Nature* 325: 276–279.

Kashiwabuchi N, Ikeda K, Araki K, et al. (1995) Impairment of motor coordination, Purkinje cell synapse formation, and cerebellar long-term depression in GluRδ2 mutant mice. *Cell* 81: 245–252.

Kasono K and Hirano T (1995) Involvement of inositol trisphosphate in cerebellar long-term depression. *NeuroReport* 6: 569–572.

Katsuki H, Izumi Y, and Zorumski CF (1997) Noradrenergic regulation of synaptic plasticity in the hippocampal CA1 region. *J. Neurophysiol.* 77: 3013–3020.

Kelso SR, Ganong AH, and Brown T (1986) Hebbian synapses in the hippocampus. *Proc. Natl. Acad. Sci. USA* 83: 5326–5330.

Kemp N and Bashir ZI (1997a) NMDA receptor-dependent and -independent long-term depression in the CA1 region of the adult rat hippocampus *in vitro*. *Neuropharmacology* 36: 397–399.

Kemp N and Bashir ZI (1997b) A role for adenosine in the regulation of long-term depression in the adult rat hippocampus *in vitro*. *Neurosci. Lett.* 225: 189–192.

Khodakhah K and Armstrong CM (1997) Induction of long-term depression and rebound potentiation by inositol triphosphate in cerebellar Purkinje neurons. *Proc. Natl. Acad. Sci. USA* 94: 14009–14014.

Khodakhah K and Ogden D (1993) Functional heterogeneity of calcium release by inositol trisphosphate in single Purkinje neurones, cultured cerebellar astrocytes, and peripheral tissues. *Proc. Natl. Acad. Sci. USA* 90: 4976–4980.

Kim JJ, Foy MR, and Thompson RF (1994) Behavioral stress enhances LTD in rat hippocampus. *Soc. Neurosci. Abstr.* 20: 1769.

Kim JJ and Thompson RF (1997) Cerebellar circuits and synaptic mechanisms involved in classical eyeblink conditioning. *Trends Neurosci.* 20: 177–181.

Kimura T, Sugimori M, and Llinas RR (2005) Purkinje cell long-term depression is prevented by T-588, a neuroprotective compound that reduces cytosolic calcium release from internal stores. *Proc. Natl. Acad. Sci. USA* 102: 17160–17165.

Kirkwood A and Bear MF (1994) Homosynaptic long-term depression in the visual cortex. *J. Neurosci.* 14: 3404–3412.

Kirkwood A, Dudek SM, Gold JT, Aizenman CD, and Bear MF (1993) Common forms of synaptic plasticity in the hippocampus and neocortex *in vitro*. *Science* 260: 1518–1521.

Kirkwood A, Rioult MG, and Bear MF (1996) Experience-dependent modification of synaptic plasticity in visual cortex. *Nature* 381: 526–528.

Kirkwood A, Rozas C, Kirkwood J, Perez F, and Bear MF (1999) Modulation of long-term synaptic depression in visual cortex by acetylcholine and norepinephrine. *J. Neurosci.* 19: 1599–1609.

Knopfel T, Vranesic I, Staub C, and Gahwiler BH (1990) Climbing fibre responses in olive-cerebellar slice cultures. II. Dynamics of cytosolic calcium in Purkinje cells. *Eur. J. Neurosci.* 3: 343–348.

Kobayashi K, Manabe T, and Takahashi T (1996) Presynaptic long-term depression at the hippocampal mossy fiber–CA3 synapse. *Science* 273: 648–650.

Koekkoek SKE, Hulscher HC, Dortland BR, et al. (2003) Cerebellar LTD and learning-dependent timing of conditioned eyelid responses. *Science* 301: 1736–1739.

Koester HJ and Sakmann B (1998) Calcium dynamics in single spines during coincident pre- and postsynaptic activity depend on relative timing of back-propagating action potentials and subthreshold excitatory postsynaptic potentials. *Proc. Natl. Acad. Sci. USA* 95: 9596–9601.

Kohda K, Inoue T, and Mikoshiba K (1995) Ca release from Ca stores, particularly from ryanodine-sensitive Ca stores, is required for the induction of LTD in cultured cerebellar Purkinje cells. *J. Neurophysiol.* 74: 2184–2188.

Konnerth A, Dreessen J, and Augustine GJ (1992) Brief dendritic calcium signals initiate long-lasting synaptic depression in cerebellar Purkinje cells. *Proc. Natl. Acad. Sci. USA* 89: 7051–7055.

Krupa DJ and Thompson RF (1995) Inactivation of the superior cerebellar peduncle blocks expression but not acquisition of the rabbit's classically conditioned eye-blink response. *Proc. Natl. Acad. Sci. USA* 92: 5097–5101.

Krupa DJ and Thompson RF (1997) Reversible inactivation of the cerebellar interpositus nucleus completely prevents acquisition of the classically conditioned eye-blink response. *Learn. Mem.* 3: 545–556.

Krupa DJ, Thompson JK, and Thompson RF (1993) Localization of a memory trace in the mammalian brain. *Science* 260: 989–991.

Kumoi K, Saito N, Kuno T, and Tanaka C (1988) Immunohistochemical localization of gamma-amino butyric acid- and aspartate-containing neurons in the rat deep cerebellar nuclei. *Brain Res.* 439: 302–310.

Kurihara H, Hashimoto K, Kano M, et al. (1997) Impaired parallel fiber–Purkinje cell synapse stabilization during cerebellar development of mutant mice lacking the glutamate receptor delta2 subunit. *J. Neurosci.* 17: 9613–9623.

Kushner SA, Elgersma Y, Murphy GG, et al. (2005) Modulation of presynaptic plasticity and learning by the H-ras/extracellular signal-regulated kinase/synapsin I signaling pathway. *J. Neurosci.* 25: 9721–9734.

Larson J, Xiao P, and Lynch G (1993) Reversal of LTP by theta frequency stimulation. *Brain Res.* 600: 97–102.

Lavond DG and Steinmetz JE (1989) Acquisition of classical conditioning without cerebellar cortex. *Behav. Brain Res.* 33: 113–164.

Lee H-K, Barbarosie M, Kameyama K, Bear MF, and Huganir RL (2000) Regulation of distinct AMPA receptor phosphorylation sites during bidirectional synaptic plasticity. *Nature* 405: 955–959.

Lee HK, Kameyama K, Huganir RL, and Bear MF (1998) NMDA induces long-term synaptic depression and dephosphorylation of the GluR1 subunit of AMPA receptors in hippocampus. *Neuron* 21: 1151–1162.

Lee HK, Takamiya K, Han JS, et al. (2003) Phosphorylation of the AMPA receptor GluR1 subunit is required for synaptic plasticity and retention of spatial memory. *Cell* 112: 631–643.

Leitges M, Kovac J, Plomann M, and Linden DJ (2004) A unique PDZ ligand in PKCα confers induction of cerebellar long-term synaptic depression. *Neuron* 44: 585–594.

Lev-Ram V, Jiang T, Wood J, Lawrence DS, and Tsien RY (1997a) Synergies and coincidence requirements between NO, cGMP, and Ca in the induction of cerebellar long-term depression. *Neuron* 18: 1025–1038.

Lev-Ram V, Makings LR, Keitz PF, Kao JPY, and Tsien RY (1995) Long-term depression in cerebellar Purkinje neurons results from coincidence of nitric oxide and depolarization-induced Ca transients. *Neuron* 15: 407–415.
Lev-Ram V, Nebyelul Z, Ellisman MH, Huang PL, and Tsien RY (1997b) Absence of cerebellar long-term depression in mice lacking neuronal nitric oxide synthase. *Learn. Mem.* 4: 169–177.
Lev-Ram V, Wong ST, Storm DR, and Tsien RY (2002) A new form of cerebellar long-term potentiation is postsynaptic and depends on nitric oxide but not cAMP. *Proc. Natl. Acad. Sci. USA* 99: 8389–8393.
Li H, Weiss SR, Chuang DM, Post RM, and Rogawski MA (1998) Bidirectional synaptic plasticity in the rat basolateral amygdala: Characterization of an activity-dependent switch sensitive to the presynaptic metabotropic glutamate receptor antagonist 2S-alpha-ethylglutamic acid. *J. Neurosci.* 18: 1662–1670.
Linden DJ (1994) Input-specific induction of cerebellar long-term depression does not require presynaptic alteration. *Learn. Mem.* 1: 121–128.
Linden DJ (1997) Long-term potentiation of glial synaptic currents in cerebellar culture. *Neuron* 18: 983–994.
Linden DJ (1999) The return of the spike: Postsynaptic action potentials and the induction of LTP and LTD. *Neuron* 22: 661–666.
Linden DJ (2001) The expression of cerebellar LTD in culture is not associated with changes in AMPA-receptor kinetics, agonist affinity, or unitary conductance. *Proc. Natl. Acad. Sci. USA* 98: 14066–14071.
Linden DJ and Ahn S (1999) Activation of presynaptic cAMP-dependent protein kinase is required for induction of cerebellar long-term potentiation. *J. Neurosci.* 19: 10221–10227.
Linden DJ and Connor JA (1991) Participation of postsynaptic PKC in cerebellar long-term depression in culture. *Science* 254: 1656–1659.
Linden DJ and Connor JA (1992) Long-term depression of glutamate currents in cultured cerebellar Purkinje neurons does not require nitric oxide signalling. *Eur. J. Neurosci.* 4: 10–15.
Linden DJ, Dawson TM, and Dawson VL (1995) An evaluation of the nitric oxide/cGMP/cGMP-dependent protein kinase cascade in the induction of cerebellar long-term depression in culture. *J. Neurosci.* 15: 5098–5105.
Linden DJ, Dickinson MH, Smeyne M, and Connor JA (1991) A long-term depression of AMPA currents in cultured cerebellar Purkinje neurons. *Neuron* 7: 81–89.
Linden DJ, Smeyne M, and Connor JA (1993) Induction of cerebellar long-term depression in culture requires postsynaptic action of sodium ions. *Neuron* 11: 1093–1100.
Ling DSF, Benardo LS, and Sacktor TC (2006) Protein kinase Mζ enhances excitatory synaptic transmission by increasing the number of active postsynaptic AMPA receptors. *Hippocampus* 16: 443–452.
Lisman J (1989) A mechanism for the Hebb and the anti-Hebb processes underlying learning and memory. *Proc. Natl. Acad. Sci. USA* 86: 9574–9578.
Lisman J and Zhabotinsky AM (2001) A model of synaptic memory: A CaMKII/PP1 switch that potentiates transmission by organizing an AMPA receptor anchoring assembly. *Neuron* 31: 191–201.
Lledo PM, Hjelmstad GO, Mukherji S, Soderling TR, Malenka RC, and Nicoll RA (1995) Calcium/calmodulin-dependent kinase II and long-term potentiation enhance synaptic transmission by the same mechanism. *Proc. Natl. Acad. Sci. USA* 92: 11175–11179.
Lonart G, Schoch S, Kaeser PS, Larkin J, Südhof TC, and Linden DJ (2003) Phosphorylation of RIM1α by PKA triggers presynaptic long-term potentiation at cerebellar parallel fiber synapses. *Cell* 115: 49–60.
Lovinger DM, Tyler EC, and Merritt A (1993) Short- and long-term synaptic depression in rat neostriatum. *J. Neurophysiol.* 70: 1937–1949.
Lüscher C, Xia H, Beattie EC, et al. (1999) Role of AMPA receptor cycling in synaptic transmission and plasticity. *Neuron* 24: 649–658.
Luthi A, Chittajallu R, Duprat F, et al. (1999) Hippocampal LTD expression involves a pool of AMPARs regulated by the NSF-GluR2 Interaction. *Neuron* 24: 389–399.
Malenka R, Kauer J, Perkel D, et al. (1989) An essential role for postsynaptic calmodulin and protein kinase activity in long-term potentiation. *Nature* 340: 554–557.
Malinow R (2003) AMPA receptor trafficking and long-term potentiation. *Philos. Trans. R. Soc. Lond. B Biol. Sci.* 358: 707–714.
Malinow R and Miller JP (1986) Postsynaptic hyperpolarization during conditioning reversibly blocks induction of long-term potentiation. *Nature* 320: 529–530.
Malinow R, Schulman H, and Tsien RW (1989) Inhibition of postsynaptic PKC or CaMKII blocks induction but not expression of LTP. *Nature* 245: 862–865.
Malleret G, Haditsch U, Genoux D, et al. (2001) Inducible and reversible enhancement of learning, memory, and long-term potentiation by genetic inhibition of calcineurin. *Cell* 104: 675–686.
Mammen AL, Kameyama K, Roche KW, and Huganir RL (1997) Phosphorylation of the alpha-amino-3-hydroxy-5-methylisoxazole4-propionic acid receptor GluR1 subunit by calcium/calmodulin-dependent kinase II. *J. Biol. Chem.* 272: 32528–32533.
Man YH, Lin YW, Ju WH, et al. (2000) Regulation of AMPA receptor-mediated synaptic transmission by clathrin-dependent receptor internalization. *Neuron* 25: 649–662.
Manahan-Vaughan D (1997) Group 1 and 2 metabotropic glutamate receptors play differential roles in hippocampal long-term depression and long-term potentiation in freely moving rats. *J. Neurosci.* 17: 3303–3311.
Manahan-Vaughan D (1998) Priming of group 2 metabotropic glutamate receptors facilitates induction of long-term depression in the dentate gyrus of freely moving rats. *Neuropharmacology* 37: 1459–1464.
Manahan-Vaughan D and Braunewell KH (1999) Novelty acquisition is associated with induction of hippocampal long-term depression. *Proc. Natl. Acad. Sci. USA* 96: 8739–8744.
Margrie TW, Brecht M, and Sakmann B (2002) *In vivo*, low-resistance, whole-cell recordings from neurons in the anaesthetized and awake mammalian brain. *Pflugers Arch.* 444: 491–498.
Markram H, Lubke J, Frotscher M, and Sakmann B (1997) Regulation of synaptic efficacy by coincidence of postsynaptic APs and EPSPs. *Science* 275: 213–215.
Marr D (1969) A theory of cerebellar cortex. *J. Physiol.* 202: 437–470.
Martin LJ, Blackstone CD, Huganir RL, and Price DL (1992) Cellular localization of a metabotropic glutamate receptor in rat brain. *Neuron* 9: 259–270.
Marty A and Llano I (1995) Modulation of inhibitory synapses in the mammalian brain. *Curr. Opin. Neurobiol.* 5: 335–341.
Mauk MD (1997) Roles of cerebellar cortex and nuclei in motor learning: Contradictions or clues? *Neuron* 18: 343–346.
Mauk MD and Donegan NH (1997) A model of Pavlovian eyelid conditioning based on the synaptic organization of the cerebellum. *Learn. Mem.* 3: 130–158.
Mauk MD, Steinmetz JE, and Thompson RF (1986) Classical conditioning using stimulation of the inferior olive as the unconditioned stimulus. *Proc. Natl. Acad. Sci. USA* 83: 5349–5353.
Mayford M, Wang J, Kandel E, and O'Dell T (1995) CaMKII regulates the frequency-response function of hippocampal

synapses for the production of both LTD and LTP. *Cell* 81: 1–20.
McCormack SG, Stornetta RL, and Zhu JJ (2006) Synaptic AMPA receptor exchange maintains bidirectional plasticity. *Neuron* 50: 75–88.
McCormick DA, Clark GA, Lavond DG, and Thompson RF (1982) Initial localization of the memory trace for a basic form of learning. *Proc. Natl. Acad. Sci. USA* 79: 2731–2735.
McCormick DA and Thompson RF (1984a) Cerebellum: Essential involvement in the classically conditioned eyelid response. *Science* 223: 296–299.
McCormick DA and Thompson RF (1984b) Neuronal responses of the rabbit cerebellum during acquisition and performance of a classically conditioned nictitating membrane-eyelid response. *J. Neurosci.* 4: 2811–2822.
Medina JF and Mauk MD (1999) Simulations of cerebellar motor learning: Computational analysis of plasticity at the mossy fiber to deep nucleus synapse. *J. Neurosci.* 19: 7140–7151.
Medina JF, Repa JC, Mauk MD, and LeDoux JE (2002) Parallels between cerebellum- and amygdala-dependent conditioning. *Nat. Rev. Neurosci.* 3: 122–131.
Merlin LR, Bergold PJ, and Wong RKS (1998) Requirement of protein synthesis for group 1 mGluR-mediated induction of eplileptiform discharges. *J. Neurophys.* 80: 989–993.
Migaud M, Charlesworth P, Dempster M, et al. (1998) Enhanced long-term potentiation and impaired learning in mice with mutant postsynaptic density-95 protein. *Nature* 396: 433–439.
Miyata M, Okada D, Hashimoto K, Kano M, and Ito M (1999) Corticotropin-releasing factor plays a permissive role in cerebellar long-term depression. *Neuron* 22: 763–775.
Monsivais P, Clark BA, Roth A, and Häusser M (2005) Determinants of action potential propagation in cerebellar Purkinje cell axons. *J. Neurosci.* 25: 464–472.
Morishita W, Connor JH, Xia H, Qinlan EM, Shenolikar S, and Malenka RC (2001) Regulation of synaptic strength by protein phosphatase 1. *Neuron* 32: 1133–1148.
Moult PR, Gladding CM, Sanderson TM, et al. (2006) Tyrosine phosphatases regulate AMPA receptor trafficking during metabotropic glutamate receptor-mediated long-term depression. *J. Neurosci.* 26: 2544–2554.
Mulkey RM, Endo S, Shenolikar S, and Malenka RC (1994) Calcineurin and inhibitor-1 are components of a protein-phosphatase cascade mediating hippocampal LTD. *Nature* 369: 486–488.
Mulkey RM, Herron CE, and Malenka RC (1993) An essential role for protein phosphatases in hippocampal long-term depression. *Science* 261: 1051–1055.
Mulkey RM and Malenka RC (1992) Mechanisms underlying induction of homosynaptic long-term depression in area CA1 of the hippocampus. *Neuron* 9: 967–975.
Mutoh H, Yuan Q, and Knöpfel T (2005) Long-term depression at olfactory nerve synapses. *J. Neurosci.* 25: 4252–4259.
Nairn AC and Shenolikar S (1992) The role of protein phosphatases in synaptic transmission, plasticity and neuronal development. *Curr. Opin. Neurobiol.* 2: 296–301.
Nakanishi S, Maeda N, and Mikoshiba K (1991) Immunohistochemical localization of an inositol 1,4,5-trisphosphate receptor, P400, in neural tissue: Studies in developing and adult mouse brain. *J. Neurosci.* 11: 2075–2086.
Narasimhan K and Linden DJ (1996) Defining a minimal computational unit for cerebellar long-term depression. *Neuron* 17: 333–341.
Narasimhan K, Pessah IN, and Linden DJ (1998) Inositol-1,4,5-trisphosphate receptor-mediated Ca mobilization is not required for the induction of cerebellar long-term depression in reduced preparations. *J. Neurophysiol.* 80: 2963–2974.
Neveu D and Zucker RS (1996) Postsynaptic levels of $[Ca^{2+}]i$ needed to trigger LTD and LTP. *Neuron* 16: 619–629.
Nicoll RA, Tomita S, and Bredt DS (2006) Auxiliary subunits assist AMPA-type glutamate receptors. *Science* 311: 1253–1256.
Nishimune A, Isaac JT, Molnar E, et al. (1998) NSF binding to GluR2 regulates synaptic transmission. *Neuron* 21: 87–97.
Noel J, Ralph GS, Pickard L, et al. (1999) Surface expression of AMPA receptors in hippocampal neurons is regulated by an NSF-dependent mechanism. *Neuron* 23: 365–376.
Nosyreva ED and Huber KM (2005) Developmental switch in synaptic mechanisms of hippocampal metabotropic glutamate receptor-dependent long-term depression. *J. Neurosci.* 25: 2992–3001.
Nouranifar R, Blitzer RD, Wong T, and Landau E (1998) Metabotropic glutamate receptors limit adenylyl cyclase-mediated effects in rat hippocampus via protein kinase C. *Neurosci. Lett.* 244: 101–105.
Oberdick J, Smeyne RJ, Mann JR, Zackson S, and Morgan JI (1990) A promoter that drives transgene expression in cerebellar Purkinje and retinal bipolar neurons. *Science* 248: 223–226.
O'Dell TJ and Kandel ER (1994) Low-frequency stimulation erases LTP through an NMDA receptor-mediated activation of protein phosphatases. *Learn. Mem.* 1: 129–139.
Oliet SH, Malenka RC, and Nicoll RA (1996) Bidirectional control of quantal size by synaptic activity in the hippocampus. *Science* 271: 1294–1297.
Oliet SH, Malenka RC, and Nicoll RA (1997) Two distinct forms of long-term depression coexist in CA1 hippocampal pyramidal cells. *Neuron* 18: 969–982.
Osten P, Srivastava S, Inman GJ, et al. (1998) The AMPA receptor GluR2 C terminus can mediate a reversible, ATP-dependent interaction with NSF and alpha- and beta-SNAPs. *Neuron* 21: 99–110.
Otani S and Connor JA (1998) Requirement of rapid Ca entry and synaptic activation of metabotropic glutamate receptors for the induction of long-term depression in adult rat hippocampus. *J. Physiol. (Lond)* 511: 761–770.
Perrett S and Mauk M (1995) Extinction of conditioned eyelid response requires the anterior lobe of the cerebellar cortex. *J. Neurosci.* 15: 2074–2080.
Perrett S, Ruiz B, and Mauk M (1993) Cerebellar cortex lesions disrupt learning-dependent timing of conditioned eyelid responses. *J. Neurosci.* 13: 1708–1718.
Pettit DL, Perlman S, and Malinow R (1994) Potentiated transmission and prevention of further LTP by increased CaMKII activity in postsynaptic hippocampal slice neurons. *Science* 266: 1881–1885.
Pin JP and Bockaert J (1995) Get receptive to metabotropic glutamate receptors. *Curr. Opin. Neurobiol.* 5: 342–349.
Pugh JR and Raman IM (2006) Potentiation of mossy fiber EPSCs in the cerebellar nuclei by NMDA receptor activation followed by postinhibitory rebound current. *Neuron* 51: 113–123.
Qi M, Zhuo M, Skalhegg BS, et al. (1996) Impaired hippocampal plasticity in mice lacking the Cbeta1 catalytic subunit of cAMP-dependent protein kinase. *Proc. Natl. Acad. Sci. USA* 93: 1571–1576.
Quinlan EM, Olstein DH, and Bear MF (1999) Bidirectional, experience-dependent regulation of NMDA subunit composition in rat visual cortex during postnatal development. *Proc. Natl. Acad. Sci. USA* 96: 12876–12880.
Ramakers GM, McNamara RK, Lenox RH, and De GP (1999) Differential changes in the phosphorylation of the protein kinase C substrates myristoylated alanine-rich C kinase substrate and growth- associated protein-43/B-50 following Schaffer collateral long-term potentiation and long-term depression. *J. Neurochem.* 73: 2175–2183.

Ramnani N and Yeo CH (1996) Reversible inactivations of the cerebellum prevent the extinction of conditioned nictitating membrane responses in rabbits. *J. Physiol*. 495: 159–168.

Raymond CR, Thompson VL, Tate WP, and Abraham WC (2000) Metabotropic glutamate receptors trigger homosynaptic protein synthesis to prolong long-term potentiation. *J. Neurosci*. 20(3): 969–976.

Raymond JL, Lisberger SG, and Mauk MD (1996) The cerebellum: A neuronal learning machine? *Science* 272: 1126–1131.

Reyes HM, Potter BV, Galione A, and Stanton PK (1999) Induction of hippocampal LTD requires nitric-oxide-stimulated PKG activity and Ca release from cyclic ADP-ribose-sensitive stores. *J. Neurophysiol*. 82: 1569–1576.

Reyes M and Stanton PK (1996) Induction of hippocampal long-term depression requires release of Ca from separate pre-synaptic and postsynaptic intracellular stores. *J. Neurosci*. 16: 5951–5960.

Reyes HM and Stanton PK (1998) Postsynaptic phospholipase C activity is required for the induction of homosynaptic long-term depression in rat hippocampus. *Neurosci. Lett*. 252: 155–158.

Riedel G, Micheau J, Lam AG, et al. (1999) Reversible neural inactivation reveals hippocampal participation in several memory processes. *Nat. Neurosci*. 2: 898–905.

Rittenhouse CD, Shouval HZ, Paradiso MA, and Bear MF (1999) Monocular deprivation induces homosynaptic long-term depression in visual cortex. *Nature* 397: 347–350.

Roche KW, O'Brien RJ, Mammen AL, Bernhardt J, and Huganir RL (1996) Characterization of multiple phosphorylation sites on the AMPA receptor GluR1 subunit. *Neuron* 16: 1179–1188.

Rosenmund C, Legendre P, and Westbrook GL (1992) Expression of NMDA channels on cerebellar Purkinje cells acutely dissociated from newborn rats. *J. Neurophysiol*. 68: 1901–1905.

Ross WN and Werman R (1987) Mapping calcium transients in the dendrites of Purkinje cells from the guinea-pig cerebellum *in vitro*. *J. Physiol*. 389: 319–336.

Sakurai M (1990) Calcium is an intracellular mediator of the climbing fiber in induction of cerebellar long-term depression. *Proc. Natl. Acad. Sci. USA* 87: 3383–3385.

Salin PA, Malenka RC, and Nicoll RA (1996) Cyclic AMP mediates a presynaptic form of LTP at cerebellar parallel fiber synapses. *Neuron* 16: 797–806.

Sastry RB, Goh JW, and Auyeung A (1986) Associative induction of posttetanic and long-term potentiation in CA1 neurons of rat hippocampus. *Science* 232: 988.

Sawtell NB, Huber KM, Roder JC, and Bear MF (1999) Induction of NMDA receptor-dependent long-term depression in visual cortex does not require metabotropic glutamate receptors. *J. Neurophysiol*. 82: 3594–3597.

Schmahmann JD (1997) *International Review of Neurobiology, Vol. 41: The Cerebellum and Cognition*. San Diego, CA: Academic Press.

Schmolesky MT, De Ruiter MM, De Zeeuw CI, and Hausel C (2007) The neuropeptide corticotropin-releasing factor regulates excitatory transmission and plasticity at the climbing fibre-Purkinje cell synapse. *Eur. J. Neurosci*. 25: 1460–1466.

Schmolesky MT, De Zeeuw CI, and Hansel C (2005) Climbing fiber synaptic plasticity and modifications in Purkinje cell excitability. *Prog. Brain Res*. 148: 81–94.

Schmolesky MT, Weber JT, De Zeeuw CI, and Hansel C (2002) The making of a complex spike: Ionic composition and plasticity. *Ann. N.Y. Acad. Sci*. 978: 359–390.

Schreurs BG and Alkon DL (1993) Rabbit cerebellar slice analysis of long-term depression and its role in classical conditioning. *Brain Res*. 631: 235–240.

Schreurs BG, Oh MM, and Alkon DL (1996) Pairing-specific long-term depression of Purkinje cell excitatory postsynaptic potentials results from a classical conditioning procedure in the rabbit cerebellar slice. *J. Neurophysiol*. 75: 1051–1060.

Seeburg PH (1993) The TINS/TiPS Lecture. The molecular biology of mammalian glutamate receptor channels. *Trends Neurosci*. 16: 359–365.

Seidenman KJ, Steinberg JP, Huganir RL, and Malinow R (2003) Glutamate receptor subunit 2 serine 880 phosphorylation modulates synaptic transmission and mediates plasticity in CA1 pyramidal cells. *J. Neurosci*. 23: 9220–9228.

Selig DK, Hjelmstad GO, Herron C, Nicoll RA, and Malenka RC (1995a) Independent mechanisms for long-term depression of AMPA and NMDA responses. *Neuron* 15: 417–426.

Selig DK, Lee H-K, Bear MF, and Malenka RC (1995b) Reexamination of the effects of MCPG on hippocampal LTP, LTD, and depotentiation. *J. Neurophys*. 74: 1075–1082.

Shen Y, Hansel C, and Linden DJ (2002) Glutamate release during LTD at cerebellar climbing fiber–Purkinje cell synapses. *Nat. Neurosci*. 5, 725–726.

Shibuki K, Gomi H, Chen L, et al. (1996) Deficient cerebellar long-term depression, impaired eyeblink conditioning and normal motor coordination in GFAP mutant mice. *Neuron* 16: 587–599.

Shibuki K and Okada D (1991) Endogenous nitric oxide release required for long-term synaptic depression in the cerebellum. *Nature* 349: 326–328.

Shibuki K and Okada D (1992) Cerebellar long-term potentiation under suppressed postsynaptic Ca activity. *NeuroReport* 3: 231–234.

Shigemoto R, Nakanishi S, and Hirano T (1994) Antibodies inactivating mGluR1 metabotropic glutamate receptor block long-term depression in cultured Purkinje cells. *Neuron* 12: 1245–1255.

Shin JH and Linden DJ (2005) An NMDA receptor/nitric oxide cascade is involved in cerebellar LTD but is not localized to the parallel fiber terminal. *J. Neurophysiol* 94: 4281–4289.

Singer W (1995) Development and plasticity of cortical processing architectures. *Science* 270: 758–764.

Silva AJ (2003) Molecular and cellular cognitive studies of the role of synaptic plasticity in memory. *J. Neurobiol*. 54: 224–237.

Silva AJ, Stevens CF, Tonegawa S, and Wang Y (1992) Deficient hippocampal long-term potentiation in alpha-calcium/calmodulin kinase II mutant mice. *Science* 257: 201–206.

Song I and Huganir RL (2002) Regulation of AMPA receptors during synaptic plasticity. *Trends Neurosci*. 25, 578–588.

Song I, Kamboj S, Xia J, Dong H, Liao D, and Huganir RL (1998) Interaction of the N-ethylmaleimide-sensitive factor with AMPA receptors. *Neuron* 21: 393–400.

Stanton PK (1995) Transient protein kinase C activation primes long-term depression and suppresses long-term potentiation of synaptic transmission in hippocampus. *Proc. Natl. Acad. Sci. USA* 92: 1724–1728.

Staubli U and Chun D (1996) Proactive and retrograde effects on LTP produced by theta pulse stimulation: Mechanisms and characteristics of LTP reversal *in vitro*. *Learn. Mem*. 3: 96–105.

Staubli U and Lynch G (1990) Stable depression of potentiated synaptic responses in the hippocampus with 1–5 Hz stimulation. *Brain Res*. 513: 113–118.

Staubli U and Scafidi J (1997) Studies on long-term depression in area CA1 of the anesthetized and freely moving rat. *J. Neurosci*. 17: 4820–4828.

Steele PM and Mauk MD (1999) Inhibitory control of LTP and LTD: Stability of synapse strength. *J. Neurophysiol*. 81: 1559–1566.

Steinberg JP, Takamiya K, Shen Y, et al. (2006) Targeted *in vivo* mutations of the AMPA receptor subunit GluR2 and its interacting protein PICK1 eliminate cerebellar long-term depression. *Neuron* 49: 845–860.

Steinmetz JE, Lavond DG, Ivkovich D, Logan CG, and Thompson RF (1992) Disruption of classical eyelid conditioning after cerebellar lesions: Damage to a memory trace system or a simple performance deficit? *J. Neurosci.* 12: 4403–4426.

Steinmetz JE, Lavond DG, and Thompson RF (1989) Classical conditioning in rabbits using pontine nucleus stimulation as a conditioned stimulus and inferior olive stimulation as an unconditioned stimulus. *Synapse* 3: 225–233.

Steinmetz JE, Rosen DJ, Chapman PF, Lavond DG, and Thompson RF (1986) Classical conditioning of the rabbit eyelid response with a mossy-fiber stimulation CS: I. Pontine nuclei and middle cerebellar peduncle stimulation. *Behav. Neurosci.* 100: 878–887.

Stevens CF and Wang Y (1994) Changes in reliability of synaptic function as a mechanism for plasticity. *Nature* 371: 704–707.

Steward O, Davis L, Dotti C, Phillips LL, Rao A, and Banker G (1988) Protein synthesis and processing in cytoplasmic microdomains beneath postsynaptic sites on CNS neurons. A mechanism for establishing and maintaining a mosaic postsynaptic receptive surface. *Mol. Neurobiol.* 2: 227–261.

Storm DR, Hansel C, Hacker B, Parent A, and Linden DJ (1998) Impaired cerebellar long-term potentiation in type I adenylyl cyclase mutant mice. *Neuron* 20: 1199–1210.

Strata P and Rossi F (1998) Plasticity of the olivocerebellar pathway. *Trends Neurosci.* 21: 407–413.

Stuart G and Häusser M (1994) Initiation and spread of sodium action potentials in cerebellar Purkinje cells. *Neuron* 13: 703–712.

Tang YP, Shimizu E, Dube GR, et al. (1999) Genetic enhancement of learning and memory in mice. *Nature* 401: 63–69.

Tempia F, Kano M, Schneggenburger R, et al. (1996) Fractional calcium current through neuronal AMPA-receptor channels with a low calcium permeability. *J. Neurosci.* 16: 456–466.

Teune TM, van der Burg J, De Zeeuw CI, Voogd J, and Ruigrok TJH (1998) Single Purkinje cells can innervate multiple classes of projection neurons in the cerebellar nuclei of the rat: A light microscopic and ultrastructural triple-tracer study in the rat. *J. Comp. Neurol.* 392: 164–178.

Thiels E, Barrionuevo G, and Berger TW (1994) Excitatory stimulation during postsynaptic inhibition induces long-term depression in hippocampus *in vivo*. *J. Neurophysiol.* 71: 3009–3016.

Thiels E, Norman ED, Barrionuevo G, and Klann E (1998) Transient and persistent increases in protein phosphtase activity during long-term depression in the adult hippocampus *in vivo*. *Neuroscience* 86: 1023–1029.

Thomas MJ, Moody TD, Makhinson M, and O'Dell TJ (1996) Activity-dependent beta-adrenergic modulation of low frequency stimulation induced LTP in the hippocampal CA1 region. *Neuron* 17: 475–482.

Tsumoto T (1993) Long-term depression in cerebral cortex: A possible substrate of "forgetting" that should not be forgotten. *Neurosci. Res.* 16: 263–270.

Vincent SR and Kimura H (1992) Histochemical mapping of nitric oxide synthase in the rat brain. *Neuroscience* 46: 755–784.

Volk LJ, Daly CA, and Huber KM (2006) Differential roles for group I mGluR subtypes in induction and expression of chemically induced hippocampal long-term depression. *J. Neurophysiol.* 95: 2427–2438.

Wagner JJ and Alger BE (1995a) GABAergic and developmental influences on homosynaptic LTD and depotentiation in rat hippocampus. *J. Neurosci.* 15: 1577–1586.

Wang H and Wagner JJ (1999) Priming-induced shift in synaptic plasticity in the rat hippocampus. *J. Neurophysiol.* 82: 2024–2028.

Wang SJ and Gean PW (1999) Long-term depression of excitatory synaptic transmission in the rat amygdala. *J. Neurosci.* 19: 10656–10663.

Wang SS and Augustine GJ (1995) Confocal imaging and local photolysis of caged compounds; dual probes of synaptic function. *Neuron* 15: 755–760.

Wang SSH, Denk W, and Häusser M (2000) Coincidence detection in single dendritic spines mediated by calcium release. *Nat. Neurosci.* 3: 1266–1273.

Wang Y-T and Linden DJ (2000) Expression of cerebellar long-term depression requires postsynaptic clathrin-mediated endocytosis. *Neuron* 25: 635–647.

Weber JT, De Zeeuw CI, Linden DJ, and Hansel C (2003) Long-term depression of climbing fiber–evoked calcium transients in Purkinje cell dendrites. *Proc. Natl. Acad. Sci. USA* 100: 2878–2883.

Weiler IJ and Greenough WT (1993) Metabotropic glutamate receptors trigger postsynaptic protein synthesis. *Proc. Natl. Acad. Sci. USA* 90: 7168–7171.

Weiler IJ, Irwin SA, Klintsova AY, et al. (1997) Fragile X mental retardation protein is translated near synapses in response to neurotransmitter activation. *Proc. Natl. Acad. Sci. USA* 94: 5395–5400.

Welsh JP and Harvey JA (1989) Cerebellar lesions and the nictitating membrane reflex: Performance deficits of the conditioned and unconditioned response. *J. Neurosci.* 9: 299–311.

Welsh JP, Yamaguchi H, Zeng XH, et al. (2005) Normal motor learning during pharmacological prevention of Purkinje cell long-term depression. *Proc. Natl. Acad. Sci. USA* 102: 17166–176171.

Wenthold RJ, Petralia RS, Blahos J, and Niedzielski AS (1996) Evidence for multiple AMPA receptor complexes in hippocampal CA1/CA2 neurons. *J. Neurosci.* 16: 1982–1989.

Wigstrom M and Gustafsson B (1985) On long-lasting potentiation in the hippocampus: A proposed mechanism for its dependence on coincident pre- and postsynaptic activity. *Acta Physiol. Scand.* 123: 519–522.

Wilson M and McNaughton B (1993) Dynamics of the hippocampal ensemble that codes for space. *Science* 261: 1055–1058.

Xia J, Chung HJ, Wihler C, Huganir RL, and Linden DJ (2000) Cerebellar long-term depression requires PKC-regulated interactions between GluR2/3 and PDZ domain containing proteins. *Neuron* 28: 499–510.

Xia J, Zhang X, Staudinger J, and Huganir RL (1999) Clustering of AMPA receptors by the synaptic PDZ domain-containing protein PICK1. *Neuron* 22: 179–187.

Xiang JZ and Brown MW (1998) Differential neuronal encoding of novelty, familiarity and recency in regions of the anterior temporal lobe. *Neuropharmacology* 37: 657–676.

Xiao MY, Karpefors M, Gustafsson B, and Wigstrom H (1995) On the linkage between AMPA and NMDA receptor-mediated EPSPs in homosynaptic long-term depression in the hippocampal CA1 region of young rats. *J. Neurosci.* 15: 4496–4506.

Xiao MY, Niu YP, and Wigstrom H (1996) Activity-dependent decay of early LTP revealed by dual EPSP recording in hippocampal slices from young rats. *Eur. J. Neurosci.* 8: 1916–1923.

Xiao MY, Wigstrom H, and Gustafsson B (1994) Long-term depression in the hippocampal CA1 region is associated with equal changes in AMPA and NMDA receptor-mediated synaptic potentials. *Eur. J. Neurosci.* 6: 1055–1057.

Xu L, Anwyl R, and Rowan MJ (1997) Behavioural stress facilitates the induction of long-term depression in the hippocampus. *Nature* 387: 497–500.

Xu L, Anwyl R, and Rowan MJ (1998a) Spatial exploration induces a persistent reversal of long-term potentiation in rat hippocampus. *Nature* 394: 891–894.

Xu L, Holscher C, Anwyl R, and Rowan MJ (1998b) Glucocorticoid receptor and protein/RNA synthesis-dependent mechanisms underlie the control of synaptic plasticity by stress. *Proc. Natl. Acad. Sci. USA* 95: 3204–3208.

Yang SN, Tang YG, and Zucker RS (1999) Selective induction of LTP and LTD by postsynaptic [Ca^{2+}]i elevation. *J. Neurophysiol*. 81: 781–787.

Yeo CH and Hardiman MJ (1992) Cerebellar cortex and eyeblink conditioning: A reexamination. *Exp. Brain Res*. 88: 623–638.

Yeo CH, Hardiman MJ, and Glickstein M (1985a) Classical conditioning of the nictitating membrane response of the rabbit I. Lesions of the cerebellar nuclei. *Exp. Brain Res*. 60: 87–98.

Yeo CH, Hardiman MJ, and Glickstein M (1985b) Classical conditioning of the nictitating membrane response of the rabbit II. Lesions of the cerebellar cortex. *Exp. Brain Res*. 60: 99–113.

Yuzaki M (2004) The δ2 glutamate receptor: A key molecule controlling synaptic plasticity and structure in Purkinje cells. *Cerebellum* 3: 89–93.

Zeng H, Chattarji S, Barbarosie M, et al. (2001) *Cell* 107: 617–629.

Zhang W and Linden DJ (2006) Long-term depression at the mossy fiber–deep cerebellar nucleus synapse. *J. Neurosci*. 26: 6935–6944.

Zhuo M, Zhang W, Son H, et al. (1999) A selective role of calcineurin Aalpha in synaptic depotentiation in hippocampus. *Proc. Natl. Acad. Sci. USA* 96: 4650–4655.

Zucker RS (1999) Calcium- and activity-dependent synaptic plasticity. *Curr. Opin. Neurobiol*. 9: 305–313.

Zuo J, De Jager PL, Takahashi K, Jiang W, Linden DJ, and Heintz N (1997) Neurodegeneration in Lurcher mice results from a mutation in the δ2 receptor gene. *Nature* 388: 769–772.

13 Activity-Dependent Structural Plasticity of Dendritic Spines

C. A. Chapleau and L. Pozzo-Miller, University of Alabama at Birmingham, Birmingham, AL, USA

13.1 Introduction

Neuroscientists have long been fascinated by the problem of how memory is formed, stored, and recalled, not only because learning and remembering are at the core of our human experience, but also for the evolutionary significance to adapt behaviorally by learning about and making predictions in response to our surroundings. As early as the later part of the nineteenth century and around the time when the cellular basis of brain structure was still hotly debated, Cajal and Tanzi speculated that the improvement of existing skills and the acquisition of new ones required structural changes in nerve cells. Current cellular and molecular models of learning and memory are deeply rooted in these pioneering ideas, whereby biochemical modifications and morphological remodeling of existing synaptic junctions, as well as the formation of new ones, lead to enduring functional changes in neuronal networks. This chapter will review the experimental evidence in support of the activity-dependent structural plasticity of dendritic spines, the small processes extending from the surface of dendrites where most excitatory synapses of the central nervous system (CNS) are formed. We will focus on the morphological consequences of environmental enrichment and behavioral learning of associative tasks, as well as *in vitro* manipulations of neuronal activity resulting in long-term synaptic plasticity in the hippocampus, a brain region critical for memory formation. We will review the actions of neurotrophins and hormones on dendritic spines in the context of hippocampal-dependent learning and memory. Since several developmental disorders associated with mental retardation present with abnormal dendritic spines, we will also discuss the potential implications of such structural differences in cognition as well as in learning and memory.

13.2 Brief Historical Perspective

The cellular and molecular mechanisms of memory acquisition, consolidation, and subsequent recall have been intensely studied by neuroscientists for more than a century. The first ideas about the possibility that experience can modify the structure of the brain, including its comprising nerve cells and their junctions, can be traced back to the later part of the nineteenth century (Bain, 1872; James, 1890; Cajal, 1893; Tanzi, 1893; Foster and Sherringhton, 1897). Eugenio Tanzi and Santiago Ramón y Cajal postulated that the improvement of learned habits and skills by 'mental exercise' arises from the growth of existing synapses, whereas learning new ones requires the formation of new nerve cell connections. Despite the appeal of these remarkably intuitive ideas, it was later realized that the mature nervous system might not be as plastic as it is during development and that neuronal growth may be too slow to account for learning. Later, Donald Hebb proposed a 'dual trace mechanism' to address the discrepancy between the rapidity of learning and the time required for structural growth, whereby

> ... a reverbatory trace might cooperate with the structural change, and carry the memory until the growth change is made... (Hebb, 1949).

Hebb's more famous contribution is a cellular mechanism for associative learning postulating that coincident activity at given synaptic junctions modifies the properties of those synapses, thereby increasing their efficiency (Hebb, 1949). Together with the pioneering ideas of Tanzi and Cajal, this 'Hebbian' principle dominates the current thinking of how use-dependent changes at synapses occur during learning.

Research into the mechanisms underlying learning has thus primarily focused on the computational unit of the nervous system, the synapse. It is now well known that synapses are not static: the cellular mechanisms of learning and memory, triggered by experience, involve molecular modifications and morphological remodeling of existing synapses, as well as genesis of new synapses, resulting in activity-dependent functional changes. The vast majority of the studies on the mechanisms underlying changes in synaptic strength as a consequence of behavioral experience have focused on one of the brain regions most relevant to learning and memory, the hippocampus. The study of synaptic plasticity in the hippocampus and its relationship to learning and memory has uncovered a labyrinth of molecular, cellular, and biophysical mechanisms that have been extensively reviewed (Martin et al., 2000; Abel and Lattal, 2001) (*See* Chapter 11).

13.3 The Structure and Function of Dendritic Spines

The acquisition, consolidation, and storage of information are dynamic processes that involve constant modification of synapses. A dynamic structure that makes up one half of the synapse long thought to be critical for learning and memory is the dendritic spine (**Figure 1**). Spines were first described by Cajal as small protrusions extending from the surface of dendrites (Cajal, 1891), likely representing the points of reception of nerve impulses (Cajal, 1909). It is now well known that these micron-long dendritic projections are the main postsynaptic site of excitatory synapses in the CNS, whereby approximately 90% of spines are innervated by a single

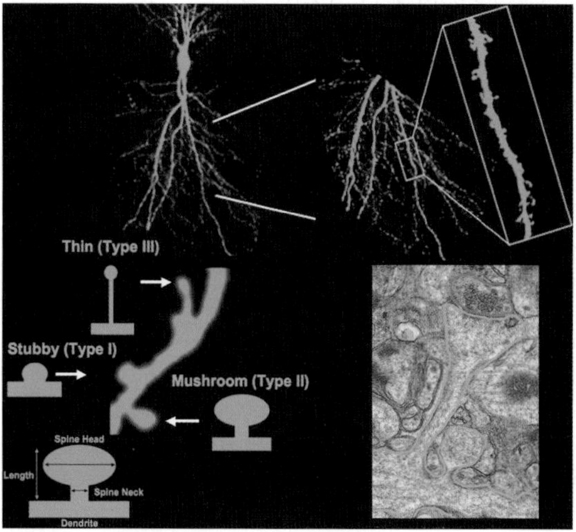

Figure 1 The structure of dendritic spines of hippocampal pyramidal neurons. Using particle-mediated gene transfer (a.k.a. gene gun), organotypic slice cultures were transfected with cDNA coding for enhanced yellow fluorescent protein. *Top panels:* Laser-scanning confocal microscopy images of a pyramidal neuron in area CA1 are shown at different magnifications to illustrate the complexity of their dendritic arbor and the abundance of dendritic spines in secondary and tertiary branches. *Bottom left panel:* A maximum-intensity projection of *z*-stacks shows a dendritic segment studded with the most common spine morphologies (i.e., stubby, mushroom, and thin). The cartoon illustrates the geometrical dimensions measured in individual spines to categorize them. *Bottom right panel:* A mushroom dendritic spine (outlined in green) forms an asymmetric synapse with a single presynaptic terminal (outlined in red) in *stratum radiatum* of area CA1 in organotypic slice culture. Bottom left panel adapted from Tyler WJ and Pozzo-Miller L (2003) Miniature synaptic transmission and BDNF modulate dendritic spine growth and form in rat CA1 neurones. *J. Physiol.* 553: 497–509, with permission.

presynaptic terminal (Gray, 1959b). Furthermore, 'naked' spines lacking a presynaptic partner are hardly observed in serial electron microscopy (EM) reconstructions of the hippocampus (Harris and Stevens, 1989). In some occasions, two or more spines from the same dendrite share the same presynaptic terminal, the so-called multiple synapse bouton. Structurally, a spine consists of a spherical head connected by a neck to its parent dendrite. In the hippocampus, the morphology of individual spines varies widely due to differences in their length, head shape, and neck diameter (Sorra and Harris, 2000). Simple spines can be characterized into three major types: (1) stubby, or Type-I spines, which lack obvious necks; (2) mushroom, Type-II spines, which have large heads and short narrow necks; and (3) thin, Type-III spines, which have small heads and long narrow necks (Peters and Kaiserman-Abramof, 1970). More complex morphological variations have also been observed, including bifurcated spines with multiple heads sharing the same neck (Harris, 1999). Time-lapse imaging of live spines has vividly demonstrated that dendritic spines are not static structures, but rather motile processes, especially during development (Matus, 2000; Dunaevsky and Mason, 2003). Thus, the aforementioned morphological types need to be considered as arbitrary snapshots of an underlying continuous distribution of possible geometrical forms, likely morphing from one another (Parnass et al., 2000). In the following sections, we will further discuss the intriguing possibility that spine geometry is modulated by synaptic activity, and how this structural modification may have functional consequences for synaptic transmission and plasticity.'

At the most distal region of the spine head facing the active zone (i.e., release site) of the apposing presynaptic terminal, a noticeable electron dense thickening is observed in EM micrographs, termed the postsynaptic density (PSD) (Kennedy, 1997; Ziff, 1997; Sheng and Sala, 2001). The PSD contains cytoskeletal components, scaffolding, and regulatory proteins, as well as neurotransmitter receptors. Simple dendritic spines do not contain mitochondria or microtubules, and the main cytoskeletal components are F-actin microfilaments (Peters et al., 1991). Notably, some spines will exhibit polyribosomes at the base of their necks (Spacek, 1985), suggesting that protein synthesis can occur locally near synapses. Approximately half of the spines of hippocampal pyramidal neurons contain one or several cisterns of smooth endoplasmic reticulum (SER) within their heads, a structure sometimes called the spine apparatus (Spacek and Harris, 1997; Cooney et al., 2002). Intriguingly, spine SER cisterns are not static but can dynamically interact with those within the parent dendrite (Toresson and Grant, 2005). Together with the role of SER as a Ca^{2+} source and sink (Berridge, 1998; Pozzo-Miller et al., 2000), the presence of Ca^{2+}-permeable ligand and voltage-gated channels in the spine membrane supports one of the most recognized functions of dendritic spines, i.e., a biochemical compartment for intracellular Ca^{2+} signaling (Muller and Connor, 1991; Petrozzino et al., 1995; Yuste and Denk, 1995; reviewed by Connor et al., 1994; Yuste et al., 2000; Sabatini et al., 2001).

It is becoming increasingly clear that the particular morphology of a dendritic spine may play an important role in determining its function, a concept that has been extensively reviewed (Shepherd, 1996; Yuste and Majewska, 2001; Nimchinsky et al., 2002). Two morphological features of dendritic spines seem to be critical for their role as biochemical compartments: the geometrical dimensions of the head and neck. If one formally considers a dendritic spine in terms of an electrical resistor and relates Ohm's law to diffusional resistance, the electrical coupling between the spine head and the dendritic shaft can be estimated from the diffusion of small fluorescence molecules from the spine to the parent dendrite. Using this approach, it was initially shown that diffusional coupling depends on the length and diameter of the neck (Svoboda et al., 1996). Furthermore, different levels of synaptic activity are able to regulate the diffusional isolation of individual spines (Bloodgood and Sabatini, 2005). Chronic blockade of excitatory synaptic transmission enhanced the diffusion of a photoactivatable green fluorescent protein (GFP) from the spine into the parent dendrite, while increasing excitatory transmission enhanced spine diffusional isolation. Notably, patterns of coincident synaptic activation and postsynaptic action potentials known to induce long-term potentiation (LTP) rapidly restricted diffusion across the spine neck. However, no correlation was found between spine geometry and diffusional isolation. These changes may be relevant for the induction and input specificity of Ca^{2+}-dependent forms of synaptic plasticity (i.e., long-term potentiation), because the diffusional coupling of individual spines affects the spatiotemporal profile of Ca^{2+} signals within spine heads (Korkotian and Segal, 2000; Majewska et al., 2000a). Indeed, a few experimental and modeling studies have shown that the spine neck can function as a diffusional barrier for Ca^{2+} ions flowing between the spine head and the parent dendrite, whereby short spines facilitated the Ca^{2+} flux from the head to the dendrite and long spines prevented it (Volfovsky et al., 1999; Korkotian et al., 2004). Using two-photon uncaging of methoxy nitroindolino glutamate (MNI-glutamate) to activate *N*-methyl-D-aspartate-type glutamate receptors (NMDARs) in individual spines, it has been shown that larger spines permitted greater efflux of Ca^{2+} into the dendritic shaft, whereas smaller spines manifested a larger increase in Ca^{2+} within the spine compartment as a result of a smaller Ca^{2+} flux through the neck (Noguchi et al., 2005). However, this view has been challenged based on the observations that the spatio-temporal profile of intracellular Ca^{2+} signals within spine heads is primarily determined by sequestration and extrusion, likely within the head or neck (Nimchinsky et al., 2002; Sabatini et al., 2002). Additional confounding factors include the perturbation of the intrinsic Ca^{2+} buffering capacity by the Ca^{2+} indicator dyes, the apparent increased diffusion of Ca^{2+} ions bound to the highly mobile indicator dyes, and the temperature dependence of the sequestration and extrusion processes.

Despite the difficulty of determining the role of spine morphology in the coupling of spine Ca^{2+} signals with the parent dendrite (Majewska et al., 2000a; Nimchinsky et al., 2002), recent evidence supports an early suggestion that spine morphology and size correlate with synaptic strength (Pierce and Lewin, 1994). For example, the volume of the spine head is directly proportional to the number of docked vesicles at the active zone of presynaptic terminals (Harris and Sultan, 1995; Boyer et al., 1998; Schikorski and Stevens, 1999) and to the number of alpha-amino-3-hydroxy-5-methyl-4-isoxazolepropionate-type glutamate receptors (AMPARs) (Nusser et al., 1998). These observations indicate that larger spines bear larger synapses, which are more reliable and stronger in terms of probability of release and postsynaptic sensitivity, respectively (Murthy et al., 2001). Another measure of synaptic strength is the expression of AMPARs at individual excitatory spine synapses, as observed during brain development and after induction of LTP, the most studied cellular model of learning and memory (Malinow and Malenka, 2002). The expression of AMPARs within individual spines of different morphologies was mapped by two-photon uncaging of MNI-glutamate, revealing that mushroom (Type-II) spines show larger AMPAR-mediated responses than thin (Type-III) spines (Matsuzaki et al., 2001). These studies provide functional evidence that larger spines represent stronger synapses, as defined by their expression of AMPARs (Kasai et al., 2003). As we will discuss later, it has been shown that the induction of LTP leads to an increase in spine head size, while long-term depression (LTD) causes spine shrinkage and retraction.

Other functions beyond that of compartmentalization of Ca^{2+} signals have been proposed for dendritic spines (Shepherd, 1996). These include (1) providing additional neuronal surface area to increase synapse density, (2) isolation of cytoplasmic biochemical/molecular signals to activated synaptic inputs, (3) neuroprotection by isolating large Ca^{2+} elevations from parent dendrites, (4) amplification of synaptic potentials, and (5) enhancing the spatial spread of back-propagating action potentials. Because some of these functional properties have been observed in nonspiny neurons, it is still currently unclear what, if any, is the functional advantage of producing and maintaining dendritic spines. Besides the function/structure relationship of dendritic spines, a number of physiological, pathophysiological, and experimental conditions modify spine density and morphology, including behavioral learning, hormonal state, levels of excitatory synaptic activity, growth factors (including neurotrophins), aging, malnutrition, poisoning, and several neurological disorders, such as schizophrenia and mental retardation (Fiala et al., 2002). Before we consider each of the physiological factors that modify dendritic spine number and form, we begin discussing the development of dendritic spines.

13.4 The Development of Dendritic Spines

The dendrites of pyramidal neurons in neonatal mammals are initially smooth, devoid of dendritic spines (Cajal, 1909; Marin-Padilla, 1972a; Purpura, 1975b). Spine density in pyramidal neurons seems to follow a developmental pattern similar to synapse formation, where an initial overproduction is followed by an activity-dependent pruning of excess synapses. In addition, spine morphology also changes during brain development. The majority of spines in the developing hippocampus are stubby, although the most frequent dendritic processes are filopodia. Because dendritic spines represent the postsynaptic compartment of the vast majority of excitatory synapses in the CNS, the study of their formation and evolution during brain development has been recently reviewed (Sorra and Harris, 2000; Yuste and Bonhoeffer, 2004).

Spine synapses were initially thought to originate from established synapses formed first on the dendritic shaft by the extension and narrowing of a neck and the appearance of a spine head (Miller and Peters, 1981). Alternatively, and due to their predominance and motility in the developing brain, dendritic filopodia have been considered as precursors of mature dendritic spines. Considering that approximately 90% of spines have a presynaptic partner (Gray, 1959a; Harris and Kater, 1994), it has been speculated that dendritic filopodia actively search for presynaptic axon terminals to form synapses, giving rise to spines with more mature morphologies after the initial contact (Jontes and Smith, 2000; Yuste and Bonhoeffer, 2004). This model was initially supported by studies showing that dendritic filopodia lacking presynaptic partners populate the dendrites of 1-week-old neurons, which later acquire shorter spines always associated with a presynaptic terminal (Papa et al., 1995). Time-lapse observations in organotypic cultures of hippocampal slices later demonstrated that filopodia are extremely dynamic, extending and retracting in short periods of time (Dailey and Smith, 1996). Furthermore, some filopodia of cultured neurons were shown to make contact with axons at their tips, and the number of filopodia decreased in parallel with an increase in the number of spines (Ziv and Smith, 1996). These observations led to the proposal that the initial contact with axons triggers the formation of spines from filopodia. Serial EM reconstructions in the developing hippocampus *in situ* also support the role of filopodia as the site of initial axon contact, but only after their complete retraction and morphing into a shaft synapse, which will then serve as the emerging site of a mature spine with a synapse on its head (Fiala et al., 1998). Lastly, longitudinal *in vivo* multiphoton imaging of dendritic spines in the neocortex of developing and even adult animals supports the view that spines constantly form by seeking out presynaptic partners in the surrounding neuropil and stabilizing into functional spines of 3-varied morphology, a process driven by sensory experience (Lendvai et al., 2000; Trachtenberg et al., 2002; Holtmaat et al., 2005; Knott et al., 2006).

Regardless of the specific model of spine synapse formation, the highly dynamic behavior of filopodia during synatogenesis and the continuous rapid motility of dendritic spines require a careful orchestration and modulation of the dendritic cytoskeleton (Matus, 2000). The mechanism responsible for filopodia and spine motility is based on actin polymerization (Fischer et al., 1998; Dunaevsky et al., 1999; Korkotian and Segal, 2001; Zito et al., 2004) and seems to involve the Rho family of small GTPases (GTP: guanosine triphosphate) (Nakayama et al., 2000; Tashiro et al., 2000; Hering and Sheng, 2001). Moreover, spine motility is not only modulated by intracellular Ca^{2+} levels (Oertner and Matus, 2005), but may also affect Ca^{2+} compartmentalization within individual spines (Majewska et al., 2000b). Actin-based rapid spine motility, whereby the spine head and neck are in a seemingly constant process of movement, is not only critical for spine formation and synaptogenesis during brain development, but has also been proposed to be fundamental throughout lifetime (Matus, 2005; Harms and Dunaevsky, 2006). As we shall discuss in the following sections, actin-based motility allows dendritic spines to be malleable structures sensitive to ongoing levels of neuronal activity, underlying activity-dependent structural plasticity during experience-driven behavioral learning.

13.5 Structural Plasticity of Dendritic Spines Induced by Synaptic Activity: Homeostatic Plasticity, LTP, and LTD

Despite speculation by Cajal and Tanzi more than 100 years ago that the improvement of learned skills by 'mental exercise' arises from the growth of existing synapses, whereas acquiring new ones requires the formation of new neuronal connections, it was not until the 1960s that such structural plasticity was observed in response to the amount of afferent synaptic activity. In these early studies, dendritic spines of pyramidal neurons in the visual cortex were lost when afferent input was deprived by either surgical lesions (Globus and Scheibel, 1966) or by rearing mice in total darkness (Valverde, 1967). Moreover, deafferentation-induced spine loss was reversible and not pathological, as spine density could recover after only a few days of exposure to normal lighting conditions (Valverde, 1971). On the other hand, rearing rats in continuous illumination led to an increase in spine density in visual cortical neurons (Parnavelas et al., 1973), suggesting that morphological changes induced by deafferentation were bidirectional. It was later shown that these effects were not exclusive of the visual cortex. Surgical lesions of the perforant path – the afferent fibers from the entorhinal cortex into the dentate gyrus – caused an initial loss of dendritic spines of granule cells, which was followed by a recovery to prelesion levels due to subsequent axonal sprouting (Parnavelas et al., 1974). These early observations consolidated the concept that changes in the levels of afferent input evoked an adaptive response in terms of dendritic spine density in several brain regions.

13.5.1 Ongoing Synaptic Activity

Because dendritic spines represent the postsynaptic compartment of excitatory synapses, the aforementioned *in vivo* studies were followed by varied manipulations of glutamatergic synaptic transmission in brain slices and cultured neurons. Long-term exposure to gamma-aminobutyric acid$_A$ (GABA$_A$) receptor antagonists, which increases neuronal excitability and thus excitatory synaptic drive, caused a significant reduction in spine density in pyramidal neurons within organotypic cultures of hippocampal slices (Muller et al., 1993; Thompson et al., 1996). Due to the excessive recurrent innervation in long-term hippocampal slice cultures (Gutierrez and Heinemann, 1999), this manipulation may have evoked pathological levels of excitability, leading to spine loss as described in epilepsy patients (Scheibel et al., 1974). On the other hand, exposing cultured hippocampal neurons to GABA$_A$ receptor antagonists for shorter periods led to an increase in dendritic spine density (Papa and Segal, 1996). Additional studies in cultured neurons support the hypothesis that moderate levels of excitatory synaptic transmission promotes spine growth and formation while excessive levels cause spine shrinkage and loss, representing an adaptive response mediated by intracellular Ca^{2+} levels (Korkotian and Segal, 1999a,b; Segal et al., 2000). In fact, dendritic spines are rapidly formed and orient themselves toward a local source of glutamate (Richards et al., 2005). On the other side of the coin, weeklong pharmacological blockade of NMDARs or Na^+-dependent action potentials reduced spine density in CA1 pyramidal neurons in slice cultures (Collin et al., 1997). Furthermore, spontaneous quantal excitatory synaptic transmission, i.e., miniature synaptic currents or 'minis,' seemed to be sufficient for the maintenance of spines, as long-term blockade of AMPARs or inhibition of vesicular neurotransmitter release with *Botulinum* neurotoxins led to a decrease in spine density in hippocampal pyramidal neurons maintained in organotypic slice cultures (McKinney et al., 1999). The spine loss in these chronic blockade experiments may result from the prolonged absence of excitatory synaptic input (7 days *in vitro*), because shorter periods of inactivity (48 h) did not cause spine loss but rather a change in the proportion of morphological spine types (Tyler and Pozzo-Miller, 2003). In fact, even shorter inactivity (~8 h) induced filopodia and immature synapse formation in CA1 pyramidal neurons of acute hippocampal slices (Kirov and Harris, 1999; Petrak et al., 2005). Such brief periods of inactivity actually promote the active searching of presynaptic partners by filopodia and immature dendritic spines (Richards et al., 2005) that, if unsuccessful, would lead to the collapse and pruning of spines. It has been proposed that highly motile immature dendritic spines containing only NMDARs (i.e., silent synapses) (Isaac et al., 1995; Liao et al., 1995) may later stabilize by the acquisition of AMPARs (Shi et al., 1999). Taken together, these observations provide a physiological mechanism for deafferentation-induced spine loss and support the early notion that the levels of afferent synaptic input directly influence neuronal morphology, e.g., spine synapse density.

13.5.2 Homeostatic Plasticity

Due to the duration (days to weeks) and generalized extent of the experimental manipulations of synaptic activity, the aforementioned experiments may reflect cell-wide global adaptations as thought to occur during homeostatic synaptic plasticity. Homeostatic mechanisms maintain an 'optimal' level of input to a neuron by regulating the strength of afferent excitatory and inhibitory synapses, by modulating intrinsic neuronal excitability, and by altering synapse number (Turrigiano and Nelson, 2004; Davis, 2006). Despite the lack of changes in spine density in cultured developing neurons after activity blockade (Davis and Bezprozvanny, 2001; Burrone and Murthy, 2003), CA1 pyramidal neurons in acute slices exhibit more – and longer – spines after blockade of synaptic transmission (Kirov and Harris, 1999). In addition to the duration of the activity blockade (hours in acute slices vs. days in cultures), the developmental age of the neurons in these studies was different. The absence of synaptic activity during the critical period of synaptogenesis and pruning in the hippocampus (postnatal day 6 through postnatal day 16) did not evoke an homeostatic modulation in spine number (Kirov et al., 2004a), despite the well-characterized changes in quantal scaling of glutamate receptors and neuronal excitability in developing cultured neurons (Turrigiano, 1999). Instead, homeostatic plasticity of spine density seems to appear once the adult-like dendritic complement of spines is achieved (Kirov et al., 2004a). Complementary studies focused on the morphological consequences of activity-dependent manipulations of glutamatergic synaptic transmission with 'Hebbian' features resembling associative learning (Hebb, 1949), such as LTP and LTD of excitatory synaptic transmission (Malenka and Bear, 2004). Since this topic has been reviewed extensively over the years (e.g., Wallace et al., 1991; Geinisman, 2000; Yuste and Bonhoeffer, 2001; Segal, 2005), we will briefly discuss the main classical findings in addition to the most recent observations employing state-of-the-art imaging technologies.

13.5.3 Long-Term Potentiation

Instead of reflecting an adaptive response to prolonged and widespread changes in synaptic input, LTP is induced and expressed by a small number of activated synapses. Due to several of its properties (e.g., input specificity, associativity, cooperativity), LTP has become the most recognized synaptic model of associative learning and memory (Bliss and Collingridge, 1993). As pointed out earlier, the need for a structural change to underlie the longevity of memories has been repeatedly speculated (Cajal, 1893; Tanzi, 1893; Hebb, 1949). In fact, this possibility was explicitly proposed as one of the potential mechanisms for the enhancement of excitatory transmission in the very first description of LTP (Bliss and Lomo, 1973). In this groundbreaking paper, Bliss and Lomo quoted Rall, stating that

> . . . a reduction in the resistance of the narrow stem by which spines are attached to the parent dendrite . . .

may change the relative weight of synapses and thus contribute to the observed potentiation of excitatory transmission (Rall, 1970, as cited in Bliss and Lomo, 1973; Rall and Segev, 1987; Diamond et al., 1970, as cited in Rall and Segev, 1987). Soon thereafter, Van Harreveld and Fifkova tested this hypothesis by using pioneering rapid freezing methods of tissue preparation for EM following *in vivo* stimulation protocols described in the first LTP papers. In these studies, dendritic spines within the outer two thirds of the dentate molecular layer – which received the stimulated perforant path fibers – had larger heads as well as wider and shorter necks, features observed as early as 2 min and lasting as long as 23 h from the stimulation (Van Harreveld and Fifkova, 1975; Fifkova and Van Harreveld, 1977; Fifkova and Anderson, 1981). The layer specificity and time course of these changes strongly suggest that they are directly correlated with the potentiation of synaptic responses, despite the lack of electrophysiological confirmation of LTP induction and the identification of activated synapses.

The pioneering ultrastructural studies by Van Harreveld and Fifkova were followed by a series of EM observations after LTP-inducing afferent stimulation both *in vivo* and in the more amenable *in vitro* brain slice preparation, which sometimes included contradicting observations:

1. Increase in the proportion of shaft synapses, without changes in spine number, size, or form in area CA1 *in vivo* and *in vitro*, although much of these observations might have come from relatively aspiny inhibitory interneurons (Lee et al., 1979, 1980).
2. Layer-specific increases in the proportion of spines with concave heads and larger PSDs, without net changes in the total number density of spine or shaft synapses on dentate gyrus granule cells (Desmond and Levy, 1983, 1986a,b, 1990).
3. Increase in the number of 'sessile' (likely stubby spines) and shaft synapses in area CA1 of *in vitro* hippocampal slices, without detectable changes in the number of spines or in the dimensions of their heads and necks, although typical cup-shaped spines seemed to have been replaced by more flat spine profiles (Chang and Greenough, 1984).
4. Decrease in the number of spine synapses and a parallel increase in shaft synapses on dentate granule cells after high-frequency stimulation of the perforant path in acute hippocampal slices (Gomez et al., 1990). Intriguingly, these changes were correlated with the magnitude and success rate of LTP induction observed in rats with different inborn learning capacity.
5. Increase in the ratio of perforated to nonperforated spines synapses in the dentate molecular layer in chronically implanted rats 1 h after perforant path stimulation, without changes in the total number of spine synapses (Geinisman et al., 1991). These studies were later followed by the observation of an increase in the number of spine synapses with multiple, completely partitioned transmission zones (Geinisman et al., 1993).
6. Increase in spine number in dentate gyrus after *in vivo* stimulation of perforant path fibers, as well as the proportion of 'bifurcated' spines (Trommald

et al., 1996), thought to originate from the splitting of spine synapses bearing perforated PSDs (Peters and Kaiserman-Abramof, 1969).

7. Increase in multiple-bouton spine synapses with perforated PSDs in area CA1 of slice cultures, which were known to have been activated during LTP-inducing afferent stimulation (Buchs and Muller, 1996; Toni et al., 1999, 2001). In these studies, synapses activated during the high-frequency conditioning stimulus – and thus presumably potentiated – were identified at the EM level using a Ca^{2+} precipitate protocol (Buchs et al., 1994).

8. No changes in the absolute number of spine synapses in area CA1 of acute slices (Sorra and Harris, 1998). However, these and other observations in acute hippocampal slices may be confounded by the fact that spine density is increased by temperature changes during slice preparation (Kirov et al., 1999, 2004b; Bourne et al., 2006).

9. Increase in spine synapses with perforated PSDs in dentate granule cells after successfully maintained LTP in aged rats, while spine branching was only observed after high-frequency stimulation without sustained potentiation (Dhanrajan et al., 2004).

10. Increase in the number of spines with perforated PSDs and of multiple-synapse boutons in area CA1 after chemically induced LTP in acute slices (Stewart et al., 2005).

Despite the increasing sophistication of the morphological studies at the EM level listed above, especially with regard to the confirmation of LTP induction and the identification of potentiatied synapses, it was clear from the beginning that time-lapse imaging of live neurons before, during, and after LTP induction would yield more consistent results. To this aim, repeated laser-scanning confocal microscopy was performed in live acute hippocampal slices to follow spine morphology during chemically induced LTP, a procedure that would ensure that most synapses in the slice are potentiatied (Hosokawa et al., 1995). The appearance of new dendritic spines in these DiI-labeled (DiI is a long-chain dialkylcarbocyanines dye) CA1 pyramidal neurons was a rare – and statistically insignificant – event. However, small spines were seen to extend, and others appeared to change their orientation with respect to the parent dendrite. Circumventing the optical limitations of confocal microscopy applied to acute slices, imaging live neurons within organotypic slice cultures (Gahwiler, 1981; Stoppini et al., 1991; Pozzo Miller et al., 1993) by multiphoton excitation microscopy – a.k.a. two-photon microscopy (Denk and Svoboda, 1997) – yielded a much clearer picture. High-frequency afferent stimulation was shown to induce the formation of protrusions that resembled dendritic filopodia in CA1 pyramidal neurons expressing enhanced GFP (eGFP) (Maletic-Savatic et al., 1999). Some of these synaptically induced filopodia persisted for the duration of the imaging session (up to 1 h) and later acquired a bulbous head – suggesting that they developed into spines – and their appearance required NMDAR activity, as LTP induction does. Similar spine formation associated with successful LTP induction was observed in CA1 pyramidal neurons injected with the fluorescent dye calcein (Engert and Bonhoeffer, 1999). These studies further showed that spine growth occurred selectively within a synaptically active region, which was restricted to a ~30-μm area, while some spines were seen to randomly disappear in distant regions where synaptic transmission was blocked, suggesting an homeostatic balance in spine number. Similar filopodia and spine formation was also shown to occur in CA1 pyramidal neurons after the intracellular application of autophosphorylated Ca^{2+}/calmodulin-dependent protein kinase II (CaMKII), an enzyme implicated in LTP induction (Jourdain et al., 2003).

In addition to spine number, time-lapse imaging by multiphoton excitation microscopy during and after LTP induction in hippocampal slices also revealed rapid changes in spine morphology, which resembled the spine head swelling initially described by Van Harreveld and Fifkova at the EM level (Van Harreveld and Fifkova, 1975). Induction of LTP by high-frequency stimulation in acute slices from eGFP-expressing mice caused a transient expansion of activated CA1 neuron spines, which were identified by synaptically mediated Ca^{2+} elevations (Lang et al., 2004). The predicted increase in spine volume observed in these studies was detected as early as 30 s after stimulation and lasted for 10–20 min. On the other hand, repetitive (1 min at 1 Hz) miniature excitatory postsynaptic current (mEPSC)-like two-photon uncaging of MNI-glutamate on individual CA1 neuron spines led to equally rapid (1–5 min) and selective enlargement of stimulated spines that was transient in large mushroom spines but persistent in small spines, lasting up to 100 min (Matsuzaki et al., 2004). Furthermore, the enduring spine enlargement was associated with an increase in AMPAR-mediated currents and required NMDAR activity, CaMKII, and actin polymerization. A similar photorelease approach – but using ultraviolet (UV) uncaging and wide-field fluorescence imaging in thinner slice cultures – failed to reveal any morphological changes in spines during the potentiation of AMPAR-mediated currents (Bagal et al., 2005). However, the potentiation of uncaging currents in the latter studies was induced by a single UV flash paired with postsynaptic depolarization, suggesting that structural remodeling of dendritic spines may require repeated activation of NMDARs, as during LTP of synaptic responses. Further support to this idea comes from spine size changes after a global induction of LTP in slice cultures. CA1 pyramidal neurons were transfected with the fluorescent protein tDimer-dsRed and glutamate receptor subunits tagged with pH-sensitive GFP to monitor morphological changes and receptor trafficking simultaneously (Kopec et al., 2006). Generalized induction of 'chemical' LTP (Otmakhov et al., 2004) caused a significant increase in spine volume that was maximum by 2 min after the application of the chemical LTP-inducing cocktail. Furthermore, the observed spine enlargement preceded the membrane insertion of AMPA receptor subunits, suggesting that different mechanisms mediate structural and functional changes at individual spines after synaptic potentiation.

Regarding the molecular machinery responsible for the structural plasticity of dendritic spines, it was originally proposed that the actin cytoskeleton plays a critical role (Crick, 1982; Fifkova and Delay, 1982). Only recently it was shown that LTP-inducing stimulus enlarged spine heads in parallel with an increase in their content of filamentous actin relative to globular actin as imaged by fluorescence resonance energy transfer (FRET) (Okamoto et al., 2004). Furthermore, the latter studies in CA1 neurons in slice cultures showed that LTD-inducing stimulus led to the opposite results, namely a reduction in F-actin relative to G-actin and a reduction in spine size, suggesting that spine structural plasticity is bidirectional. In addition to multiple signaling pathways, in particular the one mediated by Rho and Rac small GTPases (Nakayama et al., 2000; Tashiro et al., 2000), several scaffold proteins and actin binding proteins converge on the actin cytoskeleton to regulate spine morphology and dynamics, an issue that has been recently reviewed (Tada and Sheng, 2006).

13.5.4 Long-Term Depression

Further evidence of the bidirectional nature of spine structural plasticity is beginning to emerge. GFP-expressing CA1 pyramidal neurons in slice cultures of Thy-1-GFP mice rapidly and persistently lost their dendritic spines after their afferent inputs were stimulated at low frequency (900 pulses at 1 Hz) (Nagerl et al., 2004), a protocol well known to induce NMDAR-dependent LTD (Dudek and Bear, 1992; Mulkey and Malenka, 1992). In addition, CA1 neurons individually filled with the fluorescent dye calcein showed spine shrinkage leading to spine retraction in response to low-frequency stimulation (Zhou et al., 2004). Similar to the requirements for LTD induction, spine retraction and pruning were also sensitive to NMDAR antagonists and calcineurin, an inhibitor of protein phosphatases (Nagerl et al., 2004; Zhou et al., 2004), strengthening the view that dendritic spines are formed and eliminated in an activity-dependent manner that correlates with bidirectional changes in synaptic efficacy.

13.6 Structural Plasticity of Dendritic Spines Induced by Experience and Behavioral Learning

The seminal ideas proposed by Hebb regarding associative learning sparked experimental research not only at the cellular level, but also on the structural consequences of behavioral training, spatial learning, or differential experience (Bailey and Kandel, 1993). Apparently inspired by Hebb's anecdotal report of the enhanced learning ability of laboratory rats when housed as home pets during their development (Hebb, 1949), Rosenzweig and colleagues showed that raising rodents in 'enriched' environments led to neurochemical and anatomical changes in the cerebral cortex (reviewed in Rosenzweig and Bennett, 1996). Among the anatomical consequences of rearing rodents in enriched environments was an increase in dendritic spine number in the visual cortex (Globus et al., 1973; Greenough and Volkmar, 1973), an observation in keeping with the concept that continuous use is critical for the maintenance and even the formation of new synaptic contacts on dendritic spines (e.g., Globus and Scheibel, 1966; Valverde, 1967).

Because these enriched complex environments were initially considered as visual and motor challenges, the majority of the studies focused in those brain regions thought to be engaged in such behaviors (e.g., somatosensory, motor, and visual cortices). It was later realized that a complex environment also represents a challenge for spatial navigation abilities, likely engaging the hippocampus, a region well known for the functional and structural plasticity of its excitatory spine synapses. Indeed, rats that were repeatedly trained in a complex environment (up to 5 floors connected by ladders, 4 h per day for 14–30 days) exhibit higher spine density in basal dendrites of CA1 pyramidal neurons, an observation that correlated with an improved performance in the Morris water maze compared to untrained littermates (Moser et al., 1994, 1997). Similar increases in spine density were also observed in the CA1 region of mice (Rampon et al., 2000) and marmosets, New World monkeys (Kozorovitskiy et al., 2005). However, an 'enriched' environment consists of a combination of enhanced social interactions, cognitive stimulation, and physical exercise in addition to requiring spatial navigation abilities. Not surprisingly then, environmental enrichment enhances several aspects of hippocampal function, including neurogenesis, LTP, and spatial learning (van Praag et al., 2000). It remains to be established which features of the enriched environment are more important for those lasting functional outcomes.

Learning-specific hippocampal-dependent associative tasks, such as trace eye blink conditioning or odor discrimination, were also correlated with increases in spine density on CA1 neurons, although on their apical dendrites (Leuner et al., 2003; Knafo et al., 2004). In contrast, unbiased stereological analyses failed to detect differences in spine synapse number on CA1 pyramidal neurons after Morris water maze training (Rusakov et al., 1997; Miranda et al., 2006) or trace eye blink conditioning (Geinisman et al., 2000). However, the latter study did reveal an increase in the area of the PSD of nonperforated spine synapses (Geinisman et al., 2000). These discrepancies may originate from 'snapshot' observations of likely transient changes made at different time points through a continuous distribution of morphological states. Indeed, learning-induced increases in spine density of dentate gyrus granule cells were transient, with maximum levels observed 6–9 h after passive avoidance (O'Malley et al., 1998) or spatial water maze training (O'Malley et al., 2000; Eyre et al., 2003), and returning to control levels after 24–72 h. Despite the attractiveness of the possibility that dendritic spines and memory formation mutually interact – i.e., "learning makes more spines" and "more spines promotes learning" – their causal relationship, if any, has eluded more than 100 years of intensive research and continues to raise alternative interpretations (Moser, 1999; Segal, 2005).

Although we have focused on the structural plasticity of dendritic spines in the hippocampus, it should be noted that recent advances in multiphoton excitation microscopy have allowed the study of dendritic spines in cortical regions of the intact brain *in vivo*. Due to the obvious limitation of accessibility, most of the work so far has focused in the cerebral cortex, where long-term imaging has demonstrated that subpopulations of spines appear and disappear while others remain for months (Grutzendler et al., 2002; Trachtenberg et al., 2002; Holtmaat et al., 2005). Furthermore, spines in the somatosensory barrel cortex are modulated by sensory experience (Trachtenberg et al., 2002; Zuo et al., 2005; Holtmaat et al., 2006), and such experience-driven spine formation precedes synapse formation (Knott et al., 2006). However, the only report of dendritic spine imaging in the hippocampus *in vivo* showed a remarkable stability, at least for up to 4 h, even after induction of epileptic seizures with the muscarinic agonist pilocarpine or the $GABA_A$ antagonist bicuculline (Mizrahi et al., 2004). However, the conditions used in this study for imaging spines in the intact hippocampus *in vivo* (e.g., halothane anesthesia and blunt resection of the overlaying cerebral cortex) may have affected their physiological behavior. Thus, it remains to be determined whether dendritic spines in the intact hippocampus *in vivo* display the types of rapid structural rearrangements they are capable of *in vitro* in response to varying levels of afferent synaptic activity. A further challenge will be to relate synaptic activity-dependent rapid spine plasticity with the morphological remodeling described after experience-driven hippocampal-dependent learning.

13.7 Structural Plasticity of Dendritic Spines Induced by Neuromodulators: Ovarian Hormones and Neurotrophins

In addition to the ongoing levels of excitatory afferent input, exposure to enriched environments and learning spatial navigation tasks, dendritic spines of hippocampal neurons are also sensitive to slow-acting neuromodulators. Due to their established role during brain development and throughout aging, some of the most attractive molecular candidates for modulating spine structural plasticity include the ovarian steroid hormones (i.e., estradiol and progesterone) and members of the family of neurotrophins, such as brain-derived neurotrophic factor (BDNF). As we shall discuss below, the interplay between estradiol and BDNF actions on hippocampal neurons is reflected not only in the modulation of dendritic spine density, but also in the modulation of hippocampal synaptic plasticity thought to underlie associative learning and memory.

13.7.1 Estradiol

Traditionally, the effects of steroid ovarian hormones have been defined as 'organizational' and 'activational.' Organizational effects are permanent structural changes induced by hormones during a critical period of brain development, while activational effects represent the initiation or termination of previously established neuronal circuits (Arnold and Gorski, 1984). Initial studies of the effects of steroid hormones on neuronal and synaptic structure focused in sexually dimorphic brain regions that control reproductive behaviors, such as the arcuate and ventromedial nuclei of the hypothalamus (Matsumoto and Arai, 1979, 1986; Carrer and Aoki, 1982; Frankfurt et al., 1990; Pozzo Miller and Aoki, 1991, 1992). Relevant to learning and memory, several studies had shown that elevations in the circulating levels of estradiol induced experimentally, or those achieved during the proestrus in rodents, resulted in enhanced neuronal excitability in the hippocampus (Woolley and Timiras, 1962; Terasawa and Timiras, 1968; Kawakami et al., 1970). Inspired by the growing literature reporting that enhanced afferent synaptic activity promoted dendritic spine growth in several brain regions, McEwen and colleagues first demonstrated that ovariectomized female rats had reduced spine density in CA1 pyramidal neurons compared to sham-operated controls (Gould et al., 1990). Later they showed that this effect was reversible upon treatment with estradiol and progesterone (Gould et al., 1990; Woolley and McEwen, 1993), and that in fact spine density fluctuated during the estrous cycle in a manner that is consistent with the effects of estrogen and progesterone (Woolley et al., 1990). Similar effects of estradiol were observed in cultured hippocampal neurons (Murphy and Segal, 1996) and CA1 pyramidal neurons maintained in organotypic slice culture (Pozzo-Miller et al., 1999b). Furthermore, CA1 pyramidal neurons in the hippocampus of young and aged nonhuman primates (African green monkeys and Rhesus monkeys) also lose their spines after ovariectomy, an effect that is reversed by estrogen-replacement therapy (Leranth et al., 2002; Hao et al., 2003). Curiously, hippocampal CA1 neurons in ovariectomized mice of the C57BL/6J strain commonly used for genetic knockout and transgenic approaches did not exhibit changes in spine density after estrogen exposure, although the proportion of their mushroom Type-II spines was increased (Li et al., 2004). Since mushroom spines are thought to represent 'potentiated' spines (Kasai et al., 2003), these observations suggest a role of estrogen in dendritic spine structural plasticity during activity-dependent synaptic potentiation.

The changes in spine density induced experimentally by estradiol or during the estrous cycle were accompanied by increases in the binding sites for NMDARs (Weiland, 1992), enhanced immunofluorescence of the NR1 receptor subunit (Gazzaley et al., 1996), upregulation of NMDAR-mediated synaptic potentials (Woolley et al., 1997; Foy et al., 1999), and enhanced synaptic NMDAR-mediated Ca^{2+} elevations in spines of CA1 pyramidal neurons (Pozzo-Miller et al., 1999b). This enhancement of NMDAR-mediated synaptic transmission has consequences for long-term synaptic plasticity. Indeed, the likelihood for the induction of LTP is elevated at proestrous (when estradiol is highest) (Warren et al., 1995) and by estradiol treatment *in vivo* (Cordoba Montoya and Carrer, 1997), as well as in acute brain slices (Foy et al., 1999). The functional consequences of estradiol-replacement therapy in ovariectomized rats may also involve changes in the ratio of NMDAR-to AMPAR-mediated synaptic responses (Smith and McMahon, 2005). In these experiments, the magnitude of LTP after estradiol treatment was larger only when spine density increased simultaneously with an elevation in NMDAR transmission relative to AMPAR transmission, suggesting that the increase in functional synapse density alone is not sufficient to support heightened plasticity. Rather, estradiol may increase LTP via enhancing NMDAR transmission, likely through receptor insertion into newly formed or preexisting synapses. The mechanisms of estradiol action leading to spine formation resemble other forms of activity-dependent plasticity due to the requirement of NMDARs (Woolley and McEwen, 1994; Murphy and Segal, 1996), as well as activation of cyclic adenosine monophosphate (cAMP) response element binding protein (CREB) and CREB binding protein (CBP) (Murphy and Segal, 1997).

Parallel to these cellular and molecular studies, clinical studies in postmenopausal women receiving estrogen-replacement therapy initially reported improvements in mood and cognitive functions (Sherwin, 1996), although some lingering issues remain unanswered (Sherwin, 2005). The similarities in downstream signaling and cellular effects between ovarian hormones and neurotrophins such as BDNF

(Toran-Allerand, 1996) have suggested a potential neuroprotective role for estrogens in age-related memory loss and Alzheimer's disease dementia (Gibbs and Aggarwal, 1998; Lee and McEwen, 2001). BDNF is a polypeptide related to nerve growth factor (NGF) that has been shown to provide neurotrophic support for cholinergic (Knusel et al., 1992; Widmer et al., 1993), serotonergic (Mamounas et al., 1995), and dopaminergic (Hyman et al., 1994; Yurek et al., 1996) neurons. Thus, BDNF may influence hippocampal function by maintaining the innervation of one or more of these neurotransmitter systems. In addition, the expression of BDNF mRNA in the hippocampus fluctuates during the estrous cycle and is increased after estrogen replacement in ovariectomized rats (Gibbs, 1998). Hence, increases in BDNF expression following estrogen treatment may help to enhance and maintain proper hippocampal function. However, estradiol was shown to downregulate BDNF levels in cultured hippocampal neurons, leading to spine formation by reduced GABAergic inhibition and increased excitation (Murphy et al., 1998). BDNF itself blocked the effects of estradiol on spine formation, and BDNF depletion with selective antisense oligonucleotides or with anti-BDNF antibodies mimicked the effects of estradiol, increasing spine density (Murphy et al., 1998). As we shall see in the next section, the interplay between estrogen and BDNF may be more complex than initially proposed. We next discuss the actions of BDNF on the structure and function of hippocampal neurons, with particular attention to dendritic spines and their role in synaptic plasticity.

13.7.2 Brain-Derived Neurotrophic Factor

Neurotrophins are secretory proteins involved in neuronal survival and differentiation (Barde, 1989). Four neurotrophins have been identified in mammals, and all are widely expressed in the CNS: NGF, BDNF, neurotrophin-3 (NT3), and NT4/5 (Lewin and Barde, 1996). They exert their effects by binding to pan-neurotrophin $p75^{NTR}$ receptors and to specific tyrosine kinase receptors, members of the *trk* family of proto-oncogenes related to insulin and epidermal growth factor receptors (Barbacid, 1993). NGF binds selectively to tyrosine kinase A (TrkA), BDNF and NT4/5 to TrkB, and NT3 to TrkC and, with a lower affinity, to TrkB as well (Chao, 1992). Binding of a neurotrophin to a specific Trk receptor stimulates its kinase activity, leading to the activation of phosphatidylinositol 3-kinase (PI3K), mitogen-activated protein kinase (MAPK, also known as ERK), and phospholipase C-γ (PLC-γ) (Segal and Greenberg, 1996; Huang and Reichardt, 2003). Interaction of neurotrophins with $p75^{NTR}$ results in the activation of different signaling cascades mostly involved in the regulation of cell fate, such as nuclear factor kappa B (NF-κB) or c-*jun* N-terminal kinase (Kaplan and Miller, 2000). In addition to their well-established role in neuronal survival and differentiation during development, neurotrophins are strong candidates for providing the molecular signaling pathways that mediate the complex interactions between internal developmental programs and external environmental factors, ultimately leading to the appropriate development of dendrites and synapses (McAllister et al., 1999). Furthermore, BDNF has recently emerged as a fundamental modulator of hippocampal function, where its levels are amongst the highest in the brain (Murer et al., 2001). Together with the dendritic localization of GFP-tagged BDNF to dendritic process in cultured hippocampal neurons (Hartmann et al., 2001; Kojima et al., 2001; Brigadski et al., 2005), the significant release of native (i.e., endogenous) BDNF in response to stimulus patterns most amenable for LTP induction (Balkowiec and Katz, 2002; Gartner and Staiger, 2002; Aicardi et al., 2004) strongly supports the role of this prominent neurotrophin in activity-dependent functional and structural plasticity of hippocampal synapses. In the remaining paragraphs of this chapter we will focus on the morphological actions of BDNF, as its role in hippocampal synaptic transmission and plasticity in the context of learning and memory has been extensively reviewed (Lo, 1995; Thoenen, 1995, 2000; Black, 1999; Schinder and Poo, 2000; Poo, 2001; Tyler et al., 2002a,b; Vicario-Abejon et al., 2002; Lu, 2003; Bramham and Messaoudi, 2005).

Neurotrophins were shown to increase the length and complexity of dendrites of cortical pyramidal neurons when applied to slice cultures of ferret visual cortex (McAllister et al., 1995). Cortical pyramidal neurons in slice cultures treated with Trk 'receptor-bodies' to scavenge endogenous neurotrophins showed limited dendritic growth and even dendritic retraction (McAllister et al., 1997), confirming that endogenous neurotrophins play a critical role in dendritic development. In addition, cortical pyramidal neurons that overexpress BDNF exhibit increased dendritic arborization, as well as enhanced rates of spine retraction and formation (Horch et al., 1999; Horch and Katz, 2002). More relevant to hippocampal function, BDNF increases spine density in CA1 pyramidal neurons, an effect blocked by the scavenger TrkB-immunoglobulin G, the receptor tyrosine kinase inhibitor k-252a, and inhibitors of the MAPK/ERK signaling cascade (Tyler and Pozzo-Miller, 2001; Alonso et al., 2004). Sustained Ca^{2+} elevations set off by BDNF-induced Ca^{2+} mobilization from inositol triphosphate (IP_3)-sensitive intracellular stores followed by transient receptor potential, canonical subfamily (TRPC)-mediated capacitative Ca^{2+} entry (Amaral and Pozzo-Miller, 2005) may play a critical role in BDNF-induced increase in spine density. Indeed, inhibition or siRNA-mediated knockdown of TRPC channels prevented not only the BDNF-induced sustained depolarization and dendritic Ca^{2+} elevation, but also the increase in spine density (Amaral and Pozzo-Miller, 2007). Moreover, the BDNF-induced structural remodeling of spiny dendrites of CA1 pyramidal neurons has consequences for Ca^{2+} signals evoked by coincident pre- and postsynaptic activity. Dendritic Ca^{2+} signals evoked by coincident excitatory postsynaptic potentials (EPSPs) and backpropagating action potentials (bAPs) were always larger than those triggered by bAPs in CA1 neurons exposed to BDNF (Pozzo-Miller, 2006), representing a potential consequence of neurotrophin-mediated dendritic remodeling of hippocampal neurons. BDNF promoted spine formation also in granule cells of the dentate gyrus (Danzer et al., 2002) and in cultured hippocampal neurons, where the effect was 'gated' by cAMP (Ji et al., 2005); but see earlier discussion of the opposite effect of BDNF in the context of estradiol-induced spine formation reported by Murphy et al. (1998).

In addition to increasing spine density *per se*, BDNF also increased the proportion of stubby spines (Type-I) under conditions of *both* action potential-dependent *and* independent synaptic transmission (Tyler and Pozzo-Miller, 2003). Even when SNARE (soluble N-ethylmaleimide-sensitive-factor attachment protein receptor)-dependent vesicular synaptic transmission was abolished with *Botulinum* neurotoxin C, BDNF was still capable of inducing spine formation. Under these conditions, however, BDNF selectively increased the proportion of thin spines (Type-III), while decreasing the proportion of stubby spines (Type-I). Consistent with an activity-dependent process of morphological differentiation of synapses, the effects of BDNF on hippocampal spines suggest that it cooperates with spontaneous miniature synaptic activity to sculpt the fine structure of CA1 pyramidal neurons in the postnatal hippocampus. Since BDNF also increases quantal transmitter release from presynaptic terminals (Tyler and Pozzo-Miller, 2001; Tyler et al., 2002b; Tyler et al., 2006), its role in spine growth and their morphological sculpting spans the synaptic cleft.

The activation of membrane-bound $p75^{NTR}$ and Trk receptors by neurotrophin binding – in addition to physical interactions between them – organizes precise signaling cascades that control their varied actions throughout development, such as cell survival, differentiation, neurite outgrowth, and synaptic function (Patapoutian and Reichardt, 2001; Hempstead, 2002; Roux and Barker, 2002; Chao, 2003; Huang and Reichardt, 2003; Nykjaer et al., 2005). Recent observations regarding the differential role of the two types of membrane receptors have uncovered an intriguing level of complexity in neurotrophin signaling, namely opposing functional actions of $p75^{NTR}$ and Trk receptors (Lu et al., 2005). For example, while Trk receptors are essential for neuronal survival, $p75^{NTR}$ has been implicated in neuronal death. Similarly, $p75^{NTR}$ signaling has been linked to the inhibition of axonal growth, an opposing effect to that of Trk receptors. Lastly, while TrkB receptors have been shown to be critical for the role of BDNF in hippocampal LTP (Minichiello et al., 1999, 2002; Xu et al., 2000), recent reports indicate that $p75^{NTR}$ is necessary for the induction and/or expression of hippocampal LTD (Rosch et al., 2005; Woo et al., 2005). With regard to dendritic organization, $p75^{NTR}$ and Trk receptors also seem to have functional antagonisms. TrkB activity has been shown to modulate dendritic growth (Yacoubian and Lo, 2000), while a recent report using $p75^{NTR}$ knockout and $p75^{NTR}$ overexpressing mice indicates that these receptors negatively modulate dendritic morphology in hippocampal pyramidal neurons (Zagrebelsky et al., 2005), further strengthening the 'yin and yang' model of functional antagonism between Trk and $p75^{NTR}$ signaling (Lu et al., 2005).

What is the contribution of these receptors to BDNF-induced changes in spine morphology and density? It is tempting to extend the 'yin and yang' model of functional antagonism also to the modulation of spine number and form. Indeed, dendritic spine density in hippocampal pyramidal neurons was higher in $p75^{NTR}$ knockout mice, which also showed a reduction in the proportion of stubby (Type-I) spines (Zagrebelsky et al., 2005). On the other hand, mice with a conditional deletion of the TrkB receptor have reduced spine density and a higher proportion of long spines (Luikart et al., 2005; von Bohlen und Halbach et al., 2006). In addition, the proportion of stubby (Type-I) spines was reduced in CA1 pyramidal neurons of adult transgenic mice expressing a dominant-negative TrkB (Chakravarthy et al., 2006). Intriguingly, brief exposures to k-252a, an inhibitor of receptor tyrosine kinases such as TrkS, caused a significant increase in spine density in CA1 pyramidal neurons expressing enhanced yellow fluorescent protein (eYFP) (Chapleau and Pozzo-Miller, unpublished data). However, most of these spines are of the long and thin Type-III, known to be highly motile and unstable structures (Dailey and Smith, 1996; Dunaevsky et al., 1999) and characteristic of immature synapses (Sorra and Harris, 2000). The fact that longer exposures to k-252a by itself caused spine loss (Tyler and Pozzo-Miller, 2001; Alonso et al., 2004) suggests that an initial increase in long and thin spines may precede spine regression leading to spine pruning (Segal et al., 2000). Alternatively, these observations may reflect the functional antagonism between $p75^{NTR}$ and Trk receptor signaling for dendritic spine formation and maintenance (Lu et al., 2005). In this interpretation, preferential activation of $p75^{NTR}$ by spontaneously released BDNF under conditions of Trk receptor inhibition (i.e., in the presence of k252a) leads to an initial and transient increase in thin and unstable spines, followed by a persistent spine loss. Further complexity was uncovered by the outgrowth of dendritic filopodia through the interaction of the truncated TrkB receptor (TrkB.T1) with $p75^{NTR}$, intriguingly enough, in the absence of neurotrophin binding (Hartmann et al., 2004). The combination of all these structural and physiological effects in the hippocampus may underlie the role of BDNF in the consolidation of synaptic plasticity and hippocampal-dependent learning and memory (Tyler et al., 2002a; Bramham and Messaoudi, 2005).

13.8 BDNF, MeCP2, and Dendritic Spine Pathologies in Rett Syndrome

Neurological disorders associated with mental retardation (MR) are characterized by a prevalent deficit in cognitive function and adaptive behavior that range in phenotype severity and are often accompanied by specific symptoms. MR-associated disorders that have environmental, neurodegenerative, or genetic origins have long been associated with structural anomalies of dendritic spines that are a common feature of various neurological disorders (Fiala et al., 2002). The pioneering studies by Huttenlocher (1970, 1974), Marin-Padilla (1972b, 1976), and Purpura (1974, 1975a) described strikingly similar abnormalities in the dendritic organization of cortical neurons from human patients with unclassified MR-associated disorders. Pyramidal neurons of the cerebral cortex showed a reduction in the number and length of dendritic branches, a significant loss of dendritic spines, and a predominance of long 'tortuous' spines. Interestingly, no other neuropathologies were found in these patients. Since then, similar features of dendritic branching, as well as spine density and morphology, have been described in other MR-associated genetic developmental disorders, ranging from autosomal genetic forms of MR (e.g., Down syndrome, Angelman syndrome) to X chromosome–linked forms of MR (e.g., Rett syndrome, fragile X syndrome) (Kaufmann and Moser, 2000; Fiala et al., 2002; Newey et al., 2005). Thus, it seems that dendritic and spine anomalies are the major brain pathologies underlying the cognitive impairments observed in humans with MR, because such dendritic and spine changes will reduce postsynaptic surface area and the density of mature excitatory synapses.

One MR-associated disorder with an intriguing link to BDNF signaling is Rett syndrome (RTT) (*See also* Chapter 36). RTT is an X-linked neurodevelopmental disorder and the leading cause of severe mental retardation in females, affecting 1:10,000–20,000 births worldwide without predisposition to a particular racial or ethnic group (Percy, 2002; Neul and Zoghbi, 2004). Patients with RTT are born healthy and achieve standard developmental milestones until 6–18 months of age, when they begin a regression period associated with loss of acquired cognitive, social, and motor skills (Armstrong, 1997). Later symptoms and deficits include irregularities in motor activity, characterized by a stereotypic hand movement or useless hand movements, altered breathing patterns, gait and motor imbalance, and continued cognitive decline. As the period of regression concludes, the individuals are often left in a severely impaired condition, with a majority of children developing seizure activity, although seizure frequency diminishes with age. As the children get older, a period of stabilization occurs where they develop greater communication abilities with their eyes, yet motor function continues to regress gradually (Percy and Lane, 2005). Loss-of-function mutations in the gene encoding methyl-CpG-binding protein 2 (MeCP2) have been recently identified in RTT patients (Amir et al., 1999). MeCP2 binds specifically to CpG-methylated DNA and is thought to inhibit gene transcription by recruiting corepressor and histone deacetylase complexes and altering the structure of genomic DNA (Nan et al., 1998). Because other neurodevelopmental disorders with autistic features have also been associated with MeCP2 dysfunction, the role of MeCP2 in neuronal function may extend beyond RTT (Percy, 2002). Intriguingly, one of the targets of MeCP2-mediated transcriptional repression is the gene encoding BDNF, whereby MeCP2 binds to and represses the transcription of the promoter region of the *BDNF* gene (Chen et al., 2003; Martinowich et al., 2003).

The neuropathology of RTT reveals several areas of abnormal brain development (Armstrong et al., 1995; Bauman et al., 1995a,b). Several studies reported abnormal dendritic structure in the frontal cortex (Jellinger et al., 1988), and pyramidal neuron dendritic area and growth are significantly decreased in the frontal and motor cortices, as well as in the *subiculum*, while dendritic length was not affected in the hippocampus (Armstrong et al., 1995). Another group reported a similar dendritic appearance; in addition, they observed a thickening of dendrites (Cornford et al., 1994). Finally, a reduction in the levels of microtubule-associated protein-2 (MAP-2), a dendritic protein involved in microtubule stabilization, was found throughout the neocortex of RTT brains (Kaufmann et al., 1995, 2000). Relevant to the role of neurotrophins in dendritic spine formation and maturation, RTT brains have reduced spine density in dendrites of the frontal cortex (Belichenko et al., 1994). In addition, the levels of cyclooxygenase-2, a protein enriched in dendritic spines, are reduced in the frontal cortex in RTT (Kaufmann et al., 1997). With regard to synapse density, reduced levels of the synaptic vesicle protein synaptophysin were detected in the motor, frontal, and temporal cortices by immunofluorescence (Belichenko et al., 1997), although another study reported unaltered synaptophysin levels in frontal cortex and cerebellum (Cornford et al., 1994).

To further the understanding of RTT, a number of different mouse models have been generated, either carrying a null deletion of *MECP2* (Chen et al., 2001; Guy et al., 2001) or expressing a truncated, nonfunctional form of the wild-type MeCP2 protein (*MECP2^{308}*) (Shahbazian et al., 2002). These mice have common phenotypes, including delayed onset of symptoms (at approximately 5 weeks of age) and motor impairment and abnormal gait, whereby the null *MECP2* mice have hindlimb irregularities, while the *MECP2^{308}* mice have forelimb impairment (Shahbazian and Zoghbi, 2002; Armstrong, 2005). In addition, null *MECP2* mice have altered synaptic transmission and plasticity, including impaired hippocampal LTP (Asaka et al., 2006), and reduced excitatory transmission in the hippocampus (Nelson et al., 2006) and neocortex (Dani et al., 2005). Deficits in hippocampal LTP and hippocampal-dependent learning and memory were also observed in the *MECP2^{308}* mice expressing the truncated protein (Moretti et al., 2006). On the other hand, transgenic mice that mildly overexpress wild-type MeCP2 (~2 times wild-type levels) display a higher rate of hippocampal-dependent learning and enhanced LTP, though they developed a neurological phenotype that included seizures after 20 weeks of age (Collins et al., 2004).

Intriguingly, observations regarding neuronal and synaptic morphology in these mouse models of RTT have produced varying results, sometimes inconsistent with the neuropathology found in RTT patients (Armstrong et al., 1995; Bauman et al., 1995a,b). Pyramidal neurons of layer II/III of the neocortex of null *MECP2* hemizygous mice (MECP2$^{-/y}$) are smaller and have reduced dendritic branching as observed in RTT brains, although no differences were found in dendritic spine density (Kishi and Macklis, 2004), a distinctive feature observed in one study of the cortex of RTT patients (Belichenko et al., 1994). Another study of the somatosensory cortex of null *MECP2* hemizygous mice (MECP2$^{-/y}$) reported that dendrites of layer II/III neurons were thinner and had fewer spines than those of wild-type littermates (Fukuda et al., 2005). On the other hand, transient overexpression of wildtype MeCP2 in cultured cortical neurons led to a significant increase in dendritic and axonal length and arborization, while neurons overexpressing a nonfunctional, truncated form of MeCP2 (*MECP2^{293}*) only showed increases in dendritic and axonal branching (Jugloff et al., 2005). Quantitative analyses of dendritic morphology in neurons from layers III and V of the frontal cortex of *MECP2^{308}* mice, which express a truncated *MECP2* allele, reported no major abnormalities in dendritic branching (Moretti et al., 2006). Further analyses at the EM level in area CA1 of the hippocampus yielded no differences in the density of asymmetric synapses and in the number of synaptic vesicles, either docked at the active zone or in the main vesicle cluster within the terminals. However, the mean length of the PSD was smaller in *MECP2^{308}* mice, driven by a concomitant increase in the smaller PSDs and a decrease in the larger ones (>150 nm) (Moretti et al., 2006). Since the size of the active zone is tightly correlated with the size of the PSD across the synaptic cleft (Harris and Sultan, 1995; Boyer et al., 1998; Schikorski and Stevens, 1999), the observation of smaller PSDs and similar numbers of docked vesicles in the *MECP2*^{308} mice suggests that the density of docked vesicles is increased in the mutant active zone. These apparent discrepancies clearly warrant further investigations of the role of wild-type and mutant MeCP2 on dendritic and synaptic morphology in specific brain regions as a potential underlying mechanism for the functional impairments observed in animal models and RTT patients.

The molecular pathways contributing to the pathogenesis of Rett syndrome remain unclear. Considering that the best-characterized function of MeCP2 is as transcriptional repressor, numerous gene expression profiles have been conducted on RTT patients and in the available mouse models of RTT (Colantuoni et al., 2001; Tudor et al., 2002; Ballestar et al., 2005; Nuber et al., 2005; Delgado et al., 2006). However, these studies identified several genes that are either upregulated or downregulated, but their contribution to the disease remains unknown. A more targeted approach, such as chromatin immunoprecipitation, has identified the promoter region of the *BDNF* gene as a target of MeCP2 transcriptional control (Chen et al., 2003; Martinowich et al., 2003). These studies demonstrated that MeCP2 binds to and represses the transcription of mouse *BDNF* promoter IV, equivalent to the rat *BDNF* III promoter, which is well known to be activated by neuronal activity and the ensuing voltage-gated Ca^{2+} influx (Tao et al., 1998). As expected, the levels of *BDNF* exon IV transcript were low in cultured cortical neurons from wildtype mice in the absence of neuronal activity (i.e., in the presence of tetrodotoxin, TTX). On the other hand, neurons from *MECP2* null mice showed a twofold increase in their basal levels of *BDNF* exon IV transcript, as predicted from its transcriptional repressor function. Furthermore, *BDNF* exon IV transcript levels induced by a strong depolarizing stimulus (i.e., KCl) were similar between control and mutant cells, due to the large increase observed in wild-type neurons and the already elevated levels in *MECP2* null neurons, which were unresponsive to KCl depolarization (Chen et al., 2003). Considering that BDNF is a positive modulator of excitatory synaptic function (Thoenen, 2000; Poo, 2001; Tyler et al., 2002a,b; Lu, 2003; Bramham and Messaoudi, 2005), the observation of elevated BDNF levels (at least in terms of its activity-dependent mRNA transcripts) was unexpected and somewhat puzzling. However, BDNF protein levels measured by enzyme-linked immunosorbent assay (ELISA) were found to be lower in brain samples of *MECP2* null mice at 6–8 weeks of age compared to wild-type controls, a difference not observed at 2 weeks (Chang et al., 2006). In addition, conditional deletion of the *BDNF* gene in *MECP2* null mice exacerbated the onset of the RTT-associated phenotypes of the *MECP2* null animals, which included hypoactivity in the running wheel and reduced action potential frequency in pyramidal neurons of acute cortical slices *in vitro*. Surprisingly, overexpression of *BDNF* slowed down the disease progression in *MECP2* null mice, with increased wheel running behavior and augmented action potential firing in cortical neurons (Chang et al., 2006). Since BDNF mRNA and protein levels are tightly regulated by neuronal activity, the reduced firing frequency of neurons from *MECP2* null mice (Dani et al., 2005) may cause the reduced BDNF protein levels measured by ELISA (Chang et al., 2006). The discrepancy between the elevated basal levels of *BDNF* exon IV transcripts in cultured *MECP2* neurons (Chen et al., 2003) and the reduced BDNF protein levels in *MECP2* brain tissue (Chang et al., 2006) likely originates from different basal conditions (TTX in culture vs. naive fresh brain samples), developmental age (embryonic vs. postnatal), or the modulation of mRNA translation into protein. Whether direct or indirect, the relationship between MeCP2 function and BDNF-mediated signaling seems potentially relevant to the speculated impairments in Rett syndrome, especially with regard to synaptic function (Dani et al., 2005; Asaka et al., 2006; Moretti et al., 2006; Nelson et al., 2006).

Unfortunately, the few available studies of neurotrophin levels in RTT patients have not yielded results consistent with the 'BDNF hypothesis of Rett,' at least at a first approximation. First, reduced NGF levels were observed in cerebrospinal fluid (CSF) of RTT patients, a difference not found in blood serum levels, while BDNF was unaffected in CSF or blood serum RTT samples (Lappalainen et al., 1996; Vanhala et al., 1998; Riikonen and Vanhala, 1999; Riikonen, 2003). Second, the expression levels of NGF and its receptor TrkA were reduced in postmortem RTT brains, as assessed by immunohistochemistry (Lipani et al., 2000), while the number of basal forebrain neurons expressing $p75^{NTR}$ was unaffected in RTT brains (Wenk and Hauss-Wegrzyniak, 1999). Third, NGF serum levels tend to decrease with age in RTT patients, opposite to the characteristic developmental increase in healthy individuals (Calamandrei et al., 2001). Taken together, these few reports reveal our incomplete understanding of the potential and intriguing role of neurotrophin signaling in the pathogenesis of Rett syndrome. Furthermore, they underscore the need for further cellular and molecular studies, perhaps at the single-cell level, of the consequences of mutant MeCP2 expression on neurotrophin expression, targeting, and/or release, as well as signaling through its $p75^{NTR}$ and Trk receptors.

13.9 Final Considerations

The observations reviewed in this chapter provide strong evidence that dendritic spines are highly specialized neuronal compartments that are exquisitely tuned to sense ongoing and fluctuating levels of afferent synaptic activity, which likely play a fundamental role in synaptic integration and plasticity. However, most of the experimental evidence is so far correlative: for example, while LTP or behavioral learning cause structural changes, those changes may not contribute to the synaptic potentiation or the formation of the engram. On the other hand, the new spines formed after LTP induction may not initially participate in synaptic transmission, but rather may be the sites of future synaptic plasticity (i.e., NMDA-only silent synapses). In any case, dendritic spines are prime examples that function affects structure and vice versa in a global and ongoing homeostatic balance (i.e., negative feedback), which can be locally modified by rapid 'Hebbian' positive-feedback changes. After more than a century of their discovery and the speculation that 'mental exercise' may promote their formation and growth, dendritic spines still represent a truly fascinating 'thorny' issue in our quest for the neurobiological basis of learning and memory.

Acknowledgments

The work from the Pozzo-Miller lab discussed here was supported by NIH grants NS40593 (LP-M), P30-HD38985 (UAB Mental Retardation Research Center), the Evelyn F. McKnight Brain Research Foundation, and the Civitan International Foundation. LP-M is a McNulty Civitan Scientist.

References

Abel T and Lattal KM (2001) Molecular mechanisms of memory acquisition, consolidation and retrieval. *Curr. Opin. Neurobiol.* 11: 180–187.

Aicardi G, Argilli E, Cappello S, et al. (2004) Induction of long-term potentiation and depression is reflected by corresponding changes in secretion of endogenous brain-derived neurotrophic factor. *Proc. Natl. Acad. Sci. USA* 101: 15788–15792.

Alonso M, Medina JH, and Pozzo-Miller L (2004) ERK1/2 activation is necessary for BDNF to increase dendritic spine density in hippocampal CA1 pyramidal neurons. *Learn. Mem.* 11: 172–178.

Amaral MD and Pozzo-Miller L (2005) On the role of neurotrophins in dendritic calcium signaling: Implications for hippocampal transsynaptic plasticity. Stanton PK, Bramham CR, and Scharfman HE (eds.) *Synaptic Plasticity and Transsynaptic Signaling*, pp. 185–200. New York: Springer Science and Business Media.

Amaral MD and Pozzo-Miller L (2007) TRPC3 channels are necessary for brain-derived neurotrophic factor to activate a non-selective cationic current and to induce dendritic spine formation. *J. Neurosci.* 27: 5179–5189.

Amir RE, Van den Veyver IB, Wan M, Tran CQ, Francke U, and Zoghbi HY (1999) Rett syndrome is caused by mutations in X-linked MECP2, encoding methyl-CpG-binding protein 2. *Nat. Genet.* 23: 185–188.

Armstrong D, Dunn JK, Antalffy B, and Trivedi R (1995) Selective dendritic alterations in the cortex of Rett syndrome. *J. Neuropathol. Exp. Neurol.* 54: 195–201.

Armstrong DD (1997) Review of Rett syndrome. *J. Neuropathol. Exp. Neurol.* 56: 843–849.

Armstrong DD (2005) Can we relate MeCP2 deficiency to the structural and chemical abnormalities in the Rett brain? *Brain Dev.* 27(supplement 1): S72–S76.

Arnold AP and Gorski RA (1984) Gonadal steroid induction of structural sex differences in the central nervous system. *Annu. Rev. Neurosci.* 7: 413–442.

Asaka Y, Jugloff DG, Zhang L, Eubanks JH, and Fitzsimonds RM (2006) Hippocampal synaptic plasticity is impaired in the Mecp2-null mouse model of Rett syndrome. *Neurobiol. Dis.* 21: 217–227.

Bagal AA, Kao JP, Tang CM, and Thompson SM (2005) Long-term potentiation of exogenous glutamate responses at single dendritic spines. *Proc. Natl. Acad. Sci. USA* 102: 14434–14439.

Bailey CH and Kandel ER (1993) Structural changes accompanying memory storage. *Annu. Rev. Physiol.* 55: 397–426.

Bain A (1872) *Mind and Body: The Theories of Their Relation*. London: Henry S. King.

Balkowiec A and Katz DM (2002) Cellular mechanisms regulating activity-dependent release of native brain-derived neurotrophic factor from hippocampal neurons. *J. Neurosci.* 22: 10399–10407.

Ballestar E, Ropero S, Alaminos M, et al. (2005) The impact of MECP2 mutations in the expression patterns of Rett syndrome patients. *Hum. Genet.* 116: 91–104.

Barbacid M (1993) Nerve growth factor: A tale of two receptors. *Oncogene* 8: 2033–2042.

Barde YA (1989) Trophic factors, and neuronal survival. *Neuron* 2: 1525–1534.

Bauman ML, Kemper TL, and Arin DM (1995a) Microscopic observations of the brain in Rett syndrome. *Neuropediatrics* 26: 105–108.

Bauman ML, Kemper TL, and Arin DM (1995b) Pervasive neuroanatomic abnormalities of the brain in three cases of Rett's syndrome. *Neurology* 45: 1581–1586.

Belichenko PV, Hagberg B and Dahlstrom A (1997) Morphological study of neocortical areas in Rett syndrome. *Acta Neuropathol. (Berl.)* 93: 50–61.

Belichenko PV, Oldfors A, Hagberg B, and Dahlstrom A (1994) Rett syndrome: 3-D confocal microscopy of cortical pyramidal dendrites, and afferents. *Neuroreport* 5: 1509–1513.

Berridge MJ (1998) Neuronal calcium signaling. *Neuron* 21: 13–26.

Black IB (1999) Trophic regulation of synaptic plasticity. *J. Neurobiol.* 41: 108–118.

Bliss TV and Collingridge GL (1993) A synaptic model of memory: Long-term potentiation in the hippocampus. *Nature* 361: 31–39.

Bliss TV and Lomo T (1973) Long-lasting potentiation of synaptic transmission in the dentate area of the anaesthetized rabbit following stimulation of the perforant path. *J. Physiol.* 232: 331–356.

Bloodgood BL and Sabatini BL (2005) Neuronal activity regulates diffusion across the neck of dendritic spines. *Science* 310: 866–869.

Bourne JN, Kirov SA, Sorra KE, and Harris KM (2006) Warmer preparation of hippocampal slices prevents synapse proliferation that might obscure LTP-related structural plasticity. *Neuropharmacology* 52: 55–59.

Boyer C, Schikorski T, and Stevens CF (1998) Comparison of hippocampal dendritic spines in culture, and in brain. *J. Neurosci.* 18: 5294–5300.

Bramham CR and Messaoudi E (2005) BDNF function in adult synaptic plasticity: The synaptic consolidation hypothesis. *Prog. Neurobiol.* 76: 99–125.

Brigadski T, Hartmann M, and Lessmann V (2005) Differential vesicular targeting and time course of synaptic secretion of the mammalian neurotrophins. *J. Neurosci.* 25: 7601–7614.

Buchs PA and Muller D (1996) Induction of long-term potentiation is associated with major ultrastructural changes of activated synapses. *Proc. Natl. Acad. Sci. USA* 93: 8040–8045.

Buchs PA, Stoppini L, Parducz A, Siklos L, and Muller D (1994) A new cytochemical method for the ultrastructural localization of calcium in the central nervous system. *J. Neurosci. Methods* 54: 83–93.

Burrone J and Murthy VN (2003) Synaptic gain control and homeostasis. *Curr. Opin. Neurobiol.* 13: 560–567.

Cajal SR (1891) Sur la structure de l'ecorce cérébrale de quelques mammifères. *La Cellule* 7: 125–176.

Cajal SR (1893) Neue Darstellung vom histologischen Bau des Zentralnervensystem. *Arch. Anat. Entwick.* 319–418.

Cajal SR (1909) *Histologie du Systeme Nerveux de l'Homme et des Vertebres*. Paris: Maloine (reprinted in 1952 by Consejo Superior de Investigaciones Científicas, Instituto Ramón y Cajal, Madrid.).

Calamandrei G, Aloe L, Hajek J, and Zappella M (2001) Developmental profile of serum nerve growth factor levels in Rett complex. *Ann. Ist. Super. Sanita* 37: 601–605.

Carrer HF and Aoki A (1982) Ultrastructural changes in the hypothalamic ventromedial nucleus of ovariectomized rats after estrogen treatment. *Brain Res.* 240: 221–233.

Chakravarthy S, Saiepour MH, Bence M, et al. (2006) Postsynaptic TrkB signaling has distinct roles in spine maintenance in adult visual cortex and hippocampus. *Proc. Natl. Acad. Sci. USA* 103: 1071–1076.

Chang FL and Greenough WT (1984) Transient and enduring morphological correlates of synaptic activity and efficacy change in the rat hippocampal slice. *Brain Res.* 309: 35–46.

Chang Q, Khare G, Dani V, Nelson S, and Jaenisch R (2006) The disease progression of mecp2 mutant mice is affected by the level of BDNF expression. *Neuron* 49: 341–348.

Chao MV (1992) Neurotrophin receptors: A window into neuronal differentiation. *Neuron* 9: 583–593.

Chao MV (2003) Neurotrophins and their receptors: A convergence point for many signalling pathways. *Nat. Rev. Neurosci.* 4: 299–309.

Chen RZ, Akbarian S, Tudor M, and Jaenisch R (2001) Deficiency of methyl-CpG binding protein-2 in CNS neurons results in a Rett-like phenotype in mice. *Nat. Genet.* 27: 327–331.

Chen WG, Chang Q, Lin Y, et al. (2003) Derepression of BDNF transcription involves calcium-dependent phosphorylation of MeCP2. *Science* 302: 885–889.

Colantuoni C, Jeon OH, Hyder K, et al. (2001) Gene expression profiling in postmortem Rett Syndrome brain: Differential gene expression and patient classification. *Neurobiol. Dis.* 8: 847–865.

Collin C, Miyaguchi K, and Segal M (1997) Dendritic spine density and LTP induction in cultured hippocampal slices. *J. Neurophysiol.* 77: 1614–1623.

Collins AL, Levenson JM, Vilaythong AP, et al. (2004) Mild overexpression of MeCP2 causes a progressive neurological disorder in mice. *Hum. Mol. Genet.* 13: 2679–2689.

Connor JA, Miller LD, Petrozzino J, and Muller W (1994) Calcium signaling in dendritic spines of hippocampal neurons. *J. Neurobiol.* 25: 234–242.

Cooney JR, Hurlburt JL, Selig DK, Harris KM, and Fiala JC (2002) Endosomal compartments serve multiple hippocampal dendritic spines from a widespread rather than a local store of recycling membrane. *J. Neurosci.* 22: 2215–2224.

Cordoba Montoya DA and Carrer HF (1997) Estrogen facilitates induction of long term potentiation in the hippocampus of awake rats. *Brain Res.* 778: 430–438.

Cornford ME, Philippart M, Jacobs B, Scheibel AB, and Vinters HV (1994) Neuropathology of Rett syndrome: Case report with neuronal and mitochondrial abnormalities in the brain. *J. Child Neurol.* 9: 424–431.

Crick F (1982) Do dendritic spines twitch? *Trends Neurosci.* 5: 44.

Dailey ME and Smith SJ (1996) The dynamics of dendritic structure in developing hippocampal slices. *J. Neurosci.* 16: 2983–2994.

Dani VS, Chang Q, Maffei A, Turrigiano GG, Jaenisch R, and Nelson SB (2005) Reduced cortical activity due to a shift in the balance between excitation and inhibition in a mouse model of Rett syndrome. *Proc. Natl. Acad. Sci. USA* 102: 12560–12565.

Danzer SC, Crooks KR, Lo DC, and McNamara JO (2002) Increased expression of brain-derived neurotrophic factor induces formation of basal dendrites and axonal branching in dentate granule cells in hippocampal explant cultures. *J. Neurosci.* 22: 9754–9763.

Davis GW (2006) Homeostatic control of neural activity: From phenomenology to molecular design. *Annu. Rev. Neurosci.* 29: 307–323.

Davis GW and Bezprozvanny I (2001) Maintaining the stability of neural function: A homeostatic hypothesis. *Annu. Rev. Physiol.* 63: 847–869.

Delgado IJ, Kim DS, Thatcher KN, LaSalle JM, and Van den Veyver IB (2006) Expression profiling of clonal lymphocyte cell cultures from Rett syndrome patients. *BMC Med. Genet.* 7: 61.

Denk W and Svoboda K (1997) Photon upmanship: Why multiphoton imaging is more than a gimmick. *Neuron* 18: 351–357.

Desmond NL and Levy WB (1983) Synaptic correlates of associative potentiation/depression: An ultrastructural study in the hippocampus. *Brain Res.* 265: 21–30.

Desmond NL and Levy WB (1986a) Changes in the numerical density of synaptic contacts with long-term potentiation in the hippocampal dentate gyrus. *J. Comp. Neurol.* 253: 466–475.

Desmond NL and Levy WB (1986b) Changes in the postsynaptic density with long-term potentiation in the dentate gyrus. *J. Comp. Neurol.* 253: 476–482.

Desmond NL and Levy WB (1990) Morphological correlates of long-term potentiation imply the modification of existing synapses, not synaptogenesis, in the hippocampal dentate gyrus. *Synapse* 5: 139–143.

Dhanrajan TM, Lynch MA, Kelly A, Popov VI, Rusakov DA, and Stewart MG (2004) Expression of long-term potentiation in aged rats involves perforated synapses but dendritic spine branching results from high-frequency stimulation alone. *Hippocampus* 14: 255–264.

Dudek SM and Bear MF (1992) Homosynaptic long-term depression in area CA1 of hippocampus and effects of NMDA receptor blockade. *Proc. Natl. Acad. Sci. USA* 89: 4363–4367.

Dunaevsky A and Mason CA (2003) Spine motility: A means towards an end? *Trends Neurosci.* 26: 155–160.

Dunaevsky A, Tashiro A, Majewska A, Mason C, and Yuste R (1999) Developmental regulation of spine motility in the mammalian central nervous system. *Proc. Natl. Acad. Sci. USA* 96: 13438–13443.

Engert F and Bonhoeffer T (1999) Dendritic spine changes associated with hippocampal long-term synaptic plasticity. *Nature* 399: 66–70.

Eyre MD, Richter-Levin G, Avital A, and Stewart MG (2003) Morphological changes in hippocampal dentate gyrus synapses following spatial learning in rats are transient. *Eur. J. Neurosci.* 17: 1973–1980.

Fiala JC, Feinberg M, Popov V, and Harris KM (1998) Synaptogenesis via dendritic filopodia in developing hippocampal area CA1. *J. Neurosci.* 18: 8900–8911.

Fiala JC, Spacek J and Harris KM (2002) Dendritic spine pathology: Cause or consequence of neurological disorders? *Brain Res. Brain Res. Rev.* 39: 29–54.

Fifkova E and Anderson CL (1981) Stimulation-induced changes in dimensions of stalks of dendritic spines in the dentate molecular layer. *Exp. Neurol.* 74: 621–627.

Fifkova E and Delay RJ (1982) Cytoplasmic actin in neuronal processes as a possible mediator of synaptic plasticity. *J. Cell Biol.* 95: 345–350.

Fifkova E and Van Harreveld A (1977) Long-lasting morphological changes in dendritic spines of dentate granular cells following stimulation of the entorhinal area. *J. Neurocytol.* 6: 211–230.

Fischer M, Kaech S, Knutti D, and Matus A (1998) Rapid actin-based plasticity in dendritic spines. *Neuron* 20: 847–854.

Foster M and Sherringhton CS (1897) *A Text Book of Physiology. Part III. The Central Nervous System*. London: Macmillan.

Foy MR, Xu J, Xie X, Brinton RD, Thompson RF, and Berger TW (1999) 17beta-estradiol enhances NMDA receptor-mediated EPSPs and long-term potentiation. *J. Neurophysiol.* 81: 925–929.

Frankfurt M, Gould E, Woolley CS, and McEwen BS (1990) Gonadal steroids modify dendritic spine density in ventromedial hypothalamic neurons: A Golgi study in the adult rat. *Neuroendocrinology* 51: 530–535.

Fukuda T, Itoh M, Ichikawa T, Washiyama K, and Goto Y (2005) Delayed maturation of neuronal architecture and synaptogenesis in cerebral cortex of Mecp2-deficient mice. *J. Neuropathol. Exp. Neurol.* 64: 537–544.

Gahwiler BH (1981) Organotypic monolayer cultures of nervous tissue. *J. Neurosci. Methods* 4: 329–342.

Gartner A and Staiger V (2002) Neurotrophin secretion from hippocampal neurons evoked by long-term-potentiation-inducing electrical stimulation patterns. *Proc. Natl. Acad. Sci. USA* 99: 6386–6391.

Gazzaley AH, Weiland NG, McEwen BS, and Morrison JH (1996) Differential regulation of NMDA R1 mRNA and protein by estradiol in the rat hippocampus. *J. Neurosci.* 16: 6830–6838.

Geinisman Y (2000) Structural synaptic modifications associated with hippocampal LTP and behavioral learning. *Cereb. Cortex* 10: 952–962.

Geinisman Y, de Toledo-Morrell L, Morrell F, Heller RE, Rossi M, and Parshall RF (1993) Structural synaptic correlate of long-term potentiation: Formation of axospinous synapses with multiple, completely partitioned transmission zones. *Hippocampus* 3: 435–445.

Geinisman Y, deToledo-Morrell L, and Morrell F (1991) Induction of long-term potentiation is associated with an increase in the number of axospinous synapses with segmented postsynaptic densities. *Brain Res.* 566: 77–88.

Geinisman Y, Disterhoft JF, Gundersen HJ, et al. (2000) Remodeling of hippocampal synapses after hippocampus-dependent associative learning. *J. Comp. Neurol.* 417: 49–59.

Gibbs RB (1998) Levels of trkA and BDNF mRNA, but not NGF mRNA, fluctuate across the estrous cycle and increase in response to acute hormone replacement. *Brain Res.* 787: 259–268.

Gibbs RB and Aggarwal P (1998) Estrogen and basal forebrain cholinergic neurons: Implications for brain aging and Alzheimer's disease-related cognitive decline. *Horm. Behav.* 34: 98–111.

Globus A, Rosenzweig MR, Bennett EL, and Diamond MC (1973) Effects of differential experience on dendritic spine counts in rat cerebral cortex. *J. Comp. Physiol. Psychol.* 82: 175–181.

Globus A and Scheibel AB (1966) Loss of dendrite spines as an index of pre-synaptic terminal patterns. *Nature* 212: 463–465.

Gomez RA, Pozzo Miller LD, Aoki A, and Ramirez OA (1990) Long-term potentiation-induced synaptic changes in hippocampal dentate gyrus of rats with an inborn low or high learning capacity. *Brain Res.* 537: 293–297.

Gould E, Woolley CS, Frankfurt M, and McEwen BS (1990) Gonadal steroids regulate dendritic spine density in hippocampal pyramidal cells in adulthood. *J. Neurosci.* 10: 1286–1291.

Gray E (1959a) Electron microscopy of synaptic contacts on dendritic spines of the cerebral cortex. *Nature* 183: 1592–1594.

Gray EG (1959b) Axo-somatic and axo-dendritic synapses of the cerebral cortex: An electron microscope study. *J. Anat.* 93: 420–433.

Greenough WT and Volkmar FR (1973) Pattern of dendritic branching in occipital cortex of rats reared in complex environments. *Exp. Neurol.* 40: 491–504.

Grutzendler J, Kasthuri N, and Gan WB (2002) Long-term dendritic spine stability in the adult cortex. *Nature* 420: 812–816.

Gutierrez R and Heinemann U (1999) Synaptic reorganization in explanted cultures of rat hippocampus. *Brain Res.* 815: 304–316.

Guy J, Hendrich B, Holmes M, Martin JE, and Bird A (2001) A mouse Mecp2-null mutation causes neurological symptoms that mimic Rett syndrome. *Nat. Genet.* 27: 322–326.

Hao J, Janssen WG, Tang Y, et al. (2003) Estrogen increases the number of spinophilin-immunoreactive spines in the hippocampus of young and aged female rhesus monkeys. *J. Comp. Neurol.* 465: 540–550.

Harms KJ and Dunaevsky A (2006) Dendritic spine plasticity: Looking beyond development. *Brain Res.* (doi:10.1016/j.brainres.2006.02.094).

Harris KM (1999) Structure, development, and plasticity of dendritic spines. *Curr. Opin. Neurobiol.* 9: 343–348.

Harris KM and Kater SB (1994) Dendritic spines: Cellular specializations imparting both stability and flexibility to synaptic function. *Annu. Rev. Neurosci.* 17: 341–371.

Harris KM and Stevens JK (1989) Dendritic spines of CA1 pyramidal cells in the rat hippocampus: Serial electron microscopy with reference to their biophysical characteristics. *J. Neurosci.* 9: 2982–2997.

Harris KM and Sultan P (1995) Variation in the number, location and size of synaptic vesicles provides an anatomical basis for the nonuniform probability of release at hippocampal CA1 synapses. *Neuropharmacology* 34: 1387–1395.

Hartmann M, Brigadski T, Erdmann KS, et al. (2004) Truncated TrkB receptor-induced outgrowth of dendritic filopodia involves the p75 neurotrophin receptor. *J. Cell Sci.* 117: 5803–5814.

Hartmann M, Heumann R, and Lessmann V (2001) Synaptic secretion of BDNF after high-frequency stimulation of glutamatergic synapses. *EMBO J.* 20: 5887–5897.

Hebb DO (1949) *The Organization of Behavior*. New York: John Wiley & Sons.

Hempstead BL (2002) The many faces of p75NTR. *Curr. Opin. Neurobiol.* 12: 260–267.

Hering H and Sheng M (2001) Dendritic spines: Structure, dynamics and regulation. *Nat. Neurosci. Rev.* 2: 880–888.

Holtmaat A, Wilbrecht L, Knott GW, Welker E, and Svoboda K (2006) Experience-dependent and cell-type-specific spine growth in the neocortex. *Nature* 441: 979–983.

Holtmaat AJ, Trachtenberg JT, Wilbrecht L, et al. (2005) Transient and persistent dendritic spines in the neocortex in vivo. *Neuron* 45: 279–291.

Horch HW and Katz LC (2002) BDNF release from single cells elicits local dendritic growth in nearby neurons. *Nat. Neurosci.* 5: 1177–1184.

Horch HW, Kruttgen A, Portbury SD, and Katz LC (1999) Destabilization of cortical dendrites and spines by BDNF. *Neuron* 23: 353–364.

Hosokawa T, Rusakov DA, Bliss TV, and Fine A (1995) Repeated confocal imaging of individual dendritic spines in the living hippocampal slice: Evidence for changes in length and orientation associated with chemically induced LTP. *J. Neurosci.* 15: 5560–5573.

Huang EJ and Reichardt LF (2003) Trk receptors: Roles in neuronal signal transduction. *Annu. Rev. Biochem.* 72: 609–642.

Huttenlocher PR (1970) Dendritic development and mental defect. *Neurology* 20: 381.

Huttenlocher PR (1974) Dendritic development in neocortex of children with mental defect and infantile spasms. *Neurology* 24: 203–210.

Hyman C, Juhasz M, Jackson C, Wright P, Ip NY, and Lindsay RM (1994) Overlapping and distinct actions of the neurotrophins BDNF, NT-3, and NT-4/5 on cultured dopaminergic and GABAergic neurons of the ventral mesencephalon. *J. Neurosci.* 14: 335–347.

Isaac JT, Nicoll RA, and Malenka RC (1995) Evidence for silent synapses: Implications for the expression of LTP. *Neuron* 15: 427–434.

James W (1890) *Principles of Psychology*. New York: Henry Holt.

Jellinger K, Armstrong D, Zoghbi HY, and Percy AK (1988) Neuropathology of Rett syndrome. *Acta Neuropathol. (Berl.)* 76: 142–158.

Ji Y, Pang PT, Feng L, and Lu B (2005) Cyclic AMP controls BDNF-induced TrkB phosphorylation and dendritic spine formation in mature hippocampal neurons. *Nat. Neurosci.* 8: 164–172.

Jontes JD and Smith SJ (2000) Filopodia, spines, and the generation of synaptic diversity. *Neuron* 27: 11–14.

Jourdain P, Fukunaga K, and Muller D (2003) Calcium/calmodulin-dependent protein kinase II contributes to activity-dependent filopodia growth and spine formation. *J. Neurosci.* 23: 10645–10649.

Jugloff DG, Jung BP, Purushotham D, Logan R, and Eubanks JH (2005) Increased dendritic complexity and axonal length in cultured mouse cortical neurons overexpressing methyl-CpG-binding protein MeCP2. *Neurobiol. Dis.* 19: 18–27.

Kaplan DR and Miller FD (2000) Neurotrophin signal transduction in the nervous system. *Curr. Opin. Neurobiol.* 10: 381–391.

Kasai H, Matsuzaki M, Noguchi J, Yasumatsu N, and Nakahara H (2003) Structure-stability-function relationships of dendritic spines. *Trends Neurosci.* 26: 360–368.

Kaufmann WE, MacDonald SM, and Altamura CR (2000) Dendritic cytoskeletal protein expression in mental retardation: An immunohistochemical study of the neocortex in Rett syndrome. *Cereb. Cortex* 10: 992–1004.

Kaufmann WE and Moser HW (2000) Dendritic anomalies in disorders associated with mental retardation. *Cereb. Cortex* 10: 981–991.

Kaufmann WE, Naidu S, and Budden S (1995) Abnormal expression of microtubule-associated protein 2 (MAP-2) in neocortex in Rett syndrome. *Neuropediatrics* 26: 109–113.

Kaufmann WE, Worley PF, Taylor CV, Bremer M, and Isakson PC (1997) Cyclooxygenase-2 expression during rat neocortical development and in Rett syndrome. *Brain Dev.* 19: 25–34.

Kawakami M, Terasawa E, and Ibuki T (1970) Changes in multiple unit activity of the brain during the estrous cycle. *Neuroendocrinology* 6: 30–48.

Kennedy MB (1997) The postsynaptic density at glutamatergic synapses. *Trends Neurosci.* 20: 264–268.

Kirov SA, Goddard CA, and Harris KM (2004a) Age-dependence in the homeostatic upregulation of hippocampal dendritic spine number during blocked synaptic transmission. *Neuropharmacology* 47: 640–648.

Kirov SA and Harris KM (1999) Dendrites are more spiny on mature hippocampal neurons when synapses are inactivated. *Nat. Neurosci.* 2: 878–883.

Kirov SA, Petrak LJ, Fiala JC, and Harris KM (2004b) Dendritic spines disappear with chilling but proliferate excessively upon rewarming of mature hippocampus. *Neuroscience* 127: 69–80.

Kirov SA, Sorra KE, and Harris KM (1999) Slices have more synapses than perfusion-fixed hippocampus from both young and mature rats. *J. Neurosci.* 19: 2876–2886.

Kishi N and Macklis JD (2004) MECP2 is progressively expressed in post-migratory neurons and is involved in neuronal maturation rather than cell fate decisions. *Mol. Cell. Neurosci.* 27: 306–321.

Knafo S, Ariav G, Barkai E, and Libersat F (2004) Olfactory learning-induced increase in spine density along the apical dendrites of CA1 hippocampal neurons. *Hippocampus* 14: 819–825.

Knott GW, Holtmaat A, Wilbrecht L, Welker E, and Svoboda K (2006) Spine growth precedes synapse formation in the adult neocortex in vivo. *Nat. Neurosci.* 9: 1117–1124.

Knusel B, Beck KD, Winslow JW, et al. (1992) Brain-derived neurotrophic factor administration protects basal forebrain cholinergic but not nigral dopaminergic neurons from degenerative changes after axotomy in the adult rat brain. *J. Neurosci.* 12: 4391–4402.

Kojima M, Takei N, Numakawa T, et al. (2001) Biological characterization and optical imaging of brain-derived neurotrophic factor-green fluorescent protein suggest an activity-dependent local release of brain-derived neurotrophic factor in neurites of cultured hippocampal neurons. *J. Neurosci. Res.* 64: 1–10.

Kopec CD, Li B, Wei W, Boehm J, and Malinow R (2006) Glutamate receptor exocytosis and spine enlargement during chemically induced long-term potentiation. *J. Neurosci.* 26: 2000–2009.

Korkotian E, Holcman D, and Segal M (2004) Dynamic regulation of spine-dendrite coupling in cultured hippocampal neurons. *Eur. J. Neurosci.* 20: 2649–2663.

Korkotian E and Segal M (1999a) Bidirectional regulation of dendritic spine dimensions by glutamate receptors. *Neuroreport* 10: 2875–2877.

Korkotian E and Segal M (1999b) Release of calcium from stores alters the morphology of dendritic spines in cultured hippocampal neurons. *Proc. Natl. Acad. Sci. USA* 96: 12068–12072.

Korkotian E and Segal M (2000) Structure-function relations in dendritic spines: Is size important? *Hippocampus* 10: 587–595.

Korkotian E and Segal M (2001) Regulation of dendritic spine motility in cultured hippocampal neurons. *J. Neurosci.* 21: 6115–6124.

Kozorovitskiy Y, Gross CG, Kopil C, et al. (2005) Experience induces structural and biochemical changes in the adult primate brain. *Proc. Natl. Acad. Sci. USA* 102: 17478–17482.

Lang C, Barco A, Zablow L, Kandel ER, Siegelbaum SA, and Zakharenko SS (2004) Transient expansion of synaptically connected dendritic spines upon induction of hippocampal long-term potentiation. *Proc. Natl. Acad. Sci. USA* 101: 16665–16670.

Lappalainen R, Lindholm D, and Riikonen R (1996) Low levels of nerve growth factor in cerebrospinal fluid of children with Rett syndrome. *J. Child Neurol.* 11: 296–300.

Lee K, Oliver M, Schottler F, Creager R, and Lynch G (1979) Ultrastructural effects of repetitive synaptic stimulation in the hippocampal slice preparation: A preliminary report. *Exp. Neurol.* 65: 478–480.

Lee KS, Schottler F, Oliver M, and Lynch G (1980) Brief bursts of high-frequency stimulation produce two types of structural change in rat hippocampus. *J. Neurophysiol.* 44: 247–258.

Lee SJ and McEwen BS (2001) Neurotrophic and neuroprotective actions of estrogens and their therapeutic implications. *Annu. Rev. Pharmacol. Toxicol.* 41: 569–591.

Lendvai B, Stern EA, Chen B, and Svoboda K (2000) Experience-dependent plasticity of dendritic spines in the developing rat barrel cortex in vivo. *Nature* 404: 876–881.

Leranth C, Shanabrough M, and Redmond DE Jr. (2002) Gonadal hormones are responsible for maintaining the integrity of spine synapses in the CA1 hippocampal subfield of female nonhuman primates. *J. Comp. Neurol.* 447: 34–42.

Leuner B, Falduto J, and Shors TJ (2003) Associative memory formation increases the observation of dendritic spines in the hippocampus. *J. Neurosci.* 23: 659–665.

Lewin GR and Barde YA (1996) Physiology of the neurotrophins. *Annu. Rev. Neurosci.* 19: 289–317.

Li C, Brake WG, Romeo RD, et al. (2004) Estrogen alters hippocampal dendritic spine shape and enhances synaptic protein immunoreactivity and spatial memory in female mice. *Proc. Natl. Acad. Sci. USA* 101: 2185–2190.

Liao D, Hessler NA, and Malinow R (1995) Activation of postsynaptically silent synapses during pairing-induced LTP in CA1 region of the hippocampal slice. *Nature* 375: 400–404.

Lipani JD, Bhattacharjee MB, Corey DM, and Lee DA (2000) Reduced nerve growth factor in Rett syndrome postmortem brain tissue. *J. Neuropathol. Exp. Neurol.* 59: 889–895.

Lo DC (1995) Neurotrophic factors and synaptic plasticity. *Neuron* 15: 979–981.

Lu B (2003) BDNF and activity-dependent synaptic modulation. *Learn. Mem.* 10: 86–98.

Lu B, Pang PT, and Woo NH (2005) The yin and yang of neurotrophin action. *Nat. Rev. Neurosci.* 6: 603–614.

Luikart BW, Nef S, Virmani T, et al. (2005) TrkB has a cell-autonomous role in the establishment of hippocampal Schaffer collateral synapses. *J. Neurosci.* 25: 3774–3786.

Majewska A, Brown E, Ross J, and Yuste R (2000a) Mechanisms of calcium decay kinetics in hippocampal spines: Role of spine calcium pumps and calcium diffusion through the spine neck in biochemical compartmentalization. *J. Neurosci.* 20: 1722–1734.

Majewska A, Tashiro A, and Yuste R (2000b) Regulation of spine calcium dynamics by rapid spine motility. *J. Neurosci.* 20: 8262–8268.

Malenka RC and Bear MF (2004) LTP and LTD: An embarrassment of riches. *Neuron* 44: 5–21.

Maletic-Savatic M, Malinow R, and Svoboda K (1999) Rapid dendritic morphogenesis in CA1 hippocampal dendrites induced by synaptic activity. *Science* 283: 1923–1927.

Malinow R and Malenka RC (2002) AMPA receptor trafficking and synaptic plasticity. *Annu. Rev. Neurosci.* 25: 103–126.

Mamounas LA, Blue ME, Siuciak JA, and Altar CA (1995) Brain derived neurotrophic factor promotes the survival and sprouting of serotonergic axons in rat brain. *J. Neurosci.* 15: 7929–7939.

Marin-Padilla M (1972a) Prenatal ontogenetic history of the principal neurons of the neocortex of the cat (Felis domestica). A Golgi study. II. Developmental differences and their significances. *Z. Anat. Entwicklungsgesch.* 136: 125–142.

Marin-Padilla M (1972b) Structural abnormalities of the cerebral cortex in human chromosomal aberrations: A Golgi study. *Brain Res.* 44: 625–629.

Marin-Padilla M (1976) Pyramidal cell abnormalities in the motor cortex of a child with Down's syndrome. A Golgi study. *J. Comp. Neurol.* 167: 63–81.

Martin SJ, Grimwood PD, and Morris RG (2000) Synaptic plasticity and memory: An evaluation of the hypothesis. *Annu. Rev. Neurosci.* 23: 649–711.

Martinowich K, Hattori D, Wu H, et al. (2003) DNA methylation-related chromatin remodeling in activity-dependent BDNF gene regulation. *Science* 302: 890–893.

Matsumoto A and Arai Y (1979) Synaptogenic effect of estrogen on the hypothalamic arcuate nucleus of the adult female rat. *Cell Tissue Res.* 198: 427–433.

Matsumoto A and Arai Y (1986) Male-female difference in synaptic organization of the ventromedial nucleus of the hypothalamus in the rat. *Neuroendocrinology* 42: 232–236.

Matsuzaki M, Ellis-Davies GC, Nemoto T, Miyashita Y, Iino M, and Kasai H (2001) Dendritic spine geometry is critical for AMPA receptor expression in hippocampal CA1 pyramidal neurons. *Nat. Neurosci.* 4: 1086–1092.

Matsuzaki M, Honkura N, Ellis-Davies GC, and Kasai H (2004) Structural basis of long-term potentiation in single dendritic spines. *Nature* 429: 761–766.

Matus A (2000) Actin-based plasticity in dendritic spines. *Science* 290: 754–758.

Matus A (2005) Growth of dendritic spines: A continuing story. *Curr. Opin. Neurobiol.* 15: 67–72.

McAllister AK, Katz LC, and Lo DC (1997) Opposing roles for endogenous BDNF and NT-3 in regulating cortical dendritic growth. *Neuron* 18: 767–778.

McAllister AK, Katz LC, and Lo DC (1999) Neurotrophins and synaptic plasticity. *Annu. Rev. Neurosci.* 22: 295–318.

McAllister AK, Lo DC, and Katz LC (1995) Neurotrophins regulate dendritic growth in developing visual cortex. *Neuron* 15: 791–803.

McKinney RA, Capogna M, Durr R, Gahwiler BH, and Thompson SM (1999) Miniature synaptic events maintain dendritic spines via AMPA receptor activation. *Nat. Neurosci.* 2: 44–49.

Miller M and Peters A (1981) Maturation of rat visual cortex. II. A combined Golgi-electron microscope study of pyramidal neurons. *J. Comp. Neurol.* 203: 555–573.

Minichiello L, Calella AM, Medina DL, Bonhoeffer T, Klein R, and Korte M (2002) Mechanism of TrkB-mediated hippocampal long-term potentiation. *Neuron* 36: 121–137.

Minichiello L, Korte M, Wolfer D, et al. (1999) Essential role for TrkB receptors in hippocampus-mediated learning. *Neuron* 24: 401–414.

Miranda R, Blanco E, Begega A, Santin LJ, and Arias JL (2006) Reversible changes in hippocampal CA1 synapses associated with water maze training in rats. *Synapse* 59: 177–181.

Mizrahi A, Crowley JC, Shtoyerman E, and Katz LC (2004) High-resolution in vivo imaging of hippocampal dendrites and spines. *J. Neurosci.* 24: 3147–3151.

Moretti P, Levenson JM, Battaglia F, et al. (2006) Learning and memory and synaptic plasticity are impaired in a mouse model of Rett syndrome. *J. Neurosci.* 26: 319–327.

Moser MB (1999) Making more synapses: A way to store information? *Cell. Mol. Life Sci.* 55: 593–600.

Moser MB, Trommald M, and Andersen P (1994) An increase in dendritic spine density on hippocampal CA1 pyramidal cells following spatial learning in adult rats suggests the formation of new synapses. *Proc. Natl. Acad. Sci. USA* 91: 12673–12675.

Moser MB, Trommald M, Egeland T, and Andersen P (1997) Spatial training in a complex environment and isolation alter the spine distribution differently in rat CA1 pyramidal cells. *J. Comp. Neurol.* 380: 373–381.

Mulkey RM and Malenka RC (1992) Mechanisms underlying induction of homosynaptic long-term depression in area CA1 of the hippocampus. *Neuron* 9: 967–975.

Muller M, Gahwiler BH, Rietschin L, and Thompson SM (1993) Reversible loss of dendritic spines and altered excitability after chronic epilepsy in hippocampal slice cultures. *Proc. Natl. Acad. Sci. USA* 90: 257–261.

Muller W and Connor JA (1991) Dendritic spines as individual neuronal compartments for synaptic Ca2+ responses. *Nature* 354: 73–76.

Murer MG, Yan Q, and Raisman-Vozari R (2001) Brain-derived neurotrophic factor in the control human brain, and in Alzheimer's disease and Parkinson's disease. *Prog. Neurobiol.* 63: 71–124.

Murphy DD, Cole NB, and Segal M (1998) Brain-derived neurotrophic factor mediates estradiol-induced dendritic spine formation in hippocampal neurons. *Proc. Natl. Acad. Sci. USA* 95: 11412–11417.

Murphy DD and Segal M (1996) Regulation of dendritic spine density in cultured rat hippocampal neurons by steroid hormones. *J. Neurosci.* 16: 4059–4068.

Murphy DD and Segal M (1997) Morphological plasticity of dendritic spines in central neurons is mediated by activation of cAMP response element binding protein. *Proc. Natl. Acad. Sci. USA* 94: 1482–1487.

Murthy VN, Schikorski T, Stevens CF, and Zhu Y (2001) Inactivity produces increases in neurotransmitter release and synapse size. *Neuron* 32: 673–682.

Nagerl UV, Eberhorn N, Cambridge SB, and Bonhoeffer T (2004) Bidirectional activity-dependent morphological plasticity in hippocampal neurons. *Neuron* 44: 759–767.

Nakayama AY, Harms MB, and Luo L (2000) Small GTPases Rac and Rho in the maintenance of dendritic spines and branches in hippocampal pyramidal neurons. *J. Neurosci.* 20: 5329–5338.

Nan X, Ng HH, Johnson CA, et al. (1998) Transcriptional repression by the methyl-CpG-binding protein MeCP2 involves a histone deacetylase complex. *Nature* 393: 386–389.

Nelson ED, Kavalali ET, and Monteggia LM (2006) MeCP2-dependent transcriptional repression regulates excitatory neurotransmission. *Curr. Biol.* 16: 710–716.

Neul JL and Zoghbi HY (2004) Rett syndrome: A prototypical neurodevelopmental disorder. *Neuroscientist* 10: 118–128.

Newey SE, Velamoor V, Govek EE, and Van Aelst L (2005) Rho GTPases, dendritic structure, and mental retardation. *J. Neurobiol.* 64: 58–74.

Nimchinsky EA, Sabatini BL, and Svoboda K (2002) Structure and function of dendritic spines. *Annu. Rev. Physiol.* 64: 313–353.

Noguchi J, Matsuzaki M, Ellis-Davies GC, and Kasai H (2005) Spine-neck geometry determines NMDA receptor-dependent Ca2+ signaling in dendrites. *Neuron* 46: 609–622.

Nuber UA, Kriaucionis S, Roloff TC, et al. (2005) Up-regulation of glucocorticoid-regulated genes in a mouse model of Rett syndrome. *Hum. Mol. Genet.* 14: 2247–2256.

Nusser Z, Lujan R, Laube G, Roberts JD, Molnar E, and Somogyi P (1998) Cell type and pathway dependence of synaptic AMPA receptor number and variability in the hippocampus. *Neuron* 21: 545–559.

Nykjaer A, Willnow TE, and Petersen CM (2005) p75NTR—Live or let die. *Curr. Opin. Neurobiol.* 15: 49–57.

O'Malley A, O'Connell C, Murphy KJ, and Regan CM (2000) Transient spine density increases in the mid-molecular layer of hippocampal dentate gyrus accompany consolidation of a spatial learning task in the rodent. *Neuroscience* 99: 229–232.

O'Malley A, O'Connell C, and Regan CM (1998) Ultrastructural analysis reveals avoidance conditioning to induce a transient increase in hippocampal dentate spine density in the 6 hour post-training period of consolidation. *Neuroscience* 87: 607–613.

Oertner TG and Matus A (2005) Calcium regulation of actin dynamics in dendritic spines. *Cell Calcium* 37: 477–482.

Okamoto K, Nagai T, Miyawaki A, and Hayashi Y (2004) Rapid and persistent modulation of actin dynamics regulates postsynaptic reorganization underlying bidirectional plasticity. *Nat. Neurosci.* 7: 1104–1112.

Otmakhov N, Khibnik L, Otmakhova N, et al. (2004) Forskolin-induced LTP in the CA1 hippocampal region is NMDA receptor dependent. *J. Neurophysiol.* 91: 1955–1962.

Papa M, Bundman MC, Greenberger V, and Segal M (1995) Morphological analysis of dendritic spine development in primary cultures of hippocampal neurons. *J. Neurosci.* 15: 1–11.

Papa M and Segal M (1996) Morphological plasticity in dendritic spines of cultured hippocampal neurons. *Neuroscience* 71: 1005–1011.

Parnass Z, Tashiro A, and Yuste R (2000) Analysis of spine morphological plasticity in developing hippocampal pyramidal neurons. *Hippocampus* 10: 561–568.

Parnavelas JG, Globus A, and Kaups P (1973) Continuous illumination from birth affects spine density of neurons in the visual cortex of the rat. *Exp. Neurol.* 40: 742–747.

Parnavelas JG, Lynch G, Brecha N, Cotman CW, and Globus A (1974) Spine loss and regrowth in hippocampus following deafferentation. *Nature* 248: 71–73.

Patapoutian A and Reichardt LF (2001) Trk receptors: Mediators of neurotrophin action. *Curr. Opin. Neurobiol.* 11: 272–280.

Percy AK (2002) Rett syndrome. Current status and new vistas. *Neurol. Clin.* 20: 1125–1141.

Percy AK and Lane JB (2005) Rett syndrome: Model of neurodevelopmental disorders. *J. Child Neurol.* 20: 718–721.

Peters A and Kaiserman-Abramof I (1970) The small pyramidal neuron of the rat cerebral cortex. The perikarion, dendrites and spines. *J. Anat.* 127: 321–356.

Peters A and Kaiserman-Abramof IR (1969) The small pyramidal neuron of the rat cerebral cortex. The synapses upon dendritic spines. *Z. Zellforsch. Mikrosk. Anat.* 100: 487–506.

Peters A, Palay SL, and Webster H (1991) *The Fine Structure of the Nervous System. Neurons and Their Supporting Cells.* New York: Oxford University Press.

Petrak LJ, Harris KM, and Kirov SA (2005) Synaptogenesis on mature hippocampal dendrites occurs via filopodia and immature spines during blocked synaptic transmission. *J. Comp. Neurol.* 484: 183–190.

Petrozzino JJ, Pozzo Miller LD, and Connor JA (1995) Micromolar Ca2+ transients in dendritic spines of hippocampal pyramidal neurons in brain slice. *Neuron* 14: 1223–1231.

Pierce JP and Lewin GR (1994) An ultrastructural size principle. *Neuroscience* 58: 441–446.

Poo MM (2001) Neurotrophins as synaptic modulators. *Nat. Rev. Neurosci.* 2: 24–32.

Pozzo Miller LD and Aoki A (1991) Stereological analysis of the hypothalamic ventromedial nucleus. II. Hormone-induced changes in the synaptogenic pattern. *Brain Res. Dev. Brain Res.* 61: 189–196.

Pozzo Miller LD and Aoki A (1992) Postnatal development of the hypothalamic ventromedial nucleus: Neurons and synapses. *Cell. Mol. Neurobiol.* 12: 121–129.

Pozzo Miller LD, Petrozzino JJ, Mahanty NK, and Connor JA (1993) Optical imaging of cytosolic calcium, electrophysiology, and ultrastructure in pyramidal neurons of organotypic slice cultures from rat hippocampus. *Neuroimage* 1: 109–120.

Pozzo-Miller L (2006) BDNF enhances dendritic Ca2+ signals evoked by coincident EPSPs and back-propagating action potentials in CA1 pyramidal neurons. *Brain Res.* 1104: 45–54.

Pozzo-Miller LD, Connor JA, and Andrews SB (2000) Microheterogeneity of calcium signalling in dendrites. *J. Physiol.* 525: 53–61.

Pozzo-Miller LD, Gottschalk W, Zhang L, et al. (1999a) Impairments in high-frequency transmission, synaptic vesicle docking, and synaptic protein distribution in the hippocampus of BDNF knockout mice. *J. Neurosci.* 19: 4972–4983.

Pozzo-Miller LD, Inoue T, and Murphy DD (1999b) Estradiol increases spine density and N-methyl-D-aspartate-dependent Ca2+ transients in spines of CA1 pyramidal neurons from hippocampal slices. *J. Neurophysiol.* 81: 1404–1411.

Purpura DP (1974) Dendritic spine "dysgenesis" and mental retardation. *Science* 186: 1126–1128.

Purpura DP (1975a) Dendritic differentiation in human cerebral cortex: Normal and aberrant developmental patterns. *Adv. Neurol.* 12: 91–134.

Purpura DP (1975b) Normal and aberrant neuronal development in the cerebral cortex of human fetus and young infant. *UCLA Forum Med. Sci.* 141–169.

Rall W and Segev I (1987) Functional possibilities for synapses on dendrites and dendritic spines. Edelman GM, Gall WE, and Cowan WM (eds.) *Synaptic Function*, pp. 605–636. New York: John Wiley & Sons.

Rampon C, Tang YP, Goodhouse J, Shimizu E, Kyin M, and Tsien JZ (2000) Enrichment induces structural changes and recovery from nonspatial memory deficits in CA1 NMDA R1-knockout mice. *Nat. Neurosci.* 3: 238–244.

Richards DA, Mateos JM, Hugel S, et al. (2005) Glutamate induces the rapid formation of spine head protrusions in hippocampal slice cultures. *Proc. Natl. Acad. Sci. USA* 102: 6166–6171.

Riikonen R (2003) Neurotrophic factors in the pathogenesis of Rett syndrome. *J. Child Neurol.* 18: 693–697.

Riikonen R and Vanhala R (1999) Levels of cerebrospinal fluid nerve-growth factor differ in infantile autism and Rett syndrome. *Dev. Med. Child Neurol.* 41: 148–152.

Rosch H, Schweigreiter R, Bonhoeffer T, Barde YA, and Korte M (2005) The neurotrophin receptor p75NTR modulates long-term depression and regulates the expression of AMPA receptor subunits in the hippocampus. *Proc. Natl. Acad. Sci. USA* 102: 7362–7367.

Rosenzweig MR and Bennett EL (1996) Psychobiology of plasticity: Effects of training and experience on brain and behavior. *Behav. Brain. Res.* 78: 57–65.

Roux PP and Barker PA (2002) Neurotrophin signaling through the p75 neurotrophin receptor. *Prog. Neurobiol.* 67: 203–233.

Rusakov DA, Davies HA, Harrison E, et al. (1997) Ultrastructural synaptic correlates of spatial learning in rat hippocampus. *Neuroscience* 80: 69–77.

Sabatini BL, Maravall M, and Svoboda K (2001) Ca(2+) signaling in dendritic spines. *Curr. Opin. Neurobiol.* 11: 349–356.

Sabatini BL, Oertner TG, and Svoboda K (2002) The life cycle of Ca(2+) ions in dendritic spines. *Neuron* 33: 439–452.

Scheibel ME, Crandall PH, and Scheibel AB (1974) The hippocampal-dentate complex in temporal lobe epilepsy. A Golgi study. *Epilepsia* 15: 55–80.

Schikorski T and Stevens CF (1999) Quantitative fine-structural analysis of olfactory cortical synapses. *Proc. Natl. Acad. Sci. USA* 96: 4107–4112.

Schinder AF and Poo M (2000) The neurotrophin hypothesis for synaptic plasticity. *Trends Neurosci.* 23: 639–645.

Segal I, Korkotian I, and Murphy DD (2000) Dendritic spine formation and pruning: Common cellular mechanisms? *Trends Neurosci.* 23: 53–57.

Segal M (2005) Dendritic spines and long-term plasticity. *Nat. Rev. Neurosci.* 6: 277–284.

Segal RA and Greenberg ME (1996) Intracellular signaling pathways activated by neurotrophic factors. *Annu. Rev. Neurosci.* 19: 463–489.

Shahbazian M, Young J, Yuva-Paylor L, et al. (2002) Mice with truncated MeCP2 recapitulate many Rett syndrome features and display hyperacetylation of histone H3. *Neuron* 35: 243–254.

Shahbazian MD and Zoghbi HY (2002) Rett syndrome and MeCP2: Linking epigenetics and neuronal function. *Am. J. Hum. Genet.* 71: 1259–1272.

Sheng M and Sala C (2001) PDZ domains and the organization of supramolecular complexes. *Annu. Rev. Neurosci.* 24: 1–29.

Shepherd GM (1996) The dendritic spine: A multifunctional integrative unit. *J. Neurophysiol.* 75: 2197–2210.

Sherwin BB (1996) Hormones, mood, and cognitive functioning in postmenopausal women. *Obstet. Gynecol.* 87: 20S–26S.

Sherwin BB (2005) Estrogen and memory in women: How can we reconcile the findings? *Horm. Behav.* 47: 371–375.

Shi SH, Hayashi Y, Petralia RS, et al. (1999) Rapid spine delivery and redistribution of AMPA receptors after synaptic NMDA receptor activation. *Science* 284: 1811–1816.

Smith CC and McMahon LL (2005) Estrogen-induced increase in the magnitude of long-term potentiation occurs only when the ratio of NMDA transmission to AMPA transmission is increased. *J. Neurosci.* 25: 7780–7791.

Sorra KE and Harris KM (1998) Stability in synapse number and size at 2 hr after long-term potentiation in hippocampal area CA1. *J. Neurosci.* 18: 658–671.

Sorra KE and Harris KM (2000) Overview on the structure, composition, function,development, and plasticity of hippocampal dendritic spines. *Hippocampus* 10: 501–511.

Spacek J (1985) Three-dimensional analysis of dendritic spines. II. Spine apparatus and other cytoplasmic components. *Anat. Embryol.* 171: 235–243.

Spacek J and Harris KM (1997) Three-dimensional organization of smooth endoplasmic reticulum in hippocampal CA1 dendrites and dendritic spines of the immature and mature rat. *J. Neurosci.* 17: 190–203.

Stewart MG, Medvedev NI, Popov VI, et al. (2005) Chemically induced long-term potentiation increases the number of perforated and complex postsynaptic densities but does not alter dendritic spine volume in CA1 of adult mouse hippocampal slices. *Eur. J. Neurosci.* 21: 3368–3378.

Stoppini L, Buchs PA, and Muller D (1991) A simple method for organotypic cultures of nervous tissue. *J. Neurosci. Methods* 37: 173–182.

Svoboda K, Tank DW, and Denk W (1996) Direct measurement of coupling between dendritic spines and shafts. *Science* 272: 716–719.

Tada T and Sheng M (2006) Molecular mechanisms of dendritic spine morphogenesis. *Curr. Opin. Neurobiol.* 16: 95–101.

Tanzi E (1893) I fatti e le induzioni nell'odierna isologia del sistema nervosa. *Rivista Sperimentale di Freniatria e di Medicina Legale* 19: 419–472.

Tao X, Finkbeiner S, Arnold DB, Shaywitz AJ, and Greenberg ME (1998) Ca2+ influx regulates BDNF transcription by a CREB family transcription factor-dependent mechanism. *Neuron* 20: 709–726.

Tashiro A, Minden A, and Yuste R (2000) Regulation of dendritic spine morphology by the Rho family of small GTPases: Antagonistic roles of Rac and Rho. *Cereb. Cortex* 10: 927–938.

Terasawa E and Timiras PS (1968) Electrical activity during the estrous cycle of the rat: Cyclic changes in limbic structures. *Endocrinology* 83: 207–216.

Thoenen H (1995) Neurotrophins and neuronal plasticity. *Science* 270: 593–598.

Thoenen H (2000) Neurotrophins and activity-dependent plasticity. *Prog. Brain. Res.* 128: 183–191.

Thompson SM, Fortunato C, McKinney RA, Muller M, and Gahwiler BH (1996) Mechanisms underlying the neuropathological consequences of epileptic activity in the rat hippocampus in vitro. *J. Comp. Neurol.* 372: 515–528.

Toni N, Buchs PA, Nikonenko I, Bron CR, and Muller D (1999) LTP promotes formation of multiple spine synapses between a single axon terminal and a dendrite. *Nature* 402: 421–425.

Toni N, Buchs PA, Nikonenko I, Povilaitite P, Parisi L, and Muller D (2001) Remodeling of synaptic membranes after induction of long-term potentiation. *J. Neurosci.* 21: 6245–6251.

Toran-Allerand CD (1996) Mechanisms of estrogen action during neural development: Mediation by interactions with the neurotrophins and their receptors? *J. Steroid Biochem. Mol. Biol.* 56: 169–178.

Toresson H and Grant SG (2005) Dynamic distribution of endoplasmic reticulum in hippocampal neuron dendritic spines. *Eur. J. Neurosci.* 22: 1793–1798.

Trachtenberg JT, Chen BE, Knott GW, et al. (2002) Long-term in vivo imaging of experience-dependent synaptic plasticity in adult cortex. *Nature* 420: 788–794.

Trommald M, Hulleberg G, and Andersen P (1996) Long-term potentiation is associated with new excitatory spine synapses on rat dentate granule cells. *Learn. Mem.* 3: 218–228.

Tudor M, Akbarian S, Chen RZ, and Jaenisch R (2002) Transcriptional profiling of a mouse model for Rett syndrome reveals subtle transcriptional changes in the brain. *Proc. Natl. Acad. Sci. USA* 99: 15536–15541.

Turrigiano GG (1999) Homeostatic plasticity in neuronal networks: The more things change, the more they stay the same. *Trends Neurosci.* 22: 221–227.

Turrigiano GG and Nelson SB (2004) Homeostatic plasticity in the developing nervous system. *Nat. Rev. Neurosci.* 5: 97–107.

Tyler WJ, Alonso M, Bramham CR, and Pozzo-Miller LD (2002a) From acquisition to consolidation: On the role of brain-derived neurotrophic factor signaling in hippocampal-dependent learning. *Learn. Mem.* 9: 224–237.

Tyler WJ, Perrett SP, and Pozzo-Miller LD (2002b) The role of neurotrophins in neurotransmitter release. *Neuroscientist* 8: 524–531.

Tyler WJ and Pozzo-Miller L (2003) Miniature synaptic transmission and BDNF modulate dendritic spine growth and form in rat CA1 neurones. *J. Physiol.* 553: 497–509.

Tyler WJ and Pozzo-Miller LD (2001) BDNF enhances quantal neurotransmitter release and increases the number of docked vesicles at the active zones of hippocampal excitatory synapses. *J. Neurosci.* 21: 4249–4258.

Tyler WJ, Zhang XL, Hartman K, et al. (2006) BDNF increases release probability and the size of a rapidly recycling vesicle pool within rat hippocampal excitatory synapses. *J. Physiol.* 574: 787–803.

Valverde F (1967) Apical dendritic spines of the visual cortex and light deprivation in the mouse. *Exp. Brain Res.* 3: 337–352.

Valverde F (1971) Rate and extent of recovery from dark rearing in the visual cortex of the mouse. *Brain Res.* 33: 1–11.

Van Harreveld A and Fifkova E (1975) Swelling of dendritic spines in the fascia dentata after stimulation of the perforant fibers as a mechanism of post-tetanic potentiation. *Exp. Neurol.* 49: 736–749.

van Praag H, Kempermann G, and Gage FH (2000) Neural consequences of environmental enrichment. *Nat. Rev. Neurosci.* 1: 191–198.

Vanhala R, Korhonen L, Mikelsaar M, Lindholm D, and Riikonen R (1998) Neurotrophic factors in cerebrospinal fluid and serum of patients with Rett syndrome. *J. Child Neurol.* 13: 429–433.

Vicario-Abejon C, Owens D, McKay R, and Segal M (2002) Role of neurotrophins in central synapse formation and stabilization. *Nat. Rev. Neurosci.* 3: 965–974.

Volfovsky N, Parnas H, Segal M, and Korkotian E (1999) Geometry of dendritic spines affects calcium dynamics in hippocampal neurons: Theory and experiments. *J. Neurophysiol.* 81: 450–462.

von Bohlen und Halbach O, Krause S, Medina D, Sciarretta C, Minichiello L, and Unsicker K (2006) Regional- and age-dependent reduction in trkB receptor expression in the hippocampus is associated with altered spine morphologies. *Biol. Psychiatry* 59: 793–800.

Wallace CS, Hawrylak N, and Greenough WT (1991) Studies of synaptic structural modifications after long-term potentiation and kindling: Contex for a molecular morphology. Baudry M and Davis JL (eds.) *Long-Term Potentiation. A Debate of Current Issues*, pp. 189–232. Cambridge, MA: The MIT Press.

Warren SG, Humphreys AG, Juraska JM, and Greenough WT (1995) LTP varies across the estrous cycle: Enhanced synaptic plasticity in proestrus rats. *Brain Res.* 703: 26–30.

Weiland NG (1992) Estradiol selectively regulates agonist binding sites on the NMDA receptor complex in the CA1 region of the hippocampus. *Endocrinology* 131: 662–668.

Wenk GL and Hauss-Wegrzyniak B (1999) Altered cholinergic function in the basal forebrain of girls with Rett syndrome. *Neuropediatrics* 30: 125–129.

Widmer HR, Knusel B, and Hefti F (1993) BDNF protection of basal forebrain cholinergic neurons after axotomy: Complete protection of p75NGFR-positive cells. *Neuroreport* 4: 363–366.

Woo NH, Teng HK, Siao CJ, et al. (2005) Activation of p75NTR by proBDNF facilitates hippocampal long-term depression. *Nat. Neurosci.* 8: 1069–1077.

Woolley CS, Gould E, Frankfurt M, and McEwen BS (1990) Naturally occurring fluctuation in dendritic spine density on adult hippocampal pyramidal neurons. *J. Neurosci.* 10: 4035–4039.
Woolley CS and McEwen BS (1993) Roles of estradiol and progesterone in regulation of hippocampal dendritic spine density during the estrous cycle in the rat. *J. Comp. Neurol.* 336: 293–306.
Woolley CS and McEwen BS (1994) Estradiol regulates hippocampal dendritic spine density via an NMDA receptor-dependent mechanism. *J. Neurosci.* 14: 7680–7687.
Woolley CS, Weiland NG, McEwen BS, and Schwartzkroin PA (1997) Estradiol increases the sensitivity of hippocampal CA1 pyramidal cells to NMDA receptor-mediated synaptic input: Correlation with dendritic spine density. *J. Neurosci.* 17: 1848–1859.
Woolley DE and Timiras PS (1962) The gonad-brain relationship: Effects of female sex hormones on electroshock convulsions in the rat. *Endocrinology* 70: 196–209.
Xu B, Gottschalk W, Chow A, et al. (2000) The role of brain-derived neurotrophic factor receptors in the mature hippocampus: Modulation of long-term potentiation through a presynaptic mechanism involving TrkB. *J. Neurosci.* 20: 6888–6897.
Yacoubian TA and Lo DC (2000) Truncated and full-length TrkB receptors regulate distinct modes of dendritic growth. *Nat. Neurosci.* 3: 342–349.
Yurek DM, Lu W, Hipkens S, and Wiegand SJ (1996) BDNF enhances the functional reinnervation of the striatum by grafted fetal dopamine neurons. *Exp. Neurol.* 137: 105–118.
Yuste R and Bonhoeffer T (2001) Morphological changes in dendritic spines associated with long-term synaptic plasticity. *Annu. Rev. Neurosci.* 24: 1071–1089.
Yuste R and Bonhoeffer T (2004) Genesis of dendritic spines: Insights from ultrastructural and imaging studies. *Nat. Rev. Neurosci.* 5: 24–34.
Yuste R and Denk W (1995) Dendritic spines as basic functional units of neuronal integration. *Nature* 375: 682–684.
Yuste R and Majewska A (2001) On the function of dendritic spines. *Neuroscientist* 7: 387–395.
Yuste R, Majewska A, and Holthoff K (2000) From form to function: Calcium compartmentalization in dendritic spines. *Nat. Neurosci.* 3: 653–659.
Zagrebelsky M, Holz A, Dechant G, Barde YA, Bonhoeffer T, and Korte M (2005) The p75 neurotrophin receptor negatively modulates dendrite complexity and spine density in hippocampal neurons. *J. Neurosci.* 25: 9989–9999.
Zhou Q, Homma KJ, and Poo MM (2004) Shrinkage of dendritic spines associated with long-term depression of hippocampal synapses. *Neuron* 44: 749–757.
Ziff EB (1997) Enlightening the postsynaptic density. *Neuron* 19: 1163–1174.
Zito K, Knott G, Shepherd GM, Shenolikar S, and Svoboda K (2004) Induction of spine growth and synapse formation by regulation of the spine actin cytoskeleton. *Neuron* 44: 321–334.
Ziv NE and Smith SJ (1996) Evidence for a role of dendritic filopodia in synaptogenesis and spine formation. *Neuron* 17: 91–102.
Zuo Y, Yang G, Kwon E, and Gan WB (2005) Long-term sensory deprivation prevents dendritic spine loss in primary somatosensory cortex. *Nature* 436: 261–265.

14 Plasticity of Intrinsic Excitability as a Mechanism for Memory Storage

R. Mozzachiodi and J. H. Byrne, The University of Texas Medical School at Houston, Houston, TX, USA

14.1 Introduction

During the past several decades, the analysis of the cellular and molecular mechanisms underlying learning and memory revealed two major targets for learning-dependent neuronal modulation: synaptic efficacy and intrinsic excitability (for review see Byrne, 1987).

The efficacy of a synapse is highly plastic and can be modified by neuronal activity in different ways. Indeed, different patterns of neuronal activity can lead to distinct and enduring changes in synaptic strength associated with phenomena such as long-term potentiation (LTP) and long-term depression (LTD). In addition, several behavioral training tasks, capable of inducing nonassociative and associative forms of learning, alter synaptic efficacy, thus supporting a role for synaptic plasticity in the storage of memory (e.g., Martin and Morris, 2002). Because of the extremely large number of individual synaptic contacts that neurons can form with other neurons as well as because of some computational properties that synapses exhibit such as associativity and input specificity, a memory storage system based on changes in synaptic strength has a potentially massive storage capacity (Poirazi and Mel, 2001). Consequently, theories based on persistent experience-driven changes in synaptic function have been extensively used to explain the storage of information (e.g., Fusi et al., 2005).

Nevertheless, an accumulating body of work indicates that learning also leads to persistent changes in intrinsic neuronal excitability (e.g., Brons and Woody, 1980; Crow and Alkon, 1980; Moyer et al., 1996; Cleary et al., 1998; Antonov et al., 2001; Brembs et al., 2002; Lorenzetti et al., 2006). These changes are due to modifications of membrane conductances and can affect electrophysiological properties including the resting potential, the input resistance, the shape and the threshold of the action potential, and the discharge frequency (for reviews see Daoudal and Debanne, 2003; Debanne et al., 2003; Zhang and Linden, 2003). What is the functional relevance of changes in intrinsic neuronal excitability to memory storage?

In this chapter, we will review some of the earlier work illustrating plasticity of intrinsic excitability produced by experience together with some more recent findings. In addition, we will discuss the implications of these results and the extent to which changes in synaptic efficacy and changes in intrinsic excitability can both contribute to memory storage.

14.2 Changes in Intrinsic Excitability Produced by Learning and Experience

Research over the past three decades has discovered modifications in the intrinsic membrane properties occurring in invertebrates and vertebrates following different forms of nonassociative and associative learning.

14.2.1 Invertebrate Models

Crow and Alkon (1980) were the first to report that classical conditioning (i.e., the learned ability to associate a predictive stimulus with a subsequent salient event) altered the excitability of the photoreceptors in the nudibranch mollusk *Hermissenda crassicornis*. The positive phototaxis that the animal normally exhibits in response to illumination was reduced when the animal was trained with multiple paired presentations of light (conditioned stimulus, CS) and rotation (unconditioned stimulus, US), which activates the vestibular system (Crow and Alkon, 1978). This form of learning was associative, and the suppression of phototaxis, the conditioned response, persisted for several days (Crow and Alkon, 1978). Classical conditioning produced changes in several membrane properties of the type B photoreceptors, which are the primary sensory neurons of the CS pathway. The type B photoreceptors are excited by light and also by synaptic drive from the statocyst cells, which are part of the vestibular system activated by rotation. The changes produced by classical conditioning included increases in input resistance, spontaneous firing and spike activity in response to light presentation or current injection, and generator potentials evoked by the CS (Crow and Alkon, 1980). Importantly, these changes persisted when the synaptic input to the photoreceptors was removed. Voltage-clamp analysis of the type B photoreceptors revealed that pairing-specific changes in several ionic currents were the biophysical substrate of the aforementioned altered membrane properties. Classical conditioning decreased two K^+ currents, a rapidly activating and inactivating K^+ current (I_A) and a Ca^{2+}-activated K^+ current ($I_{K,Ca}$) (Alkon et al., 1982, 1985; Farley, 1988), and also altered a voltage-dependent Ca^{2+} current (Collin et al., 1988). These biophysical changes were consistent with the increase in excitability observed in the type B photoreceptors following classical conditioning because a reduction of I_A and $I_{K,Ca}$ would tend to produce an enhanced depolarization and increased spike activity in the photoreceptors in response to the presentation of light. The pairing-specific increase in intrinsic excitability was observed for several days following conditioning. Also, the magnitude of the increase in excitability was positively correlated with the degree of phototactic suppression, thus suggesting a causal relationship between the biophysical changes in the type B photoreceptors and the expression of the conditioned response (Crow and Alkon, 1980).

Following the results observed in *Hermissenda*, other learning-related changes in intrinsic excitability were identified in other invertebrates including annelids and mollusks. In the leech *Hirudo medicinalis*, habituation and sensitization, two forms of nonassociative learning, altered in opposite directions the intrinsic excitability of an identified neuron. *Hirudo* exhibits a defensive withdrawal reflex that consists of whole-body shortening in response to light touch of the skin (Sahley, 1995). This reflex can be habituated, when it is repetitively evoked, or sensitized, when a strong, noxious stimulus is delivered (Sahley, 1995). Sensitization, which is mediated by serotonin (5-HT), requires the activity of a group of electrically coupled interneurons called the S-cells (Sahley et al., 1994). Sensitization increased the input resistance of the S-cells as well as their spike threshold and the number of action potentials evoked by intracellular depolarization (Burrell et al., 2001). These effects were mimicked by exogenous application of 5-HT (Burrell and Sahley, 2005). Conversely, habituation produced a decrease in intrinsic excitability (Burrell et al., 2001). These results indicate that in the leech bidirectional changes in intrinsic excitability represent cellular correlates of two distinct forms of nonassociative learning.

The marine mollusk *Aplysia californica* has been probably the most extensively used invertebrate model to study the cellular and molecular mechanisms of learning and memory. Several examples of experience-dependent changes in intrinsic excitability have been reported in *Aplysia* following both nonassociative and associative learning of simple defensive reflexes as well as associative learning of more complex behaviors such as feeding. Long-term (24-h) sensitization was associated with facilitation of the sensorimotor neuron synapse (Cleary et al., 1998) as well as changes in the biophysical properties of the tail sensory neurons (Cleary et al., 1998). The intrinsic changes included increases in the excitability and in the afterdepolarization following either a single spike or a burst of action potentials (Cleary et al., 1998). Voltage-clamp analysis revealed that long-term sensitization reduced the net outward current in the tail sensory neurons, which is consistent with the increased excitability observed in these neurons following learning (Scholz and Byrne, 1987). Interestingly, long-term sensitization training also altered the biophysical properties of tail motor neurons. These changes included a more hyperpolarized resting membrane potential and a decrease in the threshold for spike initiation (Cleary et al., 1998). The changes produced by long-term sensitization in the sensory neurons resembled those induced by short-term sensitization, thus suggesting that the phenotype of the expression mechanism for the short-term memory is preserved for the long-term memory. However, this is not always the case. Indeed, a more robust sensitization training protocol, which produced morphological changes in the sensory neurons and long-term synaptic facilitation of the sensorimotor neuron synapse (Wainwright et al., 2002), did not change the intrinsic excitability of the sensory neurons (Wainwright et al., 2004), but instead it induced narrowing of their action potentials (Antzoulatos and Byrne, 2007).

In *Aplysia*, classical conditioning also produced changes in the intrinsic excitability of sensory neurons. In a simplified preparation of the *Aplysia* siphon-withdrawal reflex, classical conditioning led to an increased input resistance and excitability of the siphon sensory neurons (Antonov et al., 2001, 2003). The changes in intrinsic excitability, as well as the pairing-specific strengthening of the sensorimotor neuron synapses, were restricted to the sensory neurons that were activated by mechanical stimulation of the siphon (i.e., on-field neurons), thus providing CS specificity to the expression of the conditioned response (Antonov et al., 2001, 2003). The presence of biophysical as well as synaptic changes following both nonassociative and associative learning suggested the intriguing hypothesis that the same cellular phenotype underlying nonassociative learning may also serve as the physiological substrate for associative memory (Byrne, 1987; Lechner and Byrne, 1998).

In *Aplysia*, the cellular mechanisms of associative learning were also studied using a more complex behavior (for a review see Baxter and Byrne, 2006). Appetitive forms of classical and operant conditioning (i.e., the ability to learn the consequences of a behavior) both increased the frequency of feeding behavior after training (Lechner et al., 2000a,b; Brembs et al., 2002; Baxter and Byrne, 2006; Lorenzetti et al., 2006). Also, both operant and classical conditioning changed the biophysical properties of neuron B51, a key element of the feeding neural circuitry, but the changes were remarkably different. Operant conditioning induced changes in B51 membrane properties (i.e., increased input resistance and decreased burst threshold), suggesting an increase in intrinsic excitability, which can contribute to the increased activity in B51 observed after training (Nargeot et al., 1999a,b; Brembs et al., 2002; Mozzachiodi et al., 2006). In contrast to operant conditioning, classical conditioning did not alter the input resistance, but increased the burst threshold of B51, resulting in a decreased intrinsic excitability (Lorenzetti et al., 2006).

These findings provided a biophysical substrate for the hypothesis that at the cellular level operant and classical conditioning are mediated by fundamentally different mechanisms (for a review see Baxter and Byrne, 2006). The decreased excitability in B51 was counterintuitive because classical conditioning enhances feeding in response to the CS and also strengthens the CS-evoked excitatory drive to B51 (Lorenzetti et al., 2006). However, the analysis of the responsiveness of B51 to the CS after training revealed that classical conditioning indeed facilitated the recruitment of B51, indicating that the factors that enhanced the recruitment of B51 overpowered the diminished excitability (Lorenzetti et al., 2006). Although experimental evidence is needed, the pairing-specific decrease in the excitability of B51 might represent an adaptive mechanism to help shape the CS specificity produced by classical conditioning.

Although most of the effects of learning on the membrane properties involved changes in input resistance and/or intrinsic excitability, other forms of intrinsic modifications were described as a result of experience in mollusks. For example, as mentioned above, long-term sensitization in *Aplysia* was associated with an increase in the resting potential of the motor neurons (Cleary et al., 1998). In the pond snail *Lymnaea stagnalis*, long-term memory for appetitive classical conditioning of feeding, induced by repetitive paired presentations of mechanical stimulation of the lips (CS) and application of sucrose as a feeding stimulant (US; for a review see Benjamin et al., 2000), was associated with a persistent depolarization in the modulatory neuron CV1a involved in the initiation of feeding movements (Jones et al., 2003). The pairing-specific depolarization of CV1a was positively correlated with the fictive feeding response to the CS in reduced preparations from conditioned animals, but it was not associated with any change in other membrane properties such as input resistance, spike threshold, or spike frequency (Jones et al., 2003). The time course of the persistent depolarization also mirrored the duration of retention of long-term memory (Jones et al., 2003). This pairing-specific depolarization would render CV1a more likely to fire in response to the CS and allow the CS to more effectively generate feeding responses.

14.2.2 Vertebrate Models

The first evidence of experience-dependent changes in neuronal excitability in a vertebrate model system was reported by Brons and Woody in 1980.

These authors used a conditioning paradigm in the cat in which repetitive paired presentations of an auditory click (CS) and a glabella tap (US), which evoked an eyeblink response, led to the appearance of the conditioned response consisting of a combined eyeblink and nose twitch (Brons and Woody, 1980). Cellular analysis conducted in the sensory-motor cortical areas and in the facial nucleus of awake cats revealed that classical conditioning was associated with an increased excitability as measured by the minimum amount of injected current necessary to evoke an action potential (Brons and Woody, 1980). An increase in input resistance was also measured in neurons of the facial nucleus. The persistence of the increased excitability, once the conditioned response was extinguished, indicated that this mechanism was not directly implicated in the formation and retention of the conditioned response (Brons and Woody, 1980). A detailed analysis of the biophysical substrate of the increased excitability has not been pursued.

Several other examples of experience-dependent changes in intrinsic excitability were identified in vertebrate models. In the rabbit, delay eyelid conditioning, which is performed using a tone as CS and a co-terminating air puff as US, depends on the activation of both the cerebellar cortex and cerebellar deep nuclei (for reviews see Kim and Thompson, 1997; Christian and Thompson, 2003). Recordings from Purkinje cells revealed a reduced spike threshold and a reduced afterhyperpolarization (AHP) evoked by bursts of spikes in slices from conditioned animals when compared to control animals (Schreurs et al., 1998). The AHP that follows action potentials is an important determinant for the firing activity of neurons, and a pairing-specific reduction of its amplitude is consistent with an increased excitability observed following classical conditioning. Importantly, these changes were long-lasting (up to 30 days), restricted to defined microzones of the cerebellar lobule HVI and the degree of reduction in spike threshold positively correlated with the conditioned response in the paired animals (Schreurs et al., 1997, 1998). Another form of classical conditioning is trace eyelid conditioning, which requires the hippocampus and occurs when a trace interval is imposed between the CS offset and the US onset. Cellular analysis of trace eyelid conditioning revealed that hippocampal pyramidal neurons in the CA1 and CA3 areas from conditioned animals exhibited a greater number of spikes evoked by depolarizing current injections (Moyer et al., 1996; Thompson et al., 1996) and a decreased AHP due to a reduction in the Ca^{2+}-dependent K^+ current underlying the AHP as compared to control animals (Coulter et al., 1989; Moyer et al., 1996; Thompson et al., 1996). These changes were consistent with a pairing-specific increase in excitability. Although the increased excitability was similar to that found following delay conditioning, it was not restricted to a specific area, but it was instead widespread through the dorsal hippocampus and also could not be detected 7 days after training when the memory for trace eyelid conditioning was still retained (Moyer et al., 1996; Thompson et al., 1996). These findings indicate that it is unlikely that this transient increased excitability in hippocampal neurons constitutes a part of the memory trace itself, but it could represent a mechanism through which the hippocampal circuit is set in a more permissive state for input-specific synaptic modification to occur during memory formation. A similar learning-dependent reduction in AHP also occurred in CA1 pyramidal neurons in the dorsal hippocampus following a spatial learning task that depends on the hippocampus (Oh et al., 2003).

In rats, pairing-specific enhancements in both CS-evoked synaptic drive and neuronal excitability (i.e., increased input resistance and a reduced amount of injected current necessary to elicit an action potential) were measured *in vivo* in neurons from the lateral nucleus of the amygdala of anesthetized rats trained with a conditioning paradigm during which an odor (CS) was repetitively paired with a foot shock (US; Rosenkranz and Grace, 2002). The synaptic and the intrinsic changes were both prevented when dopamine signaling, which is relevant for amygdala-dependent forms of learning, was pharmacologically blocked in the lateral nucleus of the amygdala (Rosenkranz and Grace, 2002). These results are consistent with the aforementioned studies of *Aplysia* withdrawal reflexes in which both synaptic and intrinsic plasticity occur together during memory formation.

Changes in intrinsic excitability have also been found in vertebrates following operant conditioning tasks. In monkeys, operant conditioning of the spinal stretch reflex is associated with changes in the intrinsic properties of the motor neurons. The spinal stretch reflex is among the simplest vertebrate reflexes and is largely mediated by a monosynaptic pathway between Ia afferent neurons and alpha motor neurons (Wolpaw, 1997). Because this reflex is influenced by descending activity from supraspinal structures, it can be operantly conditioned and animals can learn to gradually increase or decrease this reflex or its electrical analog, the H-reflex (Wolpaw, 1997). In particular, operantly conditioned decrease in the H-reflex in monkeys was associated with an increase in the depolarization needed for the spinal motor neuron to fire and a decrease in its conduction velocity (Carp and Wolpaw, 1994). These apparently intrinsic changes were consistent with the hypothesis that a positive shift in motor neuron firing threshold and a consequent increase in the depolarization needed to reach that threshold could contribute to weaken the magnitude of the H-reflex following operant conditioning. Modeling studies proposed that a positive shift in the activation of voltage dependence of Na^+ channels might represent the biophysical substrate for the operantly conditioned decrease in the H-reflex (Halter et al., 1995).

Changes in excitability were also reported in rats following an olfactory discrimination task (for a review see Saar and Barkai, 2003). Rats were trained to discriminate pairs of odors for a water reward. Several consecutive days of training were required for a rat to successfully discriminate between a first pair of odors, but once the rat reached good performance, its ability to learn to discriminate between a new pair of odors improved dramatically and only 1 day was needed to achieve good performance (Saar and Barkai, 2003). Cellular analysis revealed that both spike frequency adaptation and AHP amplitude were reduced in pyramidal neurons of the rat olfactory cortex following olfactory discrimination training when compared to naive or pseudo-trained animals (Saar et al., 1998, 2001). These changes were detected 1–3 days after training, but they decayed to baseline values by 5–7 days after training (Saar et al., 1998, 2001). It has been speculated that this example of increased excitability is not *per se* a mechanism of memory storage, but it might be involved in rule learning, setting the neural circuits in the piriform cortex in an excitable, more permissive state for activity-dependent synaptic modifications to occur (Saar and Barkai, 2003).

14.3 Activity-Dependent Modulation of Intrinsic Excitability

In addition to learning tasks *in vivo*, intrinsic excitability can be modulated by patterns of electrical stimulation of neurons and neural pathways. Depending on the protocol of stimulation, some of these patterns of neuronal activity may induce either an enhancement or a reduction of synaptic strength, or LTP (for a review see Lynch, 2004) and LTD (for a review see Ito, 2001), respectively. LTP, which is probably the most studied example of activity-dependent modulation of synaptic efficacy, can be induced in several areas of the vertebrate brain, including the hippocampus, the amygdala, the neocortex, and the cerebellar cortex, and is commonly considered to be a mechanism underlying aspects of learning and memory (for reviews see Bliss and Collingridge, 1993; Martin and Morris, 2002). Because several forms of LTP and LTD can be induced in isolated brain slices, the biochemical cascades underlying these forms of neuronal plasticity can be analyzed.

Although most of the work on LTP has focused on the mechanisms underlying the persistent augmentation of synaptic efficacy, several lines of evidence indicate that, at least in some cases, LTP is also accompanied by modifications in intrinsic excitability. Bliss and Lømo, who first described LTP in the dentate area of the rabbit hippocampus in 1973, also reported an increase in the population spike (i.e., the extracellularly recorded signal representing the summation of the evoked action potentials in postsynaptic neurons) accompanying LTP, which could not be entirely explained by the LTP-evoked increase in the population excitatory postsynaptic potential (EPSP). This nonsynaptic component of LTP was termed E-S potentiation, or E-S potentiation (Bliss and Lømo, 1973). The mechanisms underlying E-S potentiation are still subject to some debate. Two hypotheses have been developed to explain this phenomenon: an LTP-induced decrease in the ratio of inhibitory to excitatory drive (e.g., Abraham et al., 1987; Chavez-Noriega et al., 1989) and an LTP-induced increase in the intrinsic excitability of the postsynaptic neurons through modulation of voltage-dependent channels (e.g., Taube and Schwartzkroin, 1988; Bernard and Wheal, 1995). Several lines of evidence indicate that a reduction in the ratio of inhibitory to excitatory drive is not sufficient to account for the E-S potentiation, thus pointing to a role for LTP-induced intrinsic plasticity, the consequence of which would lead to a higher efficiency of E-S coupling (e.g., Wathey et al., 1992). One example, which suggests the modulation of voltage-dependent channels as a mechanism underlying the increased excitability accompanying synaptic LTP, has been reported in hippocampal CA1 pyramidal neurons. In these neurons, a pattern of synaptic inputs paired with postsynaptic spikes induced a long-term increase of intrinsic excitability concurring with synaptic LTP (Xu et al., 2005). The increased excitability was manifested as a decrease in the action potential threshold that was attributable to a shift in the activation curve of voltage-gated Na^+ channels (Xu et al., 2005). This form of enduring increase of intrinsic excitability shared a similar signaling pathway with the late phase of synaptic LTP, which included the requirement of activation of glutamate receptors of the *N*-methyl-D-aspartate (NMDA) type, the influx of Ca^{2+}, the activity of Ca^{2+}/calmodulin-dependent protein kinase II (CaMKII), and changes in protein synthesis (Xu et al., 2005).

The modulation of the E-S coupling appears to be bidirectional. In the CA1 region of the hippocampus, LTD, normally induced by low-frequency patterns of electrical stimulation, was accompanied by a reduction of the E-S coupling (Daoudal et al., 2002). This reduction of the E-S coupling was largely due to a decrease in the intrinsic excitability of hippocampal cells (Daoudal et al., 2002). Therefore, opposite modulation of the synaptic strength is associated with bidirectional changes in E-S coupling, which reflect bidirectional modifications of intrinsic excitability.

Other examples of activity-dependent changes in intrinsic excitability produced by synaptic activation have been reported in different brain areas. For example, in the rat entorhinal cortex, persistent graded increases in firing frequency were induced in pyramidal neurons by repetitive excitatory synaptic activation (Egorov et al., 2002). These sustained levels of firing could be either increased or decreased in an input-specific manner and relied on activity-dependent changes of Ca^{2+}-dependent cationic current (Egorov et al., 2002). This intrinsic ability of the neurons in the entorhinal cortex to generate graded persistent activity has been proposed as a cellular mechanism for working memory (Egorov et al., 2002). Another example of modulation of intrinsic excitability induced by synaptic activation has been reported in the cerebellar cortex. High-frequency stimulation of the mossy fiber-to-granule cells pathway led to LTP and was also accompanied by a persistent enhancement of intrinsic excitability of granule cells, which was associated with increased input resistance and decreased spike threshold (Armano et al., 2000). Neurons of the cerebellar deep nuclei also exhibited a rapid, synaptically driven, increase in their intrinsic excitability, which required Ca^{2+} influx through activation of NMDA-type glutamate receptors (Aizemann and Linden, 2000). However, in this case, the pattern of synaptic stimulation used to activate these neurons did not produce any facilitation of the synaptic input (Aizemann and Linden, 2000). This last example indicates that modulation of intrinsic excitability can be expressed without the occurrence of changes in synaptic function, thus providing a contribution to the information storage independent from synaptic plasticity.

Recent findings indicate that changes in intrinsic excitability may not require synaptic activation. For example, a train of high-frequency intracellular depolarizations delivered to pyramidal neurons in layer V of the primary visual cortex produced an enduring increase in intrinsic excitability (Cudmore and Turrigiano, 2004). This change in excitability required Ca^{2+} entry during neuronal activity and did not affect the passive membrane properties, thus suggesting the involvement of voltage-dependent channels (Cudmore and Turrigiano, 2004). Another example of synaptic-independent modulation of intrinsic excitability has been reported in hippocampal CA1 pyramidal neurons (Fan et al., 2005). A pattern of suprathreshold repeated intracellular stimulation (i.e., theta-burst firing) produced a decrease in somatic excitability, which was due to an upregulation of the hyperpolarization-activated cationic current I_h (Fan et al., 2005). This decrease in excitability was prevented by Ca^{2+} chelators; by low concentrations of tetrodotoxin, which blocked back propagation of action potentials from the soma to the dendrites; and by NMDA receptor antagonists even in the absence of synaptic activation (Fan et al., 2005). These findings suggest that during theta-burst firing, back-propagating action potentials would lead to Ca^{2+} influx through the NMDA receptor, which, in turn, would increase the I_h via a mechanism mediated by CaM kinase II.

Recent findings indicate that the synaptic drive does not need to be excitatory to induce an increase in intrinsic excitability. In the medial vestibular nucleus, brief periods of inhibitory synaptic input, or direct membrane hyperpolarization, triggered a long-lasting increase in both the spontaneous firing rate and firing responses to intracellular depolarization (Nelson et al., 2003). This increase in excitability, termed firing rate potentiation, was due to a decrease in cytosolic Ca^{2+}, which reduced CaM kinase II activity and, in turn, downregulated BK-type $I_{K,Ca}$ (Nelson et al., 2005). This novel form of neuronal plasticity might contribute to motor learning in the vestibulo-ocular reflex.

The intrinsic changes produced by patterns of neuronal activity are not restricted to ion channels and can include modulation of the activity of membrane transporters. For example, interneurons of the rat dentate gyrus exhibited a long-term depolarization of their resting membrane potential after high-frequency stimulation of the perforant path that was attributed to an activity-dependent change in the rate of the electrogenic Na^+ pump (Ross and Soltesz, 2001). This activity-dependent depolarization, which occurred in the absence of any potentiation of the excitatory synaptic input, required the rise of intracellular Ca^{2+} and the activation of alpha-amino-3-hydroxy-5-methyl-4-isoxazole propionic acid (AMPA), but not NMDA receptors (Ross and Soltesz, 2001). As a result of the depolarization, the interneurons of the dentate gyrus responded with action potential discharge to previously subthreshold EPSPs even in the absence of synaptic potentiation, thus indicating an increase in the E-S coupling (Ross and Soltesz, 2001). Activity-dependent changes in the function of the electrogenic Na^+ pump have been found also in invertebrate neurons. In the leech, low-frequency repetitive stimulation of touch (T) sensory neurons led to a lasting increase in the amplitude of the AHP produced by the firing discharge, which is due to an increase in the activity of the electrogenic Na^+ pump (Scuri et al., 2002). The modulation of the Na^+ pump activity was regulated by both the influx of Ca^{2+} during neural activity and the release of Ca^{2+} from intracellular stores. In addition, phospholipase A2 and the downstream activation of arachidonic acid metabolites, derived from the 5-lipoxygenase pathway, were necessary for the increase of the AHP amplitude (Scuri et al., 2005). The increase of the AHP amplitude was associated with a persistent depression of the synaptic connection between T cells and their follower neurons (Scuri et al., 2002). This synaptic depression may be a cellular mechanism contributing to short-term habituation. Since 5-HT mediates sensitization in the leech (e.g., Catarsi et al., 1990; Sahley et al., 1994; Zaccardi et al., 2004), it has effects on the amplitude of the AHP in T neurons opposite those produced by repetitive stimulation. Indeed, 5-HT reduced the AHP amplitude by inhibiting the Na^+ pump (Catarsi and Brunelli, 1991) in a cyclic adenosine monophosphate (cAMP)-dependent manner (Catarsi et al., 1993). Injection of cAMP into a T neuron enhanced the synaptic connection between the T cell and its follower neurons (Scuri et al., 2007). Together these findings indicate that bidirectional changes in the AHP amplitude that alter synaptic efficacy may represent cellular mechanisms underlying habituation and sensitization, two simple forms of learning.

14.4 Plasticity of Intrinsic Excitability as a Mechanism for Memory Storage: Hypotheses and Lines of Evidence

The general motif that emerges from the examples above is that several different learning tasks, nonassociative and associative, as well as activation of neurons and neural pathways, induce changes in the biophysical properties of neurons in both invertebrates and vertebrates. These neurophysiological correlates have been identified at the level of sensory neurons, interneurons, and motor neurons.

What is the functional relevance of these changes? In some cases, a direct role for the intrinsic plasticity in memory storage appears straightforward. For example, in *Aplysia* and *Hermissenda*, because the loci of plasticity induced by classical conditioning were found at the level of the first central relay in the circuits controlling the responses, neuron-wide changes in intrinsic excitability in response to the conditioned stimuli appear to be an appropriate memory mechanism to express and retain the conditioned response. However, in other cases the changes in intrinsic excitability failed to correlate, or correlated poorly, with the learned behavioral changes, thus making it difficult to assess their contribution to the storage of memory (e.g., Cleary et al., 1998). Although additional results are required, one hypothesis is that some of the intrinsic changes may not function as part of the engram itself, but they may represent either adaptive mechanisms to shape the stimulus specificity of the learned response (as in the case of classical conditioning of feeding in *Aplysia* (Baxter and Byrne, 2006; Lorenzetti et al., 2006), or mechanisms through which a neural circuit is set to a permissive state to facilitate the occurrence of the synaptic modifications necessary for memory formation (as in the case of trace eyelid conditioning in rabbits (Moyer et al., 1996; Thompson et al., 1996) or olfactory operant conditioning in rats (Saar and Barkai, 2003).

Another issue that requires more investigation is the extent to which the changes in intrinsic excitability are complementary to experience-dependent modifications in synaptic efficacy. The majority of theoretical models of memory storage have been largely based on persistent experience-driven changes in synaptic function (Poirazi and Mel, 2001; Fusi et al., 2005). Certain unique properties of the synapses such as associativity and input specificity cause systems of memory storage based on changes in synaptic strength to have a potentially massive storage capacity (Poirazi and Mel, 2001; Fusi et al., 2005). In contrast, global changes in intrinsic excitability would theoretically alter the throughput of all the synaptic inputs impinging on a given neuron. If this is the case, memory mechanisms based on neuron-wide altered intrinsic excitability would have a lower storage capacity and would be less versatile than systems of memory storage based on changes in synaptic strength.

Some recent results may help to reconcile differences between models of memory storage based on synaptic plasticity and models based on intrinsic plasticity. Patch-clamp techniques and simultaneous Ca^{2+} imaging that allow for recordings from individual dendrites (for a review see Magee and Johnston, 2005) have revealed that the induction of LTP was accompanied by a local increase in dendritic excitability that favored back propagation of action potentials into that dendritic region with a subsequent boost in the Ca^{2+} influx (Frick et al., 2004). A shift in the inactivation curve of a transient A-type K^+ current was found to account for the enhanced excitability (Frick et al., 2004). Importantly, the activity-dependent increase in dendritic excitability was localized at, or in the vicinity of, the synaptic site, which was potentiated in an input-specific manner following electrical stimulation (Frick et al., 2004). A local increase in dendritic excitability could facilitate enhanced propagation of synaptic potentials toward the site of action potential initiation (for a review see Magee and Johnston, 2005). Therefore, enhancement of local excitability could contribute to the higher efficiency of coupling between synaptic potentials and spike as observed following LTP induction.

Although validation in *in vivo* preparations is required, these findings indicate that changes in intrinsic excitability can be induced in restricted membrane compartments and can be co-expressed with changes in synaptic efficacy in a manner that affects signal integration locally and can preserve input specificity.

14.5 Summary

Data collected over the past decades in both vertebrate and invertebrate model systems indicate that learning and memory as well as patterns of electrical stimulation of neurons and neural pathways not only alter synaptic function but also produce changes in intrinsic excitability. These changes in intrinsic excitability can be neuron-wide or restricted to specific membrane compartments such as the dendrites, thus affecting neuronal function and signal integration either globally or locally. Although the functional relevance of certain changes in intrinsic excitability in the context of a given form of learning has not been fully elucidated, it is becoming clear that experience-dependent changes in intrinsic excitability may function as part of the engram itself, as adaptive mechanisms to shape the stimulus specificity of the learned response or also as mechanisms through which a neural circuit is set to a permissive state to facilitate the occurrence of the synaptic modifications necessary for memory formation and retrieval.

References

Abraham WC, Gustafsson B, and Wigstrom H (1987) Long-term potentiation involves enhanced synaptic excitation relative to synaptic inhibition in guinea-pig hippocampus. *J. Physiol.* 394: 367–380.

Aizenman CD and Linden DJ (2000) Rapid, synaptically driven increases in the intrinsic excitability of cerebellar deep nuclear neurons. *Nat. Neurosci.* 3: 109–111.

Alkon DL, Lederhendler I, and Shoukimas JJ (1982) Primary changes of membrane currents during retention of associative learning. *Science* 215: 693–695.

Alkon DL, Sakakibara M, Forman R, Harrigan J, Lederhendler I, and Farley J (1985) Reduction of two voltage-dependent K^+ currents mediates retention of a learned association. *Behav. Neural Biol.* 44: 278–300.

Antonov I, Antonova I, Kandel ER, and Hawkins RD (2001) The contribution of activity-dependent synaptic plasticity to classical conditioning in *Aplysia*. *J. Neurosci.* 21: 6413–6422.

Antonov I, Antonova I, Kandel ER, and Hawkins RD (2003) Activity-dependent presynaptic facilitation and Hebbian LTP are both required and interact during classical conditioning *Aplysia*. *Neuron* 37: 135–147.

Antzoulatos E and Byrne JH (2007) Long-term sensitization training produces spike narrowing in *Aplysia* sensory neurons. *J. Neurosci.* 27: 676–683.

Armano S, Rossi P, Taglietti V, and D'Angelo E (2000) Long-term potentiation of intrinsic excitability at the mossy fiber-granule cell synapse of rat cerebellum. *J. Neurosci.* 20: 5208–5216.

Baxter DA and Byrne JH (2006) Feeding behavior of *Aplysia:* A model system for comparing cellular mechanisms of classical and operant conditioning. *Learn. Mem.* 13: 669–680.

Benjamin PR, Staras K, and Kemenes G (2000) A system approach to the cellular analysis of associative learning in the pond snail *Lymnaea*. *Learn. Mem.* 7: 124–131.

Bernard C and Wheal HV (1995) Simultaneous expression of excitatory postsynaptic potential/spike potentiation and excitatory postsynaptic potential/spike depression in the hippocampus. *Neuroscience* 67: 73–82.

Bliss TV and Collingridge GL (1993) A synaptic model of memory: Long-term potentiation in the hippocampus. *Nature* 361: 31–39.

Bliss TV and Lømo T (1973) Long-lasting potentiation of synaptic transmission in the dentate area of the anaesthetized rabbit following stimulation of the perforant path. *J. Physiol.* 232: 331–356.

Brembs B, Lorenzetti FD, Reyes FD, Baxter DA, and Byrne JH (2002) Operant reward learning in *Aplysia:* Neuronal correlates and mechanisms. *Science* 296: 1706–1709.

Brons JF and Woody CD (1980) Long-term changes in excitability of cortical neurons after Pavlovian conditioning and extinction. *J. Neurophysiol.* 44: 605–615.

Burrell BD and Sahley CL (2005) Serotonin mediates learning-induced potentiation of excitability. *J. Neurophysiol.* 94: 4002–4010.

Burrell BD, Sahley CL, and Muller KJ (2001) Non-associative learning and serotonin induce similar bi-directional changes in excitability of a neuron critical for learning in the medicinal leech. *J. Neurosci.* 21: 1401–1412.

Byrne JH (1987) Cellular analysis of associative learning. *Physiol. Rev.* 67: 329–439.

Carp JS and Wolpaw JR (1994) Motoneuron plasticity underlying operantly conditioned decrease in primate H reflex. *J. Neurophysiol.* 72: 431–442.

Catarsi S and Brunelli M (1991) Serotonin depresses the after-hyperpolarization through the inhibition of the Na+/K+ electrogenic pump in T sensory neurones of the leech. *J. Exp. Biol.* 155: 261–273.

Catarsi S, Garcia-Gil M, Traina G, and Brunelli M (1990) Seasonal variation of serotonin content and nonassociative learning of swim induction in the leech *Hirudo medicinalis*. *J. Comp. Physiol. A* 167: 469–474.

Catarsi S, Scuri R, and Brunelli M (1993) Cyclic AMP mediates inhibition of the Na(+)-K+ electrogenic pump by serotonin in tactile sensory neurones of the leech. *J. Physiol.* 462: 229–242.

Chavez-Noriega LE, Bliss TV, and Halliwell JV (1989) The EPSP-spike (E-S) component of long-term potentiation in the rat hippocampal slice is modulated by GABAergic but not cholinergic mechanisms. *Neurosci. Lett.* 104: 58–64.

Christian KM and Thompson RF (2003) Neural substrates of eyeblink conditioning: Acquisition and retention. *Learn. Mem.* 10: 427–455.

Cleary LJ, Lee WL, and Byrne JH (1998) Cellular correlates of long-term sensitization in *Aplysia*. *J. Neurosci.* 18: 5988–5998.

Collin C, Ikeno H, Harrigan JF, Lederhendler I, and Alkon DL (1988) Sequential modification of membrane currents with classical conditioning. *Biophys. J.* 54: 955–960.

Coulter DA, Lo Turco JJ, Kubota M, Disterhoft JF, Moore JW, and Alkon DL (1989) Classical conditioning reduces amplitude and duration of calcium-dependent afterhyperpolarization in rabbit hippocampal pyramidal cells. *J. Neurophysiol.* 61: 971–981.

Crow TJ and Alkon DL (1978) Retention of an associative behavioral change in *Hermissenda*. *Science* 201: 1239–1241.

Crow TJ and Alkon DL (1980) Associative behavioral modification in *Hermissenda:* Cellular correlates. *Science* 209: 412–414.

Cudmore RH and Turrigiano GG (2004) Long-term potentiation of intrinsic excitability in LV visual cortical neurons. *J. Neurophysiol.* 92: 341–348.

Daoudal G and Debanne D (2003) Long-term plasticity of intrinsic excitability: Learning rules and mechanisms. *Learn. Mem.* 10: 456–465.

Daoudal G, Hanada Y, and Debanne D (2002) Bidirectional plasticity of excitatory postsynaptic potential (EPSP)-spike coupling in CA1 hippocampal pyramidal neurons. *Proc. Natl. Acad. Sci. USA* 99: 14512–14517.

Debanne D, Daoudal G, Sourdet V, and Russier M (2003) Brain plasticity and ion channels. *J. Physiol. Paris* 97: 403–414.

Egorov AV, Hamam BN, Fransen E, Hasselmo ME, and Alonso AA (2002) Graded persistent activity in entorhinal cortex neurons. *Nature* 420: 173–178.

Fan Y, Fricker D, Brager DH, et al. (2005) Activity-dependent decrease of excitability in rat hippocampal neurons through increases in I_h. *Nat. Neurosci.* 8: 1542–1551.

Farley J (1988) Associative training results in persistent reductions in a calcium-activated potassium current in *Hermissenda* type B photoreceptors. *Behav. Neurosci.* 102: 784–802.

Frick A, Magee J, and Johnston D (2004) LTP is accompanied by an enhanced local excitability of pyramidal neuron dendrites. *Nat. Neurosci.* 7: 126–135.

Fusi S, Drew PJ, and Abbott LF (2005) Cascade models of synaptically stored memories. *Neuron* 45: 599–611.

Halter JA, Carp JS, and Wolpaw JR (1995) Operantly conditioned motoneuron plasticity: Possible role of sodium channels. *J. Neurophysiol.* 73: 867–871.

Ito M (2001) Cerebellar long-term depression: Characterization, signal transduction, and functional roles. *Physiol. Rev.* 81: 1143–1195.

Jones NG, Kemenes I, Kemenes G, and Benjamin PR (2003) A persistent cellular change in a single modulatory neuron contributes to associative long-term memory. *Curr. Biol.* 13: 1064–1069.

Kim JJ and Thompson RF (1997) Cerebellar circuits and synaptic mechanisms involved in classical eyeblink conditioning. *Trends Neurosci.* 20: 177–181.

Lechner HA and Byrne JH (1998) New perspectives on classical conditioning: A synthesis of Hebbian and non-Hebbian mechanisms. *Neuron* 20: 355–358.

Lechner HA, Baxter DA, and Byrne JH (2000a) Classical conditioning of feeding behavior in *Aplysia:* I. Behavioral analysis. *J. Neurosci.* 20: 3369–3376.

Lechner HA, Baxter DA, and Byrne JH (2000b) Classical conditioning of feeding behavior in *Aplysia:* II. Neurophysiological correlates. *J. Neurosci.* 20: 3377–3386.

Lorenzetti FD, Mozzachiodi R, Baxter DA, and Byrne JH (2006) Classical and operant conditioning differentially modify the intrinsic properties of an identified neuron. *Nat. Neurosci.* 9: 17–19.

Lynch MA (2004) Long-term potentiation and memory. *Physiol. Rev.* 84: 87–136.

Magee JC and Johnston D (2005) Plasticity of dendritic function. *Curr. Opin. Neurobiol.* 15: 334–342.

Martin SJ and Morris RG (2002) New life in an old idea: The synaptic plasticity and memory hypothesis revisited. *Hippocampus* 12: 609–636.

Mozzachiodi R, Baxter DA, and Byrne JH (2006) Enduring changes in the intrinsic excitability of an identified neuron contribute to long-term memory following operant conditioning. Program No. 669.9. 2006 *Abstract Viewer/Itinerary Planner.* Washington, DC: Society for Neuroscience.

Moyer JR, Thompson LT, and Disterhoft JF (1996) Trace eyeblink conditioning increases CA1 excitability in a transient and learning specific manner. *J. Neurosci.* 16: 5536–5546.

Nargeot R, Baxter DA, and Byrne JH (1999a) *In vitro* analog of operant conditioning in *Aplysia*. I. Contingent reinforcement modifies the functional dynamics of an identified neuron. *J. Neurosci.* 19: 2247–2260.

Nargeot R, Baxter DA, and Byrne JH (1999b). *In vitro* analog of operant conditioning in *Aplysia*. II. Modifications of the functional dynamics of an identified neuron contribute to motor pattern selection. *J. Neurosci.* 19: 2261–2272.

Nelson AB, Krispel CM, Sekirnjak C, and du Lac S (2003) Long-lasting increases in intrinsic excitability triggered by inhibition. *Neuron* 40: 609–620.

Nelson AB, Gittis AH, and du Lac S (2005) Decreases in CaMKII activity trigger persistent potentiation of intrinsic excitability in spontaneously firing vestibular nucleus neurons. *Neuron* 46: 623–631.

Oh MM, Kuo AG, Wu WW, Sametsky EA, and Disterhoft JF (2003) Watermaze learning enhances excitability of CA1 pyramidal neurons. *J. Neurophysiol.* 90: 2171–2179.

Poirazi P and Mel BW (2001) Impact of active dendrites and structural plasticity on the memory capacity of neural tissue. *Neuron* 29: 779–796.

Rosenkranz JA and Grace AA (2002) Dopamine-mediated modulation of odour-evoked amygdala potentials during pavlovian conditioning. *Nature* 417: 282–287.

Ross ST and Soltesz I (2001) Long-term plasticity in interneurons of the dentate gyrus. *Proc. Natl. Acad. Sci. USA* 98: 8874–8879.

Saar D and Barkai E (2003) Long-term modifications in intrinsic neuronal properties and rule learning in rats. *Eur. J. Neurosci.* 17: 2727–2734.

Saar D, Grossman Y, and Barkai E (1998) Reduced after-hyperpolarization in rat piriform cortex pyramidal neurons is associated with increased learning capability during operant conditioning. *Eur. J. Neurosci.* 10: 1518–1523.

Saar D, Grossman Y, and Barkai E (2001) Long-lasting cholinergic modulation underlies rule learning in rats. *J. Neurosci.* 21: 1385–1392.

Sahley CL (1995) What we have learned from the study of learning in the leech. *J. Neurobiol.* 27: 434–445.

Sahley CL, Modney BK, Boulis NM, and Muller KJ (1994) The S cell: An interneuron essential for sensitization and full dishabituation of leech shortening. *J. Neurosci.* 14: 6715–6721.

Scholz KP and Byrne JH (1987) Long-term sensitization in *Aplysia:* Biophysical correlates in tail sensory neurons. *Science* 235: 685–687.

Schreurs BG, Tomsic D, Gusev PA, and Alkon DL (1997) Dendritic excitability microzones and occluded long-term depression after classical conditioning of the rabbit's nictitating membrane response. *J. Neurophysiol.* 77: 86–92.

Schreurs BG, Gusev PA, Tomsic D, Alkon DL, and Shi T (1998) Intracellular correlates of acquisition and long-term memory of classical conditioning in Purkinje cell dendrites in slices of rabbit cerebellar lobule HVI. *J. Neurosci.* 18: 5498–5507.

Scuri R, Mozzachiodi R, and Brunelli M (2002) Activity-dependent increase of the AHP amplitude in T sensory neurons of the leech. *J. Neurophysiol.* 88: 2490–2500.

Scuri R, Mozzachiodi R, and Brunelli M (2005) Role of calcium signaling and arachidonic acid metabolites in the activity-dependent increase of AHP amplitude in leech T sensory neurons. *J. Neurophysiol.* 94: 1066–1073.

Scuri R, Lombardo P, Cataldo E, Ristori C, and Brunelli M (2007) The inhibition of the Na/K ATPase potentiates synaptic transmission in T sensory neurons of the leech. *Eur. J. Neurosci.* 25: 159–167.

Taube JS and Schwartzkroin PA (1988) Mechanisms of long-term potentiation: EPSP/spike dissociation, intradendritic recordings, and glutamate sensitivity. *J. Neurosci.* 8: 1632–1644.

Thompson LT, Moyer JR, and Disterhoft JF (1996) Transient changes in excitability of rabbit CA3 neurons with a time course appropriate to support memory consolidation. *J. Neurophysiol.* 76: 1836–1849.

Wainwright ML, Zhang H, Byrne JH, and Cleary LJ (2002) Localized neuronal outgrowth induced by long-term sensitization training in *Aplysia*. *J. Neurosci.* 22: 4132–4141.

Wainwright ML, Byrne JH, and Cleary LJ (2004) Dissociation of morphological and physiological changes associated with long-term memory in *Aplysia*. *J. Neurophysiol.* 92: 2628–2632.

Wathey JC, Lytton WW, Jester JM, and Sejnowski TJ (1992) Computer simulations of EPSP-spike (E-S) potentiation in hippocampal CA1 pyramidal cells. *J. Neurosci.* 12: 607–618.

Wolpaw JR (1997) The complex structure of a simple memory. *Trends Neurosci.* 20: 588–894.

Xu J, Kang N, Jiang L, Nedergaard M, and Kang J (2005) Activity-dependent long-term potentiation of intrinsic excitability in hippocampal CA1 pyramidal neurons. *J. Neurosci.* 25: 1750–1760.

Zaccardi ML, Traina G, Cataldo E, and Brunelli M (2004) Sensitization and dishabituation of swim induction in the *Hirudo medicinalis:* Role of serotonin and cyclic AMP. *Behav. Brain Res.* 153: 317–326.

Zhang W and Linden DJ (2003) The other side of the engram: Experience-driven changes in neuronal intrinsic excitability. *Nat. Rev. Neurosci.* 4: 885–900.

15 Neural Computation Theories of Learning

S. B. Moldakarimov, Salk Institute for Biological Studies, La Jolla, CA, USA

T. J. Sejnowski, Salk Institute for Biological Studies and University of California at San Diego, La Jolla, CA, USA

15.1 Introduction

The anatomical discoveries in the nineteenth century and the physiological studies in the twentieth century showed that brains were networks of neurons connected through synapses. This led to the theory that learning could be the consequence of changes in the strengths of the synapses.

The best-known theory of learning based on synaptic plasticity is that proposed by Donald Hebb, who postulated that connection strengths between neurons are modified based on neural activities in the presynaptic and postsynaptic cells:

> When an axon of cell A is near enough to excite cell B and repeatedly or persistently takes part in firing it, some growth process or metabolic change takes place in one or both cells such that A's efficiency, as one of the cells firing B, is increased. (Hebb, 1949)

This postulate was experimentally confirmed in the hippocampus with high-frequency stimulation of a presynaptic neuron that caused long-term potentiation (LTP) in the synapses connecting it to the postsynaptic neuron (Bliss and Lomo, 1973). LTP takes place only if the postsynaptic cell is also active and sufficiently depolarized (Kelso et al., 1986). This is due to the *N*-methyl-D-aspartate (NMDA) type of glutamate receptor, which opens when glutamate is bound to the receptor, and the postsynaptic cell is sufficiently depolarized at the same time (*See* Chapter 16).

Hebb's postulate has served as the starting point for studying the learning capabilities of artificial neural networks (ANN) and for the theoretical analysis and computational modeling of biological neural systems. The architecture of an ANN determines its behavior and learning capabilities. The architecture of a network is defined by the connections among the artificial neural units and the function that each unit performs on its inputs. Two general classes are feedforward and recurrent architecture.

The simplest feedforward network has one layer of input units and one layer of output units (**Figure 1**, left). All connections are unidirectional and project from the input units to the output units. The perceptron is an example of a simple feedforward network (Rosenblatt, 1958). It can learn to classify patterns from examples. It turned out that the perceptron can only classify patterns that are linearly separable – that is, if the positive patterns can be separated from all negative patterns by a plane in the space of input patterns. More powerful multilayer feedforward networks can discriminate patterns that are not linearly separable. In a multilayer feedforward network, the 'hidden' layers of units between the input and output layers allow more flexibility in learning features. Multilayer feedforward networks have also been applied to solve some other difficult problems (Rumelhart and McClelland, 1986).

In contrast to strictly feedforward network models, recurrent networks also have feedback connections

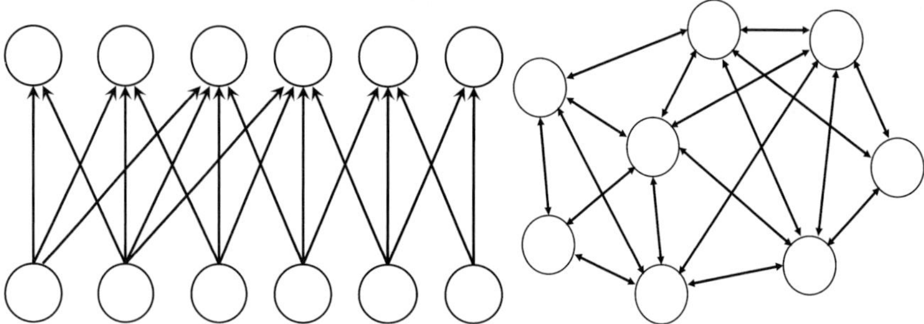

Figure 1 Network architectures. Left: Feedforward network. Right: Recurrent network. Open circles represent neuronal units, and arrowhead lines represent synaptic connections.

among units in the network (**Figure 1**, right). A simple recurrent network can have a uniform architecture such as all-to-all connectivity combined with symmetric weights between units, as in a Hopfield network (Hopfield, 1982), or it can be a network with specific connections designed to model a particular biological system.

Modeling learning processes in networks implies that the strengths of connections and other parameters are adjusted according to a learning rule (*See* Chapter 16). Other parameters that may change include the threshold of the unit, time constants, and other dynamical variables. A learning rule is a dynamical equation that governs changes in the parameters of the network. There are three main categories of learning rules: unsupervised, supervised, and reinforcement. Unsupervised learning rules are those that require no feedback from a teaching signal. Supervised learning rules require a teacher, who provides detailed information on the desired values of the output units of the network, and connections are adjusted based on discrepancies between the actual output and the desired one. Reinforcement learning is also error correcting but involves a single scalar signal about the overall performance of the network. Thus, reinforcement learning requires less-detailed information than supervised learning.

A learning algorithm specifies how and under what conditions a learning rule or a combination of learning rules should be applied to adjust the network parameters. For a simple task, it is possible to invent an algorithm that includes only one type of learning rule, but for more complex problems, an algorithm may involve a combination of several different learning rules.

In the following sections, we give an overview of basic learning rules and examples of learning algorithms used in neural network models, and describe specific problems solved by neural networks with adjustable parameters.

15.2 Hebbian Learning

Implementations of Hebb's rule can take different forms (Sejnowski and Tesauro, 1988). Simple associative Hebbian learning is based on the coincidence of activities in presynaptic and postsynaptic neurons. The dynamics of Hebbian learning are governed by a differential equation:

$$\frac{\mathrm{d}w_{ij}}{\mathrm{d}t} = \alpha \cdot v_i \cdot u_j$$

where w_{ij} is the weight of a connection from an input unit j with activity u_j to an output unit i with activity v_i, and α is a learning rate.

The Hebbian learning rule has been used to model a wide variety of problems, including feature selectivity and cortical map development.

Cortical neurons respond selectively to particular feature stimuli, such as selectivity for ocular dominance and orientation in the visual cortex. To understand challenges of modeling the development of feature selectivity, consider a network with many input units and one output unit. We would like to explore under what conditions the output unit will respond well to few input units and less to the others. If we apply a stimulus to the input units and allow the connections to develop according to the Hebbian learning rule, then all connections will grow and eventually saturate, and no selectivity will emerge. To develop selectivity, some dependencies among weights are needed, so that changes at one connection will influence the others. There are many different ways to introduce dependencies. One approach is to introduce weight normalization (Miller and Mackay, 1994). A different approach, based on competition among input patterns, called the BCM (Bienenstock, Cooper, and Munro) rule (Bienenstock et al., 1982), has been used to model the development of orientation selectivity and ocular dominance in neural networks.

Neuronal response selectivity varies across the cortex in regular patterns called cortical maps. Although some aspects of cortical map formation during development are activity independent, neuronal activity can modify the maps. Hebbian learning rules have also been applied to model the effects of cortical activity on map formations. For comprehensive overviews of neural network models that develop orientation selectivity maps and ocular dominance columns, see Swindale (1996) and Ferster and Miller (2000).

Models of cortical map formation can become extremely complex when multiple features, such as retinotopic location, ocular dominance, orientation preference, and others, are considered simultaneously. To deal with such problems, a more abstract class of models was developed by Kohonen (1982). The Kohonen algorithm is usually applied to two-layer networks with feedforward connections from an input layer to an output layer. The input layer is an N-dimensional vector layer. The output layer is normally a one- or two-dimensional array. There are no lateral connections in the output layer, but the algorithm can accomplish what models with lateral connections can achieve at less computational cost. The algorithm does this by a weight updating procedure that involves neighboring units. At every step, it chooses a 'winner' among output units whose weights are closest to the input pattern. Then it updates the weights of the winner and the nearby neighbors of the winner. The number of neighbors that participate in weight updating is controlled through a neighborhood function, which is dynamically changed during learning to ensure convergence. The neighborhood function starts out long range and is reduced as learning proceeds. This allows the network to organize a map rapidly and then refine it more slowly with subsequent learning.

Models based on the Kohonen algorithm perform dimensionality reduction, which facilitates data analysis, taking input vectors from a high-dimensional feature space and projecting them onto a low-dimensional representation.

15.3 Unsupervised Hebbian Learning

If the goal of learning is to discover the statistical structure in unlabeled input data, then the learning is said to be unsupervised. A common method for unsupervised learning is principal component analysis (PCA). Suppose the data are a set of N-dimensional input vectors. The task is to find an $M < N$ dimensional representation of N-dimensional input vectors that contains as much information as possible of the input data. This is an example of dimensionality reduction, which can significantly simplify subsequent data analysis.

A simple network that can extract the first principal component (the one with the maximal variance) is a network with N input units and one output unit. At each time step an N-dimensional input vector is applied to the input layer. If we allow the connections to be modified according to the Hebbian learning rule, then in the case of zero mean value of the input vector, the weights will form an N-dimensional vector, along which the variance will be the largest. This is the principal eigenvector or component. A network with N input and M output units, augmented with a generalized Hebbian learning rule, can learn first M components. The projections of the input data onto the components give us M-dimensional representation of the N-dimensional input data.

PCA is appropriate when the data obey Gaussian statistics, but images, audio recordings, and many types of scientific data often do not have Gaussian distributions. As an example of such a problem, consider a room where a number of people are talking simultaneously (cocktail party), and the task is to focus on one of the speakers. The human brain can, to some extent, solve this auditory source separation problem by using knowledge of the speaker, but this becomes a more difficult problem when the signals are arbitrary. The goal of blind source separation (BSS) is to recover source signals given only sensor signals that are linear mixtures of the independent source signals. Independent component analysis (ICA) is a method that solves the BSS problem for non-Gaussian signals. In contrast to correlation-based algorithms such as PCA and factor analysis, ICA finds a nonorthogonal linear coordinate system such that the resulting signals are as statistically independent from each other as possible.

One approach to BSS derives unsupervised learning rules based on information theory. The input is assumed to be N mixtures of N independent sources, and the goal is to maximize the mutual information between the inputs and the outputs of a two-layer neural network. The resulting stochastic gradient learning rules are highly effective in the blind separation and deconvolution of hundreds of non-Gaussian sources (Bell and Sejnowski, 1995).

ICA is particularly effective at analyzing electroencephalograms (EEG) and functional magnetic resonance imaging (fMRI) data (Jung et al., 2001). Consider, for example, electrical recordings of brain activity at many different locations on the scalp. These EEG potentials are generated by underlying components of brain activity and various muscle and eye movements. This is similar to the cocktail-party problem: We would like to recover the original components of the brain activity, but we can only observe mixtures of the components. ICA can reveal interesting information of the brain activity by giving access to its independent components. ICA also gives useful insights into task-related human brain activity from fMRI recordings when the underlying temporal structure of the sources is unknown.

Another application of ICA is feature extraction (Lee, 1998). A fundamental problem in signal processing is to find suitable representations for images, audio recordings, and other kinds of data. Standard linear transformations used in image and auditory processing, such the Fourier transforms and cosine transforms, may not be optimal, and but it would be useful to find the most efficient linear transformation, based on the statistics of the data, to optimally compress the data.

15.4 Supervised Learning

Consider the problem of learning to retrieve an output pattern given an input pattern. To remember the patterns, the Hebbian rule can be applied to adjust weights between input and output units. As mentioned earlier, however, the associative Hebbian learning rule will lead to saturation with multiple repetitions, which reduces the capacity of the network. To resolve this problem, one can augment the Hebbian rule with a weight normalization algorithm as in the case of unsupervised learning algorithms.

Another disadvantage of using the associative Hebbian learning rule is that weight adjustments do not depend on the actual performance of the network. An effective way to adjust weights would be by using information of the actual performance of the network. Supervised learning can do this. Supervised learning requires a teacher, who provides detailed information of the desired outputs of the network and adjusts the connections based on discrepancies between the actual outputs and the desired ones.

The perceptron uses a supervised learning rule to learn to classify input patterns (Rosenblatt, 1958). The perceptron is a two-layer network with one output unit that can classify input patterns into two categories. The Hebbian learning rule can be used to solve the task, but the perceptron with the Hebbian learning rule works well only if the number of input patterns is significantly less than the number of input units. An error-correcting supervised learning algorithm for weight adjustments is more effective for a large number of input patterns:

$$\frac{\mathrm{d}w_{ij}}{\mathrm{d}t} \propto u_j \cdot (R_i - v_i)$$

where w_{ij} is a weight of a connection from the input unit j with activity u_j to an output unit i with activity v_i, R_i is a target value of the output unit, and

$$v_i = \sum_j w_{ij} \cdot u_j$$

The perceptron learning rule uses the performance of the network to decide how much adjustment is needed and in which direction the weights should be changed to decrease the discrepancy between the actual network outputs and the desired ones. If input patterns are linearly separable, then the perceptron learning rule guarantees to find a set of weights that allow pattern classification.

A simple unsupervised Hebbian learning rule adjusts synaptic weights based on correlations between presynaptic and postsynaptic neurons. However, this approach is inefficient when the goal of the network is to perform a specific function, rather than simply represent data. To perform a specific task, the network should receive some information about the task.

An example of how Hebbian plasticity can be incorporated into a supervised learning framework is a two-layer network that was trained to perform a function approximation task (Swinehart and Abbott, 2005). The feedforward connections from input units to output units were modified according to an unsupervised Hebbian rule, and a supervised learning mechanism was used to adjust connections from a supervisor to the network. The supervisor is a network that assesses the performance of the training network and, based on that information, modifies the gains of the input units using an error-correcting learning rule. The purpose of the supervised modulation was to enhance connections between the input and the output units to facilitate the synaptic plasticity needed to learn the task. Thus, Hebbian plasticity did not have direct access to the supervision, and the supervised modulations did not produce any permanent changes. Nonetheless, this network could learn to approximate different functions. In the initial phase the improvement in the network performance was mostly due to the gain modulation, and the synaptic adjustments were minimal. But later, the synaptic adjustments and the gain modulation were equally involved in shaping the performance. Once the network learned the task with the supervisor, it was possible to turn off the supervision, relying only on further Hebbian plasticity to refine the approximation.

The role of the supervisor in the model was to compute an error by comparing the actual and the desired output of the network and to use this error to direct the modification of network parameters such that the network performance improves. Conventionally, the major targets of this process were the synaptic weights. The novel feature of this supervised learning scheme was that supervision took place at the level of neuronal responsiveness rather than synaptic plasticity.

A simple two-layer perceptron cannot solve higher-order problems, but adding additional layers to the feedforward network provides more representational power. Then new learning algorithms are needed to train multilayer networks. The simple error-correcting learning rule was effective for training two-layer networks. With the rule, the connections from the input layer to the output one are adjusted based on discrepancies between the desired output and the actual output produced by the network. In a multilayer network, however, there are intermediate 'hidden' layers that also need to be trained. The back-propagation learning algorithm was developed to train multilayer networks (Rumelhart and McClelland, 1986). The learning rule relies on passing an error from the output layer back to the input layer. Multilayer networks trained with the back-propagation learning rule have been effective in solving many difficult problems.

An example of a multilayer network that was trained using a back-propagation algorithm is a model of song learning in songbirds (Fiete et al., 2004). Juvenile male songbirds learn their songs from adult male tutors of the same species. Birdsong is a learned complex motor behavior driven by a discrete set of premotor brain nuclei with well-studied anatomy. Syringeal and respiratory motor neurons responsible for song production are driven by precisely executed sequences of neural activity in the premotor nucleus robustus archistriatalis (RA) of songbirds (**Figure 2**). Activity in RA is driven by excitatory feedforward inputs from the forebrain nucleus high vocal center (HVC), whose RA-projecting neural population displays temporally sparse, precise, and stereotyped sequential activity. Individual RA-projecting HVC neurons burst just once in an entire song motif and fire almost no spikes elsewhere in the motif. The temporal sparseness of HVC activity implies that these HVC–RA synapses are used in a special way during song; that is, each synapse is used only once during the motif. The goal of the work was to study the effect of HVC sparseness on the learning speed of the network. They studied multilayer feedforward network with an HVC layer that provides input to a 'hidden' RA layer and RA

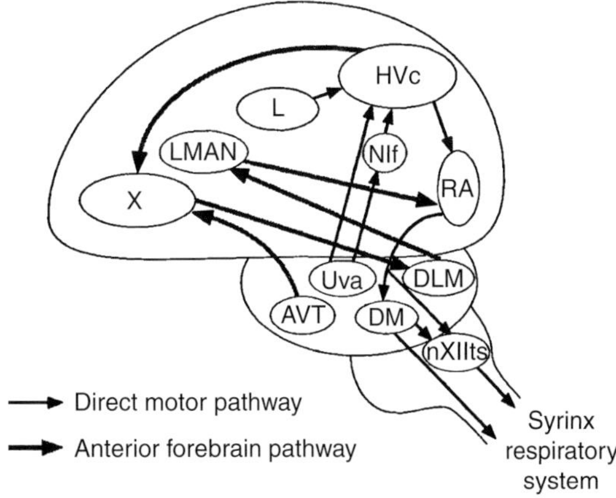

Figure 2 Schematic diagram of the major songbird brain nuclei involved in song control. The thinner arrows show the direct motor pathway, and the thicker arrows show the anterior forebrain pathway. Abbreviations: Uva, nucleus uvaeformis of the thalamus; NIf, nucleus interface of neostriatum; L, field L (primary auditory area of the forebrain); HVc, higher vocal center; RA, robust nucleus of the archistriatum; DM, dorsomedial part of the nucleus intercollicularis; nXIIts, tracheosyringeal part of the hypoglossal nucleus; AVT, ventral area of Tsai of the midbrain; X, area X of lobus parolfactorius; DLM, medial part of the dorsolateral nucleus of the thalamus; LMAN, lateral magnocellular nucleus of the anterior neostriatum. From Doya K and Sejnowski TJ (2000) A computational model of avian song learning. In: Gazzaninga MS (ed.) *The New Cognitive Neurosciences*, 2nd edn., p. 469. Cambridge, MA: MIT Press; used with permission.

projecting to an output layer of motor units. Song learning is thought to involve plasticity of synapses from HVC to RA because these synapses display extensive synaptic growth and redistribution during the critical period. So in the model, the weights from HVC layer to RA layer were modified. Because there is no evidence of plasticity in the synapses from RA to motor neurons, those connections in the model were kept fixed. For learning, the connections from HVC to RA were adjusted to minimize discrepancy between the desired outputs and the actual outputs produced by the network. They used the back-propagation gradient descent rule and varied the number of bursts in HVC neurons per motif. The network learned the motif for any number of bursts in HVC neurons, but the learning time for two bursts per motif nearly doubled compared to the one burst case and increased rapidly with the number of bursts. Based on these simulations, they concluded that the observed sparse coding in HVC minimized interference and the time needed for learning. It is important to note here that the back-propagation learning algorithm was not used to model the biological learning process itself, but rather to determine if the network architecture can solve the problem and what constraints the representation may have on the speed of learning.

15.5 Reinforcement Learning

Learning about stimuli or actions based solely on rewards and punishments is called reinforcement learning. Reinforcement learning is minimally supervised because animals are not told explicitly what actions to take in a particular situation. The reinforcement learning paradigm has attracted considerable interest because of the notion that the learner is able to learn from its own experience at attempting to perform a task without the aid of an intelligent 'teacher.' In contrast, in the more commonly employed paradigm of supervised learning, a detailed 'teacher signal' is required that explicitly tells the learner what the correct output pattern is for every input pattern.

A computational model of birdsong learning based on reinforcement learning has been proposed (Doya and Sejnowski, 2000). A young male songbird learns to sing by imitating the song of a tutor, which is usually the father or other adult males in the colony. If a young bird does not hear a tutor song during a critical period, it will sing short, poorly structured songs. If a bird is deafened during the period when it practices vocalization, it develops highly abnormal songs. Thus, there are two phases in song learning – the sensory learning phase, when a young bird memorizes song templates, and the sensorimotor learning phase, in which the bird establishes the motor programs using auditory feedback. These two phases can be separated by several months in some species, implying that birds have remarkable capability for memorizing complex temporal sequences. Once a song is crystallized, its pattern is very stable. Even deafening the bird has little immediate effect.

The anterior forebrain pathway, which is not involved in song production, is necessary for song learning. In the previously discussed model (Fiete et al., 2004), it was assumed that HVC is a locus of pattern memorization during the first phase of learning, song acquisition, and RA is a motor command area. Therefore, the patterns stored in HVC serve as inputs to RA to produce motor commands. It was also assumed that evaluation of the similarity of the produced song to the memorized tutor song takes place in area X in the anterior forebrain. This assumption is supported by a finding that area X receives dopaminergic input. Depending on how closely the produced song is to the tutor's song, the connections from HVC to RA are modulated via the lateral magnocellular nucleus (LMAN).

The learning algorithm consisted of making small random changes in the HVC to RA synapses and keeping the new weights only if overall performance was improved. The network learned artificial song motifs and was even able to replicate realistic birdsongs within the number of trials that birds take to learn their songs.

Reinforcement learning has thus far had few practical successes in solving large-scale complex real-world problems. In the case of reinforcement learning with delay, the temporal credit assignment aspect of the problem has made learning very slow. However, a method called temporal difference (TD) learning has overcome some of these limitations (Sutton and Barto, 1998). The basic idea of TD learning is to compute the difference between temporally successive predictions. In other words, the goal of learning is to make the learner's current prediction for the current input pattern more closely match the prediction at the next time step. One of the most effective of these TD methods is an algorithm called TD(λ), in which there is an exponentially decaying feedback of the error in time, so that previous estimates for previous states are also corrected. The time scale of the exponential decay is governed by the λ parameter.

Perhaps the most successful application of TD(λ) is TD-Gammon, which was designed for networks to learn to play backgammon (Tesauro, 1995). Backgammon is an ancient two-player game that is played on an effectively one-dimensional track. The players take turns rolling dice and moving their checkers in opposite directions along the track as allowed by the dice roll. The first player to move all his checkers all the way forward and off his end of the board is the winner.

At the heart of TD-Gammon is a neural network with a standard multilayer architecture. Its output is computed by a feedforward flow of activation from the input nodes, representing the game position, to the output node, which evaluates the strength of the position. Each of the connections in the network is parameterized by a real valued weight. Each of the nodes in the network outputs a real number equal to a weighted linear sum of inputs feeding into it, followed by a nonlinear sigmoid operation. At each time step, the TD(λ) algorithm is applied to the output, which is then back-propagated to change the network's weights.

During training, the neural network selects moves for both sides. At each time step during the course of a game, the neural network scores every possible legal move. The move that is then selected is the move with maximum expected outcome for the side making the move. In other words, the neural network learns by playing against itself. At the start of self-play, the network's weights are random, and hence its initial strategy is random. But after a few hundred thousand games, TD-Gammon played significantly better than any previous backgammon program, equivalent to an advanced level of play. In particular, it is not dependent on a human teacher, which would limit the level of play it can achieve (Tesauro and Sejnowski, 1989). After one million games, TD-Gammon was playing at a championship level.

One of the essential features of reinforcement learning is a trade-off between exploration and exploitation. The learning system should exploit a successful strategy to reach the goal of the task it learns, but it should also explore other strategies to find out if there is a better one. In models, exploration has been implemented by stochasticity. The source of such stochasticity in the brain remains unclear. A model implementing this trade-off between exploration and exploitation has been proposed (Seung, 2003). The model is based on the probabilistic nature of synaptic release by a presynaptic terminal when an action potential arrives at the terminal. The model combines this local synaptic release-failure event and a global reward signal received outside based on the output of the model. The main assumption is that synapses are hedonistic: they increase their probabilities of release or failure depending on which action immediately preceded reward. This concept of the hedonistic synapse is potentially relevant to any brain area in which a global reinforcement signal is received (Klopf, 1982).

This version of reinforcement learning was used to address the matching law phenomenon (Seung, 2003). When animals are presented with repeated choices between competing alternatives, they distribute their choices so that returns from two alternatives are approximately the same. A return is the total reward obtained from an alternative divided by the number of times it was chosen. Before trials, the alternatives are baited with unequal probabilities. The network had to learn a probabilistic strategy in which one alternative is favored over the other one. The network started from equal choices for both alternatives, but over time, it learned a preference that satisfied the matching law.

In the present model, stochastic vesicle release was assumed to be a source of stochasticity in the brain. However, there might be many other possible sources of noise, such as fluctuations in quantal size, irregular action potential firing, and on a slower time scale, the stochastic creation and destruction of synapses. Thus, identifying specific sources of randomness is essential for connecting mathematical models and neurobiology.

15.6 Spike-Timing Dependent Plasticity

The traditional coincidence version of the Hebbian learning rule implies simply that the correlation of activities of presynaptic and postsynaptic neurons drives learning. This approach has been implemented in many types of neural network models using average firing rate or average membrane potentials of neurons. Although Hebb's formulation implicitly recognized the idea of causality and relative spike timing (Hebb, 1949; Sejnowski, 1999), this was not appreciated by a generation of modelers because rate coding was generally accepted as the primary form of information processing, and high-frequency stimulation protocols were used to induce plasticity at synapses. More recently, the relative timing of spikes has been shown to be critical for the direction and magnitude of synaptic plasticity in the cortex as well as the hippocampus (Markram et al., 1997; Bi and Poo, 1998). Potentiation of a synapse takes place if the presynaptic spike precedes the postsynaptic spike, and depression occurs when presynaptic spike follows the postsynaptic spike. This spike-timing dependent plasticity (STDP) is an asymmetric function of relative spike times in the presynaptic and postsynaptic neurons. The time window for the plasticity can be as short as 10 ms and as long as 100 ms, depending on the synapse.

A natural application for STDP is temporal sequence learning (*See* Chapter 15). If neurons are activated in a sequential manner then, due to the asymmetry of the learning rule, synapses from previously activated neurons to following active neurons will be strengthened. For example, such a spike-timing dependent learning algorithm has been used to train a network to link sequential hippocampal place cells while a rat navigates a maze (Blum and Abbott, 1996). The goal was to predict the direction of a future motion on the basis of a previous experience. Asymmetric synaptic weights develop in the model because of the temporal asymmetry of LTP induction and because place fields are activated sequentially during locomotion. This learning algorithm closely resembles the STDP learning rule. The only essential difference is time scale, which in the model was 200 ms, longer than the STDP windows found in cortical or hippocampal neurons.

This model of a navigational map was based on three observations. First, NMDA-dependent LTP in hippocampal slices occurs only if presynaptic activity precedes postsynaptic activity by less than approximately 200 ms. Presynaptic activity following postsynaptic firing produces either no LTP or long-term depression (LTD). Second, place cells are broadly tuned and make synaptic connections with each other both within the CA3 region and between CA3 and CA1. Third, a spatial location can be determined by appropriately averaging the activity of an ensemble of hippocampal place cells. These three observations imply that when an animal travels through its environment, causing different sets of place cells to fire, information about both temporal and spatial aspects of its motion will be reflected in changes of the strengths of synapses between place cells. Because this LTP affects a subsequent place cell firing, it can shift the spatial location coded by the place cell activity. These shifts suggest that an animal could navigate by heading from its present location toward the position coded by the place cell activity. To illustrate both how a spatial map arises and how it can be used to guide movement, these ideas were applied to navigation in the Morris maze. The network was trained using this spike-timing dependent learning algorithm to form a direction map, which improved with training.

Timing is important in auditory processing, and a number of perceptual tasks, such as sound localization, explicitly use temporal information. Sound localization is important to the survival of many species, in particular to those that hunt in the dark. Interaural time differences (ITD) are often used as a spatial cue. However, the question of how temporal information from both ears can be transmitted to a site of comparison, where neurons are tuned to ITDs, and how those ITD-tuned neurons can be organized in a map remains unclear. A network model based on STDP can successfully account for a fine precision of barn owl sound localization (Kempter et al., 2001). The model converts ITDs into a place code by combining axonal delay lines from both ears and STDP in synapses with distributed delays. The neurons are organized as a single-layer network for each frequency and receive inputs from both ears through axonal arbors. The axons have different time delays. After training, each neuron adjusts its connections to axons with the appropriate time delays in agreement with the neuron's spatial position. In this way, a map with neurons tuned to particular ITDs can be formed.

There is an interesting connection between STDP and TD learning at the computational level (Rao and Sejnowski, 2003). If, consistent with TD learning, synaptic weights between Hodgkin–Huxley type spiking neurons are updated based on the difference in the postsynaptic voltage at time $t + \Delta t$ and at time t, where t is the time when the presynaptic neuron fired a spike, and Δt is a fixed time interval, then the learning rule resembles the conventional STDP learning rule. Networks with this spike-dependent TD learning rule are able to learn and predict temporal sequences, as demonstrated by the development of direction selectivity in a recurrent cortical network. The network consisted of a single chain of recurrently connected excitatory neurons. Each neuron initially received symmetric excitatory and inhibitory inputs of the same magnitude. For training, the neurons in the network were exposed to 100 trials of retinotopic sensory inputs consisting of moving pulses of excitation in the rightward direction.

The effect of learning on the network was in developing a profound asymmetry in the pattern of excitatory connections from preceding and successor neurons. The synaptic conductances of excitatory connections from the left side were strengthened, whereas the ones from the right side were weakened. Because neurons on the left side fired (on average) a few milliseconds before a considered neuron, whereas neurons on the right side fired (on average) a few milliseconds after, as a result, the synaptic strengths of connections from the left side were increased, whereas the synaptic strengths for connections from the right side were decreased. As expected from the learned pattern of connections, the neuron responded vigorously to rightward motion but not to leftward motion.

To investigate the question of how selectivity for different directions of motion may emerge simultaneously, they also simulated a network comprising two parallel chains of neurons, with mutual inhibition between corresponding pairs of neurons along the two chains. As in the previous simulation, a given excitatory neuron received both excitation and inhibition from its predecessors and successors. To break the symmetry between the two chains, they provided a slight bias in the recurrent excitatory connections, so that neurons in one chain fired slightly earlier than neurons in the other chain for a given motion direction. To evaluate the consequences of spike-based TD learning in the two-chain network, the model neurons were exposed alternately to leftward- and rightward-moving stimuli for a total of 100 trials. As in the previous simulation, the excitatory and inhibitory connections to a neuron in one chain showed asymmetry after training, with stronger excitatory connections from the left neurons and stronger inhibitory connections from the right neurons. A corresponding neuron in the other chain exhibited the opposite pattern, and as expected from the learned patterns of connectivity, neurons in one chain were selective to rightward motion, and neurons in the other chain were selective to the leftward motion. This explanation was consistent with the development of directionally selective neurons in the visual cortex of kittens.

15.7 Plasticity of Intrinsic Excitability

Several lines of evidence argue for the presence of activity-dependent modification of intrinsic neuronal excitability during development and learning (Daoudal and Debanne, 2003; *See* Chapter 14). In the dentate gyrus of the hippocampus, for example, in addition to homosynaptic LTP of excitatory synaptic transmission, the probability of discharge of the postsynaptic neurons to a fixed excitatory synaptic input is enhanced by high-frequency stimulation (HFS, 100 Hz) of the afferent fibers (Bliss et al., 1973). This second component has been called excitatory postsynaptic potential (EPSP)-to-spike potentiation (E-S potentiation) (Frick et al., 2004). Synaptic plasticity (LTP) and nonsynaptic E-S potentiation are complementary. As in LTP, E-S potentiation requires the activation of NMDA receptor (NMDAR) for its induction. These two forms of plasticity may share common induction pathways. In a recent study of deep cerebellar nuclei neurons, tetanization of inputs to these neurons produces a rapid and long-lasting increase in intrinsic excitability that depends on NMDAR activation (Aizenman and Linden, 2000). These studies suggest that plasticity of intrinsic excitability may be important in developmental plasticity and information storage.

Another form of plasticity in intrinsic excitability has been demonstrated in spontaneously firing vestibular nucleus neurons, which may be responsible for learning of the vestibuloocular reflex. Purkinje cells, which are inhibitory, contact a subset of the neuron in the vestibular nucleus, which receive direct vestibular input and project to the oculomotor nuclei. Brief periods of synaptic inhibition or membrane hyperpolarization produced a dramatic increase in both spontaneous firing rate and responses to intracellularly injected current (Gittis and du Lac, 2006). A similar change occurred after silencing the vestibular nerve. Neurons in the vestibular system fire at remarkably high rates in the intact animal, with resting rates on the order of 50–100 spikes/s and responses to head movements ranging up to 300 spikes/s. Loss of peripheral vestibular function silences the vestibular nerve, resulting in a significant loss of spontaneous firing in the neurons of the vestibular nucleus, which then returns to control values within about a week, even in the absence of vestibular nerve recovery. This plasticity of intrinsic excitability could potentially contribute either to adaptive changes in vestibular function during recovery from peripheral damage or to oculomotor learning in intact animals.

A similar phenomenon has been demonstrated in cultured neocortical pyramidal neurons (Desai et al., 1999). Prolonged activity blockade lowers the threshold for spike generation, and neurons fire at a higher frequency for any given level of current injection. These changes occurred through selective modifications in the magnitude of voltage-dependent currents: sodium currents increase and persistent potassium currents decrease, whereas calcium currents and transient potassium currents are unaltered. Increase of neuronal excitability in response to reduced activity may contribute to the activity-dependent stabilization of firing rates. The stability in neuronal firing rates is maintained through many mechanisms, and regulation of neuronal excitability may be one of them.

Information about the outside world is transformed into spike trains in the nervous system. How do the neurons learn to represent the information, and do they change their behavior based on changing external stimuli? In the discussion of unsupervised learning and the ICA algorithm, it was shown that information theoretical approaches can be effective in solving real-world problems. A similar information theoretical approach can be implemented to search for an optimal representation. A Hodgkin–Huxley type model of a neuron that can adjust its membrane conductances to maximize information transfer has been proposed (Stemmler and Koch, 1999). The slope of the neuronal gain function should line up with the peak of the input to maximize information transfer. The learning rules they implemented in the model performed this matchup by adjusting the membrane conductances. The conductance modulations did not require calculation of mutual information but were based solely on local characteristics of the neuron. They showed that for different input distributions the model could successfully line up the gain function and the input distributions leading to maximization of information transfer. Thus, the ability of activity-dependent selective modification of the gain functions based on the active balance of inward and outward ion channels could serve a number of important functions, including fine-tuning of the output properties of neurons to match the properties of their inputs.

Plasticity of intrinsic excitability can also participate in regulating the conventional synaptic plasticity. For details, see the previously discussed model, which combines Hebbian and supervised learning (Swinehart and Abbott, 2005), in the section titled 'Supervised learning.'

15.8 Homeostatic Plasticity

Correlation-based Hebbian plasticity is thought to be crucial for information storage because it produces associative changes in the strength of individual synaptic connections. However, correlation-based learning in neural networks can be unstable. According to the Hebb rule, if a presynaptic neuron participates in firing of a postsynaptic neuron, it leads to strengthening the synapses between the neurons. This makes it more likely that next time the presynaptic neuron fires, it will cause firing in the postsynaptic neuron, which leads to further strengthening of the synapse. Simple associative Hebbian algorithm causes instability in the network by increasing the total activity of the network and losing selectivity among synapses. To keep the network stable and maintain the selectivity of the network, an additional mechanism must stabilize the properties of neuronal networks.

Homeostatic plasticity is a mechanism by which the neurons regulate the network's activity (Turrigiano and Nelson, 2000). There are many different ways neural activities could be regulated to keep them within a functional dynamical range. One mechanism that could maintain relatively constant activity levels is to increase the strength of all excitatory connections into a neuron in response to a prolonged drop in firing rates, and vice versa. This form of homeostatic plasticity is called synaptic scaling.

Regulating synaptic strength is not the only mechanism by which homeostatic activity can be maintained. Previously discussed plasticity of intrinsic excitability also contributes to the homeostatic regulation by controlling the firing rates of the neurons.

All theoretical models implementing associative Hebbian learning rule have to deal with the instability problem. For example, the BCM learning rule deals with unconstrained growth of synaptic weights by dynamically adjusting the threshold between potentiation and depression (Bienenstock et al., 1982). This algorithm is biologically plausible and reflects experimental findings indicating that calcium level is crucial for the direction of plasticity. The dynamical threshold modulation implemented in the BCM rule not only prevents the synapses from unconstrained growth but also maintains the activity level of the units at the appropriate value (*See* Chapter 16).

In the next section we present some other examples of learning algorithms involving homeostatic plasticity as a critical element of learning.

15.9 Complexity of Learning

The learning paradigms discussed earlier were based on a single mechanism for plasticity (e.g., STDP versus homeostatic and synaptic versus intrinsic neuronal). However, many difficult tasks cannot be solved using a single learning rule, but require combinations of several learning rules working together. Another essential element of modeling learning processes is the time scale of learning. There are multiple time scales for plasticity, from milliseconds to years, and depending on the demands of the task, different mechanisms for plasticity with different time scales may be involved.

Long-term memory is vulnerable to degradation from passive decay of the memory trace and ongoing formation of new memories. Memory based on synapses with two states shows exponential decay, but experimental data shows that forgetting (memory degradation) follows a power law. A cascade model was developed to address this problem (Fusi et al., 2005). In the model, synapses had two states, weak and strong, but in addition to transition between these two states, there were metaplastic transitions within each state. Based on the stage of metaplasticity, the synapses showed the range of behavior from being highly plastic to being resistant to any plasticity at all. The metaplastic transitions effectively introduced multiple time scales into the model.

The cascade model outperformed alternative models and exhibited a power law for the decay of memory as a function of time. The dependence of memory lifetime on the number of synapses in the model is also a power law function. Memory lifetimes diminish when the balance between excitation and inhibition is disturbed, but the effect is much less severe in the cascade model than in noncascade models.

The function of homeostatic plasticity is to maintain the activity of the cortex at a functional level. But are there any other computational or functional advantages of such plasticity? One study has shown that a combination of Hebbian and homeostatic plasticity can lead to temporal sharpening in response to multiple applications of transient sensory stimuli (Moldakarimov et al., 2006). The model included two types of homeostatic mechanisms, fast and slow. Relatively fast plasticity was responsible for maintaining the average activity of the units. To maintain activity in the excitatory neurons at a target homeostatic level, they implemented a learning rule, according to which inhibitory connections have been adjusted. The slow plasticity was used to determine the value of the target average activities. Thus, the model had three time scales for synaptic adjustments: Hebbian, fast homeostatic, and slow homeostatic mechanisms. Repeated presentations of a transient signal taught the network to respond to the signal with a high amplitude and short duration, in agreement with experimental findings. This sharpening enhances the processing of transients and may also be relevant for speech perception.

A standard approach in models of self-organized map (SOM) formation is the application of Hebbian plasticity augmented with a mechanism of weight normalization. A conventional way to normalize weights is based on a sum of weights coming into each neuron: The soma collects information on every weight, sums them, and then decides on the amount of normalization. An alternative approach to weight normalization has been proposed (Sullivan and de Sa, 2006). The normalization algorithm did not need information from every synapse but rather was based on the average activities of the units and homeostatic plasticity. When Hebbian and homeostatic mechanisms were combined, the average activities of the units were better maintained compared to the standard Hebbian models.

Dimensionality reduction facilitates the classification, the visualization, and the storage of high-dimensional data. A simple and widely used method is PCA, which finds the directions of greatest variance in the data set and represents each data point by its coordinates along each of these directions. A new deep network model has been proposed to transform the high-dimensional data into a low-dimensional code (Hinton and Salakhutdinov, 2006). The adaptive multilayer network consisted of two subnetworks, an encoder and decoder. The encoder transformed high-dimensional data into a low-dimensional code. The code layer was then used as the input layer to the decoder network to reconstruct the original input pattern.

The two networks were trained together to minimize the discrepancy between the original data and its reconstruction. The required gradients were obtained using the chain rule to back-propagate error derivatives, first through the decoder network and then through the encoder network. In general, it is difficult to optimize the weights in a multilayer network with many hidden layers. Large initial weights typically lead to poor local minima; with small initial weights, the gradients in the early layers are tiny, making it impossible to train. But if the initial weights are close to a good solution, gradient descent back-propagation works well. A good initial network was obtained with unsupervised learning based on Restricted Boltzmann Machine (RBM) learning algorithm. First, the input layer of the multilayer network was used as a visible layer of RBM, and the next layer served as a feature layer. After learning one layer of feature detectors, the weights were fixed and used for learning a second layer of feature detectors. This layer-by-layer learning was repeated many times. After pretraining multiple layers of feature detectors, the model was unfolded to produce the encoder and decoder networks that initially used the same weights. The global fine-tuning stage used back-propagation through the whole network to adjust the weights for optimal reconstruction.

They applied the algorithm to multiple tasks including handwritten digits visualization, grayscale images, and documents generalization. In all these tasks, the new algorithm outperformed different approaches based on PCA and other supervised algorithms.

15.10 Conclusions

We have discussed learning rules and learning algorithms designed for neural network models and described some problems that can be solved by neural networks with modifiable connections. Neural computation is a broad field that continues to grow; only a few selected studies have been used to illustrate general principles.

Although early modeling efforts focused mainly on traditional synaptic plasticity, such as LTP and LTD, relatively new homeostatic plasticity mechanisms are also being explored. Although synaptic plasticity was once presumed to be the primary neural mechanism of learning, recent models have incorporated changes of intrinsic properties of the neurons as well.

Most experimental studies of learning have studied the mechanisms of synaptic plasticity in reduced preparations. Recently the focus has shifted to relating the changes in the synapses with behavioral learning. For example, inhibitory avoidance learning in rats produced the same changes in hippocampal glutamate receptors as induction of LTP with HFS (Whitlock et al., 2006). Because the learning-induced synaptic potentiation occluded HFS-induced LTP, they concluded that inhibitory avoidance training induced LTP in hippocampus.

Theoretical approaches can integrate local mechanisms with whole system behavior. Even after locating particular sites where changes occur, it is still not clear to what degree those changes are directly related to the learning. Building a computational model that integrates learning mechanisms allows one to evaluate the importance of different sites of plasticity. The observed plasticity for some sites may be secondary, or compensatory to the primary sites of learning (Lisberger and Sejnowski, 1992).

References

Aizenman CD and Linden DJ (2000) Rapid, synaptically driven increases in the intrinsic excitability of cerebellar deep nuclear neurons. *Nature Neurosci.* 3: 109–111.

Bell AJ and Sejnowski TJ (1995) An information maximization approach to blind separation and blind deconvolution. *Neural Comput.* 7: 1129–1159.

Bi G-Q and Poo M-M (1998) Synaptic modifications in cultured hippocampal neurons: Dependence on spike timing, synaptic strength, and postsynaptic cell type. *J. Neurosci.* 18: 10464–10472.

Bienenstock E, Cooper LN, and Munro PW (1982) Theory for the development of neuron selectivity: Orientation specificity and binocular interaction in visual cortex. *J. Neurosci.* 2: 32–48.

Bliss TV and Lomo T (1973) Long-lasting potentiation of synaptic transmission in the dentate area of the anaesthetized rabbit following stimulation of the perforant path. *J. Physiol.* 232: 331–356.

Bliss TV, Lomo T, and Gardner-Medwin AR (1973) Synaptic plasticity in the hippocampal formation. In: Ansell G and Bradley PB (eds.) *Macromolecules and Behavior*, pp. 192–303. London: Macmillan.

Blum KI and Abbott LF (1996) A model of spatial map formation in the hippocampus of the rat. *Neural Comput.* 8: 85–93.

Daoudal G and Debanne D (2003) Long-term plasticity of intrinsic excitability: Learning rules and mechanisms. *Learn. Mem.* 10: 456–465.

Desai NS, Rutherford LC, and Turrigiano GG (1999) Plasticity in the intrinsic excitability of cortical pyramidal neurons. *Nature Neurosci.* 2: 515–520.

Doya K and Sejnowski TJ (2000) A computational model of avian song learning. In: Gazzaninga MS (ed.) *The New Cognitive Neurosciences,* 2nd edn., p. 469. Cambridge, MA: MIT Press.

Ferster D and Miller KD (2000) Neural mechanisms of orientation selectivity in the visual cortex. *Annu. Rev. Neurosci.* 23: 441–471.

Fiete IR, Hahnloser RHR, Fee MS, and Seung HS (2004) Temporal sparseness of the premotor drive is important for rapid learning in a neural network model of birdsong. *J. Neurophysiol.* 92: 2274–2282.

Frick A, Magee J, and Johnston D (2004) LTP is accompanied by an enhanced local excitability of pyramidal neuron dendrites. *Nature Neurosci.* 7: 126–135.

Fusi S, Drew PJ, and Abbott LF (2005) Cascade models of synaptically stored memories. *Neuron* 45: 599–611.

Gittis AH and du Lac S (2006) Intrinsic and synaptic plasticity in the vestibular system. *Curr. Opin. Neurobiol.* 16: 385–390.

Hebb DO (1949) *Organization of Behavior: A Neuropsychological Theory.* New York: Wiley.

Hinton GE and Salakhutdinov RR (2006) Reducing the dimensionality of data with neural networks. *Science* 313: 504–507.

Hopfield JJ (1982) Neural networks and physical systems with emergent collective computational abilities. *Proc. Natl. Acad. Sci. USA* 79: 2554–2558.
Jung T-P, Makeig S, McKeown MJ, Bell AJ, Lee T-W, and Sejnowski TJ (2001) Imaging brain dynamics using independent component analysis. *Proc. IEEE* 89: 1107–1122.
Kelso SR, Ganong AH, and Brown TH (1986) Hebbian synapses in hippocampus. *Proc. Natl. Acad. Sci. USA* 83: 5326–5330.
Kempter R, Leibold C, Wagner H, and van Hemmen JL (2001) Formation of temporal-feature maps by axonal propagation of synaptic learning. *Proc. Natl. Acad. Sci. USA* 98: 4166–4171.
Klopf AH (1982) *The Hedonistic Neuron: A Theory of Memory, Learning and Intelligence.* Washington, DC: Hemisphere.
Kohonen T (1982) Self-organized formation of topologically correct feature maps. *Biol. Cybern.* 43: 59–69.
Lee T-W (1998) *Independent Component Analysis. Theory and Applications.* Boston: Kluwer Academic Publishers.
Lisberger SG and Sejnowski TJ (1992) Motor learning in a recurrent network model based on the vestibule-ocular reflex. *Nature* 360: 159–161.
Markram H, Lubke J, Frotscher M, and Sakmann B (1997) Regulation of synaptic efficacy by coincidence of postsynaptic APs and EPSPs. *Science* 275: 213–215.
Miller KD and Mackay DJC (1994) The role of constraints on Hebbian learning. *Neural Comput.* 6: 100–109.
Moldakarimov SB, McClelland JL, and Ermentrout GB (2006) A homeostatic rule for inhibitory synapses promotes temporal sharpening and cortical reorganization. *Proc. Natl. Acad. Sci. USA* 103: 16526–16531.
Rao RP and Sejnowski TJ (2003) Self-organizing neural systems based on predictive learning. *Philos. Trans. R. Soc. Lond.* 361: 1149–1175.
Rosenblatt F (1958) The perceptron: A probabilistic model for information storage and organization in the brain. *Psychol. Rev.* 65: 386–408.
Rumelhart DE and McClelland JL (1986) *Parallel Distributed Processing, Vol. 1: Foundations.* Cambridge, MA: MIT Press.
Sejnowski TJ (1999) The book of Hebb. *Neuron* 24: 773–776.
Sejnowski TJ and Tesauro G (1988) The Hebb rule for synaptic plasticity: Algorithms and implementations. In: Byrne J and Berry WO (eds.) *Neural Models of Plasticity*, pp. 94–103. New York: Academic Press.
Seung HS (2003) Learning in spiking neural networks by reinforcement of stochastic synaptic transmission. *Neuron* 40: 1063–1073.
Stemmler M and Koch C (1999) How voltage-dependent conductances can adapt to maximize the information encoded by neuronal firing rate. *Nature Neurosci.* 2: 521–527.
Sullivan TJ and de Sa VR (2006) Homeostatic synaptic scaling in self-organizing maps. *Neural Networks* 19: 734–743.
Sutton RS and Barto AG (1998) *Reinforcement Learning. An Introduction.* Cambridge, MA: MIT Press.
Swindale NV (1996) The development of topography in the visual cortex: A review of models. *Network* 7: 161–247.
Swinehart CD and Abbott LF (2005) Supervised learning through neuronal responses modulation. *Neural Comput.* 17: 609–631.
Tesauro G (1995) Temporal difference learning and TD-Gammon. *Comm. ACM* 38: 58–68.
Tesauro G and Sejnowski TJ (1989) A parallel network that learns to play backgammon *J. Artif. Intell.* 39: 357–390.
Turrigiano GG and Nelson SB (2000) Hebb and homeostasis in neural plasticity. *Curr. Opin. Neurobiol.* 10: 358–364.
Whitlock JR, Heynen AJ, Shuler MG, and Bear MF (2006) Learning induces long-term potentiation in the hippocampus. *Science* 313: 1093–1097.

16 Computational Models of Hippocampal Functions

E. T. Rolls, University of Oxford, Oxford, UK

16.1 Introduction

In this chapter, a computational approach to the function of the hippocampus in memory is described and compared to other approaches. The theory is quantitative and takes into account the internal and systems-level connections of the hippocampus, the effects on memory of damage to different parts of the hippocampus, and the responses of hippocampal neurons recorded during memory tasks. The theory was developed by Rolls (1987, 1989a,b,c, 1996b, 2007), Treves and Rolls (1992, 1994), and with other colleagues (Rolls et al., 2002; Rolls and Stringer, 2005; Rolls and Kesner, 2006). The theory was preceded by the work of Marr (1971), who developed a mathematical model, which, although not applied to particular networks within the hippocampus and dealing with binary neurons and binary synapses that utilized heavily the properties of the binomial distribution, was important in utilizing computational concepts and in considering how recall could occur in a network with recurrent collateral connections. Analyses of these autoassociation or attractor networks developed rapidly (Gardner-Medwin, 1976; Kohonen, 1977; Hopfield, 1982; Amit, 1989; Treves and Rolls, 1991; Rolls and Treves, 1998). Rolls (1987, 1989b) produced a theory of the hippocampus in which the CA3 neurons operated as an autoassociation memory to store episodic memories including object and place memories, and the dentate granule cells operated as a preprocessing stage for this by performing pattern separation so that the mossy fibers could act to set up different representations for each memory to be stored in the CA3 cells. He suggested that the CA1 cells operate as a recoder for the information recalled from the CA3 cells to a partial memory cue, so that the recalled information would be represented more efficiently to enable recall, via the backprojection synapses, of activity in the neocortical areas similar to that which had been present during the original episode. At about the same time, McNaughton and Morris (1987) suggested that the CA3 network might be an autoassociation network, and that the mossy fiber–to-CA3 connections might implement detonator synapses. The concepts that the diluted mossy fiber connectivity might implement selection of a new random set of CA3 cells for each new memory and that a direct perforant path input to CA3 was needed to initiate retrieval were introduced by Treves and Rolls (1992). Since then, many investigators have contributed to our understanding of hippocampal computation, with some of these approaches described in the section titled 'Comparison with other theories of hippocampal function' and throughout the chapter.

16.2 A Theory of Hippocampal Function

16.2.1 Systems-Level Functions of the Hippocampus

Any theory of the hippocampus must state at the systems level what is computed by the hippocampus. Some of the relevant evidence comes from the effects of damage to the hippocampus, the responses of neurons in the hippocampus during behavior, and the systems-level connections of the hippocampus, described in more detail elsewhere (Rolls and Kesner, 2006; Rolls, 2007).

16.2.1.1 Evidence from the effects of damage to the hippocampus

Damage to the hippocampus or to some of its connections such as the fornix in monkeys produces deficits in learning about the places of objects and about the places where responses should be made (Buckley and Gaffan, 2000). For example, macaques and humans with damage to the hippocampal system or fornix are impaired in object–place memory tasks in which not only the objects seen but where they were seen must be remembered (Gaffan, 1994; Burgess et al., 2002; Crane and Milner, 2005). Posterior parahippocampal lesions in macaques impair even a simple type of object-place learning in which the memory load is just one pair of trial-unique stimuli (Malkova and Mishkin, 2003). Further, neurotoxic lesions that selectively damage the primate hippocampus impair spatial scene memory, tested by the ability to remember where in a scene to touch to obtain reward (Murray et al., 1998). Rats with hippocampal lesions are impaired in using environmental spatial cues to remember particular places (O'Keefe and Nadel, 1978; Jarrard, 1993; Cassaday and Rawlins, 1997; Martin et al., 2000; Kesner et al., 2004). These memory functions are important in event or episodic memory, in which the ability to remember what happened where on typically a single occasion is important.

It will be suggested below that an autoassociation memory implemented by the CA3 neurons enables event or episodic memories to be formed by enabling associations to be formed between spatial and other including object representations.

16.2.1.2 The necessity to recall information from the hippocampus

Information stored in the hippocampus will need to be retrieved and affect other parts of the brain in order to be used. The information about episodic events recalled from the hippocampus could be used to help form semantic memories (Rolls, 1989b,d, 1990a; Treves and Rolls, 1994). For example, remembering many particular journeys could help to build a geographic cognitive map in the neocortex. The hippocampus and neocortex would thus be complementary memory systems, with the hippocampus being used for rapid, on-the-fly, unstructured storage of information involving activity potentially arriving from many areas of the neocortex, while the neocortex would gradually build and adjust the semantic representation on the basis of much accumulating information (Rolls, 1989b; Treves and Rolls, 1994; McClelland et al., 1995; Moscovitch et al., 2005). The present theory shows how information could be retrieved within the hippocampus and how this retrieved information could enable the activity in neocortical areas that was present during the original storage of the episodic event to be reinstated, thus implementing recall, by using hippocampo-neocortical backprojections (see **Figure 1**).

16.2.1.3 Systems-level neurophysiology of the primate hippocampus

The systems-level neurophysiology of the hippocampus shows what information could be stored or processed by the hippocampus. To understand how the hippocampus works, it is not sufficient to state just that it can store information – one needs to know what information. The systems-level neurophysiology of the primate hippocampus has been reviewed recently by Rolls and Xiang (2006), and a brief summary is provided here because it provides a perspective relevant to understanding the function of the human hippocampus that is somewhat different from that provided by the properties of place cells in rodents, which have been reviewed elsewhere (see McNaughton et al., 1983; O'Keefe, 1984; Muller et al., 1991; Jeffery et al., 2004; Jeffery and Hayman, 2004).

The primate hippocampus contains spatial cells that respond when the monkey looks at a certain part of space, for example, at one quadrant of a video monitor, while the monkey is performing an object–place memory task in which he must remember where on the monitor he has seen particular images (Rolls et al., 1989). Approximately 9% of the hippocampal neurons have such spatial view fields, and about 2.4% combine information about the position in space with information about the object that is in that position in space (Rolls et al., 1989). The representation of space is for the majority of hippocampal

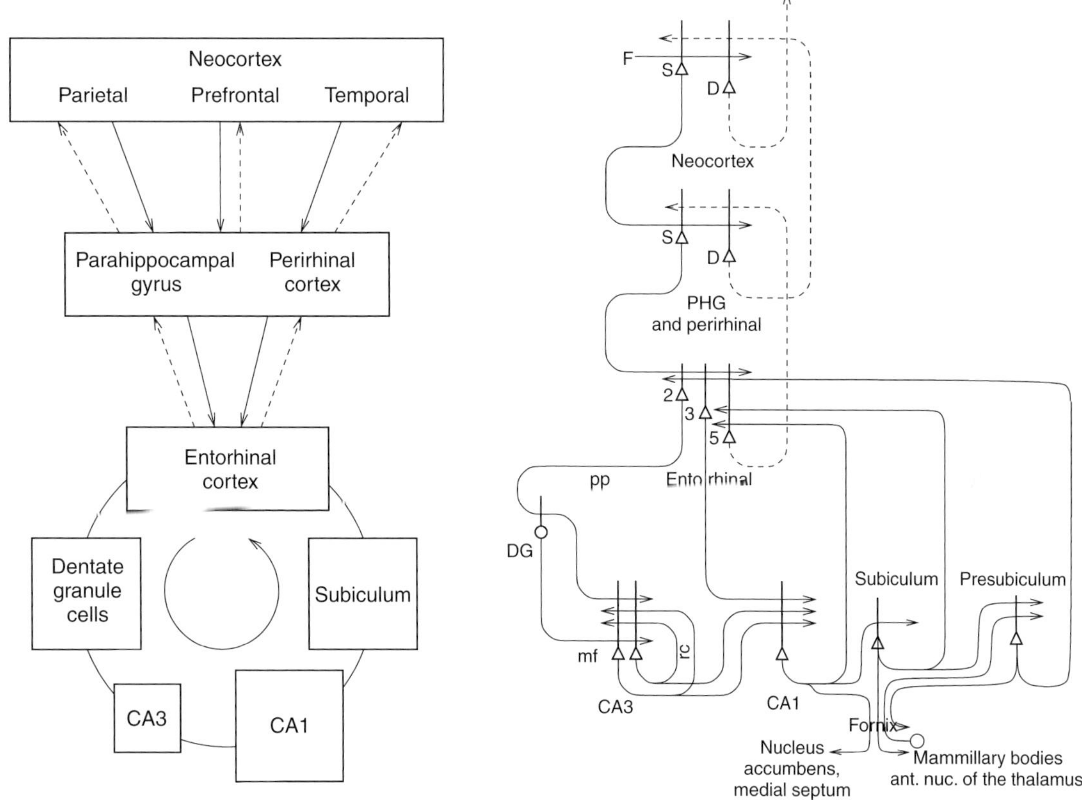

Figure 1 Forward connections (solid lines) from areas of cerebral association neocortex via the parahippocampal gyrus and perirhinal cortex, and entorhinal cortex, to the hippocampus; and backprojections (dashed lines) via the hippocampal CA1 pyramidal cells, subiculum, and parahippocampal gyrus to the neocortex. There is great convergence in the forward connections down to the single network implemented in the CA3 pyramidal cells and great divergence again in the backprojections. Left: block diagram. Right: more detailed representation of some of the principal excitatory neurons in the pathways. Abbreviations: D, deep pyramidal cells; DG, dentate granule cells; F, forward inputs to areas of the association cortex from preceding cortical areas in the hierarchy; mf, mossy fibers. PHG, parahippocampal gyrus and perirhinal cortex; pp, perforant path; rc, recurrent collateral of the CA3 hippocampal pyramidal cells; S, superficial pyramidal cells; 2, pyramidal cells in layer 2 of the entorhinal cortex; 3, pyramidal cells in layer 3 of the entorhinal cortex. The thick lines above the cell bodies represent the dendrites.

neurons in allocentric – not egocentric – coordinates (Feigenbaum and Rolls, 1991). These spatial view cells can be recorded while monkeys move themselves round the test environment by walking (or running) on all fours (Rolls et al., 1997a, 1998; Robertson et al., 1998; Georges-François et al., 1999). These hippocampal spatial view neurons respond significantly differently for different allocentric spatial views, and have information about spatial view in their firing rate, but do not respond differently just on the basis of eye position, head direction, or place. If the view details are obscured by curtains and darkness, then some spatial view neurons (especially those in CA1 and less those in CA3) continue to respond when the monkey looks toward the spatial view field, showing that these neurons can be updated for at least short periods by idiothetic (self-motion) cues including eye position and head direction signals (Rolls et al., 1997b; Robertson et al., 1998).

A fundamental question about the function of the primate including human hippocampus is whether object as well as allocentric spatial information is represented. To investigate this, Rolls et al. (2005) made recordings from single hippocampal formation neurons while macaques performed an object–place memory task that required the monkeys to learn associations between objects, and where they were shown in a room. Some neurons (10%) responded differently to different objects independently of location; other neurons (13%) responded to the spatial view independently of which object was present at the location; and some neurons (12%) responded to a combination of a particular object and the place where it was shown in the room. These results show that there are separate as well as combined representations of objects and their locations in space in the primate hippocampus. This is a property required in an episodic memory system, for which associations between objects and the places where they are seen are prototypical. The results thus show that a requirement for a human episodic memory system, separate and combined neuronal representations of objects and where they are seen out there in the environment, are present in the primate hippocampus (Rolls et al., 2005). What may be a corresponding finding in rats is that some rat hippocampal neurons respond on the basis of the conjunction of location and odor (Wood et al., 1999).

Primate hippocampal neuronal activity has also been shown to be related to the recall of memories. In a one–trial object place recall task, images of an object in one position on a screen and of a second object in a different position on the screen were shown successively. Then one of the objects was shown at the top of the screen, and the monkey had to recall the position in which it had been shown earlier in the trial and to touch that location (Rolls and Xiang, 2006). In addition to neurons that responded to the objects or places, a new type of neuronal response was found in which 5% of hippocampal neurons had place-related responses when a place was being recalled by an object cue.

The primate anterior hippocampus (which corresponds to the rodent ventral hippocampus) receives inputs from brain regions involved in reward processing such as the amygdala and orbitofrontal cortex (Pitkanen et al., 2002). To investigate how this affective input may be incorporated into primate hippocampal function, Rolls and Xiang (2005) recorded neuronal activity while macaques performed a reward-place association task in which each spatial scene shown on a video monitor had one location, which if touched yielded a preferred fruit juice reward, and a second location that yielded a less preferred juice reward. Each scene had different locations for the different rewards. Of 312 hippocampal neurons analyzed, 18% responded more to the location of the preferred reward in different scenes, and 5% to the location of the less preferred reward (Rolls and Xiang, 2005). When the locations of the preferred rewards in the scenes were reversed, 60% of 44 neurons tested reversed the location to which they responded, showing that the reward–place associations could be altered by new learning in a few trials. The majority (82%) of these 44 hippocampal reward–place neurons tested did not respond to object–reward associations in a visual discrimination object–reward association task. Thus the primate hippocampus contains a representation of the reward associations of places out there being viewed, and this is a way in which affective information can be stored as part of an episodic memory, and how the current mood state may influence the retrieval of episodic memories. There is consistent evidence that rewards available in a spatial environment can influence the responsiveness of rodent place neurons (Hölscher et al., 2003; Tabuchi et al., 2003).

16.2.1.4 Systems-level anatomy

The primate hippocampus receives inputs via the entorhinal cortex (area 28) and the highly developed parahippocampal gyrus (areas TF and TH) as well as the perirhinal cortex from the ends of many processing streams of the cerebral association cortex, including the visual and auditory temporal lobe association cortical areas, the prefrontal cortex, and the parietal cortex (Van Hoesen, 1982; Amaral, 1987; Amaral et al., 1992; Suzuki and Amaral, 1994b; Witter et al., 2000b; Lavenex et al., 2004) (see **Figure 1**). The hippocampus is thus by its connections potentially able to associate together object and spatial representations. In addition, the entorhinal cortex receives inputs from the amygdala and the orbitofrontal cortex, which could provide reward-related information to the hippocampus (Suzuki and Amaral, 1994a; Carmichael and Price, 1995; Stefanacci et al., 1996; Pitkanen et al., 2002).

The primary output from the hippocampus to neocortex originates in CA1 and projects to subiculum, entorhinal cortex, and parahippocampal structures (areas TF-TH), as well as prefrontal cortex (Van Hoesen, 1982; Witter, 1993; Delatour and Witter, 2002; van Haeften et al., 2003) (see **Figure 1**), though there are other outputs (Rolls and Kesner, 2006).

16.2.2 The Operation of Hippocampal Circuitry as a Memory System

16.2.2.1 Hippocampal circuitry

(see Figure 1; Amaral and Witter, 1989; Storm-Mathiesen et al., 1990; Amaral, 1993; Witter et al., 2000b; Naber et al., 2001; Lavenex et al., 2004)

Projections from the entorhinal cortex layer 2 reach the granule cells (of which there are 10^6 in the rat) in the dentate gyrus (DG), via the perforant path (pp) (Witter, 1993). The granule cells project to CA3 cells via the mossy fibers (mf), which provide a sparse but possibly powerful connection to the $3 \cdot 10^5$

CA3 pyramidal cells in the rat. Each CA3 cell receives approximately 50 mf inputs, so that the sparseness of this connectivity is thus 0.005%. By contrast, there are many more – possibly weaker – direct perforant path inputs also from layer 2 of the entorhinal cortex onto each CA3 cell, in the rat on the order of $4 \cdot 10^3$. The largest number of synapses (approximately $1.2 \cdot 10^4$ in the rat) on the dendrites of CA3 pyramidal cells is, however, provided by the (recurrent) axon collaterals of CA3 cells themselves (rc) (see **Figure 2**). It is remarkable that the recurrent collaterals are distributed to other CA3 cells throughout the hippocampus (Amaral and Witter, 1989; Amaral et al., 1990; Ishizuka et al., 1990; Amaral and Witter, 1995), so that effectively the CA3 system provides a single network, with a connectivity of approximately 2% between the different CA3 neurons given that the connections are bilateral. The neurons that comprise CA3, in turn, project to CA1 neurons via the Schaffer collaterals. In addition, projections that terminate in the CA1 region originate in layer 3 of the entorhinal cortex (see **Figure 1**).

16.2.2.2 Dentate granule cells

The theory is that the dentate granule cell stage of hippocampal processing that precedes the CA3 stage acts in a number of ways to produce during learning

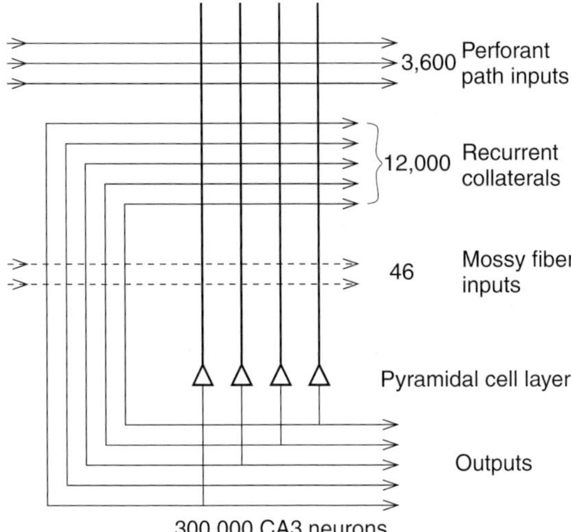

Figure 2 The numbers of connections from three different sources onto each CA3 cell from three different sources in the rat. After Treves A and Rolls ET (1992) Computational constraints suggest the need for two distinct input systems to the hippocampal CA3 network. *Hippocampus* 2: 189–199; Rolls ET and Treves A (1998) *Neural Networks and Brain Function.* Oxford: Oxford University Press.

the sparse yet efficient (i.e., nonredundant) representation in CA3 neurons that is required for the autoassociation implemented by CA3 to perform well (Rolls, 1989b; Treves and Rolls, 1992; Rolls and Kesner, 2006; Rolls et al., 2006).

The first way is that the perforant path – the dentate granule cell system with its Hebb-like modifiability is suggested to act as a competitive learning network to remove redundancy from the inputs producing a more orthogonal, sparse, and categorized set of outputs (Rolls, 1987, 1989a,b,d, 1990a,b, Rolls and Treves, 1998; Rolls, 2007). (Competitive networks are described elsewhere: Hertz et al., 1991; Rolls and Treves, 1998; Rolls and Deco, 2002; Rolls, 2008). The nonlinearity in the *N*-methyl-D-aspartate (NMDA) receptors may help the operation of such a competitive net, for it ensures that only the most active neurons left after the competitive feedback inhibition have synapses that become modified and thus learn to respond to that input (Rolls, 1989a). Because of the feedback inhibition, the competitive process may result in a relatively constant number of strongly active dentate neurons relatively independently of the number of active perforant path inputs to the dentate cells. The operation of the dentate granule cell system as a competitive network may also be facilitated by a Hebb rule of the form:

$$\delta w_{ij} = k \,.\, r_i\,(r'_j - w_{ij}), \qquad [1]$$

where k is a constant, r_i is the activation of the dendrite (the postsynaptic term), r'_j is the presynaptic firing rate, w_{ij} is the synaptic weight, and r'_j and w_{ij} are in appropriate units (Rolls, 1989a). Incorporation of a rule such as this which implies heterosynaptic long-term depression (LTD) as well as long-term potentiation (LTP) (see Levy and Desmond, 1985; Levy et al., 1990) makes the sum of the synaptic weights on each neuron remain roughly constant during learning (cf. Oja, 1982; see Rolls, 1989a; Rolls and Treves, 1998; Rolls, 2008; Rolls and Deco, 2002).

This functionality could be used to help build hippocampal place cells in rats from the grid cells present in the medial entorhinal cortex (Hafting et al., 2005). Each grid cell responds to a set of places in a spatial environment, with the places to which a cell responds set out in a regular grid. Different grid cells have different phases (positional offsets) and grid spacings (or frequencies) (Hafting et al., 2005). We (Rolls et al., 2006) have simulated the dentate granule cells as a system that receives as inputs the activity of a population of entorhinal cortex grid cells as the animal traverses a spatial environment and have shown that the competitive net builds dentate-like place cells from such entorhinal grid cell inputs (see **Figure 3**). This occurs because the firing states of entorhinal cortex cells that are active at the same time when the animal is in one place become associated together by the learning in the competitive net, yet each dentate cell represents primarily one place because the dentate representation is kept sparse, thus helping to implement symmetry breaking (Rolls et al., 2006).

The second way is also a result of the competitive learning hypothesized to be implemented by the dentate granule cells (Rolls, 1987, 1989a,b,d, 1990a,b, 1994). It is proposed that this allows overlapping (or very similar) inputs to the hippocampus to be separated in the following way (see also Rolls, 1996b). Consider three patterns B, W, and BW, where BW is a linear combination of B and W. (To make the example very concrete, we could consider binary patterns where B = 10, W = 01, and BW = 11.) Then the memory system is required to associate B with reward and W with reward, but BW with punishment. Without the hippocampus, rats might have more difficulty in solving such problems, particularly when they are spatial, for

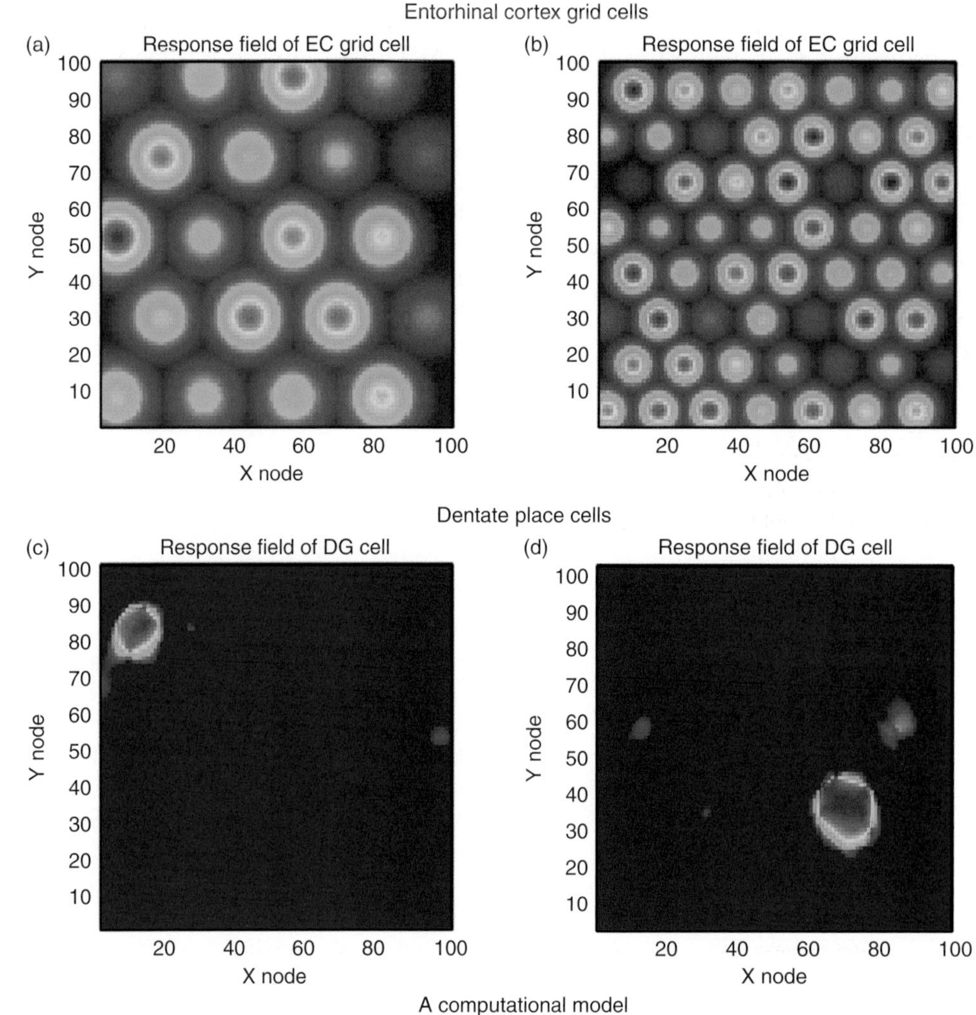

Figure 3 Simulation of competitive learning in the dentate gyrus to produce place cells from the entorhinal cortex grid cell inputs. (a), (b). Firing rate profiles of two entorhinal cortex grid cells with frequencies of four and seven cycles. In the simulation, cells with frequencies of four to seven cycles were used, and with 25 phases or spatial offsets. (A phase is defined as an offset in the X and Y directions, and five offset values were used in each direction.) The standard deviation of the peak heights was set to 0.6. (c), (d): Firing rate profiles of two dentate gyrus cells after competitive network training with the Hebb rule. After Rolls ET, Stringer SM, and Elliot T (2006) Entorhinal cortex grid cells can map to hippocampal place cells by competitive learning. *Netw. Comput. Neural Sys.* 17: 447–465.

the dentate/CA3 system in rodents is characterized by being implicated in spatial memory. However, it is a property of competitive neuronal networks that they can separate such overlapping patterns, as has been shown elsewhere (Rolls, 1989a; Rolls and Treves, 1998; Rolls, 2008); normalization of synaptic weight vectors is required for this property. It is thus an important part of hippocampal neuronal network architecture that there is a competitive network that precedes the CA3 autoassociation system. Without the dentate gyrus, if a conventional autoassociation network were presented with the mixture BW having learned B and W separately, then the autoassociation network would produce a mixed output state and would therefore be incapable of storing separate memories for B, W, and BW. It is suggested, therefore, that competition in the DG is one of the powerful computational features of the hippocampus and could enable it to help solve spatial pattern separation tasks (Rolls and Kesner, 2006).

This computational hypothesis and its predictions have been tested. Rats with DG lesions are impaired at a metric spatial pattern separation task (Gilbert et al., 2001; Goodrich-Hunsaker et al., 2005) (see **Figure 4**). The recoding of grid cells in the entorhinal cortex (Hafting et al., 2005) into small place field cells in the dentate granule cells that has been modeled (Rolls et al., 2006) can also be considered to be a case where overlapping inputs must be recoded so that different spatial components can be treated

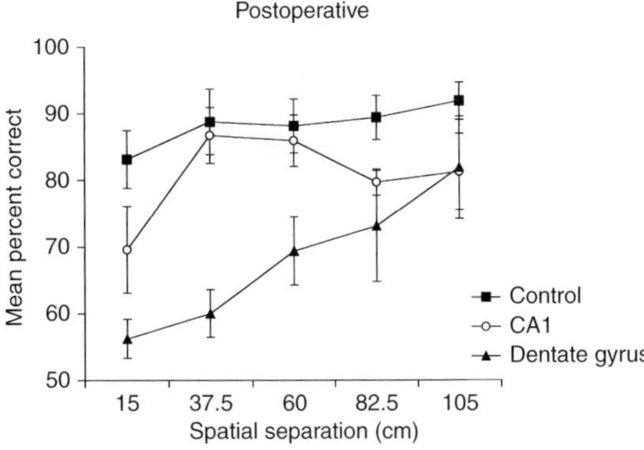

Figure 4 Pattern separation impairment produced by dentate gyrus lesions. Mean percent correct performance as a function of spatial separation of control group, CA1 lesion group, and dentate gyrus lesion group on postoperative trials. A graded impairment was found as a function of the distance between the places only following dentate gyrus lesions. After Gilbert PE, Kesner RP, and Lee I (2001) Dissociating hippocampal subregions: Double dissociation between dentate gyrus and CA1. *Hippocampus* 11: 626–636.

differently. I note that Sutherland and Rudy's configural learning hypothesis was similar but was not tested with spatial pattern separation. Instead, when tested with, for example, tone and light combinations, it was not consistently found that the hippocampus was important (Sutherland and Rudy, 1991; O'Reilly and Rudy, 2001). I suggest that application of the configural concept, but applied to spatial pattern separation, may capture part of what the DG – acting as a competitive network – could perform, particularly when a large number of such overlapping spatial memories must be stored and retrieved.

The third way in which the DG is hypothesized to contribute to the sparse and relatively orthogonal representations in CA3 arises because of the very low contact probability in the mf–CA3 connections and is described in the section titled 'Mossy fiber inputs to the CA3 cells' and by Treves and Rolls (1992).

A fourth way is that, as suggested and explained in the section titled 'Mossy fiber inputs to the CA3 cells,' the dentate granule cell–mf input to the CA3 cells may be powerful, and its use, particularly during learning, would be efficient in forcing a new pattern of firing onto the CA3 cells during learning.

In the ways just described, the dentate granule cells could be particularly important in helping to build and prepare spatial representations for the CA3 network. The actual representation of space in the primate hippocampus includes a representation of spatial view, whereas in the rat hippocampus it is of the place where the rat is. The representation in the rat may be related to the fact that with a much less developed visual system than the primate, the rat's representation of space may be defined more by the olfactory and tactile as well as distant visual cues present and may thus tend to reflect the place where the rat is. However, the spatial representations in the rat and primate could arise from essentially the same computational process as follows (Rolls, 1999; de Araujo et al., 2001). The starting assumption is that in both the rat and the primate, the dentate granule cells (and the CA3 and CA1 pyramidal cells) respond to combinations of the inputs received. In the case of the primate, a combination of visual features in the environment will, because of the fovea providing high spatial resolution over a typical viewing angle of perhaps 10°–20°, result in the formation of a spatial view cell, the effective trigger for which will thus be a combination of visual features within a relatively small part of space. In contrast, in the rat, given the very extensive visual field subtended by the rodent retina, which may extend over 180°–270°, a combination of visual features formed over such a wide visual angle would effectively define a position in space that is a place (de Araujo et al., 2001).

Although spatial view cells are present in the parahippocampal areas (Rolls et al., 1997a, 1998; Robertson et al., 1998; Georges-François et al., 1999), and neurons with place-like fields (though in some cases as a grid [Hafting et al., 2005]) are found in the medial entorhinal cortex (Moser and Moser, 1998; Brun et al., 2002; Fyhn et al., 2004; Moser, 2004), there are backprojections from the hippocampus to the entorhinal cortex and thus to parahippocampal areas, and these backprojections could enable the hippocampus to influence the spatial representations found in the entorhinal cortex and parahippocampal gyrus. On the other hand, as described above, the grid-like place cells in the medial entorhinal cortex could, if transformed by the competitive net functionality of the dentate cells, result in the place cell activity (without a repeating grid) that is found in dentate and rat hippocampal neurons.

16.2.2.3 CA3 as an autoassociation memory

16.2.2.3.(i) Arbitrary associations and pattern completion in recall Many of the synapses in the hippocampus show associative modification as shown by long-term potentiation, and this synaptic modification appears to be involved in learning (see Morris, 1989, 2003; Morris et al., 2003; Lynch, 2004). On the basis of the evidence summarized above, Rolls (1987, 1989a,b,d, 1990a,b, 1991) and others (McNaughton and Morris, 1987; Levy, 1989; McNaughton, 1991) have suggested that the CA3 stage acts as an autoassociation memory that enables episodic memories to be formed and stored in the CA3 network, and that subsequently the extensive recurrent collateral connectivity allows for the retrieval of a whole representation to be initiated by the activation of some small part of the same representation (the cue). The crucial synaptic modification for this is in the recurrent collateral synapses. A description of the operation of autoassociative networks is provided by Hertz et al. (1991), Rolls and Treves (1998), Rolls and Deco (2002), and Rolls (2007). The architecture of an autoassociation network is shown in **Figure 2**, and the learning rule is as shown in eqn [1], except that the subtractive term could be the presynaptic firing rate (Rolls and Treves, 1998; Rolls and Deco, 2002).

The hypothesis is that because the CA3 operates effectively as a single network, it can allow arbitrary associations between inputs originating from very different parts of the cerebral cortex to be formed. These might involve associations between information originating in the temporal visual cortex about the presence of an object, as well as information originating in the parietal cortex about where it is. I note that although there is some spatial gradient in the CA3 recurrent connections, so that the connectivity is not fully uniform (Ishizuka et al., 1990), nevertheless the network will still have the properties of a single interconnected autoassociation network allowing associations between arbitrary neurons to be formed, given the presence of many long-range connections that overlap from different CA3 cells.

Crucial issues include how many memories could be stored in this system (to determine whether the autoassociation hypothesis leads to a realistic estimate of the number of memories that the hippocampus could store); whether the whole of a memory could be completed from any part; whether the autoassociation memory can act as a short-term memory, for which the architecture is inherently suited, and whether the system could operate with spatial representations, which are essentially continuous because of the continuous nature of space. These and related issues are considered in the remainder of this section and in more detail elsewhere (Rolls and Kesner, 2006; Rolls, 2008).

16.2.2.3.(i).(a) Storage capacity We have performed quantitative analyses of the storage and retrieval processes in the CA3 network (Treves and Rolls, 1991, 1992). We have extended previous formal models of autoassociative memory (see Amit, 1989) by analyzing a network with graded response units, so as to represent more realistically the continuously variable rates at which neurons fire, and with incomplete connectivity (Treves, 1990; Treves and Rolls, 1991). We have found that in general, the maximum number $p_{\max}$ of firing patterns that can be (individually) retrieved is proportional to the number C^{RC} of (associatively) modifiable recurrent collateral synapses per cell, by a factor that increases roughly with the inverse of the sparseness a of the neuronal representation (Each memory is precisely defined in the theory: It is a set of firing rates of the population of neurons – which represent a memory – that can be stored and later retrieved, with retrieval being possible from a fraction of the originally stored set of neuronal firing rates.) The sparseness of response (or selectivity) of a single cell to a set of stimuli (which in the brain has approximately the same value as the sparseness of the response of the population of neurons to any one stimulus, which can in turn be thought of as the proportion of neurons that is active to any one stimulus if the neurons had binary responses; see Franco et al., 2007) is defined as

$$a = \left(\sum_{i=1,n} r_i/n\right)^2 / \sum_{i=1,n} (r_i^2/n), \qquad [2]$$

where r_i is the firing rate to the *i*th stimulus in the set of n stimuli. The sparseness ranges from $1/n$, when the cell responds to only one stimulus, to a maximal value of 1.0, attained when the cell responds with the same rate to all stimuli. Approximately,

$$p_{\max} \cong \frac{C^{\mathrm{RC}}}{a \ln(1/a)} k, \qquad [3]$$

where k is a factor that depends weakly on the detailed structure of the rate distribution, on the connectivity pattern, and so on, but is roughly on the order of 0.2–0.3 (Treves and Rolls, 1991). The sparseness a in this equation is strictly the population sparseness (Treves and Rolls, 1991; Franco et al., 2007). The population sparseness a^{p} would be measured by measuring the distribution of firing rates of all neurons to a single stimulus at a single time. The single-cell sparseness or selectivity a^{s} would be measured by the distribution of firing rates to a set of stimuli, which would take a long time. These concepts are elucidated by Franco et al. (2007). The sparseness estimates obtained by measuring early gene changes, which are effectively population sparsenesses, would thus be expected to depend greatly on the range of environments or stimuli in which these were measured. If the environment was restricted to one stimulus, this would reflect the population sparseness. If the environment was changing, the measure from early gene changes would be rather undefined, as all the populations of neurons activated in an undefined number of testing situations would be likely to be activated. For example, for $C^{\mathrm{RC}} = 12{,}000$ and $a = 0.02$, $p_{\max}$ is calculated to be approximately 36,000. This analysis emphasizes the utility of having a sparse representation in the hippocampus, for this enables many different memories to be stored. Third, in order for most associative networks to store information efficiently, heterosynaptic LTD (as well as LTP) is required (Fazeli and Collingridge, 1996; Rolls and Deco, 2002; Rolls and Treves, 1990, 1998; Treves and Rolls, 1991). Simulations that are fully consistent with the analytic theory are provided by Simmen et al. (1996) and Rolls et al. (1997b).

We have also indicated how to estimate I, the total amount of information (in bits per synapse) that can be retrieved from the network. I is defined with respect to the information i_{p} (in bits per cell) contained in each stored firing pattern, by subtracting the amount i_{l} lost in retrieval and multiplying by p/C^{RC}:

$$I = \frac{p}{C^{\mathrm{RC}}} (i_p - i_l) \qquad [4]$$

The maximal value $I_{\max}$ of this quantity was found (Treves and Rolls, 1991) to be in several interesting cases around 0.2–0.3 bits per synapse, with only a mild dependency on parameters such as the sparseness of coding a.

We may then estimate (Treves and Rolls, 1992) how much information has to be stored in each pattern for the network to efficiently exploit its information retrieval capacity $I_{\max}$. The estimate is expressed as a requirement on i_{p}:

$$i_p > a \ln(1/a) \qquad [5]$$

As the information content of each stored pattern i_{p} depends on the storage process, we see how the retrieval capacity analysis, coupled with the notion that the system is organized so as to be an efficient memory device in a quantitative sense, leads to a constraint on the storage process.

A number of points that arise are treated elsewhere (Rolls and Kesner, 2006; Rolls, 2007). Here I note that given that the memory capacity of the hippocampal CA3 system is limited, it is necessary to have some form of forgetting in this store, or another mechanism to ensure that its capacity is not exceeded. (Exceeding the capacity can lead to a loss of much of the information retrievable from the network.) Heterosynaptic LTD could help this forgetting, by enabling new memories to overwrite old memories (Rolls, 1996a, 2007). The limited capacity of the CA3 system does also provide one of the arguments that some transfer of information from the hippocampus to neocortical memory stores may be useful (see Treves and Rolls, 1994). Given its limited capacity, the hippocampus might be a useful store for only a limited period, which might be on the order of days, weeks, or months. This period may well depend on the acquisition rate of new episodic memories. If the animal were in a constant and limited environment, then as new information is not being added to the hippocampus, the representations in the hippocampus would remain stable and persistent. These hypotheses have clear experimental implications, both for recordings from single neurons and for the gradient of retrograde amnesia, both of which might be expected to depend on whether the environment is stable or frequently changing. They show that the conditions under which a gradient of retrograde amnesia might be demonstrable would be when large numbers of new memories are being acquired, not when only a few memories (few in the case of the hippocampus being less than a few hundred) are being learned.

16.2.2.3.(i).(b) Recall A fundamental property of the autoassociation model of the CA3 recurrent collateral network is that the recall can be symmetric, that is, the whole of the memory can be retrieved from any part. For example, in an object–place autoassociation memory, an object could be recalled from a place retrieval cue, and vice versa. This is not the case with a pattern association network. If, for example, the CA3 activity represented a place–spatial view, and perforant path inputs with associative synapses to CA3 neurons carried object information (consistent with evidence that the lateral perforant path [LPP] may reflect inputs from the perirhinal cortex connecting via the lateral entorhinal cortex [Hargreaves et al., 2005]), then an object could recall a place, but a place could not recall an object.

A prediction of the theory is thus that the CA3 recurrent collateral associative connections enable arbitrary associations to be formed between whatever is represented in the hippocampus, in that, for example, any place could be associated with any object, and in that the object could be recalled with a spatial recall cue, or the place with an object recall cue.

In one test of this, Day et al. (2003) trained rats in a study phase to learn in one trial an association between two flavors of food and two spatial locations. During a recall test phase they were presented with a flavor that served as a cue for the selection of the correct location. They found that injections of an NMDA blocker (AP5) or alpha-amino-3-hydroxy-5-methyl-isoxazole-4-propionic acid (AMPA) blocker (CNQX) to the dorsal hippocampus prior to the study phase impaired encoding, but injections of AP5 prior to the test phase did not impair the place recall, whereas injections of CNQX did impair the place recall. The interpretation is that somewhere in the hippocampus NMDA receptors are necessary for forming one-trial odor–place associations, and that recall can be performed without further involvement of NMDA receptors.

In a hippocampus subregion test of this, rats in a study phase are shown one object in one location, and then a second object in another location. (There are 50 possible objects and 48 locations.) In the test phase, the rat is shown one object in the start box and then after a 10-s delay must go to the correct location (choosing between two marked locations). CA3 lesions made after training in the task produced chance performance on this one-trial object–place recall task. A control, fixed visual conditional-to-place task (Rolls and Kesner, 2006) with the same delay was not impaired, showing that it is recall after one-trial (or rapid) learning that is impaired. In the context of arbitrary associations between whatever is represented in CA3, the theory also predicts that cued place–object recall tasks and cued place–odor recall tasks should be impaired by CA3 lesions.

Evidence that the CA3 system is not necessarily required during recall in a reference memory spatial task, such as the water maze spatial navigation for a single spatial location task, is that CA3-lesioned rats are not impaired during recall of a previously learned water maze task (Brun et al., 2002; Florian and Roullet, 2004). However, if completion from an incomplete cue is needed, then CA3 NMDA receptors are necessary (presumably to ensure satisfactory CA3–CA3 learning), even in a reference memory task (Nakazawa et al., 2002). Thus, the CA3 system appears to be especially needed in rapid, one-trial object–place recall and when completion from an incomplete cue is required.

In a neurophysiological investigation of one-trial object–place learning followed by recall of the spatial position in which to respond when shown the object, Rolls and Xiang (2005) showed that some primate hippocampal (including CA3) neurons respond to an object cue with the spatial position in which the object had been shown earlier in the trial. Thus, some hippocampal neurons appear to reflect spatial recall given an object recall cue.

16.2.2.3.(i).(c) Completion Another fundamental property is that the recall can be complete even from a small fragment. Thus, it is a prediction that when an incomplete retrieval cue is given, CA3 may be especially important in the retrieval process. Tests of this prediction of a role for CA3 in pattern completion have been performed, as follows.

Rats were tested on a cheese board with a black curtain with four extramaze cues surrounding the apparatus. (The cheese board is like a dry-land water maze with 177 holes on a 119-cm-diameter board.) Rats were trained to move a sample phase object covering a food well that could appear in one of five possible spatial locations. During the test phase of the task, following a 30-s delay, the animal needs to find the same food well in order to receive reinforcement with the object now removed. After reaching stable performance in terms of accuracy to find the correct location, rats received lesions in CA3. During postsurgery testing, four extramaze cues were always available during the sample phase. However, during the test phase zero, one, two, or three cues were removed in different combinations. The results indicate that controls performed well on the task regardless of the availability of one, two, three, or all cues, suggesting intact spatial pattern completion. Following the CA3 lesion, however, there was an impairment in accuracy compared to the controls especially when only one or two cues were available, suggesting impairment in spatial pattern completion in CA3-lesioned rats (Gold and Kesner, 2005) (see **Figure 5**). A useful aspect of this task is that the test

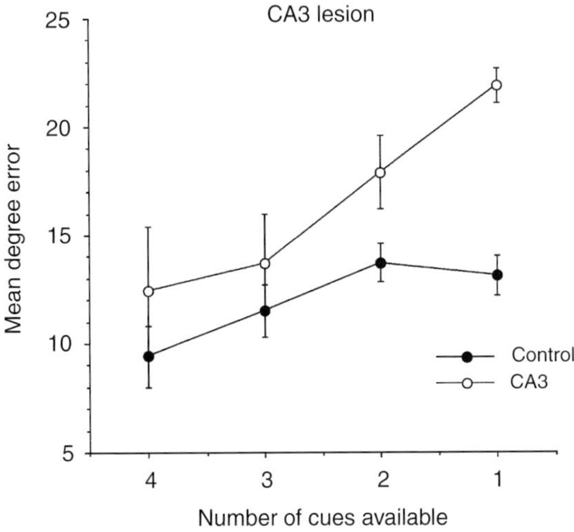

Figure 5 Pattern completion impairment produced by CA3 lesions. The mean (and SEM) degree of error in finding the correct place in the cheeseboard task when rats were tested with 1, 2, 3, or 4 of the cues available. A graded impairment in the CA3 lesion group as a function of the number of cues available was found. The task was learned in the study phase with the four cues present. The performance of the control group is also shown. After Gold AE and Kesner RP (2005) The role of the CA3 subregion of the dorsal hippocampus in spatial pattern completion in the rat. *Hippocampus* 15: 808–814.

for the ability to remember a spatial location learned in one presentation can be tested with a varying number of available cues, and many times in which the locations vary, to allow for accurate measurement of pattern completion ability when the information stored on the single presentation must be recalled.

In another study, Nakazawa et al. (2002) trained CA3 NMDA receptor-knockout mice in an analogous task, using the water maze. When the animals were required to perform the task in an environment where some of the familiar cues were removed, they were impaired in performing the task. The result suggests that the NMDA receptor–dependent synaptic plasticity mechanisms in CA3 are critical to perform the pattern completion process in the hippocampus.

16.2.2.3.(ii) Continuous spatial patterns and CA3 representations The fact that spatial patterns, which imply continuous representations of space, are represented in the hippocampus has led to the application of continuous attractor models to help understand hippocampal function. This has been necessary because space is inherently continuous, because the firing of place and spatial view cells is approximately Gaussian as a function of the distance away from the preferred spatial location, because these cells have spatially overlapping fields, and because the theory is that these cells in CA3 are connected by Hebb-modifiable synapses. This specification would inherently lead the system to operate as a continuous attractor network. Continuous attractor network models have been studied by Amari (1977), Zhang (1996), Taylor (1999), Samsonovich and McNaughton (1997), Battaglia and Treves (1998), Stringer et al. (2002a,b, 2004), Stringer and Rolls (2002), and Rolls and Stringer (2005) (see Rolls, 2007; Rolls and Deco, 2002) and are described next.

A continuous attractor neural network (CANN) can maintain the firing of its neurons to represent any location along a continuous physical dimension such as spatial position and head direction. It uses excitatory recurrent collateral connections between the neurons (as are present in CA3) to reflect the distance between the neurons in the state space of the animal (e.g., place or head direction). These networks can maintain the bubble of neural activity constant for long periods wherever it is started, to represent the current state (head direction, position, etc.) of the animal, and are likely to be involved in many aspects of spatial processing and memory, including spatial vision. Global inhibition is used to keep the number

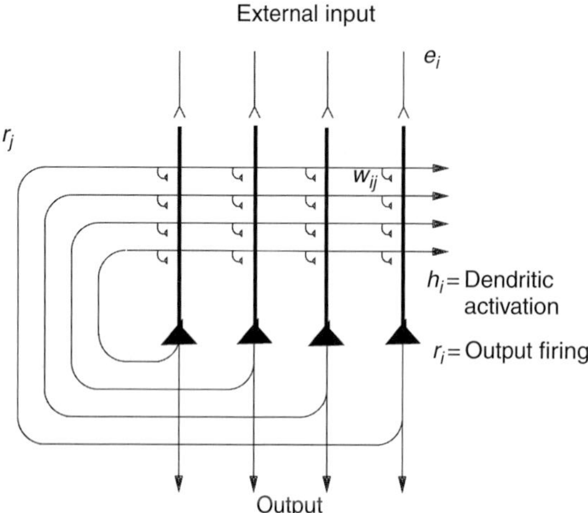

Figure 6 The architecture of a continuous attractor neural network. The architecture is the same as that of a discrete attractor neural network.

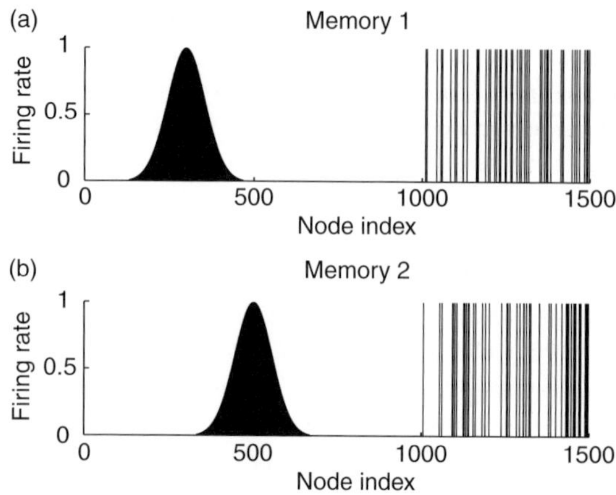

Figure 7 The types of firing patterns stored in continuous attractor networks are illustrated for the patterns present on neurons 1–1000 for Memory 1 (when the firing is that produced when the spatial state represented is that for location 300), and for Memory 2 (when the firing is that produced when the spatial state represented is that for location 500). The continuous nature of the spatial representation results from the fact that each neuron has a Gaussian firing rate that peaks at its optimal location. This particular mixed network also contains discrete representations that consist of discrete subsets of active binary firing rate neurons in the range 1001–1500. The firing of these latter neurons can be thought of as representing the discrete events that occur at the location. Continuous attractor networks by definition contain only continuous representations, but this particular network can store mixed continuous and discrete representations, and is illustrated to show the difference of the firing patterns normally stored in separate continuous attractor and discrete attractor networks. For this particular mixed network, during learning, Memory 1 is stored in the synaptic weights, then Memory 2, etc., and each memory contains a part that is continuously distributed to represent physical space and a part that represents a discrete event or object.

of neurons in a bubble or packet of actively firing neurons relatively constant and to help to ensure that there is only one activity packet. Continuous attractor networks can be thought of as very similar to autoassociation or discrete attractor networks (see Rolls and Deco, 2002) and have the same architecture, as illustrated in **Figure 6**. The main difference is that the patterns stored in a CANN are continuous patterns, with each neuron having broadly tuned firing that decreases with, for example, a Gaussian function as the distance from the optimal firing location of the cell is varied, and with different neurons having tuning that overlaps throughout the space. Such tuning is illustrated in **Figure 7**. For comparison, autoassociation networks normally have discrete (separate) patterns (each pattern implemented by the firing of a particular subset of the neurons), with no continuous distribution of the patterns throughout the space (see **Figure 7**). A consequent difference is that the CANN can maintain its firing at any location in the trained continuous space, whereas a discrete attractor or autoassociation network moves its population of active neurons toward one of the previously learned attractor states, and thus implements the recall of a particular previously learned pattern from an incomplete or noisy (distorted) version of one of the previously learned patterns.

The energy landscape of a discrete attractor network (see Rolls and Deco, 2002) has separate energy minima, each one of which corresponds to a learned pattern, whereas the energy landscape of a continuous attractor network is flat, so that the activity packet remains stable with continuous firing wherever it is started in the state space. (The state space refers to the set of possible spatial states of the animal in its environment, e.g., the set of possible places in a room.)

So far we have said that the neurons in the continuous attractor network are connected to each other by synaptic weights w_{ij} that are a simple function, for example, Gaussian, of the distance between the states of the agent in the physical world (e.g., head directions, spatial views, etc.) represented by the neurons. In many simulations, the weights are set by formula to have weights with these appropriate Gaussian values. However, Stringer et al. (2002b) showed how the appropriate weights could be set up by learning. They started with the fact that since the neurons have broad tuning that may be Gaussian in shape, nearby neurons in the state space will have overlapping spatial fields, and will thus be coactive to a degree that depends on the distance between them. The authors postulated that therefore the synaptic weights could be set up by associative learning based on the coactivity of the neurons produced by external stimuli as the animal moved in the state space. For example, head direction cells are forced to fire during learning by visual cues in the environment that produces Gaussian firing as a function of head direction from an optimal head direction for each cell. The learning rule is simply that the weights w_{ij} from head direction cell j with firing rate r_j^{HD} to head direction cell i with firing rate r_i^{HD} are updated according to an associative (Hebb) rule:

$$\delta w_{ij} = k r_i^{\mathrm{HD}} r_j^{\mathrm{HD}}, \qquad [6]$$

where δw_{ij} is the change of synaptic weight and k is the learning rate constant. During the learning phase, the firing rate r_i^{HD} of each head direction cell i might be the following the Gaussian function of the displacement of the head from the optimal firing direction of the cell:

$$r_i^{\mathrm{HD}} = e^{-s_{\mathrm{HD}}^2/2\sigma_{\mathrm{HD}}^2}, \qquad [7]$$

where s_{HD} is the difference between the actual head direction x (in degrees) of the agent and the optimal head direction x_i for head direction cell i, and σ_{HD} is the standard deviation. Stringer et al. (2002b) showed that after training at all head directions, the synaptic connections develop strengths that are an almost Gaussian function of the distance between the cells in head direction space.

16.2.2.3.(iii) Combined continuous and discrete memory representations in the same (e.g., CA3) network, and episodic memory Space is continuous, and object representations are discrete. If these representations are to be combined in, for example, an object–place memory, then we need to understand the operation of networks that combine these representations. It has now been shown that attractor networks can store both continuous patterns and discrete patterns (as illustrated in **Figure** 7) and can thus be used to store, for example, the location in (continuous, physical) space (e.g., the place out there in a room represented by spatial view cells) where an object (a discrete item) is present (Rolls et al., 2002).

16.2.2.3.(iv) The capacity of a continuous attractor network, and multiple charts If spatial representations are stored in the hippocampus, the important issue arises in terms of understanding memories that include a spatial component or context of how many such spatial representations could be stored in a continuous attractor network. The very interesting result is that because there are in general low correlations between the representations of places in different maps or charts (where each map or chart might be of one room or locale), very many different maps can be simultaneously stored in a continuous attractor network (Battaglia and Treves, 1998a).

16.2.2.3.(v) Idiothetic update by path integration We have considered how spatial representations could be stored in continuous attractor networks and how the activity can be maintained at any location in the state space in a form of short-term memory when the external (e.g., visual) input is removed. However, many networks with spatial representations in the brain can be updated by internal, self-motion (i.e., idiothetic) cues even when there is no external (e.g., visual) input. The way in which path integration could be implemented in recurrent networks such as the CA3 system in the hippocampus or in related systems is described next.

Single-cell recording studies have shown that some neurons represent the current position along a continuous physical dimension or space even when no inputs are available, for example, in darkness. Examples include neurons that represent the positions of the eyes (i.e., eye direction with respect to the head), the place where the animal is looking in space, head direction, and the place where the animal is located. In particular, examples of such classes of cells include head direction cells in rats (Ranck, 1985; Taube et al., 1990; Muller et al., 1996; Taube et al., 1996) and primates (Robertson et al., 1999), which respond maximally when the animal's head is facing in a particular preferred direction; place cells in rats (O'Keefe and Dostrovsky, 1971; McNaughton et al., 1983; O'Keefe, 1984; Muller et al., 1991; Markus et al., 1995) that fire maximally when the animal is in a particular location; and spatial view cells in primates that respond when the monkey is looking toward a particular location in space (Rolls et al., 1997a; Robertson et al., 1998; Georges-François et al., 1999).

One approach to simulating the movement of an activity packet produced by idiothetic cues (which is a form of path integration whereby the current location is calculated from recent movements) is to employ a look-up table that stores (taking head direction cells as an example), for every possible head direction and head rotational velocity input generated by the vestibular system, the corresponding new head direction (Samsonovich and McNaughton, 1997). An analogous approach has been described for entorhinal cortex grid cells (McNaughton et al., 2006). Another approach involves modulating the strengths of the recurrent synaptic weights in the continuous attractor on one but not the other side of a currently represented position, so that the stable position of the packet of activity, which requires symmetric connections in different directions from each node, is lost, and the packet moves in the direction of the temporarily increased weights, although no possible biological implementation was proposed of how the appropriate dynamic synaptic weight changes might be achieved (Zhang, 1996). Another mechanism (for head direction cells) (Skaggs et al., 1995) relies on a set of cells, termed (head) rotation cells, which are coactivated by head direction cells and vestibular cells and drive the activity of the attractor network by anatomically distinct connections for clockwise and counterclockwise rotation cells, in what is effectively a look-up table. However, these proposals did not show how the synaptic weights for this path integration could be achieved by a biologically plausible learning process.

Stringer et al. (2002b) introduced a proposal with more biological plausibility about how the synaptic connections from idiothetic inputs to a continuous attractor network can be learned by a self-organizing learning process. The mechanism associates a short-term memory trace of the firing of the neurons in the attractor network reflecting recent movements in the state space (e.g., of places) with an idiothetic velocity of movement input (see **Figure 8**). This has been applied to head direction cells (Stringer et al., 2002b), rat place cells (Stringer et al., 2002a,b), and primate spatial view cells (Stringer et al., 2004, 2005; Rolls and Stringer, 2005). These attractor networks provide a basis for understanding cognitive maps and how they are updated by learning and by self-motion. The implication is that to the extent that path integration of place or spatial view representations is performed within the hippocampus itself, then the CA3 system is the most likely part of the hippocampus to be involved in this, because it has the appropriate recurrent collateral connections. Consistent with this, Whishaw and colleagues (Maaswinkel et al., 1999; Whishaw et al., 2001; Wallace and Whishaw, 2003) have shown that path integration is impaired by hippocampal lesions. Path integration of head direction is reflected in the firing of neurons in the presubiculum, and mechanisms outside the hippocampus probably implement path integration for head direction.

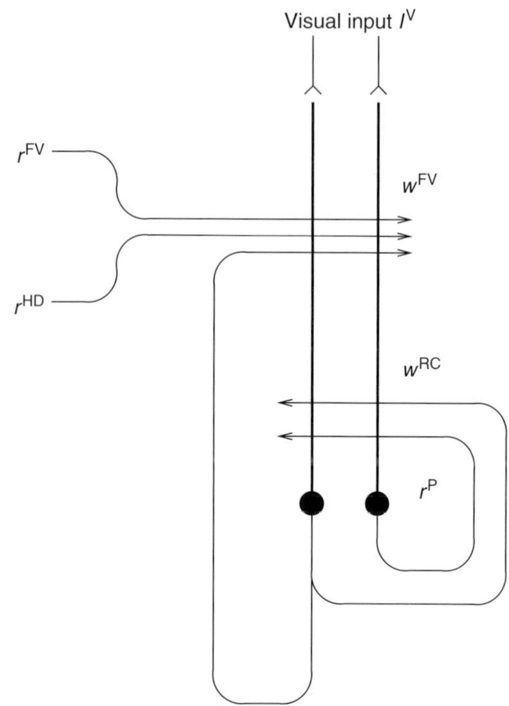

Figure 8 Neural network architecture for two-dimensional continuous attractor models of place cells. There is a recurrent network of place cells with firing rates r^P, which receives external inputs from three sources: (i) the visual system I^V, (ii) a population of head direction cells with firing rates r^{HD}, and (iii) a population of forward velocity cells with firing rates r^{FV}. The recurrent weights between the place cells are denoted by w^{RC}, and the idiothetic weights to the place cells from the forward velocity cells and head direction cells are denoted by w^{FV}.

16.2.2.3.(vi) The dynamics of the recurrent network The analysis described earlier of the capacity of a recurrent network such as the CA3 considered steady-state conditions of the firing rates of the neurons. The question arises of how quickly the recurrent network would settle into its final state. With reference to the CA3 network, how long does it take before a pattern of activity, originally evoked in

CA3 by afferent inputs, becomes influenced by the activation of recurrent collaterals? In a more general context, recurrent collaterals between the pyramidal cells are an important feature of the connectivity of the cerebral neocortex. How long would it take these collaterals to contribute fully to the activity of cortical cells? If these settling processes took on the order of hundreds of milliseconds, they would be much too slow to contribute usefully to cortical activity, whether in the hippocampus or the neocortex (Rolls, 1992; Panzeri et al., 2001; Rolls and Deco, 2002; Rolls, 2003).

It has been shown that if the neurons are not treated as McCulloch-Pitts neurons, which are simply updated at each iteration, or cycle of time steps (and assume the active state if the threshold is exceeded), but instead are analyzed and modeled as integrate-and-fire neurons in real continuous time, then the network can effectively relax into its recall state very rapidly in one or two time constants of the synapses (Treves, 1993; Battaglia and Treves, 1998b; Rolls and Treves, 1998; Rolls and Deco, 2002). This corresponds to perhaps 20 ms in the brain. One factor in this rapid dynamics of autoassociative networks with brain-like integrate-and-fire membrane and synaptic properties is that with some spontaneous activity, some of the neurons in the network are close to threshold already before the recall cue is applied, and hence some of the neurons are very quickly pushed by the recall cue into firing, so that information starts to be exchanged very rapidly (within 1–2 ms of brain time) through the modified synapses by the neurons in the network. The progressive exchange of information starting early on within what would otherwise be thought of as an iteration period (of perhaps 20 ms, corresponding to a neuronal firing rate of 50 spikes/s) is the mechanism accounting for rapid recall in an autoassociative neuronal network made biologically realistic in this way. Further analysis of the fast dynamics of these networks if they are implemented in a biologically plausible way with integrate-and-fire neurons, is provided in Section 7.7 of Rolls and Deco (2002), in Appendix A5 of Rolls and Treves (1998), by Treves (1993), and by Panzeri et al. (2001).

16.2.2.3.(vii) Mossy fiber inputs to the CA3 cells We hypothesize that the mf inputs force efficient information storage by virtue of their strong and sparse influence on the CA3 cell firing rates (Rolls, 1987, 1989b,d; Treves and Rolls, 1992). (The strong effects likely to be mediated by the mfs were also emphasized by McNaughton and Morris [1987] and McNaughton and Nadel [1990].) We hypothesize that the mf input appears to be particularly appropriate in several ways.

First of all, the fact that mf synapses are large and located very close to the soma makes them relatively powerful in activating the postsynaptic cell. (This should not be taken to imply that a CA3 cell can be fired by a single mf excitatory postsynaptic potential [EPSP].)

Second, the firing activity of dentate granule cells appears to be very sparse (Jung and McNaughton, 1993), and this, together with the small number of connections on each CA3 cell, produces a sparse signal, which can then be transformed into an even sparser firing activity in CA3 by a threshold effect. For example, if only one granule cell in 100 were active in the dentate gyrus, and each CA3 cell received a connection from 50 randomly placed granule cells, then the number of active mf inputs received by CA3 cells would follow a Poisson distribution of average $50/100 = 1/2$, that is, 60% of the cells would not receive any active input, 30% would receive only one, 7.5% two, little more than 1% would receive three, and so on. (It is easy to show from the properties of the Poisson distribution and our definition of sparseness that the sparseness of the mf signal as seen by a CA3 cell would be $x/(1+x)$, with $x = C^{MF}a_{DG}$, assuming equal strengths for all mf synapses.) If three mf inputs were required to fire a CA3 cell and these were the only inputs available, we see that the activity in CA3 would be roughly as sparse, in the example, as in the dentate gyrus. C^{MF} is the number of mf connections to a CA3 neuron, and a_{DG} is the sparseness of the representation in the dentate granule cells.

Third, nonassociative plasticity of mfs (see Brown et al., 1989, 1990) might have a useful effect in enhancing the signal-to-noise ratio, in that a consistently firing mf would produce nonlinearly amplified currents in the postsynaptic cell, which would not happen with an occasionally firing fiber (Treves and Rolls, 1992). This plasticity, and also learning in the dentate, would also have the effect that similar fragments of each episode (e.g., the same environmental location) recurring on subsequent occasions would be more likely to activate the same population of CA3 cells, which would have potential advantages in terms of economy of use of the CA3 cells in different memories, and in making some link between different episodic memories with a common feature, such as the same location in space.

Fourth, with only a few, and powerful, active mf inputs to each CA3 cell, setting a given sparseness of the representation provided by CA3 cells would be simplified, for the EPSPs produced by the mfs would be Poisson distributed with large membrane potential differences for each active mf. Setting the average firing rate of the dentate granule cells would effectively set the sparseness of the CA3 representation, without great precision being required in the threshold setting of the CA3 cells (Rolls et al., 1997b). Part of what is achieved by the mf input may be setting the sparseness of the CA3 cells correctly, which, as shown above, is very important in an autoassociative memory store.

Fifth, the nonassociative and sparse connectivity properties of the mf connections to CA3 cells may be appropriate for an episodic memory system that can learn very fast, in one trial. The hypothesis is that the sparse connectivity would help arbitrary relatively uncorrelated sets of CA3 neurons to be activated for even somewhat similar input patterns without the need for any learning of how best to separate the patterns, which in a self-organizing competitive network would take several repetitions (at least) of the set of patterns.

The mf solution may thus be adaptive in a system that must learn in one trial, and for which the CA3 recurrent collateral learning requires uncorrelated sets of CA3 cells to be allocated for each (one-trial) episodic memory. The hypothesis is that the mf sparse connectivity solution performs the appropriate function without the mf system having to learn by repeated presentations of how best to separate a set of training patterns. The perforant path input would, the quantitative analysis shows, not produce a pattern of firing in CA3 that contains sufficient information for learning (Treves and Rolls, 1992).

On the basis of these points, we predict that the mfs may be necessary for new learning in the hippocampus but may not be necessary for recall of existing memories from the hippocampus. Experimental evidence consistent with this prediction about the role of the mfs in learning has been found in rats with disruption of the dentate granule cells (Lassalle et al., 2000).

As acetylcholine turns down the efficacy of the recurrent collateral synapses between CA3 neurons (Hasselmo et al., 1995), then cholinergic activation also might help to allow external inputs rather than the internal recurrent collateral inputs to dominate the firing of the CA3 neurons during learning, as the current theory proposes. If cholinergic activation at the same time facilitated LTP in the recurrent collaterals (as it appears to in the neocortex), then cholinergic activation could have a useful double role in facilitating new learning at times of behavioral activation, when presumably it may be particularly relevant to allocate some of the limited memory capacity to new memories.

16.2.2.3.(viii) Perforant path inputs to CA3 cells By calculating the amount of information that would end up being carried by a CA3 firing pattern produced solely by the perforant path input and by the effect of the recurrent connections, we have been able to show (Treves and Rolls, 1992) that an input of the perforant path type, alone, is unable to direct efficient information storage. Such an input is too weak, it turns out, to drive the firing of the cells, as the dynamics of the network are dominated by the randomizing effect of the recurrent collaterals. This is the manifestation, in the CA3 network, of a general problem affecting storage (i.e., learning) in all autoassociative memories. The problem arises when the system is considered to be activated by a set of input axons making synaptic connections that have to compete with the recurrent connections, rather than having the firing rates of the neurons artificially clamped into a prescribed pattern.

An autoassociative memory network needs afferent inputs also in the other mode of operation, that is, when it retrieves a previously stored pattern of activity. We have shown (Treves and Rolls, 1992) that the requirements on the organization of the afferents are in this case very different, implying the necessity of a second, separate input system, which we have identified with the perforant path to CA3. In brief, the argument is based on the notion that the cue available to initiate retrieval might be rather small, that is, the distribution of activity on the afferent axons might carry a small correlation, $q \ll 1$, with the activity distribution present during learning. In order not to lose this small correlation altogether, but rather transform it into an input current in the CA3 cells that carries a sizable signal – which can then initiate the retrieval of the full pattern by the recurrent collaterals – one needs a large number of associatively modifiable synapses. This is expressed by the formulas that give the specific signal S produced by sets of associatively modifiable synapses, or by nonassociatively modifiable synapses: If C^{AFF} is the number of afferents per cell,

$$S_{\mathrm{ASS}} \sim \frac{\sqrt{C^{\mathrm{AFF}}}}{\sqrt{p}}\, q \qquad S_{\mathrm{NONASS}} \sim \frac{1}{\sqrt{C^{\mathrm{AFF}}}}\, q. \tag{8}$$

Associatively modifiable synapses are therefore needed and are needed in a number C^{AFF} of the same order as the number of concurrently stored patterns p, so that small cues can be effective, whereas nonassociatively modifiable synapses – or even more so, nonmodifiable ones – produce very small signals, which decrease in size the larger the number of synapses. In contrast with the storage process, the average strength of these synapses does not play now a crucial role. This suggests that the perforant path system is the one involved in relaying the cues that initiate retrieval.

16.2.2.4 CA1 cells

16.2.2.4.(i) Associative retrieval at the CA3 to CA1 (Schaffer collateral) synapses The CA3 cells connect to the CA1 cells by the Schaeffer collateral synapses. The following arguments outline the advantage of this connection being associatively modifiable and apply independently of the relative extent to which the CA3 or the direct entorhinal cortex inputs to CA1 drive the CA1 cells during the learning phase.

The amount of information about each episode retrievable from CA3 has to be balanced against the number of episodes that can be held concurrently in storage. The balance is regulated by the sparseness of the coding. Whatever the amount of information per episode in CA3, one may hypothesize that the organization of the structures that follow CA3 (i.e., CA1, the various subicular fields, and the return projections to neocortex) should be optimized so as to preserve and use this information content in its entirety. This would prevent further loss of information, after the massive but necessary reduction in information content that has taken place along the sensory pathways and before the autoassociation stage in CA3. We have proposed (Treves and Rolls, 1994; Treves, 1995) that the need to preserve the full information content present in the output of an autoassociative memory requires an intermediate recoding stage (CA1) with special characteristics. In fact, a calculation of the information present in the CA1 firing pattern, elicited by a pattern of activity retrieved from CA3, shows that a considerable fraction of the information is lost if the synapses are nonmodifiable, and that this loss can be prevented only if the CA3 to CA1 synapses are associatively modifiable. Their modifiability should match the plasticity of the CA3 recurrent collaterals. The additional information that can be retrieved beyond that retrieved by CA3 because the CA3 to CA1 synapses are associatively modifiable is strongly demonstrated by the hippocampal simulation described by Rolls (1995) and is quantitatively analyzed by Schultz and Rolls (1999).

16.2.2.4.(ii) Recoding in CA1 to facilitate retrieval to the neocortex If the total amount of information carried by CA3 cells is redistributed over a larger number of CA1 cells, less information needs to be loaded onto each CA1 cell, rendering the code more robust to information loss in the next stages. For example, if each CA3 cell had to code for two bits of information, for example, by firing at one of four equiprobable activity levels, then each CA1 cell (if there were twice as many as there are CA3 cells) could code for just 1 bit, for example, by firing at one of only two equiprobable levels. Thus, the same information content could be maintained in the overall representation while reducing the sensitivity to noise in the firing level of each cell. In fact, there are more CA1 cells than CA3 cells in rats (2.5×10^5). There are even more CA1 cells (4.6×10^6) in humans (and the ratio of CA1 to CA3 cells is greater). The CA1 cells may thus provide the first part of the expansion for the return projections to the enormous numbers of neocortical cells in primates, after the bottleneck of the single network in CA3, the number of neurons in which may be limited because it has to operate as a single network.

Another argument on the operation of the CA1 cells is also considered to be related to the CA3 autoassociation effect. In this, several arbitrary patterns of firing occur together on the CA3 neurons and become associated together to form an episodic or whole scene memory. It is essential for this CA3 operation that several different sparse representations are present conjunctively in order to form the association. Moreover, when completion operates in the CA3 autoassociation system, all the neurons firing in the original conjunction can be brought into activity by only a part of the original set of conjunctive events. For these reasons, a memory in the CA3 cells consists of several different simultaneously active ensembles of activity. To be explicit, the parts A, B, C, D, and E of a particular episode would each be represented, roughly speaking, by its own population of CA3 cells, and these five populations would be linked together by autoassociation. It is suggested that the CA1 cells, which receive these groups of simultaneously active ensembles, can detect the conjunctions of firing of the different ensembles that represent the episodic memory and allocate by competitive learning neurons to represent at least larger parts of each episodic memory (Rolls, 1987, 1989a,b,d, 1990a,b). In relation to the simple example above, some CA1 neurons might code for ABC, and others for BDE, rather than having to maintain independent representations in CA1 of A, B, C, D, and E. This implies a more efficient representation, in the sense that when eventually, after many further stages, neocortical neuronal activity is recalled (as discussed later), each neocortical cell need not be accessed by all the axons carrying each component A, B, C, D, and E but, instead, by fewer axons carrying larger fragments, such as ABC and BDE. This process is performed by competitive networks, which self-organize to find categories in the input space, where each category is represented by a set of simultaneously active inputs (Rolls and Treves, 1998; Rolls, 2000; Rolls and Deco, 2002).

16.2.2.4.(iii) CA1 inputs from CA3 vs direct entorhinal inputs Another feature of the CA1 network is its double set of afferents, with each of its cells receiving most synapses from the Schaeffer collaterals coming from CA3, but also a proportion (about 1/6; Amaral et al., 1990) from direct perforant path projections from entorhinal cortex. Such projections appear to originate mainly in layer 3 of entorhinal cortex (Witter et al., 1989) from a population of cells only partially overlapping with that (mainly in layer 2) giving rise to the perforant path projections to DG and CA3. This suggests that it is useful to include in CA1 not only what it is possible to recall from CA3 but also the detailed information present in the retrieval cue itself (see Treves and Rolls, 1994).

Another possibility is that the perforant path input provides the strong forcing input to the CA1 neurons during learning and that the output of the CA3 system is associated with this forced CA1 firing during learning (McClelland et al., 1995). During recall, an incomplete cue could then be completed in CA3, and the CA3 output would then produce firing in CA1 that would correspond to that present during the learning. This suggestion is essentially identical to that of Treves and Rolls (1994) about the backprojection system and recall, except that McClelland et al. (1995) suggest that the output of CA3 is associated at the CA3 to CA1 (Schaeffer collateral) synapses with the signal present during training in CA1, whereas in the theory of Treves and Rolls (1994), the output of the hippocampus consists of CA1 firing, which is associated in the entorhinal cortex and earlier cortical stages with the firing present during learning, providing a theory of how the correct recall is implemented at every backprojection stage though the neocortex (see the next section).

16.2.2.5 Backprojections to the neocortex – a hypothesis

The need for information to be retrieved from the hippocampus to affect other brain areas was noted in the introduction. The way in which this could be implemented via backprojections to the neocortex is now considered.

It is suggested that the modifiable connections from the CA3 neurons to the CA1 neurons allow the whole episode in CA3 to be produced in CA1. This may be assisted as described above by the direct perforant path input to CA1. This might allow details of the input key for the recall process, as well as the possibly less information-rich memory of the whole episode recalled from the CA3 network, to contribute to the firing of CA1 neurons. The CA1 neurons would then activate, via their termination in the deep layers of the entorhinal cortex, at least the pyramidal cells in the deep layers of the entorhinal cortex (see **Figure 1**). These entorhinal cortex layer 5 neurons would then, by virtue of their backprojections (Lavenex and Amaral, 2000; Witter et al., 2000a) to the parts of cerebral cortex that originally provided the inputs to the hippocampus, terminate in the superficial layers (including layer 1) of those neocortical areas, where synapses would be made onto the distal parts of the dendrites of the (superficial and deep) cortical pyramidal cells (Rolls, 1989a, 1989b, 1989d). The areas of cerebral neocortex in which this recall would be produced could include multimodal cortical areas (e.g., the cortex in the superior temporal sulcus, which receives inputs from temporal, parietal, and occipital cortical areas, and from which it is thought that cortical areas such as 39 and 40, related to language, developed), and also areas of unimodal association cortex (e.g., inferior temporal visual cortex). The backprojections, by recalling previous episodic events, could provide information useful to the neocortex in the building of new representations in the multimodal and unimodal association cortical areas, which by building new long-term representations can be considered as a form of memory consolidation (Rolls, 1989a,b,d, 1990a,b), or in organizing actions.

The hypothesis of the architecture with which this would be achieved is shown in **Figure 1**. The feedforward connections from association areas of the cerebral neocortex (solid lines in **Figure 1**) show major convergence as information is passed to CA3, with the CA3 autoassociation network having the smallest number of neurons at any stage of the processing. The backprojections allow for divergence back to neocortical areas. The way in which I suggest that the backprojection synapses are set up to have the appropriate strengths for recall is as follows (Rolls, 1989a,b,d). During the setting up of a new episodic memory, there would be strong feedforward activity progressing toward the hippocampus. During the episode, the CA3 synapses would be modified, and via the CA1 neurons and the subiculum, a pattern of activity would be produced on the backprojecting synapses to the entorhinal cortex. Here the backprojecting synapses from active backprojection axons onto pyramidal cells being activated by the forward inputs to entorhinal cortex would be associatively modified. A similar process would be implemented at preceding stages of neocortex, that is, in the parahippocampal gyrus/perirhinal cortex stage, and in association cortical areas, as shown in **Figure 1**.

The concept is that during the learning of an episodic memory, cortical pyramidal cells in at least one of the stages would be driven by forward inputs but would simultaneously be receiving backprojected activity (indirectly) from the hippocampus, which would, by pattern association from the backprojecting synapses to the cortical pyramidal cells, become associated with whichever cortical cells were being made to fire by the forward inputs. Then, later on, during recall, a recall cue from perhaps another part of cortex might reach CA3, where the firing during the original episode would be completed. The resulting backprojecting activity would then, as a result of the pattern association learned previously, bring back the firing in any cortical area that was present during the original episode. Thus, retrieval involves reinstating the activity that was present in different cortical areas during the learning of an episode. (The pattern association is also called heteroassociation, to contrast it with autoassociation. The pattern association operates at multiple stages in the backprojection pathway, as made evident in **Figure 1**.) If the recall cue was an object, this might result in recall of the neocortical firing that represented the place in which that object had been seen previously. As noted elsewhere in this chapter and by McClelland et al. (1995), that recall might be useful to the neocortex to help it build new semantic memories, which might inherently be a slow process and is not part of the theory of recall.

16.2.2.6 Backprojections to the neocortex – quantitative aspects

A plausible requirement for a successful hippocampus-directed recall operation is that the signal generated from the hippocampally retrieved pattern of activity, and carried backward toward neocortex, remains undegraded when compared to the noise due, at each stage, to the interference effects caused by the concurrent storage of other patterns of activity on the same backprojecting synaptic systems. That requirement is equivalent to that used in deriving the storage capacity of such a series of heteroassociative memories, and it was shown in Treves and Rolls (1991) that the maximum number of independently generated activity patterns that can be retrieved is given, essentially, by the same formula as eqn (3) above where, however, a is now the sparseness of the representation at any given stage and C is the average number of (back)projections each cell of that stage receives from cells of the previous one. (k' is a similar, slowly varying factor to that introduced above.) If p is equal to the number of memories held in the hippocampal memory, it is limited by the retrieval capacity of the CA3 network, p_{max}. Putting together the formula for the latter with that shown here, one concludes that, roughly, the requirement implies that the number of afferents of (indirect) hippocampal origin to a given neocortical stage (C^{HBP}), must be $C^{HBP} = C^{RC} a_{nc}/a_{CA3}$, where C^{RC} is the number of recurrent collaterals to any given cell in CA3, the average sparseness of a representation is a_{nc}, and a_{CA3} is the sparseness of memory representations there in CA3.

This requirement is very strong: Even if representations were to remain as sparse as they are in CA3, which is unlikely, to avoid degrading the signal, C^{HBP} should be as large as C^{RC}, that is, 12,000 in the rat. If then C^{HBP} has to be of the same order as C^{RC}, one is led to a very definite conclusion: A mechanism of the type envisaged here could not possibly rely on a set of monosynaptic CA3-to-neocortex backprojections. This would imply that, to make a sufficient number of synapses on each of the vast number of neocortical cells, each cell in CA3 has to generate a disproportionate number of synapses (i.e., C^{HBP} times the ratio between the number of neocortical and the number of CA3 cells). The required divergence can be kept within reasonable limits only by assuming that the backprojecting system is polysynaptic, provided that the number of cells involved grows gradually at each stage, from CA3 back to neocortical association areas (Treves and Rolls, 1994) (cf. **Figure 1**).

The theory of recall by the backprojections thus provides a quantitative account of why the cerebral cortex has as many backprojection as forward projection connections. Further aspects of the operation of the backprojecting systems are described elsewhere (Rolls, 2008).

16.3 Comparison with Other Theories of Hippocampal Function

The overall theory described here is close in different respects to those of a number of other investigators (Marr, 1971; Brown and Zador, 1990; McNaughton and Nadel, 1990; Eichenbaum et al., 1992; Gaffan, 1992; Squire, 1992; Moscovitch et al., 2005), and of course priority is not claimed on all the propositions put forward here.

Some theories postulate that the hippocampus performs spatial computation. The theory of O'Keefe and Nadel (1978), that the hippocampus implements a cognitive map, placed great emphasis on spatial function. It supposed that the hippocampus at least holds information about allocentric space in a form that enables rats to find their way in an environment even when novel trajectories are necessary, that is, it permits an animal to 'go from one place to another independent of particular inputs (cues) or outputs (responses), and to link together conceptually parts of the environment which have never been experienced at the same time' (O'Keefe and Nadel, 1978). O'Keefe (1990) extended this analysis and produced a computational theory of the hippocampus as a cognitive map, in which the hippocampus performs geometric spatial computations. Key aspects of the theory are that the hippocampus stores the centroid and slope of the distribution of landmarks in an environment and stores the relationships between the centroid and the individual landmarks. The hippocampus then receives as inputs information about where the rat currently is and where the rat's target location is and computes geometrically the body turns and movements necessary to reach the target location. In this sense, the hippocampus is taken to be a spatial computer, which produces an output that is very different from its inputs. This is in contrast to the present theory, in which the hippocampus is a memory device that is able to recall what was stored in it, using as input a partial cue. A prototypical example in Rolls' theory is the learning of object–place association memory and the recall of the whole memory from a part, which can be used as a model of event or episodic memory. O'Keefe's theory postulates that the hippocampus actually performs a spatial computation. A later theory (Burgess et al., 1994, 2000) also makes the same postulate, but now the firing of place cells is determined by the distance and approximate bearing to landmarks, and the navigation is performed by increasing the strength of connections from place cells to goal cells and then performing a gradient-ascent style search for the goal using the network.

McNaughton et al. (1991) have also proposed that the hippocampus is involved in spatial computation. They propose a compass solution to the problem of spatial navigation along novel trajectories in known environments, postulating that distances and bearings (i.e., vector quantities) from landmarks are stored, and that computation of a new trajectory involves vector subtraction by the hippocampus. They postulate that a linear associative mapping is performed, using as inputs a cross-feature (combination) representation of (head) angular velocity and (its time integral) head direction, to produce as output the future value of the integral (head direction) after some specified time interval. The system can be reset by learned associations between local views of the environment and head direction, so that when later a local view is seen, it can lead to an output from the network that is a (corrected) head direction. They suggest that some of the key signals in the computational system can be identified with the firing of hippocampal cells (e.g., local view cells) and subicular cells (head direction cells). It should be noted that this theory requires a (linear) associative mapping with an output (head direction) different in form from the inputs (head angular velocity over a time period, or local view). This is pattern association (with the conditioned stimulus local view and the unconditioned stimulus head direction), not autoassociation, and it has been postulated that this pattern association can be performed by the hippocampus (cf. McNaughton and Morris, 1987). This theory is again in contrast to the present theory, in which the hippocampus operates as a memory to store events that occur at the same time and can recall the whole memory from any part of what was stored. (A pattern associator uses a conditioned stimulus to map an input to a pattern of firing in an output set of neurons, which is like that produced in the output neurons by the unconditioned stimulus. A description of pattern associations and autoassociators in a neurobiological context is provided by Rolls (1996a, 2007) and Rolls and Treves (1998). The present theory is fully consistent with the presence of spatial view cells and whole-body motion cells in the primate hippocampus (Rolls, 1999; Rolls and O'Mara, 1993; Rolls and Xiang, 2006) (or place or local view cells in the rat hippocampus, and head direction cells in the presubiculum), for it is often important to store and later recall where one has been (views of the environment, body turns made, etc.), and indeed such (episodic) memories are required for navigation by dead reckoning in small environments.

The present theory thus holds that the hippocampus is used for the formation of episodic memories using autoassociation. This function is often necessary for successful spatial computation but is not itself spatial computation. Instead, I believe that spatial computation is more likely to be performed in the neocortex (utilizing information if necessary recalled from the hippocampus). Consistent with this view, hippocampal damage impairs the ability to learn new environments but not to perform spatial computations such as finding one's way to a place in a familiar environment, whereas damage to the parietal cortex and parahippocampal cortex can lead to problems such as topographical and other spatial agnosias in humans (see Gruesser and Landis, 1991; Kolb and Whishaw, 2003). This is consistent with spatial computations normally being performed in the neocortex. In monkeys, there is evidence for a role of the parietal cortex in allocentric spatial computation. For example, monkeys with parietal cortex lesions are impaired at performing a landmark task in which the object to be chosen is signified by the proximity to it of a landmark (another object; Ungerleider and Mishkin, 1982).

A theory closely related to the present theory of how the hippocampus operates has been developed by McClelland et al. (1995). It is very similar to the theory we have developed (Rolls, 1987, 1989a,b,d; Treves and Rolls, 1992, 1994; Rolls, 2007) at the systems level, except that it takes a stronger position on the gradient of retrograde amnesia, emphasizes that recall from the hippocampus of episodic information is used to help build semantic representations in the neocortex, and holds that the last set of synapses that are modified rapidly during the learning of each episode are those between the CA3 and the CA1 pyramidal cells, as described above (see **Figure 1**). It also emphasizes the important point that the hippocampal and neocortical memory systems may be quite different, with the hippocampus specialized for the rapid learning of single events or episodes and the neocortex for the slower learning of semantic representations, which may necessarily benefit from the many exemplars needed to shape the semantic representation.

Lisman and colleagues (2005) have considered how the memory of sequences could be implemented in the hippocampus. This theory of sequential recall within the hippocampus is inextricably linked to the internal timing within the hippocampus imposed, he believes, by the theta and gamma oscillations, and this makes it difficult to recall each item in the sequence as it is needed. It is not specified how one would read out the sequence information, given that the items are only 12 ms apart. The Jensen and Lisman (1996) model requires short, time constant NMDA channels and is therefore unlikely to be implemented in the hippocampus. Hasselmo and Eichenbaum (2005) have taken up some of these sequence ideas and incorporated them into their model, which has its origins in the Rolls and Treves model (Rolls, 1989b; Treves and Rolls, 1992, 1994), but proposes, for example, that sequences are stored in entorhinal cortex layer III. The proposal that acetylcholine could be important during encoding by facilitating CA3–CA3 LTP, and should be lower during retrieval (Hasselmo et al., 1995), is an important concept.

Another type of sequence memory uses synaptic adaptation to effectively encode the order of the items in a sequence (Deco and Rolls, 2005). This could be implemented in recurrent networks such as the CA3 or the prefrontal cortex.

In this chapter, we have seen that quantitative approaches to the functions of the hippocampus in memory are being developed by a number of investigators and that these theories are consistent with the quantitative circuitry of the hippocampus as well as with neuronal recordings and the effects of lesions. Moreover, we have seen that the predictions of these theories are now being tested.

Acknowledgments

Different parts of the research described here were supported by Programme Grants from the Medical Research Council, a Human Frontier Science program grant, an EEC BRAIN grant, the MRC Oxford Interdisciplinary Research Centre in Cognitive Neuroscience, and the Oxford McDonnell-Pew Centre in Cognitive Neuroscience.

References

Amaral DG (1987) Memory: Anatomical organization of candidate brain regions. In: Mountcastle VB (ed.) *Handbook of Physiology. Section 1, The Nervous System*, pp. 211–294. Washington DC: American Physiological Society.

Amaral DG (1993) Emerging principles of intrinsic hippocampal organisation. *Curr. Opin. Neurobiol.* 3: 225–229.

Amaral DG and Witter MP (1989) The three-dimensional organization of the hippocampal formation: A review of anatomical data. *Neuroscience* 31: 571–591.

Amaral DG and Witter MP (1995) The hippocampal formation. In: Paxinos G (ed.) *The Rat Nervous System*, pp. 443–493. San Diego: Academic Press.

Amaral DG, Ishizuka N, and Claiborne B (1990) Neurons, numbers, and the hippocampal network. *Prog. Brain Res.* 83: 1–11.

Amaral DG, Price JL, Pitkanen A, and Carmichael ST (1992) Anatomical organization of the primate amygdaloid complex. In: Aggleton JP (ed.) *The Amygdala*, pp. 1–66. New York: Wiley-Liss.

Amari S (1977) Dynamics of pattern formation in lateral-inhibition type neural fields. *Biol. Cybern.* 27: 77–87.

Amit DJ (1989) *Modeling Brain Function*. Cambridge University Press: Cambridge.

Battaglia FP and Treves A (1998a) Attractor neural networks storing multiple space representations: A model for hippocampal place fields. *Phys. Rev.* 58: 7738–7753.

Battaglia FP and Treves A (1998b) Stable and rapid recurrent processing in realistic auto-associative memories. *Neural Comput.* 10: 431–450.

Brown TH and Zador A (1990) The hippocampus. In: Shepherd G (ed.) *The Synaptic Organisation of the Brain*, pp. 346–388. New York: Oxford University Press.

Brown TH, Ganong AH, Kairiss EW, Keenan CL, and Kelso SR (eds.) (1989) *Long-Term Potentiation in Two Synaptic Systems of the Hippocampal Brain Slice*. San Diego: Academic Press.

Brown TH, Kairiss EW, and Keenan CL (1990) Hebbian synapses: Biophysical mechanisms and algorithms. *Annu. Rev. Neurosci.* 13: 475–511.

Brun VH, Otnass MK, Molden S, et al. (2002) Place cells and place recognition maintained by direct entorhinal-hippocampal circuitry. *Science* 296: 2243–2246.

Buckley MJ and Gaffan D (2000) The hippocampus, perirhinal cortex, and memory in the monkey. In: Bolhuis JJ (ed.) *Brain Perception, and Memory: Advances in Cognitive Neuroscience*, pp. 279–298. Oxford: Oxford University Press.

Burgess N, Recce M, and O'Keefe J (1994) A model of hippocampal function. *Neural Netw.* 7: 1065–1081.

Burgess N, Jackson A, Hartley T, and O'Keefe J (2000) Predictions derived from modelling the hippocampal role in navigation. *Biol. Cybern.* 83: 301–312.

Burgess N, Maguire EA, and O'Keefe J (2002) The human hippocampus and spatial and episodic memory. *Neuron* 35: 625–641.

Carmichael ST and Price JL (1995) Limbic connections of the orbital and medial prefrontal cortex in macaque monkeys. *J. Comp. Neurol.* 346: 403–434.

Cassaday HJ and Rawlins JN (1997) The hippocampus, objects, and their contexts. *Behav. Neurosci.* 111: 1228–1244.

Crane J and Milner B (2005) What went where? Impaired object-location learning in patients with right hippocampal lesions. *Hippocampus* 15: 216–231.

Day M, Langston R, and Morris RG (2003) Glutamate-receptor-mediated encoding and retrieval of paired-associate learning. *Nature* 424: 205–209.

de Araujo IET, Rolls ET, and Stringer SM (2001) A view model which accounts for the spatial fields of hippocampal primate spatial view cells and rat place cells. *Hippocampus* 11: 699–706.

Deco G and Rolls ET (2005) Sequential memory: A putative neural and synaptic dynamical mechanism. *J. Cogn. Neurosci.* 17: 294–307.

Delatour B and Witter MP (2002) Projections from the parahippocampal region to the prefrontal cortex in the rat: Evidence of multiple pathways. *Eur. J. Neurosci.* 15: 1400–1407.

Eichenbaum H, Otto T, and Cohen NJ (1992) The hippocampus – What does it do? *Behav. Neural Biol.* 57: 2–36.

Fazeli MS and Collingridge GL (eds.) (1996) *Cortical Plasticity: LTP and LTD*. Oxford: Bios Scientific.

Feigenbaum JD and Rolls ET (1991) Allocentric and egocentric spatial information processing in the hippocampal formation of the behaving primate. *Psychobiology* 19: 21–40.

Florian C and Roullet P (2004) Hippocampal CA3-region is crucial for acquisition and memory consolidation in Morris water maze task in mice. *Behav. Brain Res.* 154: 365–374.

Franco L, Rolls ET, Aggelopoulos NC, and Jerez JM (2007) *Neuronal Selectivity, Population Sparseness, and Ergodicity in the Inferior Temporal Visual Cortex*. New York: Springer-Verlag.

Fyhn M, Molden S, Witter MP, Moser EI, and Moser MB (2004) Spatial representation in the entorhinal cortex. *Science* 305: 1258–1264.

Gaffan D (1992) The role of hippocampo-fornix-mammillary system in episodic memory. In: Squire LR and Butters N (eds.) *Neuropsychology of Memory*, pp. 336–346. New York: Guilford.

Gaffan D (1994) Scene-specific memory for objects: A model of episodic memory impairment in monkeys with fornix transection. *J. Cogn. Neurosci.* 6: 305–320.

Gardner-Medwin AR (1976) The recall of events through the learning of associations between their parts. *Proc. R. Soc. Lond. B* 194: 375–402.

Georges-François P, Rolls ET, and Robertson RG (1999) Spatial view cells in the primate hippocampus: Allocentric view not head direction or eye position or place. *Cereb. Cortex* 9: 197–212.

Gilbert PE, Kesner RP, and Lee I (2001) Dissociating hippocampal subregions: Double dissociation between dentate gyrus and CA1. *Hippocampus* 11: 626–636.

Gold AE and Kesner RP (2005) The role of the CA3 subregion of the dorsal hippocampus in spatial pattern completion in the rat. *Hippocampus* 15: 808–814.

Goodrich-Hunsaker NJ, Hunsaker MR, and Kesner RP (2005) Effects of hippocampus sub-regional lesions for metric and topological spatial information processing. *Soc. Neurosci. Abst.* 647.1.

Gruesser O-J and Landis T (1991) *Visual Agnosias*. London: Macmillan.

Hafting T, Fyhn M, Molden S, Moser MB, and Moser EI (2005) Microstructure of a spatial map in the entorhinal cortex. *Nature* 436: 801–806.

Hargreaves EL, Rao G, Lee I, and Knierim JJ (2005) Major dissociation between medial and lateral entorhinal input to dorsal hippocampus. *Science* 308: 1792–1794.

Hasselmo ME and Eichenbaum HB (2005) Hippocampal mechanisms for the context-dependent retrieval of episodes. *Neural Netw.* 18: 1172–1190.

Hasselmo ME, Schnell E, and Barkai E (1995) Dynamics of learning and recall at excitatory recurrent synapses and cholinergic modulation in rat hippocampal region CA3. *J. Neurosci.* 15: 5249–5262.

Hertz J, Krogh A, and Palmer RG (1991) *An Introduction to the Theory of Neural Computation*. Wokingham: Addison-Wesley.

Hölscher C, Jacob W, and Mallot HA (2003) Reward modulates neuronal activity in the hippocampus of the rat. *Behav. Brain Res.* 142: 181–191.

Hopfield JJ (1982) Neural networks and physical systems with emergent collective computational abilities. *Proc. Natl. Acad. Sci. USA* 79: 2554–2558.

Ishizuka N, Weber J, and Amaral DG (1990) Organization of intrahippocampal projections originating from CA3 pyramidal cells in the rat. *J. Comp. Neurol.* 295: 580–623.

Jarrard EL (1993) On the role of the hippocampus in learning and memory in the rat. *Behav. Neural Biol.* 60: 9–26.

Jeffery KJ and Hayman R (2004) Plasticity of the hippocampal place cell representation. *Rev. Neurosci.* 15: 309–331.

Jeffery KJ, Anderson MI, Hayman R, and Chakraborty S (2004) A proposed architecture for the neural representation of spatial context. *Neurosci. Biobehav. Rev.* 28: 201–218.

Jensen O and Lisman JE (1996) Theta/gamma networks with slow NMDA channels learn sequences and encode episodic memory: Role of NMDA channels in recall. *Learn. Mem.* 3: 264–278.

Jung MW and McNaughton BL (1993) Spatial selectivity of unit activity in the hippocampal granular layer. *Hippocampus* 3: 165–182.

Kesner RP, Lee I, and Gilbert P (2004) A behavioral assessment of hippocampal function based on a subregional analysis. *Rev. Neurosci.* 15: 333–351.

Kohonen T (1977) *Associative Memory: A System Theoretical Approach*. New York: Springer.

Kolb B and Whishaw IQ (2003) *Fundamentals of Human Neuropsychology*. New York: Worth.

Lassalle JM, Bataille T, and Halley H (2000) Reversible inactivation of the hippocampal mossy fiber synapses in mice impairs spatial learning, but neither consolidation nor memory retrieval in the Morris navigation task. *Neurobiol. Learn. Mem.* 73: 243–257.

Lavenex P and Amaral DG (2000) Hippocampal-neocortical interaction: A hierarchy of associativity. *Hippocampus* 10: 420–430.

Lavenex P, Suzuki WA, and Amaral DG (2004) Perirhinal and parahippocampal cortices of the macaque monkey: Intrinsic projections and interconnections. *J. Comp. Neurol.* 472: 371–394.

Levy WB (1989) A computational approach to hippocampal function. In: Hawkins RD and Bower GH (eds.) *Computational Models of Learning in Simple Neural Systems*, pp. 243–305. San Diego: Academic Press.

Levy WB and Desmond NL (1985) The rules of elemental synaptic plasticity. In: Levy WB, Anderson JA, and Lehmkuhle S (eds.) *Synaptic Modification Neuron Selectivity, and Nervous System Organization*, pp. 105–121. Hillsdale, NJ: Erlbaum.

Levy WB, Colbert CM, and Desmond NL (1990) Elemental adaptive processes of neurons and synapses: A statistical/computational perspective. In: Gluck MA and Rumelhart DE (eds.) *Neuroscience and Connectionist Theory*, pp. 187–235. Hillsdale, NJ: Erlbaum.

Lisman JE, Talamini LM, and Raffone A (2005) Recall of memory sequences by interaction of the dentate and CA3: A revised model of the phase precession. *Neural Netw.* 18: 1191–1201.

Lynch MA (2004) Long-term potentiation and memory. *Physiol. Rev.* 84: 87–136.

Maaswinkel H, Jarrard LE, and Whishaw IQ (1999) Hippocampectomized rats are impaired in homing by path integration. *Hippocampus* 9: 553–561.

Malkova L and Mishkin M (2003) One-trial memory for object-place associations after separate lesions of hippocampus and posterior parahippocampal region in the monkey. *J. Neurosci.* 23: 1956–1965.

Markus EJ, Qin YL, Leonard B, Skaggs W, McNaughton BL, and Barnes CA (1995) Interactions between location and task affect the spatial and directional firing of hippocampal neurons. *J. Neurosci.* 15: 7079–7094.

Marr D (1971) Simple memory: A theory for archicortex. *Phil. Trans. Roy. Soc. Lond. B* 262: 23–81.

Martin SJ, Grimwood PD, and Morris RG (2000) Synaptic plasticity and memory: An evaluation of the hypothesis. *Annu. Rev. Neurosci.* 23: 649–711.

McClelland JL, McNaughton BL, and O'Reilly RC (1995) Why there are complementary learning systems in the hippocampus and neocortex: Insights from the successes and failures of connectionist models of learning and memory. *Psychol. Rev.* 102: 419–457.

McNaughton BL (1991) Associative pattern completion in hippocampal circuits: New evidence and new questions. *Brain Res. Rev.* 16: 193–220.

McNaughton BL and Morris RG M (1987) Hippocampal synaptic enhancement and information storage within a distributed memory system. *Trends Neurosci.* 10: 408–415.

McNaughton BL, Barnes CA, and O'Keefe J (1983) The contributions of position, direction, and velocity to single unit activity in the hippocampus of freely-moving rats. *Exp. Brain Res.* 52: 41–49.

McNaughton BL and Nadel L (1990) Hebb-Marr networks and the neurobiological representation of action in space. In: Gluck MA and Rumelhart DE (eds.) *Neuroscience and Connectionist Theory*, pp. 1–63. Hillsdale, NJ: Erlbaum.

McNaughton BL, Chen LL, and Markus EJ (1991) "Dead reckoning", landmark learning, and the sense of direction: A neurophysiological and computational hypothesis. *J. Cogn. Neurosci.* 3: 190–202.

McNaughton BL, Battaglia FP, Jensen O, Moser EI, and Moser M-B (2006) Path integration and the neural basis of the "cognitive map." *Nat. Rev. Neurosci.* 7: 663–678.

Morris RG (2003) Long-term potentiation and memory. *Philos. Trans. R. Soc. Lond. B Biol. Sci.* 358: 643–647.

Morris RGM (1989) Does synaptic plasticity play a role in information storage in the vertebrate brain? In: Morris RGM (ed.) *Parallel Distributed Processing: Implications for Psychology and Neurobiology*, pp. 248–285. Oxford: Oxford University Press.

Morris RG, Moser EI, Riedel G, et al. (2003) Elements of a neurobiological theory of the hippocampus: The role of activity-dependent synaptic plasticity in memory. *Philos. Trans. R. Soc. Lond. B Biol. Sci.* 358: 773–786.

Moscovitch M, Rosenbaum RS, Gilboa A, et al. (2005) Functional neuroanatomy of remote episodic, semantic and spatial memory: A unified account based on multiple trace theory. *J. Anat.* 207: 35–66.

Moser EI (2004) Hippocampal place cells demand attention. *Neuron* 42: 183–185.

Moser MB and Moser EI (1998) Functional differentiation in the hippocampus. *Hippocampus* 8: 608–619.

Muller RU, Kubie JL, Bostock EM, Taube JS, and Quirk GJ (1991) Spatial firing correlates of neurons in the hippocampal formation of freely moving rats. In: Paillard J (ed.) *Brain and Space*, pp. 296–333. Oxford: Oxford University Press.

Muller RU, Ranck JB Jr, and Taube JS (1996) Head direction cells: Properties and functional significance. *Curr. Opin. Neurobiol.* 6: 196–206.

Murray EA, Baxter MG, and Gaffan D (1998) Monkeys with rhinal cortex damage or neurotoxic hippocampal lesions are impaired on spatial scene learning and object reversals. *Behav. Neurosci.* 112: 1291–1303.

Naber PA, Lopes da Silva FH, and Witter MP (2001) Reciprocal connections between the entorhinal cortex and hippocampal fields CA1 and the subiculum are in register with the

projections from CA1 to the subiculum. *Hippocampus* 11: 99–104.
Nakazawa K, Quirk MC, Chitwood RA, et al. (2002) Requirement for hippocampal CA3 NMDA receptors in associative memory recall. *Science* 297: 211–218.
Oja E (1982) A simplified neuron model as a principal component analyser. *J. Math. Biol.* 15: 267–273.
O'Keefe J (1984) Spatial memory within and without the hippocampal system. In: Seifert W (ed.) *Neurobiology of the Hippocampus*, pp. 375–403. London: Academic Press.
O'Keefe J (1990) A computational theory of the hippocampal cognitive map. *Prog. Brain Res.* 83: 301–312.
O'Keefe J and Dostrovsky J (1971) The hippocampus as a spatial map: Preliminary evidence from unit activity in the freely moving rat. *Brain Res.* 34: 171–175.
O'Keefe J and Nadel L (1978) *The Hippocampus as a Cognitive Map*. Oxford: Clarendon Press.
O'Reilly RC and Rudy JW (2001) Conjunctive representations in learning and memory: Principles of cortical and hippocampal function. *Psychol. Rev.* 108: 311–345.
Panzeri S, Rolls ET, Battaglia F, and Lavis R (2001) Speed of information retrieval in multilayer networks of integrate-and-fire neurons. *Netw. Comput. Neural Sys.* 12: 423–440.
Pitkanen A, Kelly JL, and Amaral DG (2002) Projections from the lateral, basal, and accessory basal nuclei of the amygdala to the entorhinal cortex in the macaque monkey. *Hippocampus* 12: 186–205.
Ranck JBJ (1985) Head direction cells in the deep cell layer of dorsolateral presubiculum in freely moving rats. In: Buzaki G and Vanderwolf CH (eds.) *Electrical Activity of the Archicortex*. Budapest: Akademiai Kiado.
Robertson RG, Rolls ET, and Georges-François P (1998) Spatial view cells in the primate hippocampus: Effects of removal of view details. *J. Neurophysiol.* 79: 1145–1156.
Robertson RG, Rolls ET, Georges-François P, and Panzeri S (1999) Head direction cells in the primate pre-subiculum. *Hippocampus* 9: 206–219.
Rolls ET (1987) Information representation, processing and storage in the brain: Analysis at the single neuron level. In: Changeux J-P and Konishi M (eds.) *The Neural and Molecular Bases of Learning*, pp. 503–540. Chischester: Wiley.
Rolls ET (1989a) Functions of neuronal networks in the hippocampus and cerebral cortex in memory. In: Cotterill RMJ (ed.) *Models of Brain Function*, pp. 15–33. Cambridge: Cambridge University Press.
Rolls ET (1989b) Functions of neuronal networks in the hippocampus and neocortex in memory. In: Byrne JH and Berry WO (eds.) *Neural Models of Plasticity: Experimental and Theoretical Approaches*, pp. 240–265. San Diego: Academic Press.
Rolls ET (1989c) Parallel distributed processing in the brain: Implications of the functional architecture of neuronal networks in the hippocampus. In: Morris RGM (ed.) *Parallel Distributed Processing: Implications for Psychology and Neurobiology*, pp. 286–308. Oxford: Oxford University Press.
Rolls ET (1989d) The representation and storage of information in neuronal networks in the primate cerebral cortex and hippocampus. In: Durbin R, Mlall C, and Mitchison G (eds.) *The Computing Neuron*, pp. 125–159. Wokingham, UK: Addison-Wesley.
Rolls ET (1990a) Functions of the primate hippocampus in spatial processing and memory. In: Olton DS and Kesner RP (eds.) *Neurobiology of Comparative Cognition*, pp. 339–362. Hillsdale, NJ: Erlbaum.
Rolls ET (1990b) Theoretical and neurophysiological analysis of the functions of the primate hippocampus in memory. *Cold Spring Harb. Symp. Quant. Biol.* 55: 995–1006.
Rolls ET (1991) Functions of the primate hippocampus in spatial and non-spatial memory. *Hippocampus* 1: 258–261.
Rolls ET (1992) Neurophysiological mechanisms underlying face processing within and beyond the temporal cortical visual areas. *Philos. Trans. R. Soc. Lond. B* 335: 11–21.
Rolls ET (1994) Neurophysiological and neuronal network analysis of how the primate hippocampus functions in memory. In: Delacour J (ed.) *The Memory System of the Brain*, pp. 713–744. London: World Scientific.
Rolls ET (1995) A model of the operation of the hippocampus and entorhinal cortex in memory. *Int. J. Neural Sys.* 6: 51–70.
Rolls ET (1996a) Roles of long term potentiation and long term depression in neuronal network operations in the brain. In: Fazeli GL and Collingridge GL (eds.) *Cortical Plasticity*, pp. 223–250. Oxford: Bios Scientific.
Rolls ET (1996b) A theory of hippocampal function in memory. *Hippocampus* 6: 601–620.
Rolls ET (1999) Spatial view cells and the representation of place in the primate hippocampus. *Hippocampus* 9: 467–480.
Rolls ET (2000) Memory systems in the brain. *Annu. Rev. Psychol.* 51: 599–630.
Rolls ET (2003) Consciousness absent and present: A neurophysiological exploration. *Prog. Brain Res.* 144: 95–106.
Rolls ET (2008) *Memory Attention, and Decision-Making: A Unifying Computational Neuroscience Approach*. Oxford: Oxford University Press.
Rolls ET and Deco G (2002) *Computational Neuroscience of Vision*. Oxford: Oxford University Press.
Rolls ET and Kesner RP (2006) A computational theory of hippocampal function, and empirical tests of the theory. *Prog. Neurobiol.* 79: 1–48.
Rolls ET and O'Mara S (1993) Neurophysiological and theoretical analysis of how the primate hippocampus functions in memory. In: Ono T, Squire LR, Raichle ME, Perret DI, and Fukuda M (eds.) *Brain Mechanisms of Perception and Memory: From Neuron to Behavior*, pp. 276–300. New York: Oxford University Press.
Rolls ET and Stringer SM (2005) Spatial view cells in the hippocampus, and their idiothetic update based on place and head direction. *Neural Netw.* 18: 1229–1241.
Rolls ET and Treves A (1990) The relative advantages of sparse versus distributed encoding for associative neuronal networks in the brain. *Network* 1: 407–421.
Rolls ET and Treves A (1998) *Neural Networks and Brain Function*. Oxford: Oxford University Press.
Rolls ET and Xiang J-Z (2005) Reward-spatial view representations and learning in the hippocampus. *J. Neurosci.* 25: 6167–6174.
Rolls ET and Xiang J-Z (2006) Spatial view cells in the primate hippocampus, and memory recall. *Rev. Neurosci.* 17: 175–200.
Rolls ET, Miyashita Y, Cahusac PMB, et al. (1989) Hippocampal neurons in the monkey with activity related to the place in which a stimulus is shown. *J. Neurosci.* 9: 1835–1845.
Rolls ET, Robertson RG, and Georges-François P (1997a) Spatial view cells in the primate hippocampus. *Eur. J. Neurosci.* 9: 1789–1794.
Rolls ET, Treves A, Foster D, and Perez-Vicente C (1997b) Simulation studies of the CA3 hippocampal subfield modelled as an attractor neural network. *Neural Netw.* 10: 1559–1569.
Rolls ET, Treves A, Robertson RG, Georges-François P, and Panzeri S (1998) Information about spatial view in an ensemble of primate hippocampal cells. *J. Neurophysiol.* 79: 1797–1813.
Rolls ET, Stringer SM, and Trappenberg TP (2002) A unified model of spatial and episodic memory. *Proc. R. Soc. Lond. B* 269: 1087–1093.

Rolls ET, Xiang J-Z, and Franco L (2005) Object, space and object-space representations in the primate hippocampus. *J. Neurophysiol.* 94: 833–844.
Rolls ET, Stringer SM, and Elliot T (2006) Entorhinal cortex grid cells can map to hippocampal place cells by competitive learning. *Netw. Comput. Neural Sys.* 17: 447–465.
Samsonovich A and McNaughton BL (1997) Path integration and cognitive mapping in a continuous attractor neural network model. *J. Neurosci.* 17: 5900–5920.
Schultz S and Rolls ET (1999) Analysis of information transmission in the Schaffer collaterals. *Hippocampus* 9: 582–598.
Simmen MW, Treves A, and Rolls ET (1996) Pattern retrieval in threshold-linear associative nets. *Network* 7: 109–122.
Skaggs WE, Knierim JJ, Kudrimoti HS, and McNaughton BL (1995) A model of the neural basis of the rat's sense of direction. In: Tesauro G, Touretzky DS, and Leen TK (eds.) *Advances in Neural Information Processing Systems*, pp. 173–180. Cambridge, MA: MIT Press.
Squire LR (1992) Memory and the hippocampus: A synthesis from findings with rats, monkeys and humans. *Psychol. Rev.* 99. 195–231.
Stefanacci L, Suzuki WA, and Amaral DG (1996) Organization of connections between the amygdaloid complex and the perirhinal and parahippocampal cortices in macaque monkeys. *J. Comp. Neurol.* 375: 552–582.
Storm-Mathiesen J, Zimmer J, and Ottersen OP Eds. (1990) *Understanding the Brain Through the Hippocampus*. Oxford: Elsevier.
Stringer SM and Rolls ET (2002) Invariant object recognition in the visual system with novel views of 3D objects. *Neural Comput.* 14: 2585–2596.
Stringer SM, Rolls ET, Trappenberg TP, and Araujo IE T (2002a) Self-organizing continuous attractor networks and path integration. Two-dimensional models of place cells. *Netw. Comput. Neural Sys.* 13: 429–446.
Stringer SM, Trappenberg TP, Rolls ET, and Araujo IE T (2002b) Self-organizing continuous attractor networks and path integration: One-dimensional models of head direction cells. *Netw. Comput. Neural Sys.* 13: 217–242.
Stringer SM, Rolls ET, and Trappenberg TP (2004) Self-organising continuous attractor networks with multiple activity packets, and the representation of space. *Neural Netw.* 17: 5–27.
Stringer SM, Rolls ET, and Trappenberg TP (2005) Self-organizing continuous attractor network models of hippocampal spatial view cells. *Neurobiol. Learn. Mem.* 83: 79–92.
Sutherland RJ and Rudy JW (1991) Exceptions to the rule of space. *Hippocampus* 1: 250–252.
Suzuki WA and Amaral DG (1994a) Perirhinal and parahippocampal cortices of the macaque monkey – cortical afferents. *J. Comp. Neurol.* 350: 497–533.
Suzuki WA and Amaral DG (1994b) Topographic organization of the reciprocal connections between the monkey entorhinal cortex and the perirhinal and parahippocampal cortices. *J. Neurosci.* 14: 1856–1877.
Tabuchi E, Mulder AB, and Wiener SI (2003) Reward value invariant place responses and reward site associated activity in hippocampal neurons of behaving rats. *Hippocampus* 13: 117–132.
Taube JS, Muller RU, and Ranck JB J (1990) Head-direction cells recorded from the postsubiculum in freely moving rats 1: Description and quantitative analysis. *J. Neurosci.* 10: 420–435.
Taube JS, Goodridge JP, Golob EJ, Dudchenko PA, and Stackman RW (1996) Processing the head direction signal: A review and commentary. *Brain Res. Bull.* 40: 477–486.
Taylor JG (1999) Neural "bubble" dynamics in two dimensions: Foundations. *Biol. Cybern.* 80: 393–409.
Treves A (1990) Graded-response neurons and information encodings in autoassociative memories. *Phys. Rev.* A 42: 2418–2430.
Treves A (1993) Mean-field analysis of neuronal spike dynamics. *Network* 4: 259–284.
Treves A (1995) Quantitative estimate of the information relayed by Schaffer collaterals. *J. Comp. Neurosci.* 2: 259–272.
Treves A and Rolls ET (1991) What determines the capacity of autoassociative memories in the brain? *Network* 2: 371–397.
Treves A and Rolls ET (1992) Computational constraints suggest the need for two distinct input systems to the hippocampal CA3 network. *Hippocampus* 2: 189–199.
Treves A and Rolls ET (1994) A computational analysis of the role of the hippocampus in memory. *Hippocampus* 4: 374–391.
Ungerleider LG and Mishkin M (1982) Two cortical visual systems. In: Ingle DJ, goodale MA, and Mansfield RJW (eds.) *Analysis of Visual Behavior*, pp. 549–586. Cambridge, MA: MIT Press.
van Haeften T, Baks-te-Bulte L, Goede PH, Wouterlood FG, and Witter MP (2003) Morphological and numerical analysis of synaptic interactions between neurons in deep and superficial layers of the entorhinal cortex of the rat. *Hippocampus* 13: 943–952.
Van Hoesen GW (1982) The parahippocampal gyrus. New observations regarding its cortical connections in the monkey. *Trends Neurosci.* 5: 345–350.
Wallace DG and Whishaw IQ (2003) NMDA lesions of Ammon's horn and the dentate gyrus disrupt the direct and temporally paced homing displayed by rats exploring a novel environment: Evidence for a role of the hippocampus in dead reckoning. *Eur. J. Neurosci.* 18: 513–523.
Whishaw IQ, Hines DJ, and Wallace DG (2001) Dead reckoning (path integration) requires the hippocampal formation: Evidence from spontaneous exploration and spatial learning tasks in light (allothetic) and dark (idiothetic) tests. *Behav. Brain Res.* 127: 49–69.
Witter MP (1993) Organization of the entorhinal-hippocampal system: A review of current anatomical data. *Hippocampus* 3: 33–44.
Witter MP, Van Hoesen GW, and Amaral DG (1989) Topographical organisation of the entorhinal projection to the dentate gyrus of the monkey. *J. Neurosci.* 9: 216–228.
Witter MP, Naber PA, van Haeften T, et al. (2000a) Cortico-hippocampal communication by way of parallel parahippocampal-subicular pathways. *Hippocampus* 10: 398–410.
Witter MP, Wouterlood FG, Naber PA, and Van Haeften T (2000b) Anatomical organization of the parahippocampal-hippocampal network. *Ann. NY Acad. Sci.* 911: 1–24.
Wood ER, Dudchenko PA, and Eichenbaum H (1999) The global record of memory in hippocampal neuronal activity. *Nature* 397: 613–616.
Zhang K (1996) Representation of spatial orientation by the intrinsic dynamics of the head-direction cell ensemble: A theory. *J. Neurosci.* 16: 2112–2126.

17 Neurobiology of Procedural Learning in Animals

M. G. Packard, Texas A&M University, College Station, TX, USA

17.1 Introduction

Research investigating learning and memory from a neurobiological perspective provides support for the hypothesis that multiple memory systems exist in the mammalian brain (for reviews, see Eichenbaum and Cohen, 2001; White and McDonald, 2002). Several theories outlining the psychological operating principles that define different types of memory have been proposed (e.g., Hirsh, 1974; O'Keefe and Nadel, 1978; Olton and Papas, 1979; Cohen and Squire, 1980; Mishkin and Petri, 1984; Graf and Schacter, 1985). In lower animals in particular, theoretical development of the sets of psychological mechanisms that distinguish different types of memory has been significantly influenced by the classic debate between cognitive (e.g., Tolman, 1932) and stimulus-response (e.g., Thorndike, 1933; Hull, 1943) learning theorists. One prominent dual-memory theory draws a distinction between declarative and procedural memory (Cohen and Squire, 1980; Squire and Zola-Morgan, 1991; Eichenbaum and Cohen, 2001). In lower animals, declarative memory involves the acquisition, consolidation, and retrieval of relational representations that allow for flexibility during behavioral expression (Eichenbaum and Cohen, 2001) in a manner analogous to the cognitive (Tolman, 1932) view of learning and memory. Declarative memory relies largely on a neuroanatomical system composed of the hippocampus and related structures in the medial temporal lobe (Squire et al., 1993; Eichenbaum and Cohen, 2001). In contrast, procedural memory involves the acquisition, consolidation, and retrieval of individual representations that are behaviorally expressed in an inflexible manner (Eichenbaum and Cohen, 2001), analogous, at least in part, to the stimulus-response or habit (Hull, 1943) view of learning and memory.

In rats, numerous findings from studies employing lesion, pharmacological, molecular, and electrophysiological approaches provide converging evidence supporting the hypothesis that the dorsal striatum (i.e., caudate-putamen) mediates the formation of stimulus–response habits. The goals of the present chapter are to provide a brief historical perspective to the development of this hypothesis and to summarize evidence of the role of the dorsal striatum in this form of procedural learning. Studies employing brain lesion techniques and pharmacological approaches in rats are emphasized, particularly in those instances in which dorsal striatal involvement in procedural and declarative memory tasks has been directly compared. However, it should be noted that neurobehavioral findings from electrophysiological (e.g., Graybiel et al., 1994; Rolls, 1994; Graybiel, 1998; Jog et al., 1999) and molecular (e.g., Colombo et al., 2003; Teather et al., 2005; Pittenger et al., 2006) experiments in rats and nonhuman primates also implicate the dorsal striatum in procedural learning.

In addition to dorsal striatal-dependent stimulus-response memory, learning that is selectively mediated by other brain structures might also be considered procedural in nature, at least to the extent that they involve acquisition, consolidation, and retrieval of information that is behaviorally expressed in a relatively inflexible, stimulus-bound manner (Eichenbaum and Cohen, 2001). For example, under this definition, cerebellar-dependent classical conditioning of skeletal musculature (for review, see Thompson, 2005) and basolateral amygdala-dependent stimulus-affect learning (for review, see McDonald and White, 2002) might also be broadly construed as forms of procedural learning (Squire and Zola-Morgan, 1991). Findings of several studies have dissociated the roles of the dorsal striatum and basolateral amygdala in learning and memory. Therefore, following a consideration of dorsal striatal involvement in stimulus-response learning, data suggesting that learning based on stimulus-affect associations is mediated by the basolateral amygdala is briefly discussed.

17.2 The Neural Bases of Procedural Learning: Emergence of the Dorsal Striatal Hypothesis

In lower animals, the hypothesis that multiple memory systems exist was derived from an analysis of the effects of damage to the hippocampal system on behavior across a wide range of learning tasks (for reviews, see Hirsh, 1974; O'Keefe and Nadel, 1978; Olton, 1979). Similar to the selective behavioral pattern that is observed in rats, lesions of the hippocampal system in monkeys impair behavior in tasks requiring declarative/cognitive memory and spare acquisition of tasks that can be acquired by a putative procedural or habit learning mechanism (for review, see Mishkin and Appenzeller, 1987). In an attempt to identify the neural bases of this spared learning, the hypothesis that the primate dorsal striatum and associated putamen mediate procedural learning that involves the formation of stimulus–response habits was introduced (Mishkin et al., 1984; Mishkin and Petri, 1984; Mahut et al., 1984). At the time that it was originally proposed, this hypothesis was based largely on anatomical considerations. Specifically, the dorsal striatum receives sensory stimulus input from all regions of the cortex via topographically arranged corticostriatal projections and can readily influence motor output via downstream projections to brainstem structures and/or via corticothalamic-basal ganglia loops (e.g., Webster, 1961; Van Hoesen et al., 1981; Alexander et al., 1986). Thus, it was suggested that the dorsal striatum is anatomically well situated to mediate S-R habit learning across various sensory modalities (Mishkin and Petri, 1984; Mahut et al., 1984), although the behavioral evidence implicating the striatum in procedural learning in nonhuman primates was fairly meager (Divac et al., 1967; Buerger et al., 1974).

As noted by Iversen (1979), researchers interested in the neurobiology of learning and memory were not likely encouraged to examine a potential role for the dorsal striatum in view of Karl Lashley's premature conclusion that "the evidence seems conclusive that in mammals the basal ganglia are not an essential link in the patterning of learned activities" (Lashley, 1950, p. 454). Nonetheless, prior to the advent of multiple memory system theories, several experiments examining the effects of lesions of the dorsal striatum on learning were conducted in rats. When considered in retrospect, the findings of many of these studies are consistent with the hypothesized role of this structure in procedural learning and memory. For example, dorsal striatal lesions impair acquisition of various conditioned avoidance behaviors that can be readily acquired using a procedural learning mechanism (e.g., Kirkby and Kimble, 1968; Winocur and Mills, 1969; Neill and Grossman, 1971; Mitcham and Thomas, 1972; Allen and Davidson, 1973; Kirkby and Polgar, 1974). In addition, by the mid-1970s several studies in rats had demonstrated a modulatory effect of posttraining electrical stimulation of the dorsal striatum on memory consolidation using various tasks that could conceivably be acquired using a procedural learning mechanism (for review, see Kesner and Wilburn, 1974).

17.3 Dorsal Striatum and Procedural Learning: Dissociation Lesion Experiments

The impairments observed following dorsal striatal lesions in simultaneous discrimination learning in monkeys (Divac et al., 1967; Buerger et al., 1974) and in conditioned avoidance behaviors in rats (for review, see Oberg and Divac, 1979) are consistent with a putative role for this brain structure in procedural learning and memory. However, rather than impairing learning or memory processes per se, a lesion-induced deficit in acquisition of a single type of task may reflect an influence on nonmnemonic factors that are involved in task performance (e.g., sensory, motor, or motivational processes).

Dissociation methodology provides an experimental design that more directly addresses the question of whether a particular brain structure plays a selective role in learned behavior. In a single dissociation design, the role of a single brain structure (X) in behavior is contrasted using a pair of behavioral tasks (A, B). For example, lesions of the dorsal striatum impair retention of an egocentric left-right discrimination in a radial maze but do not impair retention of an allocentric place learning task (Cook and Kesner, 1988). In addition, dorsal striatal lesions impair acquisition of a tactile discrimination procedural learning task in a T maze but do not impair declarative memory guiding goal-arm alternation (Colombo et al., 1989). These examples of single dissociations provide evidence consistent with a selective role of the dorsal striatum in procedural learning and are clearly more compelling than studies using only one behavioral task. Nonetheless, the presence of single dissociations may not reflect a strict functional independence of procedural and declarative memory systems in the brain (Eichenbaum and Cohen, 2001; Packard, 2002).

A more stringent test of the hypothesis that the dorsal striatum selectively mediates procedural learning employs double dissociation methodology. In this experimental design, the function of two brain structures in behavior is contrasted in two behavioral tasks. Ideally, this approach involves the use of a pair of tasks that possess similar nonmnemonic (e.g., sensory, motor, motivational) characteristics but that differ in terms of the type of learning and memory processes required. The first study to implement this design to investigate the role of the dorsal striatum in learning employed two radial maze tasks to compare the effects of dorsal striatum and hippocampal system lesions on procedural and declarative memory in rats (Packard et al., 1989). In a declarative or cognitive memory version of the task, rats obtained food rewards by visiting each arm of the radial maze once within a daily training session, and reentries into maze arms that were previously visited are scored as errors. This task requires rats to remember which maze arms have been previously visited within a trial and is essentially a test of declarative knowledge that may involve spatial working memory (Olton, 1979) and/or the use of a cognitive mapping strategy (O'Keefe and Nadel, 1978). In a procedural memory version of the task, rats obtained food rewards by visiting four randomly selected and illuminated maze arms twice within a daily training session, and visits to unlit maze arms are scored as errors. Every visit to an illuminated maze arm was reinforced, and thus there was no requirement to use declarative memory to remember specific arm entries. Rather, this task can be acquired by a procedural or habit learning mechanism by which a light cue (i.e., a stimulus) evokes approach behavior (i.e., a response). Pretraining electrolytic lesions of the dorsal striatum produce a dissociation in behavior in these two radial maze tasks, impairing acquisition of the procedural task and leaving acquisition of the declarative task unaffected (**Figure 1**). In contrast, lesions of the fimbria-fornix (a major input/output pathway of the hippocampus) selectively impaired acquisition of the declarative radial maze task, resulting in a double dissociation of the effects of dorsal striatal and hippocampal system lesions on learning (Packard et al., 1989). These findings were later replicated in a study examining the effects of neurotoxic lesions of the dorsal striatum and hippocampus (McDonald and White, 1993).

Although lesions of the dorsal striatum selectively impair acquisition of visual discrimination behavior in a procedural learning version of the radial maze task (Packard et al., 1989; McDonald and White, 1993), it is possible that this deficit reflects disruption of a stimulus–stimulus (light–food) association, rather than a stimulus–response (light–approach) association. The nature of the association guiding the expression of learned behavior can be assessed in a reinforcer devaluation paradigm (Adams and Dickinson, 1981). Rats exposed to reinforcer devaluation following acquisition of the dorsal striatal-dependent radial maze task continue to approach illuminated maze arms, indicating that performance of the task involves expression of a stimulus-response/habit form of procedural memory (Sage and Knowlton, 2000).

A second study used two water maze tasks to demonstrate that the selective role of the dorsal striatum in procedural learning generalizes to aversively motivated behavior (Packard and McGaugh, 1992). In these tasks, two rubber balls differing in visual appearance (vertical vs. horizontal black and white stripes) served as visual cues. One ball (correct) was located on top of a platform that could be used to escape the water, and the other ball (incorrect) was located on top of a thin rod that did not provide escape. In a declarative version of the task, the correct platform was located in the same spatial location on every trial. However, the visual pattern on the ball associated

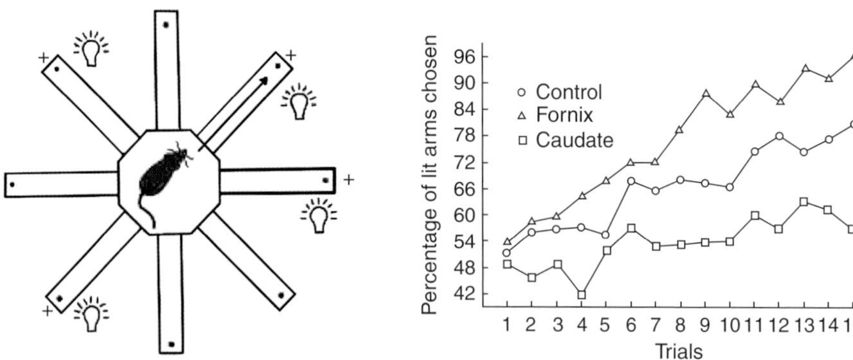

Figure 1 (a) In a radial maze task that can be acquired using a procedural learning mechanism, rats obtain eight food pellets by visiting each of four randomly selected and illuminated maze arms twice within a daily training session (Packard et al., 1989). This task can be acquired using a stimulus (light)–response (approach) form of procedural learning. Consistent with this suggestion, rats trained in this task and exposed to reinforcer devaluation continue to approach illuminated maze arms (Sage and Knowlton, 2000). Radial maze illustration used with permission from Eichenbaum H and Cohen NJ (2001) *From Conditioning to Conscious Recollection: Memory Systems of the Brain*. Oxford Psychology Series, no. 35. New York: Oxford University Press. (b) Lesions of the caudate (i.e., dorsal striatum) severely impair acquisition, consistent with the hypothesis that the dorsal striatum mediates procedural learning and memory. Note that lesions of the hippocampal system (i.e., fornix) actually enhance acquisition. This finding suggests that in some learning situations, hippocampus-dependent declarative memory interferes with dorsal striatal–dependent procedural memory (for a review of competitive interactions among multiple memory systems, see Poldrack and Packard, 2003). Data/graph used with permission from Packard MG, Hirsh R, and White NM (1989) Differential effects of fornix and caudate nucleus lesions on two radial maze tasks: Evidence for multiple memory systems. *J. Neurosci.* 9: 1465–1472.

with the correct platform varied across trials, and thus acquisition of this task required animals to use a spatial form of declarative memory. In a procedural version of the task, the visual pattern on the ball associated with the correct platform was consistent, but the platform was located in different spatial locations across trials. Therefore, this task can be acquired by a procedural learning mechanism that involved performing an approach response to a specific visual cue. Pretraining lesions of the dorsal striatum impair acquisition of the procedural task without affecting acquisition of the declarative task (**Figure 2**). An analogous dissociation is observed using a single-platform water maze task in which rats are trained to swim to a visible escape platform that is always located in the same spatial location. In this situation,

Habit water maze task

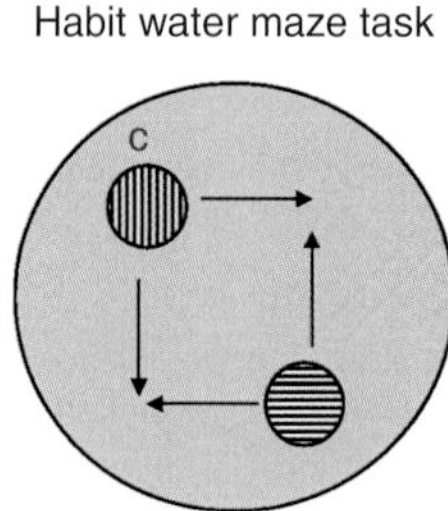

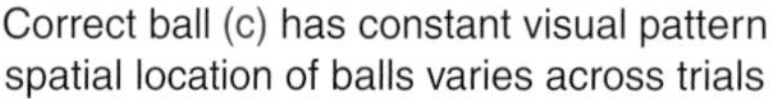

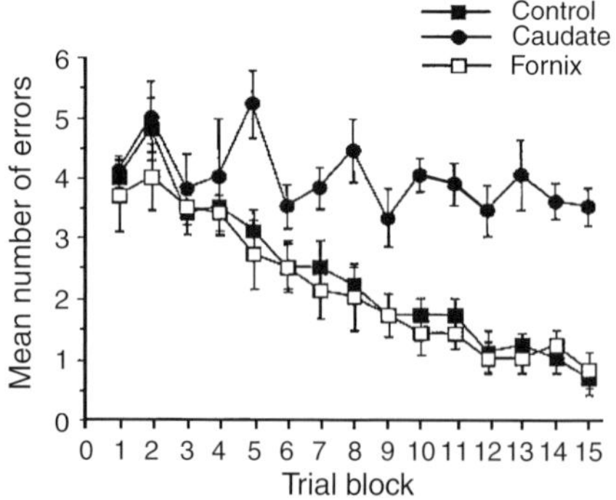

Figure 2 (a) A two-platform water maze task that can be acquired using a stimulus (visual pattern)–response (approach) form of procedural learning (Packard and McGaugh, 1992). Rats learn to swim to a correct (C) escape platform with a distinct visual pattern (ball with vertical stripes). Contact with an incorrect and inescapable platform (ball with horizontal stripes) is scored as an error. The spatial location of both balls varies across trials, and therefore a spatial form of declarative memory is not adequate for task acquisition. (b) Lesions of the caudate (i.e., dorsal striatum) severely impair acquisition, consistent with the hypothesis that the dorsal striatum mediates procedural learning and memory. Note that lesions of the hippocampal system (i.e., fornix) have no effect on acquisition. Data/graph used with permission from Packard MG and McGaugh JL (1992) Double dissociation of fornix and caudate nucleus lesions on acquisition of two water maze tasks: Further evidence for multiple memory systems. *Behav. Neurosci.* 106: 439–446.

when the visible platform is moved to a new spatial location following training, rats with pretraining lesions of the dorsal striatum exhibit a declarative/cognitive strategy and swim to the spatial location that the platform was previously located in, whereas control rats exhibit a procedural/habit strategy and swim to the visible platform in its new location (McDonald and White, 1994).

A third example of a lesion study providing evidence of a selective role for the dorsal striatum in procedural learning employed a plus-maze task that was originally introduced as a means of distinguishing between cognitive and stimulus-response habit theories of learning (Tolman et al., 1946, 1947). The plus-maze apparatus is arranged so that a goal box (e.g., east or west) can be approached from one of two start boxes (e.g., north or south). In a dual-solution version of the task, rats are trained to obtain food from a consistently baited goal box (e.g., east) from the same start box (e.g., north). According to a declarative or cognitive view of learning, rats trained in this task learn the spatial location of the reinforcer, and this relational information can be used to guide an approach response to the baited goal box. In contrast, according to a procedural or stimulus-response view of learning, rats can learn to approach the baited goal box by acquiring a response tendency (i.e., a specific body turn) at the choice point of the maze. Note that either a declarative or a procedural learning mechanism can be used to successfully acquire this dual-solution task. Following acquisition, a probe trial in which rats are given a trial starting from the opposite start box (e.g., north) can be used to assess the type of learning acquired. Thus, rats with declarative knowledge of the spatial location of the reinforcer should continue to approach the baited goal box on the probe trial (i.e., termed place learning), whereas rats that have learned a specific body turn should choose the opposite goal box on the probe trial (i.e., termed response learning). The hypothesis that the dorsal striatum may play a selective role in the expression of procedural/response learning in the plus-maze was examined using a reversible brain lesion technique (Packard and McGaugh, 1996). In this study, rats were trained in a daily session to obtain food from a consistently baited goal box and were allowed to approach this maze arm from the same start box on each trial. Following 7 days of training (i.e., on day 8), rats were given a probe trial to determine whether they had acquired the task using place information or had learned a specific body turn response. Prior to the probe trial, a localized and reversible brain lesion was produced via intradorsolateral striatal injections of the sodium channel blocker lidocaine. On the day 8 probe trial, rats receiving lidocaine or saline vehicle injections into the dorsal striatum were predominantly place learners. Thus, consistent with the findings from the radial and water maze studies described above, infusions of lidocaine into the dorsal striatum did not impair the expression of declarative/place learning. With extended training in the dual-solution plus-maze, intact rats eventually switch from the use of place learning to a response-learning tendency (Ritchie et al., 1950; Hicks, 1964). Therefore, the rats were trained for an additional 7 days, given a second probe trial on day 16, and again received intracerebral injections of lidocaine prior to the probe trial. On this second probe trial, rats receiving vehicle injections into the dorsal striatum were now predominantly response learners. However, rats receiving intradorsal striatal injections of lidocaine prior to the second probe trial exhibited place learning, indicating a blockade of the expression of response learning (**Figure 3**). The selective impairment in expression of response learning in the plus-maze following neural inactivation of the dorsolateral striatum is consistent with other evidence implicating this brain region in egocentric learning (e.g., Potegal. 1969; Cook and Kesner, 1988; Kesner et al., 1993). The results also suggest that the shift or transition from the use of place learning to response learning in a dual-solution plus-maze task involves the gradual recruitment of a dorsal striatal-based procedural learning system to guide behavior. The functional integrity of the dorsolateral striatum is also necessary for the acquisition of a single-solution plus-maze task that requires rats to use procedural response learning by varying the start point on each trial and reinforcing the same body turn at the choice point (Chang and Gold, 2004).

It is important to note that in the radial maze (Packard et al., 1989; McDonald and White, 1993), water maze (Packard and McGaugh, 1992; McDonald and White, 1994), and plus-maze, (Packard and McGaugh, 1996) tasks described above, lesions of the hippocampal system produce the opposite effect of dorsal striatal lesions. Specifically, hippocampal damage impairs acquisition of the declarative/cognitive versions of the tasks and spares (or in some cases enhances) acquisition of procedural learning. Moreover, the individual pairs of maze tasks used in these studies possess the same motivational, sensory, and motoric characteristics, suggesting that the double dissociations observed reflect differential roles of

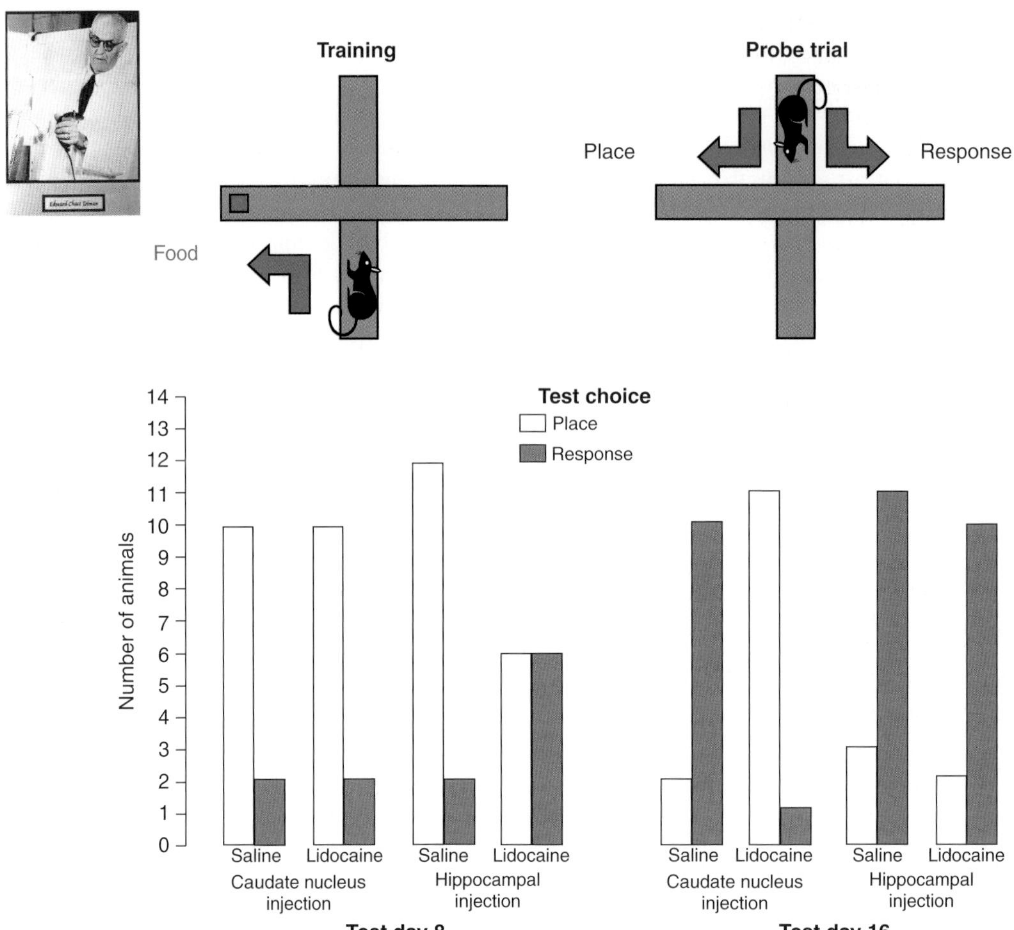

Figure 3 (a) In a dual-solution plus-maze task (Tolman et al., 1946), rats are trained to obtain food from a consistently baited goal box (e.g., west) from the same start box (e.g., south). Either a declarative (i.e., place) or a procedural (i.e., response) memory mechanism can be used to acquire this task. Following acquisition, a probe trial starting from the opposite start box (e.g., north) is used to assess the type of learning strategy employed. Rats approaching the maze arm that was baited during training are designated place learners, whereas rats that perform the specific body turn that was reinforced during training are designated response learners. Photograph of E.C. Tolman provided courtesy of James L. McGaugh. (b) On an initial probe trial (day 8), rats receiving intrastriatal saline or lidocaine are predominantly place learners, indicating that inactivation of the striatum does not impair expression of declarative memory. On a second probe trial given after additional training (day 16), rats receiving saline have switched to the use of response learning. In contrast, rats receiving intrastriatal lidocaine display place learning, indicating a blockade of the expression of procedural learning. Note that hippocampal injections of lidocaine produce the opposite effect, blocking expression of place (day 8), but not response learning (day 16). Thus, the transition to response learning involves an anatomical shift from the use of the hippocampus to the dorsal striatum. In rats receiving intrastriatal lidocaine, the use of place at the time point at which saline-treated rats have transitioned to response learning indicates a continued functional independence of declarative and procedural memory. Data/graph used with permission from Packard MG and McGaugh JL (1996) Inactivation of the hippocampus or caudate nucleus with lidocaine differentially affects expression of place and response learning. *Neurobiol. Learn. Mem.* 65: 65–72.

the hippocampus and dorsal striatum in declarative and procedural memory, rather than lesion-induced deficits in non-mnemonic factors. The observed double dissociations also allow for a more compelling argument that deficits in task acquisition following dorsal striatal lesions in studies employing a single task reflect a selective impairment of procedural learning. Examples include one-way and two-way active avoidance (e.g., Kirkby and Kimble, 1968; Neill and Grossman, 1971; Kirkby and Polgar, 1974; Mitcham and Thomas, 1972; Winocur, 1974), auditory discrimination learning (Adams et al., 2001), and straight-alley runway behavior (Kirkby et al., 1981; Salinas and White, 1998).

17.4 The Dorsal Striatum and Procedural Memory Revisited: Functional Heterogeneity

Although extensive evidence supports a role for the dorsal striatum in a stimulus–response form of procedural learning (for reviews, see White, 1997; Packard and Knowlton, 2002; Yin and Knowlton, 2006), increasing evidence from brain lesion studies in rats suggests that this function does not involve the entirety of this brain structure. Rather, lateral, but not medial, regions of the dorsal striatum may be particularly critical in procedural learning that results in the formation of stimulus–response habits. The hypothesis that functional heterogeneity exists in the learning and memory processes mediated by the dorsal striatum is based in part on recognition that this brain structure receives input from all areas of the neocortex (e.g., Webster, 1961; Carman et al., 1963; Webster, 1965; Kemp and Powell, 1970; Veening et al., 1980; McGeorge and Faull, 1989). This idea was explored behaviorally in several early lesion experiments investigating the functional relationship between the frontal cortex and the anteromedial regions of the dorsal striatum in delayed alternation behavior and reversal learning (Rosvold, 1968; Divac, 1968, 1972; Kolb, 1977; for reviews, see Iversen, 1979; Oberg and Divac, 1979).

In rats, damage to the medial dorsal striatum can in some cases produce cognitive learning deficits fairly similar to those observed following hippocampal system damage (e.g., Divac, 1968; Kolb, 1977; Whishaw et al., 1987; Devan et. al., 1999; Devan and White, 1999; but see also Packard and McGaugh, 1992; DeCoteau and Kesner, 2000; Adams et al., 2001; Sakamoto and Okaichi, 2001). Consistent with the idea that medial and lateral regions of the dorsal striatum are differentially involved in learning and memory, lesions of the posterior dorsomedial, but not the dorsolateral striatum, block the ability of reinforcer devaluation to reduce instrumental responding (Yin et. al., 2004, 2005, 2006). These findings suggest that the dorsomedial striatum selectively mediates expression of behavior based on action-outcome associations in instrumental conditioning, whereas the dorsolateral striatum selectively mediates stimulus–response habit formation. In addition, pretraining lesions of a posterior region of the dorsomedial striatum, but not the dorsolateral striatum, result in the predominant use of response learning in the dual-solution plus-maze (Yin and Knowlton, 2004). Further examples of dissociations between the role of medial and lateral regions of the dorsal striatum in learning include evidence that neurotoxic lesions of the dorsolateral, but not dorsomedial striatum, impair acquisition of an operant visual discrimination task (Reading et al., 1991) and of a conditional discrimination task that presumably involves stimulus-response procedural learning (Featherstone and McDonald, 2004a,b).

In addition to evidence suggesting that lateral, but not medial, regions of the rat dorsal striatum mediate procedural learning involving stimulus–response habit formation, other findings indicate that mnemonic function of the lateral dorsal striatum is organized based on the nature of the sensory information provided by cortical input. For example, lesions of the ventrolateral dorsal striatum, an area that receives olfactory cortical input, impairs procedural learning involving olfactory, but not visual sensory, information (Viaud and White, 1989). In contrast, lesions of the posteroventrolateral dorsal striatum, an area that receives visual cortical input, impairs procedural learning involving visual but not olfactory sensory information (Viaud and White, 1989). Similarly, the impairing effect of lesions of the dorsolateral striatum on response learning in the plus-maze may reflect a role for the vestibular/kinesthetic information that this striatal region receives from the somatosensory cortex.

In summary, modification of the hypothesis that stimulus-response procedural learning is mediated by the dorsal striatum is likely necessary to account for evidence indicating functional heterogeneity in the mnemonic functions of this brain structure. At least two levels of functional heterogeneity in the mnemonic functions of the dorsal striatum may exist. Specifically, a medial-to-lateral anatomical gradient may exist in the dorsal striatum that corresponds to a differential functional involvement in declarative and procedural memory, respectively. Second, within the lateral regions of the dorsal striatum, stimulus-response procedural learning appears to be organized based on the nature of the specific sensory input that is received from different cortical regions.

17.5 Dorsal Striatum and Procedural Learning: Pharmacological Experiments

The dorsal striatum contains several different neurotransmitters and neuropeptides (for review, see Graybiel, 1990). With regard to the function of this brain structure in procedural learning and memory, several studies have focused on the role of dopaminergic, glutamatergic, and cholinergic neurotransmission. Dopaminergic projections to the dorsal striatum originate in the substantia nigra (Moore and Bloom, 1978; Gerfen and Wilson, 1996) and may provide a reinforcing signal that is critical in the initial formation of stimulus–response associations (White 1989a; White et al., 1994). Corticostriatal projections are primarily glutamatergic in nature (Fonnum et al., 1981) and are hypothesized to provide sensory or stimulus information embedded in stimulus–response associations (White 1989; White et al., 1994). Acetylcholine is present in the dorsal striatum within a substantial population of interneurons (Lynch et al., 1972) and can interact with dopaminergic transmission to modulate habit memory (White et al., 1994). In addition, the proportional amounts of acetylcholine release in the hippocampus and dorsal striatum may influence the use of habit memory relative to other available learning strategies (for review, see Gold, 2004).

Evidence implicating each of these three neurotransmitters in dorsal striatal-dependent procedural learning and memory is briefly described here. Particular emphasis is placed on studies investigating the effects of posttraining manipulations of neurotransmission in the dorsal striatum on the consolidation of procedural memory. This experimental approach is based on evidence that memory is in a labile state following early exposure(s) to new information (Muller and Pilzecker 1900) and can therefore be either strengthened or weakened by experimental manipulations (e.g., Duncan, 1949; Breen and McGaugh, 1961; McGaugh, 1966). Importantly, this approach avoids several potential nonmnemonic confounds that arise in interpretation of drug effects on memory when pretraining pharmacological treatments are administered (for review, see McGaugh, 1989).

17.5.1 Dopamine

Impairments in the acquisition of various conditioned avoidance behaviors following depletion of dopamine in the nigrostriatal pathway memory provided the initial evidence of a possible role for striatal dopamine in procedural learning and memory (Neill et al., 1974; Zis et al., 1974). Subsequent research demonstrated that posttraining electrical stimulation of the nigrostriatal bundle enhances memory (Major and White, 1978), and this effect is blocked by administration of the dopamine receptor antagonist pimozide (White and Major, 1978). An enhancement of procedural memory is also observed following posttraining injections of the indirect catecholamine agonist amphetamine directly into the dorsal striatum (Carr and White, 1984). Moreover, in a manner analogous to the double dissociation produced by irreversible lesions, posttraining intracerebral infusions of amphetamine (Viaud and White, 1989) or the dopamine D2 receptor agonist quinpirole (White and Viaud, 1991) into the ventrolateral dorsal striatum selectively enhance procedural memory involving olfactory sensory information, whereas infusion of these drugs into the posteroventrolateral dorsal striatum selectively enhances procedural memory involving visual sensory information. The latter findings suggest that dopamine release in the dorsal striatum enhances memory consolidation underlying procedural memory in a site-specific manner that is dependent on the nature of the sensory input provided by corticostriatal projections.

The first study to directly compare the role of dopaminergic function in the dorsal striatum in declarative and procedural learning and memory utilized versions of the two radial maze tasks described earlier (Packard and White, 1991). In a declarative memory version of the task, rats were first allowed to obtain food from four of eight randomly selected maze arms. They were then removed from the maze and received an intradorsal striatal injection of saline vehicle, amphetamine, the dopamine D1 receptor agonist SKF 38393, or the dopamine D2 receptor agonist quinpirole. Eighteen hours later, the rats were returned to the maze for a retention test with all eight maze arms open, and only the four arms that had not been visited prior to the delay contained food. In a procedural memory version of the task, rats obtained food rewards by visiting four randomly selected and illuminated maze arms. Rats were removed from the maze following training on day 5 and received an intradorsal striatal injection of either vehicle, amphetamine, SKF 38393, or quinpirole and were returned for a retention test 24 h later. Posttraining injection of all three dopamine agonists enhanced memory in the procedural memory radial maze task but had no effect on memory in the declarative memory radial maze task (Packard and White, 1991). Similarly, in a cued water maze task in which a visible escape platform is moved to a new spatial location on each trial, procedural memory consolidation is enhanced by posttraining peripheral injections of amphetamine and quinpirole

(Packard and McGaugh, 1994) and by intradorsal striatum infusions of amphetamine (Packard et al., 1994; Packard and Teather, 1998). In contrast, posttraining intradorsal striatal infusions of amphetamine have no effect on memory in a declarative/cognitive version of the water maze task in which rats are trained to swim to a hidden escape platform that is located in the same spatial location across trials.

In each of the above studies, posttraining intradorsal striatal infusions of amphetamine or direct dopamine agonists that were delayed until 2 h after training did not enhance memory. The time-dependent nature of the effects of the posttraining infusions suggest that the drug treatments enhanced the consolidation of procedural memory and argue against the possibility that the drugs affected behavior by influencing nonmnemonic factors (McGaugh, 1989). Posttraining intradorsal striatal injection of the dopamine receptor antagonist cis-flupenthixol impairs procedural memory in the radial maze (Legault et al., 2006), suggesting that intact dopamine function is a necessary component of habit formation.

Whereas extensive evidence implicates dorsal striatal dopamine in the initial consolidation of procedural memory, other findings suggest that dopaminergic function in this brain region may not be necessary for the expression of stimulus–response habits after they have been acquired (but see also Aosaki et al., 1994). For example, 6-hydroxydopamine lesions of the nigrostriatal pathway impair acquisition of active avoidance conditioning but do not affect task performance when the lesions are produced after acquisition has occurred (Zis et al., 1974). In addition, relative to early stages of training, significant decreases in neuronal responses of midbrain dopamine neurons are observed in monkeys following extended habit training (Ljungberg et al., 1992), and peripheral administration of dopamine receptor antagonists impair performance of a simple appetitive response only during early stages of training (Choi et al., 2005).

Taken together, evidence indicating a role for dorsal striatal dopamine in memory consolidation but not the expression of procedural memory is consistent with the hypothesis that dopamine release may act as a reinforcing signal in the initial formation of stimulus–response habits (White, 1989a). According to this view, dopamine release in the dorsolateral striatum may function as the proverbial stamp or glue (e.g., Thorndike, 1933) that binds stimulus–response associations rather than providing a representation of a specific stimulus or response. Note that the hypothesized reinforcing effect of dopamine on habit formation in the dorsal striatum is active in both appetitively and aversively motivated habit learning tasks (Packard and White, 1991; Packard and McGaugh, 1994; Packard and Teather, 1998). Therefore, this dopaminergic function is conceptually different (White, 1989b) than the putative reward signal often associated with dopamine release in the nucleus accumbens. In contrast to the stimulus–response learning mediated by the dorsal striatum, the nucleus accumbens has been implicated in stimulus-reward learning (for review, see Cador et al., 1989) and hippocampus-dependent declarative memory (for review, see Setlow, 1997).

17.5.2 Glutamate

Glutamatergic input to the dorsal striatum is supplied primarily via corticostriatal projections (Fonnum et al., 1981). Glutamate release in the dorsal striatum resulting from activation of corticostriatal pathways is hypothesized to provide sensory input critical to the formation of stimulus–response habits (White, 1989; White et al., 1994), and behavioral evidence is consistent with a role for this transmitter in procedural learning. For example, in a cued water maze task in which rats are trained to swim to a visible escape platform, procedural memory consolidation is impaired by posttraining intradorsal striatal injection of the glutamatergic *N*-methyl-D-aspartate (NMDA) receptor antagonist AP5 (Packard and Teather, 1997) and enhanced by injection of glutamate (Packard and Teather, 1999). In contrast, posttraining intradorsal striatal infusions of AP5 or glutamate have no effect on memory in a declarative version of the water maze task in which rats are trained to swim to a hidden escape platform that is located in the same spatial location across trials. The role of dorsal striatal glutamate in procedural memory is not limited to the fast excitatory neurotransmission mediated by NMDA receptor activation, as posttraining intrastriatal infusions of metabotropic glutamate receptor antagonists (i.e., MCPG, ACPD) also impair memory consolidation in procedural, but not declarative, memory water maze tasks (Packard et al., 2001).

Further evidence of a selective role for dorsal striatal glutamate in procedural learning and memory was obtained using the dual-solution plus-maze task (Packard, 1999). As described previously, rats that are given extended training in this task eventually transition from the use of hippocampus-dependent place learning to dorsal striatal-dependent response learning

(Packard and McGaugh, 1996). Interestingly, the transition to procedural learning can be facilitated by posttraining intradorsal striatal injections of glutamate. Specifically, intradorsal striatal injections of glutamate following initial training trials in the plus-maze result in the predominant use of response learning during an early probe trial on which control rats predominantly display place learning. Thus, in a task for which a declarative and a procedural learning strategy each provide an adequate solution, an increase in glutamatergic tone in the dorsolateral striatum during early learning appears to favor a more rapid adoption of procedural/response learning. In contrast, posttraining intrahippocampal infusions of glutamate following early training in the plus-maze prevents the transition to procedural learning that is normally produced by extended training. This finding suggests that a relative increase in glutamatergic tone in the hippocampus during early training is detrimental to the development of dorsal striatal-dependent procedural memory.

Consistent with an enhancing function of glutamate on memory consolidation underlying procedural learning (Packard, 1999), infusions of the NMDA receptor antagonist AP5 into the dorsolateral striatum impair acquisition of response learning in a plus-maze (Palencia and Raggozino, 2005). The region of the dorsal striatum targeted in these two latter studies receives glutamatergic input from somatosensory cortex (Fonnum et al., 1981; McGeorge and Faull, 1989). Therefore, similar to dopamine (Viaud and White, 1989, 1991), glutamatergic input to lateral regions of the dorsal striatum may enhance procedural memory in a site-specific manner that is organized based on the nature of the sensory information provided by the cortex. Moreover, infusions of AP5 into the dorsomedial striatum do not impair acquisition of response learning in the plus-maze (Palencia and Ragozzino, 2004), consistent with evidence from the lesion studies reviewed earlier indicating that this region of the dorsal striatum does not mediate procedural learning.

17.5.3 Acetylcholine

Prominent cholinergic systems (e.g., the basal forebrain cholinergic system) provide diffuse projections to widespread regions of the mammalian brain. In contrast, acetylcholine within the dorsal striatum is contained within a population of interneurons (Lynch et al., 1972). Numerous studies examining the effects of posttraining intracerebral injections of acetylcholine agonist and antagonist drugs on avoidance behavior implicate dorsal striatal cholinergic activity in consolidation of procedural memory (Haycock et al., 1973; Prado-Alcala and Cobos-Zapian, 1977, 1979; Prado-Alcala et al., 1981; Packard et al., 1996). Taken together, these several findings indicate that posttraining intrastriatal infusions of cholinergic agonists (e.g., oxotremorine, choline) enhance procedural memory consolidation in a time-dependent manner, whereas cholinergic antagonists (e.g., atropine, scopolamine) impair memory. In addition, immunotoxin-induced ablation of striatal cholinergic neurons impairs acquisition of a tone-cued T maze task but does not impair declarative memory in a hidden platform water maze task (Kitabatake et. al., 2003), suggesting that the facilitatory role of striatal acetylcholine may be selective for procedural memory.

A series of experiments using intracerebral microdialysis to monitor neurotransmitter release in the hippocampus and dorsolateral striatum during performance of the dual-solution plus-maze task suggests that the relative amount of acetylcholine release in these two brain regions influences the use of striatal-dependent procedural learning (for review, see Gold, 2004). For example, following training in the plus-maze, rats that exhibit response learning on a subsequent probe trial also display a higher ratio of acetylcholine release in the dorsolateral striatum relative to the hippocampus, whereas the opposite pattern of acetylcholine release is observed in rats displaying place learning (McIntyre et al., 2003). In addition, the transition from hippocampus-dependent place learning to dorsal-striatal response learning that occurs with extended training in the plus-maze (e.g., Packard and McGaugh, 1996; Packard, 1999) coincides temporally with an asymptotic value of acetylcholine release in the dorsolateral striatum (Chang and Gold, 2003). A similar relationship between increases in acetylcholine release and transition from a spatial strategy to a response learning strategy was observed in rats trained in a food-rewarded Y maze task (Pych et al., 2005).

Finally, the cholinergic interneurons in the striatum appear to correspond to the tonically active neurons (TANs) that have been identified in this brain structure using *in vivo* electrophysiological recordings (for review, see Zhou et al., 2002). During procedural sensorimotor learning, striatal TANs develop responsiveness to conditioned stimuli (reflected in part as a brief pause in tonic firing) and are hypothesized to integrate dopaminergic and cholinergic transmission in the striatum and ultimately influence the activity of afferent projection neurons (Aosaki et al., 1994). The idea that dopamine and acetylcholine interact to influence striatal-dependent procedural learning is supported by several pharmacological studies in rats (for reviews, see Beninger, 1983; White et al., 1994).

In summary, several lines of evidence implicate dorsal striatal dopamine, glutamate, and acetylcholine in stimulus–response procedural learning. Similar to the effects of irreversible and reversible brain lesions, posttraining pharmacological manipulations also result in a double dissociation of dorsal striatal and hippocampal involvement in procedural and declarative memory, respectively. For example, in the radial maze, water maze, and plus-maze, intra-hippocampal infusions of dopaminergic and glutamatergic drugs selectively affect consolidation underlying declarative memory. Thus, as multiple memory systems evolved in the vertebrate brain (Sherry and Schacter, 1987), a role for specific neurotransmitters in different types of memory appears to have been conserved. A challenge for future research is to understand how activity of essentially the same neurotransmitters can differentially influence the type of information acquired in multiple memory systems. The relative activation of transmitter systems produced by engaging in a particular learning task appears to shape the participation of different brain structures in guiding learned behavior (Packard, 1999; Gold, 2004; Korol, 2004). However, future research investigating potential differences in the physiological characteristics of the various forms of synaptic plasticity that have been observed in brain structures mediating declarative and procedural memory (e.g., long-term potentiation and long-term depression; Garcia-Munoz et al., 1992; Lovinger et al., 1993; Charpier and Deniau, 1997; Fino et al., 2005) may ultimately help define the neural mechanisms that allow independent brain systems to acquire different types of information in a given learning situation.

17.6 Procedural Learning Beyond the Dorsal Striatum: Amygdala and Stimulus-Affect Associations

In addition to findings implicating the dorsal striatum in procedural learning involving stimulus–response habits, other research suggests that the amygdala may mediate a form of procedural learning in which stimulus–affect associations are acquired. This hypothesis is consistent with extensive evidence indicating involvement of the amygdala in specific fear conditioning paradigms (for reviews, see Davis, 1992; LeDoux, 1995). However, the role of the amygdala in stimulus–affect procedural learning is clearly not limited to aversively motivated tasks (e.g., Cador et al., 1989). For example, the functional integrity of the basolateral amygdala is necessary for acquisition of conditioned place preference behavior for both natural rewards (e.g., food, McDonald and White, 1993; Schroeder and Packard, 2002) and addictive drugs (e.g., amphetamine; Hiroi and White, 1991; Hsu et al., 2002). In a conditioned place preference task, rats are confined on alternating days to one distinct environmental context paired with natural or drug rewards and a second context that is not paired with the rewarding treatment. On a reward-free test session given following training, the amount of time spent in the two environments is measured, and rats demonstrate a reliable preference for the environment previously paired with the rewarding stimulus. The conditioned place preference task has been used to demonstrate a double dissociation between the roles of the basolateral amygdala and dorsal striatum in stimulus–affect and stimulus–response procedural learning (McDonald and White, 1993). Specifically, lesions of the basolateral amygdala but not dorsal striatum impair acquisition of stimulus–affect learning underlying conditioned place preference behavior. In contrast, lesions of the dorsal striatum but not basolateral amygdala impair acquisition of stimulus–response learning underlying simultaneous visual discrimination behavior.

Finally, activation of efferent basolateral amygdala projections can act to modulate memory consolidation occurring in other brain structures, including declarative memory processes mediated by the hippocampus and procedural learning mediated by the dorsal striatum (e.g., Packard et al., 1994; for review, see Cahill and McGaugh, 1998; McGaugh, 2002). The modulatory role of the basolateral amygdala on memory consolidation is associated in part with hormonal influences on emotional arousal (for review, see McGaugh, 2004; *See* Chapter 27). Moreover, an organism's emotional state may interact with amygdala function to influence the relative use of multiple memory systems. For example, peripheral and intrabasolateral amygdala injections of anxiogenic drugs result in a predominant use of dorsal striatal-dependent procedural learning in the dual-solution plus-maze task (Packard and

Wingard, 2004). Finally, the memory storage and modulation views have at times been contrasted as mutually exclusive and competing theories of amygdala function (e.g., Cahill et al., 1999; Fanselow and LeDoux, 1999). However, a time-limited modulatory role for the basolateral amygdala in some types of learning and memory (e.g., hippocampus-dependent declarative or dorsal striatal-dependent habit memory) does not necessarily rule out a possible long-term role for this structure in stimulus–affect procedural learning and memory (or vice versa).

17.7 Conclusions

Significant progress has been made in identifying the neuroanatomical and neurochemical bases of stimulus–response habit learning in lower animals. Extensive evidence supports the hypothesis that this form of procedural learning is mediated by a neural system that contains the dorsal striatum as a primary component. Studies employing irreversible and reversible brain lesion techniques have dissociated the role of the dorsal striatum in procedural and declarative memory. In addition, pharmacological experiments indicate a selective role for dorsal striatal dopamine, acetylcholine, and glutamate in memory consolidation underlying stimulus–response procedural learning.

Finally, although the present chapter focused on studies involving rats, it is important to note that similar evidence for the role of the dorsal striatum in procedural learning also exists in nonhuman primates (e.g., Teng et al., 2000; Fernandez-Ruiz. et al., 2001) and humans (e.g., Knowlton et al., 1996; for reviews, see Packard and Knowlton, 2002). Understanding the influence of the dorsal striatal habit learning system on human behavior ranging from adaptive social interaction and self-regulation (e.g., Lieberman, 2000; Wood et al., 2002) to maladaptive psychopathology (e.g., White, 1996; McDonald et al., 2004; Marsh et al., 2004; Everitt and Robbins, 2005) is an exciting and challenging prospect for future research.

References

Adams CD (1981) Variations in the sensitivity of instrumental responding to reinforcer devalaution. *Q. J. Exp. Psychol.* 34B: 77–98.

Adams S, Kesner RP, and Ragozzino ME (2001) Role of the medial and lateral caudate-putamen in mediating an auditory conditional response association. *Neurobiol. Learn. Mem.* 76: 106–116.

Alexander GE, DeLong MR, and Strick PL (1986) Parallel organization of functionally segregated circuits linking basal ganglia and cortex. *Annu. Rev. Neurosci.* 9: 357–381.

Allen JD and Davidson CS (1973) Effects of caudate lesions on signaled and nonsignaled Sidman avoidance in the rat. *Behav. Biol.* 8: 239–250.

Aosaki T, Graybiel AM, and Kimura M (1994) Effect of the nigrostriatal dopamine system on acquired neural responses in the striatum of behaving monkeys. *Science* 265: 412–415.

Beninger RJ (1983) The role of dopamine in locomotor activity and learning. *Brain Res.* 287(2): 173–196.

Breen RA and McGaugh JL (1961) Facilitation of maze learning with post-trial injections of picrotoxin. *J. Comp. Physiol. Psychol.* 54: 495–501.

Buerger AA, Gross CG, and Rocha-Miranda CE (1974) Effects of ventral putamen lesions on discrimination learning by monkeys. *J. Comp. Physiol. Psychol.* 86: 440–446.

Cador M, Robbins TW, and Everitt BJ (1989) Involvement of the amygdala in stimulus-reward associations: Interaction with the ventral striatum. *Neuroscience* 30: 77–86.

Cahill L and McGaugh JL (1998) Mechanisms of emotional arousal and lasting declarative memory. *Trends Neurosci.* 21: 294–299.

Cahill L, Weinberger NM, Roozendaal B, and McGaugh JL (1999) Is the amygdala a locus of "conditioned fear"? Some questions and caveats. *Neuron* 23(2): 227–228.

Calabresi P, Maj R, Pisani A, Mercuri NB, and Bernardi G (1992) Long-term synaptic depression in the rat striatum: Physiological and pharmacological characterization. *J. Neurosci.* 12: 4224–4433.

Carman JB, Cowan WM, and Powell TP (1963) The organization of cortico-striatal connections in the rabbit. *Brain* 86: 525–562.

Carr GD and White NM (1984) The relationship between stereotypy and memory improvement produced by amphetamine. *Psychopharmacology* 82: 203–209.

Chang Q and Gold PE (2003) Switching memory systems during learning: Changes in patterns of brain acetylcholine release in the hippocampus and striatum in rats. *J. Neurosci.* 23(7): 3001–3005.

Charpier S and Deniau JM (1997) In vivo activity-dependent plasticity at cortico-striatal connections: Evidence for physiological long-term potentiation. *Proc. Natl. Acad. Sci. USA* 94: 7036–7040.

Choi WY, Balsam PD, and Horvitz JC (2005) Extended habit training reduces dopamine mediation of appetitive response expression. *J. Neurosci.* 25(29): 6729–6733.

Cohen NJ and Squire LR (1980) Preserved learning and retention of pattern analyzing skill in amnesics: Dissociation of knowing how and knowing that. *Science* 210: 207–210.

Colombo PJ, Davis HP, and Volpe BT (1989) Allocentric spatial and tactile memory impairments in rats with dorsal caudate lesions are affected by preoperative behavioral training. *Behav. Neurosci.* 103: 1242–1250.

Colombo PJ, Brightwell JJ, and Countryman RA (2003) Cognitive strategy-specific increases in phosphorylated cAMP response element-binding protein and c-Fos in the hippocampus and dorsal striatum. *J. Neurosci.* 23(8): 3547–3554.

Cook D and Kesner RP (1988) Caudate nucleus and memory for egocentric localization. *Behav. Neural Biol.* 49: 332–343.

Davis M (1992) The role of the amygdala in fear and anxiety. *Annu. Rev. Neurosci.* 15: 353–375.

DeCoteau WE and Kesner RP (2000) A double dissociation between the rat hippocampus and medial caudoputamen in processing two forms of knowledge. *Behav. Neurosci.* 114: 1096–1108.

Devan BD and White NM (1999) Parallel information processing in the dorsal striatum: Relation to hippocampal function. *J. Neurosci.* 19: 2789–2798.

Devan BD, McDonald RJ, and White NM (1999) Effects of medial and lateral caudate-putamen lesions on place- and cue-guided behaviors in the water maze: Relation to thigmotaxis. *Behav. Brain Res.* 100: 5–14.

Divac I (1968) Functions of the caudate nucleus. *Acta Neurobiol. Exp. (Warsz.)* 28: 107–120.

Divac I (1972) Neostriatum and functions of the prefrontal cortex. *Acta. Neurobiol. Exp.* 32: 461–477.

Divac I, Rosvold HE, and Szwarcbart MK (1967) Behavioral effects of selective ablation of the caudate nucleus. *J. Comp. Physiol. Psychol.* 63: 183–190.

Duncan CP (1949) The retroactive effect of electroshock on learning. *J. Comp. Physiol. Psychol.* 42: 32–44.

Eichenbaum H and Cohen NJ (2001) *From Conditioning to Conscious Recollection: Memory Systems of the Brain*. Oxford Psychology Series, no. 35. New York: Oxford University Press.

Everitt BJ and Robbins TW (2005) Neural systems of reinforcement for drug addiction: From actions to habits to compulsion. *Nat. Neurosci.* 8(11): 1481–1489.

Fanselow MS and LeDoux JE (1999) Why we think plasticity underlying Pavlovian fear conditioning occurs in the basolateral amygdala. *Neuron* 23(2): 229–232.

Featherstone RE and McDonald RJ (2004a) Dorsal striatum and stimulus-response learning: Lesions of the dorsolateral, but not dorsomedial, striatum impair acquisition of a simple discrimination task. *Behav. Brain Res.* 150(1–2): 15–23.

Featherstone RE and McDonald RJ (2004b) Dorsal striatum and stimulus-response learning: Lesions of the dorsolateral, but not dorsomedial, striatum impair acquisition of a stimulus-response-based instrumental discrimination task, while sparing conditioned place preference learning. *Neuroscience* 124(1): 23–31.

Fernandez-Ruiz J, Wang J, Aigner TG, and Mishkin M (2001) Visual habit formation in monkeys with neurotoxic lesions of the ventrocaudal neostriatum. *Proc. Natl. Acad. Sci. USA* 98: 4196–4201.

Fino E, Glowinski J, and Venance L (2005) Bidirectional activity-dependent plasticity at corticostriatal synapses. *J. Neurosci.* 25(49): 11279–11287.

Fonnum F, Storm-Mathisen J, and Divac I (1981) Biochemical evidence for glutamate as neurotransmitter in corticostriatal and corticothalamic fibres in rat brain. *Eur. J. Pharm.* 6: 863–873.

Garcia-Munoz M, Young SJ, and Groves PM (1992) Presynaptic long-term changes in excitability of the corticostriatal pathway. *Neuroreport* 3: 357–360.

Gerfen CR and Wilson CJ (1996) The basal ganglia. In: Swanson LW, Bjorkland A, and Hokfelt T (eds.) *Handbook of Chemical Neuroanatomy, Integrated Systems of the CNS, Part III*, pp. 371–468. New York: Elsevier.

Gold PE (2004) Coordination of multiple memory systems. *Neurobiol. Learn. Mem.* 82(3): 230–242.

Graf P and Schacter DL (1985) Implicit and explicit memory for new associations in normal and amnesic subjects. *J. Exp. Psychol. Learn. Mem. Cog.* 11(3): 501–518.

Graybiel AM (1990) Neurotransmitters and neuromodulators in the basal ganglia. *Trends Neurosci.* 13: 244–254.

Graybiel AM (1998) The basal ganglia and chunking of action repertories. *Neurobiol. Learn. Mem.* 70: 119–136.

Graybiel AM, Aosaki T, Flaherty AW, and Kimura M (1994) The basal ganglia and adaptive motor control. *Science* 265: 1826–1831.

Haycock JW, Deadwyler SA, Sideroff SI, and McGaugh JL (1973) Retrograde amnesia and cholinergic systems in the caudate-putamen complex and dorsal hippocampus of the rat. *Exp. Neurol.* 41: 201–213.

Hicks LH (1964) Effects of overtraining on acquisition and reversal of place and response learning. *Psychol. Report.* 15: 459–462.

Hiroi N and White NM (1991) The lateral nucleus of the amygdala mediates expression of the amphetamine-produced conditioned place preference. *J. Neurosci.* 11(7): 2107–2116.

Hirsh R (1974) The hippocampus and contextual retrieval of information from memory: A theory. *Behav. Biol.* 12: 421–444.

Hsu EH, Schroeder JP, and Packard MG (2002) The amygdala mediates memory consolidation for an amphetamine conditioned place preference. *Behav. Brain Res.* 129: 93–100.

Hull CL (1943) *Principles of Behavior*. New York: Appleton-Century Crofts.

Iversen SD (1979) Behaviour after neostriatal lesions in animals. In: Divac I and Oberg RGE (eds.) *The Neostriatum*, pp. 291–313. Oxford: Permagon Press.

Jog MS, Kubota Y, Connolly CI, Hillegaart V, and Graybiel AM (1999) Building neural representations of habits. *Science* 286: 1745–1749.

Kemp JM and Powell TP (1970) The cortico-striate projection in the monkey. *Brain* 93(3): 525–546.

Kesner RP and Wilburn MW (1974) A review of electrical stimulation of the brain in context of learning and retention. *Behav. Biol.* 10: 259–293.

Kesner RP, Bolland BL, and Dakis M (1993) Memory for spatial locations, motor responses, and objects: Triple dissociation among the hippocampus, caudate nucleus, and extrastriate visual cortex. *Exp. Brain Res.* 93: 462–470.

Kim JJ, Lee H, Han JS, and Packard MG (2001) Amygdala is critical for stress-induced modulation of hippocampal LTP and learning. *J. Neurosci.* 21: 5222–5228.

Kimura M (1995) Role of the basal ganglia in behavioral learning. *Neurosci. Res.* 22: 353–358.

Kirkby RJ and Kimble DP (1968) Avoidance and escape behavior following striatal lesions in the rat. *Exp. Neurol.* 20: 215–227.

Kirkby RJ and Polgar S (1974) Active avoidance in the laboratory rats following lesions of the dorsal or ventral caudate nucleus. *Physiol. Psychol.* 2: 301–306.

Kirkby RJ, Polgar S, and Coyle IR (1981) Caudate nucleus lesions impair the ability of rats to learn a simple straight-alley task. *Percep. Mot. Skills* 52: 499–502.

Kitabatake Y, Hikida T, Watanabe D, Pastan I, and Nakanishi S (2003) Impairment of reward-related learning by cholinergic cell ablation in the striatum. *Proc. Natl. Acad. Sci. USA* 100(13): 7965–7670.

Knowlton BJ, Mangels JA, and Squire LR (1996) A neostriatal habit learning system in humans. *Science* 273: 1399–1402.

Kolb B (1977) Studies on the caudate-putamen and the dorsomedial thalamic nucleus of the rat: Implications for mammalian frontal-lobe functions. *Physiol. Behav.* 18: 237–244.

Korol DL (2004) Role of estrogen in balancing contributions from multiple memory systems. *Neurobiol. Learn. Mem.* 82(3): 309–323.

Lashley KS (1950) S.E.B. Symposium IV, pp. 545–582.

LeDoux JE (1995) Emotion: clues from the brain. *Ann. Rev. Psychol.* 46: 209–235.

Legault G, Smith CT, and Beninger RJ (2006) Post-training intra-striatal scopolamine or flupenthixol impairs radial maze learning in rats. *Behav. Brain Res.* 170(1): 148–155.

Lieberman MD (2000) Intuition: A social cognitive neuroscience approach. *Psychol. Bull.* 126(1): 109–137.

Ljungberg T, Apicella P, and Schultz W (1992) Responses of monkey dopamine neurons during learning of behavioral reactions. *J. Neurophysiol.* 67(1): 145–163.

Lovinger DM, Tyler EC, and Marritt A (1993) Short and long term depression in the rat neostriatum. *J. Neurophysiol.* 70: 1937–1949.

Lynch GS, Lucas PA, and Deadwyler SA (1972) The demonstration of acetylcholinesterase containing neurones within the caudate nucleus of the rat. *Brain Res.* 45: 617–621.

Mahut HS, Zola-Morgan S, and Moss M (1984) Consolidation of Memory: The hippocampus revisited. In: Butters N and Squire LR (eds.) *The Neuropsychology of Memory*, pp. 297–315. New York: Guilford.

Major R and White NM (1978) Memory facilitation produced by self-stimulation reinforcement mediated by the nigro-neostriatal bundle. *Physiol. Behav.* 20: 723–733.

Marsh R, Alexander GM, Packard MG, et al. (2004) Habit learning in Tourette syndrome: A translational neuroscience approach to a developmental psychopathology. *Arch. Gen. Psychiatry* 61(12): 1259–1268.

McDonald RJ and White NM (1993) A triple dissociation of memory systems: Hippocampus, amygdala, and dorsal striatum. *Behav. Neurosci.* 107: 3–22.

McDonald RJ and White NM (1994) Parallel information processing in the water maze: Evidence for independent memory systems involving the dorsal striatum and hippocampus. *Behav. Neural Biol.* 61: 260–270.

McDonald RJ, Devan BD, and Hong NS (2004) Multiple memory systems: The power of interactions. *Neurobiol. Learn. Mem.* 82(3): 333–346.

McGaugh JL (1966) Time-dependent processes in memory storage. *Science* 153: 1351–1358.

McGaugh JL (1989) Dissociating learning and performance: Drug and hormone enhancement of memory storage. *Brain Res. Bull.* 23: 339–345.

McGaugh JL (2002) Memory consolidation and the amygdala: A systems perspective. *Trends Neurosci.* 25(9): 456.

Mc Gaugh JL (2004) The amygdala modulates the consolidation of memories of emotionally arousing experiences. *Ann. Rev. Neurosci.* 27: 1–28.

McGeorge AJ and Faull RLM (1989) The organization of the projection from the cerebral cortex to the striatum in the rat. *Neuroscience* 29: 503–537.

McIntyre CK, Marriott LK, and Gold PE (2003) Patterns of brain acetylcholine release predict individual differences in preferred learning strategies in rats. *Neurobiol. Learn. Mem.* 79(2): 177–183.

Mishkin M and Appenzeller T (1987) The anatomy of memory. *Sci. Am.* 256(6): 80–89.

Mishkin M and Petri HL (1984) Memories and habits: Some implications for the analysis of learning and retention. In: Squire LR and Butters N (eds.) *Neuropsychology of Memory*, pp. 287–96. New York: Guilford.

Mishkin M, Malamut BL, and Bachevalier J (1984) Memories and habits: Two neural systems. In: McGaugh JL, Lynch G, and Weinberger NM (eds.) *The Neurobiology of Learning and Memory*, pp. 65–77. New York: Guilford Press.

Mitcham JC and Thomas RK Jr (1972) Effects of substantia nigra and caudate nucleus lesions on avoidance learning in rats. *J. Comp. Physiol. Psychol.* 81(1): 101–107.

Moore RY and Bloom FE (1978) Central catecholamine neuron systems: Anatomy and physiology of the dopamine systems. *Ann. Rev. Neurosci.* 1: 129–169.

Muller GE and Pilzecker A (1900) Experimentelle Beitrage zur Lehre vom Gedachtnis. *Zeitschrift Psychol.* (Suppl 1).

Neill DB and Grossman SP (1971) Behavioral effects of lesions or cholinergic blockade of the dorsal and ventral caudate of rats. *J. Comp. Physiol. Psychol. Neurosci.* 6: 863–873.

Neill DB, Boggan WO, and Grossman SP (1974) Impairment of avoidance performance by intrastriatal administration of 6-hydroxydopamine. *Pharm. Biochem. Behav.* 2: 97–103.

O'Keefe J and Nadel L (1978) *The Hippocampus as a Cognitive Map*. Oxford: Oxford University Press.

Oberg RGE and Divac I (1979) "Cognitive" functions of the neostriatum. In: Divac I and Oberg RGE (eds.) *The Neostriatum*, pp. 291–313. Oxford: Permagon Press.

Olton DS and Papas BC (1979) Spatial memory and hippocampal function. *Neuropsychologia* 17: 669–682.

Packard MG (1999) Glutamate infused posttraining into the hippocampus or caudate-putamen differentially strengthens place and response learning. *Proc. Natl. Acad. Sci. USA* 96: 12881–12886.

Packard MG (2002) Dissociation Methodology. In: Nadel L (ed.) *Encyclopedia of Cognitive Science*, London: Nature Publishing Group.

Packard MG and Knowlton BJ (2002) Learning and memory functions of the basal ganglia. *Ann. Rev. Neurosci.* 25: 563–593.

Packard MG and McGaugh JL (1992) Double dissociation of fornix and caudate nucleus lesions on acquisition of two water maze tasks: Further evidence for multiple memory systems. *Behav. Neurosci.* 106: 439–446.

Packard MG and McGaugh JL (1994) Post-training quinpirole and d-amphetamine administration enhances memory on spatial and cued water maze tasks. *Psychobiology* 22: 54–60.

Packard MG and McGaugh JL (1996) Inactivation of the hippocampus or caudate nucleus with lidocaine differentially affects expression of place and response learning. *Neurobiol. Learn. Mem.* 65: 65–72.

Packard MG and Teather LA (1997) Double dissociation of hippocampal and dorsal striatal memory systems by post-training intracerebral injections of 2-amino-phosphonopentanoic acid. *Behav. Neurosci.* 111: 543–551.

Packard MG and Teather LA (1998) Amygdala modulation of multiple memory systems: Hippocampus and caudate-putamen. *Neurobiol. Learn. Mem.* 69: 163–203.

Packard MG and Teather LA (1999) Dissociation of multiple memory systems by posttraining intracerebral injections of glutamate. *Psychobiology* 27: 40–50.

Packard MG and White NM (1991) Dissociation of hippocampus and caudate nucleus memory systems by posttraining intracerebral injection of dopamine agonists. *Behav. Neurosci.* 105: 295–306.

Packard MG and Wingard JC (2004) Amygdala and "emotional" modulation of the relative use of multiple memory systems. *Neurobiol. Learn. Mem.* 82(3): 243–252.

Packard MG, Hirsh R, and White NM (1989) Differential effects of fornix and caudate nucleus lesions on two radial maze tasks: Evidence for multiple memory systems. *J. Neurosci.* 9: 1465–1472.

Packard MG, Cahill L, and McGaugh JL (1994) Amygdala modulation of hippocampal-dependent and caudate nucleus-dependent memory processes. *Proc. Natl. Acad. Sci. USA* 91: 8477–8481.

Packard MG, Introini-Collison IB, and McGaugh JL (1996) Stria terminalis lesions attenuate memory enhancement produced by intra-caudate nucleus injections of oxotremorine. *Neurobiol. Learn. Mem.* 65: 278–282.

Packard MG, Vecchioli SF, Schroeder JP, and Gasbarri A (2001) Task-dependent role for dorsal striatum metabotropic glutamate receptors in memory. *Learn. Mem.* 8: 96–103.

Palencia CA and Ragozzino ME (2004) The influence of NMDA receptors in the dorsomedial striatum on response reversal learning. *Neurobiol. Learn. Mem.* 82(2): 81–89.

Palencia CA and Ragozzino ME (2005) The contribution of NMDA receptors in the dorsolateral striatum to egocentric response learning. *Behav. Neurosci.* 119(4): 953–960.

Pittenger C, Fasano S, Mazzocchi-Jones D, Dunnett SB, Kandel ER, and Brambilla R (2006) Impaired bidirectional synaptic plasticity and procedural memory formation in striatum-specific cAMP response element-binding protein-deficient mice. *J. Neurosci.* 26(10): 2808–2813.

Potegal M (1972) The caudate nucleus egocentric localization system. *Acta Neurobiol. Exp. (Warsz.).* 32: 479–494.

Prado-Alcala RA and Cobos-Zapiain GC (1977) Learning deficits induced by cholinergic blockade of the caudate nucleus as a function of experience. *Brain Res.* 138: 190–196.

Prado-Alcala RA and Cobos-Zapiain GG (1979) Improvement of learned behavior through cholinergic stimulation of the caudate nucleus. *Neurosci. Lett.* 14: 253–258.

Prado-Alcala RA, Grinberg ZJ, Arditti ZL, et al. (1975) Learning deficits produced by chronic and reversible lesions of the corpus striatum in rats. *Physiol. Behav.* 15: 283–287.

Prado-Alcala RA, Signoret L, and Figueroa M (1981) Time-dependent retention deficits induced by post-training injections of atropine into the caudate nucleus. *Pharm. Biochem. Behav.* 15: 633–636.

Pych JC, Chang Q, Colon-Rivera C, and Gold PE (2005) Acetylcholine release in hippocampus and striatum during testing on a rewarded spontaneous alternation task. *Neurobiol. Learn. Mem.* 84(2): 93–101.

Reading PJ, Dunnett SB, and Robbins TW (1991) Dissociable roles of the ventral, medial and lateral striatum on the acquisition and performance of a complex visual stimulus response habit. *Behav. Brain Res.* 45: 147–161.

Ritchie BF, Aeschliman B, and Pierce P (1950) Studies in spatial learning: VIII. Place performance and acquisition of place dispositions. *J. Comp. Physiol. Psychol.* 43: 73–85.

Rolls ET (1994) Neurophysiology and cognitive functions of the striatum. *Rev. Neurolog.* 150(8–9): 648–660.

Rosvold HE (1968) The prefrontal cortex and caudate nucleus: A system for effecting correction in response mechanisms. In: Rupp C (ed.) *Mind as Tissue*, pp. 21–38. New York: Harper and Row.

Sage JR and Knowlton BJ (2000) Effects of US devaluation on win-stay and win-shift radial arm maze performance in rats. *Behav. Neurosci.* 114: 295–306.

Sakamoto T and Okaichi H (2001) Use of win-stay and win-shift strategies in place and cue tasks by medial caudate putamen (MCPu) lesioned rats. *Neurobiol. Learn. Mem.* 76: 192–208.

Salinas JA and White NM (1998) Contributions of the hippocampus, amygdala, and dorsal striatum to the response elicited by reward reduction. *Behav. Neurosci.* 112: 812–826.

Schroeder JP and Packard MG (2002) Posttraining intra-basolateral amygdala scopolamine impairs food- and amphetamine-induced conditioned place preferences. *Behav. Neurosci.* 116(5): 922–927.

Setlow B (1997) The nucleus accumbens and learning and memory. *J. Neurosci. Res.* 49: 515–521.

Sherry DF and Schacter DL (1987) Evolution of multiple memory systems. *Psychol. Rev.* 94(4): 439–454.

Squire LR and Zola-Morgan S (1991) The medial temporal lobe memory system. *Science* 253(5026): 1380–1386.

Squire LR, Knowlton B, and Musen G (1993) The structure and organization of memory. *Ann. Rev. Psychol.* 44: 453–495.

Teather LA, Packard MG, Smith DE, Ellis-Behnke RG, and Bazan NG (2005) Differential induction of c-Jun and Fos-like proteins in rat hippocampus and dorsal striatum after training in two water maze tasks. *Neurobiol. Learn. Mem.* 84(2): 75–84.

Teng E, Stefanacci L, Squire LR, and Zola SM (2000) Contrasting effects on discrimination learning after hippocampal lesions and conjoint hippocampal-caudate lesions in monkeys. *J. Neurosci.* 20: 3853–3863.

Thompson RF (2005) In search of memory traces. *Annu. Rev. Psychol.* 56: 1–23.

Thorndike EL (1933) A proof of the law of effect. *Science* 77: 173–175.

Tolman EC (1932) *Purposive Behavior in Animals and Men*. New York: Appleton-Century Crofts.

Tolman EC, Ritchie BF, and Kalish D (1946) Studies in spatial learning II. Place versus response learning. *J. Exp. Psychol.* 36(3): 221–229.

Tolman EC, Ritchie BF, and Kalish D (1947) Studies in spatial learning V. Response vs. place learning by the non-correction method. *J. Exp. Psychol.* 37(4): 285–292.

Van Hoesen GW, Yeterian EH, and Lavizzo-Mourey R (1981) Widespread corticostriate projections from temporal cortex of the rhesus monkey. *J. Comp. Neurol.* 199(2): 205–219.

Veening JG, Cornelissen FM, and Lieven JM (1980) The topical organization of the afferents to the caudatoputamen of the rat. A horseradish peroxidase study. *Neuroscience* 5: 1253–1268.

Viaud MD and White NM (1989) Dissociation of visual and olfactory conditioning in the neostriatum of rats. *Behav. Brain Res.* 32: 31–42.

Webster KE (1961) Cortico-striate interrelations in the albino rat. *J. Anatomy* 95: 532–544.

Webster KE (1065) The corticostriatal projection in the cat. *J. Anatomy* 99: 329–337.

Whishaw IQ, Mittlemann G, Bunch ST, and Dunnett SB (1987) Impairments in the acquisition, retention, and selection of spatial navigation strategies after medial caudate-putamen lesions in rats. *Behav. Brain Res.* 24: 125–138.

White NM (1989a) A functional hypothesis concerning the striatal matrix and patches: Mediation of S-R memory and reward. *Life Sci.* 45: 1943–1957.

White NM (1989b) Reward or reinforcement: What's the difference? *Neurosci. Biobehav. Rev.* 13: 181–186.

White NM (1996) Addictive drugs as reinforcers: Multiple partial actions on memory systems. *Addiction* 91(7): 921–949.

White NM (1997) Mnemonic functions of the basal ganglia. *Curr. Opin. Neurobiol.* 7: 164–169.

White NM and Major R (1978) Effect of pimozide on the improvement in learning produced by self-stimulation and water reinforcement. *Pharm. Biochem. Behav.* 8: 565–571.

White NM and McDonald RJ (2002) Multiple parallel memory systems in the brain of the rat. *Neurobiol. Learn. Mem.* 77(2): 125–184.

White NM and Viaud M (1991) Localized intracaudate dopamine D2 receptor activation during the post-training period improves memory for visual or olfactory conditioned emotional responses in rats. *Behav. Neural Biol.* 55(3): 255–269.

White NM, Viaud M, and Packard MG (1994) Dopaminergic-cholinergic function in neo-striatal memory function: Role of nigro-striatal terminals. In: Palomo T, Archer T, and Beninger R (eds.) *Strategies for Studying Brain Disorders, Vol. 2, Schizophrenia, Movement Disorders, and Age-Related Cognitive Disorders*, pp. 299–312. Madrid: Editorial Complutense.

Winocur G (1974) Functional dissociation within the caudate nucleus of rats. *J. Comp. Physiol. Psychol.* 86: 432–439.

Winocur G and Mills JA (1969) Effects of caudate lesions on avoidance behavior in rats. *J. Comp. Physiol. Psychol.* 65: 552–557.

Wood W, Quinn JM, and Kashy DA (2002) Habits in everyday life: Thought, emotion, and action. *J. Pers. Soc. Psychol.* 83(6): 1281–1297.

Yin HH and Knowlton BJ (2004) Contributions of striatal subregions to place and response learning. *Learn. Mem.* 11(4): 459–463.

Yin HH and Knowlton BJ (2006) The role of the basal ganglia in habit formation. *Nat. Rev. Neurosci.* 7(6): 464–476.

Yin HH, Knowlton BJ, and Balleine BW (2004) Lesions of dorsolateral striatum preserve outcome expectancy but

disrupt habit formation in instrumental learning. *Eur. J. Neurosci.* 19(1): 181–189.
Yin HH, Ostlund SB, Knowlton BJ, and Balleine BW (2005) The role of the dorsomedial striatum in instrumental conditioning. *Eur. J. Neurosci.* 22(2): 513–523.
Yin HH, Knowlton BJ, and Balleine BW (2006) Inactivation of dorsolateral striatum enhances sensitivity to changes in the action-outcome contingency in instrumental conditioning. *Behav. Brain Res.* 166(2): 189–196.
Zhou FM, Wilson CJ, and Dani JA (2002) Cholinergic interneuron characteristics and nicotinic properties in the striatum. *J. Neurobiol.* 53(4): 590–605.
Zis AP, Fibiger HC, and Phillips AG (1974) Reversal by l-dopa of impaired learning due to destruction of the dopaminergic nigro-striatal projection. *Science* 185: 960–963.

18 Sensitization and Habituation: Invertebrate

D. Fioravante, E. G. Antzoulatos, and J. H. Byrne, The University of Texas Medical School at Houston, Houston, TX, USA

18.1 Introduction

Survival of animals is dependent on their capacity to adapt to their environment by modifying their behavior. The experience-induced modification of behavior is a manifestation of learning, whereas memory is the retention of a learned behavior over time. A conceptual scheme that has driven the investigation of learning for the largest part of the twentieth century rests on the distinction between associative and nonassociative forms of learning. Nonassociative learning is best exemplified by habituation and sensitization. Habituation is defined as the gradual waning of a behavioral response to a weak or moderate stimulus that is presented repeatedly. Following habituation, the response may be restored to its initial state either passively with time (i.e., spontaneous recovery), or with the presentation of a novel stimulus (i.e., dishabituation). Sensitization is defined as the enhancement of a behavioral response elicited by a weak stimulus following another, usually noxious stimulus. Sensitization can also develop in response to a moderate stimulus that is presented repeatedly at relatively short intervals.

Associative learning refers to the formation of an association either between two stimuli (i.e., classical conditioning), or between a behavior and a stimulus (i.e., operant conditioning). In classical conditioning, a novel or weak stimulus (conditioned stimulus; CS) is paired with a stimulus that generally elicits a reflexive response (unconditioned stimulus and response, respectively; US and UR). After sufficient training with contingent CS-US presentations (which may be a single trial), the CS comes to elicit a learned response (conditioned response; CR), which often resembles the UR (or some aspect of it). Operant conditioning is an experimental procedure in which the behavior of an animal may be followed by either a desirable or an aversive stimulus, arranged by the experimenter. The desirable stimulus (e.g., food) will typically increase the future occurrence of this behavior (a process called positive reinforcement). An aversive stimulus (e.g., a noxious electric shock) will tend to decrease the future probability of this behavior (a process called punishment). A behavior can also be reinforced when it becomes contingent with the removal of an aversive stimulus from the animal's environment (i.e., negative reinforcement). Thus, through the processes of operant conditioning an animal learns the consequences of its behavior.

Humans and other animals are capable of displaying more complex forms of learning than the four types described above. However, these four types are likely to constitute the building blocks for more complex forms of learning. Thus, a major goal of neurobiologists is to explain the anatomical, biophysical, and molecular processes of the nervous system that underlie simple forms of learning and memory. Specifically, what parts of the nervous system are critical for learning? How is information about a learned event acquired and encoded in neuronal terms? How is information stored, and, once stored, how is it retrieved? Most neuroscientists believe that the answers to these questions lie in understanding the ways in which the properties of individual nerve cells in general, and synaptic connections, in particular, change when learning occurs. To that end, the investigation of neuronal mechanisms of learning and memory in invertebrates has been very fruitful over the past 40 years. This chapter will focus on mechanisms of habituation and sensitization in *Aplysia* and other invertebrates. A detailed discussion of mechanisms of associative learning in *Aplysia* and other invertebrates can be found in the next chapter (*See* Chapter 19).

18.2 Habituation and Sensitization in *Aplysia*

18.2.1 *Aplysia* Withdrawal Reflexes and Underlying Neural Circuits

One animal that is well suited for the examination of the molecular, cellular, morphological, and network mechanisms underlying neuronal plasticity and learning and memory is the marine mollusc *Aplysia.* This animal has a relatively simple nervous system with large, identifiable neurons that are accessible for detailed anatomical, biophysical, and biochemical studies. Neurons and neural circuits that mediate many behaviors in *Aplysia* have been identified. In several cases, these behaviors can be modified by learning. Moreover, specific loci within neural circuits at which modifications occur during learning have been identified and aspects of the cellular mechanisms underlying these modifications have been analyzed.

Two withdrawal reflexes of *Aplysia* have been used extensively to analyze the neuronal mechanisms contributing to nonassociative and associative learning (for reviews, see Hawkins and Kandel, 1984; Carew and Sahley, 1986; Byrne, 1987; Byrne et al., 1991, 1993). The first behavior is the siphon–gill withdrawal reflex. Within the mantle cavity is the respiratory organ of the animal, the gill, and protruding from the mantle cavity is the siphon (**Figure 1**). The

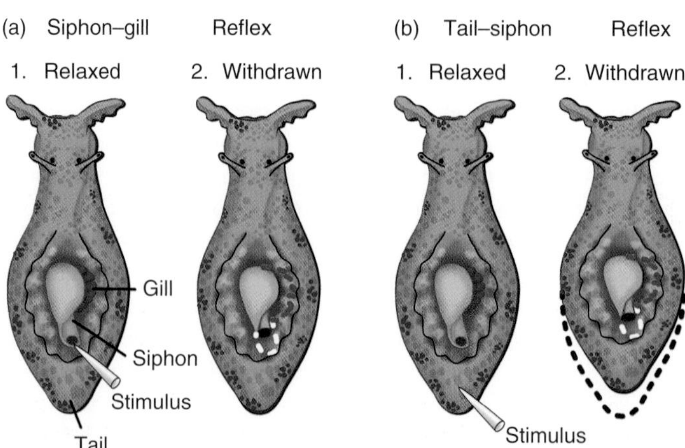

Figure 1 Siphon–gill and tail–siphon withdrawal reflexes of *Aplysia*. (a) Siphon–gill withdrawal. Dorsal view of *Aplysia* (1) Relaxed position. (2) A stimulus (e.g., a water jet, brief touch, or weak electric shock) applied to the siphon causes the siphon and the gill to withdraw into the mantle cavity. (b) Tail–siphon withdrawal reflex. (1) Relaxed position. (2) A stimulus applied to the tail elicits a reflex withdrawal of the tail and siphon.

siphon–gill withdrawal reflex is elicited when a tactile or electrical stimulus is delivered to the siphon and results in withdrawal of the siphon and gill (**Figure 1(a)**). A second behavior that has been examined extensively is the tail–siphon withdrawal reflex. Tactile or electrical stimulation of the tail elicits a coordinated set of defensive responses, two components of which are a reflex withdrawal of the tail and the siphon (**Figure 1(b)**).

A prerequisite for the analysis of the neural and molecular basis of learning is an understanding of the neural circuit that controls the behavior. The afferent limb of the siphon–gill withdrawal reflex consists of sensory neurons with somata in the abdominal ganglion. The siphon sensory neurons (SN) monosynaptically excite gill and siphon motor neurons (MN) that are also located in the abdominal ganglion (**Figure 2**). Activation of the gill and siphon motor neurons leads to contraction of the gill and siphon. Excitatory, inhibitory, and modulatory interneurons (IN) in the withdrawal circuit have also been identified, although only excitatory interneurons are illustrated in **Figure 2**. The afferent limb of the tail–siphon withdrawal reflex consists of a bilaterally symmetric cluster of sensory neurons that are located in the left and right pleural ganglia (Walters et al., 1983a). These sensory neurons make monosynaptic excitatory connections with motor neurons in the adjacent pedal ganglion, which produce withdrawal of the tail (**Figure 2**). In addition, the tail sensory neurons form synapses with various identified excitatory and inhibitory interneurons (Buonomano et al., 1992; Cleary and Byrne, 1993; Xu et al., 1994). Some of these interneurons activate motor neurons in the abdominal ganglion, which control reflex withdrawal of the siphon. Moreover, several additional neurons modulate the tail–siphon withdrawal reflex (Raymond and Byrne, 1994; Cleary et al., 1995) (**Figure 3(a1)**).

The sensory neurons for both the siphon–gill and tail–siphon withdrawal reflexes are similar and appear to be important plastic elements in the neural circuits. Changes in their membrane properties and the strength of their synaptic connections (synaptic efficacy) are associated with learning and memory. Moreover, the properties of these neurons are modulated by *in vitro* analogs of behavioral training.

18.2.2 Habituation

Habituation, perhaps the simplest form of nonassociative learning, refers to the gradual waning of the responses elicited by a repeatedly presented stimulus. Repeated presentation of a relatively weak stimulus will most probably lead to habituation, whereas repeated presentation of a relatively strong stimulus

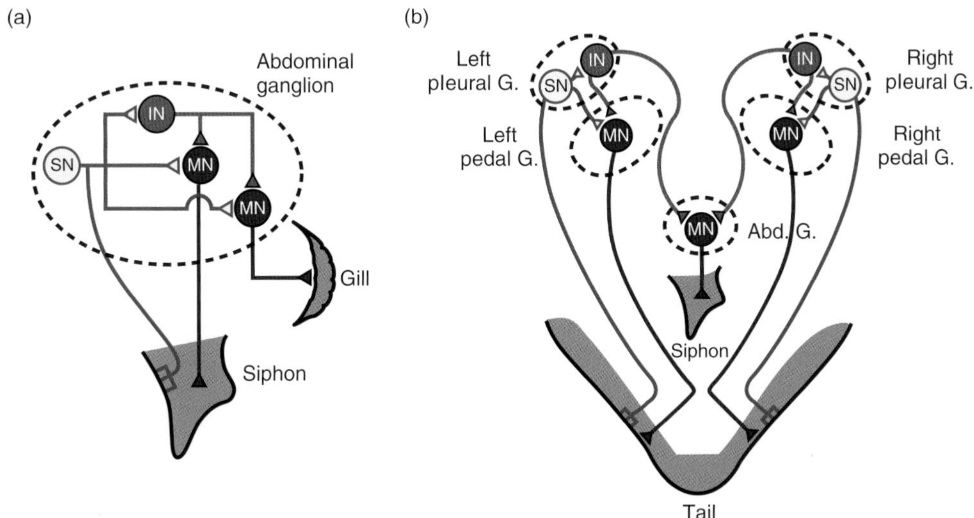

Figure 2 Simplified circuit diagrams of the siphon–gill (a) and tail–siphon (b) withdrawal reflexes. Stimuli activate the afferent terminals of mechanoreceptor sensory neurons (SN) whose somata are located in central ganglia. The sensory neurons make excitatory synaptic connections (triangles) with interneurons (IN) and motor neurons (MN). The excitatory interneurons provide a parallel pathway for excitation of the motor neurons. Action potentials elicited in the motor neurons, triggered by the combined input from the SNs and INs, propagate out peripheral nerves to activate muscle cells and produce the subsequent reflex withdrawal of the organs. Modulatory neurons (not shown here but see **Figure 3(a1)**), such as those containing serotonin (5-HT), regulate the properties of the circuit elements, and, consequently, the strength of the behavioral responses.

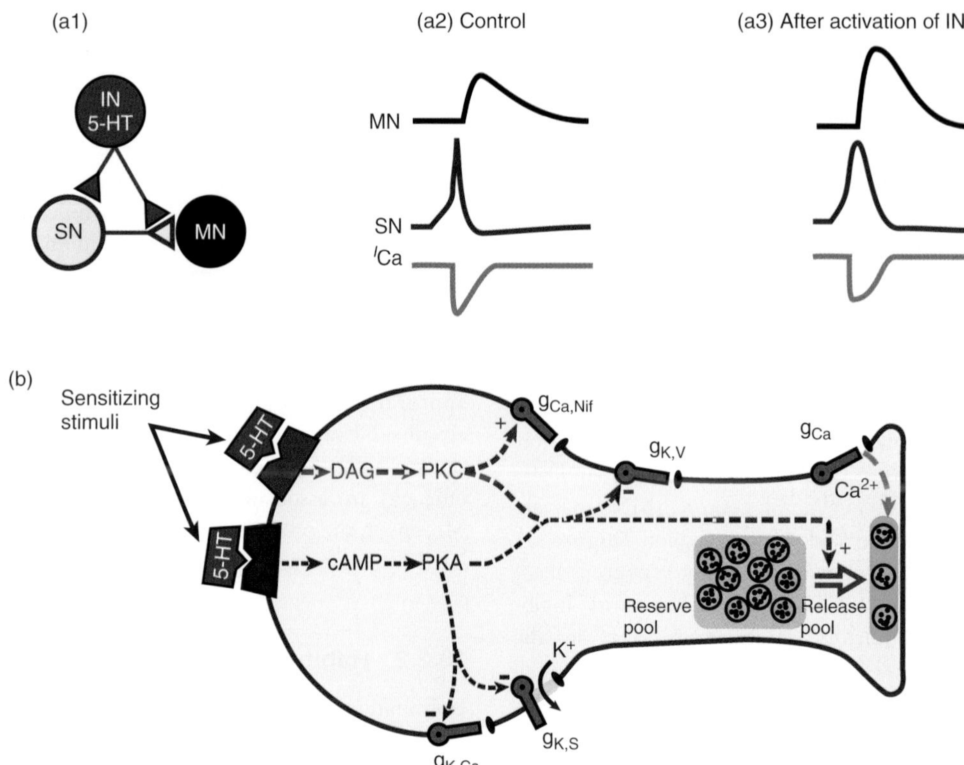

Figure 3 Model of heterosynaptic facilitation of the sensorimotor connection that contributes to short-term sensitization in *Aplysia*. (a1) Sensitizing stimuli activate facilitatory interneurons (IN) that release modulatory transmitters, one of which is 5-HT. The modulator leads to an alteration of the properties of the sensory neuron (SN). (a2, a3) An action potential in a SN after the sensitizing stimulus results in greater transmitter release and hence a larger postsynaptic potential in the motor neuron (MN) than an action potential prior to the sensitizing stimulus. For short-term sensitization the enhancement of transmitter release is due, at least in part, to broadening of the action potential and an enhanced flow of Ca^{2+} into the sensory neuron. (b) Molecular events in the sensory neuron. 5-HT released from the facilitatory interneuron (Part a1) binds to at least two distinct classes of receptors on the outer surface of the membrane of the sensory neuron, which leads to the transient activation of two intracellular second messengers: DAG and cAMP. These second messengers, acting though their respective protein kinases, affect multiple cellular processes, the combined effects of which lead to enhanced transmitter release when a subsequent action potential is fired in the sensory neuron. See section 18.2.3.1 for abbreviation definitions.

may lead to sensitization, which is discussed in the next section of the chapter. Habituation is generally distinguished from simple fatigue or sensory adaptation because responsiveness can be rapidly restored (dishabituated) by the presentation of a novel stimulus to the animal. The parametric features of habituation have been previously described in detail by Thompson and Spencer (1966).

Habituation shares some features with more complex forms of learning. First, habituation has a temporal gradient. Similar to most forms of learning, each trial has only a transient effect, which necessitates the presentation of multiple trials. Second, the interval at which training trials are presented is critical. Massing many trials together may lead to faster, albeit only short-lived habituation. In contrast, spacing trials too far apart may lead to little or no habituation. Therefore, an optimal intertrial interval exists, which is determined by the stimulus features and the response system. Third, the effects of habituation training are reversible. As mentioned above, they can be reversed spontaneously with the passage of time (spontaneous recovery), or they may be reversed by the presentation of a novel stimulus (dishabituation). Fourth, habituation learning is stimulus-specific. Although habituation can generalize to novel stimuli, this generalization is limited and depends on the degree of physical similarity between the trained and novel stimuli. Habituation is an indispensable form of learning. It is probably the earliest manifestation of the ability of all animals to store and retrieve the memory of a stimulus, as well as the ability to filter out stimuli that are inconsequential. The latter is a necessary element of selective attention, which places behavior under the dynamic control of stimuli that carry important behavioral contingencies.

A major step in the understanding of neural mechanisms of habituation was made in the early 1970s (Pinsker et al., 1970; Carew and Kandel, 1973). In a group of three seminal articles, it was reported that the siphon–gill withdrawal reflex of *Aplysia* can display habituation, that habituation was accompanied by a decrease in the spike activity of gill motor neurons in response to tactile stimulation of the siphon, and that an activity-induced decrease in the efficacy of sensorimotor synapses could be responsible for the reduced responsiveness of motor neurons and for behavioral habituation (Castellucci et al., 1970, Kupfermann et al., 1970; Pinsker et al., 1970). Starting with those early reports, behavioral habituation of withdrawal reflexes became tightly linked to homosynaptic depression of sensorimotor synapses. Since then, the vast majority of research studies that aimed at understanding the mechanisms of habituation focused on understanding the mechanisms of synaptic depression, which, similar to habituation, can appear in both short- and long-term forms.

18.2.2.1 Short-term depression of Aplysia sensorimotor synapses

Quantal analysis of sensorimotor synapses suggested that short-term homosynaptic depression involves primarily a decrease in presynaptic transmitter release (Castellucci and Kandel, 1974). The presynaptic nature of synaptic depression was also supported by a more recent report that repeated application of exogenous glutamate to the postsynaptic neuron did not result in depression, that blockade of postsynaptic glutamate receptors did not block depression, and that synaptic depression did not correlate with changes in the amplitude of miniature excitatory postsynaptic potentials (mEPSPs) (Armitage and Siegelbaum, 1998). To account for the depressive effect of repeated activity of sensory neurons on transmitter release, an early model of depression relied on cumulative inactivation of calcium channels and decline in the calcium entering the presynaptic terminal and triggering release (Klein et al., 1980).

Extensive parametric analysis of the kinetics of depression and recovery from depression as a function of the stimulation frequency revealed that the mechanisms must be more complex than just a decrease in calcium influx or a depletion of presynaptic vesicles (Byrne, 1982). A quantitative model of transmission at the sensorimotor synapse suggested that the inactivation kinetics of presynaptic calcium channels cannot account for the kinetics of depression; neither does simple depletion of releasable vesicles (Gingrich and Byrne, 1985). Rather, the model suggested the existence of dynamic interactions between use-dependent depletion of readily releasable vesicles and calcium-dependent mobilization of stored vesicles to supply the releasable ones. This model of synaptic depression was supported by morphological studies of the sensorimotor synapse, which indicated that the fraction of readily releasable vesicles decreased with activity, parallel to synaptic depression (Bailey and Chen, 1988b).

A subsequent study of spontaneous release from cultured sensory neurons revealed that synaptic depression was accompanied by a decrease in the frequency of mEPSPs (Eliot et al., 1994). However, the change in mini EPSP frequency did not parallel the synaptic depression in magnitude or in duration. This finding argued against the depletion of presynaptic terminals with releasable vesicles as the sole mechanism of depression, and suggested that depression may be due to a change in excitation–secretion coupling as well. However, this decrease in excitation–secretion coupling does not appear to be due to the decrease in calcium influx that had been previously suggested (Klein et al., 1980): Calcium imaging of cultured sensory neurons revealed that the calcium transients are unaffected by repetitive activity (Armitage and Siegelbaum, 1998).

Based on theoretical and statistical analyses of transmission at the sensorimotor synapse, another model of synaptic depression put forth the activity-dependent inactivation of individual release sites, proposing the transient switching off of presynaptic release machinery following an action potential (Royer et al., 2000). A similar model of synaptic depression arising from inactivation of release sites was suggested by Gover et al. (2002). Finally, the comparison of transmitter release from cultured sensory neurons stimulated by hypertonic solutions versus electrical activity revealed that both types of stimuli draw transmitter from the same presynaptic pool, and suggested that depression is mediated by both depletion of releasable transmitter and a change in excitation–secretion coupling (Zhao and Klein, 2002). Thus, the most recently proposed model of depression of sensorimotor synapses relies again on activity-dependent depletion of releasable vesicles, acknowledging though that there must be at least one other process that contributes as well.

Despite their differences, the studies outlined in this section have two common elements. First, they all supported the presynaptic nature of depression. Second, they all employed repetitive stimulation of the synapse at intervals at least as long as 1 s. However, when the sensorimotor synapse is stimulated at 10 Hz (100-ms interval), but not at 1 Hz, depression of evoked excitatory postsynaptic potentials (EPSPs) partly results from desensitization of the postsynaptic receptors (Antzoulatos et al., 2003). Therefore, both the kinetics of synaptic depression (Byrne, 1982; Eliot et al., 1994) and the mechanisms underlying it depend on the stimulation regime.

Another form of short-term depression of *Aplysia* sensorimotor synapses can be elicited by brief exposure to the neuropeptide Phe-Met-Arg-Phe-NH_2 (FMRFa). Because activation of a third type of synapse, a modulatory one, and release of a neuromodulator are required, this form of plasticity is termed heterosynaptic. In contrast, depression arising exclusively from intrinsic activity is termed homosynaptic depression. FMRFa-immunoreactive inhibitory interneurons have been identified that innervate tail and siphon sensory neurons (Mackey et al., 1987; Small et al., 1992; Xu et al., 1994). These interneurons are activated by shock to nerves that innervate the tail, and stimulation of these neurons inhibits sensorimotor synapses. However, the extent to which activation of these FMRFa-immunoreactive neurons contributes to habituation has not been determined.

Applying FMRFa to sensory neurons leads to a hyperpolarization of the membrane potential, a decrease in the duration of the action potential, and inhibition of synaptic transmission via the modulation of potassium conductances (Abrams et al., 1984; Ocorr and Byrne, 1985; Belardetti et al., 1987; Critz et al., 1991; Pieroni and Byrne, 1992). Moreover, FMRFa directly affects presynaptic Ca^{2+} currents (Blumenfeld et al., 1990; Edmonds et al., 1990) and the release machinery itself, as indicated by a decrease in the frequency of mEPSPs (Dale and Kandel, 1990). The second messenger mediating the actions of FMRFa seems to be arachidonic acid (AA) produced by phospholipid metabolism (Piomelli et al., 1987) and its downstream metabolite 12-hydroperoxyeicosatetraenoic acid (12-HPETE) (Buttner et al., 1989). Recently, FMRFa was found to inhibit one member of the MAP kinase family, extracellular signal-regulated protein kinase (ERK), but activate another, p38 mitogen-activated protein kinase (p38 MAPK) (Guan et al., 2003; Fioravante et al., 2006). The latter probably activates a phospholipase A2 molecule, which in turn can release AA from phospholipids (Piomelli, 1991). FMRFa also engages protein phosphatases in regulating the outward potassium currents (Ichinose and Byrne, 1991), in particular protein phosphatase 1 (PP1). In other systems, p38 MAPK can activate PP1 (Westermarck et al., 2001), raising the interesting possibility that FMRFa exercises its actions on sensory neuron conductances through a p38 MAPK-PP1 pathway.

18.2.2.2 Long-term depression of Aplysia *sensorimotor synapses*

Repetitive stimulation of *Aplysia* withdrawal reflexes can lead to both short- and long-term habituation (Pinsker et al., 1970; Carew and Kandel, 1973; Stopfer et al., 1996). Short- and long-term habituation share aspects of a common mechanism, synaptic depression. However, whereas short-term synaptic depression arises primarily from transient changes in release, long-term depression has been attributed to persistent structural changes in sensory neurons (Bailey and Chen, 1988a). Extensive morphological analyses of sensory neurons from habituated animals have revealed that the number of synaptic contacts is reduced compared to controls. Moreover, the structure of presynaptic terminals is affected, with fewer synaptic vesicles and reduced size of active zones (the sites of transmitter release).

In addition, activation of sensory neurons at 2 Hz for 15 min induces prolonged (at least 80 min) homosynaptic depression (long-term depression; LTD) of isolated *Aplysia* sensorimotor synapses in cell culture (Lin and Glanzman, 1996). This form of depression relies on activation of postsynaptic *N*-methyl-D-aspartate (NMDA)-like receptors and is sensitive to postsynaptic Ca^{2+}, because infusion of the calcium chelator BAPTA into the postsynaptic motor neuron blocks induction of LTD, but not short-term synaptic depression. Similarly, prolonged habituation of the siphon-elicited gill withdrawal reflex in reduced preparations was recently shown to depend on activity of postsynaptic glutamate receptors both of the NMDA and non-NMDA type (Ezzeddine and Glanzman, 2003).

A more extensively studied form of long-term synaptic depression in *Aplysia* is elicited by repeated application of the neuropeptide FMRFa (Montarolo et al., 1988; Guan et al., 2003). FMRFa-induced LTD requires transcription, translation (Montarolo et al., 1988; Bailey et al., 1992), but also gene silencing (Guan et al., 2002). Inducing events in FMRFa-mediated LTD include activation of p38 MAPK and recruitment of the transcription repressor CREB2 (cAMP response element binding protein) to the promoter region of genes such as *c/ebp* (Guan et al., 2003; Fioravante et al., 2006).

Little is known about the mechanisms underlying consolidation of LTD. Two genes that are regulated by FMRFa and could be important in the consolidation of LTD are sensorin (Sun et al., 2001) and *Aplysia* cell adhesion molecule (Schacher et al., 2000), even though the requirement of their regulation for LTD has not been demonstrated. Finally, expression of heterosynaptic LTD is accompanied by morphological changes, including loss of presynaptic varicosities and retraction of neurites (Schacher and Montarolo, 1991).

18.2.3 Sensitization

Sensitization refers to the augmentation of the behavioral response elicited by a test stimulus. Sensitization to a test stimulus can be induced in one of two ways. First, it can be induced by presentation of another, usually strong stimulus. An example of such sensitization is pseudoconditioning, where an increase in responsiveness to the CS in a classical conditioning procedure may not be due to associative learning (as in classical conditioning), but instead due to the sensitization induced by the strong US. Second, sensitization can be induced by the mere repetition of the test stimulus. As mentioned above, the repetition of a weak stimulus will lead to habituation of the behavioral response, whereas repetition of a moderate to strong stimulus may lead to sensitization. This form of sensitization can sometimes appear as a transient rise in response magnitude before habituation eventually ensues.

Both forms of sensitization have been studied in *Aplysia*, with major emphasis on the former one described above. Similar to habituation, sensitization was also attributed early on to plasticity of the sensorimotor synapse (see next section). Although habituation was attributed to homosynaptic depression of the synapse, sensitization was attributed to heterosynaptic facilitation, induced by the diffuse release of neuromodulators, such as serotonin. Also similar to habituation, sensitization can appear both in short- and long-term forms, which have been extensively studied in their neuronal analogs, short and long-term synaptic facilitation.

18.2.3.1 Short-term sensitization

In *Aplysia*, sensitization of withdrawal reflexes can be induced by electric shocks to the tail or the lateral body wall of the animal (Carew et al., 1971). Peripheral electric shock has been shown to modulate transmission at the sensorimotor synapse through heterosynaptic facilitation (Carew et al., 1971; Walters et al., 1983a,b).

Several lines of evidence suggest that serotonin (5-HT) is the neurotransmitter involved in heterosynaptic facilitation. First, 5-HT is present in *Aplysia* hemolymph, and its concentration increases in sensitized animals (Levenson et al., 1999). Recent studies also indicated that 5-HT concentration increases in several regions of the *Aplysia* CNS in response to nerve stimulation (Marinesco and Carew, 2002). Second, serotonergic cells are present (Hawkins, 1989; Nolen and Carew, 1994) and serotonergic fibers are in close proximity to sensory neurons (SNs) (Zhang et al., 1991; Marinesco and Carew, 2002; Zhang et al., 2003). Third, depletion of endogenous 5-HT by addition of a neurotoxin (5,7-DHT) blocks the ability of tail stimuli to sensitize the gill-withdrawal reflex (Glanzman et al., 1989). Along the same lines, application of the 5-HT receptor antagonist cyproheptadine blocks facilitation induced by nerve stimulation (Mercer et al., 1991). Finally, exogenously applied 5-HT mimics the actions of tail stimulation both in facilitating the strength of synaptic connections and in increasing the strength of reflex responses (Brunelli et al., 1976; Walters et al., 1983a, b; Abrams et al., 1984; Zhang et al., 1997), and nerve shock-induced 5-HT release correlates with synaptic plasticity (Marinesco et al., 2006).

The conclusions drawn from studies conducted in the 1970s and 1980s led to the formulation of a model for short-term sensitization, according to which sensitizing stimuli activate serotonergic facilitatory interneurons, releasing 5-HT and activating a serial cascade of events in the sensory neurons. The binding of 5-HT to one class of receptors on the outer surface of the membrane of the sensory neurons leads to the activation of adenylyl cyclase, which in turn, leads to an elevation of the intracellular level of the second messenger adenosine-3′,5′-monophosphate (cyclic AMP, cAMP) in sensory neurons. When cAMP binds to the regulatory subunit of cAMP-dependent protein kinase (protein kinase A, PKA), the catalytic subunit is freed and can now add phosphate groups to specific substrate proteins and, hence, alter their functional properties (Bernier et al., 1982; Ocorr and Byrne, 1985; Pollock et al., 1985; Ocorr and Byrne, 1986; Ocorr et al., 1986; Sweatt et al., 1989). One effect of activated PKA is phosphorylation of a class of membrane channels (S-K^+ channels, named for their ability to be modulated by serotonin) and reduction of the S-K^+ conductance ($G_{K,S}$) (Klein and Kandel, 1980; Klein et al., 1982; Siegelbaum et al., 1982). Consequently, a test stimulus triggers a greater number of action potentials in the sensory neuron after sensitization. Each of these spikes is broader, leading to increased Ca^{2+} influx and enhanced transmitter release. As a result, the follower motor neuron is more intensely activated, and the behavioral response is enhanced (i.e., sensitized). Thus, it was previously believed that serotonin (5-HT) exerted all of its actions in the sensory neurons via the cAMP-mediated reduction of $G_{K,S}$.

Later studies, however, indicated that the effects of 5-HT are more complex than originally suggested. Not only $G_{K,S}$ is modulated by 5-HT, but also at least three other conductances: 5-HT increases a dihydropyridine-sensitive Ca^{2+} current ($G_{Ca,Nif}$) (Braha et al., 1990; Edmonds et al., 1990), decreases a component of the Ca^{2+}-activated K^+ current ($G_{K,Ca}$) (Walsh and Byrne, 1989), and modulates a voltage-dependent K^+ current ($G_{K,V}$) (Baxter and Byrne, 1989, 1990a; Goldsmith and Abrams, 1992; Hochner and Kandel, 1992; Sugita et al., 1994; White et al., 1994). The effects of channel modulation appear to be synergistic, favoring increased sensory neuron excitability or transmitter release. Spike broadening, which has a major impact on transmitter release, is probably due to modulation of $G_{K,V}$ rather than $G_{K,S}$, whereas $G_{K,S}$ and $G_{K,Ca}$ appear to be critical for regulating membrane excitability, with modest effects on spike duration (Baxter and Byrne, 1990a, b). The 5-HT-induced increase in $G_{Ca,Nif}$ does not appear to contribute to enhanced transmitter release, as this conductance is not directly responsible for triggering exocytosis of synaptic vesicles, although it may contribute to accumulation of presynaptic calcium during intense activity (Edmonds et al., 1990).

Two of the three 5-HT-induced effects on K^+ conductances (modulation of $G_{K,S}$ and $G_{K,Ca}$) are mediated exclusively by PKA. The effects of 5-HT on $G_{K,V}$ appear to be caused by activation of two second messenger pathways, only one of which is the cAMP pathway mentioned above (Hochner and Kandel, 1992). Serotonin also appears to act through another class of receptors to increase the level of the second messenger diacylglycerol (DAG). DAG activates protein kinase C (PKC), leading to its translocation (Sossin, 2007). PKC, like PKA, is involved in the spike-duration-dependent process of facilitation (Sugita et al., 1992, 1994). In addition, a nifedipine-sensitive Ca^{2+} conductance ($G_{Ca,Nif}$) and the delayed K^+ conductance ($G_{K,V}$) are regulated by PKC. The modulation of $G_{K,V}$ contributes importantly to the increase in duration of the action potential (**Figure 3(a3)**). Because of its small magnitude, the modulation of $G_{Ca,Nif}$ appears to play a minor role in the facilitatory process.

The role of ionic conductances in modulation of synaptic transmission is relatively well understood. Less well understood is a second process that has a profound effect on synaptic transmission, but which is independent of spike duration (spike-duration independent process; SDI). The existence of the second process was first postulated based on a mathematical model of a sensory neuron (Gingrich and Byrne, 1985, 1987). Experimental studies have provided support for the SDI process (Hochner et al., 1986; Braha et al., 1990; Pieroni and Byrne, 1992; Klein, 1993, 1994). Although the mechanism is poorly understood, the SDI process is likely to include mobilization of vesicles into a readily releasable pool. This process appears to be particularly important when the sensory neuron is depressed by previous low frequency (ISI = 10 s) stimulation (Braha et al., 1990; Ghirardi et al., 1992; Pieroni and Byrne, 1992; Klein, 1993; Sugita et al., 1997), making the SDI process an attractive candidate for dishabituation mechanisms and for maintaining synaptic strength during high levels of release (see below). The relative contribution of PKA and PKC to facilitation of previously depressed synapses varies as a function of the extent of preexisting depression. In nondepressed synapses, 5-HT produces short-term facilitation that can be blocked completely by inhibitors of PKA but is not affected by H7, an inhibitor of PKC. In contrast, as synapses become more depressed, the inhibitor of PKC becomes progressively more effective in blocking 5-HT-induced short-term facilitation (Braha et al., 1990; Ghirardi et al., 1992; Sugita et al., 1997).

Nevertheless, it has only recently become clear that, apart from dishabituation, sensitization may also involve facilitation of depressed synapses, because a moderate stimulus does not trigger a single spike in the sensory neuron, but a burst of spikes (Phares et al., 2003). By the end of this burst, the motor neuron responses depress substantially, regardless of the state of the first response. Enhancement of these depressed responses by sensitization is likely to involve the SDI process.

Progress has been made in understanding the second-messenger cascades involved in the SDI process and identified synaptic terminal proteins as downstream targets. These targets include synapsin and SNAP-25, highly conserved synaptic proteins that appear to regulate homosynaptic depression and short-term heterosynaptic facilitation. Synapsin is localized in presynaptic nerve terminals, where it interacts with synaptic vesicles, actin and spectrin (Jovanovic et al., 1996; Matsubara et al., 1996; Hosaka et al., 1999; Zimmer et al., 2000). Because the interaction of synapsin with actin and synaptic vesicles is regulated by phosphorylation, synapsin is believed to reversibly tether synaptic vesicles in a reserve pool, thereby regulating vesicle availability and mobilization (Hilfiker et al., 1998, 1999). The *Aplysia* isoform of synapsin (apSyn) contains the same domain arrangement as other vertebrate and invertebrate synapsins (Angers et al., 2002). Several potential regulatory sites have been identified throughout the sequence of apSyn. In addition to the PKA/CAMK I consensus phosphorylation site in the A-domain, two potential MAPK sites and several PKC sites are detected. In ganglia and in cultured cells, synapsin localizes in presynaptic varicosities and forms distinct puncta, presumably due to the aggregation of protein and its interaction with vesicle membranes (Angers et al., 2002).

ApSyn is phosphorylated following application of 5-HT, which results in short-term facilitation of the sensorimotor synapse. This phosphorylation requires PKA and MAPK. Also, 5-HT results in a reduction in the number of apSyn puncta, which represents the dissociation of the protein from synaptic vesicles (and probably the cytoskeleton) upon phosphorylation. The reduction of apSyn puncta after 5-HT is dynamic and reversible, and it requires PKA and MAPK activity (Angers et al., 2002). Finally, recent results from apSyn overexpression experiments indicated that synapsin regulates basal synaptic strength, homosynaptic depression and 5-HT-induced recovery from depression (Fioravante et al., 2007).

Based on the results described above, the following model has been proposed (Angers et al., 2002): At rest, most vesicles are clustered in a filamentous protein network forming the reserve pool, and 5-HT can modulate the function of apSyn by altering its phosphorylation state via PKA and MAPK. Upon phosphorylation, apSyn molecules dissociate from the vesicles and the cytoskeleton, allowing vesicles to be mobilized to release sites when they become depleted.

Another highly conserved synaptic protein, SNAP-25, has recently been implicated in the regulation of short-term facilitation, especially in previously depressed synapses. In these synapses, PKC, rather than PKA, predominantly mediates 5-HT-induced dedepression (Ghirardi et al., 1992; Dumitriu et al., 2006) through phosphorylation of SNAP-25 (Houeland et al., 2007) and probably other, yet unidentified synaptic targets.

18.2.3.2 Long-term sensitization

Whereas short-term sensitization can be induced by a single brief stimulus, the induction of long-term sensitization, whose memory can persist for days to weeks, requires a more extensive training regime (e.g., repeating the sensitizing stimuli over a 1.5-h period). Compared with short-term sensitization, less is known about the cellular mechanisms underlying long-term sensitization. One simplifying hypothesis is that the mechanisms underlying the expression of long-term sensitization are the same as those of short-term sensitization, but extended in time. Some evidence supports this hypothesis. For example, similar to short-term sensitization, K^+ conductances and excitability of sensory neurons are also modified by long-term sensitization (Scholz and Byrne, 1987; Cleary et al., 1998).

Biophysical properties of neurons mediating the *Aplysia* withdrawal reflexes have been examined following long-term sensitization induced by a single 1.5-h-long training session (1-day protocol), or by four such sessions repeated at 24-h intervals (4-day protocol). Twenty-four hours following the 1-day protocol of long-term sensitization training, three biophysical properties of tail sensory neurons are altered: Neuronal excitability, the after-depolarization following long current pulses, and the after-depolarization following short current pulses (Cleary et al., 1998). In addition to the biophysical properties of sensory neurons, 1-day training affects two properties of motor neurons: The resting membrane potential is increased and the spike threshold is decreased (Cleary et al., 1998). Long-term sensitization also correlates with facilitation of the sensorimotor synapses, both after 1-day training and after 4-day training (Frost et al., 1985; Cleary et al., 1998; Wainwright et al., 2004; Antzoulatos and Byrne, 2007). Surprisingly, although short-term sensitization is associated with spike broadening in sensory neurons (see above), long-term sensitization is associated with spike narrowing in sensory neurons (Antzoulatos and Byrne, 2007). The functional effects of the spike narrowing are not clear, but narrowing of the spike may be related to a decrease in spike propagation failures that occurs in response to high-frequency peripheral stimulation after long-term sensitization.

Another branch of the research on long-term sensitization has focused on the morphological effects of sensitization training on sensory neurons. One-day training for long-term sensitization does not induce gross structural changes in sensory neuron morphology, even though it does induce long-term changes in excitability and synaptic strength (Cleary et al., 1998). In contrast to 1-day training, 4-day training is more effective at inducing outgrowth when compared to untrained controls (Bailey and Chen, 1983; Wainwright et al., 2002;, 2004). This outgrowth includes an increase in the total arborization length of sensory neuron branches, in the number of sensory neuron branch points and varicosities, and in the number of synaptic contacts between sensory and motor neurons (Wainwright et al., 2002, 2004).

Biochemical correlates of long-term sensitization have also been examined. Most of these studies have focused on the induction phase, identifying changes in levels of the second messenger cAMP and regulation of several proteins (Barzilai et al., 1989; Eskin et al., 1989; Muller and Carew, 1998; Zwartjes et al., 1998). Progress has been made in identifying biochemical changes related to the consolidation or expression of long-term sensitization. Recently, long-term training was observed to produce enhanced uptake of glutamate (Levenson et al., 2000), the putative transmitter of sensory neurons (Antzoulatos and Byrne, 2004). This increase in uptake occurred in sensory neurons and appeared to be caused by an increased number of glutamate transporters. Although the functional role of this enhanced uptake is presently unclear, it indicates that clearance of glutamate from the cleft may be an important factor in the regulation of synaptic efficacy (Chin et al., 2002b). A change in glutamate uptake could potentially exert a significant effect on synaptic efficacy by regulating the amount of transmitter available for release, the rate of clearance from the cleft, and thereby the duration of the EPSP and the degree of receptor desensitization (Antzoulatos et al., 2003).

A substantial amount of data indicates that the induction of both short- and long-term sensitization partly share common cellular pathways (**Figure 4**). For example, both forms of sensitization activate the cAMP/PKA cascade. In the long-term form, however, activation is prolonged and sufficient to induce gene transcription and new protein synthesis (Castellucci et al., 1989; Levenson et al., 1999). This finding is consistent with the relatively long duration of the training period required for inducing long-term sensitization and the lasting duration of the effects. cAMP presumably exerts its major effects by activation of PKA (Schacher et al., 1988; Scholz and Byrne, 1988; O'Leary et al., 1995; Muller and Carew, 1998). Activated PKA translocates to the nucleus,

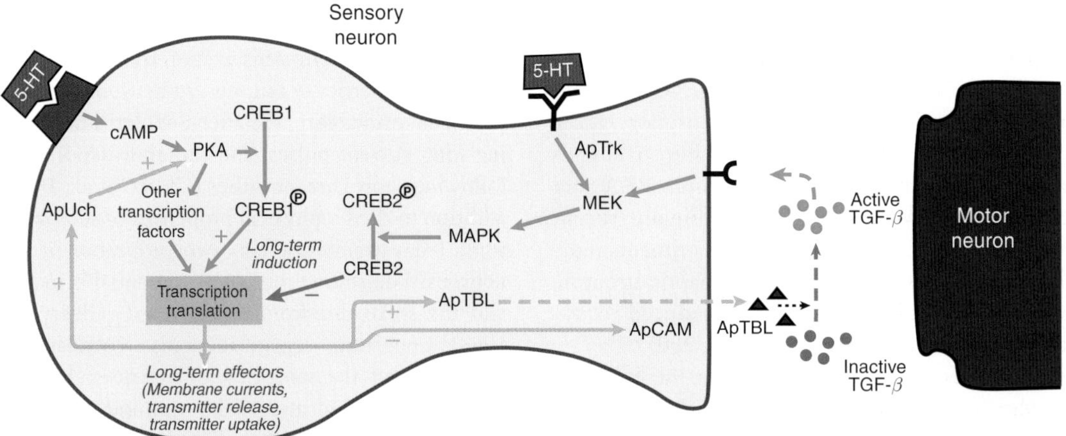

Figure 4 Simplified scheme of the mechanisms in sensory neurons that contribute to long-term sensitization. Sensitization training leads to release of 5-HT, which activates the cAMP/PKA cascade and the ERK MAPK cascade. PKA phosphorylates and activates CREB1, whereas ERK phosphorylates and inhibits CREB2. CREB1 acts as an initiator of gene transcription and CREB2 acts as a repressor of gene transcription. The combined effects of activation of CREB1 and inhibition of CREB2 lead to regulation of the synthesis of at least ten proteins, only three of which (apTBL, apUCH, apCAM) are shown. ApTBL is believed to activate latent forms of TGF-β, which can then bind to receptors on the sensory neuron and further activate MAPK. See section 18.2.3.2 for abbreviation definitions.

where it phosphorylates and activates the transcription factor CREB1. Activated CREB1, which is necessary for long-term facilitation (LTF), binds to the promoter region of responsive genes, and induces their expression (Dash et al., 1990, 1991; Bartsch et al., 1998; Guan et al., 2002). A prolonged increase in cAMP also leads to the induction and subsequent expression of a gene encoding the protein ubiquitin C-terminal hydrolase (Ap-Uch). This neuron-specific enzyme enhances the degradation of certain proteins including the regulatory subunits of PKA (Hegde et al., 1997). With fewer regulatory subunits of PKA to bind to catalytic subunits, the catalytic subunits are persistently active and may contribute to long-term facilitation of transmitter release (Muller and Carew, 1998).

In addition to the cAMP/PKA cascade, sensitization training and prolonged 5-HT application also activate MAPK (Sacktor and Schwartz, 1990; Sossin and Schwartz, 1992, 1993; Sossin et al., 1994; Sossin and Schwartz, 1994; Martin et al., 1997a; Sharma et al., 2003; Sharma and Carew, 2004). Prolonged application of 5-HT results in persistent phosphorylation (and subsequent activation) of MAPK though activation of a tyrosine receptor kinase-like molecule (ApTrk) (Ormond et al., 2004), cAMP (Martin et al., 1997b; Michael et al., 1998) (but see Dyer et al., 2003), and/or the neuropeptide sensorin (Hu et al., 2004b). Activated MAPK translocates to the nucleus (Martin et al., 1997b) where it may regulate gene transcription, possibly through inhibition of the transcription factor CREB2 (Bartsch et al., 1995). Since under basal conditions CREB2 acts as a repressor of gene transcription, its inhibition may lead to derepression and net gene expression in concert with CREB1 (**Figure 4**). The involvement of additional transcription factors such as ApAF (*Aplysia* activating factor) (Bartsch et al., 2000; Lee et al., 2006) and ApLLP (*Aplysia* LAPS18-like protein) (Kim et al., 2003a, 2006) in learning-induced gene expression is currently being investigated.

Recently, it has become clear that the role of transcription factors in long-term memory formation is not limited to the induction phase but may also extend to the consolidation phase. For example, prolonged treatment with 5-HT leads to the binding of CREB1 to the promoter of its own gene and induces CREB1 synthesis (Mohamed et al., 2005). The newly synthesized CREB1 appears to be necessary for LTF (Liu et al., 2008). This observation agrees well with earlier findings that the requirement for gene expression is not limited to the induction phase. The necessity of prolonged transcription and translation for LTF observed at 24 h persists for at least 7–9 h after induction (Alberini et al., 1994; O'Leary et al., 1995). These results suggest that CREB1 can regulate its own level of expression, giving rise to a CREB1 positive feedback loop that is necessary for memory consolidation.

In addition to CREB1, several other proteins are regulated during LTF. One of the newly synthesized proteins, intermediate filament protein (IFP) (Noel et al., 1993), is thought to contribute to the new growth observed after prolonged treatment with 5-HT. Increased synthesis of calmodulin (CaM) (Zwartjes et al., 1998) also occurs, but the functional significance of this effect has not been determined. The neuropeptide sensorin is also upregulated by 5-HT and is thought to contribute to the formation and stabilization of new synapses (Hu et al., 2004a,b).

Aplysia tolloid/BMP-like protein (apTBL-1) (Liu et al., 1997) is also synthesized in response to increases in cAMP. Tolloid and the related molecule BMP-1 appear to function as secreted Zn^{2+} proteases. A signal sequence at the amino terminal indicates that apTBL-1 is secreted to the extracellular space where one of its actions may be to activate members of the TGF-β family of growth factors (**Figure 4**). Indeed, in sensory neurons, TGF-β mimics the effects of 5-HT in that it produces long-term increases in synaptic strength and excitability of the sensory neurons (Zhang et al., 1997; Farr et al., 1999). Interestingly, TGF-β activates the MEK/MAPK pathway in the sensory neurons and induces MAPK translocation to the nucleus (Chin et al., 2002a, 2006), where it phosphorylates CREB1 (Chin et al., 2006). This activation could yield another round of protein synthesis to further consolidate long-term sensitization.

LTF involves not only increased synthesis but also downregulation of proteins such as the regulatory subunit of PKA (discussed earlier in this section) and a homolog of neuronal cell adhesion molecule (NCAM). Downregulation of NCAM alters the interaction of the neuron with other cells and allows the restructuring of the axon arbor (Mayford et al., 1992; Bailey et al., 1997). The sensory neuron could then form additional connections with the same postsynaptic target or make new connections with other cells.

18.2.3.3 Other temporal domains for the memory of sensitization

Operationally, memory has frequently been divided into two temporal domains, short-term and long-term. It has become increasingly clear from studies of a number of memory systems that this distinction is overly restrictive. For example, in *Aplysia*, Carew and his colleagues (Sutton et al., 2001) and Kandel and his colleagues (Ghirardi et al., 1995) discovered an intermediate phase of memory that has distinctive temporal characteristics and a unique molecular signature. The intermediate-phase memory (ITM) for sensitization is expressed approximately 30 min to 3 h after the beginning of training. It declines completely prior to the onset of long-term memory. Like long-term sensitization, its induction requires protein synthesis, but unlike long-term memory, it does not require mRNA synthesis. The expression of the intermediate-phase memory requires the persistent activation of PKA (Muller and Carew, 1998; Sutton and Carew, 2000; Sutton et al., 2001).

An intermediate-term facilitation (ITF) of the sensorimotor synapse, which is produced by application of five pulses of 5-HT (an analog of sensitization training), corresponds to the ITM as it displays similar temporal dynamics and requires protein synthesis but not RNA synthesis (Ghirardi et al., 1995; Sutton and Carew, 2000). This latter feature of ITF distinguishes it from short-term facilitation, which requires neither protein nor RNA synthesis, and long-term facilitation, which requires both (see above). Depending on the induction protocol, ITF may require intermediate-term activation of PKA or PKC (Sossin et al., 1994; Sutton and Carew, 2000; Pepio et al., 2002; Lim and Sossin, 2006). These kinases can be activated for hours following prolonged treatment with 5-HT (Muller and Carew, 1998; Sutton and Carew, 2000). Finally, activation of previously silent release sites has also been implicated in ITF and could be a mechanism for memory consolidation (Kim et al., 2003b).

In addition to the intermediate-phase memory, it is likely that *Aplysia* has different phases of long-term memory. For example, at 24 h after sensitization training there is increased synthesis of a number of proteins, some of which are different from those whose synthesis is increased during and immediately after training (Noel et al., 1993). These results suggest that the memory for sensitization that persists for more than 24 h may be dependent on the synthesis of proteins occurring at 24 h and may have a different molecular signature than the 24-h memory.

Based on the experimental results reviewed above, a synthesis of the sensitization mechanisms in *Aplysia* can now be attempted. A brief sensitizing experience can affect the animal transiently (i.e., short-term sensitization), through an increase in the excitability of sensory neurons and in the efficacy of sensory neuron synapses. Short-term facilitation is achieved through spike-broadening-mediated and spike-duration-independent increases in transmitter release. These modifications, lasting up to several minutes, are mediated by phosphorylation of K^+ channels and other effector molecules, such as synapsin. More prolonged training, which typically involves multiple, appropriately timed stages of sensitization, can lead to modifications lasting 24 h or more. A single day of sensitization training leads to persistent increases in the efficacy of sensory neuron synapses and in the excitability of sensory neurons. Long-term facilitation after a single day of training does not involve gross structural changes of sensory neurons or changes in the number of synaptic varicosities. With 4 days of training, long-term sensitization is still accompanied by synaptic facilitation, but changes in sensory neuron excitability are not as prominent as they are after short-term training or after a single session of long-term training. After 4 days of training, long-term synaptic facilitation is achieved through an increase in the number of synaptic contacts. Collectively, these results indicate that facilitation of sensory neuron synapses is a ubiquitous feature of sensitization. However, the mechanisms that support the facilitation vary over time and with the extent of training. The conversion of one type of long-term expression mechanism to another is interesting, as it presumably reflects the engagement of a distinct set of genes that are part of an overall program for the expression of particularly enduring forms of long-term memory.

18.3 Habituation and Sensitization in Other Invertebrates

18.3.1 Gastropod Molluscs

18.3.1.1 Tritonia

To escape a noxious stimulus, the opisthobranch *Tritonia diomedea* initiates stereotypical oscillatory swimming. This escape swim can be dissected into several components, including number of cycles per swim, latency to swim onset, and swim cycle period. The various swim components can exhibit habituation, dishabituation, and/or sensitization (Frost et al., 1996). In particular, the escape swim undergoes habituation and dishabituation of the number of cycles per swim (Mongeluzi and Frost, 2000). Swimming probability can also decrease as a result of habituation (Brown,

1998). This habituation is accompanied by sensitization of the latency to swim onset (Frost et al., 1998).

The neural circuit underlying swim consists of sensory neurons, precentral pattern generating (CPG) neurons, and motor neurons. This circuit can be studied in the isolated perfused brain of *Tritonia*, where electrical stimulation of a nerve can elicit fictive swimming patterns (Dorsett et al., 1973). Habituation of fictive swimming correlates with a decrease in the cycle number and cycle period of swim motor programs (Frost et al., 1996; Brown, 1997) and appears to involve plasticity at multiple loci, including decrement at the first afferent synapse. Sensitization appears to involve enhanced excitability and synaptic strength in one of the CPG interneurons. Modulation of interneurons can be mediated by 5-HT, which has diverse effects on multiple loci of the circuit (Sakurai et al., 2006).

18.3.1.2 *Land snail* (Helix)

Land snails withdraw in response to weak tactile stimulation. The withdrawal behavior is mediated by a neuronal circuit involving four groups of nerve cells: Sensory neurons, motor neurons, modulatory neurons, and command neurons (Balaban, 2002). This withdrawal can be habituated or sensitized, depending on the intensity of stimulation. Habituation of the withdrawal behavior emerges from depletion of neurotransmitter at sensory cell synapses as well as heterosynaptic inhibition mediated by FMRFa-containing neurons (Balaban et al., 1991). Sensitization appears to be mediated by serotonergic modulatory cells whose spiking frequency increases following noxious stimulation (Balaban, 2002). These serotonergic cells are electrically coupled so that they get recruited and fire synchronously in response to strong excitatory input. One gene that is upregulated by external noxious input is the *Helix* Command Specific #2 (HCS2) (Balaban et al., 2001). The *HCS2* gene encodes a precursor protein whose processed products may function as neuromodulators or neurotransmitters mediating the withdrawal reactions of the snail (Korshunova et al., 2006). Application of neurotransmitters and second messengers known to be involved in withdrawal behavior result in upregulation of *HCS2* gene (Balaban, 2002).

The mechanisms underlying habituation and sensitization in the *Helix* can be further investigated by reconstructing behaviorally relevant synapses in culture. Using this approach, mechanosensory neuron-withdrawal interneuron synapses were found to display several forms of short-term synaptic plasticity such as facilitation, augmentation, and posttetanic potentiation (Fiumara et al., 2005).

18.3.2 Arthropods

18.3.2.1 *Crayfish* (Procambarus clarkii)

A crayfish escapes from noxious stimuli by flipping its tail. A key component of the tail-flip circuit is a pair of large neurons called the lateral giants (LGs), which run the length of the animal's nerve cord. The LGs are the decision and command cells for the tail-flip. The crayfish tail-flip response exhibits habituation (Wine et al., 1975) and sensitization (Krasne and Glanzman, 1986). Plastic changes induced during learning involve modulation of the strength of synaptic input driving the LGs (Edwards et al., 1999). A diminution of transmitter release with repeated activation of afferents is thought to underlie habituation (Krasne and Roberts, 1967; Zucker, 1972). An inhibitory pathway was also identified that can tonically inhibit the LGs (Krasne and Wine, 1975; Vu and Krasne, 1992, 1993; Vu et al., 1993). This putatively GABAergic (Vu and Krasne, 1993) (but see Heitler et al., 2001) inhibitory pathway also plays a major role in habituation (Krasne and Teshiba, 1995). In addition to the regulation of synaptic strength, habituation also results in decreased excitability of LGs (Araki and Nagayama, 2005). Bath application of the endogenous neuromodulators 5-HT and octopamine decrease the rate of LG habituation to repetitive sensory stimulation (Araki et al., 2005). Octopamine is also thought to at least partly mediate sensitization, because it mimics the sensitizing effects of strong stimulation on the tail-flip (Glanzman and Krasne, 1986; Krasne and Glanzman, 1986).

18.3.2.2 *Honeybee* (Apis mellifera)

Honeybees, like other insects, are superb at learning. For example, classical conditioning of feeding behavior can be produced by pairing a visual or olfactory stimulus with sugar solution to the antennae. Numerous studies described the molecular mechanisms underlying memory formation, which involve upregulation of the cAMP pathway and activation of PKA resulting in CREB-mediated transcription of downstream genes (Menzel, 2001). Nonassociative learning has also been studied in the honeybee, albeit to a lesser extent. Habituation of the proboscis extension reflex can be elicited by repeatedly touching one antenna with a droplet of sugar water (Braun and Bicker, 1992) and lasts for at least 10 min (Bicker and Hahnlein, 1994). Following habituation, the proboscis extension response can be restored spontaneously with time (spontaneous recovery) (Bicker and Hahnlein, 1994) or by stimulating the contralateral antenna (dishabituation) (Braun and Bicker, 1992). Application of tyramine, a metabolic precursor of the endogenous neuromodulator octopamine, accelerates the rate of habituation of the reflex (Braun and Bicker, 1992). Recently, activation of PKA was implicated in habituation of the reflex, but not dishabituation or spontaneous recovery, suggesting that the cellular mechanisms mediating habituation, dishabituation, and spontaneous recovery are distinct (Muller and Hildebrandt, 2002). With repeated training sessions over 2 days, long-term memory for habituation lasting for 24 h can be demonstrated (Bicker and Hahnlein, 1994). Finally, sensitization of the antenna reflex can be produced as a result of presenting gustatory stimuli to the antennae (Mauelshagen, 1993; Menzel et al., 1999).

18.3.2.3 Drosophila melanogaster

Because the neural circuitry in the fruit fly is both complex and inaccessible, the fly might seem to be an unpromising subject for studying the neural basis of learning. However, the ease with which genetic studies are performed compensates for the difficulty in performing electrophysiological studies (DeZazzo and Tully, 1995). A multitude of behaviors have been used as a model system to study nonassociative learning in *Drosophila*, including proboscis extension (Duerr and Quinn, 1982), thoracic bristle-elicited cleaning reflex (Corfas and Dudai, 1989), landing response (Rees and Spatz, 1989; Asztalos et al., 1993), jump-and-flight escape response (Engel and Wu, 1996), and odor-elicited startle response (Cho et al., 2004). Habituation has been demonstrated in all of these behaviors and molecular pathways underlying this form of learning have been identified and include the cAMP/PKA pathway (dunce and rutabaga mutants) (Duerr and Quinn, 1982; Corfas and Dudai, 1989; Engel and Wu, 1996; Cho et al., 2004), protein phosphatase 1 (Asztalos et al., 1993), and cGMP-dependent protein kinase (PKG) (Engel et al., 2000). In flies carrying the rutabaga mutation, which leads to diminished cAMP synthesis, habituation of the cleaning reflex is abnormally short-lived but dishabituation is unaffected (Corfas and Dudai, 1989). Moreover, in flies carrying the dunce mutation, which results in elevated cAMP levels, habituation rates of the jump-and-flight reflex are moderately increased but spontaneous recovery and dishabituation are not affected (Engel and Wu, 1996). These results reinforce the idea that the processes underlying habituation, dishabituation, and spontaneous recovery are distinct (also see the section titled 'Honeybee (*Apis mellifera*)'). Finally, in the dunce and rutabaga flies, sensitization of the proboscis-extension reflex dissipates more rapidly compared to wild-type controls (Duerr and Quinn, 1982).

18.3.3 Annelids

18.3.3.1 Leech

In the leech *Hirudo medicinalis*, nonassociative learning has been studied in several well characterized behaviors: Movements in response to light and water currents (Ratner, 1972), bending (Lockery and Kristan, 1991), shortening reflex to repeated light (Lockery et al., 1985) or tactile stimulation (Belardetti et al., 1982; Boulis and Sahley, 1988; Sahley et al., 1994), and swimming (Catarsi et al., 1993; Zaccardi et al., 2001).

In the shortening reflex of the leech, the neuronal changes underlying habituation and sensitization occur in the pathway from mechanosensory neurons to electrically coupled neurons, the S cells (Bagnoli and Magni, 1975; Sahley et al., 1994). Habituation of this reflex can reach asymptotic levels after 20 training trials and correlates with decreased S-cell excitability (Burrell et al., 2001). The reflex can be restored following application of a single noxious stimulus (dishabituation) (Boulis and Sahley, 1988). The potentiation of the shortening reflex observed during sensitization requires the S neurons, as their ablation disrupts sensitization (Sahley et al., 1994). This potentiation is mediated by 5-HT through an increase of cAMP (Belardetti et al., 1982), which also increases S-cell excitability (Burrell et al., 2001). Depletion of 5-HT disrupts sensitization (Sahley et al., 1994). Interestingly, ablation of the S cells only partly disrupts dishabituation, indicating that separate processes contribute to dishabituation and sensitization (Ehrlich et al., 1992; Sahley et al., 1994).

An additional mechanism that could potentially contribute to habituation of the shortening reflex involves depression of the synapses of touch (T) sensory neurons onto their follower target neurons. This synaptic depression has been associated with an increase in the amplitude of the T-cell after-hyperpolarizing potential (AHP) that follows their discharge (Brunelli et al., 1997; Scuri et al., 2002). The lasting increase in AHP amplitude, following low-frequency stimulation of T cells, has been attributed, in turn, to increased activity of the electrogenic Na^{+} pump, and requires activation of phospholipase A2 and the downstream arachidonic acid metabolites (Scuri et al., 2005).

18.3.4 Nematoda

18.3.4.1 Caenorhabditis elegans

C. elegans is a valuable model system for cellular and molecular studies of learning. Its principal advantages are threefold. First, its nervous system is extremely simple. It has a total of 302 neurons, the anatomical connectivity of which has been described at the electron microscopy level. Second, the developmental lineage of each neuron is completely specified. Third, its entire genome has been sequenced, making it highly amenable to a number of genetic and molecular manipulations. *C. elegans* responds to a vibratory stimulus applied to the medium in which they locomote by swimming backwards. This reaction, known as the tap withdrawal reflex, exhibits habituation, dishabituation, sensitization, and long-term (24-h) retention of habituation training (Rankin et al., 1990). Laser ablation studies have been used to elucidate the neural circuitry supporting the tap withdrawal reflex and to identify likely sites of plasticity within the network. Plastic changes during habituation appear to occur at the chemical synapses between presynaptic sensory neurons and postsynaptic command interneurons (Wicks and Rankin, 1997). Analysis of several *C. elegans* mutants has revealed that synapses at the locus of plasticity in the network may be glutamatergic (Rose and Rankin, 2001). Mutation of the gene coding for the brain-specific inorganic phosphate transporter *eat-4* results in more rapid habituation compared to wild-type worms and slower recovery (Rankin and Wicks, 2000). The protein coded by *eat-4* is involved in the regulation of glutamatergic transmission and is homologous to the mammalian vesicular glutamate transporter VGLUT1 (Bellocchio et al., 2000). *Eat-4* worms also do not display dishabituation, suggesting that neurotransmitter regulation plays a role in habituation and dishabituation (Rankin and Wicks, 2000). Moreover, worms that carry a mutation in glr-1, an excitatory glutamate receptor expressed in postsynaptic command interneurons, do not display long-term memory for habituation (Rose et al., 2003). In general, the study of behavioral genetics in the worm has provided significant insights into the ways in which genes regulate behavior (Rankin, 2002).

18.4 Emerging Principles

As a result of research on several invertebrate model systems, some general principles have emerged. A list of these principles might include the following: (1) short-term and long-term forms of learning and memory require changes in existing neural circuits, (2) these changes may involve multiple cellular mechanisms within single neurons, (3) second messenger systems play a role in mediating cellular changes, (4) changes in the properties of membrane channels are commonly correlated with learning and memory, (5) changes in intrinsic excitability (*See* Chapter 14) and synaptic efficacy are correlated with short- and long-term memory, and (6) long-term memory requires new protein synthesis and growth, whereas short-term memory does not.

References

Abrams TW, Castellucci VF, Camardo JS, Kandel ER, and Lloyd PE (1984) Two endogenous neuropeptides modulate the gill and siphon withdrawal reflex in *Aplysia* by presynaptic facilitation involving cAMP-dependent closure of a serotonin-sensitive potassium channel. *Proc. Natl. Acad. Sci. USA* 81: 7956–7960.

Alberini CM, Ghirardi M, Metz R, and Kandel ER (1994) C/EBP is an immediate-early gene required for the consolidation of long-term facilitation in *Aplysia*. *Cell* 76: 1099–1114.

Angers A, Fioravante D, Chin J, Cleary LJ, Bean AJ, and Byrne JH (2002) Serotonin stimulates phosphorylation of *Aplysia* synapsin and alters its subcellular distribution in sensory neurons. *J. Neurosci.* 22: 5412–5422.

Antzoulatos EG and Byrne JH (2004) Learning insights transmitted by glutamate. *Trends Neurosci.* 27: 555–560.

Antzoulatos EG and Byrne JH (2007) Long-term sensitization training produces spike narrowing in *Aplysia* sensory neurons. *J. Neurosci.* 27: 676–683.

Antzoulatos EG, Cleary LJ, Eskin A, Baxter DA, and Byrne JH (2003) Desensitization of postsynaptic glutamate receptors contributes to high-frequency homosynaptic depression of *Aplysia* sensorimotor connections. *Learn. Mem.* 10: 309–313.

Araki M and Nagayama T (2005) Decrease in excitability of LG following habituation of the crayfish escape reaction. *J. Comp. Physiol. A Neuroethol. Sens. Neural Behav. Physiol.* 191: 481–489.

Araki M, Nagayama T, and Sprayberry J (2005) Cyclic AMP mediates serotonin-induced synaptic enhancement of lateral giant interneuron of the crayfish. *J. Neurophysiol.* 94: 2644–2652.

Armitage BA and Siegelbaum SA (1998) Presynaptic induction and expression of homosynaptic depression at *Aplysia* sensorimotor neuron synapses. *J. Neurosci.* 18: 8770–8779.

Asztalos Z, von Wegerer J, Wustmann G, et al. (1993) Protein phosphatase 1-deficient mutant *Drosophila* is affected in habituation and associative learning. *J. Neurosci.* 13: 924–930.

Bagnoli P and Magni F (1975) Synaptic inputs to Retzius' cells in the leech. *Brain Res.* 96: 147–152.

Bailey CH and Chen M (1983) Morphological basis of long-term habituation and sensitization in *Aplysia*. *Science* 220: 91–93.

Bailey CH and Chen M (1988a) Long-term memory in *Aplysia* modulates the total number of varicosities of single identified sensory neurons. *Proc. Natl. Acad. Sci. USA* 85: 2373–2377.

Bailey CH and Chen M (1988b) Morphological basis of short-term habituation in *Aplysia*. *J. Neurosci.* 8: 2452–2459.

Bailey CH, Montarolo P, Chen M, Kandel ER, and Schacher S (1992) Inhibitors of protein and RNA synthesis block structural changes that accompany long-term heterosynaptic plasticity in *Aplysia*. *Neuron* 9: 749–758.

Bailey CH, Kaang BK, Chen M, et al. (1997) Mutation in the phosphorylation sites of MAP kinase blocks learning-related internalization of apCAM in *Aplysia* sensory neurons. *Neuron* 18: 913–924.

Balaban PM (2002) Cellular mechanisms of behavioral plasticity in terrestrial snail. *Neurosci. Biobehav. Rev.* 26: 597–630.

Balaban PM, Bravarenko NI, and Zakharov IS (1991) The neurochemical basis of recurrent inhibition in the reflex arch of the defensive reaction. *Zh. Vyssh. Nerv. Deiat. Im. I. P. Pavlova* 41: 1033–1038.

Balaban PM, Poteryaev DA, Zakharov IS, Uvarov P, Malyshev A, and Belyavsky AV (2001) Up- and down-regulation of *Helix* command-specific 2 (HCS2) gene expression in the nervous system of terrestrial snail *Helix lucorum*. *Neuroscience* 103: 551–559.

Bartsch D, Ghirardi M, Skehel PA, et al. (1995) *Aplysia* CREB2 represses long-term facilitation: relief of repression converts transient facilitation into long-term functional and structural change. *Cell* 83: 979–992.

Bartsch D, Casadio A, Karl KA, Serodio P, and Kandel ER (1998) CREB1 encodes a nuclear activator, a repressor, and a cytoplasmic modulator that form a regulatory unit critical for long-term facilitation. *Cell* 95: 211–223.

Bartsch D, Ghirardi M, Casadio A, et al. (2000) Enhancement of memory-related long-term facilitation by ApAF, a novel transcription factor that acts downstream from both CREB1 and CREB2. *Cell* 103: 595–608.

Barzilai A, Kennedy TE, Sweatt JD, and Kandel ER (1989) 5-HT modulates protein synthesis and the expression of specific proteins during long-term facilitation in *Aplysia* sensory neurons. *Neuron* 2: 1577–1586.

Baxter DA and Byrne JH (1989) Serotonergic modulation of two potassium currents in the pleural sensory neurons of *Aplysia*. *J. Neurophysiol.* 62: 665–679.

Baxter DA and Byrne JH (1990a) Differential effects of cAMP and serotonin on membrane current, action-potential duration, and excitability in somata of pleural sensory neurons of *Aplysia*. *J. Neurophysiol.* 64: 978–990.

Baxter DA and Byrne JH (1990b) Reduction of voltage-activated K+ currents by forskolin is not mediated via cAMP in pleural sensory neurons of *Aplysia*. *J. Neurophysiol.* 64: 1474–1483.

Belardetti F, Biondi C, Colombaioni L, Brunelli M, and Trevisani A (1982) Role of serotonin and cyclic AMP on facilitation of the fast conducting system activity in the leech *Hirudo medicinalis*. *Brain Res.* 246: 89–103.

Belardetti F, Kandel ER, and Siegelbaum SA (1987) Neuronal inhibition by the peptide FMRFamide involves opening of S K+ channels. *Nature* 325: 153–156.

Bellocchio EE, Reimer RJ, Fremeau RT Jr., and Edwards RH (2000) Uptake of glutamate into synaptic vesicles by an inorganic phosphate transporter. *Science* 289: 957–960.

Bernier L, Castellucci VF, Kandel ER, and Schwartz JH (1982) Facilitatory transmitter causes a selective and prolonged increase in adenosine 3′: 5′-monophosphate in sensory neurons mediating the gill and siphon withdrawal reflex in *Aplysia*. *J. Neurosci.* 2: 1682–1691.

Bicker G and Hahnlein I (1994) Long-term habituation of an appetitive reflex in the honeybee. *Neuroreport* 6: 54–56.

Blumenfeld H, Spira ME, Kandel ER, and Siegelbaum SA (1990) Facilitatory and inhibitory transmitters modulate calcium influx during action potentials in *Aplysia* sensory neurons. *Neuron* 5: 487–499.

Boulis NM and Sahley CL (1988) A behavioral analysis of habituation and sensitization of shortening in the semi-intact leech. *J. Neurosci.* 8: 4621–4627.

Braha O, Dale N, Hochner B, Klein M, Abrams TW, and Kandel ER (1990) Second messengers involved in the two processes of presynaptic facilitation that contribute to sensitization and dishabituation in *Aplysia* sensory neurons. *Proc. Natl. Acad. Sci. USA* 87: 2040–2044.

Braun G and Bicker G (1992) Habituation of an appetitive reflex in the honeybee. *J. Neurophysiol.* 67: 588–598.

Brown GD (1997) Isolated-brain parallels to simple types of learning and memory in *Tritonia*. *Physiol. Behav.* 62: 509–518.

Brown GD (1998) Nonassociative learning processes affecting swimming probability in the seaslug *Tritonia diomedea*: Habituation, sensitization and inhibition. *Behav. Brain Res.* 95: 151–165.

Brunelli M, Castellucci V, and Kandel ER (1976) Synaptic facilitation and behavioral sensitization in *Aplysia*: Possible role of serotonin and cyclic AMP. *Science* 194: 1178–1181.

Brunelli M, Garcia-Gil M, Mozzachiodi R, Scuri R, and Zaccardi ML (1997) Neurobiological principles of learning and memory. *Arch. Ital. Biol.* 135: 15–36.

Buonomano DV, Cleary LJ, and Byrne JH (1992) Inhibitory neuron produces heterosynaptic inhibition of the sensory-to-motor neuron synapse in *Aplysia*. *Brain Res.* 577: 147–150.

Burrell BD, Sahley CL, and Muller KJ (2001) Non-associative learning and serotonin induce similar bi-directional changes in excitability of a neuron critical for learning in the medicinal leech. *J. Neurosci.* 21: 1401–1412.

Buttner N, Siegelbaum SA, and Volterra A (1989) Direct modulation of *Aplysia* S-K^+ channels by a 12-lipoxygenase metabolite of arachidonic acid. *Nature* 342: 553–555.

Byrne JH (1982) Analysis of synaptic depression contributing to habituation of gill-withdrawal reflex in *Aplysia californica*. *J. Neurophysiol.* 48: 431–438.

Byrne JH (1987) Cellular analysis of associative learning. *Physiol. Rev.* 67: 329–439.

Byrne JH, Baxter DA, Buonomano DV, et al. (1991) Neural and molecular bases of nonassociative and associative learning in *Aplysia*. *Ann. NY Acad. Sci.* 627: 124–149.

Byrne JH, Zwartjes R, Homayouni R, Critz SD, and Eskin A (1993) Roles of second messenger pathways in neuronal plasticity and in learning and memory. Insights gained from *Aplysia*. *Adv. Second Messenger Phosphoprotein Res.* 27: 47–108.

Byrne JH, Fioravante D, and Liu R (2006) The CREB1 feedback loop is necessary for consolidation of long-term facilitation in *Aplysia.* In: Program No. 669.6. 2006 Neuroscience Meeting Planner. Atlanta, GA: Society for Neuroscience.

Carew TJ and Kandel ER (1973) Acquisition and retention of long-term habituation in *Aplysia*: correlation of behavioral and cellular processes. *Science* 182: 1158–1160.

Carew TJ and Sahley CL (1986) Invertebrate learning and memory: From behavior to molecules. *Annu. Rev. Neurosci.* 9: 435–487.

Carew TJ, Castellucci VF, and Kandel ER (1971) An analysis of dishabituation and sensitization of the gill-withdrawal reflex in *Aplysia*. *Int. J. Neurosci.* 2: 79–98.

Castellucci VF and Kandel ER (1974) A quantal analysis of the synaptic depression underlying habituation of the gill-withdrawal reflex in *Aplysia*. *Proc. Natl. Acad. Sci. USA* 71: 5004–5008.

Castellucci V, Pinsker H, Kupfermann I, and Kandel ER (1970) Neuronal mechanisms of habituation and dishabituation of the gill-withdrawal reflex in *Aplysia*. *Science* 167: 1745–1748.

Castellucci VF, Blumenfeld H, Goelet P, and Kandel ER (1989) Inhibitor of protein synthesis blocks long-term behavioral sensitization in the isolated gill-withdrawal reflex of *Aplysia*. *J. Neurobiol.* 20: 1–9.

Catarsi S, Scuri R, and Brunelli M (1993) Cyclic AMP mediates inhibition of the Na(+)- K+ electrogenic pump by serotonin in tactile sensory neurones of the leech. *J. Physiol.* 462: 229–242.

Chin J, Angers A, Cleary LJ, Eskin A, and Byrne JH (2002a) Transforming growth factor beta1 alters synapsin distribution and modulates synaptic depression in *Aplysia*. *J. Neurosci.* 22: RC220.

Chin J, Burdohan JA, Eskin A, and Byrne JH (2002b) Inhibitor of glutamate transport alters synaptic transmission at sensorimotor synapses in *Aplysia*. *J. Neurophysiol.* 87: 3165–3168.

Chin J, Liu RY, Cleary LJ, Eskin A, and Byrne JH (2006) TGF-beta1-induced long-term changes in neuronal excitability in *Aplysia* sensory neurons depend on MAPK. *J. Neurophysiol.* 95: 3286–3290.

Cho W, Heberlein U, and Wolf FW (2004) Habituation of an odorant-induced startle response in *Drosophila*. *Genes Brain Behav.* 3: 127–137.

Cleary LJ and Byrne JH (1993) Identification and characterization of a multifunction neuron contributing to defensive arousal in *Aplysia*. *J. Neurophysiol.* 70: 1767–1776.

Cleary LJ, Byrne JH, and Frost WN (1995) Role of interneurons in defensive withdrawal reflexes in *Aplysia*. *Learn. Mem.* 2: 133–151.

Cleary LJ, Lee WL, and Byrne JH (1998) Cellular correlates of long-term sensitization in *Aplysia*. *J. Neurosci.* 18: 5988–5998.

Corfas G and Dudai Y (1989) Habituation and dishabituation of a cleaning reflex in normal and mutant *Drosophila*. *J. Neurosci.* 9: 56–62.

Critz SD, Baxter DA, and Byrne JH (1991) Modulatory effects of serotonin, FMRFamide, and myomodulin on the duration of action potentials, excitability, and membrane currents in tail sensory neurons of *Aplysia*. *J. Neurophysiol.* 66: 1912–1926.

Dale N and Kandel ER (1990) Facilitatory and inhibitory transmitters modulate spontaneous transmitter release at cultured *Aplysia* sensorimotor synapses. *J. Physiol.* 421: 203–222.

Dash PK, Hochner B, and Kandel ER (1990) Injection of the cAMP-responsive element into the nucleus of *Aplysia* sensory neurons blocks long-term facilitation. *Nature* 345: 718–721.

Dash PK, Karl KA, Colicos MA, Prywes R, and Kandel ER (1991) cAMP response element-binding protein is activated by Ca2+/calmodulin- as well as cAMP-dependent protein kinase. *Proc. Natl. Acad. Sci. USA* 88: 5061–5065.

DeZazzo J and Tully T (1995) Dissection of memory formation: From behavioral pharmacology to molecular genetics. *Trends Neurosci.* 18: 212–218.

Dorsett DA, Willows AO, and Hoyle G (1973) The neuronal basis of behavior in *Tritonia*. IV. The central origin of a fixed action pattern demonstrated in the isolated brain. *J. Neurobiol.* 4: 287–300.

Duerr JS and Quinn WG (1982) Three *Drosophila* mutations that block associative learning also affect habituation and sensitization. *Proc. Natl. Acad. Sci. USA* 79: 3646–3650.

Dumitriu B, Cohen JE, Wan Q, Negroiu AM, and Abrams TW (2006) Serotonin receptor antagonists discriminate between PKA- and PKC-mediated plasticity in *Aplysia* sensory neurons. *J. Neurophysiol.* 95: 2713–2720.

Dyer JR, Manseau F, Castellucci VF, and Sossin WS (2003) Serotonin persistently activates the extracellular signal-related kinase in sensory neurons of *Aplysia* independently of cAMP or protein kinase C. *Neuroscience* 116: 13–17.

Edmonds B, Klein M, Dale N, and Kandel ER (1990) Contributions of two types of calcium channels to synaptic transmission and plasticity. *Science* 250: 1142–1147.

Edwards DH, Heitler WJ, and Krasne FB (1999) Fifty years of a command neuron: The neurobiology of escape behavior in the crayfish. *Trends Neurosci.* 22: 153–161.

Ehrlich JS, Boulis NM, Karrer T, and Sahley CL (1992) Differential effects of serotonin depletion on sensitization and dishabituation in the leech, *Hirudo medicinalis*. *J. Neurobiol.* 23: 270–279.

Eliot LS, Kandel ER, and Hawkins RD (1994) Modulation of spontaneous transmitter release during depression and posttetanic potentiation of *Aplysia* sensory-motor neuron synapses isolated in culture. *J. Neurosci.* 14: 3280–3292.

Engel JE and Wu CF (1996) Altered habituation of an identified escape circuit in *Drosophila* memory mutants. *J. Neurosci.* 16: 3486–3499.

Engel JE, Xie XJ, Sokolowski MB, and Wu CF (2000) A cGMP-dependent protein kinase gene, foraging, modifies habituation-like response decrement of the giant fiber escape circuit in *Drosophila*. *Learn. Mem.* 7: 341–352.

Eskin A, Garcia KS, and Byrne JH (1989) Information storage in the nervous system of *Aplysia*: Specific proteins affected by serotonin and cAMP. *Proc. Natl. Acad. Sci. USA* 86: 2458–2462.

Ezzeddine Y and Glanzman DL (2003) Prolonged habituation of the gill-withdrawal reflex in *Aplysia* depends on protein synthesis, protein phosphatase activity, and postsynaptic glutamate receptors. *J. Neurosci.* 23: 9585–9594.

Farr M, Mathews J, Zhu DF, and Ambron RT (1999) Inflammation causes a long-term hyperexcitability in the nociceptive sensory neurons of *Aplysia*. *Learn. Mem.* 6: 331–340.

Fioravante D, Smolen PD, and Byrne JH (2006) The 5-HT- and FMRFa-activated signaling pathways interact at the level of the Erk MAPK cascade: Potential inhibitory constraints on memory formation. *Neurosci. Lett.* 396: 235–240.

Fioravante D, Liu RY, Netek A, Cleary LJ, and Byrne JH (2007) Synapsin regulates basal synaptic strength, synaptic depression and serotonin-induced facilitation of sensorimotor synapses in *Aplysia*. *J. Neurophysiology* 98: 3568–3580.

Fiumara F, Leitinger G, Milanese C, Montarolo PG, and Ghirardi M (2005) In vitro formation and activity-dependent plasticity of synapses between *Helix* neurons involved in the neural control of feeding and withdrawal behaviors. *Neuroscience* 134: 1133–1151.

Frost WN, Castellucci VF, Hawkins RD, and Kandel ER (1985) Mono-synaptic connections made by the sensory neurons of the gill-withdrawal and siphon-withdrawal reflex in *Aplysia* Participate in the storage of long-term-memory for sensitization. *Proc. Natl. Acad. Sci. USA* 82: 8266–8269.

Frost WN, Brown GD, and Getting PA (1996) Parametric features of habituation of swim cycle number in the marine mollusc *Tritonia diomedea*. *Neurobiol. Learn. Mem.* 65: 125–134.

Frost WN, Brandon CL, and Mongeluzi DL (1998) Sensitization of the *Tritonia* escape swim. *Neurobiol. Learn. Mem.* 69: 126–135.

Ghirardi M, Braha O, Hochner B, Montarolo PG, Kandel ER, and Dale N (1992) Roles of PKA and PKC in facilitation of evoked and spontaneous transmitter release at depressed and nondepressed synapses in *Aplysia* sensory neurons. *Neuron* 9: 479–489.

Ghirardi M, Montarolo PG, and Kandel ER (1995) A novel intermediate stage in the transition between short- and long-term facilitation in the sensory to motor neuron synapse of *Aplysia*. *Neuron* 14: 413–420.

Gingrich KJ and Byrne JH (1985) Simulation of synaptic depression, posttetanic potentiation, and presynaptic facilitation of synaptic potentials from sensory neurons mediating gill-withdrawal reflex in *Aplysia*. *J. Neurophysiol.* 53: 652–669.

Gingrich KJ and Byrne JH (1987) Single-cell neuronal model for associative learning. *J. Neurophysiol.* 57: 1705–1715.

Glanzman DL and Krasne FB (1986) 5,7-Dihydroxytryptamine lesions of crayfish serotonin-containing neurons: Effect on the lateral giant escape reaction. *J. Neurosci.* 6: 1560–1569.

Glanzman DL, Mackey SL, Hawkins RD, Dyke AM, Lloyd PE, and Kandel ER (1989) Depletion of serotonin in the nervous system of *Aplysia* reduces the behavioral enhancement of gill withdrawal as well as the heterosynaptic facilitation produced by tail shock. *J. Neurosci.* 9: 4200–4213.

Goldsmith BA and Abrams TW (1992) cAMP modulates multiple K^+ currents, increasing spike duration and excitability in *Aplysia* sensory neurons. *Proc. Natl. Acad. Sci. USA* 89: 11481–11485.

Gover TD, Jiang XY, and Abrams TW (2002) Persistent, exocytosis-independent silencing of release sites underlies homosynaptic depression at sensory synapses in *Aplysia*. *J. Neurosci.* 22: 1942–1955.

Guan Z, Giustetto M, Lomvardas S, et al. (2002) Integration of long-term-memory-related synaptic plasticity involves bidirectional regulation of gene expression and chromatin structure. *Cell* 111: 483–493.

Guan Z, Kim JH, Lomvardas S, Holick K, Xu S, Kandel ER, and Schwartz JH (2003) p38 MAP kinase mediates both short-term and long-term synaptic depression in *Aplysia*. *J. Neurosci.* 23: 7317–7325.

Hawkins RD (1989) Localization of potential serotonergic facilitator neurons in *Aplysia* by glyoxylic acid histofluorescence combined with retrograde fluorescent labeling. *J. Neurosci.* 9: 4214–4226.

Hawkins RD and Kandel ER (1984) Is there a cell-biological alphabet for simple forms of learning? *Psychol. Rev.* 91: 375–391.

Hegde AN, Inokuchi K, Pei W, et al. (1997) Ubiquitin C-terminal hydrolase is an immediate-early gene essential for long-term facilitation in *Aplysia*. *Cell* 89: 115–126.

Heitler WJ, Watson AH, Falconer SW, and Powell B (2001) Glutamate is a transmitter that mediates inhibition at the rectifying electrical motor giant synapse in the crayfish. *J. Comp. Neurol.* 430: 12–26.

Hilfiker S, Schweizer FE, Kao HT, Czernik AJ, Greengard P, and Augustine GJ (1998) Two sites of action for synapsin domain E in regulating neurotransmitter release. *Nat. Neurosci.* 1: 29–35.

Hilfiker S, Pieribone VA, Czernik AJ, Kao HT, Augustine GJ, and Greengard P (1999) Synapsins as regulators of neurotransmitter release. *Philos. Trans. R. Soc. Lond. B Biol. Sci.* 354: 269–279.

Hochner B and Kandel ER (1992) Modulation of a transient K+ current in the pleural sensory neurons of *Aplysia* by serotonin and cAMP: Implications for spike broadening. *Proc. Natl. Acad. Sci. USA* 89: 11476–11480.

Hochner B, Klein M, Schacher S, and Kandel ER (1986) Additional component in the cellular mechanism of presynaptic facilitation contributes to behavioral dishabituation in *Aplysia*. *Proc. Natl. Acad. Sci. USA* 83: 8794–8798.

Hosaka M, Hammer RE, and Sudhof TC (1999) A phospho-switch controls the dynamic association of synapsins with synaptic vesicles. *Neuron* 24: 377–387.

Houeland G, Nakhost A, Sossin WS, and Castellucci VF (2007) PKC modulation of transmitter release by SNAP-25 at sensory-to-motor synapses in *Aplysia*. *J. Neurophysiol.* 97: 134–143.

Hu JY, Glickman L, Wu F, and Schacher S (2004a) Serotonin regulates the secretion and autocrine action of a neuropeptide to activate MAPK required for long-term facilitation in *Aplysia*. *Neuron* 43: 373–385.

Hu JY, Goldman J, Wu F, and Schacher S (2004b) Target-dependent release of a presynaptic neuropeptide regulates the formation and maturation of specific synapses in *Aplysia*. *J. Neurosci.* 24: 9933–9943.

Ichinose M and Byrne JH (1991) Role of protein phosphatases in the modulation of neuronal membrane currents. *Brain Res.* 549: 146–150.

Jovanovic JN, Benfenati F, Siow YL, et al. (1996) Neurotrophins stimulate phosphorylation of synapsin I by MAP kinase and regulate synapsin I-actin interactions. *Proc. Natl. Acad. Sci. USA* 93: 3679–3683.

Kim H, Chang DJ, Lee JA, Lee YS, and Kaang BK (2003a) Identification of nuclear/nucleolar localization signal in *Aplysia* learning associated protein of slug with a molecular mass of 18 kDa homologous protein. *Neurosci. Lett.* 343: 134–138.

Kim JH, Udo H, Li HL, et al. (2003b) Presynaptic activation of silent synapses and growth of new synapses contribute to intermediate and long-term facilitation in *Aplysia*. *Neuron* 40: 151–165.

Kim H, Lee SH, Han JH, et al. (2006) A nucleolar protein ApLLP induces ApC/EBP expression required for long-term synaptic facilitation in *Aplysia* neurons. *Neuron* 49: 707–718.

Klein M (1993) Differential cyclic AMP dependence of facilitation at *Aplysia* sensorimotor synapses as a function of prior stimulation: Augmentation versus restoration of transmitter release. *J. Neurosci.* 13: 3793–3801.

Klein M (1994) Synaptic augmentation by 5-HT at rested *Aplysia* sensorimotor synapses: Independence of action potential prolongation. *Neuron* 13: 159–166.

Klein M and Kandel ER (1980) Mechanism of calcium current modulation underlying presynaptic facilitation and behavioral sensitization in *Aplysia*. *Proc. Natl. Acad. Sci. USA* 77: 6912–6916.

Klein M, Shapiro E, and Kandel ER (1980) Synaptic plasticity and the modulation of the Ca2+ current. *J. Exp. Biol.* 89: 117–157.

Klein M, Camardo J, and Kandel ER (1982) Serotonin modulates a specific potassium current in the sensory neurons that show presynaptic facilitation in *Aplysia*. *Proc. Natl. Acad. Sci. USA* 79: 5713–5717.

Korshunova TA, Malyshev AY, Zakharov IS, Ierusalimskii VN, and Balaban PM (2006) Functions of peptide CNP4, encoded by the HCS2 gene, in the nervous system of *Helix lucorum*. *Neurosci. Behav. Physiol.* 36: 253–260.

Krasne FB and Glanzman DL (1986) Sensitization of the crayfish lateral giant escape reaction. *J. Neurosci.* 6: 1013–1020.

Krasne FB and Roberts A (1967) Habituation of the crayfish escape response during release from inhibition induced by picrotoxin. *Nature* 215: 769–770.

Krasne FB and Teshiba TM (1995) Habituation of an invertebrate escape reflex due to modulation by higher centers rather than local events. *Proc. Natl. Acad. Sci. USA* 92: 3362–3366.

Krasne FB and Wine JJ (1975) Extrinsic modulation of crayfish escape behaviour. *J. Exp. Biol.* 63: 433–450.

Kupfermann I, Castellucci V, Pinsker H, and Kandel E (1970) Neuronal correlates of habituation and dishabituation of the gill-withdrawal reflex in *Aplysia*. *Science* 167: 1743–1745.

Lee JA, Lee SH, Lee C, et al. (2006) PKA-activated ApAF-ApC/EBP heterodimer is a key downstream effector of ApCREB and is necessary and sufficient for the consolidation of long-term facilitation. *J. Cell Biol.* 174: 827–838.

Levenson J, Byrne JH, and Eskin A (1999) Levels of serotonin in the hemolymph of *Aplysia* are modulated by light/dark cycles and sensitization training. *J. Neurosci.* 19: 8094–8103.

Levenson J, Endo S, Kategaya LS, et al. (2000) Long-term regulation of neuronal high-affinity glutamate and glutamine uptake in *Aplysia*. *Proc. Natl. Acad. Sci. USA* 97: 12858–12863.

Lim T and Sossin WS (2006) Phosphorylation at the hydrophobic site of protein kinase C Apl II is increased during intermediate term facilitation. *Neuroscience* 141: 277–285.

Lin XY and Glanzman DL (1996) Long-term depression of *Aplysia* sensorimotor synapses in cell culture: Inductive role of a rise in postsynaptic calcium. *J. Neurophysiol.* 76: 2111–2114.

Liu QR, Hattar S, Endo S, et al. (1997) A developmental gene (Tolloid/BMP-1) is regulated in *Aplysia* neurons by treatments that induce long-term sensitization. *J. Neurosci.* 17: 755–764.

Liu RY, Fioravante D, Shah S, and Byrne JH (2008) CREB1 feedback loop is necessary for consolidation of long-term synaptic facilitation in *Aplysia*. *J. Neuroscience,* in press.

Lockery SR and Kristan WB Jr (1991) Two forms of sensitization of the local bending reflex of the medicinal leech. *J. Comp. Physiol. [A]* 168: 165–177.

Lockery SR, Rawlins JN, and Gray JA (1985) Habituation of the shortening reflex in the medicinal leech. *Behav. Neurosci.* 99: 333–341.

Mackey SL, Glanzman DL, Small SA, Dyke AM, Kandel ER, and Hawkins RD (1987) Tail shock produces inhibition as well as sensitization of the siphon-withdrawal reflex of *Aplysia*: Possible behavioral role for presynaptic inhibition mediated by the peptide Phe-Met-Arg-Phe-NH2. *Proc. Natl. Acad. Sci. USA* 84: 8730–8734.

Marinesco S and Carew TJ (2002) Serotonin release evoked by tail nerve stimulation in the CNS of *Aplysia*: Characterization and relationship to heterosynaptic plasticity. *J. Neurosci.* 22. 2299–2312.

Marinesco S, Wickremasinghe N, and Carew TJ (2006) Regulation of behavioral and synaptic plasticity by serotonin release within local modulatory fields in the CNS of *Aplysia*. *J. Neurosci.* 26: 12682–12693.

Martin KC, Casadio A, Zhu H, et al. (1997a) Synapse-specific, long-term facilitation of *Aplysia* sensory to motor synapses: A function for local protein synthesis in memory storage. *Cell* 91: 927–938.

Martin KC, Michael D, Rose JC, et al. (1997b) MAP kinase translocates into the nucleus of the presynaptic cell and is required for long-term facilitation in *Aplysia*. *Neuron* 18: 899–912.

Matsubara M, Kusubata M, Ishiguro K, Uchida T, Titani K, and Taniguchi H (1996) Site-specific phosphorylation of synapsin I by mitogen-activated protein kinase and Cdk5 and its effects on physiological functions. *J. Biol. Chem.* 271: 21108–21113.

Mauelshagen J (1993) Neural correlates of olfactory learning paradigms in an identified neuron in the honeybee brain. *J. Neurophysiol.* 69: 609–625.

Mayford M, Barzilai A, Keller F, Schacher S, and Kandel ER (1992) Modulation of an NCAM-related adhesion molecule with long-term synaptic plasticity in *Aplysia*. *Science* 256: 638–644.

Menzel R (2001) Searching for the memory trace in a mini-brain, the honeybee. *Learn. Mem.* 8: 53–62.

Menzel R, Heyne A, Kinzel C, Gerber B, and Fiala A (1999) Pharmacological dissociation between the reinforcing, sensitizing, and response-releasing functions of reward in honeybee classical conditioning. *Behav. Neurosci.* 113: 744–754.

Mercer AR, Emptage NJ, and Carew TJ (1991) Pharmacological dissociation of modulatory effects of serotonin in *Aplysia* sensory neurons. *Science* 254: 1811–1813.

Michael D, Martin KC, Seger R, Ning MM, Baston R, and Kandel ER (1998) Repeated pulses of serotonin required for long-term facilitation activate mitogen-activated protein kinase in sensory neurons of *Aplysia*. *Proc. Natl. Acad. Sci. USA* 95: 1864–1869.

Mohamed HA, Yao W, Fioravante D, Smolen PD, and Byrne JH (2005) cAMP-response elements in *Aplysia* creb1, creb2, and Ap-uch promoters: Implications for feedback loops modulating long term memory. *J. Biol. Chem.* 280: 27035–27043.

Mongeluzi DL and Frost WN (2000) Dishabituation of the *Tritonia* escape swim. *Learn. Mem.* 7: 43–47.

Montarolo PG, Goelet P, Castellucci VF, Morgan J, Kandel ER, and Schacher S (1986) A critical period for macromolecular synthesis in long-term heterosynaptic facilitation in *Aplysia. Science* 234: 1249–1254.

Montarolo PG, Kandel ER, and Schacher S (1988) Long-term heterosynaptic inhibition in *Aplysia*. *Nature* 333: 171–174.

Muller U and Carew TJ (1998) Serotonin induces temporally and mechanistically distinct phases of persistent PKA activity in *Aplysia* sensory neurons. *Neuron* 21: 1423–1434.

Muller U and Hildebrandt H (2002) Nitric oxide/cGMP-mediated protein kinase A activation in the antennal lobes plays an important role in appetitive reflex habituation in the honeybee. *J. Neurosci.* 22: 8739–8747.

Noel F, Nunez-Regueiro M, Cook R, Byrne JH, and Eskin A (1993) Long-term changes in synthesis of intermediate filament protein, actin and other proteins in pleural sensory neurons of *Aplysia* produced by an in vitro analogue of sensitization training. *Brain Res. Mol. Brain Res.* 19: 203–210.

Nolen TG and Carew TJ (1994) Ontogeny of serotonin-immunoreactive neurons in juvenile *Aplysia californica*: Implications for the development of learning. *Behav. Neural Biol.* 61: 282–295.

Ocorr KA and Byrne JH (1985) Membrane responses and changes in cAMP levels in *Aplysia* sensory neurons produced by serotonin, tryptamine, FMRFamide and small cardioactive peptideB (SCPB). *Neurosci. Lett.* 55: 113–118.

Ocorr KA and Byrne JH (1986) Evidence for separate receptors that mediate parallel effects of serotonin and small cardioactive peptideB (SCPB) on adenylate cyclase in *Aplysia californica*. *Neurosci. Lett.* 70: 283–288.

Ocorr KA, Tabata M, and Byrne JH (1986) Stimuli that produce sensitization lead to elevation of cyclic AMP levels in tail sensory neurons of *Aplysia*. *Brain Res.* 371: 190–192.

O'Leary FA, Byrne JH, and Cleary LJ (1995) Long-term structural remodeling in *Aplysia* sensory neurons requires de novo protein synthesis during a critical time period. *J. Neurosci.* 15: 3519–3525.

Ormond J, Hislop J, Zhao Y, et al. (2004) ApTrkl, a Trk-like receptor, mediates serotonin-dependent ERK activation and long-term facilitation in *Aplysia* sensory neurons. *Neuron* 44: 715–728.

Pepio AM, Thibault GL, and Sossin WS (2002) Phosphoinositide-dependent kinase phosphorylation of protein kinase C Apl II increases during intermediate facilitation in *Aplysia*. *J. Biol. Chem.* 277: 37116–37123.

Phares GA, Antzoulatos EG, Baxter DA, and Byrne JH (2003) Burst-induced synaptic depression and its modulation contribute to information transfer at *Aplysia* sensorimotor synapses: Empirical and computational analyses. *J. Neurosci.* 23: 8392–8401.

Pieroni JP and Byrne JH (1992) Differential effects of serotonin, FMRFamide, and small cardioactive peptide on multiple, distributed processes modulating sensorimotor synaptic transmission in *Aplysia*. *J. Neurosci.* 12: 2633–2647.

Pinsker H, Kupfermann I, Castellucci V, and Kandel E (1970) Habituation and dishabituation of the gill-withdrawal reflex in *Aplysia*. *Science* 167: 1740–1742.

Piomelli D (1991) Metabolism of arachidonic acid in nervous system of marine mollusk *Aplysia californica*. *Am. J. Physiol.* 260: R844–R848.

Piomelli D, Volterra A, Dale N, et al. (1987) Lipoxygenase metabolites of arachidonic acid as second messengers for presynaptic inhibition of *Aplysia* sensory cells. *Nature* 328: 38–43.

Pollock JD, Bernier L, and Camardo JS (1985) Serotonin and cyclic adenosine 3′: 5′-monophosphate modulate the potassium current in tail sensory neurons in the pleural ganglion of *Aplysia*. *J. Neurosci.* 5: 1862–1871.

Rankin CH (2002) From gene to identified neuron to behaviour in *Caenorhabditis elegans*. *Nat. Rev. Genet.* 3: 622–630.

Rankin CH and Wicks SR (2000) Mutations of the *Caenorhabditis elegans* brain-specific inorganic phosphate transporter eat-4 affect habituation of the tap-withdrawal response without affecting the response itself. *J. Neurosci.* 20: 4337–4344.

Rankin CH, Beck CD, and Chiba CM (1990) *Caenorhabditis elegans*: A new model system for the study of learning and memory. *Behav. Brain Res.* 37: 89–92.

Ratner SC (1972) Habituation and retention of habituation in the leech (*Macrobdella decora*). *J. Comp. Physiol. Psychol.* 81: 115–121.

Raymond JL and Byrne JH (1994) Distributed input to the tail-siphon withdrawal circuit in *Aplysia* from neurons in the J cluster of the cerebral ganglion. *J. Neurosci.* 14: 2444–2454.

Rees CT and Spatz HC (1989) Habituation of the landing response of *Drosophila* wild-type and mutants defective in olfactory learning. *J. Neurogenet.* 5: 105–118.

Rose JK and Rankin CH (2001) Analyses of habituation in *Caenorhabditis elegans*. *Learn. Mem.* 8: 63–69.

Rose JK, Kaun KR, Chen SH, and Rankin CH (2003) GLR-1, a non-NMDA glutamate receptor homolog, is critical for long-term memory in *Caenorhabditis elegans*. *J. Neurosci.* 23: 9595–9599.

Royer S, Coulson RL, and Klein M (2000) Switching off and on of synaptic sites at *Aplysia* sensorimotor synapses. *J. Neurosci.* 20: 626–638.

Sacktor TC and Schwartz JH (1990) Sensitizing stimuli cause translocation of protein kinase C in *Aplysia* sensory neurons. *Proc. Natl. Acad. Sci. USA* 87: 2036–2039.

Sahley CL, Modney BK, Boulis NM, and Muller KJ (1994) The S cell: An interneuron essential for sensitization and full dishabituation of leech shortening. *J. Neurosci.* 14: 6715–6721.

Sakurai A, Darghouth NR, Butera RJ, and Katz PS (2006) Serotonergic enhancement of a 4-AP-sensitive current mediates the synaptic depression phase of spike timing-dependent neuromodulation. *J. Neurosci.* 26: 2010–2021.

Schacher S and Montarolo PG (1991) Target-dependent structural changes in sensory neurons of *Aplysia* accompany long-term heterosynaptic inhibition. *Neuron* 6: 679–690.

Schacher S, Castellucci VF, and Kandel ER (1988) cAMP evokes long-term facilitation in *Aplysia* sensory neurons that requires new protein synthesis. *Science* 240: 1667–1669.

Schacher S, Wu F, Sun ZY, and Wang D (2000) Cell-specific changes in expression of mRNAs encoding splice variants of *Aplysia* cell adhesion molecule accompany long-term synaptic plasticity. *J. Neurobiol.* 45: 152–161.

Scholz KP and Byrne JH (1987) Long-term sensitization in *Aplysia*: Biophysical correlates in tail sensory neurons. *Science* 235: 685–687.

Scholz KP and Byrne JH (1988) Intracellular injection of cAMP induces a long-term reduction of neuronal $K+$ currents. *Science* 240: 1664–1666.

Scuri R, Mozzachiodi R, and Brunelli M (2002) Activity-dependent increase of the AHP amplitude in T sensory neurons of the leech. *J. Neurophysiol.* 88: 2490–2500.

Scuri R, Mozzachiodi R, and Brunelli M (2005) Role for calcium signaling and arachidonic acid metabolites in the activity-dependent increase of AHP amplitude in leech T sensory neurons. *J. Neurophysiol.* 94: 1066–1073.

Sharma SK and Carew TJ (2004) The roles of MAPK cascades in synaptic plasticity and memory in *Aplysia*: Facilitatory effects and inhibitory constraints. *Learn. Mem.* 11: 373–378.

Sharma SK, Sherff CM, Shobe J, Bagnall MW, Sutton MA, and Carew TJ (2003) Differential role of mitogen-activated protein kinase in three distinct phases of memory for sensitization in *Aplysia*. *J. Neurosci.* 23: 3899–3907.

Siegelbaum SA, Camardo JS, and Kandel ER (1982) Serotonin and cyclic AMP close single $K+$ channels in *Aplysia* sensory neurones. *Nature* 299: 413–417.

Small SA, Cohen TE, Kandel ER, and Hawkins RD (1992) Identified FMRFamide-immunoreactive neuron LPL16 in the left pleural ganglion of *Aplysia* produces presynaptic inhibition of siphon sensory neurons. *J. Neurosci.* 12: 1616–1627.

Sossin WS (2007) Isoform specificity of protein kinase Cs in synaptic plasticity. *Learn. Mem.* 14: 236–246.

Sossin WS and Schwartz JH (1992) Selective activation of Ca(2+)-activated PKCs in *Aplysia* neurons by 5-HT. *J. Neurosci.* 12: 1160–1168.

Sossin WS and Schwartz JH (1994) Translocation of protein kinase Cs in *Aplysia* neurons: Evidence for complex regulation. *Brain Res. Mol. Brain Res.* 24: 210–218.

Sossin WS, Diaz-Arrastia R, and Schwartz JH (1993) Characterization of two isoforms of protein kinase C in the nervous system of *Aplysia californica*. *J. Biol. Chem.* 268: 5763–5768.

Sossin WS, Sacktor TC, and Schwartz JH (1994) Persistent activation of protein kinase C during the development of long-term facilitation in *Aplysia*. *Learn. Mem.* 1: 189–202.

Stopfer M, Chen X, Tai YT, Huang GS, and Carew TJ (1996) Site specificity of short-term and long-term habituation in the tail-elicited siphon withdrawal reflex of *Aplysia*. *J. Neurosci.* 16: 4923–4932.

Sugita S, Goldsmith JR, Baxter DA, and Byrne JH (1992) Involvement of protein kinase C in serotonin-induced spike broadening and synaptic facilitation in sensorimotor connections of *Aplysia. J Neurophysiol* 68: 643–651.

Sugita S, Baxter DA, and Byrne JH (1994) Activators of protein kinase C mimic serotonin-induced modulation of a voltage-dependent potassium current in pleural sensory neurons of *Aplysia*. *J. Neurophysiol.* 72: 1240–1249.

Sugita S, Baxter DA, and Byrne JH (1997) Differential effects of 4-aminopyridine, serotonin, and phorbol esters on facilitation of sensorimotor connections in *Aplysia*. *J. Neurophysiol.* 77: 177–185.

Sun ZY, Wu F, and Schacher S (2001) Rapid bidirectional modulation of mRNA expression and export accompany long-term facilitation and depression of *Aplysia* synapses. *J. Neurobiol.* 46: 41–47.

Sutton MA and Carew TJ (2000) Parallel molecular pathways mediate expression of distinct forms of intermediate-term facilitation at tail sensory-motor synapses in *Aplysia*. *Neuron* 26: 219–231.

Sutton MA, Masters SE, Bagnall MW, and Carew TJ (2001) Molecular mechanisms underlying a unique intermediate phase of memory in *Aplysia*. *Neuron* 31: 143–154.

Sweatt JD, Volterra A, Edmonds B, Karl KA, Siegelbaum SA, and Kandel ER (1989) FMRFamide reverses protein phosphorylation produced by 5-HT and cAMP in *Aplysia* sensory neurons. *Nature* 342: 275–278.

Thompson RF and Spencer WA (1966) Habituation: A model phenomenon for the study of neuronal substrates of behavior. *Psychol. Rev.* 73: 16–43.

Vu ET and Krasne FB (1992) Evidence for a computational distinction between proximal and distal neuronal inhibition. *Science* 255: 1710–1712.

Vu ET and Krasne FB (1993) Crayfish tonic inhibition: Prolonged modulation of behavioral excitability by classical GABAergic inhibition. *J. Neurosci.* 13: 4394–4402.

Vu ET, Lee SC, and Krasne FB (1993) The mechanism of tonic inhibition of crayfish escape behavior: Distal inhibition and its functional significance. *J. Neurosci.* 13: 4379–4393.

Wainwright ML, Zhang H, Byrne JH, and Cleary LJ (2002) Localized neuronal outgrowth induced by long-term sensitization training in *Aplysia*. *J. Neurosci.* 22: 4132–4141.

Wainwright ML, Byrne JH, and Cleary LJ (2004) Dissociation of morphological and physiological changes associated with long-term memory in *Aplysia*. *J. Neurophysiol.* 92: 2628–2632.

Walsh JP and Byrne JH (1989) Modulation of a steady-state Ca2+-activated, K+ current in tail sensory neurons of *Aplysia*: Role of serotonin and cAMP. *J. Neurophysiol.* 61: 32–44.

Walters ET, Byrne JH, Carew TJ, and Kandel ER (1983a) Mechanoafferent neurons innervating tail of *Aplysia*. I. Response properties and synaptic connections. *J. Neurophysiol.* 50: 1522–1542.

Walters ET, Byrne JH, Carew TJ, and Kandel ER (1983b) Mechanoafferent neurons innervating tail of *Aplysia*. II. Modulation by sensitizing stimulation. *J. Neurophysiol.* 50: 1543–1559.

Westermarck J, Li SP, Kallunki T, Han J, and Kahari VM (2001) p38 mitogen-activated protein kinase-dependent activation of protein phosphatases 1 and 2A inhibits MEK1 and MEK2 activity and collagenase 1 (MMP-1) gene expression. *Mol. Cell. Biol.* 21: 2373–2383.

White JA, Baxter DA, and Byrne JH (1994) Analysis of the modulation by serotonin of a voltage-dependent potassium current in sensory neurons of *Aplysia*. *Biophys. J.* 66: 710–718.

Wicks SR and Rankin CH (1997) Effects of tap withdrawal response habituation on other withdrawal behaviors: The localization of habituation in the nematode *Caenorhabditis elegans*. *Behav. Neurosci.* 111: 342–353.

Wine JJ, Krasne FB, and Chen L (1975) Habituation and inhibition of the crayfish lateral giant fibre escape response. *J. Exp. Biol.* 62: 771–782.

Xu Y, Cleary LJ, and Byrne JH (1994) Identification and characterization of pleural neurons that inhibit tail sensory neurons and motor neurons in *Aplysia*: Correlation with FMRFamide immunoreactivity. *J. Neurosci.* 14: 3565–3577.

Zaccardi ML, Traina G, Cataldo E, and Brunelli M (2001) Nonassociative learning in the leech *Hirudo medicinalis*. *Behav. Brain Res.* 126: 81–92.

Zhang F, Endo S, Cleary LJ, Eskin A, and Byrne JH (1997) Role of transforming growth factor-beta in long-term synaptic facilitation in *Aplysia*. *Science* 275: 1318–1320.

Zhang H, Wainwright M, Byrne JH, and Cleary LJ (2003) Quantitation of contacts among sensory, motor, and serotonergic neurons in the pedal ganglion of *Aplysia*. *Learn. Mem.* 10: 387–393.

Zhang ZS, Fang B, Marshak DW, Byrne JH, and Cleary LJ (1991) Serotoninergic varicosities make synaptic contacts with pleural sensory neurons of *Aplysia*. *J. Comp. Neurol.* 311: 259–270.

Zhao Y and Klein M (2002) Modulation of the readily releasable pool of transmitter and of excitation-secretion coupling by activity and by serotonin at *Aplysia* sensorimotor synapses in culture. *J. Neurosci.* 22: 10671–10679.

Zimmer WE, Zhao Y, Sikorski AF, et al. (2000) The domain of brain beta-spectrin responsible for synaptic vesicle association is essential for synaptic transmission. *Brain Res.* 881: 18–27.

Zucker RS (1972) Crayfish escape behavior and central synapses. II. Physiological mechanisms underlying behavioral habituation. *J. Neurophysiol.* 35: 621–637.

Zwartjes RE, West H, Hattar S, et al. (1998) Identification of specific mRNAs affected by treatments producing long-term facilitation in *Aplysia*. *Learn. Mem.* 4: 478–495.

19 Cellular Mechanisms of Associative Learning in *Aplysia*

F. D. Lorenzetti and J. H. Byrne, The University of Texas Medical School at Houston, Houston, TX, USA

19.1 *Aplysia* Classical Conditioning and Operant Conditioning

The simple nervous system and the relatively large identifiable neurons of the marine mollusk *Aplysia* provide a useful model system to examine the cellular and molecular mechanisms of the two major forms of associative learning, classical conditioning and operant (instrumental) conditioning. The ability to associate a predictive stimulus with a subsequent salient event (i.e., classical conditioning) and the ability to associate an expressed behavior with the consequences (i.e., operant conditioning) allow for a predictive understanding of a changing environment. Although operationally distinct, there has been considerable debate whether at some fundamental level classical and operant conditioning are mechanistically distinct or similar (e.g., Rescorla and Solomon, 1967; Gormezano and Tait, 1976; Dayan and Balleine, 2002). Studies utilizing the defensive withdrawal reflexes of *Aplysia* have provided much information on the mechanisms underlying classical conditioning. Recent studies utilizing the feeding behavior of *Aplysia* are providing for a comparative analysis of the mechanisms underlying classical and operant conditioning, using the same behavior and studying the same neuron. This comparative analysis can help to resolve the issue of whether similar or different mechanisms underlie these two forms of associative learning.

19.2 Classical Conditioning

19.2.1 Behavioral Studies

The initial studies of classical conditioning in *Aplysia* focused on defensive reflex behaviors and used aversive conditioning procedures. A tactile or electrical stimulus delivered to the siphon of the animal resulted in a reflex withdrawal of the gill and siphon, a reaction which presumably protects sensitive structures from harmful stimuli. Aversive classical conditioning in this species can be demonstrated by presenting a conditioned stimulus (CS), a brief, weak tactile stimulus to the siphon which produced a small siphon withdrawal, and an unconditioned stimulus (US), a short-duration noxious electric shock to the tail which produced a large withdrawal of the siphon (the unconditioned response, UR). After repeated pairings of the CS and US, the CS alone produced a large siphon withdrawal (the conditioned response, CR). This withdrawal was enhanced beyond that produced by the US alone (sensitization control) or unpaired or random presentations of the CS or the US (Carew et al., 1981), and this conditioning persisted for as long as 4 days. Carew et al. (1983) also found that this reflex exhibited differential classical conditioning. CS (tactile stimulation) were delivered to either the siphon or to the mantle region. One CS (the CS^+) is paired with the US (electric shock to the tail) and the other is explicitly unpaired (the CS^-). After conditioning, the CS^+ produced a greater withdrawal than the CS^-.

In addition to the classical conditioning of defensive reflexes, classical conditioning can also be applied to feeding behavior. *Aplysia* feed by protracting a toothed structure called the radula into contact with seaweed. The radula grasps seaweed by closing and retracting, which results in the ingestion of the seaweed. Inedible objects can be rejected if the radula protracts while closed (grasping the object) and then opens as it retracts to release the object. Thus, the timing of radula closure determines which behavior will occur. Feeding behavior can be classically conditioned with an appetitive protocol (Colwill et al., 1997; Lechner et al., 2000a). This appetitive protocol (Lechner et al., 2000a) consisted of tactile stimulation of the lips with a fine-tipped paint brush (CS), and the US was a small piece of seaweed, which the animals were allowed to eat. The animals were trained by repeatedly pairing the CS and the US. After training, presentation of the CS elicited an increase in ingestive behavior (CR).

19.2.2 Neural Mechanisms of Aversive Classical Conditioning in *Aplysia*

A cellular mechanism called activity-dependent neuromodulation contributes to associative learning in *Aplysia* (Hawkins et al., 1983; Walters and Byrne, 1983; Antonov et al., 2001). A general cellular scheme of activity-dependent neuromodulation is illustrated in **Figure 1**. Two sensory neurons (SN1 and SN2) constitute the pathways for the conditioned stimuli (CS^+ and CS^-) and make weak subthreshold connections to a motor neuron. Delivering a reinforcing stimulus or US alone has two effects. First, the US activates the motor neuron and produces the UR. Second, the US activates a diffuse modulatory system that nonspecifically enhances transmitter release from all the sensory neurons. This nonspecific enhancement contributes to sensitization. Temporal specificity, which is characteristic of associative learning, occurs when there is pairing of the CS (spike activity in SN1) with the US, which causes a selective amplification of the modulatory effects in SN1. Unpaired activity does not amplify the effects of the US in SN2. The amplification of the modulatory effects in SN1 leads to an enhancement of the ability of SN1 to activate the motor neuron and produce the CR.

A reduced preparation for the siphon-withdrawal reflex was developed that consists of the isolated tail, siphon, and central nervous system (CNS) of the animal (Antonov et al., 2001). A classical conditioning

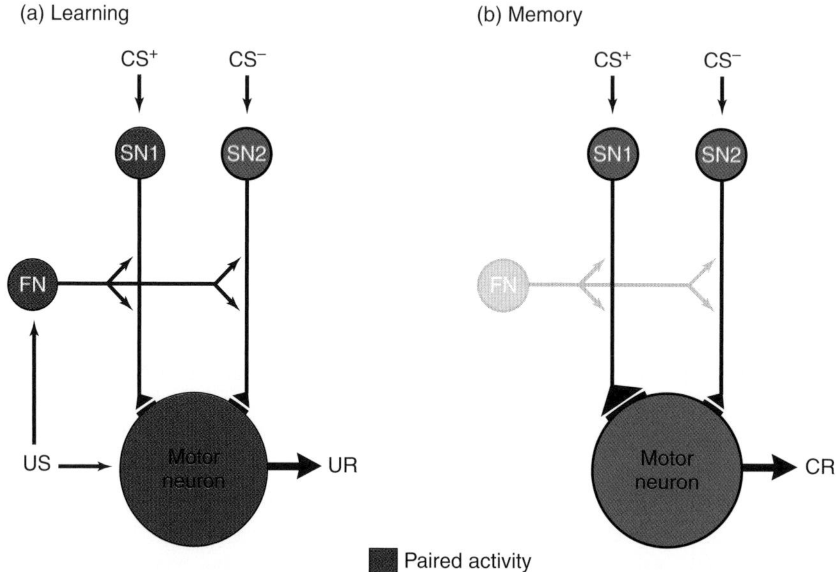

Figure 1 General model of activity-dependent neuromodulation. (a) Learning. A motivationally potent reinforcing stimulus (US) activates a motor neuron to produce the unconditioned response (UR) and a facilitatory neuron (FN) or modulatory system that regulates the strength of the connection between sensory neurons (SN1 and SN2) and the motor neuron. Increased spike activity in one sensory neuron (SN1) immediately before the modulatory signal amplifies the degree and duration of the modulatory effects, perhaps through the Ca^{+2} sensitivity of the modulatory evoked second messenger, with contributions from the postsynaptic neuron. The unpaired sensory neuron (SN2) does not show an amplification of the modulatory effects. (b) Memory: The amplified modulatory effects cause increases in transmitter release and/or excitability of the paired neuron, which in turn strengthens the functional connection between the paired sensory neuron (SN1) and the motor neuron. The associative enhancement of synaptic strength represents the conditioned response (CR).

training protocol was performed with tactile stimulation of the siphon as the CS and an electric shock to the tail as the US. Paired training significantly increased the amplitude of the siphon withdrawal, indicating successful conditioning. The classical conditioning protocol also produced a pairing-specific increase in the strength of the sensorimotor neuron synapse.

Experimental analyses of sensitization of defensive reflexes in *Aplysia* have shown that the neuromodulator released by the reinforcing stimulus, which is believed to be serotonin, activates the enzyme adenylyl cyclase in the sensory neuron. The activation of adenylyl cyclase increases the synthesis of the second messenger cyclic adenosine monophosphate (cAMP), which activates the cAMP-dependent protein kinase, and the subsequent protein phosphorylation leads to a modulation in several properties of the sensory neurons. These changes include modulation of membrane conductances and other processes which facilitate synaptic transmission. This facilitation results in the increased activation of the motor neuron and the sensitization of the reflex. The pairing specificity of the associative conditioning is at least partly due to an increase in the level of cAMP beyond that produced by serotonin alone (Ocorr et al., 1985; Abrams and Kandel, 1988). The influx of Ca^{+2} associated with the CS (spike activity) amplifies the US-mediated modulatory effect by interacting with a Ca^{+2}-sensitive component of the adenylyl cyclase (Abrams and Kandel, 1988). A critical role for Ca^{+2}-stimulated cyclase is also suggested by studies of *Drosophila* showing that the adenylyl cyclase of a mutant deficient in associative learning exhibits a loss of Ca^{+2}/calmodulin sensitivity.

The postsynaptic cell (i.e., motor neuron) also contributes to the plasticity of the synapse (Murphy and Glanzman, 1997; Bao et al., 1998). The postsynaptic membrane of the motor neuron contains *N*-methyl-D-aspartate (NMDA)-like receptors. If these receptors are blocked, then the associative modification of the synapse is disrupted. NMDA receptors require concurrent delivery of glutamate and depolarization in order to allow the entry of calcium. Activity in the sensory neuron (CS) provides the glutamate, and the US depolarizes the cell. The subsequent increase in intracellular Ca^{+2} may release a retrograde signal from the postsynaptic cell to the presynaptic terminal. This retrograde signal would then act to further enhance the cAMP cascade in the sensory neuron. Presynaptically blocking protein kinase A (PKA) by injecting a peptide inhibitor into the sensory neuron, or postsynaptically blocking Ca^{+2} by injecting BAPTA (1,2-bis-(o-aminophenoxy)-ethane-N,N,N′,N′-tetraacetic acid) into the motor neuron, also blocked the pairing-specific strengthening of the sensorimotor neuron synapse (Antonov et al., 2003) using the simplified preparation for classical conditioning mentioned earlier. The plasticity in the sensorimotor neuron synapse can be blocked by an injection to the postsynaptic motor neuron alone, suggesting that a retrograde signal is an integral part of the process.

This mechanism for associative learning appears to be an elaboration of a process already in place that mediates sensitization, which is a simpler form of learning (*See* Chapter 18 for a review of the mechanisms of sensitization). This finding raises the interesting possibility that even more complex forms of learning may use simpler forms as building blocks, an idea that has been suggested by psychologists for many years but has only recently become testable at the cellular level.

19.2.3 Neural Mechanisms of Appetitive Classical Conditioning in *Aplysia*

The feeding system of *Aplysia* has many advantages. For example, much of the cellular circuitry controlling feeding behavior has been identified, so it is possible to study neurons with known behavioral significance. The *in vivo* training protocol for classical conditioning (Lechner et al., 2000a) has been used to examine correlates of classical conditioning in several neurons that are important for the expression of feeding behavior. Classical conditioning led to the pairing-specific strengthening of the CS-evoked excitatory synaptic input to pattern-initiating neuron B31/32, although no changes were observed in the membrane properties, such as input resistance or the threshold for bursting (Lechner et al., 2000b). If B31/32 receives a greater excitatory input from the CS, then this neuron would be more likely to initiate a feeding motor pattern, and the feeding motor patterns evoked by the CS would be mostly ingestive (Lechner et al., 2000b). However, B31/32 promotes the initiation of feeding motor patterns without defining which type of pattern (i.e., ingestive or egestive) is expressed (Hurwitz et al., 1996). Thus, the pairing-specific increase in excitatory input to B31/32 alone cannot account for the specific increase in the ingestive behavior that is observed following *in vivo* classical conditioning (Lechner et al., 2000a).

Correlates of classical conditioning were measured in neuron B51 following the *in vivo* classical conditioning protocol (Lorenzetti et al., 2006). Neuron B51 is pivotal for the expression of ingestive motor patterns, and B51 exhibits a characteristic all-or-nothing sustained level of activity (i.e., plateau potential; Plummer and Kirk, 1990) during ingestive motor patterns (Nargeot et al., 1999a). Classical conditioning induced a significant pairing-specific increase in the CS-evoked excitatory synaptic input to B51, as well as an increase in the number of CS-elicited plateau potentials. The pairing-specific strengthening of the excitatory synaptic input can increase the likelihood that B51 is recruited into a motor pattern, which can contribute to the pairing-specific increase in the number of CS-evoked plateau potentials. An increase in the recruitment of B51 should bias the feeding central pattern generator (CPG) toward the expression of ingestive motor patterns (Nargeot et al., 1999b). Thus, the effects produced by classical conditioning appear to be distributed among elements of the feeding CPG such as B31/32 and B51, with the pairing-specific plasticity in B31/32 contributing to the increased number of motor patterns, while the pairing-specific plasticity in B51 is biasing the nature of the motor patterns toward ingestion.

In addition to the pairing-specific enhancement of the CS-evoked excitatory synaptic input to B51, classical conditioning can alter the intrinsic biophysical properties of B51. Classical conditioning raised the threshold for eliciting a burst (i.e., plateau potential) in B51 without affecting either the resting membrane potential or input resistance. This result adds to an increasing body of evidence that, in addition to changes in synaptic efficacy, changes in the intrinsic neuronal excitability also contribute to the storage of memory (for reviews see Daoudal and Debanne, 2003; Zhang and Linden, 2003; *See also* Chapter 14). The pairing-specific decrease in the excitability would make B51 less likely to be active, whereas the increase in the excitatory synaptic input would facilitate the recruitment of the neuron. However, the training produced more CS-evoked plateau potentials in B51 in the paired group as compared to the unpaired group. Thus, the factors that enhance the recruitment of B51 overpower the diminished excitability and bias B51 toward producing more plateau potentials, resulting in a greater number of ingestive motor patterns. This pairing-specific decrease in the excitability of B51 could be an adaptive mechanism to help shape the CS specificity produced by classical conditioning.

An *in vitro* analog of classical conditioning has been developed for the feeding system of *Aplysia* (Mozzachiodi et al., 2003). This preparation used isolated ganglia from naive animals. Stimulation of the anterior tentacular nerve was chosen as the analog of the CS. Specifically, the fourth branch of the anterior tentacular nerve was used because this branch innervates the lip region, which is the site of stimulation for the *in vivo* CS. Stimulation of the esophageal nerve was used as the analog of the US. The ganglia were trained by repeatedly pairing the CS with the US. After training, the ganglia produced more motor patterns (analogs of the CR) after CS delivery, indicating that conditioning was successful in this reduced analog. The *in vitro* analog of classical conditioning was then performed while monitoring the membrane properties and CS-elicited synaptic input to B31/32, CBI-2 (Mozzachiodi et al., 2003), and B51 (Lorenzetti et al., 2006). The *in vitro* training protocol produced an increase in the CS-elicited synaptic input to both B31/32 and to B51, an increase in the burst threshold of B51, and an increased number of CS-elicited plateau potentials in B51, similar to what was observed following *in vivo* training. In addition, *in vitro* classical conditioning led to a pairing-specific enhancement of the CS-elicited synaptic input to CBI-2 (Mozzachiodi et al., 2003), which is one of the command-like interneurons controlling the activity of the feeding CPG (Rosen et al., 1991). Synergism among these effects can help produce the pairing-specific increase in the number of CS-evoked bites observed following *in vivo* classical conditioning.

These results provide further support that memory can be distributed among multiple sites of plasticity, similar to what has been observed with other animal model systems. In *Lymnaea*, appetitive classical conditioning strengthened the CS-evoked excitatory synaptic drive to feeding motor neurons (Staras et al., 1999) and induced a persistent depolarization in the modulatory neuron CV1a (Jones et al., 2003). In *Aplysia*, empirical studies (e.g., Trudeau and Castellucci, 1993; for review see also Cleary et al., 1995) and theoretical work (White et al., 1993; Lieb and Frost, 1997) on the neural circuits controlling defensive withdrawal reflexes emphasize the role of both sensory neurons and interneurons as sites of learning-related plasticity underlying behavioral sensitization. In vertebrates, the plasticity produced by delay classical conditioning of the eyelid response is distributed between the cerebellar cortex and the deep cerebellar nuclei (for reviews see Raymond et al., 1996; Kim and Thompson, 1997). Trace classical conditioning of the same reflex can also involve the hippocampus (for review see Christian and Thompson, 2003). Therefore, studies in both invertebrate and vertebrate neural circuits support the concept that multiple sites of plasticity contribute to the storage of information for associative and non-associative forms of memory.

19.3 Operant Conditioning

19.3.1 Behavioral Studies

Feeding behavior in *Aplysia* can be modified by pairing feeding with an aversive stimulus. If food is wrapped in a tough plastic net, *Aplysia* bite and attempt to swallow the food. However, netted food cannot be swallowed, and so it is rejected. The inability to consume the food appeared to be an aversive stimulus that modified the feeding behavior, because the trained animals no longer attempted to bite the netted food (Susswein et al., 1986).

Feeding behavior can also be operantly conditioned with an appetitive stimulus (Brembs et al., 2002). The reinforcement signal for the *in vivo* training protocol was a brief shock to the esophageal nerve. The esophageal nerve is believed to be part of the pathway mediating food reward because bursts of activity in this nerve occur when the animal successfully ingests food (Brembs et al., 2002). In addition, lesions to this nerve blocked *in vivo* appetitive classical conditioning (Lechner et al., 2000a). Also, the *in vitro* analog of classical conditioning discussed earlier successfully increased the number of CS-elicited motor patterns when esophageal nerve shock was used as the US (Mozzachiodi et al., 2003). In the operant conditioning paradigm, the contingent reinforcement of biting behavior by a shock to the esophageal nerve produced an increase in the frequency of biting, when measured both immediately after training and 24 h after training, as compared to animals trained with a yoke-control procedure (Brembs et al., 2002).

19.3.2 Neural Mechanisms of Appetitive Operant Conditioning in *Aplysia*

We have previously discussed B51 (Plummer and Kirk, 1990) as being implicated in the expression of ingestive behavior and as a correlate of classical conditioning. B51 is active predominantly during the retraction phase (Nargeot et al., 1997), and when B51 is recruited into a pattern, it recruits radula closure motor neurons (see **Figure 2**).

The *in vivo* training protocol for operant conditioning was used to examine correlates in neuron B51 (Brembs et al., 2002). Operant conditioning led to changes in the membrane properties of B51. The input resistance was increased and the threshold for bursting was decreased. These changes increase the likelihood of B51 activation and thereby contribute to the conditioned increase in the ingestive response.

An *in vitro* analog of operant conditioning was developed using only the isolated buccal ganglia, which is responsible for generating the motor patterns involved in feeding (Nargeot et al., 1999a). These motor patterns can either be ingestive or egestive. In this analog of operant conditioning, motor patterns corresponding to ingestion were used as the analog of the behavior. The ingestive motor pattern was selectively reinforced by contingently shocking the esophageal nerve, which was the analog of the reinforcement. The conditioning procedure resulted in an increase in the likelihood of ingestive patterns being produced (Nargeot et al., 1999a). The contingent reinforcement also resulted in the modulation of the membrane properties of neuron B51 (Nargeot et al., 1999a). The input resistance increased and the threshold for eliciting a burst decreased in a manner similar to the *in vivo* operant conditioning protocol. These changes in the membrane properties of B51 make the cell more excitable and more likely to be recruited into a motor pattern, thus helping to explain the increase in the frequency of expression of the ingestive motor patterns following the *in vitro* analog of operant conditioning. Furthermore, these results for the membrane properties of B51 can be replicated when induced electrical activity in B51 was substituted for the analog of the behavior, instead of an ingestive motor pattern, which was then contingently reinforced with a shock to the esophageal nerve (Nargeot et al., 1999b).

The esophageal nerve, which is used to send both a reinforcement signal with operant conditioning and a US signal with classical conditioning, contains dopaminergic processes (Kabotyanski et al., 1998). Esophageal nerve stimulation produced a postsynaptic potential (PSP) in B51 and this PSP was blocked by the dopamine antagonist ergonovine (Nargeot et al., 1999c). This dopamine antagonist also blocked the acquisition of the associative changes induced by *in vitro* analogs of both operant conditioning (Nargeot et al., 1999c) and classical conditioning (Reyes et al., 2005).

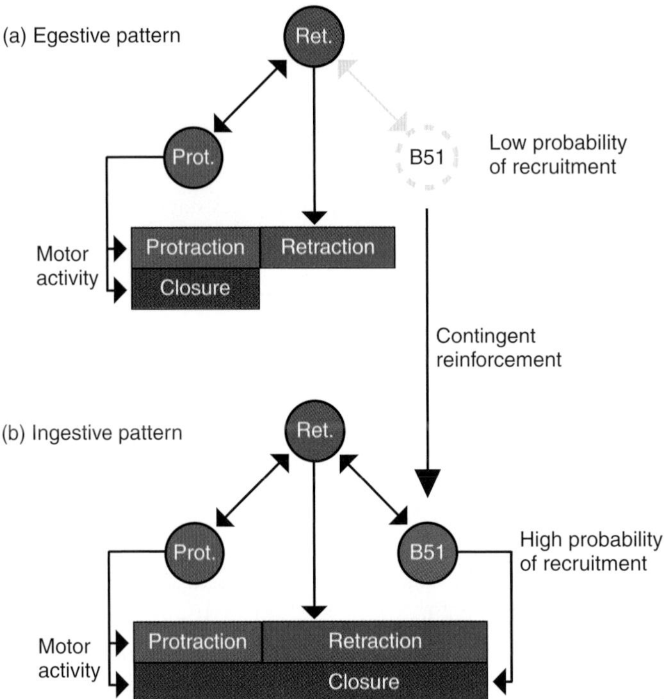

Figure 2 Model of operant conditioning of feeding in *Aplysia.* The cellular network that mediates feeding behavior is represented by the elements in circles. Motor activity comprising two basic feeding patterns is depicted below. (a) At first, the radula protraction-generating element (Prot.) is active, followed by the radula retraction element (Ret.). In the naive state, neuron B51 has a low probability for recruitment and thus does not take part in the feeding motor program. Radula closure occurs during the protraction phase. Consequently, the pattern elicited is egestive. (b) Neuron B51 now has a higher probability for recruitment following contingent reinforcement. B51 is now active during the motor program, leading to radula closure occurring primarily during the retraction phase. Thus, the pattern elicited will now be ingestive.

The analog was further reduced by removing neuron B51 from the ganglia and placing it in culture (Lorenzetti et al., 2000; Brembs et al., 2002). This single, isolated neuron was conditioned by contingently reinforcing induced electrical activity (the analog of behavior) with a direct and temporally discrete application of dopamine (the analog of reinforcement). After conditioning, the input resistance of B51 increased and the threshold for bursting decreased, similar to the *in vivo* and *in vitro* analogs of operant conditioning described above. The membrane properties of B51 were modulated such that the cell was more likely to be active in the future. Such a highly reduced preparation is a promising candidate to study the mechanisms of dopamine-mediated reward and the conditioned expression of behavior at the level of the intracellular signaling cascades.

The operant conditioning of the feeding behavior of *Aplysia* increased the expression of the ingestive responses. The excitability of B51 was also increased by the operant protocol, accounting for the bias in the output of the CPG toward ingestion. However, increasing the excitability of B51 is not likely to increase the total number of patterns expressed. Thus, another site of plasticity is probably induced by the operant protocol. A likely candidate for this additional site of plasticity is in a cell or synapse that is responsible for pattern initiation (e.g., B31). Though these possible sites of plasticity have not yet been explored, it seems likely that both operant and classical conditioning lead to the distribution of memory at multiple sites within the neural circuit.

19.4 Conclusions

The feeding system of *Aplysia,* with its relatively simple circuitry, provides a model system for a systematic comparison of the mechanisms underlying classical and operant conditioning. Some interesting similarities as well as differences are beginning to emerge (**Table 1**). One similarity is the nature of the reinforcement pathway and its neurotransmitter. The esophageal nerve mediates the reinforcement signal

Table 1 Comparative analysis between appetitive classical and operant conditioning of feeding in *Aplysia*

	Classical conditioning	*Operant conditioning*
Change in the number of bites	Increase	Increase
Pathway mediating US/reinforcement	Esophageal nerve	Esophageal nerve
Transmitter mediating US/reinforcement	Dopamine	Dopamine
B51 plateau potentials	Increase	Increase
B51 resting membrane potential	No change	No change
B51 input resistance	No change	Increase
B51 burst threshold	Increase	Decrease

for appetitive operant conditioning (Nargeot et al., 1997) and the US pathway for appetitive classical conditioning (Lechner et al., 2000a; Mozzachiodi et al., 2003). Also, this pathway appears to use dopamine as a transmitter, which is consistent with the long-held view that dopamine can mediate the US/reinforcement for appetitive forms of both classical and operant conditioning in both vertebrates and invertebrates (for review see Schultz, 2002).

Appetitive classical conditioning of feeding behavior in *Aplysia* produced two major changes in neuron B51. The synaptic input along the CS pathway into B51 was increased. This increase in the CS pathway suggests that the conditioned sensory pathway receives a preferential boost, while the other sensory pathways could remain unchanged. The second change seen with B51 was an increase in the burst threshold. This change acts on the level of the pattern generation machinery and makes the expression of ingestive feeding responses less likely. Thus, the animal would be less likely to feed unless the CS was present. Identical changes in the properties of B51 were expressed in intact animals trained with a classical conditioning protocol and in an *in vitro* analog of classical conditioning using isolated ganglia (Lorenzetti et al., 2006).

Appetitive operant conditioning of feeding behavior in *Aplysia* also produced two major changes in neuron B51. Both changes were made to the intrinsic membrane properties of the cell. First, the input resistance was increased. Second, the burst threshold was decreased. Both of these changes act in the same direction and would make B51 more likely to be active, thus accounting for the increased expression of the behavior following reinforcement. Identical changes in the membrane properties of B51 were expressed in intact animals trained with an operant conditioning protocol (Brembs et al., 2002), in an *in vitro* analog of operant conditioning using isolated ganglia (Nargeot et al., 1999a,b), and in a single-cell analog consisting of neuron B51 in culture (Brembs et al., 2002).

B51 is a cellular locus for the changes induced by both operant and classical conditioning. No pairing-specific changes in the input resistance were observed following classical conditioning, which was in contrast to the contingent-dependent increase in this parameter measured in B51 following both *in vivo* and *in vitro* operant conditioning. Both operant and classical conditioning modified the threshold level for activation of neuron B51, but in opposite directions, revealing key differences in the cellular mechanisms underlying these two forms of associative learning and suggesting a difference at the molecular level. B51 appears to be a coincidence detector for both the CS–US association (classical conditioning) and the contingency between ingestive behavior and reinforcement (operant conditioning). Because dopamine likely mediates both the US and the reinforcement, a key problem is the elucidation of the mechanisms that lead to the induction of the opposite effects on the burst threshold. One possibility is that the coincidence detector for classical conditioning involves an association between a transmitter released by the CS and dopamine, whereas for operant conditioning it involves an association between the cellular effects of B51 burst activity and dopamine.

References

Abrams TW and Kandel ER (1988) Is contiguity detection in classical conditioning a system or cellular property? Learning in *Aplysia* suggests a possible site. *Trends Neurosci.* 11: 128–135.

Antonov I, Antonova I, Kandel ER, and Hawkins RD (2001) The contribution of activity-dependent synaptic plasticity to classical conditioning in *Aplysia*. *J. Neurosci.* 21: 6413–6422.

Antonov I, Antonova I, Kandel ER, and Hawkins RD (2003) Activity-dependent presynaptic facilitation and Hebbian LTP

are both required and interact during classical conditioning in *Aplysia*. *Neuron* 37: 135–147.
Bao JX, Kandel ER, and Hawkins RD (1998) Involvement of presynaptic and postsynaptic mechanisms in a cellular analog of classical conditioning at *Aplysia* sensory-motor neuron synapses in isolated cell culture. *J. Neurosci.* 18: 458–466.
Brembs B, Lorenzetti FD, Reyes FD, Baxter DA, and Byrne JH (2002) Operant reward learning in *Aplysia*: Neuronal correlates and mechanisms. *Science* 296: 1706–1709.
Carew TJ, Walters ET, and Kandel ER (1981) Classical conditioning in a simple withdrawal reflex in *Aplysia californica*. *J. Neurosci.* 1: 1426–1437.
Carew TJ, Hawkins RD, and Kandel ER (1983) Differential classical conditioning of a defensive withdrawal reflex in *Aplysia californica*. *Science* 219: 397–400.
Christian KM and Thompson RF (2003) Neural substrates of eyeblink conditioning: Acquisition and retention. *Learn. Mem.* 10: 427–455.
Cleary LJ, Byrne JH, and Frost WN (1995) Role of interneurons in defensive withdrawal reflexes in *Aplysia*. *Learn. Mem.* 2: 133–151.
Colwill RM, Goodrum K, and Martin A (1997) Pavlovian appetitive discriminative conditioning in *Aplysia californica*. *Anim. Learn. Behav.* 25: 268–276.
Daoudal G and Debanne D (2003) Long-term plasticity of intrinsic excitability: Learning rules and mechanisms. *Learn. Mem.* 10: 456–465.
Dayan P and Balleine BW (2002) Reward, motivation, and reinforcement learning. *Neuron* 36: 285–298.
Gormezano I and Tait RW (1976) The Pavlovian analysis of instrumental conditioning. *Pavlov. J. Biol. Sci.* 11: 37–55.
Hawkins RD, Abrams TW, Carew TJ, and Kandel ER (1983) A cellular mechanism of classical conditioning in *Aplysia*: Activity-dependent amplification of presynaptic facilitation. *Science* 219: 400–405.
Hurwitz I, Neustadter D, Morton DW, Chiel HJ, and Susswein AJ (1996) Activity patterns of the B31/32 pattern initiators innervating the I2 muscle of the buccal mass during normal feeding movements in *Aplysia californica*. *J. Neurophysiol.* 75: 1309–1326.
Jones NG, Kemenes I, Kemenes G, and Benjamin PR (2003) A persistent cellular change in a single modulatory neuron contributes to associative long-term memory. *Curr. Biol.* 13: 1064–1069.
Kabotyanski EA, Baxter DA, and Byrne JH (1998) Identification and characterization of catecholaminergic neuron B65, which initiates and modifies patterned activity in the buccal ganglia of *Aplysia*. *J. Neurophysiol.* 79: 605–621.
Kim JJ and Thompson RF (1997) Cerebellar circuits and synaptic mechanisms involved in classical eyeblink conditioning. *Trends Neurosci.* 20: 177–181.
Lechner HA, Baxter DA, and Byrne JH (2000a) Classical conditioning of feeding in *Aplysia*: I. Behavioral analysis. *J. Neurosci.* 20: 3369–3376.
Lechner HA, Baxter DA, and Byrne JH (2000b) Classical conditioning of feeding in *Aplysia*: II. Neurophysiological correlates. *J. Neurosci.* 20: 3377–3386.
Lieb JR Jr. and Frost WN (1997) Realistic simulation of the *Aplysia* siphon-withdrawal reflex circuit: Roles of circuit elements in producing motor output. *J. Neurophysiol.* 77: 1249–1268.
Lorenzetti FD, Baxter DA, and Byrne JH (2000) Contingent reinforcement with dopamine modifies the properties of an individual neuron in *Aplysia*. *Soc. Neurosci. Abstr.* 26: 1524.
Lorenzetti FD, Mozzachiodi R, Baxter DA, and Byrne JH (2006) Classical and operant conditioning differentially modify the intrinsic properties of an identified neuron. *Nat. Neurosci.* 9: 17–19.
Mozzachiodi R, Lechner HA, Baxter DA, and Byrne JH (2003) In vitro analog of classical conditioning of feeding behavior in *Aplysia*. *Learn. Mem.* 10: 478–94.
Murphy GG and Glanzman DL (1997) Mediation of classical conditioning in *Aplysia californica* by long-term potentiation of sensorimotor synapses. *Science* 278: 467–71.
Nargeot R, Baxter DA, and Byrne JH (1997) Contingent-dependent enhancement of rhythmic motor patterns: An in vitro analog of operant conditioning. *J. Neurosci.* 17: 8093–8105.
Nargeot R, Baxter DA, and Byrne JH (1999a) In vitro analog of operant conditioning in *Aplysia*. I. Contingent reinforcement modifies the functional dynamics of an identified neuron. *J. Neurosci.* 19: 2247–2260.
Nargeot R, Baxter DA, and Byrne JH (1999b) In vitro analog of operant conditioning in *Aplysia*. II. Modifications of the functional dynamics of an identified neuron contribute to motor pattern selection. *J. Neurosci.* 19: 2261–2272.
Nargeot R, Baxter DA, Patterson GW, and Byrne JH (1999c) Dopaminergic synapses mediate neuronal changes in an analogue of operant conditioning. *J. Neurophysiol.* 81: 1983–1987.
Ocorr KA, Walters ET, and Byrne JH (1985) Associative conditioning analog selectively increases cAMP levels of tail sensory neurons in *Aplysia*. *Proc. Natl. Acad. Sci. USA* 82: 2548–2552.
Plummer MR and Kirk MD (1990) Premotor neurons B51 and B52 in the buccal ganglia of *Aplysia californica*: Synaptic connections, effect on ongoing motor rhythms, and peptide modulation. *J. Neurophysiol.* 63: 539–558.
Raymond JL, Lisberger SG, and Mauk MD (1996) The cerebellum: A neuronal learning machine? *Science* 272: 1126–1131.
Rescorla RA and Solomon RL (1967) Two-process learning theory: Relationships between Pavlovian conditioning and instrumental learning. *Psychol. Rev.* 74: 151–182.
Reyes FD, Mozzachiodi R, Baxter DA, and Byrne JH (2005) Reinforcement in an in vitro analog of appetitive classical conditioning of feeding behavior in *Aplysia*: Blockade by a dopamine antagonist. *Learn. Mem.* 12: 216–220.
Rosen SC, Teyke T, Miller MW, Weiss KR, and Kupfermann I (1991) Identification and characterization of cerebral-to-buccal interneurons implicated in the control of motor programs associated with feeding in *Aplysia*. *J. Neurosci.* 11: 3630–3655.
Schultz W (2002) Getting formal with dopamine and reward. *Neuron* 36: 241–263.
Susswein AJ, Schwarz M, and Feldman E (1986) Learned changes of feeding behavior in *Aplysia* in response to edible and inedible foods. *J. Neurosci.* 6: 1513–1527.
Staras K, Kemenes G, and Benjamin PR (1999) Cellular traces of behavioral classical conditioning can be recorded at several specific sites in a simple nervous system. *J. Neurosci.* 19: 347–357.
Trudeau LE and Castellucci VF (1993) Sensitization of the gill and siphon withdrawal reflex of *Aplysia*: Multiple sites of change in the neuronal network. *J. Neurophysiol.* 70: 1210–1220.
Walters ET and Byrne JH (1983) Associative conditioning of single sensory neurons suggests a cellular mechanism for learning. *Science* 219: 405–408.
White JA, Ziv I, Cleary LJ, Baxter DA, and Byrne JH (1993) The role of interneurons in controlling the tail-withdrawal reflex in *Aplysia*: A network model. *J. Neurophysiol.* 70: 1777–1786.
Zhang W and Linden DJ (2003) The other side of the engram: Experience-driven changes in neuronal intrinsic excitability. *Nat. Rev. Neurosci.* 4: 885–900.

20 Procedural Learning: Classical Conditioning

A. M. Poulos, University of California at Los Angeles, Los Angeles, CA, USA

K. M. Christian, National Institutes of Health, Bethesda, MD, USA

R. F. Thompson, University of Southern California, Los Angeles, CA, USA

20.1 Introduction

The two best understood and most extensively studied aspects of procedural learning are classical conditioning of discrete skeletal muscle responses and conditioning of fear. Indeed, more is known about the neural substrates of these two forms of learning than about any other aspects of learning and memory (*See* Chapter 21). A schema illustrating the different forms or aspects of memory is shown in **Figure 1**. The major distinction is between declarative and procedural memory (see Squire and Knowlton, 1994). Classical or Pavlovian conditioning is the *sine qua non* of procedural memory; it is defined by the procedure used. The "neutral" conditioned stimulus (CS) and the reflex-eliciting unconditioned stimulus (US) are presented paired together, with CS onset preceding US onset, and the outcome compared to various control procedures where the stimuli are not paired together. The stimuli are presented to the organism regardless of what the organism does, in contrast to instrumental or operant learning, where the organism's response can control the occurrence of the stimuli, for example, responding so as to avoid presentation of the US.

Another way of distinguishing between declarative and procedural memory is in terms of awareness – declarative memory provides the capacity for conscious recollection of facts and events, whereas procedural memory is typically not accessible to conscious recollection – it can't be brought to mind and declared. Rather, procedural memory is expressed through performance (see Clark and Thompson, in press, for a more detailed discussion and history of these concepts).

Classical conditioning provides a temporal structure where the organism learns about the causal fabric of the environment. The CS provides the organism with information concerning the subsequent occurrence of another stimulus. However, mere temporal pairings of the CS and US, simple contiguity, are not sufficient for learning. Instead, it is the contingency, the probability that the CS will be followed by the US, that determines learning. As Rescorla showed in classic studies, if there are many presentations of the US alone, as well as paired presentations of CS and US, little or nothing may be learned (see Rescorla, 1988). Indeed the learning that occurs in classical conditioning is a good predictor of the probability one stimulus will be followed by

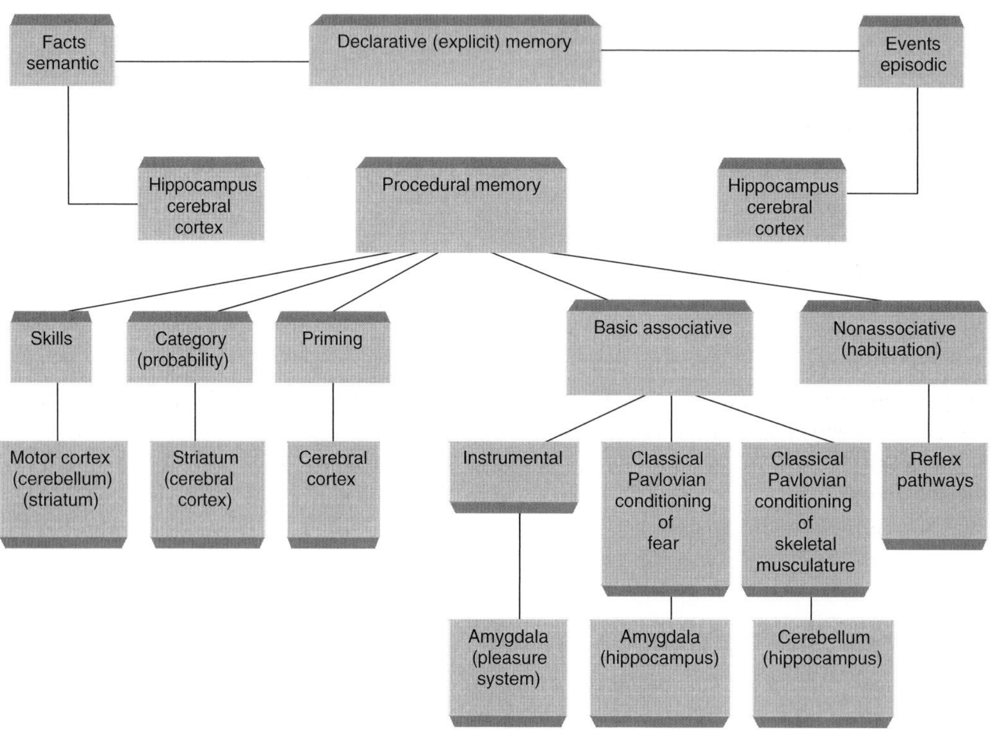

Figure 1 Taxonomy of long-term memory and the putative associated neural structures. Adapted from Squire LR (1998) Memory systems. *C. R. Acad. Sci. III* 321: 153–156, with permission.

another. This causal aspect of classical conditioning has led many to believe it is the most basic aspect of learning and memory.

Here, we focus on providing a comparative analysis of the behavioral and neurobiological mechanisms of two of the most well-understood forms of classical conditioning: eyeblink and fear conditioning.

20.2 Classical Conditioning of the Eyeblink Response

Eyeblink conditioning is perhaps the most widely studied form of procedural learning in mammals, including humans. In standard delay conditioning, a tone or a light precedes and coterminates with a reflex-eliciting stimulus such as a puff of air to the cornea. Following several presentations of these paired stimuli, an eyeblink conditioned response (CR) will develop that reflects the learned contingency between the CS and US. Extensive investigation into the neural substrates of this associative memory has resulted in perhaps the most complete description of mammalian memory formation to date (see Thompson and Krupa, 1994; Thompson and Kim, 1996; Kim and Thompson, 1997; Yeo and Hesslow, 1998; Nores et al., 2000; Steinmetz, 2000a,b; Woodruff-Pak and Steinmetz, 2000; Christian and Thompson, 2003, for reviews).

20.2.1 The Nature of the Eyeblink Conditioned Response

Gormezano et al. (1962) showed some years ago in separate studies in the rabbit that conditioned eyeball retraction, nictitating membrane (NM) extension, and external eyelid closure all had essentially identical acquisition functions. Simultaneous recording of NM extension and external eyelid closure (electromyographic (EMG) recordings from *orbicularis oculi*) during acquisition and extinction showed that they were, in essence, perfectly correlated, both within trials and over training (McCormick et al., 1982c; Lavond et al., 1990). Furthermore, some degree of conditioned contraction of facial and neck musculature also developed and was also strongly correlated with NM extension. These observations led to characterization of the CR as a "synchronous facial 'flinch' centered about closure of the eyelids and extension of the NM" (McCormick et al., 1982c: 773; see Thompson and Krupa, 1994, for overview). Substantial learning-induced increases in neuronal unit activity that correlate very closely with the conditioned NM extension response have been reported in several motor nuclei: oculomotor, trochlear, motor trigeminal, abducens, accessory abducens, and facial. These are all components of the same global CR involving, to the extent studied, essentially perfectly coordinated activity in a number of muscles and associated motor nuclei. The NM extension response is but one component of the CR. The suggestion that different motor nuclei might somehow exhibit different CR in the eyeblink conditioning paradigm (Delgado-Garcia et al., 1990) is not supported by evidence.

The CR and the unconditioned response (UR) are similar in eyeblink conditioning in the sense that, to a large extent, the same muscles and motor nuclei are engaged. However, the CR and the UR differ fundamentally in a number of respects. The minimum onset latency of the CR to a tone CS in well-trained rabbits, measured as NM extension, is about 90–100 ms; the minimum onset latency of the NM extension UR to a 3-psi corneal airpuff US in the rabbit is about 25–40 ms. Perhaps most important, the variables that determine the topographies of the UR and CR are quite different. The topography of the UR is under the control of the properties of the US: for example, stimulus intensity, rise-time, and duration. In marked contrast, the topography of the CR is substantially independent of the properties of the US and is determined primarily by the interstimulus interval (the CS-US onset interval) – the CR peaking at about the onset of the US over a wide range of effective CS-US onset intervals (Coleman and Gormezano, 1971; Steinmetz, 1990a). This key property of the CR cannot be derived from the properties of the US or the UR. The CR and the UR also differ in that certain components of the UR can be elicited separately by appropriate peripheral stimuli, but the CR always occurs as a global coordinated response (McCormick et al., 1982c). Another important difference is that the CR exhibits much greater plasticity in recovery from lesions of the motor nuclei that impair performance of the UR than does the UR itself (Disterhoft et al., 1985; Steinmetz et al., 1992a).

In sum, the conditioned eyeblink response involves highly coordinated activity in a number of motor nuclei and muscles; it is one global defensive response that is conditioned to a neutral stimulus as a result of associative training. Electrical stimulation of the small critical region of the cerebellar interpositus nucleus (see following) elicits this full complement of coordinated behaviors; it is a 'higher motor program.' The very small lesion of interpositus nucleus, which is effective in completely and permanently abolishing the conditioned NM extension response, also completely and permanently abolishes all other components of the CR that have been studied – eyeball retraction, external eyelid closure, orbicularis oculi EMG – without producing any impairment in performance of the reflex response (Steinmetz et al., 1992a).

20.2.2 Brain Systems Engaged in Eyeblink Conditioning

Electrophysiological recordings of neural activity in eyeblink conditioning indicate that a number of brain areas and systems become engaged, most prominently motor nuclei, the hippocampus, and the cerebellum (see Thompson and Kim, 1996; Steinmetz et al., 2001; Christian and Thompson, 2003, for overviews). In all these systems neuronal activity in the CS period increases over the course of learning and precedes the onset of the behavioral CR within trials. Indeed, this increased pattern of action potential discharges in the hippocampus and cerebellum predicts the occurrence and the actual temporal form of the CR (but not the reflex response). In standard delay conditioning when the CS and the US overlap, the cerebellar system is critical, but the hippocampal system is not (see below and Berger et al., 1986; Thompson and Krupa, 1994, for overviews.) Within the cerebellar system, the following regions developed the predictive response: relevant motor nuclei, a region of the fifth nucleus, various reticular brainstem regions, the cerebellar cortex (ansiform and anterior lobes), the cerebellar interpositus nucleus, the pontine nuclei, and the red nucleus (McCormick et al., 1983).

20.2.3 The Cerebellar System

20.2.3.1 Lesions

The initial discovery of the key role of the cerebellum in eyeblink conditioning involved both large aspiration lesions including cerebellar cortex and nuclei and electrolytic lesions of the dentate-interpositus nuclear region (McCormick et al., 1981). Neuronal recordings in both cortex and nuclei showed learning-induced increases of neuronal unit activity that preceded and predicted the occurrence of the behavioral CR, as noted earlier. Stimulation of the critical nuclear region elicited the eyeblink before training; the circuit is hard-wired from nuclei to behavior, as noted. In a subsequent series of studies it was found that the key nuclear region is the anterior lateral interpositus nucleus ipsilateral to the trained eye. Very large lesions of the cerebellar cortex that did not damage the interpositus nucleus did not abolish the behavioral CR, although CR latency was altered such that the eye closed and opened before the onset of the US – the timing of the behavioral response was no longer adaptive (McCormick and Thompson, 1984a,b; Logan, 1991).

In these initial studies it was shown that the interpositus lesion effect was ipsilateral – it abolished the eyeblink CR on the side of the lesion but did not impair eyeblink conditioning of the contralateral eye, providing a control for possible nonspecific or state variables (McCormick et al., 1982a). Strikingly, no recovery of the CR is observed even with extensive postlesion training (Steinmetz et al., 1992b). Furthermore, if the lesion is made before training, learning is completely prevented. These lesions had no effects at all on performance of the UR. There have now been more than 30 studies on several species of mammals showing that appropriate lesions of the anterior interpositus nucleus before training completely prevent learning of the eyeblink and other discrete responses, and completely and permanently abolish already learned responses (Christian and Thompson, 2003).

Kainic acid lesions of the interpositus as small as about 1 mm^3 in the anterior lateral region of the nucleus abolished the CR, indicating extreme localization of the critical region and ruling out the possibility that fibers of passage were involved (Lavond et al., 1984b). Finally, lesions of the output of the cerebellar nuclei, the superior cerebellar peduncle (scp), abolished the behavioral CR with no effect on the UR (McCormick et al., 1982b; Rosenfeld et al., 1985; Voneida, 2000 (limb flexion CR in cat)). It is important to emphasize that the cerebellar interpositus nucleus is essential for the learning of all discrete movements trained with an aversive US: eyeblink, limb flexion, head turn, etc. To the extent tested, the memory traces for all those learned movements are stored at separate loci in the interpositus nucleus. Eyeblink conditioning has simply been the most widely studied, although there is also considerable evidence for head turn and for limb flexion conditioning (see Voneida, 2000; Mintz and Wang-Ninio, 2001; Christian and Thompson, 2003).

Results of clinical studies of eyeblink conditioning in humans with brain damage are strikingly parallel to the infrahuman animal literature. Appropriate cerebellar lesions markedly impair or completely prevent learning of the standard delay eyeblink-conditioning task; if the cerebellar damage is unilateral, only the ipsilateral eye is affected (Daum et al., 1993; Woodruff-Pak, 1997). In general, effective lesions are large, including damage to cerebellar cortical regions and nuclei, although exact extent of damage is difficult to determine from the brain scans. Schugens et al. (2000) conclude that damage to cerebellar nuclei appears likely in most of these studies.

20.2.3.2 Recordings

As noted briefly, recordings of neuronal unit activity from the interpositus nucleus during eyeblink conditioning revealed populations of cells in the critical region of the nucleus that, as a result of training, discharged prior to the execution of the learned eyeblink response and fired in a pattern of increased frequency of response that predicted the temporal form of the behavioral CR (the 'neuronal model' of the CR in at least 20 studies to date in several species of mammals (Christian and Thompson, 2003)). Single-unit activity sampled from the interpositus and immediately adjacent regions can be categorized into several distinct response patterns (Tracy, 1995). Some cells show stimulus-evoked activity to the CS and/or the US over the course of training, a pattern that demonstrates appropriate convergence of sensory information in the interpositus but does not directly support a role for the interpositus in CR generation. Likewise, some cells show behavior-related changes in firing patterns coincident with but not prior to the onset of the CR. However, many cells, particularly in the critical region of the anterior dorsolateral interpositus, significantly increase firing in a precise temporal pattern that is delayed from the onset of the CS, occurs before the onset of the behavior, and is temporally correlated with the onset of the behavior. It is clear from recordings such as these that neurons in the interpositus are capable of contributing to the generation of the CR. While there are certainly several distinct response profiles for single cells that are likely to reflect functional subdivisions within the population of neurons in the deep nuclei, it is compelling that multiple- and single-unit activity recorded from the critical interpositus region reflects an increase in activity appropriately timed to effect the downstream motor pathway and culminate in the well-timed CR.

20.2.4 The Pathways

A large literature is in general agreement in identifying the essential circuitry for classical conditioning of eyeblink and other discrete responses. This circuitry follows closely the well-established anatomy of the cerebellar system (Brodal, 1981) and is in general accord with classical theories of cerebellar learning (Marr, 1969; Albus, 1971; Ito, 1972; Gilbert, 1975; Eccles, 1977). We summarize this work only briefly here. See Christian and Thompson (2003) for detailed citation of evidence.

20.2.4.1 The UR pathways

The eyeblink reflex in the rabbit is a coordinated response involving simultaneous and perfectly correlated external eyelid closure, eyeball retraction, and resulting passive extension of the NM, as noted.

In terms of the reflex pathways, there are direct projections from neurons in regions of the trigeminal nucleus to the accessory abducens (and abducens) nuclei and to the facial nucleus, as well as indirect projections relaying via the brainstem reticular formation, at least to the facial nucleus. Although the CR and UR share many common features, there are critical qualitative differences between the two that include both variations in the intrinsic properties and the neural substrates responsible for each response (see earlier discussion). Standard eyeblink training procedures typically result in a progressive increase in the amplitude of the UR due to both associative and nonassociative factors (Steinmetz et al., 1992a). Interpositus lesions can impair the associative component of the UR increase (Wikgren et al., 2002).

Lesions of the interpositus that are successful in abolishing the CR have only a transient depressive effect on UR amplitude in initial postlesion assays at the same US intensity level used in prelesion training (Steinmetz et al., 1992a). Subsequent training fully restored UR amplitudes to prelesion levels, demonstrating a lack of interpositus involvement in the sustained eyeblink reflex modification following conditioning. Steinmetz et al. (1992a) investigated numerous parameters of the UR including amplitude, rise time, frequency, and latency in the same animals at several US intensities and found no significant lasting effects of interpositus lesions in any of these properties. Ivkovich et al. (1993) lowered US intensity levels to threshold to equate amplitudes of prelesion CRs and URs, and it was again shown that interpositus lesions that completely abolished the CR had no significant effect on postlesion UR amplitude.

20.2.4.2 The CR pathway

Neurons in a localized region of the interpositus nucleus ipsilateral to the trained eye develop a neuronal model of the learned behavioral CR; lesions of this region selectively abolish the CR with no effect in the UR; electrical stimulation of this region evokes the eyeblink response before training (as noted). This region of the interpositus projects via the superior cerebellar peduncle to a region of the contralateral magnocellular red nucleus. Lesions of the peduncle abolish the CR, as do lesions of the key region of red nucleus, where neurons also show a model of the learned response. Stimulation of this rubral region also elicits the eyeblink response. The descending rubral pathways project contralaterally to premotor and motor nuclei, seventh for external eyelid closure, and accessory sixth and sixth for NM extension. Overwhelming evidence identifies this circuit as the efferent CR pathway for the conditioned eyeblink response (see detailed review in Thompson and Krupa, 1994). A similar pathway projecting to the spinal cord subserves classical conditioning of the limb flexion response in the cat (Voneida, 1999, 2000).

20.2.4.3 The CS pathway

The pontine nuclei send axons as mossy fibers directly to the cerebellar cortex and interpositus nucleus, mostly contralaterally. The pontine nuclei in turn receive projections from auditory, visual, somatosensory, and association systems, both cortical and subcortical. Appropriate lesions of the pontine nuclei can abolish the CR established to a tone CS but not a light CS, i.e., can be selective for CS modality (interpositus lesions abolish the CR to all modalities of CS) (Steinmetz et al., 1987). Lesions of the region of the pons receiving projections from the auditory cortex abolish the CR established with electrical stimulation of auditory cortex as a CS (Knowlton and Thompson, 1992; Knowlton et al., 1993). Extensive lesions of the middle cerebellar peduncle (mcp), which conveys mossy fibers from the pontine nuclei and other sources to the cerebellum, abolish the CR to all modalities of CS (Lewis et al., 1987).

Electrical stimulation of the pontine nuclei serves as a 'supernormal' CS, yielding more rapid learning than does a tone or light CS (Steinmetz et al., 1986; Tracy et al., 1998; Freeman and Rabinak, 2004). Stimulation of the mcp itself is an effective CS (Steinmetz, 1990a; Svensson and Ivarsson, 1999), and lesion of the interpositus nucleus abolishes the CR established with a pontine or middle peduncle stimulation CS (Steinmetz et al., 1986). When animals are trained using electrical stimulation of the pontine nuclei as a CS (corneal airpuff US), some animals show immediate and complete transfer of the behavioral CR and of the learning-induced neural responses in the interpositus nucleus to a tone CS (Steinmetz, 1990b) and complete transfer from peripheral CSs to mossy fiber stimulation in the mcp (Hesslow et al., 1999). These results indicate that the pontine–mcp stimulus and tone must activate a large number of memory circuit elements (neurons) in common. In sum, the mossy fiber system, coming mostly from the pontine nuclei, is the CS-activated pathway to the cerebellum (Thompson et al., 1997).

20.2.4.4 The US pathway

Neurons in the inferior olive (IO) send climbing fiber projections contralaterally directly to cerebellar cortex and interpositus nucleus. The critical region of the IO for eyeblink conditioning is the dorsal accessory olive (DAO), which receives predominantly somatosensory input relayed from the spinal cord and appropriate cranial nuclei, including nociceptive input (Brodal, 1981). Lesions of the critical region of the IO, the face representation in the DAO, completely prevent learning if made before training and result in extinction of the CR if made after training (McCormick et al., 1985; Mintz et al., 1994). Neurons in this critical DAO region do not respond to auditory stimuli (CS), respond only to US onset, and show no learning-related activity, and the US-evoked response decreases as animals learn (Sears and Steinmetz, 1991). Electrical microstimulation of this region serves as a very effective US (Mauk et al., 1986). All these data argue that the DAO-climbing fibers system is the essential US-reinforcing pathway for the learning of discrete responses (Thompson et al., 1998).

In a classic but largely forgotten study, Brogden and Gantt (1942) reported that stimulation of cerebellar white matter elicited discrete behavioral movements, for example, limb flexion, head turn, eyeblink, and these movements so elicited could easily be conditioned to any neutral stimulus, for example, light or sound. These observations have been replicated and extended in recent years

(Thompson et al., 2000). Swain et al. (1992) used a tone CS and showed that stimulation of cerebellar white matter in lobule HVI (rabbit) did indeed elicit movements: eyeblink, NM extension, and movements of the head and upper lip. These movements all conditioned, extinguished, and reconditioned to a tone CS in a manner identical to CRs established with aversive peripheral USs. Further, kainic acid lesions of the interpositus that spared fibers abolished both the CR and the white matter stimulation–elicited UR, thus ruling out antidromic activation via pontine nuclei or IO of the UR (Swain et al., 1999).

Shinkman et al. (1996) stimulated cerebellar cortical parallel fibers as a CS (white matter US) with similar results. In this study the parallel fiber stimulus (CS) intensity was well below movement threshold. With sufficiently intense stimulation, movements could be evoked by this parallel fiber stimulus. Interestingly, these were often quite different from the behavioral response (UR) evoked by the white matter US. However, as a result of training, the earlier subthreshold parallel fiber CS now evoked a CR that was identical to the white matter UR and often quite different from the suprathreshold response evoked by the parallel fiber stimulus prior to training. There is extraordinary plasticity in the organization of the parallel fiber actions on the cerebellar circuitry (see also Poulos and Thompson, 2004).

Evidence is consistent with stimulation of climbing fibers in cerebellar white matter as the US effective for learning. To our knowledge the IO-climbing fiber system is the only system in the brain, other than reflex afferents, where the exact response elicited by electrical stimulation can be conditioned to any neutral stimulus. Thus, such movements elicited by stimulation of the motor neocortex cannot be so conditioned (Loucks, 1935; Wagner et al., 1967; Thompson et al., 2000). We therefore argue that this system is the essential reinforcing pathway for the learning of discrete responses.

The interpositus nucleus sends direct GABAergic (GABA: gamma-aminobutyric acid) projections to the DAO (Nelson and Mugnaini, 1989). Hence, as learning-induced increases in interpositus neuron activity develop, inhibition of the DAO neurons will increase (Hesslow and Ivarsson, 1996). This accounts for the fact that US-evoked activity in the DAO decreases as learning develops (Sears and Steinmetz, 1991), consistent with the Rescorla and Wagner (1972) formulation. This also appears to serve as a part of the neural circuit essential for the behavioral learning phenomenon of 'blocking,' where prior training to one CS, for example, tone, prevents subsequent learning to a light CS when it is then presented together with the tone in paired compound stimulus training (Kamin, 1969). Infusion of picrotoxin in the DAO to block the GABA inhibition from the interpositus during compound stimulus training completely blocks the development of behavioral blocking (Kim et al., 1998).

20.2.4.5 Conjoint activation of CS and US pathways

If the aforementioned hypotheses concerning the identities of the CS and US pathways are correct, it should be possible to train behavioral conditioned responses by conjoint stimulation of these pathways. Steinmetz et al. (1989) stimulated the pontine nuclei – mossy fibers as a CS (below movement threshold) and DAO-climbing fibers as a US. Stimulus (US)-elicited movements included eyeblink, head turn, and limb flexion. The stimulus-elicited movements were learned to the mossy fiber stimulation CS just as was the case for peripheral CSs. In an even more reduced preparation, the CS was stimulation of parallel fibers by an electrode (concentric pair of ovoids) resting on the surface of the cortex of lobule HVI, and the US was a stimulation delivered through an electrode pair in the white matter directly beneath the surface electrode, as noted (Shinkman et al., 1996). Again, the movements elicited by white matter stimulation were learned in a normal fashion to the parallel fiber stimulation CS. It is tempting but premature to conclude that this procedure established a memory trace in the localized region of cortical tissue activated.

20.2.4.6 Reversible inactivation

Although the evidence cited is consistent with the interpositus nucleus being the site of the conditioned eyeblink memory trace, it does not prove this hypothesis. Predictive neuronal models of the CR develop in the interpositus nucleus, the red nucleus, and the motor nuclei, as noted. Further, lesions of the interpositus, of the scp (that conveys all the efferent projections from the interpositus), and of the red nucleus all abolish the CR with no effect on the UR. Lesions of the motor nuclei of course abolish both the CR and the UR. The technique of reversible inactivation was used to determine where within the circuit the memory trace was formed and stored (see Clark and Lavond, 1993; Thompson et al., 1993; Thompson and Krupa, 1994; Christian and Thompson, 2003, for details).

Several parts of the cerebellar circuit, illustrated in **Figure 2**, have been reversibly inactivated for the duration of training (eyeblink conditioning) in naive animals. Motor nuclei essential for generating UR and CR (primarily seventh and accessory sixth and adjacent reticular regions) were inactivated during standard tone–airpuff training. The animals showed no CRs and no URs during this inactivation training; indeed, performance was completely abolished. However, the animals exhibited asymptotic CR performance and normal UR performance from the very beginning of postinactivation training. Thus, performance of the CR and UR is completely unnecessary and makes no contribution at all to formation of the memory trace – the CR and the UR are completely efferent from the trace. Inactivation of the magnocellular red nucleus during training had no effect on the UR, but completely prevented expression of the CR. Animals showed asymptotic learned performance of the CR from the beginning of postinactivation training. Consequently, the red nucleus must be efferent from the memory trace.

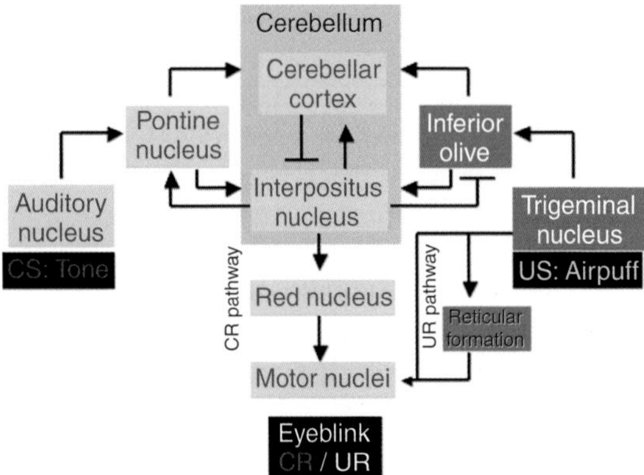

Figure 2 Simplified schemata of the neural circuits underlying Pavlovian eyeblink conditioning. In auditory eyeblink conditioning, information pertaining to a tone conditional stimulus (CS) is relayed to the cerebellar cortex and interpositus nucleus via auditory projections from the pontine nucleus, while nociceptive information about the airpuff unconditional stimulus (US) is conveyed by the trigeminal nucleus to the inferior olive, which in turn projects to both the cerebellar cortex and interpositus nucleus. Conditional eyeblink responses established and maintained within the cerebellar cortex and interpositus nucleus are relayed to the red nucleus. The final common out for both the conditional and unconditional eyeblink response is expressed via facial motor nuclei. Modified from Thompson DF and Krupa DJ (1994) Organization of memory traces in the mammalian brain. *Ann. Rev. Neurosci.* 17: 519–549, with permission.

Inactivation of the dorsal anterior interpositus and overlying cortex resulted in no expression of CRs during inactivation training and in no evidence of any learning during inactivation training. In subsequent postinactivation training, animals learned normally as though completely naive; they showed no savings at all relative to noninactivated control animals. If any part of the memory trace were established prior to the interpositus nucleus in the essential circuit, then the animals would have shown savings, but they did not. None of the methods of inactivation had any effect at all on the performance of the UR on US-alone trials. Infusions of very low doses of muscimol (1.0 nmole in 0.1 μl of vehicle) limited to the anterior lateral interpositus nucleus (with no significant ^{3}H label in cerebellar cortex) completely prevented learning of the eyeblink CR.

Finally, the output of the cerebellum was inactivated by infusion of tetrodotoxin (TTX) in the scp during training. This inactivates both descending and ascending efferent projections of the cerebellar hemisphere. TTX infusion in the scp completely prevented expression of the CR (with no effect on the UR) during training. In subsequent postinactivation training the animals immediately showed asymptotic learned performance of the CR. Collectively, these data strongly support the hypothesis that the memory trace is formed and stored in the interpositus nucleus.

20.2.5 Mechanisms of Memory Storage in the Interpositus Nucleus

Infusion of GABA antagonists, picrotoxin or bicuculline methiodide, into the interpositus in trained animals blocks performance of the behavioral eyeblink CR and the neuronal unit model of the CR in the interpositus in a dose-dependent manner with no effects on the UR (Mamounas et al., 1987). Picrotoxin infusion in the interpositus during training completely prevents learning (Bao et al., 2002). Infusion of the $GABA_B$ antagonist baclofen in the interpositus during training similarly prevents learning and performance of the CR (Ramirez et al., 1997). These results suggest that GABA and its actions on GABA receptors in the interpositus are important for both learning and performance of the CR. However, equivalent doses of strychnine had no effect on the CR or the UR, suggesting that glycine receptors are not involved (Mamounas et al., 1987). Infusion of AP5 into the interpositus markedly impaired acquisition of the eyeblink CR (Chen and Steinmetz, 2000). However, after learning, AP5 infusion had little effect on CRs. This argues for a role of glutamate *N*-methyl-D-aspartate (NMDA) receptors in the interpositus in acquisition but not performance of the CR.

Bracha et al. (1998) reported that infusion of anisomycin into the region of the interpositus nucleus impaired acquisition of the eyeblink CR but had no effect on expression of the CR. Gomi et al. (1999) reported that infusion of actinomycin D into the interpositus nucleus completely prevented acquisition of the eyeblink CR but had no effect on performance of the learned response. By the same token Chen and Steinmetz (2000) reported that infusion of the protein kinase inhibitor H7 into the interpositus markedly impaired acquisition but had no effect on performance of the learned response. Results of all these studies argue strongly that protein synthesis (both transcription and translation) in the interpositus nucleus is necessary for learning of the eyeblink CR, but not for its expression once learned. Indeed, Gomi et al. (1999) identified a kinase whose expression was increased in interpositus neurons following eyeblink conditioning. The cDNA was isolated, and the deduced amino acid sequence of the kinase contains the KKIAMRE motif, conserved among cell division cycle 2–related kinases. All these results argue for the formation of neuronal/synaptic plasticity, a memory trace, in the interpositus itself. Even with 1 month of overtraining or rest, the memory trace remains in the interpositus (Christian and Thompson, 2005).

Extremely important direct evidence for a strengthening of the mossy fiber–interpositus neuron synapses has been presented by Kleim et al. (2002), using eyeblink conditioning in the rat. They demonstrated a highly significant increase in the number of excitatory synapses in the interpositus nucleus but no change in inhibitory synapses following eyeblink conditioning, compared to unpaired stimulation control animals. We note that some years earlier Racine et al. (1986) reported the development of long-term potentiation (LTP) in interpositus following mossy fiber tetanus in the rat *in vivo,* a result recently replicated *in vitro* by Linden (Aizenman and Linden, 2000).

In sum, the evidence is now very strong from behavioral, physiological, pharmacological, anatomical, and inactivation studies that the basic associative memory trace in eyeblink conditioning is established in the interpositus nucleus. The next step is to elucidate the causal chain from behavioral training to increased synaptic efficacy and synapse formation.

20.2.6 Cerebellar Cortex

After more than two decades of research, the role of the cerebellar cortex in eyeblink conditioning is still unclear and embedded in controversy (see Yeo and Hardiman, 1992; Christian and Thompson, 2003, for reviews). However, it is clear that it plays a very important role in normal learning – animals with large cortical lesions learn more slowly than normal and not as well. In the first study to explicitly address cerebellar cortical function in eyeblink conditioning, large aspiration lesions of ansiform or ansiform and paramedian lobules in well-trained rabbits resulted in the expression of short-latency, small-amplitude CRs (McCormick and Thompson, 1984b). Yeo and associates reported that lesions of lobule HVI of cerebellar cortex abolished the conditioned eyeblink response (Yeo et al., 1984, 1985). However, subsequent studies in several laboratories, including Yeo's, have been unable to replicate this result (e.g., Lavond et al., 1987; Clark et al., 1990; Yeo and Hardiman, 1992) Harvey et al., 1993; Perrett and Mauk, 1995; .

In an experiment designed to assess the role of the cortex in acquisition, extensive unilateral lesions including complete removal of HVI and HVIIa lobules and significant portions of the anterior lobe were shown to significantly impair the rate of learning (Lavond and Steinmetz, 1989). Lesioned animals took seven times longer to reach criterion, and asymptotic levels of CR frequency were much reduced. Despite these specific learning deficits, animals were able to achieve significant levels of conditioned responding in the absence of HVI. This result was confirmed by another study in which extensive cortical lesions were shown to significantly impair the rate of acquisition but not prevent learning (Logan, 1991). Animals with complete or near-complete removal of HVI and crura I and II of the ansiform lobe took six times longer to reach criterion. Rabbits with less extensive damage to HVI and the ansiform lobe showed moderate decreases in learning rates. Both moderate and extensive lesions decreased asymptotic CR frequency, whereas extensive lesions also impaired CR magnitude and timing.

Using a different methodological approach to investigate cortical function, the HVI lobule has been temporarily inactivated via infusions of the $GABA_A$ receptor agonist muscimol, during both acquisition and retention. Muscimol acts to hyperpolarize neurons, prohibitively raising the firing threshold and thus disrupting the cortical output mediated by Purkinje cells. Muscimol inactivation restricted to the ventral HVI region has no effect on the rate of acquisition or quality of the CRs (Krupa, 1993). Extensive cortical inactivation encompassing both HVI and portions of the anterior lobe significantly impairs but does not prevent acquisition and has no effect on the CR performance once the animal reaches asymptotic levels of conditioned responding (Krupa, 1993; Thompson et al., 2001). Similarly, reversible inactivation of the HVI region achieved with a cortical cooling probe significantly decreased the learning rate but did not disrupt CR expression in well-trained animals (Clark et al., 1997).

The great difficulty in all these studies is the limitation of the permanent lesion approach. The depths of cortical tissue in lobule HVI are only a millimeter or so above the critical region of the interpositus nucleus. It is impossible to remove all relevant cerebellar cortex without damaging the interpositus nucleus. To circumvent these anatomical complications, several attempts have been made to investigate the effects of functionally inactivating the entire cerebellar cortex. The most definitive of these studies tested acquisition of eyeblink conditioning in mutant mice (pcd mice) in which Purkinje cells degenerate approximately 2 weeks postnatally (Chen et al., 1996). Elimination of these sole-output neurons in the cortex effectively eliminates the cerebellar cortex itself. pcd mice show significant deficits in both the rate of acquisition and the asymptotic level of conditioning, but nevertheless express significant levels of learning and extinction in the absence of cortical input to the interpositus. Peak latencies of the CRs in the mutants were significantly decreased compared to wild-type mice, although the effect was not great. A later study confirmed that the interpositus was responsible for the residual learning, by demonstrating that bilateral lesions of the interpositus in pcd mice completely block acquisition (Chen et al., 1999). In a recent study, OX7-saporin, an immunotoxin selective for Purkinje cells, was infused intraventricularly prior to conditioning, and deficits in both acquisition and extinction were observed which correlated with cell loss in HVI and the anterior lobe (Nolan and Freeman, 2006).

Functional and reversible lesions of the entire cerebellar cortex can also be achieved through a targeted disruption of the Purkinje cell afferents at the level of the interpositus. In one study, application of the GABA antagonist picrotoxin into the anterior interpositus nucleus resulted in short-latency, reduced-amplitude, prolonged CRs but at a frequency similar to that observed in the absence of infusion (Garcia and Mauk, 1998). These results are contradicted by other studies in which picrotoxin infusions into the interpositus blocked the expression of CRs completely (Mamounas et al., 1987; Bao et al., 2002). A much more precise elimination of cortical input can be achieved through sequential infusions of muscimol and picrotoxin. Muscimol first blocks the synaptic transmission from the cortex, and the baseline level of excitability in the interpositus neurons is restored through application of picrotoxin (Bao et al., 2002). With this procedure, onset and peak latencies were decreased in well-trained animals, CR amplitudes were increased, and no effects (i.e., no CRs) were observed in naive animals. Although studies of cerebellar patients cannot address these questions with anatomical precision, it was recently reported that damage primarily to the cerebellar cortex impaired the acquisition and timing of conditioned eyeblink responses (Gerwig et al., 2005).

In sum, it is clear that the cerebellar cortex plays a critical role in normal learning and adaptive timing of the eyeblink CR. The cortex exerts inhibitory control over the interpositus neurons; this inhibition could control precisely the timing of interpositus neurons' activation by the CS to generate the CR. Further, a decrease in this inhibition could permit the necessary activation of the interpositus neurons to express the CR. The most prominent mechanism for decreasing Purkinje neuron activity is long-term depression (LTD) at parallel fiber synapses on Purkinje dendrites, first discovered by Masao Ito (see Ito, 1984).

The majority of evidence suggesting a role for cortical LTD in learning and memory comes from behavioral assays of mutant mice with deficits in LTD expression. There is a consistent relationship between deficits in eyeblink conditioning and deficits in cerebellar cortical LTD (Kim and Thompson, 1997). It has been shown that activation of metabotropic and ionotropic glutamate receptors (mGluR and AMPAR) on the Purkinje cell dendrites is necessary for the induction of LTD (Linden and Connor, 1993; Jeromin et al., 1996). Although the downstream signaling pathway is not entirely known, several key molecules have been identified. Factors required for LTD include Ca^{2+} influx via voltage-activated channels and transient protein kinase C (PKC) activation (Hansel et al., 2001). Mutant mice in which the mGluR1 subunit is not expressed, rendering the receptor nonfunctional, have shown deficient LTD and impaired eyeblink conditioning (Aiba et al., 1994). Phospholipase Cbetas (PLCbetas) are downstream signaling molecules of mGluR activation, and the PLCbeta4 isoform is expressed selectively in Purkinje cells in the rostral cerebellum, including portions of HVI. Mutant mice deficient in PLCbeta4 also show impaired LTD and an impairment in acquisition of CRs (Kishimoto et al., 2001a; Miyata et al., 2001). Mutants lacking the $\delta 2$ subunit of the glutamate receptor exclusively in the cerebellar cortex are likewise impaired in LTD and delay eyeblink conditioning (Kishimoto et al., 2001b,c).

20.2.7 Eyeblink Conditioning and the Hippocampus

In eyeblink conditioning, neuronal unit cluster recordings in hippocampal fields CA1 and CA3 increase in discharge frequency in paired (tone CS–corneal airpuff US) training trials very rapidly, shift forward in time as learning develops, and form a predictive 'temporal model' of the learned behavioral response, both within trials and over the trials of training (Berger et al., 1976). To summarize a large body of research, the growth of the hippocampal unit response is, under normal conditions, an invariable and strongly predictive concomitant of subsequent behavioral learning (see reviews in Berger et al., 1986). This increase in neuronal activity in the hippocampus becomes significant by the second or third trial of training, long before behavioral signs of learning develop, as would be expected of a declarative memory system. This initial hippocampal unit increase is in the US period; increases in the CS period appear at about the time point in training when behavioral CRs appear. With continued training the hippocampal neuronal model eventually declines (Katz and Steinmetz, 1994).

Many neurons that could be identified as pyramidal neurons in CA1 and CA3 (antidromic stimulation and collision) showed learning-related increases in discharge frequency in the trial period. Typically, a given neuron modeled only some limited time period of the trial. Cumulating many such single pyramidal neuron responses produced the typical unit cluster model of the behavioral learned response. So the pyramidal neuron representation of the behavioral learned response is distributed over both space and time in the hippocampus. The high percentage of learning-influenced pyramidal neurons and their spatially distributed loci have been strikingly verified in studies by Disterhoft and associates (Disterhoft et al., 1986; de Jonge et al., 1990) using *in vitro* studies of hippocampal slices from trained versus control animals. The work described was all done using the basic delay paradigm, where hippocampal lesions do not impair simple acquisition (Schmaltz and Theios, 1972; Solomon and Moore, 1975). Similarly, humans with hippocampal-temporal lobe anterograde amnesia are able to learn simple acquisition of the eyeblink CR, but cannot describe it (Weiskrantz and Warrington, 1979).

20.2.7.1 Trace conditioning

Trace conditioning was first described by Pavlov; the CS terminates and there is a period of no stimulation between CS offset and US onset (as Pavlov stressed, the organism must maintain a 'trace' of the CS in the brain in order for the CS and the US to become associated). In eyeblink conditioning in animals, a typical trace interval is 500 ms. The trace CR is more difficult to learn than the standard 'delay' procedure where the CS and US overlap in time.

McEchron and Disterhoft (1997) reported marked increases in hippocampal neuronal activity in trace conditioning, as was reported earlier for delay conditioning. Further, with extensive training, the neuronal model declines. Very large bilateral removal of the dorsal plus some ventral hippocampus in rabbits markedly impaired subsequent acquisition of the 500-ms trace CR, an example of anterograde amnesia (Solomon et al., 1986; Moyer et al., 1990). Consistent with this finding, scopolamine at doses sufficiently low to have little effect on delay learning completely prevents acquisition of the trace CR (Kaneko and Thompson, 1997). If rabbits are first trained in the trace procedure, large bilateral hippocampal lesions made immediately after training completely abolish the trace CR (such immediate lesions have little effect on the delay CR). However, if these same hippocampal lesions are made a month after training, they do not impair performance of the trace CR at all (Kim et al., 1995).

To summarize, large bilateral lesions of the hippocampus made before training markedly impair learning of the trace CR. If the animals are first trained, lesions immediately after training abolish the trace CR, but lesions made 1 month after training have no effect on memory of the trace CR. These results are strikingly consistent with the literature concerned with the declarative memory deficit following damage to the hippocampal-medial temporal lobe system in humans and monkeys. These deficits have two key temporal characteristics: (1) profound and permanent anterograde amnesia, and

(2) profound but clearly time-limited retrograde amnesia. Subjects have great difficulty learning new declarative tasks/information and have substantial memory loss for events for some period just preceding brain damage (1 or more years in humans, 2–3 months for monkeys) but relatively intact memory for earlier events (Zola-Morgan and Squire, 1990). Very similar results were found for classical conditioning of fear to context in rats (Kim and Fanselow, 1992).

These results from studies on animals suggest that trace eyeblink conditioning provides a simple model of hippocampal-dependent declarative memory, a possibility strongly supported by studies of humans with hippocampal-medial temporal lobe amnesia. In brief, such patients are markedly impaired on acquisition of trace eyeblink conditioning if the trace interval is sufficiently long (see reviews by Clark and Squire, 1998; McGlinchey-Berroth, 2000). It is important to emphasize that lesions of the cerebellar interpositus nucleus completely and permanently abolish the trace conditioned eyeblink response (rabbits) (Woodruff-Pak et al., 1985).

Clark and Squire (1998, 1999) made the striking observation that awareness of the training contingencies in normal human subjects correlated highly with the degree of trace conditioning. They showed that awareness played no role in delay conditioning, that awareness does play a role in both single-cue and differential trace conditioning and that expectancy of US occurrence influenced trace but not delay conditioning (Clark and Squire, 2000; Manns et al., 2000a,b; Clark et al., 2001). They conclude that delay and trace conditioning are fundamentally different phenomena, delay inducing nondeclarative or procedural memory and trace inducing declarative memory. It would seem that this very simple procedural classical conditioning task, where the CS and US are separated by a very brief period of time, has converted the memory from a procedural memory to a declarative memory! Interestingly, new neurons persist in the dentate gyrus in trace but not delay eyeblink conditioning, and blocking formation of new neurons impairs trace but not delay conditioning (Gould et al., 1999a,b; Shors et al., 2001).

20.3 Classical Fear Conditioning

Within the past few decades Pavlovian fear conditioning has become one of the most intensely studied forms of mammalian procedural learning (*See* Chapter 21). In fear conditioning a discrete stimulus such as a tone or static features of the training context (i.e., shape, feel, lighting, and smell) is paired with an aversive stimulus. Upon return to the original training environment or presentation of the previously paired tone, fear is expressed as an array of autonomic, hormonal, and behavioral responses. The development of neurobiological, behavioral, molecular, and genetic methods and their application to rodent models of fear conditioning has yielded tremendous insight into our understanding of the neural substrates of Pavlovian fear conditioning (see Maren and Quirk, 2004; Walker and Davis, 2004; Fanselow and Poulos, 2005; Phelps and LeDoux, 2005, for reviews).

20.3.1 Nature of Conditional Fear

As described some years ago by Bolles (1970) the ability to rapidly predict impending danger is crucial for the survival of any organism; therefore mammals have evolved a series of preprogrammed species-specific defensive reactions. For example, in response to threat, the chameleon changes color, the opossum plays dead, the skunk releases an odor, the turtle retreats in its shell, and the rat or mouse freezes (Bolles, 1967).

Fear has been described as the perception and recognition of danger, the learning and remembering about dangerous experiences, and the coordination of defensive behaviors to environmental threat (Fanselow and Gale, 2003). In addition to more overt behavioral responses, conditional fear has been measured by collective changes in heart rate (Antoniadis and McDonald, 2000), body temperature (Godsil et al., 2000), defecation (Antoniadis and McDonald, 2000), cortisol release (Goldstein et al., 1996), and opiate-related analgesia (Fanselow, 1986). In rodent models of fear, arguably the most reliable measure of learned fear is freezing, a defensive posture exhibited by some mammals (e.g., rats, mice, rabbits, and deer) that is best described as the absence of movement with exception of those related to respiration. Other prominent indices of conditional fear include enhancement in startle to loud acoustic stimuli (Brown et al., 1951; Rosen and Davis, 1988) as well as suppression of previously reinforced lever press in rats (Estes and Skinner, 1941; Anglada-Figueroa and Quirk, 2005). In addition, work by McGaugh and colleagues has made tremendous strides in our understanding of the role of the amygdala in memory consolidation using an inhibitory avoidance procedure (McGaugh, 2004). Here, to limit the scope of this chapter, much of the work described will primarily focus on freezing as a measure of fear, as described in rodents, unless otherwise noted.

In contrast to eyeblink classical conditioning, the UR to footshock and the CR as measured by freezing are notably different in that footshocks evoke a reflexive burst of locomotor activity (Fanselow, 1980). Following even a single pairing of the CS and US, postfootshock freezing begins to emerge soon after the offset of the activity burst and has been used as a reliable online measure of fear learning (Fanselow, 1980).

20.3.2 Brain Systems Engaged in Fear Conditioning

The primary brain area engaged during fear conditioning is the basolateral amygdala complex (BLAc), a region composed of several heterogeneous subnuclei, including the lateral (LA), basomedial (BM), and basolateral nuclei (BL). Other brain regions that play a prominent role include the hippocampus, medial geniculate nucleus, anterior cingulate cortex, and ventral periaqueductal gray. In auditory fear conditioning, the BLAc is essential; however, under conditions in which fear to the original training context is assessed, not only is the BLAc important, but so is the hippocampus.

20.3.3 The Amygdalar System

20.3.3.1 Lesions

The primary foundation for the role of the amygdala in fear conditioning was laid by Brown and Shafer (1888) in humans and Kluver and Bucy (1937) in monkeys: damage to the medial temporal lobes that included the amygdala resulted in profound changes in emotional responsiveness and most notably a loss of fear. Later, work by Weiskrantz. (1956) showed that lesions specific to the amygdala could produce similar changes in emotional reactivity. Subsequent work by Kellicutt and Schwartzbaum (1963) showed that lesions of the amygdala attenuated fear-motivated bar-press suppression. The crucial finding for the key role of the amygdala in fear conditioning was provided by Blanchard and Blanchard (1972), who demonstrated that electrolytic lesions of the amygdala in rats prevented contextual fear conditioning as measured by freezing. In addition, McGaugh and colleagues revealed posttraining electrical stimulation of the amygdala resulted in deficits in inhibitory avoidance memory retention (Gold et al., 1973). Since then, further work in a number of laboratories has demonstrated that discrete lesions of the BLAc prior to training prevent the development of both contextual and cued fear responses (LeDoux et al., 1990; Campeau and Davis, 1995; Cousens and Otto, 1998). Conversely, similar lesions in previously trained animals completely abolish all measures of fear responding to all CS modalities tested (Phillips and LeDoux, 1992; Sananes and Davis, 1992; Campeau and Davis, 1995; Lee et al., 1996; Cousens and Otto, 1998; Koo et al., 2004). In an interesting experiment by Gale et al. (2004), lesions of the BLA 17 months following fear training, nearly equivalent to the entire life span of the rat, completely abolished the expression of conditional fear responses, suggesting that, once Pavlovian fear memories are established, they are permanently maintained by the BLAc. It should be noted that the lack of fear responding such as freezing is not due to an inability to perform the response, given that extensive overtraining (>75 footshocks) can yield significant freezing (Maren, 1999; Gale et al., 2004).

Neuropsychological studies in humans with Urbach-Weithe disease, a condition resulting in degeneration of the amygdala that leaves intact surrounding temporal lobe structures, reveal deficits in delay fear conditioning (Bechara et al., 1995). Consistent with patients with amygdala damage, magnetic resonance imaging reveals activation of the amygdala during both fear conditioning and expression (Cheng et al., 2003; Knight et al., 2005).

20.3.3.2 Measures of neuronal activity

Electrophysiological recordings and quantification of immediate early gene expression in neurons of the BLAc are consistent with lesion studies and reveal that these neurons are actively engaged during and as a result of fear conditioning. Indeed, populations of neurons in the LA nuclei respond to both the CS and US. LeDoux and colleagues have shown that responding of these individual neurons to a tone CS is enhanced as a result of fear conditioning (Quirk et al., 1995, 1997; Li et al., 1996). Similar learning-related changes have been also observed in neurons of BL nucleus (Maren and Quirk, 2004). Consistent with these findings, measurements of immediate early gene *c-fos* are elevated in regions of the amygdala (Beck and Fibiger, 1995) and interestingly show a significant lateralization within the right BLA and central nucleus of the amygdala (CeA) (Scicli et al., 2004).

20.3.3.3 The pathways

There is a general agreement within the literature that the neural circuitry underlying Pavlovian fear conditioning is centered around the BLAc (Fanselow and LeDoux, 1999; but see McGaugh, 2004) and that distinct neural efferents support the expression of different components of the conditional fear response (**Figure 3**). In contrast, examinations of pathways by which CS- and US-related information converges upon the amygdala suggest that multiple pathways are sufficient, none of which seem solely necessary for fear conditioning (Fanselow and Poulos, 2005).

20.3.3.3.1 The CS pathway In auditory fear conditioning, both the auditory cortex and medial geniculate nucleus (mGN) convey CS-related information to the lateral nucleus of the amygdala (LeDoux et al., 1990). Lesions of afferents to the LA or the LA itself disrupt the acquisition of tone-cued fear conditioning (LeDoux, et al., 1990; Romanski and LeDoux, 1992). Moreover, tone-evoked responses in the mGN occur within 12 ms, whereas learning-related increases in tone-evoked spike firing in the lateral nucleus occur around 15 ms (Li et al., 1996), suggesting that mGN activity precedes the development of learning-related LA activity.

Under conditions in which the fear response is signaled by the training context, both hippocampus and perirhinal cortex play an important role in conveying environmental cues to the BLA neurons. Either posttraining lesions of the ventral angular bundle, a primary source of hippocampal and perirhinal input to the BL, or single lesions of the hippocampus and perirhinal cortex produce deficits in the expression of contextual fear responses, but fail to disrupt tone-cued fear responses (Maren and Fanselow, 1995; Bucci et al., 2000; Burwell et al., 2004). Finally, blockade of hippocampal NMDA receptors prior to training severely attenuates contextual fear conditioning (Young et al., 1994; Quinn et al., 2005).

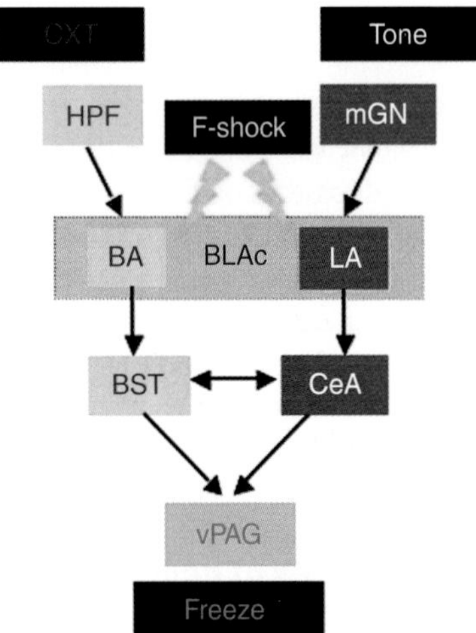

Figure 3 Simplified schemata of the neural circuits underlying Pavlovian fear conditioning. In contextual fear conditioning, information pertaining to the training context (CXT) is relayed to the basal amygdala (BA) via the hippocampal formation (HPF), where it converges with footshock-related (F-shock) information. In auditory fear conditioning, information pertaining to tone is relayed to the lateral amygdala (LA) via the medial geniculate nucleus (mGN) and converges with F-shock. Contextual and auditory fear established and maintained within the basolateral amygdala complex (BLAc) are relayed to the bed nuclei of the stria terminalis (BST) and central nucleus of the amygdala (CeA), respectively. The final common output for the generation of freezing is expressed via the ventral periaqueductal gray (vPAG).

20.3.3.3.2 The US pathway In order for the BLAc to support fear conditioning, pathways conveying information pertaining to the US must reach this region. Unlike the CS pathway, relatively less is known about how information related to the footshock is conveyed. Regions of the thalamus that respond to somatosensory information receive input from the spinothalamic tract and send projections to the lateral amygdala. In addition, insular cortex seems to play a role in relaying pain-related information as well (Shi and Davis, 1999). Interestingly, combined but not single lesions of the posterior thalamus and insular cortex attenuate tone-cued fear conditioning, but leave contextual fear conditioning intact (Brunzell and Kim, 2001). The central nucleus receives nociceptive input from the parabrachial nucleus and nucleus of the solitary tract and directly from the dorsal horn of the spinal cord (Bernard and Besson, 1990; Burstein and Potrebic, 1993; Gauriau and Bernard, 2002). The function of such inputs at the central nucleus needs further investigation, given that this region does not project back to any regions of the basolateral amygdala complex in rats (Fanselow and Poulos, 2005).

20.3.3.3.3 The CR pathway Neurons within the lateral amygdala which undergo auditory fear learning–related plasticity project to intercalated inhibitory neurons, which project to the CeA. Lesions limited to lateral amygdala or central nucleus disrupt tone-cued fear conditioning (Nader et al., 2001). In parallel, environmental cues encoded by the hippocampus in correspondence with activation by US input drive the development of learning-related plasticity among neurons of the BLA and send axonal projections which course through the central amygdala nucleus and terminate at the bed nuclei of the stria terminalis. Electrolytic lesions of the BLA, CeA, or bed nuclei of the stria terminalis disrupt the expression of contextual fear responses (Phillips and LeDoux, 1992; Sullivan et al., 2004). Excitotoxic lesions of the CeA that spare fibers of passage, as confirmed by fiber staining methods, selectively attenuate cued but not contextual fear responses (Koo et al., 2004). Whereas, if these lesions (electrolytic) include damage to fibers of passage, both context and cued-fear responses are disrupted. This suggests that projections from the lateral amygdala → central nucleus and basolateral amygdala → bed nuclei of stria terminalis may represent separate response pathways for freezing to tone and contextual fear conditioning, respectively. Conversely, both the central nucleus and bed nuclei of the stria terminalis heavily innervate the periaqueductal gray, a region critical for the expression of defensive responses such as a freezing. Lesions of the periaqueductal gray, which abolish the expression of freezing, do not disrupt the expression of other conditional fear responses, such as alterations in blood pressure, while damage to the lateral hypothalamus affects blood pressure but not freezing (LeDoux et al., 1988). Therefore, the important point here is that distinct neural pathways initialized within the BLAc mediate the expression of different components of the conditional fear responses and to the some extent the signals that predict danger.

20.3.3.4 Reversible inactivation

Although the aforementioned studies strongly implicate the BLAc in fear conditioning, they do not indicate whether effects of lesions result from learning or performance deficits or whether learning-related changes in neuronal responding are due to plasticity efferent to the BLAc. Therefore, as previously described, reversible inactivation has become a valuable tool in localizing memory traces in the brain. Reversible inactivations targeting the BLAc via direct microinfusion of the $GABA_A$ receptor agonist muscimol prior to fear conditioning prevent the development of context and cued-fear memories. Reversible inactivations of the BLAc after training and prior to tests of memory retention completely abolish the expression of cued and contextual fear responses. These results indicate that functions of BLAc neurons are vital for the development and expression of Pavlovian fear memory. In an attempt to distinguish the relative contribution of the LA and BL in cued versus contextual fear conditioning, Jaffard and colleagues demonstrated that reversible inactivation (via the sodium channel blocker lidocaine that inactivates both soma and axons) targeting the LA attenuated the acquisition of cued, but not context fear, while inactivations of the BL attenuated the acquisition of context, but not cued fear (Calandreau et al., 2005). Finally a study by Maren and colleagues showed that both development of learning-related activity in mGN and cued-fear conditioning are disrupted by reversible inactivation of the BLAc (Maren et al., 2001).

20.3.3.5 Mechanisms of storage in the basolateral amygdala complex

Since the initial demonstration of LTP by Bliss and Lomo (1973) showing that normally weak synapses in the hippocampus could be strengthened by high-frequency stimulation, LTP has become an extremely attractive cellular model of Pavlovian learning. For example, in fear conditioning, CS-generated input could be strengthened by US activation of the BLA, and thus subsequent presentations of the CS could more readily activate the amygdala and promote expression of conditional fear responses. If it were the case that amygdalar LTP represents a substrate of conditional fear memories, then manipulations that attenuate LTP should correlate with deficits in fear conditioning. A number of *in vitro* experiments have demonstrated the establishment of LTP within amygdala circuits (Racine et al., 1983; Chapman et al., 1990; Clugnet and LeDoux, 1990; Maren and Fanselow, 1995). Stimulation of previously described CS pathways, the mGN (Clugnet and LeDoux, 1990) or the hippocampus (Maren and Fanselow, 1995), are able to support LTP at BLAc synapses. Consistent with the LTP hypothesis, McKernan and Shinnick-Galagher (1997) demonstrated that brain slices taken from fear-conditioned rats with the LA and auditory nucleus intact showed larger excitatory postsynaptic potentials (EPSPs) in the LA following stimulation of the auditory nucleus than untrained control rats.

Further studies have demonstrated that, as in the hippocampus, the induction of amygdala LTP requires the activation of NMDA receptors (Bliss and Collingridge, 1993; Maren and Baudry, 1995; Fanselow and Maren, 1995; Huang and Kandel, 1998). Indeed, the induction of LTP is blocked when amygdala slices are treated with NMDA receptor antagonist aminophosphonovaleric acid (APV), whereas once LTP is established APV fails to affect its expression.

Consistent with this line of thought, Davis and colleagues demonstrated that infusion of NMDA receptor antagonist APV into the BLAc blocked the acquisition but not the expression of fear-potentiated startle (Miserendino et al., 1990). Further studies measuring freezing have yielded similar effects, with NMDA blockade disrupting the acquisition but not the expression of conditional fear (Fanselow et al., 1994; Rodrigues et al., 2001). Other forms of the glutamate receptor also implicated in LTP and fear conditioning are mGluRs, in particular mGluR5. Antagonism of this receptor not only impairs the induction of amygdala LTP, but also selectively blocks the acquisition, while leaving expression of conditional fear intact (Rodrigues et al., 2002). Both of these receptors are thought to trigger an influx of extracellular and intracellular Ca^{2+}, resulting in the activation of calcium/calmodulin-dependent protein kinase II (CaMKII). In turn, auditory fear conditioning and the induction of amygdalar LTP by stimulation of mGN result in an increased activation of αCaMKII in the lateral amygdala (Rodrigues et al., 2004). Conversely, BLAc infusion of a CaMKII blocker disrupts fear conditioning (Rodrigues et al., 2004). Along with αCaMKII, protein kinases A and C (PKA and PKC) and Akt are known signals that converge upon the microtubule-affinity regulating kinase (MARK) signaling pathway. BLA infusion of St-Ht332, which blocks PKA anchoring to scaffolding proteins, disrupts the establishment of conditional fear memory (Moita et al., 2002). In addition, blockade of tyrosine kinase B (TrkB) receptor activation of PKC signaling pathways via pharmacological blockade of brain-derived neurotrophic factor (BDNF) binding or in heterozygous BDNF knockout mice results in severe fear conditioning deficits (Liu et al., 2004; Rattiner et al., 2004). Moreover, if mitogen-activated protein kinase (MAPK) expression, which is elevated following fear conditioning, is blocked, fear memory at 24 h following training is markedly attenuated (Schafe et al., 2000). Consistent with these data, amygdala slices bathed in MAPK inhibitor U0126 have impaired LTP (Schafe et al., 2000). Both MAPK and PKA are thought to activate transcription factors such as cyclic adenosine monophosphate (cAMP) response element binding protein (CREB), which are critical for establishment of memory (Rodrigues et al., 2004). Indeed, levels of phosphorylated CREB are increased in the BLAc following fear conditioning (Hall et al., 2001; Stanciu et al., 2001), while overexpression of CREB in the amygdala enhances fear conditioning (Hall et al., 2001) and fear potentiated startle (Josselyn et al., 2001). Moreover, direct BLAc infusion of transcription inhibitor actinomycin-D blocks the acquisition of fear conditioning (Bailey et al., 1999). Further studies have demonstrated that lateral amygdala LTP results in the phosphorylation of CREB and that inhibition of protein synthesis blocks the late phase of LTP as well as the long-term fear memories (Huang et al., 2000; Schafe and LeDoux, 2000; Maren et al., 2003). Finally, *de novo* protein synthesis has been thought to promote the maintenance of both LTP and fear memory by the insertion of postsynaptic alpha-amino-3-hydroxy-5-methyl-4-isoxazole propionic acid (AMPA) receptors. Indeed, Malinow and colleagues, in a striking set of experiments, have demonstrated that both LTP and fear conditioning drive the insertion of AMPA receptors, and that if insertion of receptors is inhibited, fear memory is reduced (Hayashi et al., 2000; Rumpel et al., 2005).

20.3.4 Fear Conditioning and the Hippocampus

20.3.4.1 Contextual fear conditioning

As described earlier, the hippocampus composes part of the CS pathway, which converges with US input at the BLAc in contextual fear conditioning. A number of studies suggest that in contextual fear conditioning the hippocampus is not just a passive relay of multisensory information pertaining to the organism's immediate environment, but rather encodes a unified time-limited mnemonic representation of the context CS (Kim and Fanselow, 1992; LeDoux and Phillips, 1992; Fanselow, 2000; Anagnostaras et al., 2001; Rudy et al., 2004). Indeed, this account is in accord with other views that the hippocampus plays an important role in memory (Milner and Ettlinger, 1970; O'Keefe and Nadel, 1978; Zola-Morgan et al., 1986).

The initial study implicating the hippocampus in fear conditioning was by Blanchard and Fial (1968), demonstrating that electrolytic lesions of the hippocampus disrupted fear conditioning. Years later, Phillips and LeDoux (1992) showed that amygdala lesions disrupted both cued and context fear, while lesions of the hippocampus selectively produced anterograde amnesia of contextual fear conditioning, suggesting that the amygdala had a more general role in fear conditioning, whereas the hippocampus appeared to relay information about the training context in fear conditioning. Kim and Fanselow (1992) further showed that electrolytic lesions of the hippocampus 1 day after training abolished contextual fear, whereas lesions made at 7, 14, and 28 days showed significant contextual fear. Moreover, in the same animals, lesions failed to affect fear responses to tone at any time. Together these results were consistent with the hippocampus playing a time-dependent role in the consolidation of memory and at the same time encoding spatial cues in the animals' immediate environment. However, further studies employing excitotoxic hippocampal lesions, which continued to demonstrate retrograde memory deficits, failed to show anterograde amnesia of contextual fear (Philips and LeDoux, 1994; Maren et al., 1997; Frankland et al., 1998). A number of explanations have been posited based on these discrepancies (Anagnostaras et al., 2001). (1) Excitotoxic infusion could result in damage to neighboring areas such as the amygdala (Mintz and Knowlton, 1993). (2) Ventral hippocampal lesions could result in damage to projections that may affect normal amygdalar function (Maren and Fanselow, 1995). (3) Excitotoxic lesions may result in a sustained seizure-like activation of efferents such as the amygdala, resulting in partial damage (McCelland et al., 1995). Given this, the resulting amygdala dysfunction could result in memory deficits most apparent for recently encoded information (Anagnostaras et al., 2001). A more recent study by Fanselow and colleagues demonstrated that complete excitotoxic lesions of the hippocampus in naive rats failed to disrupt the acquisition of contextual fear, whereas in previously fear-conditioned rats, similar lesions abolish the expression of contextual fear responses (Wiltgen et al., 2006). However, these posttraining deficits could be overcome with retraining.

An alternate possibility is that under normal conditions a slowly established configural mnemonic representation of the training context is encoded by the hippocampus; however, in the absence of the hippocampus, single elements of the context, like cued conditioning, may be sufficient to produce associative plasticity within the BLAc. However, if lesions of the hippocampus are made after BLA plasticity has already been established using a configural representation, then the remaining elemental system may not be sufficient to support the retrieval of contextual fear memories (Fanselow, 2000). Indeed, a number of studies are consistent with this view. (1) Immediate delivery of footshock upon placement into the training context does not yield contextual fear conditioning (Landeira-Fernandez et al., 2006). (2) Posttraining lesions of the hippocampus are more detrimental than pretraining lesions. (3) Preexposure to the training context followed by fear conditioning 35 days later mitigates retrograde amnesia effects of hippocampal lesions (Anagnostaras et al., 1999). Moreover, an elegant study by Rudy and colleagues showed that mRNA of *Arc* and immediate early gene *c-fos* mRNA are induced in the hippocampus following context exposure or context plus shock experience, but not after immediate shock (Huff et al., 2006). However, if the BLA is inactivated, *Arc* and *c-fos* mRNA were attenuated following contextual fear training, but *Arc* mRNA levels remained unaffected by context preexposure alone. Perhaps under normal conditions hippocampal LTP may be critical for assembling elemental components of the training context into a cognitive and/or configural representation of the context (Anagnostaras et al., 2001), which is further consolidated via amygdala-dependent fear conditioning.

20.3.4.2 Trace fear conditioning

In fear conditioning, as in eyeblink conditioning, the addition of a stimulus-free period or 'trace' (>10 s) between the auditory CS and footshock requires the hippocampus (Chowdhury et al., 2005; Misane et al., 2005). Pretraining lesions of the hippocampus disrupt the acquisition of trace fear conditioning (McEchron et al., 1998; Burman et al., 2006), while posttraining lesions attenuate the expression of trace fear conditioning (Chowdhury et al., 2005; Burman et al., 2006). Subsequently Fanselow and associates revealed that blockade of dorsal hippocampal NMDA receptors disrupted the acquisition but not the expression trace fear memories (Quinn et al., 2005). Interestingly, the presentation of a visual distracter disrupts trace, but does not delay fear conditioning, suggesting that attention is required for the acquisition of trace fear memory. Finally, trace fear conditioning, which is associated with an increase in *c-fos* activation in the anterior cingulate cortex, is attenuated by lesions of this same region (Han et al., 2003).

20.3.4.3 Recent versus remote fear memories

An important question posed by the results of Kim and Fanselow (1992) is that, if the hippocampus is transiently involved in the consolidation of contextual fear memory, what brain region(s) are involved in retrieving more remotely established contextual fear memories? A series of elegant studies by Silva and colleagues suggests that a number of regions of the cortex including the anterior cingulate cortex may be required (Frankland et al., 2001, 2004, 2006). In genetically engineered mice with reduced levels of αCaMKII, recent contextual fear memory tested 24 h later is normal, whereas remote fear memory tested at 10–50 days is completely absent (Frankland et al., 2001). Interestingly these mice, which failed to show remote fear memory, revealed no changes in cortical immediate early gene expression following recent or remote memory tests, whereas wild-type mice showed correlated increases of cortical gene expression and remote context fear memory (Frankland et al., 2004). Conversely, reversible inactivation of the anterior cingulate cortex at remote, but not recent, retention intervals disrupts the retrieval of contextual fear memories. Moreover, αCaMKII mutant mice, which showed normal levels of hippocampal LTP, have impaired cortical LTP. These experiments suggest that αCaMKII expression within a number of regions, notably the anterior cingulate cortex, plays an important role in the retrieval of remote contextual fear memory.

20.4 Interactions Between Conditioned Fear and Eyeblink Conditioning: The Two-Stage Hypothesis

A number of authors have distinguished between two classes of CRs: diffuse or nonspecific preparatory CRs and precise, specific, adaptive CRs (e.g., Konorski, 1967; Rescorla and Solomon, 1967; Thompson et al., 1984). According to the 'two-stage theory,' the association between the CS and the aversive US is formed within the first few conditioning trials and results in the acquisition of emotional CRs taking the form of nonspecific, autonomic arousal. Nonspecific responses are usually autonomic but also include generalized body movements, are learned rapidly, and prepare the organism to do something. Such responses are viewed as manifestations of a 'conditioned emotional state,' for example, conditioned fear. Conditioning of specific responses, for example, eyelid closure or leg flexion, involves learning precise, adaptive CRs that deal specifically with the US and requires more extensive training. The two learning processes proceed not only at different rates but also at different brain sites.

The two-stage hypothesis suggests that the initial conditioned fear may be necessary or at least play a role in subsequent learning of discrete movements and that the learning of discrete movements may impact subsequent retention of conditioned fear. Powell and associates (1974) showed that, when heart rate and eyeblink conditioning were given simultaneously, conditioned heart rate developed very rapidly in a very few trials, but then as eyeblink conditioning developed, the conditioned heart rate diminished. As noted earlier the essential brain substrates for these two aspects of learning are quite different: amygdala for fear and cerebellum for eyeblink. Neufeld and Mintz (2001) showed that prior fear conditioning facilitated subsequent eyeblink conditioning and amygdala lesions abolished this facilitation. Weisz et al. (1992) showed that amygdala lesions could actually impair rate of learning of the eyeblink response. Lavond et al. (1984a) showed that appropriate cerebellar interpositus lesions that abolished the conditioned eyeblink response had no effect on initial acquisition of the conditioned heart rate response, as expected. However, Mintz and Wang-Ninio (2001) showed that interpositus lesions, which prevented discrete response conditioning, also prevented the subsequent decline in fear conditioning with extensive eyeblink training that normally occurs in intact animals. If the animal cannot learn to deal with the aversive US, then fear does not extinguish. Patterns of gene expression over the course of eyeblink conditioning in the interpositus nucleus (mouse) support the two-stage hypothesis (Park et al., 2006). Indeed, further work examining the relative activation of gene expression in both regions of the amygdala and cerebellum over the course of simultaneous eyeblink and heart rate conditioning could directly test the two-stage hypothesis of Pavlovian conditioning.

20.5 Conclusions

The findings described here indicate that two forms of procedural learning, eyeblink conditioning, a slowly acquired fine motor behavior, and fear conditioning, a rapidly acquired global defensive response, are established, maintained, and expressed by two different sets of neural circuits centered around the cerebellum and amygdala, respectively. Moreover, the mechanisms of plasticity within each of these brain regions at cellular and genetic levels suggest that different forms of Hebbian plasticity (LTP vs. LTD) and gene expression may be crucial for each form of procedural learning. However, at the systems level, there are similarities in eyeblink and fear conditioning in that increasing task difficulty or the interval of time between training and testing seems to differentially engage the hippocampus and regions of the neocortex. In addition, accumulating data seem to suggest that eyeblink conditioning may develop normally in a two-stage process, where initial training establishes a conditioned emotional component requiring the amygdala, which with further training facilitates the acquisition of cerebellar-dependent eyeblink responses. Collectively, these studies strongly indicate that each of these forms of procedural learning, which depend on different neural loci and mechanisms of memory, may indeed work in conjunction to promote the establishment of appropriately timed and coordinated adaptive behaviors.

References

Aiba A, Kano M, Chen C, et al. (1994) Deficient cerebellar long-term depression and impaired motor learning in mGluR1 mutant mice. *Cell* 79: 377–388.

Aizenman C and Linden DJ (2000) Rapid, synaptically-driven increases in the intrinsic excitability of cerebellar deep nuclear neurons. *Nat. Neurosci.* 3: 109–111.

Albus JS (1971) A theory of cerebellar function. *Math Biosci.* 10: 25–61.

Anagnostaras S, Gale GD, and Fanselow (2001) Hippocampus and contextual fear conditioning: Recent controversies and advances. *Hippocampus* 11(1): 8–17.

Anagnostaras SG, Maren S, and Fanselow MS (1999) Temporally graded retrograde amnesia of contextual fear after hippocampal damage in rats: Within-subjects examination. *J. Neurosci.* 19(3): 1106–1111.

Anglada-Figueroa D and Quirk GJ (2005) Lesions of the basal amygdala block expression of fear but not extinction. *J. Neurosci.* 25(42): 9680–9685.

Antoniadis EA and McDonald RJ (2000) Amygdala, hippocampus and discriminative fear conditioning to context. *Behav. Brain Res.* 108(1): 141–142.

Bailey DJ, Kim JJ, Sun W, Thompson RF, and Helmstetter FJ (1999) Acquisition of fear conditioning in rats requires the synthesis of mRNA in the amygdala. *Behav. Neurosci.* 113(2): 276–282.

Bao S, Chen L, Kim JJ, and Thompson RF (2002) Cerebellar cortical inhibition and classical eyeblink conditioning. *Proc. Natl. Acad. Sci. USA* 99: 1592–1597.

Bechara A, Tranel D, Damasio H, Adolphs R, Rockland C, and Damsio AR (1995) Double dissociation of conditioning and declarative knowledge relative to the amygdala and hippocampus in humans. *Science* 269(5227): 1115–1118.

Beck CH and Fibiger HC (1995) Conditioned fear-induced changes in behavior and in the expression of the immediate early gene c-fos: With and without diazepam pretreatment. *J. Neurosci.* 15(1 Pt 2): 709–720.

Berger TW, Alger B, and Thompson RF (1976) Neuronal substrate of classical conditioning in the hippocampus. *Science* 192: 483–485.

Berger TW, Berry SD, and Thompson RF (1986) Role of the hippocampus in classical conditioning of aversive and appetitive behaviors. In: Isaacson RL and Pribram KH (eds.) *The Hippocampus*, vol. 3–4, pp. 203–239. New York: Plenum Press.

Bernard JF and Besson JM (1990) The spino(trigemino)-pontoamygdaloid pathway: Electrophysiological evidence for an involvement in pain processes. *J. Neurophysiol.* 63(3): 473–479.

Blanchard DC and Blanchard RJ (1972) Innate and conditioned reactions to threat in rats with amygdaloid lesions. *J. Comp. Physiol. Psychol.* 81(2): 281–290.

Blanchard RJ and Fial RA (1968) Effects of limbic lesions on passive avoidance and reactivity to shock. *J. Comp. Physiol. Psychol.* 66(3): 606–612.

Bliss TV and Collingridge GL (1993) A synaptic model of memory: Long-term potentiation in the hippocampus. *Nature* 361(6407): 31–39.

Bliss TV and Lomo T (1973) Long-lasting potentiation of synaptic transmission in the dentate area of the anaesthetized rabbit following stimulation of the perforant path. *J. Physiol.* 232(2): 331–356.

Bolles RC (1967) *Theory of Motivation*. New York: Harper and Row Publishers.

Bolles RC (1970) Species-specific defense reactions and avoidance learning. *Psychol. Rev.* 77: 32–48.

Bracha V, Irwin KB, Webster ML, Wunderlich DA, Stachowiak MK, and Bloedel JR (1998) Microinjections of anisomycin into the intermediate cerebellum during learning affect the acquisition of classically conditioned responses in the rabbit. *Brain Res.* 788: 169–178.

Brodal A (1981) *Neurological Anatomy*. New York: Oxford University Press.

Brogden WJ and Gantt WH (1942) Interneural conditioning: Cerebellar conditioned reflexes. *Arch. Neurol. Psychiatry* 48: 437–455.

Brown JS, Kalish HI, and Farber IE (1951) Conditioned fear as revealed by magnitude of startle response to an auditory stimulus. *J. Exp. Psychol.* 41: 317–328.

Brown S and Schafer A (1888) An investigation into the functions of occipital and temporal lobes of the monkey's brain. *Phil. Trans. R. Soc. Lond. B* 179: 303–327.

Brunzell DH and Kim JJ (2001) Fear conditioning to tone, but not to context, is attenuated by lesions of the insular cortex and posterior extension of the intralaminar complex in rats. *Behav. Neurosci.* 115(2): 365–375.

Bucci DJ, Phillips RG, and Burwell RD (2000) Contributions of postrhinal and perirhinal cortex to contextual information processing. *Behav. Neurosci.* 114(5): 882–894.

Burman MA, Starr MJ, and Gewirtz JC (2006) Dissociable effects of hippocampus lesions on expression of fear and trace fear conditioning memories in rats. *Hippocampus* 16(2): 103–113.

Burstein R and Potrebic S (1993) Retrograde labeling of neurons in the spinal cord that project directly to the amygdala or the orbital cortex in the rat. *J. Comp. Neurol.* 335(4): 469–485.

Burwell RD, Bucci DJ, Sanborn MR, and Jutras MJ (2004) Perirhinal and postrhinal contributions to remote memory for context. *J. Neurosci.* 24(49): 11023–11028.

Calandreau L, Desmedt A, Decorte L, and Jaffard R (2005) A different recruitment of the lateral and basolateral amygdala promotes contextual or elemental conditioned association in Pavlovian fear conditioning. *Learn. Mem.* 12(40): 383–388.

Campeau S and Davis M (1995) Involvement of the central nucleus and basolateral complex of the amygdala in fear conditioning measured with fear-potentiated startle in rats trained concurrently with auditory and visual conditioned stimuli. *J. Neurosci.* 15(3 Pt 2): 2301–2311.

Chapman PF, Kairiss EW, Keenan CL, and Brown TH (1990) Long-term synaptic potentiation in the amygdala. *Synapse* 6(3): 271–278.

Chen G and Steinmetz JE (2000) Intra-cerebellar infusion of NMDA receptor antagonist AP5 disrupts classical eyeblink conditioning in rabbits. *Brain Res.* 887: 144–156.

Chen L, Bao S, Lockard JM, Kim JK, and Thompson RF (1996) Impaired classical eyeblink conditioning in cerebellar-lesioned and Purkinje cell degeneration (pcd) mutant mice. *J. Neurosci.* 16: 2829–2838.

Chen L, Bao S, and Thompson RF (1999) Bilateral lesions of the interpositus nucleus completely prevent eyeblink conditioning in Purkinje cell-degeneration mutant mice. *Behav. Neurosci.* 113: 204–210.

Cheng DT, Knight DC, Smith CN, Stein EA, and Helmstetter FJ (2003) Functional MRI of human amygdala activity during Pavlovian fear conditioning: Stimulus processing versus response expression. *Behav. Neurosci.* Feb 117(1): 3–10.

Chowdhury N, Quinn JJ, and Fanselow MS (2005) Dorsal hippocampus involvement in trace fear conditioning with long, but not short, trace intervals in mice. *Behav. Neurosci.* 119(5): 1396–1402.

Christian KM and Thompson RF (2003) Neural substrates of eyeblink conditioning: Acquisition and retention. *Learn. Mem.* 10: 427–455.

Christian KM and Thompson RF (2005) Long-term storage of an associative memory trace in the cerebellum. *Behav. Neurosci.* 119: 526–537.

Clark RE, Brown DJ, Thompson RF, and Lavond DG (1990) Reacquisition of classical conditioning after removal of cerebellar cortex in Dutch Belted rabbits. *Soc. Neurosci. Abstr.* 16: 271.

Clark RE and Lavond DG (1993) Reversible lesions of the red nucleus during acquisition and retention of a classically conditioned behavior in rabbits. *Behav. Neurosci.* 107: 264–270.

Clark RE, Manns JR, and Squire LR (2001) Trace and delay eyeblink conditioning: Contrasting phenomena of declarative and nondeclarative memory. *Psychol. Sci.* 12: 304–308.

Clark RE and Squire LR (1998) Classical conditioning and brain systems: The role of awareness. *Science* 280: 77–81.

Clark RE and Squire LR (1999) Human eyeblink classical conditioning: Effects of manipulating awareness of the stimulus contingencies. *Psychol. Sci.* 10: 14–18.

Clark RE and Squire LR (2000) Awareness and the conditioned eyeblink repsonse. In: Woodruff-Pak DS and Steinmetz JE (eds.) *Eyeblink Classical Conditioning: Applications in Humans*, vol. 1, pp. 229–251. Boston, MA: Kluwer Academic Publishers.

Clark RE and Thompson RF (in press) Procedural learning: Classical conditioning. In: Squire L, Albright T, Bloom F, Gage F, and Spitzer N (eds.) *New Encyclopedia of Neuroscience.* Oxford, UK: Elsevier.

Clark RE, Zhang AA, and Lavond DG (1997) The importance of cerebellar cortex and facial nucleus in acquisition and retention of eyeblink/NM conditioning: Evidence for critical unilateral regulation of the conditioned response. *Neurobiol. Learn. Mem.* 67: 96–111.

Clugnet MC and LeDoux JE (1990) Synaptic plasticity in fear conditioning circuits: Induction of LTP in the lateral nucleus of the amygdala by stimulation of the medial geniculate body. *J. Neurosci.* 10(8): 2818–2824.

Coleman SR and Gormezano I (1971) Classical conditioning of the rabbit's (*Oryctolagus cuniculus)* nictitating membrane response under symmetrical CS-US interval shifts. *J. Comp. Physiol. Psychol.* 77: 447–455.

Cousens G and Otto T (1998) Both pre- and posttraining excitotoxic lesions of the basolateral amygdala abolish the expression of olfactory and contextual fear conditioning. *Behav. Neurosci.* 112(5): 1092–1103.

Daum I, Schugens MM, Ackermann H, Lutzenberger W, Dichgans J, and Birbaumer N (1993) Classical conditioning after cerebellar lesions in humans. *Behav. Neurosci.* 107: 748–756.

de Jonge MC, Black J, Deyo RA, and Disterhoft JF (1990) Learning-induced afterhyperpolarization reductions in hippocampus are specific for cell type and potassium conductance. *Exp. Brain Res.* 80: 456–462.

Delgado-Garcia JM, Evinger C, Escudero M, and Baker R (1990) Behavior of accessory abducens and abducens motor neurons during eye retraction and rotation in the alert cat. *J. Neurophys.* 64: 413–422.

Disterhoft JF, Coulter DA, and Alkon DL (1986) Conditioning-specific membrane changes of rabbit hippocampal neurons measured in vitro. *Proc. Natl. Acad. Sci. USA* 83: 2733–2737.

Disterhoft JF, Quinn KJ, Weiss C, and Shipley MT (1985) Accessory abducens nucleus and conditioned eye retraction/nictitating membrane extension in rabbit. *J. Neurosci.* 5(4), 941–950.

Eccles JC (1977) An instruction-selection theory of learning in the cerebellar cortex. *Brain Res.* 127: 327–352.

Estes WK and Skinner BF (1941) Some quantitative properties of anxiety. *J. Exp. Psychol.* 29: 390–400.

Fanselow MS (1980) Conditional and unconditional components of post-shock freezing in rats. *Pavlov. J. Biol. Sci.* 15: 177–182.

Fanselow MS (1986) Conditioned fear-induced opiate analgesia: A competing motivational state theory of stress-analgesia. *Ann. N. Y. Acad. Sci.* 467: 40–54.

Fanselow MS (2000) Contextual fear, gestalt memories, and the hippocampus. *Behav. Brain Res.* 110(1–2): 73–81.

Fanselow MS and Gale GD (2003) The amygdala, fear, and memory. *Ann. N.Y. Acad. Sci.* 985: 125–134.

Fanselow MS, Kim JJ, Yipp J, and De Oca B (1994) Differential effects of the N-methyl-D-aspartate antagonist DL-2-amino-5-phosphonovalerate on acquisition of fear of auditory and contextual cues. *Behav. Neurosci.* 108: 235–240.

Fanselow MS and LeDoux JE (1999) Why we think plasticity underlying Pavlovian fear conditioning occurs in the basolateral amygdala. *Neuron* 23: 229–232.

Fanselow MS and Maren S (1995) Synaptic plasticity in the basolateral amygdala induced by hippocampal formation stimulation in vivo. *J. Neurosci.* 15(11): 7548–7564.

Fanselow MS and Poulos AM (2005) The neuroscience of mammalian associative learning. *Ann. Rev. Psychol.* 56: 207–234.

Frankland PW, Bontempi B, Talton LE, Kaczmarek L, and Silva AJ (2004) The involvement of the anterior cingulate cortex in remote contextual fear memory. *Science* 304: 881–883.

Frankland PW, Cestari V, Filipkowski RK, McDonald RJ, and Silva AJ (1998) The dorsal hippocampus is essential for context discrimination but not for contextual conditioning. *Behav. Neurosci.* 112: 863–874.

Frankland PW, Ding HK, Takahashi E, Suzuki A, Kida S, and Silva AJ (2006) Stability of recent and remote contextual fear memory. *Learn. Mem.* 13: 451–457.

Frankland PW, O'Brien C, Ohno M, Kirkwood A, and Silva AJ (2001) Alpha-CaMKII-dependent plasticity in the cortex is required for permanent memory. *Nature* 411: 309–313.

Freeman JH Jr. and Rabinak CA (2004) Eyeblink conditioning in rats using pontine stimulation as a conditioned stimulus. *Integr. Physiol. Behav. Sci.* 39(3): 180–191.

Gale GD, Anagnostaras SG, Godsil BP, et al. (2004) Role of the basolateral amygdala in the storage of fear memories across the adult lifetime of rats. *J. Neurosci.* 24: 3810–3815.

Garcia KS and Mauk MD (1998) Pharmacological analysis of cerebellar contributions to the timing and expression of conditioned eyelid responses. *Neuropharmacology* 37: 471–480.

Gauriau C and Bernard JF (2002) Pain pathways and parabrachial circuits in the rat. *Exp. Physiol.* 87(2): 251–258.

Gerwig M, Hajjar K, Dimitrova A, et al. (2005) Timing of conditioned eyeblink responses is impaired in cerebellar patients. *J. Neurosci.* 25(15): 3919–3931.

Gilbert P (1975) How the cerebellum could memorise movements. *Nature* 254: 688–689.

Godsil BP, Quinn JJ, and Fanselow MS (2000) Body temperature as a conditional response measure for Pavlovian fear conditioning. *Learn. Mem.* 7: 353–356.

Gold PE, Macri J, and McGaugh JL (1973) Retrograde amnesia produced by subseizure amygdala stimulation. *Behav. Biol.* 9: 671–680.

Goldstein LE, Rasmusson AM, Bunney BS, and Roth RH (1996) Role of the amygdala in the coordination of behavioral, neuroendocrine, and prefrontal cortical monoamine responses to psychological stress in the rat. *J. Neurosci.* 10. 4787–4798.

Gomi H, Sun W, Finch CE, Itohara S, Yoshimi K, and Thompson RF (1999) Learning induces a CDC2-related protein kinase, KKIAMRE. *J. Neurosci.* 19: 9530–9537.

Gormezano I, Schneiderman N, Deaux EG, and Fuentes J (1962) Nictitating membrane classical conditioning and extinction in the albino rabbit. *Science* 138: 33–34.

Gould E, Beylin A, Tanapat P, Reeves A, and Shors TJ (1999a) Learning enhances adult neurogenesis in the hippocampal formation. *Nat. Neurosci.* 2: 260–265.

Gould E, Tanapat P, Hastings NB, and Shors TJ (1999b) Neurogenesis in adulthood: A possible role in learning. *Trends Cogn. Sci.* 3: 186–192.

Hall J, Thomas KL, and Everitt BJ (2001) Fear memory retrieval induces CREB phosphorylation and Fos expression within the amygdala. *Eur. J. Neurosci.* 13: 1453–1458.

Han CJ, O'Tuathaigh CM, van Trigt L, et al. (2003) Trace but not delay fear conditioning requires attention and the anterior cingulate cortex. *Proc. Natl. Acad. Sci. USA* 100: 13087–13092.

Hansel C, Linden DJ, and D'Angelo E (2001) Beyond parallel fiber LTD: The diversity of synaptic and non-synaptic plasticity in the cerebellum. *Nat. Neurosci.* 4: 467–475.

Harvey JA, Welsh JP, Yeo CH, and Romano AG (1993) Recoverable and nonrecoverable deficits in conditioned responses after cerebellar cortical lesions. *J. Neurosci.* 13: 1624–1635.

Hayashi Y, Shi SH, Esteban JA, Piccini A, Poncer JC, and Malinow R (2000) Driving AMPA receptors into synapses by LTP and CaMKII: Requirement for GluR1 and PDZ domain interaction. *Science* 287: 2262–2267.

Hesslow G and Ivarsson M (1996) Inhibition of the inferior olive during conditioned responses in the decerebrate ferret. *Exp. Brain Res.* 110: 36–46.

Hesslow G, Svensson P, and Ivarsson M (1999) Learned movements elicited by direct stimulation of cerebellar mossy fiber afferents. *Neuron* 24: 179–185.

Huang YY and Kandel ER (1998) Postsynaptic induction and PKA-dependent expression of LTP in the lateral amygdala. *Neuron* 21: 169–178.

Huang YY, Martin KC, and Kandel ER (2000) Both protein kinase A and mitogen-activated protein kinase are required in the amygdala for the macromolecular synthesis-dependent late phase of long-term potentiation. *J. Neurosci.* 20: 6317–6325.

Huff NC, Frank M, Wright-Hardesty K, et al. (2006) Amygdala regulation of immediate-early gene expression in the hippocampus induced by contextual fear conditioning. *J. Neurosci.* 26: 1616–1623.

Ito M (1972) Neural design of the cerebellar motor control system. *Brain Res.* 40: 81–84.

Ito M (1984) *The Cerebellum and Neural Control*. New York: Raven Press.

Ivkovich D, Lockard JM, and Thompson RF (1993) Interpositus lesion abolition of the eyeblink conditioned response is not due to effects on performance. *Behav. Neurosci.* 107: 530–532.

Jeromin A, Huganir RL, and Linden DJ (1996) Suppression of the glutamate receptor delta 2 subunit produces a specific impairment in cerebellar long-term depression. *J. Neurophysiol.* 76: 3578–3583.

Josselyn SA, Shi C, Carlezon WA Jr., Neve RL, Nestler EJ, and Davis M (2001) Long-term memory is facilitated by cAMP response element-binding protein overexpression in the amygdala. *J. Neurosci.* 21: 2404–2412.

Kamin LJ (1969) Predictability, surprise, attention, and conditioning. In: Campbell BA and Church RM (eds.) *Punishment and Aversive Behavior*, pp. 276–296. New York: Appleton-Century-Crofts.

Kaneko T and Thompson RF (1997) Disruption of trace conditioning of the nictitating membrane response in rabbits by central cholinergic blockade. *Psychopharmacology (Berl.)* 131: 161–166.

Katz DB and Steinmetz JE (1994) How long do relational representations last in the hippocampus during classical conditioning? *Behav. Brain Sci.* 17: 484–485.

Kellicutt MH and Schwartzbaum JS (1963) Formation of a conditioned emotional response (CER) following lesions of the amygdaloid complex in rats. *Psychol. Rep.* 12: 351–358.

Kim JJ, Clark RE, and Thompson RF (1995) Hippocampectomy impairs the memory of recently, but not remotely, acquired trace eyeblink conditioned responses. *Behav. Neurosci.* 109: 195–203.

Kim JJ and Fanselow MS (1992) Modality-specific retrograde amnesia of fear. *Science* 256: 675–677.

Kim JJ, Krupa DJ, and Thompson RF (1998) Inhibitory cerebello-olivary projections and blocking effect in classical conditioning. *Science* 279: 570–573.

Kim JJ and Thompson RF (1997) Cerebellar circuits and synaptic mechanisms involved in classical eyeblink conditioning. *Trends Neurosci.* 20: 177–181.

Kishimoto Y, Hirono M, Sugiyama T, et al. (2001a) Impaired delay but normal trace eyeblink conditioning in PLCbeta4 mutant mice. *Neuroreport* 12: 2919–2922.

Kishimoto Y, Kawahara S, Fujimichi R, Mori H, Mishina M, and Kirino Y (2001b) Impairment of eyeblink conditioning in GluRdelta2-mutant mice depends on the temporal overlap between conditioned and unconditioned stimuli. *Eur. J. Neurosci.* 14: 1515–1521.

Kishimoto Y, Kawahara S, Suzuki M, Mori H, Mishina M, and Kirino Y (2001c) Classical eyeblink conditioning in glutamate receptor subunit delta 2 mutant mice is impaired in the delay paradigm but not in the trace paradigm. *Eur. J. Neurosci.* 13: 1249–1253.

Kleim JA, Freeman JH Jr., Bruneau R, et al. (2002) Synapse formation is associated with memory storage in the cerebellum. *Proc. Natl. Acad. Sci. USA* 99: 13228–13231.

Kluver H and Bucy PC (1937) "Psychic blindness" and other symptoms following bilateral temporal lobectomy in rhesus monkeys. *Am. J. Physiol.* 119: 352–353.

Knight DC, Nguyen HT, and Bandettini PA (2005) The role of the human amygdala in the production of conditioned fear responses. *Neuroimage* 26: 1193–1200.

Knowlton BJ and Squire LR (1993) The learning of categories: Parallel brain systems for item memory and category knowledge. *Science* 262: 1747–1749.

Knowlton BJ, Thompson JK, and Thompson RF (1993) Projections from the auditory cortex to the pontine nuclei in the rabbit. *Behav. Brain Res.* 56: 23–30.

Knowlton BJ and Thompson RF (1992) Conditioning using a cerebral cortical conditioned stimulus is dependent on the cerebellum and brain stem circuitry. *Behav. Neurosci.* 106: 509–517.

Konorski J (1967) *Integrative Activity of the Brain*. Chicago: University of Chicago Press.

Koo JW, Han JS, and Kim JJ (2004) Selective neurotoxic lesions of basolateral and central nuclei of the amygdala produce differential effects on fear conditioning. *J. Neurosci.* 24: 7654–7662.

Krupa DJ (1993) *Localization of the Essential Memory Trace for a Classically Conditioned Behavior.* PhD Thesis, University of Southern California.

Landeira-Fernandez J, DeCola JP, Kim JJ, and Fanselow MS (2006) Immediate shock deficit in fear conditioning: Effects of shock manipulations. *Behav. Neurosci.* 120: 873–879.

Lavond DG, Lincoln JS, McCormick DA, and Thompson RF (1984a) Effect of bilateral lesions of the dentate and interpositus cerebellar nuclei on conditioning of heart-rate and nictitating membrane/eyelid responses in the rabbit. *Brain Res.* 305: 323–330.

Lavond DG, Logan CG, Sohn JH, Garner WD, and Kanzawa SA (1990) Lesions of the cerebellar interpositus nucleus abolish both nictitating membrane and eyelid EMG conditioned responses. *Brain Res.* 514: 238–248.

Lavond DG, McCormick DA, and Thompson RF (1984b) A nonrecoverable learning deficit. *Physiol. Psychol.* 12: 103–110.

Lavond DG and Steinmetz JE (1989) Acquisition of classical conditioning without cerebellar cortex. *Behav. Brain Res.* 33: 113–164.

Lavond DG, Steinmetz JE, Yokaitis MH, and Thompson RF (1987) Reacquisition of classical conditioning after removal of cerebellar cortex. *Exp. Brain Res.* 67: 569–593.

LeDoux JE, Cicchetti P, Xagoraris A, and Romanski LM (1990) The lateral amygdaloid nucleus: Sensory interface of the amygdala in fear conditioning. *J. Neurosci.* 10: 1062–1069.

LeDoux JE, Iwata J, Cicchetti P, and Reis DJ (1988) Different projections of the central amygdaloid nucleus mediate autonomic and behavioral correlates of conditioned fear. *J. Neurosci.* 8: 2517–2529.

LeDoux and Phillips RG (1992) Differential contribution of amygdala and hippocampus to cued and contextual fear conditioning. *Behav. Neurosci.* 106(2): 274–285.

Lee Y, Walker D, and Davis M (1996) Lack of a temporal gradient of retrograde amnesia following NMDA-induced lesions of the basolateral amygdala assessed with the fear-potentiated startle paradigm. Behav. Neurosci. 110: 836–839.

Lewis JL, Lo Turco JJ, and Solomon PR (1987) Lesions of the middle cerebellar peduncle disrupt acquisition and retention of the rabbit's classically conditioned nictitating membrane response. *Behav. Neurosci.* 101: 151–157.

Li XF, Stutzmann GE, and LeDoux JE (1996) Convergent but temporally separated inputs to lateral amygdala neurons from the auditory thalamus and auditory cortex use different postsynaptic receptors: In vivo intracellular and extracellular recordings in fear conditioning pathways. *Learn. Mem.* 3: 229–242.

Liu IY, Lyons WE, Mamounas LA, and Thompson RF (2004) Brain-derived neurotrophic factor plays a critical role in contextual fear conditioning. *J. Neurosci.* 24: 7958–7963.

Linden DJ and Connor JA (1993) Cellular mechanisms of long-term depression in the cerebellum. *Curr. Opin. Neurobiol.* 3: 401–406.

Logan C (1991) *Cerebellar Cortical Involvement in Excitatory and Inhibitory Classical Conditioning.* PhD Thesis, Stanford University.

Loucks RB (1935) The experimental delimitation of neural structures essential for learning: The attempt to condition striped muscle response with faradization of the sigmoid gyri. *J. Psychol.* 1: 5–44.

Mamounas LA, Thompson RF, and Madden J (1987) Cerebellar GABAergic processes: Evidence for critical involvement in a form of simple associative learning in the rabbit. *Proc. Natl. Acad. Sci. USA* 84: 2101–2105.

Manns JR, Clark RE, and Squire LR (2000a) Awareness predicts the magnitude of single-cue trace eyeblink conditioning. *Hippocampus* 10: 181–186.

Manns JR, Clark RE, and Squire LR (2000b) Parallel acquisition of awareness and trace eyeblink classical conditioning. *Learn. Mem.* 7: 267–272.

Maren S (1999) Neurotoxic basolateral amygdala lesions impair learning and memory but not the performance of conditional fear in rats. *J. Neurosci.* 19: 8696–8703.

Maren S, Aharonov G, and Fanselow MS (1997) Neurotoxic lesions of the dorsal hippocampus and Pavlovian fear conditioning in rats. *Behav. Brain Res.* 88: 261–274.

Maren S and Baudry M (1995) Properties and mechanisms of long-term synaptic plasticity in the mammalian brain: Relationships to learning and memory. *Neurobiol. Learn. Mem.* 63: 1–18.

Maren S and Fanselow MS (1995) Synaptic plasticity in the basolateral amygdala induced by hippocampal formation stimulation in vivo. *J. Neurosci.* 15: 7548–7564.

Maren S, Ferrario CR, Corcoran KA, Desmond TJ, and Frey KA (2003) Protein synthesis in the amygdala, but not the auditory thalamus, is required for consolidation of Pavlovian fear conditioning in rats. *Eur. J. Neurosci.* 18: 3080–3088.

Maren S and Quirk GJ (2004) Neuronal signalling of fear memory. *Nat. Rev. Neurosci.* 5: 844–852.

Maren S, Yap SA, and Goosens KA (2001) The amygdala is essential for the development of neuronal plasticity in the medial geniculate nucleus during auditory fear conditioning in rats. *J. Neurosci.* 21: RC135.

Marr D (1969) A theory of cerebellar cortex. *J. Physiol.* 202: 437–470.

Mauk MD, Steinmetz JE, and Thompson RF (1986) Classical conditioning using stimulation of the inferior olive as the unconditioned stimulus. *Proc. Natl. Acad. Sci. USA* 83: 5349–5353.

McClelland JL, McNaughton BL, and O'Reilly RC (1995) Why there are complementary learning systems in the hippocampus and neocortex: Insights from the successes and failures of connectionist models of learning and memory. *Psychol. Rev.* 102: 419–457.

McCormick DA, Clark GA, Lavond DG, and Thompson RF (1982a) Initial localization of the memory trace for a basic form of learning. *Proc. Natl. Acad. Sci. USA* 79: 2731–2735.

McCormick DA, Guyer PE, and Thompson RF (1982b) Superior cerebellar peduncle lesions selectively abolish the ipsilateral classically conditioned nictitating membrane/eyelid response of the rabbit. *Brain Res.* 244: 347–350.

McCormick DA, Lavond DG, Clark GA, Kettner RE, and Thompson RF (1981) The engram found? Role of the cerebellum in classical conditioning of nictitating membrane and eyelid repsonses. *Bull. Psychon. Soc.* 28: 769–775.

McCormick DA, Lavond DG, and Thompson RF (1982c) Concomitant classical conditioning of the rabbit nictitating membrane and eyelid responses: Correlations and implications. *Physiol. Behav.* 28(5), 769–775.

McCormick DA, Lavond DG, and Thompson RF (1983) Neuronal responses of the rabbit brainstem during performance of the classically conditioned nictitating membrane (NM)/eyelid response. *Brain Res.* 271: 73–88.

McCormick DA, Steinmetz JE, and Thompson RF (1985) Lesions of the inferior olivary complex cause extinction of the classically conditioned eyeblink response. *Brain Res.* 359: 120–130.

McCormick DA and Thompson RF (1984a) Cerebellum: Essential involvement in the classically conditioned eyelid response. *Science* 223: 296–299.

McCormick DA and Thompson RF (1984b) Neuronal responses of the rabbit cerebellum during acquisition and performance of a classically conditioned nictitating membrane-eyelid response. *J. Neurosci.* 4: 2811–2822.

McEchron MD, Bouwmeester H, Tseng W, Weiss C, and Disterhoft JF (1998) Hippocampectomy disrupts auditory trace fear conditioning and contextual fear conditioning in the rat. *Hippocampus* 8: 638–646.

McEchron MD and Disterhoft JF (1997) Sequence of single neuron changes in CA1 hippocampus of rabbits during acquisition of trace eyeblink conditioned responses. *J. Neurophysiol.* 78: 1030–1044.

McGaugh JL (2004) The amygdala modulates the consolidation of memories of emotionally arousing experiences. *Ann. Rev. Neurosci.* 27: 1–28.

McGlinchey-Berroth R (2000) Eyeblink classical conditioning in amnesia. In: Woodruff-Pak DS and Steinmetz JE (eds.) *Eyeblink Classical Conditioning: Applications in Humans*, vol. 1, pp. 205–227. Boston: Kluwer Academic Publishers.

McKernan MG and Shinnick-Gallagher P (1997) Fear conditioning induces a lasting potentiation of synaptic currents in vitro. *Nature* 390: 607–611.

Milner AD and Ettlinger G (1970) Cross-modal transfer of serial reversal learning in the monkey. *Neuropsychology* 8: 251–258.

Mintz M and Knowlton BJ (1993) Dissociation of kainic acid lesion effects on the asymmetry of rotation and lateral head movements. *Brain Res. Bull.* 31: 641–647.

Mintz M, Lavond DG, Zhang AA, Yun Y, and Thompson RF (1994) Unilateral inferior olive NMDA lesion leads to unilateral deficit in acquisition and retention of eyelid classical conditioning. *Behav. Neural Biol.* 61: 218–224.

Mintz M and Wang-Ninio Y (2001) Two-stage theory of conditioning: Involvement of the cerebellum and the amygdala. *Brain Res.* 897: 150–156.

Misane I, Tovote P, Meyer M, Spiess J, Ogren SO, and Stiedl O (2005) Time-dependent involvement of the dorsal hippocampus in trace fear conditioning in mice. *Hippocampus* 15: 418–426.

Miserendino MJ, Sananes CB, Melia KR, and Davis M (1990) Blocking of acquisition but not expression of conditioned fear-potentiated startle by NMDA antagonists in the amygdala. *Nature* 345: 716–718.

Miyata M, Kim HT, Hashimoto K, et al. (2001) Deficient long-term synaptic depression in the rostral cerebellum correlated with impaired motor learning in phospholipase C beta4 mutant mice. *Eur. J. Neurosci.* 13: 1945–1954.

Moita MA, Lamprecht R, Nader K, and LeDoux JE (2002) A-kinase anchoring proteins in amygdala are involved in auditory fear memory. *Nat. Neurosci.* 5: 837–838.

Moyer JR Jr., Deyo RA, and Disterhoft JF (1990) Hippocampectomy disrupts trace eye-blink conditioning in rabbits. *Behav. Neurosci.* 104: 243–252.

Nader K, Majidishad P, Amorapanth P, and LeDoux JE (2001) Damage to the lateral and central, but not other, amygdaloid nuclei prevents the acquisition of auditory fear conditioning. *Learn. Mem.* 8(3): 156–166.

Nelson B and Mugnaini E (1989) GABAergic innervation of the inferior olivary complex and experimental evidence for its origin. In: Strata P (ed.) *The Olivocerebellar System in Motor Control*, pp. 86–107. New York: Springer-Verlag.

Neufeld M and Mintz M (2001) Involvement of the amygdala in classical conditioning of eyeblink response in the rat. *Brain Res.* 889: 112–117.

Nolan BC and Freeman JH (2006) Purkinje cell loss by OX7-saporin impairs acquisition and extinction of eyeblink conditioning. *Learn. Mem.* 13(3), 359–365.

Nores WL, Medina JF, Steele PM, and Mauk MM (2000) Relative contributions of the cerebellar cortex and cerebellar nucleus to eyelid conditioning. In: Woodruff-Pak DS and Steinmetz JE (eds.) *Eyeblink Classical Conditioning: Animal Models*, vol. 2, pp. 205–228. Boston: Kluwer Academic Publishers.

O'Keefe J and Nadel L (1978) *The Hippocampus as Cognitive Map*. Oxford: Clarendon Press.

Park J-S, Onodera T, Nishimura S, Thompson RF, and Itohara S (2006) Molecular evidence for two-stage learning and partial laterality in eyeblink conditioning of mice. *Proc. Natl. Acad. Sci. USA* 103: 5549–5554.

Perrett SP and Mauk MD (1995) Extinction of conditioned eyelid responses requires the anterior lobe of cerebellar cortex. *J. Neurosci.* 15: 2074–2080.

Phelps EA and LeDoux JE (2005) Contributions of the amygdala to emotion processing: From animal models to human behavior. *Neuron* 48: 175–187.

Phillips RG and LeDoux JE (1992) Differential contribution of amygdala and hippocampus to cued and contextual fear conditioning. *Behav. Neurosci.* 106: 274–85.

Phillips RG and LeDoux JE (1994) Lesions of the dorsal hippocampal formation interfere with background but not foreground contextual fear conditioning. *Learn. Mem.* 1: 34–44.

Poulos AM and Thompson RF (2004) Timing of conditioned responses utilizing electrical stimulation in the region of the interpositus nucleus as a CS. *Integr. Physiol. Behav. Sci.* 39(2): 83–94.

Powell DA, Kipkin M, and Milligan WL (1974) Concomitant changes in classically conditioned heart rate and corneoretinal potential discrimination in the rabbit (*Oryctolagus cuniculus*). *Learn. Motiv.* 5: 532–547.

Quinn JJ, Loya F, Ma QD, and Fanselow MS (2005) Dorsal hippocampus NMDA receptors differentially mediate trace and contextual fear conditioning. *Hippocampus* 15: 665–674.

Quirk GJ, Armony JL, and LeDoux JE (1997) Fear conditioning enhances different temporal components of tone-evoked spike trains in auditory cortex and lateral amygdala. *Neuron* 19: 613–624.

Quirk GJ, Repa C, and LeDoux JE (1995) Fear conditioning enhances short-latency auditory responses of lateral amygdala neurons: Parallel recordings in the freely behaving rat. *Neuron* 15: 1029–1039.

Racine RJ, Milgram NW, and Hafner S (1983) Long-term potentiation phenomena in the rat limbic forebrain. *Brain Res.* 260: 217–231.

Racine RJ, Wilson DA, Gingell R, and Sunderland D (1986) Long-term potentiation in the interpositus and vestibular nuclei in the rat. *Exp. Brain Res.* 63: 158–162.

Ramirez OA, Nordholm AF, Gellerman D, Thompson JK, and Thompson RF (1997) The conditioned eyeblink response: A role for the GABA-B receptor? *Pharmacol. Biochem. Behav.* 58: 127–132.

Rattiner LM, Davis M, French CT, and Ressler KJ (2004) Brain-derived neurotrophic factor and tyrosine kinase receptor B involvement in amygdala-dependent fear conditioning. *J. Neurosci.* 24: 4796–4806.

Rescorla RA (1988) Behavioral studies of Pavlovian conditioning. *Ann. Rev. Neurosci.* 11: 329–352.

Rescorla RA and Solomon RL (1967) Two-process learning theory: Relationships between Pavlovian conditioning and instrumental learning. *Psychol. Rev.* 74: 151–182.

Rescorla RA and Wagner AR (1972) A theory of Pavlovian conditioning: Variations in the effectiveness of reinforcement and nonreinforcement. In: Black AH and Prokasy WF (eds.) *Classical Conditioning II: Current Theory and Research*, pp. 64–99. New York: Appleton-Century-Crofts.

Rodrigues SM, Bauer EP, Farb CR, Schafe GE, and LeDoux JE (2002) The group I metabotropic glutamate receptor mGluR5 is required for fear memory formation and long-term potentiation in the lateral amygdala. *J. Neurosci.* 22: 5219–5229.

Rodrigues SM, Schafe GE, and LeDoux JE (2001) Intra-amygdala blockade of the NR2B subunit of the NMDA receptor disrupts the acquisition but not the expression of fear conditioning. *J. Neurosci.* 21: 6889–6896.

Rodrigues SM, Schafe GE, and LeDoux JE (2004) Molecular mechanisms underlying emotional learning and memory in the lateral amygdala. *Neuron* 44: 75–91.

Romanski LM and LeDoux (1992) Equipotentiality of thalamo-amygdala and thalamo-cortico-amygdala circuits in auditory fear conditioning. *J. Neurosci.* 12(11): 4501–4509.

Rosen JB and Davis M (1988) Enhancement of acoustic startle by electrical stimulation of the amygdala. *Behav. Neurosci.* 102: 195–202.

Rosenfield ME, Dovydaitis A, and Moore JW (1985) Brachium conjuntivum and rubrobulbar tract: Brain stem projections of red nucleus essential for the conditioned nictitating membrane response. *Physiol. Behav.* 34: 751–759.

Rudy JW, Huff NC, and Matus-Amat P (2004) Understanding contextual fear conditioning: Insights from a two-process model. *Neurosci. Biobehav. Rev.* Nov 28(7): 675–678.

Rumpel S, LeDoux J, Zador A, and Malinow R (2005) Postsynaptic receptor trafficking underlying a form of associative learning. *Science* 308: 83–88.

Sananes CB and Davis M (1992) N-methyl-D-aspartate lesions of the lateral and basolateral nuclei of the amygdala block fear-potentiated startle and shock sensitization of startle. *Behav. Neurosci.* 106: 72–80.

Schafe GE, Atkins CM, Swank MW, Bauer EP, Sweatt JD, and LeDoux JE (2000) Activation of ERK/MAP kinase in the amygdala is required for memory consolidation of Pavlovian fear conditioning. *J. Neurosci.* 20: 8177–8187.

Schafe GE and LeDoux JE (2000) Memory consolidation of auditory Pavlovian fear conditioning requires protein synthesis and protein kinase A in the amygdala. *J. Neurosci.* 20: RC96.

Schmaltz LW and Theios J (1972) Acquisition and extinction of a classically conditioned response in hippocampectomized rabbits (*Oryctolagus cuniculus*). *J. Comp. Physiol. Psychol.* 79: 328–333.

Schugens MM, Topka HR, and Daum I (2000) Eyeblink conditioning in neurological patients with motor impairments. In: Woodruff-Pak DS and Steinmetz JE (eds.) *Eyeblink Classical Conditioning: Applications in Humans*, vol. 1, pp. 191–204. Boston: Kluwer Academic Publishers.

Scicli AP, Petrovich GD, Swanson LW, and Thompson RF (2004) Contextual fear conditioning is associated with lateralized expression of the immediate early gene *c-fos* in the central and basolateral amygdalar nuclei. *Behav. Neurosci.* 118: 5–14.

Sears LL and Steinmetz JE (1991) Dorsal accessory inferior olive activity diminishes during acquisition of the rabbit classically conditioned eyelid response. *Brain Res.* 545: 114–122.

Shi C and Davis M (1999) Pain pathways involved in fear conditioning measured with fear-potentiated startle: Lesion studies. *J. Neurosci.* 19(1): 420–430.

Shinkman PG, Swain RA, and Thompson RF (1996) Classical conditioning with electrical stimulation of cerebellum as both conditioned and unconditioned stimulus. *Behav. Neurosci.* 110: 914–921.

Shors TJ, Miesegaes G, Beylin A, Zhao M, Rydel T, and Gould E (2001) Neurogenesis in the adult is involved in the formation of trace memories. *Nature* 410: 372–376.

Solomon PR and Moore JW (1975) Latent inhibition and stimulus generalization of the classically conditioned nictitating membrane response in rabbits (*Oryctolagus cuniculus*) following dorsal hippocampal ablation. *J. Comp. Physiol. Psychol.* 89: 1192–1203.

Solomon PR, Vander Schaaf ER, Thompson RF, and Weisz DJ (1986) Hippocampus and trace conditioning of the rabbit's classically conditioned nictitating membrane response. *Behav. Neurosci.* 100: 729–744.

Squire LR (1998) Memory systems. *C. R. Acad. Sci. III* 321: 153–156.

Squire LR and Knowlton BJ (1994) The learning of categories: Parallel brain systems item memory and category knowledge. *Science* 262(5140): 1747–1749.

Stanciu M, Radulovic J, and Spiess J (2001) Phosphorylated cAMP response element binding protein in the mouse brain after fear conditioning: Relationship to Fos production. *Brain Res. Mol. Brain Res.* 94: 15–24.

Steinmetz JE (1990a) Classical nictitating membrane conditioning in rabbits with varying interstimulus intervals and direct activation of cerebellar mossy fibers as the CS. *Behav. Brain Res.* 38: 97–108.

Steinmetz JE (1990b) Neural activity in the cerebellar interpositus nucleus during classical NM conditioning with a pontine stimulation CS. *Psychol. Sci.* 1: 378–382.

Steinmetz JE (2000a) Brain substrates of classical eyeblink conditioning: A highly localized but also distributed system. *Behav. Brain Res.* 110: 13–24.

Steinmetz JE (2000b) Electrophysiological recording and brain stimulation studies of eyeblink conditioning. In: Woodruff-Pak DS and Steinmetz JE (eds.) *Eyeblink Classical Conditioning: Animal Models*, vol. 2, pp. 81–103. Boston: Kluwer Academic Publishers.

Steinmetz JE, Lavond DG, Ivkovich D, Logan CG, and Thompson RF (1992a) Disruption of classical eyelid conditioning after cerebellar lesions: Damage to a memory trace system or a simple performance deficit? *J. Neurosci.* 12: 4403–4426.

Steinmetz JE, Lavond DG, and Thompson RF (1989) Classical conditioning in rabbits using pontine nucleus stimulation as a conditioned stimulus and inferior olive stimulation as an unconditioned stimulus. *Synapse* 3: 225–233.

Steinmetz JE, Logan CG, Rosen DJ, Thompson JK, Lavond DG, and Thompson RF (1987) Initial localization of the acoustic conditioned stimulus projection system to the cerebellum essential for classical eyelid conditioning. *Proc. Natl. Acad. Sci. USA* 84: 3531–3535.

Steinmetz JE, Logue SF, and Steinmetz SS (1992b) Rabbit classically conditioned eyelid responses do not reappear after interpositus nucleus lesion and extensive post-lesion training. *Behav. Brain Res.* 51: 103–114.

Steinmetz JE, Rosen DJ, Chapman PF, Lavond DG, and Thompson RF (1986) Classical conditioning of the rabbit eyelid response with a mossy-fiber stimulation CS: I. Pontine nuclei and middle cerebellar peduncle stimulation. *Behav. Neurosci.* 100: 878–887.

Steinmetz JE, Tracy JA, and Green JT (2001) Classical eyeblink conditioning: Clinical models and applications. *Integr. Physiol. Behav. Sci.* 36: 220–238.

Sullivan GM, Apergis J, Bush DE, Johnson LR, Hou M, and LeDoux JE (2004) Lesions in the bed nucleus of the stria terminalis disrupt corticosterone and freezing responses elicited by a contextual but not by a specific cue-conditioned fear stimulus. *Neuroscience* 128(1): 7–14.

Svensson P and Ivarsson M (1999) Short-lasting conditioned stimulus applied to the middle cerebellar peduncle elicits delayed conditioned eye blink responses in the decerebrate ferret. *Eur. J. Neurosci.* 11: 4333–4340.

Swain RA, Shinkman PG, Nordholm AF, and Thompson RF (1992) Cerebellar stimulation as an unconditioned stimulus in classical conditioning. *Behav. Neurosci.* 106: 739–750.

Swain RA, Shinkman PG, Thompson JK, Grethe JS, and Thompson RF (1999) Essential neuronal pathways for reflex and conditioned response initiation in an intracerebellar stimulation paradigm and the impact of unconditioned stimulus preexposure on learning rate. *Neurobiol. Learn. Mem.* 71: 167–193.

Thompson JK, Krupa DJ, Weng J, and Thompson RF (1993) Inactivation of motor nuclei blocks expression but not acquisition of rabbit's classically conditioned eyeblink response. *Soc. Neurosci. Abstr.* 19: 999.

Thompson RF, Bao S, Chen L, et al. (1997) Associative Learning. In: Schmahmann J (ed.) *The Cerebellum and Cognition, International Review of Neurobiology*, vol. 41, pp. 151–189. New York: Academic Press.

Thompson RF, Christian KM, and Krupa DJ (2001) Functional dissociation of the cerebellar cortex and interpositus nucleus during eyeblink classical conditioning. *Soc. Neurosci. Abstr.* 27: 640.11.

Thompson RF, Clark GA, Donegan NH, et al. (1984) Neuronal substrates of learning and memory: A "multiple trace" view. In: McGaugh JL, Lynch G, and Weinberger NM (eds.) *Neurobiology of Learning and Memory*, pp. 137–164. New York: Guilford Press.

Thompson RF and Kim JJ (1996) Memory systems in the brain and localization of a memory. *Proc. Natl. Acad. Sci. USA* 93: 13438–13444.

Thompson RF and Krupa DJ (1994) Organization of memory traces in the mammalian brain. *Ann. Rev. Neurosci.* 17: 519–549.

Thompson RF, Swain R, Clark R, and Shinkman P (2000) Intracerebellar conditioning – Brogden and Gantt revisited. *Behav. Brain Res.* 110: 3–11.

Thompson RF, Thompson JK, Kim JJ, Krupa DJ, and Shinkman PG (1998) The nature of reinforcement in cerebellar learning. *Neurobiol. Learn. Mem.* 70: 150–176.

Tracy JA (1995) *Brain and Behavior Correlates in Classical Conditioning of the Rabbit Eyeblink Response.* PhD Thesis, University of Southern California.

Tracy JA, Thompson JK, Krupa DJ, and Thompson RF (1998) Evidence of plasticity in the pontocerebellar conditioned stimulus pathway during classical conditioning of the eyeblink response in the rabbit. *Behav. Neurosci.* 112: 267–285.

Voneida TJ (1999) The effect of rubrospinal tractotomy on a conditioned limb response in the cat. *Behav. Brain Res.* 105(2), 151–162.

Voneida TJ (2000) The effect of brachium conjunctivum transection on a conditioned limb response in the cat. *Behav. Brain Res.* 109: 167–175.

Wagner AR, Thomas E, and Norton T (1967) Conditioning with electrical stimulation of motor cortex: Evidence of a possible source of motivation. *J. Comp. Physiol. Psychol.* 64: 191–199.

Walker DL and Davis M (2004) Are fear memories made and maintained by the same NMDA receptor-dependent mechanisms? *Neuron* 41: 680–682.

Wallace KJ and Rosen JB (2001) Neurotoxic lesions of the lateral nucleus of the amygdala decrease conditioned fear but not unconditioned fear of a predator odor: Comparison with electrolytic lesions. *J. Neurosci.* 21: 3619–3627.

Weiskrantz L (1956) Behavioral changes associated with ablation of the amygdaloid complex in monkeys. *J. Comp. Physiol. Psychol.* 49: 381–391.

Weiskrantz L and Warrington EK (1979) Conditioning in amnesic patients. *Neuropsychology* 17: 187–194.

Weisz DJ, Harden DG, and Xiang Z (1992) Effects of amygdala lesions on reflex facilitation and conditioned response acquisition during nictitating membrane response conditioning in rabbit. *Behav. Neurosci.* 106: 262–273.

Wikgren J, Ruusuvirta T, and Korhonen T (2002) Reflex facilitation during eyeblink conditioning and subsequent interpositus nucleus inactivation in the rabbit (*Oryctolagus cuniculus*). *Behav. Neurosci.* 116: 1052–1058.

Wiltgen BJ, Sanders MJ, Anagnostaras SG, Sage JR, and Fanselow MS (2006) Context fear learning in the absence of the hippocampus. *J. Neurosci.* 26: 5484–5491.

Woodruff-Pak DS (1997) Evidence for the role of cerebellum in classical conditioning in humans. In: Schmahmann JD (ed.) *The Cerebellum and Cognition*, pp. 341–366. San Diego, CA: Academic Press.

Woodruff-Pak DS, Lavond DG, and Thompson RF (1985) Trace conditioning: Abolished by cerebellar nuclear lesions but not lateral cerebellar cortex aspirations. *Brain Res.* 348: 249–260.

Woodruff-Pak DS and Steinmetz JE (2000) Past, present, and future of human eyeblink classical conditioning. In: Woodruff-Pak DS and Steinmetz JE (eds.) *Eyeblink Classical Conditioning: Applications in Humans*, vol. 1, pp. 1–17. Boston: Kluwer Academic Publishers.

Yeo CH and Hardiman MJ (1992) Cerebellar cortex and eyeblink conditioning: A reexamination. *Exp. Brain Res.* 88: 623–638.

Yeo CH, Hardiman MJ, and Glickstein M (1984) Discrete lesions of the cerebellar cortex abolish the classically conditioned nictitating membrane response of the rabbit. *Behav. Brain Res.* 13: 261–266.

Yeo CH, Hardiman MJ, and Glickstein M (1985) Classical conditioning of the nictitating membrane response of the rabbit. II. Lesions of the cerebellar cortex. *Exp. Brain Res.* 60: 99–113.

Yeo CH and Hesslow G (1998) Cerebellum and conditioned reflexes. *Trends Cogn. Sci.* 2(9): 322–330.

Young SL, Bohenek DL, and Fanselow MS (1994) NMDA processes mediate anterograde amnesia of contextual fear conditioning induced by hippocampal damage: Immunization against amnesia by context preexposure. *Behav. Neurosci.* 108(1): 19–29.

Zola-Morgan SM and Squire LR (1990) The primate hippocampal formation: Evidence for a time-limited role in memory storage. *Science* 250: 288–290.

Zola-Morgan S, Squire LR, and Amaral DG (1986) Human amnesia and the medial temporal region: Enduring memory impairment following a bilateral lesion limited to field CA1 of the hippocampus. *J. Neurosci.* 6: 2950–2967.

21 Neural and Molecular Mechanisms of Fear Memory

G. E. Schafe, Yale University, New Haven, CT, USA

J. E. LeDoux, New York University, New York, NY, USA

21.1 An Overview of Pavlovian Fear Conditioning

Classical or Pavlovian fear conditioning has long been a tool of behavioral psychology to study simple forms of associative learning in the mammal. In this paradigm, an animal (or human) learns to fear an initially emotionally neutral stimulus (the *conditioned stimulus,* CS) that acquires aversive properties after being paired with a noxious stimulus (the *unconditioned stimulus,* US). First used by J. B. Watson and his colleague Rosalie Rayner in the now infamous studies of "Little Albert" (Watson and Rayner, 2000), fear conditioning is now most widely studied in rodents, where a discrete cue (such as a tone, light, or odor; CS) is paired with a brief electric shock to the feet (US). Before conditioning, the CS does not elicit fearful behavior. After as little as one CS-US pairing, however, the animal begins to exhibit a range of *conditioned responses* (CRs), both to the tone CS and to the context in which conditioning occurs (e.g., the conditioning chamber). In rats, these CRs include 'freezing' or immobility (the rat's species-typical behavioral response to a threatening stimulus), autonomic and endocrine alterations (such as changes in heart rate and blood pressure, defecation, and increased levels of circulating stress hormones), and potentiation of reflexes like the acoustic startle response (Blanchard and Blanchard, 1969; Kapp et al., 1979; LeDoux et al., 1988; Roozendaal et al., 1991; Davis, 1997).

21.2 The Amygdala and Fear Conditioning

21.2.1 The Neuroanatomy of Fear

There are few associative learning paradigms that have been better characterized at the neuroanatomical level than Pavlovian fear conditioning (see **Figure 1**). This is particularly true for the 'auditory fear conditioning' paradigm, where an animal learns to fear a tone (CS) that is paired with foot shock (US). In this review, we will therefore emphasize the findings from the auditory fear conditioning literature, although similar mechanisms have also been proposed for conditioning to visual stimuli (Davis, 1992, 1997).

Auditory fear conditioning involves transmission of auditory CS and somatosensory US information to the lateral nucleus of the amygdala (LA), an area that lesion and functional inactivation studies have shown to be critical for learning (LeDoux et al., 1990; Helmstetter and Bellgowan, 1994; Campeau and Davis, 1995; Muller et al., 1997; Wilensky et al., 2000). Anatomical tract tracing studies have shown that cells in the LA receive direct glutamatergic projections from areas of the auditory thalamus and cortex, specifically from the medial division of the medial geniculate body and the posterior intralaminar nucleus (MGm/PIN) and cortical area TE3, respectively (LeDoux et al., 1985; LeDoux and

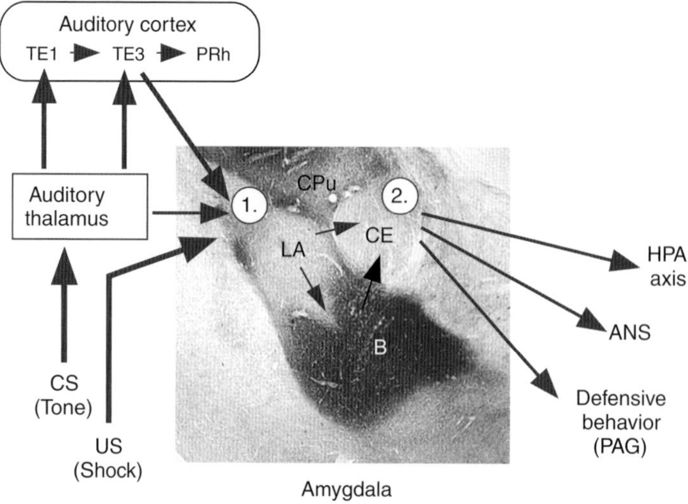

Figure 1 Anatomy of the fear system. (1) Auditory fear conditioning involves the transmission of CS sensory information from areas of the auditory thalamus and cortex to the lateral amygdala (LA), where it can converge with incoming somatosensory information from the foot shock US. It is in the LA that alterations in synaptic transmission are thought to encode key aspects of the learning. (2) During fear expression, the LA engages the central nucleus of the amygdala (CE), which projects widely to many areas of the forebrain and brainstem that control the expression of fear CRs, including freezing, hypothalamic-pituitary-adrenal (HPA) axis activation, and alterations in cardiovascular activity. CPu, caudate/putamen; B, basal nucleus of amygdala; ANS, autonomic nervous system; PRh, perirhinal cortex; PAG, periaqueductal gray.

Farb, 1991; Bordi and LeDoux, 1992; Romanski and LeDoux, 1993; McDonald, 1998; Doron and LeDoux, 1999). Neurophysiological evidence has indicated that inputs from each of these auditory areas synapse onto single neurons in the LA (Li et al., 1996), where they converge with inputs from the somatosensory US (Romanski et al., 1993). Individual cells in the LA are thus well suited to integrate CS and US information during fear conditioning, and it is here, as we will see, that alterations in synaptic transmission are thought to encode key aspects of the memory.

Thalamic and cortical inputs to the LA, while both capable of mediating fear learning (Romanski and LeDoux, 1992a), are believed to carry different types of information to the LA. The thalamic route (often called the 'low road') is believed to be critical for rapidly transmitting crude aspects of the CS to the LA, while the cortical route (known as the 'high road') is believed to carry highly refined information to the amygdala (LeDoux, 2000). Interestingly, while lesions of the MGm/PIN impair auditory fear conditioning (LeDoux et al., 1984, 1986), lesions of the auditory cortex do not (LeDoux et al., 1984; Romanski and LeDoux, 1992b). Thus, the thalamic pathway between the MGm/PIN and the LA appears to be particularly important for auditory fear conditioning. This is not to say, however, that the cortical input to the LA is not involved. Indeed, when conditioning depends on the ability of the animal to make fine discriminations between different auditory CSs, or when the CS is a complex auditory cue such as an ultrasonic vocalization, then cortical regions appear to be required (Jarrell et al., 1987; Lindquist et al., 2004).

During retrieval or expression of a fear memory, the LA, both directly and by way of the adjacent basal nucleus of the amygdala, engages the central nucleus of the amygdala (CE). The CE has traditionally been thought of as the principal output nucleus of the fear learning system, projecting to areas of the forebrain, hypothalamus, and brainstem that control behavioral, endocrine, and autonomic CRs associated with fear learning (Blanchard and Blanchard, 1969; Kapp et al., 1979; LeDoux et al., 1988; Roozendaal et al., 1991; Davis, 1997). Projections from the CE to the midbrain periaqueductal gray, for example, have been shown to be particularly important for mediating behavioral and endocrine responses such as freezing and hypoalgesia (LeDoux et al., 1988; Helmstetter and Landeira-Fernandez, 1990; Helmstetter and Tershner, 1994; De Oca et al., 1998), while projections to the lateral hypothalamus have been implicated in the control of conditioned cardiovascular responses (Iwata et al., 1986; LeDoux et al., 1988). Importantly, while lesions of these individual areas can selectively impair expression of individual CRs, damage to the CE interferes with the expression of all fear CRs (LeDoux, 2000). Thus, the CE acts to coordinate the collection of hard-wired, and typically species-specific, responses that underlie defensive behavior.

21.2.2 Synaptic Plasticity in the Amygdala and Fear Conditioning

In addition to being the recipient of CS and US information, the LA is also thought to be a critical site of synaptic plasticity underlying fear learning (LeDoux, 2000; Blair et al., 2001; Maren, 2001). In support of this view, numerous studies have shown that individual cells in the dorsal regions of the LA (LAd) alter their neurophysiological response properties when CS and US are paired during fear conditioning (**Figures 2(a)** and **2(b)**). For example, LAd neurons that are initially weakly responsive to auditory input respond vigorously to the same input after fear conditioning (Quirk et al., 1995, 1997; Rogan et al., 1997; Maren, 2000; Repa et al., 2001; Blair et al., 2003). This change in the responsiveness of LAd cells that occurs as the result of training has contributed to the view that neural plasticity in the LA encodes key aspects of fear learning and memory storage (Fanselow and LeDoux, 1999; Blair et al., 2001; Maren, 2001; Schafe et al., 2001), a topic to which we will return in a later section.

In the next several sections, we will discuss the biochemical and molecular mechanisms that likely underlie plasticity and memory formation at LA synapses. We begin with a discussion of long-term potentiation (LTP), as it has been proposed that this type of synaptic plasticity is the most likely type of mechanism that underlies memory formation in the mammalian brain (Bliss and Collingridge, 1993; Malenka and Nicoll, 1999), including in the LA (Maren, 1999; Blair et al., 2001; Schafe et al., 2001).

21.3 LTP as a Mechanism of Fear Learning

21.3.1 Why is LTP Important?

The change in the responsiveness of LA cells during fear conditioning suggests that alterations in excitatory synaptic transmission in the LA might be critical for fear conditioning. Accordingly, many of the recent studies that have examined the biochemical

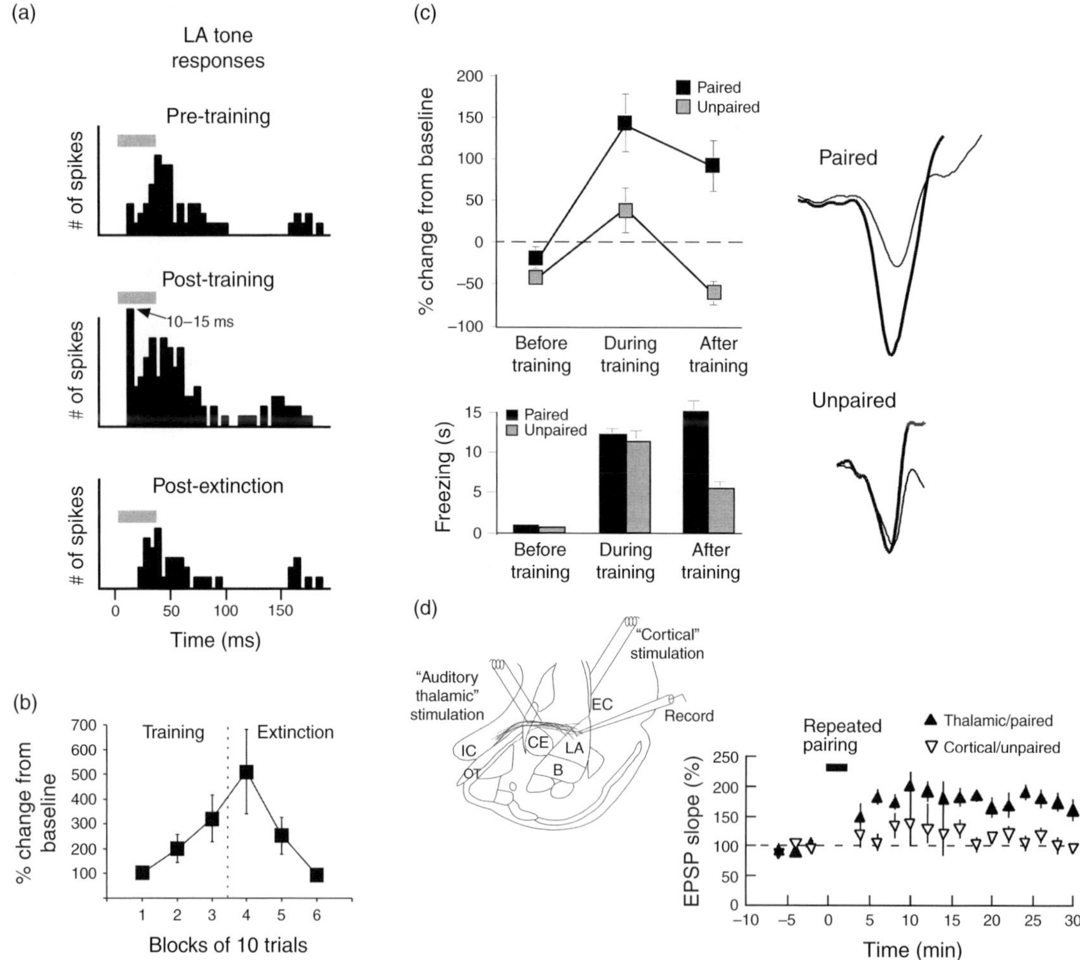

Figure 2 Synaptic plasticity in the lateral amygdala (LA) and fear conditioning. Pairing of CS and US during fear conditioning leads to changes in the responsiveness of LA cells to auditory stimuli, as measured by electrophysiological recording of single cells in the LA. (a) TOP: Prior to auditory fear conditioning, LA cells are weakly responsive to auditory stimuli. MIDDLE: Immediately after conditioning, the same cells respond vigorously, especially in the first few milliseconds of the tone (arrow). BOTTOM: Tone conditioning of LA cells decreases with extinction. In each figure, the onset of the tone stimulus is depicted by a gray bar. (b) Change in firing rate of LA cells over the course of training and extinction. The values represent averaged responses of 16 cells within the first few milliseconds of the tone stimulus and are expressed as percent change from preconditioning firing rates. (c) TOP: Fear conditioning leads to electrophysiological changes in the LA in a manner similar to long-term potentiation (LTP). The figure represents percent change in the slope of the auditory-evoked field potential in the LA before, during, and after conditioning in both paired and unpaired rats. BOTTOM: Freezing behavior across training and testing periods. Note that both paired and unpaired groups show equivalent freezing behavior during training, but only the paired group shows an enhanced neural response. Representative traces can be seen in the inset. (d) LEFT: Associative LTP is induced in the amygdala slice by pairing trains of presynaptic stimulation of fibers coming from the auditory thalamus with depolarization of LA cells. Stimulation of fibers coming from cortical areas serves as a control for input specificity. RIGHT: LTP induced by pairing as measured by the change in the slope of the excitatory postsynaptic potential (EPSP) over time. In this case, the thalamic pathway received paired stimulation, whereas the cortical pathway received unpaired stimulation (i.e., trains and depolarizations, but in a noncontingent manner). The black bar represents the duration of the pairing. IC, internal capsule; OT, optic tract; CE, central nucleus of amygdala; B, basal nucleus of amygdala; EC, external capsule.

basis of fear conditioning have drawn upon a larger literature that has focused on the biochemical events that underlie LTP, an activity-dependent form of synaptic plasticity that was initially discovered in the hippocampus (Bliss and Lømo, 1973). There are several good reasons behind this strategy, including the fact that LTP has been demonstrated in thalamic and cortical auditory input pathways to the

LA (Chapman et al., 1990; Clugnet and LeDoux, 1990; Rogan and LeDoux, 1995; Huang and Kandel, 1998; Weisskopf et al., 1999; Weisskopf and LeDoux, 1999), and that auditory fear conditioning itself has been shown to lead to neurophysiological changes in the LA that resemble artificial LTP induction (McKernan and Shinnick-Gallagher, 1997a; Rogan et al., 1997). Collectively, these findings provide strong support for the hypothesis that an LTP-like process in the LA may underlie fear conditioning (**Figures 2(c)** and **2(d)**). This, in turn, suggests that fear memory acquisition and consolidation may share a common biochemical and molecular substrate with LTP.

21.3.2 The 'Consolidation' of LTP – E-LTP Versus L-LTP

There are several pharmacologically distinct forms of LTP, most of which have been identified in the hippocampus. One form critically involves the *N*-methyl-D-aspartate receptor (NMDAR), which is normally blocked by Mg^{2+}, but which can be opened following sufficient depolarization of the postsynaptic cell during LTP induction (Malenka and Nicoll, 1993). The other, less widely studied form involves the L-type voltage-gated calcium channel (L-VGCC). Other forms require a combination of both NMDARs and L-VGCCs (Grover and Teyler, 1990; Cavus and Teyler, 1996). Importantly, both NMDAR and L-VGCC-mediated forms of LTP have been discovered in the LA (Weisskopf et al., 1999; Bauer et al., 2002).

Regardless of how it is induced, the hallmark of each form of LTP is the entry of Ca^{2+} into the postsynaptic spine, which initiates a biochemical cascade of events that leads to strengthening of the synapse. Some of these biochemical cascades lead to a transient change in synaptic strength known as early LTP (E-LTP) that is independent of *de novo* RNA and protein synthesis. This type of LTP is thought to involve the activation of protein kinase signaling pathways near the postsynaptic density and the alteration in the conductance of number of a number of key synaptic proteins involved in glutamatergic signaling, including the NMDAR and the closely related alpha-amino-3-hydroxy-5-methyl-4-isoxazole propionic acid (AMPA) receptor (Soderling and Derkach, 2000). Other intracellular cascades lead to a more permanent alteration in cell excitability known as late LTP (L-LTP). Unlike E-LTP, L-LTP requires *de novo* RNA and protein synthesis and different classes of protein kinase signaling cascades that are thought to promote long-term synaptic plasticity by engaging activators of transcription in the nucleus (Nguyen et al., 1994; Nguyen and Kandel, 1996). Thus, the two forms of LTP have features in common with the traditional phases of memory consolidation. L-LTP is conceptually similar to long-term memory (LTM) formation, which is known to be dependent on *de novo* mRNA transcription and protein synthesis, while E-LTP is conceptually similar to short-term memory (STM), which is known to be short-lasting and independent of transcription and translation (Davis and Squire, 1984; Milner et al., 1998; Schafe et al., 2000). This pattern of findings suggests, in turn, that the consolidation process can be represented at the cellular level and understood through studies of LTP (Milner et al., 1998).

An exhaustive review of the biochemical mechanisms underlying LTP is beyond the scope of this chapter (for a more exhaustive review of this topic, see Milner et al., 1998). In the next several sections, however, we will review some of the key membrane-bound receptors and intracellular signaling pathways that have been most widely implicated in LTP and in memory formation of fear conditioning.

21.4 Biochemical Mechanisms of Fear Memory Formation and Consolidation

The fact that LTP is characterized by phases that differ as a function of the requirement for transcription and translation suggests that it is an excellent cellular model by which to study the biochemical mechanisms of memory consolidation. Accordingly, inspired by the success of studies that have defined the contribution of different cellular and molecular signaling cascades underlying both E-LTP and L-LTP, a number of recent studies have asked whether these same mechanisms might underlie short- and long-term formation of fear memories in the amygdala. In this section, we will summarize these findings, beginning with recent studies that have focused on glutamatergic signaling pathways and their contribution to fear acquisition and STM formation.

21.4.1 Short-Term Fear Memory Formation – Glutamatergic Signaling, CaMKII Activation, and AMPAR Trafficking in the Amygdala

Like E-LTP, STM is a short-lasting form of memory that does not require new protein or RNA synthesis (Milner et al., 1998). While no consistent time frame of STM has been defined in the literature, it is generally tested shortly after training, usually within 1 h. Further, deficits in STM formation are typically assumed to reflect deficits in memory acquisition, although it should be emphasized that acquisition and STM formation are likely subserved by distinct molecular mechanisms (Rodrigues et al., 2004b). In this section, we will examine how glutamatergic transmission, αCaMKII, and AMPA receptor (AMPAR) regulation and trafficking might contribute to fear memory acquisition and STM formation in the LA.

21.4.1.1 NMDA receptors

The NMDAR has a long history in the fear conditioning literature. Early pharmacological studies showed that blockade of NMDARs in the LA using the NMDAR antagonist D-2-amino-5-phosphonovaleric acid (APV) reliably impaired fear conditioning (Miserendino et al., 1990; Kim et al., 1991; Campeau et al., 1992), suggesting that an NMDAR-dependent form of synaptic plasticity was critical for fear learning. Later reports, however, indicated that infusion of APV into the LA also impaired the expression of previously acquired fear responses (Maren et al., 1996). These findings are consistent with neurophysiological evidence showing that NMDARs are involved, at least in part, in routine synaptic transmission in the LA (Weisskopf and LeDoux, 1999; Bauer et al., 2002). As such, it has been difficult to conclude unambiguously that NMDARs are required for fear acquisition independently of a role in routine synaptic transmission.

Several years ago, the role of NMDARs in fear conditioning was revisited by examining the effects of selective blockade of the NR2B subunit of the NMDA receptor in the LA. NMDARs are heteromeric complexes composed of several subunits, including the NR1 subunit, which is essential for channel function, as well as a range of NR2 subunits which regulate channel function (Monyer et al., 1992; Nakanishi, 1992). *In vitro* studies have shown that the NR1-NR2B complex exhibits longer excitatory postsynaptic potentials (EPSPs) than the NR1-NR2A complex (Monyer et al., 1992). This characteristic of NR2B-containing NMDARs is thought to provide a longer time window for coincidence detection, which is thought to be especially important during synaptic plasticity (Tsien, 2000). Indeed, recent molecular genetic studies have implicated the NR2B subunit in both synaptic plasticity and memory formation; overexpression of NR2B in the forebrain of mice results in enhanced LTP and memory formation for a variety of tasks, including fear conditioning (Tang et al., 1999).

In the amygdala, blockade of the NR2B by ifenprodil, a selective antagonist of the NR2B subunit of the NMDAR, dose-dependently impairs formation of both STM and LTM of fear conditioning (Rodrigues et al., 2001); that is, memory is impaired both at 1 h and 24 h after infusion and training (**Figures 3(a)** and **3(b)**). In contrast, infusions of ifenprodil prior to testing at either time point have no effect on fear expression. These results suggest that ifenprodil lacks the nonspecific effects on routine transmission that are characteristic of the more global NMDAR antagonist APV. In support of this hypothesis, bath application of ifenprodil to amygdala slices also impairs LTP at thalamic inputs to LA neurons but has no effect on routine synaptic transmission (Bauer et al., 2002; **Figure 3(c)**). These results are also consistent with those of a recent study that examined the effects of APV on acquisition of fear-potentiated startle (Walker and Davis, 2000), showing that APV can, under certain circumstances, have selective effects on plasticity. Collectively, findings suggest that the NMDA receptor in the amygdala plays an essential role in both the acquisition and STM of conditioned fear.

21.4.1.2 Ca^{2+}/calmodulin-dependent protein kinase

One of the immediate downstream consequences of NMDAR-mediated activity-dependent increases in Ca^{2+} at the time of LTP induction is the activation of Ca^{2+}/calmodulin (CaM)-dependent protein kinase II (CaMKII). The alpha isoform of CaMKII has been widely implicated in synaptic plasticity and memory formation (Fukunaga and Miyamoto, 1999; Soderling and Derkach, 2000; Fink and Meyer, 2002; Lisman et al., 2002), in part for its ability to undergo a rapid 'autophosphorylation,' a state in which this enzyme can remain active in the absence of further Ca^{2+} entry (Soderling and Derkach, 2000). In this state, αCaMKII can phosphorylate and transiently enhance the conductance of a variety of membrane proteins, including AMPARs (Barria et al., 1997;

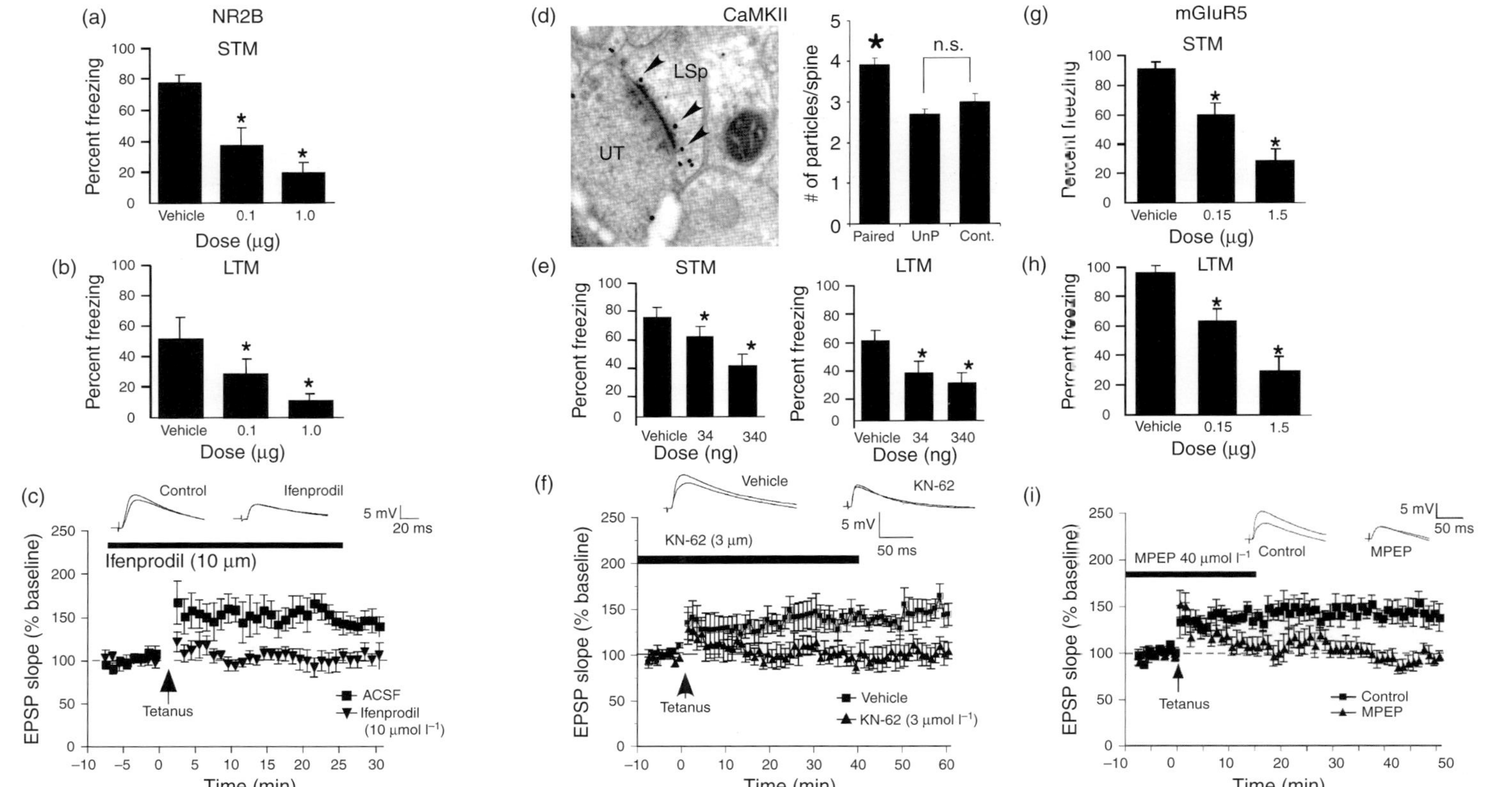

Figure 3 Glutamatergic mechanisms of fear acquisition and STM formation in the LA. (a–b) Both STM and LTM of auditory fear conditioning are dose-dependently impaired by intra-LA infusions of ifenprodil, a selective NR2B antagonist. Adapted from Rodrigues SM, Schafe GE, and LeDoux JE (2001) Intraamygdala blockade of the NR2B subunit of the NMDA receptor disrupts the acquisition but not the expression of fear conditioning. *J. Neurosci.* 21(17): 6889–6896, with permission from the Society for Neuroscience. (c) LTP at thalamic inputs to the LA is also impaired by ifenprodil. Adapted from Bauer EP, Schafe GE, and LeDoux JE (2002) NMDA receptors and L-type voltage-gated calcium channels contribute to long-term potentiation and different components of fear memory formation in the lateral amygdala. *J. Neurosci.* 22: 5239–5249, with permission from the Society for Neuroscience. (d) Fear conditioning results in an increase in autophosphorylated alpha Ca^{2+}/calmodulin-dependent protein kinase II (αCaMKII) in LA spines. Here, rats were conditioned, and activated αCaMKII was detected in LA spines using electron microscopy and an antibody against autophosphorylated αCaMKII at Thr^{286}. The image on the left shows a labeled spine (LSp) in the LA that contains numerous αCaMKII-immunogold labeled particles (arrowheads). The graph on the right shows that paired, but not unpaired (UnP), training leads to significant elevations in αCaMKII-labeled particles in LA spines. UT, unlabeled terminal. $p < .05$. (e) Both STM and LTM of auditory fear conditioning are impaired after intra-LA infusion of KN-62, a CaMKII antagonist. (f) LTP at thalamic inputs to the LA is also impaired by KN-62. (d–f) Adapted from Rodrigues SM, Farb CR, Bauer EP, LeDoux JE, and Schafe GE (2004a) Pavlovian fear conditioning regulates Thr286 autophosphorylation of Ca^{2+}/calmodulin-dependent protein kinase II at lateral amygdala synapses. *J. Neurosci.* 24: 3281–3288, with permission from the Society for Neuroscience. (g–h) Both STM and LTM of auditory fear conditioning are dose-dependently impaired by intra-LA infusions of 2-methyl-6-(phenylethynyl)-pyridine (MPEP), a selective mGluR5 antagonist. (i) LTP at thalamic inputs to the LA is also impaired by MPEP. (g–i) Adapted from Rodrigues SM, Bauer EP, Farb CR, Schafe GE, and LeDoux JE (2002) The group I metabotropic glutamate receptor mGluR5 is required for fear memory formation and long-term potentiation in the lateral amygdala. *J. Neurosci.* 22: 5219–5229, with permission from the Society for Neuroscience.

Mammen et al., 1997; Soderling and Derkach, 2000). Autophosphorylation of αCaMKII on Thr^{286}, for example, promotes the translocation of the kinase to synaptic sites (Shen and Meyer, 1999) and results in phosphorylation of the AMPAR subunit GluR1 on Ser^{831} (Barria et al., 1997; Mammen et al., 1997), an event which increases excitatory current influx into the postsynaptic cell (Derkach et al., 1999) and which is critical for LTP induction (Lee et al., 2000, 2003). Transgenic mice with a deletion of the αCaMKII gene display deficits in hippocampal LTP and hippocampal-dependent spatial memory (Silva et al., 1992a,b). Similarly, pharmacological inhibition of CaMKII blocks the induction of LTP in hippocampal area CA1 (Ito et al., 1991; Stanton and Gage, 1996) and impairs hippocampal dependent learning and memory (Tan and Liang, 1996).

Recent studies have also implicated αCaMKII in fear conditioning. Anatomical studies have shown that αCaMKII is robustly expressed in LA pyramidal neurons (McDonald et al., 2002), where it coexists with NR2B in LA spines postsynaptic to terminals that originate in the auditory thalamus (Rodrigues et al., 2004a). Fear conditioning leads to increases in the autophosphorylated form of αCaMKII at Thr^{286} in spines of LA neurons (**Figure 3(d)**). Further, intra-amygdala infusion or bath application of an inhibitor of CaMKII (KN-62) impairs acquisition and STM formation of fear conditioning and LTP at thalamic inputs to LA neurons, respectively (**Figures 3(e)** and **3(f)**). This latter finding is consistent with molecular genetic experiments indicating that induced overexpression of active αCaMKII by a transgene that replaces Thr^{286} with an aspartate residue in the amygdala and striatum results in a reversible deficit in fear conditioning (Mayford et al., 1996).

21.4.1.3 Metabotropic glutamate receptors and protein kinase C

While activation of αCaMKII and resultant GluR1 phosphorylation and receptor trafficking appears to be NMDAR dependent (Hayashi et al., 2000; Fu et al., 2004), it appears that Group I metabotropic glutamate receptors (mGluRs), including mGluR1 and mGluR5, are critical for the potentiation of NMDAR function via the Ca^{2+}/phospholipid-dependent protein kinase (PKC) (Ben-Ari et al., 1992; Kelso et al., 1992). Both mGluR1 and mGluR5, for example, are positively coupled to phospholipase C, activation of which leads to the hydrolysis of phosphatidylinositol 4,5-biphosphate into inositol 1,4,5-trisphosphate (IP3) and diacylglycerol (DAG), two substances that are directly upstream of PKC. In mGluR5 knockout mice, LTP of NMDAR currents in CA1 is absent, but can be rescued by activators of PKC (Jia et al., 1998). Further, an mGluR5 antagonist (CHPG) has been reported to induce a slowly developing, long-lasting potentiation of NMDAR currents via PKC (Doherty et al., 1997). Studies have suggested that two serine residues on the C-terminal domain of the NR2B subunit of the NMDAR, Ser^{1303} and Ser^{1323}, are the critical structural domain for PKC-mediated current potentiation (Liao et al., 2001). However, removal of all the PKC phosphorylation sites on NR1 and NR2 does not alter the PKC-induced potentiation of NMDAR currents (Zheng et al., 1999). Thus, it has been hypothesized that there is an intermediate step between PKC activation and NR2 subunit activation. One hypothesis is that this involves Src kinases (Ali and Salter, 2001; MacDonald et al., 2001). Src is the lead member of a family of protein tyrosine kinases, which also includes Fyn, Lyn, Lck, and Yes. It is thought that these kinases regulate the activity of NMDARs during LTP induction by phosphorylating tyrosine residues that, in turn, are responsible for increased channel conductance (Ali and Salter, 2001; MacDonald et al., 2001). The phosphorylation of NR2B on Tyr^{1472} is increased after tetanic stimulation in area CA1 (Nakazawa et al., 2001), and this appears to be Fyn mediated (Nakazawa et al., 2001, 2002). Further, mice lacking Fyn have impaired LTP in hippocampal area CA1 (Grant et al., 1992).

Several recent studies have examined the role of mGluRs in fear conditioning. Transgenic mice lacking mGluR5 are impaired in fear conditioning tasks (Lu et al., 1997), as are rats injected systemically with the selective mGluR5 antagonist 2-methyl-6-(phenylethynyl)-pyridine (MPEP) prior to fear conditioning (Fendt and Schmid, 2002). In a recent study, Rodrigues et al. showed that mGluR5 was localized in LA spines postsynaptic to auditory thalamic inputs and required for synaptic plasticity at thalamic inputs to LA neurons (Rodrigues et al., 2002). Further, in behavioral experiments, intra-amygdala infusion of MPEP prior to fear conditioning impaired formation of both STM and LTM of fear conditioning (Rodrigues et al., 2002; **Figures 3(g)** amd **3(h)**), and also impaired LTP at thalamic inputs to the LA (**Figure 3(i)**). Similar to the results with the NR2B antagonist ifenprodil, infusion of MPEP prior to training blocked both STM and

LTM, while infusion immediately prior to testing at either time point had no effect.

These findings suggest that mGluRs, and in particular mGluR5, are required for fear conditioning and STM formation in the amygdala. Future experiments, however, will be required to understand the exact mechanisms by which mGluRs contribute to fear conditioning. One attractive hypothesis, suggested by the LTP literature, is that activation of mGluR5 in the amygdala recruits the PKC signaling pathway and leads to modulation and trafficking of NMDARs via tyrosine phosphorylation of NR2B (Doherty et al., 1997; Anwyl, 1999; Liao et al., 2001). The role of PKC or tyrosine kinases in fear acquisition and STM formation has not been explicitly tested, although mice with a specific deletion of the β isoform of PKC have impaired fear conditioning when tested 24 h after training (Weeber et al., 2000). Additional experiments will be necessary to examine the role of mGluR5-mediated signaling in the LA in fear conditioning.

21.4.1.4 AMPA receptor regulation and trafficking

Alterations in the conductance properties of glutamatergic receptors are thought to be only one mechanism underlying LTP induction and E-LTP. Ample evidence, for example, has accumulated indicating that new AMPARs and NMDARs are trafficked and inserted into synapses during and after LTP (Grosshans et al., 2002; Malenka, 2003; Malinow, 2003). The insertion of GluR1 into synapses, for example, appears to be αCaMKII dependent, and blockade of αCaMKII-mediated synaptic delivery of GluR1 prevents LTP (Hayashi et al., 2000). Further, activation of PKC has been shown to drive NMDAR subunits into synapses, an effect which is blocked by tyrosine kinase inhibitors (Grosshans et al., 2002). Together with alterations in receptor conductance, these rapid physical alterations in the distribution of AMPARs and NMDARs represent one mechanism by which LTP might persist in the short term.

A recent study by Malinow and colleagues elegantly showed that intra-amygdala expression of a viral vector that prevents GluR1 from being inserted into synaptic sites impairs fear acquisition and synaptic plasticity in the LA (Rumpel et al., 2005). Thus, while additional studies are needed, these findings collectively suggest that activation of αCaMKII during fear acquisition may regulate the insertion of AMPARs at LA synapses and thereby contribute to the formation and maintenance of STM. It is currently unknown how long-lasting this effect is; e.g., whether it persists only over the course of hours or is also evident days after fear learning. Further, no studies have to date examined how fear conditioning might similarly regulate the trafficking of NMDARs. Additional experiments will be critical to examine each of these questions.

21.4.2 Long-Term Fear Memory Formation – Protein Kinase Signaling and Transcriptional Regulation in the Amygdala

As its name implies, LTM is a long-lasting phenomenon that can last many hours, days, weeks, or even years (Milner et al., 1998). Accordingly, LTM is typically tested at longer intervals after training, usually starting at 24 h. In this section, we discuss what is known about the mechanisms of LTM formation of fear conditioning in the amygdala. We begin with a discussion of L-VGCCs, as recent work has suggested that these channels play an essential role in promoting LTM formation in the LA.

21.4.2.1 L-VGCCs

Recent experiments have shown that LTP at thalamic input synapses to the LA is, under certain conditions, L-VGCC dependent and NMDAR independent (Weisskopf et al., 1999). These experiments used a pairing protocol in which subthreshold presynaptic stimulation of auditory afferents was paired with brief postsynaptic depolarizations (Magee and Johnston, 1997; Markram et al., 1997; Johnston et al., 1999). In this protocol, back-propagating action potentials (BPAPs) originating in the soma are thought to invade the dendrites and interact with EPSPs leading to Ca^{2+} influx through VGCCs (Magee and Johnston, 1997; Johnston et al., 1999; Stuart and Hausser, 2001). Accordingly, LTP induced by pairing in the thalamic pathway is blocked by application of the L-VGCC blockers nifedipine or verapamil (Weisskopf et al., 1999; Bauer et al., 2002).

Until recently, the contribution of L-VGCCs to fear conditioning had not been established. Bauer et al., however, examined the effect of intra-amygdala infusion of the L-VGCC blocker verapamil on the acquisition and consolidation of auditory fear conditioning (Bauer et al., 2002). The findings revealed that blockade of L-VGCCs prior to conditioning selectively impaired LTM formation of fear conditioning at 24 h after training; acquisition and STM, assessed at 1 h, were left intact. These findings, together with those of studies that examined the role of NMDAR function in fear conditioning discussed earlier, suggest that there are two sources of Ca^{2+} in the LA that are critical for fear memory formation. One, mediated by NMDARs, appears to be selectively involved in fear acquisition and STM formation of fear conditioning (Walker and Davis, 2000; Rodrigues et al., 2001). The second, mediated by L-VGCCs, is selectively involved in LTM formation. While the effects of L-VGCC blockade are not apparent in fear conditioning for many hours after training, it is important to note that this is likely due to interference with a process that is set in motion at the time of CS-US pairing and fear acquisition. Consistent with that notion, recent reports have demonstrated that L-VGCCs play a selective role in signaling to the nucleus and initiating cyclic adenosine monophosphate (cAMP) response element (CRE)-mediated transcription, which is known to be required for long-term synaptic plasticity and memory formation (Dolmetsch et al., 2001). Additional experiments will be necessary to determine the contribution of L-VGCCs to activation of protein kinases and CRE-driven gene expression in the LA following fear conditioning.

21.4.2.2 Protein kinase A and mitogen-activated protein kinase

Activity-dependent increases in intracellular Ca^{2+} in LA neurons during fear acquisition is thought to lead, either directly or indirectly, to the activation of both protein kinase A (PKA) and the extracellular signal-regulated kinase/mitogen-activated protein kinase (ERK/MAPK). There has been a great deal of recent interest in each of these kinases, in part because they have been shown to be essential for the late phase of multiple forms of synaptic plasticity and memory (Milner et al., 1998; Sweatt, 2004). Once activated by stimulation that promotes L-LTP, each of these kinases is thought to engage activators of transcription. While PKA is directly capable of regulating transcription, recent evidence suggests that PKA may play a permissive role in transcriptional regulation by promoting the activation and nuclear translocation of ERK/MAPK (Roberson et al., 1999). As a result, it has been suggested that ERK/MAPK may represent a final common pathway through which different upstream kinases regulate transcription, long-term plasticity, and memory formation (Adams and Sweatt, 2002).

Both PKA and ERK/MAPK have also been implicated in fear conditioning. Mice that overexpress an inhibitory form of PKA, R(AB), exhibit impaired L-LTP in hippocampal area CA1 and selective deficits in LTM, but not STM, of contextual fear conditioning (Abel et al., 1997). Similarly, mice that lack *Ras-GRF*, an upstream regulator of ERK/MAPK, have impaired memory consolidation of auditory and contextual fear conditioning, as well as impaired amygdala LTP (Brambilla et al., 1997).

Recent pharmacological experiments have examined the role of PKA and ERK/MAPK in amygdala LTP and in fear conditioning. Huang et al. showed that bath application of inhibitors of PKA or ERK/MAPK to amygdala slices impairs LTP at thalamic and cortical inputs to the LA but has no effect on E-LTP (Huang et al., 2000). Consistent with those findings, infusion of a PKA inhibitor or of a peptide that blocks the association of PKA with the A-kinase anchoring protein (AKAP) in the LA impairs LTM, but not STM of fear conditioning (Schafe and LeDoux, 2000; Moita et al., 2002; **Figure 4(e)**). Further, fear conditioning results in a transient activation of ERK/MAPK in the LA (**Figures 4(a)–4(c)**), and infusion of an inhibitor of MEK, an upstream regulator of ERK/MAPK, into the LA prior to fear conditioning impairs memory consolidation; that is, rats have intact STM and impaired LTM (Schafe et al., 2000; **Figure 4(d)**). Collectively, these findings support the hypothesis that both PKA and ERK/MAPK contribute to fear memory formation by engaging cellular processes, possibly those in the nucleus, that are necessary for long-term synaptic plasticity and memory formation.

21.4.2.3 Neurotrophin signaling

In addition to Ca^{2+}-mediated signaling, neurotrophins have been widely implicated in driving protein kinase signaling pathways necessary for long-term synaptic plasticity and memory formation, including fear conditioning. In hippocampal neurons, direct application of brain-derived neurotrophic factor (BDNF) produces a long-lasting, transcription-dependent form of LTP (Kang and Schuman, 1995; Figurov et al., 1996). Further, blockade or genetic deletion of BDNF or its membrane-bound receptor tyrosine kinase, TrkB, impairs L-LTP in the hippocampus (Figurov et al., 1996; Patterson et al., 1996; Korte et al., 1998; Fanselow and LeDoux, 1999), and L-LTP is impaired in hippocampal slices in mice that lack BDNF (Patterson et al., 1996; Korte et al., 1998). Consistent with the importance of ERK/MAPK signaling in long-term synaptic plasticity and memory formation, recent studies have suggested that

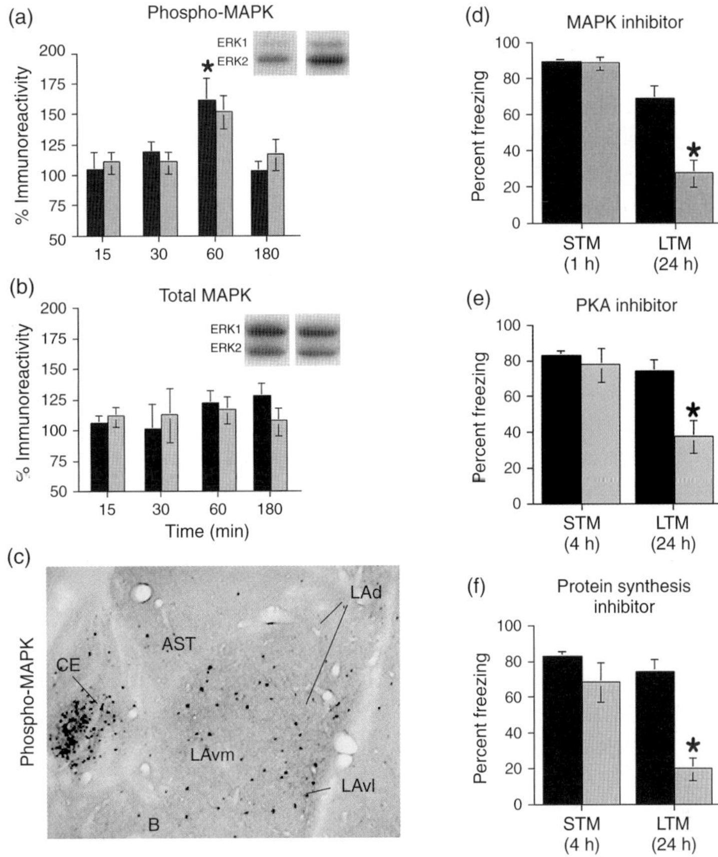

Figure 4 Protein kinase signaling pathways involved in long-term memory (LTM) formation in the lateral amygdala (LA). (a) Fear conditioning leads to an increase in phosphorylated extracellular signal-related kinase 1 (ERK1) and ERK2 at $t = 60$ min after training. In these experiments, rats were trained and sacrificed at different time points after conditioning, and LA homogenates were probed with antibodies that recognize phosphorylated ERK/mitogen-activated protein kinase (MAPK). ERK1 (black bars) and ERK2 (gray bars) are the two isoforms of ERK/MAPK recognized by the anti-phospho-ERK antibody. $p < .05$. (b) The increase in activated ERK/MAPK is not accounted for by a change in the amount of total (unphosphorylated) ERK/MAPK. (c) Immunocytochemical localization of phosphorylated ERK/MAPK in the LA after fear conditioning. The image shows ERK-labeled cells in three different regions of the LA (dorsal, LAd; ventromedial, LAvm; and ventrolateral, LAvl), with most of the label concentrated in the ventral portions of the LAd and throughout the LAvm and LAvl. Activated ERK/MAPK is also highly expressed in the nearby central nucleus (CE) and the amygdala-striatal transition zone (AST). B, basal nucleus of the amygdala. (a–c) Adapted from Schafe GE, Atkins CM, Swank MW, Bauer EP, Sweatt JD, and LeDoux JE (2000) Activation of ERK/MAP kinase in the amygdala is required for memory consolidation of Pavlovian fear conditioning. *J. Neurosci.* 20: 8177–8187, with permission from the Society for Neuroscience. (d–f) LTM, but not short-term memory (STM), in the LA requires MAPK, protein kinase A (PKA), and protein synthesis. In these studies, rats received intra-amygdala infusions of (d) U0126 (a MEK inhibitor, which is an upstream regulator of ERK/MAPK activation), (e) Rp-cAMPS (a PKA inhibitor), or (f) anisomycin (a protein synthesis inhibitor) at or around the time of training and were assayed for both STM (1–4 h later) and LTM (24 h later) of auditory fear conditioning. In each figure, vehicle-treated rats are represented by the gray bars, while drug-treated animals are represented by the black bars. $^*p < .05$ relative to vehicle controls. (d–f) Adapted from Schafe GE and LeDoux JE (2000) Memory consolidation of auditory Pavlovian fear conditioning requires protein synthesis and protein kinase A in the amygdala. *J. Neurosci.* 20: RC96, with permission from the Society for Neuroscience.

BDNF-TrkB-mediated signaling promotes long-term synaptic plasticity by engaging the ERK/MAPK signaling pathway (Patterson et al., 2001). Application of BDNF potently activates ERK/MAPK in hippocampal neurons (Ying et al., 2002), and treatment with an inhibitor of ERK/MAPK activation impairs BDNF-induced LTP (Ying et al., 2002). Collectively, these findings suggest that BDNF-induced ERK signaling plays an essential role in long-term synaptic plasticity.

A recent study has shown that BDNF-mediated signaling in the amygdala is critical to fear learning

(Rattiner et al., 2004, 2005). In that study, fear conditioning led to increases in both TrkB receptor phosphorylation and decreases in TrkB receptor immunoreactivity in the LA during the consolidation period, which is typically indicative of bound BDNF. Further, disruption of TrkB receptor signaling in the amygdala using either a Trk receptor antagonist or lentiviral overexpression of a dominant negative TrkB isoform impaired fear memory formation (Rattiner et al., 2004). While this study did not distinguish between acquisition and consolidation phases of fear learning, the assumption is that BDNF signaling in the LA plays a critical role in the establishment of long-term fear memories, possibly by promoting the activation and nuclear translocation of protein kinases such as ERK (Patterson et al., 2001; Ying et al., 2002). Additional experiments will be necessary to define the signaling pathways through which BDNF acts during fear learning.

21.4.2.4 Transcriptional regulation and macromolecular synthesis

Both L-LTP in the LA (Huang and Kandel, 1998; Huang et al., 2000) and LTM of fear conditioning (Bailey et al., 1999; Schafe and LeDoux, 2000) are known to require new RNA and protein synthesis in the LA (**Figure 4(f)**). The requirement for *de novo* RNA synthesis is particularly important, because it suggests that a nuclear event is required for the transition between short- and long-term memory formation.

As previously discussed, signaling via ERK/MAPK plays a critical role in memory formation by engaging activators of transcription in the nucleus. ERK/MAPK is thought to promote transcription by binding to and activating transcription factors, including, by way of the Rsk and MSK1 signaling pathways (Xing et al., 1996; Adams and Sweatt, 2002), the cAMP-response-element binding protein (CREB) (Impey et al., 1996, 1998a). It is the activation of CREB and CRE-mediated genes that ultimately leads to the protein and RNA synthesis-dependent functional and/or structural changes that are thought to underlie L-LTP (Frank and Greenberg, 1994; Yin and Tully, 1996; Silva et al., 1998; Stevens, 1998; Holt and Maren, 1999). While many of these genes and their functional roles remain to be elucidated, it has been suggested that the regulation of a number of CRE- and serum response element (SRE)-mediated immediate early genes (IEGs) plays a critical intermediate role in regulating the expression of late-response genes. These have included *Zif-268*, and its protein product EGR-1, and the activity-regulated cytoskeletal-associated protein (Arc). Importantly, each of these IEGs is known to be regulated by hippocampal LTP (Richardson et al., 1992; Abraham et al., 1993; Worley et al., 1993; Link et al., 1995) and required for hippocampal-dependent LTM formation (Guzowski et al., 2000; Jones et al., 2001).

Several transcription factors have been implicated in long-term synaptic plasticity and in memory formation, but CREB is perhaps the best studied. CREB is a family of transcription factors consisting of several functionally distinct isoforms. Some, known as activator isoforms, bind to DNA at CRE promoter regions and promote transcription. Others, known as repressor isoforms, compete with the binding of activator isoforms to DNA (Bartsch et al., 1995; Abel et al., 1998; Silva et al., 1998). CREB is an attractive candidate molecule for memory consolidation because it has direct interaction with the transcriptional machinery and also contains phosphorylation sites for the major protein kinase signaling pathways that are known to be involved in memory formation, including PKA, ERK/MAPK, and CaMKII (Silva et al., 1998).

The first evidence that suggested CREB might be involved in memory consolidation came from a study employing a Pavlovian conditioning task in *Drosophila.* Overexpression of a dominant negative (repressor) isoform of CREB in flies impaired LTM formation in a conditioned odor aversion task (Yin et al., 1994). Conversely, overexpression of an activator isoform of CREB facilitated LTM; that is, behavioral training that would normally produce only STM was effective at producing LTM (Yin et al., 1995).

CREB has also been implicated in fear conditioning. Mice lacking two critical isoforms of CREB, the α and δ, have impaired hippocampal L-LTP and memory consolidation for auditory and contextual fear conditioning; that is, LTM is impaired, while STM is intact (Bourtchuladze et al., 1994). Further, induced overexpression of a dominant negative isoform of CREB in the forebrain impairs LTM formation of fear conditioning (Kida et al., 2002). Conversely, overexpression of the transcription factor CREB in the LA facilitates fear memory formation (Josselyn et al., 2001). In the latter study, CREB was overexpressed locally in the LA, using viral transfection methods. Consistent with the role of CREB in long-term synaptic plasticity and memory formation, overexpression of CREB in the LA facilitated LTM of fear conditioning, but had no effect on STM.

While CRE-mediated transcription clearly supports the development of long-term plasticity and memory, the downstream targets of CREB have remained largely unknown. However, a number of studies have shown that fear conditioning induces the expression of both IEGs (Beck and Fibiger, 1995; Rosen et al., 1998; Malkani and Rosen, 2000; Scicli et al., 2004) and downstream genes (Stork et al., 2001; Ressler et al., 2002; Rattiner et al., 2004) in the LA. While the specific contributions of many of these genes to fear conditioning is still unclear, it is widely believed that learning-induced gene expression ultimately contributes to changes in cell (especially synaptic) structure that stabilizes memory (Bailey and Kandel, 1993; Woolf, 1998; Rampon et al., 2000; Sweatt, 2004), presumably by altering the actin cytoskeleton underlying synaptic organization (van Rossum and Hanisch, 1999; Matus, 2000; Kasai et al., 2003). Such changes in synaptic structure have been well documented in invertebrates, where stimulation that promotes long-term synaptic plasticity has been shown to lead to an increase in new synaptic contacts (Bailey et al., 1992, 1994; Bailey and Kandel, 1993). Further, both learning and LTP result in a number of structural changes in the hippocampus and cortex, including an increase in spine head volume and widening and shortening of the spine neck (Van Harreveld and Fifkova, 1975; Fifkova and Van Harreveld, 1977; Fifkova and Anderson, 1981), spine perforation (Toni et al., 1999), and an increase in the total number of spines (Engert and Bonhoeffer, 1999; Leuner et al., 2003).

Recent studies have suggested that fear conditioning leads to alterations in cytoskeletal proteins and to new spine formation in the LA. Fear conditioning, for example, leads to the transcription of genes involved in cytoskeletal remodeling, including the CRE-mediated gene neurofilament-light chain (NF-l) (Ressler et al., 2002). Further, interference with molecular pathways known to be involved in structural plasticity during early development, such as the Rho GTPase (GTP: guanosine triphosphate) activating protein (Rho-GAP) signaling pathway, disrupts memory formation (Lamprecht et al., 2002), and fear conditioning drives actin cytoskeleton-regulatory proteins, such as profilin, into amygdala spines shortly after training (Lamprecht et al., 2006). Finally, a recent morphological study has suggested that fear conditioning leads to an increase in spinophilin-immunoreactive dendritic spines in the LA (Radley et al., 2006).

21.4.3 A Presynaptic Component to Fear Learning?

As outlined, most recent studies have focused on postsynaptic mechanisms and their role in amygdala LTP and memory formation (for review, see Schafe et al., 2001). There is growing evidence, however, that suggests that synaptic plasticity and memory formation in the LA involves a presynaptic process. McKernan and Shinnick-Gallagher (1997), for example, showed that auditory fear conditioning occludes paired-pulse facilitation (PPF) at cortical inputs to the LA, a type of short-term plasticity that is largely believed to be presynaptic. Similarly, Huang and Kandel (1998) observed that LTP at cortical inputs to the LA occludes PPF in this pathway. Further, bath application, but not postsynaptic injection, of a PKA inhibitor impairs LTP in LA neurons (Huang and Kandel, 1998). Conversely, bath application of forskolin, a PKA activator, in the presence of antagonists of postsynaptic NMDAR and AMPAR receptors, induces LTP and occludes PPF at cortical inputs (Huang and Kandel, 1998), suggesting that the presynaptic component of LTP in this pathway is PKA dependent. More recently, Tsvetkov et al. showed that auditory fear conditioning itself, in addition to LTP, occludes PPF at cortical inputs to LA (Tsvetkov et al., 2002). It is thus clear from the available evidence that a complete understanding of memory formation and synaptic plasticity in the LA will require attention to both sides of the synapse.

21.4.3.1 Nitric oxide signaling and fear learning

Recent evidence has suggested that nitric oxide (NO) signaling in the LA is critical to fear memory formation (Schafe et al., 2005) and may represent a mechanism whereby postsynaptic induction of plasticity induced by fear conditioning in LA neurons may engage accompanying presynaptic changes. NO is a highly soluble gas generated by the conversion of L-arginine to L-citrulline by the Ca^{2+}-regulated enzyme nitric oxide synthase (NOS) (Bredt and Snyder, 1992). In other memory systems, NO is thought to serve as a 'retrograde messenger' that engages aspects of presynaptic plasticity (Schuman and Madison, 1991; Zhuo et al., 1994; Arancio et al.,

1996; Doyle et al., 1996; Son et al., 1998; Ko and Kelly, 1999; Lu et al., 1999) and memory formation (Chapman et al., 1992; Bohme et al., 1993; Bernabeu et al., 1995; Holscher et al., 1996; Suzuki et al., 1996; Zou et al., 1998). One immediate downstream effector of NO, for example, is soluble guanylyl cyclase (Bredt and Snyder, 1992; Son et al., 1998; Denninger and Marletta, 1999; Arancio et al., 2001). This enzyme directly leads to the formation of cyclic guanosine monophosphate (cGMP) and in turn to the activation of the cGMP-dependent protein kinase (PKG). PKG, in turn, can have a number of effects, including targeting and mobilization of synaptic vesicles in the presynaptic cell, leading to enhanced transmitter release (Hawkins et al., 1993, 1998). In the hippocampus, pharmacological inhibition of NOS activation, guanylyl cyclase, or PKG impairs LTP in CA1 (Zhuo et al., 1994; Doyle et al., 1996; Son et al., 1998; Lu et al., 1999; Monfort et al., 2002). Conversely, bath application of exogenous NO or pharmacological activators of cGMP or PKG combined with weak tetanic stimulation, which would not produce LTP alone, induces long-lasting LTP (Zhuo et al., 1994; Son et al., 1998; Lu et al., 1999; Lu and Hawkins, 2002). Inhibition of NOS activity is equally effective at impairing LTP, whether the NOS inhibitor is injected directly into the postsynaptic cell or perfused over the entire slice, suggesting that the critical activation of NOS occurs postsynaptically (Schuman and Madison, 1991; Arancio et al., 1996; Ko and Kelly, 1999). However, NO is thought to act presynaptically, at least in part, because bath application of membrane-impermeable scavengers of NO also impairs LTP in CA1 (Schuman and Madison, 1991; Ko and Kelly, 1999). Collectively, this pattern of findings supports the notion that LTP in area CA1 is induced postsynaptically, but maintained or expressed presynaptically, at least in part, by an NO-dependent mechanism.

In our recent experiments, we showed that neuronal nitric oxide synthase (nNOS) is localized in LA spines (**Figure 5(a)**). Further, PPF was occluded by LTP at thalamic inputs to the LA, and bath application of either a NOS inhibitor or a membrane impermeable scavenger of NO impaired LTP at thalamo–LA synapses (**Figures 5(b)–5(d)**). Finally, intra-amygdala infusion of both compounds impaired fear memory consolidation; that is, LTM was impaired, while STM was intact (Schafe et al., 2005; **Figures 5(e)** and **5(f)**). While additional studies will be necessary, these are among the first to define a role for NO signaling in fear memory formation in the LA.

21.5 Is the Lateral Amygdala an Essential Locus of Fear Memory Storage?

In the previous sections, we have discussed the findings of lesion, neurophysiological, pharmacological, and biochemical studies. Collectively, these findings suggest that fear memory formation and consolidation involve alterations in synaptic transmission at LA synapses via an LTP-like mechanism. But is the LA really a site of fear memory storage? This question has proven extremely difficult to address experimentally. Recent findings, however, have provided a fresh look at this question and provide a new strategy for revealing the location of the fear engram.

21.5.1 An Alternative View of the Amygdala and Fear Conditioning

While an ever-increasing number of studies using lesion, neurophysiological, and most recently, pharmacological/biochemical techniques have suggested that the LA is an essential site of fear memory formation and storage, an alternative view has offered alternative interpretations of each of the aforementioned findings (Cahill et al., 1999). One obvious way to ask whether a brain structure might be involved in permanent storage of a memory is to lesion that structure at different time points after training (e.g., 1 day later, 1 week later, 1 year later). If memory is impaired as the result of the lesion at each of these time points it suggests that some type of permanent storage has occurred there, *provided that* the area of interest is not involved in some way in the expression of that type of learning. In support of the memory storage hypothesis, lesions of the amygdala impair fear learning even if given years after the initial training event (Gale et al., 2004). The conclusions drawn from these studies, however, have long been called into question due to the fact that the LA and its connections with the CE are also critical for fear expression (Cahill et al., 1999, 2001). Accordingly, lesion studies alone cannot unambiguously distinguish a role for the LA in fear acquisition from that of fear expression.

Neurophysiological and pharmacological studies supporting a role for the amygdala in memory storage have also been called into question. It has been pointed out, for example, that the LA is not unique but rather one of many regions of the wider fear network to exhibit training-related neurophysiological changes during and after fear conditioning.

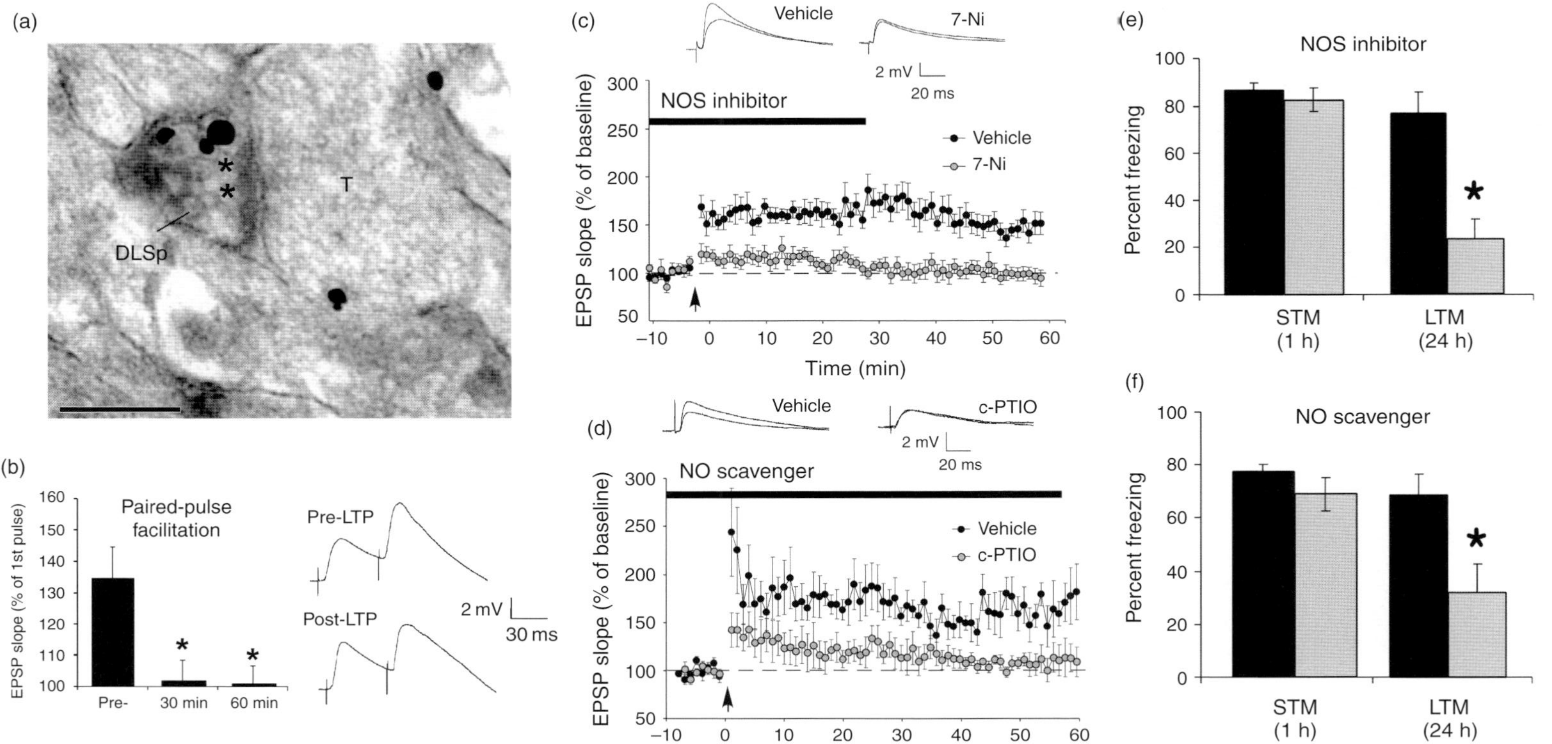

Figure 5 Nitric oxide (NO) signaling and fear memory formation. (a) Localization of neuronal NOS (nNOS) in LA spines. A terminal (T) forms an asymmetric synapse (asterisks) onto a nNOS- and αCaMKII-immunoreactivity dually labeled spine (DLSp) in the LA. The immunogold particles represent labeling of αCaMKII, while the peroxidase represents labeling of nNOS. (b) Paired-pulse facilitation at thalamic inputs to the LA before (Pre-) and 30 and 60 min after LTP induction. Each cell was given two stimulations that were spaced 50 ms apart, and the second pulse was expressed as a percentage of the first pulse. Representative traces can be seen at the right. (c–d) LTP at thalamic inputs to the LA is impaired by bath application of either (c) an inhibitor of nNOS (7-nitroindazole, 7-Ni) or (d) a membrane impermeable scavenger of NO (carboxy-PTIO, c-PTIO). (e–f) Fear memory consolidation is also impaired by 7-Ni and carboxy-PTIO. In both cases, STM is intact, while LTM is impaired. All figures adapted, with permission, from Schafe GE, Bauer EP, Rosis S, Farb CR, Rodrigues SM, and LeDoux JE (2005) Memory consolidation of Pavlovian fear conditioning requires nitric oxide signaling in the lateral amygdala. *Eur. J. Neurosci.* 22: 201–211. Copyright by Blackwell Publishing.

Auditory fear conditioning, for example, induces associative alterations in the activity of neurons not only in the LA, but also in the auditory cortex (Bakin and Weinberger, 1990; Edeline and Weinberger, 1993) and the auditory thalamus (Gabriel et al., 1975; Weinberger, 1993). Consequently, it has been difficult to argue with certainty that training-induced changes in the LA are of local origin rather than the result of a passive reflection of plasticity in these upstream regions (Cahill et al., 1999). This has been especially true of training-induced changes in the auditory thalamus (MGm/PIN), which are of short enough latency (e.g., 5–7 ms) to account for the shortest observed changes in the LA (e.g., 12–15 ms). Finally, rather than indicating that the LA is a site of storage of fear memories, it has been suggested that memory deficits observed after pharmacological manipulations may instead indicate that the LA is essential for triggering or modulating the strength of plasticity and memory storage in other regions of the wider fear network (Cahill et al., 1999). In support of this notion, recent studies have suggested that the acquisition of training-induced plasticity in the auditory thalamus is dependent on the amygdala (Maren et al., 2001; Poremba and Gabriel, 2001). Accordingly, one may argue that pharmacological manipulations of the LA that are aimed at disrupting synaptic plasticity may be doing so by modulating the strength of plasticity in regions of the wider fear network, such as the MGm/PIN, which is in turn reflected back to the LA.

21.5.2 A New Strategy for Tracking the Fear Engram

Recognizing that neurophysiological or pharmacological methods alone are unlikely to be able to answer the question of where fear memories are stored, a recent study from our lab has taken a new approach. In our studies, we combined simultaneous neurophysiological recordings from both LA and MGm/PIN with intra-LA infusion of the MAP kinase kinase (MEK) inhibitor U0126 (**Figure 6**). We reasoned that if local synaptic plasticity in the LA was necessary for fear memory formation and storage via an ERK/MAPK dependent mechanism, then local inhibition of MEK in the LA should selectively impair training-induced plasticity in the LA rather than the MGm/PIN. The findings showed that MEK inhibition in the LA impaired both memory consolidation of auditory fear conditioning (**Figures 6(a)** and **6(b)**), and also the consolidation of training-induced synaptic plasticity in the LA (**Figures 6(c)–6(e)**). That is, acquisition and short-term retention of fear learning and cellular changes were intact, whereas long-term retention was impaired. Intra-LA infusion of the MEK inhibitor had no effect, however, on training-induced neurophysiological changes in the MGm/PIN (**Figures 6(f)–6(h)**).

Together, these findings strongly indicate that ERK/MAPK-mediated signaling in the LA is required for memory consolidation of fear conditioning as well as for consolidation of conditioning-induced synaptic plasticity in the LA. Further, our findings rule out the possibility that MEK inhibition in the LA may be impairing to fear memory formation by influencing synaptic plasticity (either short- or long-term) in the MGm/PIN. Further, these findings suggest that conditioned enhancement of CS responses in the auditory thalamus is not sufficient to support memory storage of fear conditioning, whereas ERK-dependent conditioned enhancement of CS responses in LA is necessary, at least in part, for memory storage. Importantly, it should be emphasized that these recent findings do not diminish the potential importance of the auditory thalamus and other structures in the encoding of different components of the whole fear memory trace, nor do they suggest, as we will see later, that the amygdala plays no role in modulating certain types of memory storage. However, these recent findings provide strong support to the notion that long-term storage of an emotional memory trace relies, in part, on local synaptic plasticity in the LA.

21.6 Distributed Versus Local Plasticity in the Amygdala

While the LA clearly appears to be a critical locus of synaptic plasticity, fear memory acquisition, and storage, it should not be assumed that LA synapses are the only critical synapses in the amygdala which undergo changes that are essential to fear memory formation and/or consolidation. Several recent studies, for example, have suggested that a distributed, rather than localized, network of plasticity in the amygdala underlies fear learning (Medina et al., 2002; Paré et al., 2004).

21.6.1 Distributed Plasticity within the LA

The distributed view of plasticity underlying fear learning begins in the LA itself, where plasticity at two sets of synapses has been linked to fear learning,

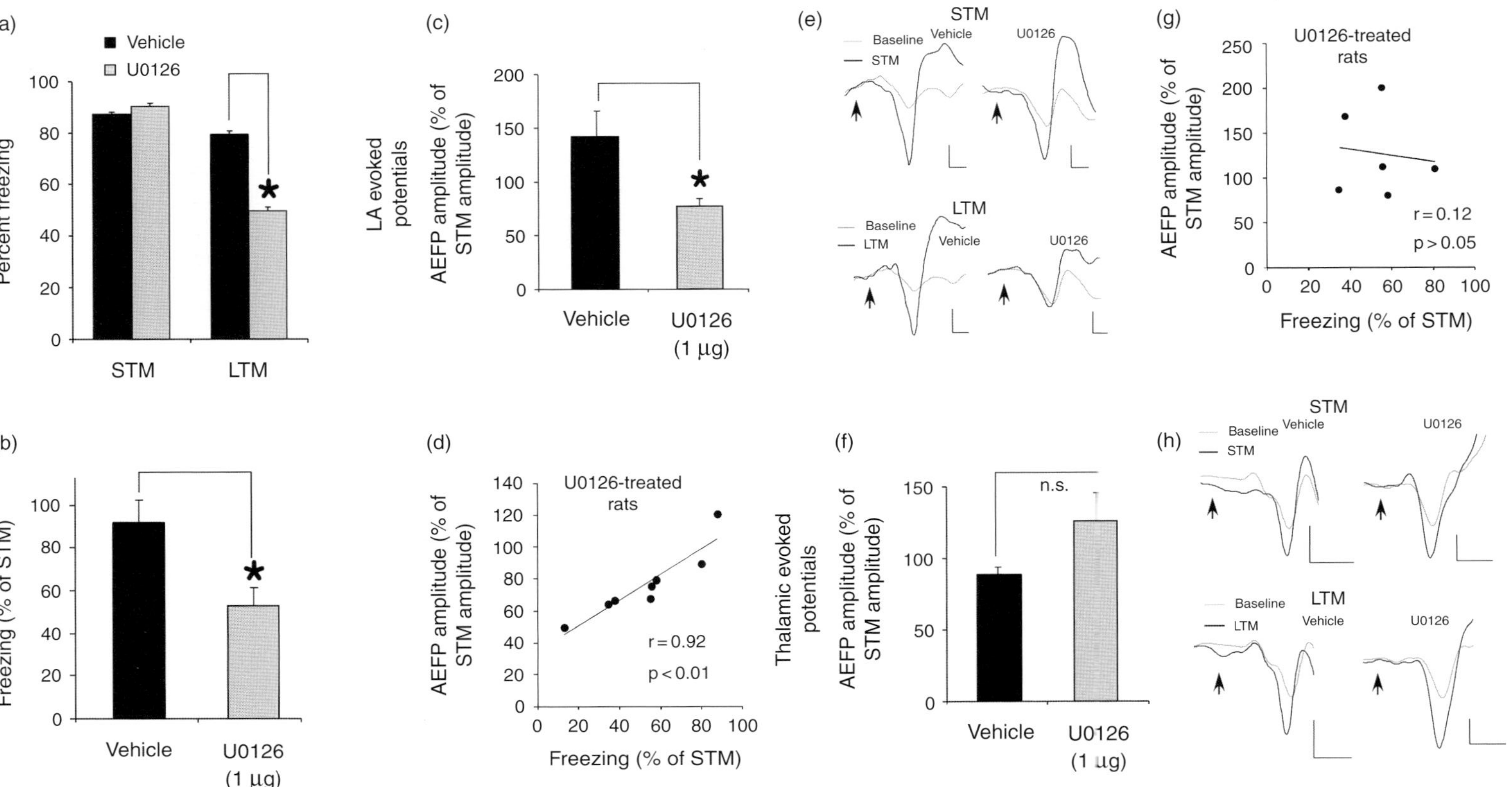

Figure 6 Local synaptic plasticity is required for fear memory consolidation in the lateral amygdala (LA). (a) Impaired fear memory in rats receiving intra-LA infusions of U0126 while neurophysiological recordings were made from both LA and the medial geniculate body and the posterior intralaminal nucleus (MGm/PIN). Mean (± SEM) percent freezing expressed during STM and LTM tests in rats treated with 50% dimethyl sulfoxide vehicle (black bars) or 1 μg U0126 (ray bars). (b) Mean (± SEM) retention of freezing in both groups; freezing during LTM is expressed as a percentage of that observed during the STM test. (c) Mean (± SEM) changes in the amplitude of LA auditory-evoked field potentials (AEFPs) during the LTM test, expressed as a percentage of that obtained during the STM test. (d) Correlation between freezing scores and LA AEFP amplitudes in U0126-treated rats (each expressed as a percentage of STM). (e) Representative AEFPs in the LA for each group (vehicle, U0126) during baseline, STM, and LTM tests. Scale = 20 μs, 5 ms. (f) Mean (± SEM) changes in the amplitude of MGm/PIN AEFPs during the LTM test, expressed as a percentage of that obtained during the STM test. (g) Correlation between freezing scores and LA AEFP amplitudes in U0126-treated rats (each expressed as a percentage of STM). (h) Representative AEFPs in the MGm/PIN for each group (vehicle, U0126) during baseline, STM, and LTM tests. Scale = 20 μs, 5 ms. Adapted from Schafe GE, Doyère V, LeDoux JE (2005b) Tracking the fear engram: The lateral amygdala is an essential locus of fear memory storage. *J. Neurosci.* 25: 10010–10015, with permission from the Society for Neuroscience.

and in unique ways. While most studies that have documented training-induced alterations in synaptic plasticity have focused on cells in the LAd (Quirk et al., 1995, 1997; Rogan et al., 1997; Maren, 2000; Blair et al., 2003), a relatively recent study has documented plastic changes in two populations of cells in the LA (Repa et al., 2001; **Figure** 7). The first is the traditionally studied dorsal population in the LAd that shows enhanced firing to the CS in the initial stages of training and testing and is sensitive to fear extinction. These so-called 'transiently plastic cells' exhibit short-latency changes (within 10–15 ms after tone onset) that are consistent with the involvement of rapid, monosynaptic thalamic input (**Figure 7(b)**). The second population of cells occupies a more ventral position in the LA. In contrast to the transiently plastic cells, these more ventral cells exhibit enhanced firing to the CS throughout training and testing and do not appear to be sensitive to extinction (**Figure 7(c)**). Further, these 'long-term plastic cells' exhibit longer latencies (within 30–40 ms after tone onset), indicative of a polysynaptic pathway. Thus, it has been hypothesized that a network of neurons within the LA is responsible for triggering and storing fear memories (Repa et al., 2001; Medina et al., 2002).

Interestingly, the cells that express activated ERK/MAPK after fear conditioning occupy a more ventral position in the LA, in the same anatomical location of cells that exhibit long-term plasticity during and after fear conditioning (Schafe et al., 2000; Repa et al., 2001; **Figure 7(d)**). In fact, very little activated ERK is observed in the dorsal region of the LA, the site of the majority of CS-US convergence and of cells that exhibit rapid, and transient, plastic changes during fear conditioning (Romanski et al., 1993; Repa et al., 2001). This pattern of findings is consistent with the hypothesis that fear conditioning induces long-term plastic change and memory formation in a ventral population of cells in the LA via the ERK/MAPK signaling cascade. It remains unknown whether this involves a rapid 'transfer' of plasticity between dorsal and ventral cells in the LA during fear conditioning, or an independent, parallel process.

21.6.2 Distributed Plasticity within Amygdala Nuclei

Recently, interest has also grown in the idea that distributed plasticity *between* amygdala nuclei may be critical for fear learning. This has been sparked, in part, by a recent study showing that the central nucleus of the amygdala may also be an important locus of fear memory acquisition and consolidation (Wilensky et al., 2006). In that study, functional inactivation restricted to *either* the LA or the CE impaired acquisition of auditory fear conditioning. Further, infusion of the protein synthesis inhibitor anisomycin into the CE impaired fear memory consolidation; that is, rats had intact STM but impaired LTM (Wilensky et al., 2006). These findings suggest that the CE plays an important role not only in fear expression, as has been previously thought, but also in the acquisition and consolidation of fear learning.

How might the CE participate in fear memory acquisition and consolidation? Since the CE, and particularly the medial division of the CE (CEm), also appears to be a recipient of somatosensory (Bernard and Besson, 1990; Jasmin et al., 1997) and possibly also auditory (LeDoux et al., 1987; Turner and Herkenham, 1991; Frankland et al., 1998; Linke et al., 2000) information, one possibility is that the CE encodes in parallel the same type of association that is encoded in the LA. In support of this possibility, a recent study showed that high-frequency stimulation of the auditory thalamus induces an NMDAR-dependent LTP in CEm neurons (Samson and Paré, 2005). If the CE were encoding memory in parallel to the LA, however, this would suggest that the CE should readily be capable of mediating fear learning when the LA is compromised, a finding which is not supported by the literature. Another possibility is that plasticity in the LA and the CE proceeds in a serial manner, such that plasticity and memory formation in the CE depends on plasticity in the LA. This view has been advocated in a recent model that proposes that plasticity in the LA enables CEm neurons to encode plasticity that is essential for fear conditioning, resulting in distributed plasticity and memory formation throughout the amygdala (Paré et al., 2004). The mechanism by which this distributed plasticity between the LA and the CE occurs is at present unknown, but likely involves projections from the LA to CEm neurons via the nearby intercalated cell masses which lie between the LA and the CE (Paré and Smith, 1993; Royer et al., 1999). Additional experiments employing single-unit recording techniques in both the LA and the CEm will be required to determine how these two regions influence one another during fear conditioning.

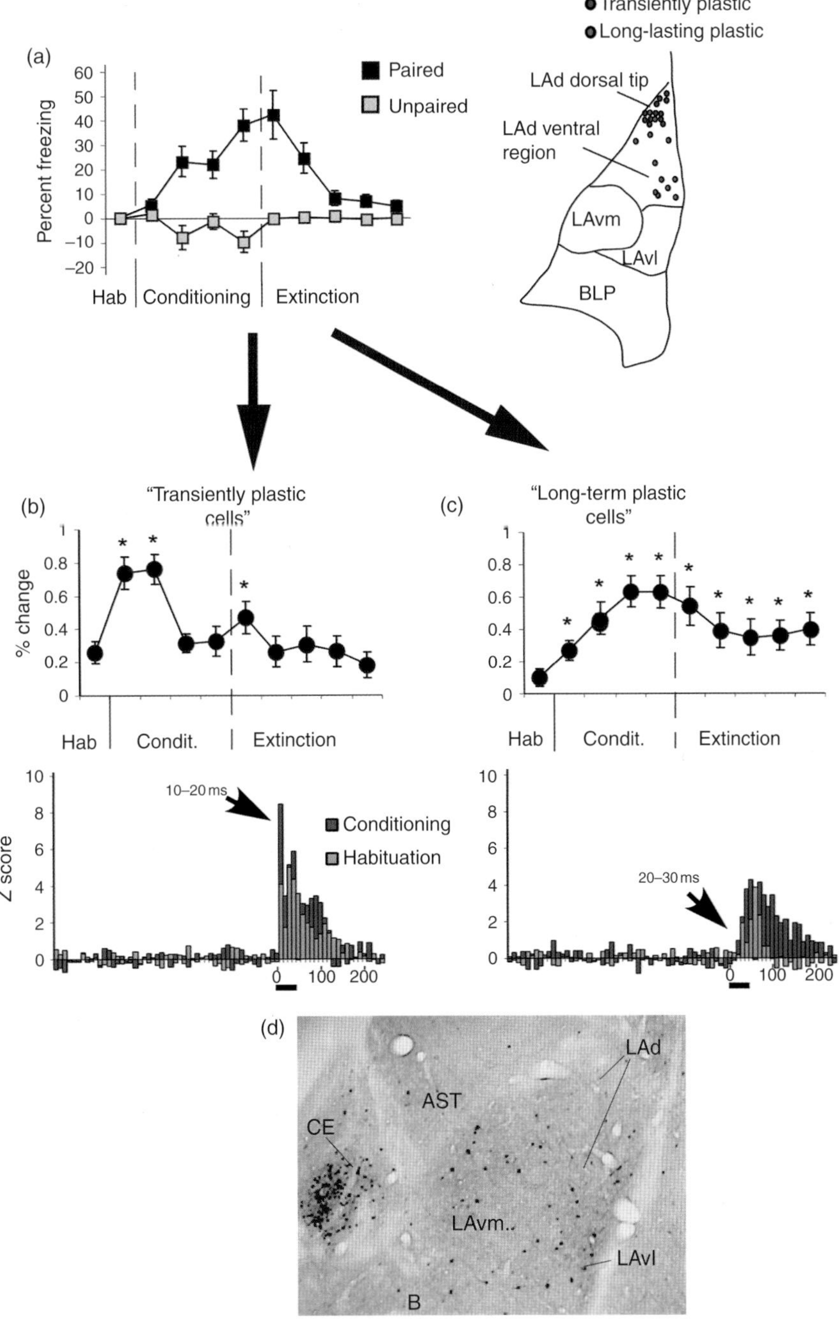

Figure 7 Distributed plasticity in the LA during fear conditioning. Pairing of CS and US during fear conditioning leads to changes in fear behavior (a) and also to changes in the responsiveness of single LA cells to auditory stimuli. During fear conditioning, there are two populations of cells that undergo plastic change. (b) 'Transiently plastic cells' are generally short latency and show enhanced firing shortly after training and during the initial phases of extinction, but not at other times. (c) 'Long-term plastic cells' are generally longer latency and show enhanced firing throughout training and extinction. INSET: 'Transiently plastic cells' are generally found in the dorsal tip of the LAd, where they may serve to trigger the initial stages of memory formation. 'Long-term plastic cells,' on the other hand, are found in the ventral regions of the LAd and may be important for long-term, extinction-resistant memory storage. (d) Location of cells expressing phospho-ERK following fear conditioning. Note the location of ERK-positive cells relative to 'long-term plastic cells.' CE, central nucleus of the amygdala; regions of the LA: LAd, dorsal; LAvm, ventromedial; LAvl, ventrolateral; AST, amygdala-striatal transition zone; B, basal nucleus of amygdala. (a–c) Adapted from Repa JC, Muller J, Apergis J, Desrochers TM, Zhou Y, and LeDoux JE (2001) Two different lateral amygdala cell populations contribute to the initiation and storage of memory. *Nat. Neurosci.* 4: 724–731, with permission from Nature Publishing Group. (d) Adapted from Schafe GE, Atkins CM, Swank MW, Bauer EP, Sweatt JD, and LeDoux JE (2000) Activation of ERK/MAP kinase in the amygdala is required for memory consolidation of Pavlovian fear conditioning. *J. Neurosci.* 20: 8177–8187, with permission from the Society for Neuroscience.

21.7 Summary: A Model of Fear Memory Acquisition and Consolidation in the Amygdala

In summary, the converging evidence from a number of recent studies supports a model of fear conditioning in which CS and US inputs converge onto individual LA neurons and initiate changes in synaptic function and/or structure (Blair et al., 2001; **Figure 8**). The convergence of CS and US inputs onto LA principal cells during training leads to Ca^{2+} influx through both NMDARs (Miserendino et al., 1990; Kim et al., 1991; Campeau et al., 1992; Walker and Davis, 2000; Rodrigues et al., 2001) and also L-VGCCs (Bauer et al., 2002). The NMDAR-mediated increase in intracellular Ca^{2+}, together with mGluR5 (Rodrigues et al., 2002), leads to the activation of a variety of local protein kinases at the postsynaptic density (PSD), including αCaMKII (Rodrigues et al., 2004a) and likely PKC, that promote STM formation by targeting and modulating the conductance and trafficking of glutamate receptors at LA synapses (Barria et al., 1997; Benke et al., 1998; Rumpel et al., 2005). The combined entry of Ca^{2+} through both NMDARs and L-VGCCs, together with signaling via the BDNF-TrkB pathway, however, may promote the activation of PKA and ERK/MAPK (Schafe et al., 2000; Schafe and LeDoux, 2000). These kinases, and particularly ERK/MAPK, appear to be exclusively involved in the formation of LTM, possibly via translocation to the cell nucleus and activation of transcription factors such as CREB (Josselyn et al., 2001). The activation of CREB by ERK/MAPK promotes CRE-mediated gene transcription (Bailey et al., 1999; Ressler et al., 2002) and the synthesis of new proteins (Schafe and LeDoux, 2000), which likely promotes LTM formation by leading to alterations in the structure of LA synapses (Lamprecht et al., 2002; Ressler et al., 2002; Radley et al., 2006). Intracellular signaling in the postsynaptic neuron, alone, however, does not appear to be sufficient for fear memory formation (McKernan and Shinnick-Gallagher, 1997b; Huang and Kandel, 1998; Tsvetkov et al., 2002). Modifications in presynaptic signaling, possibly engaged by retrograde signaling in the LA via NO and its downstream targets, also appears to be critical

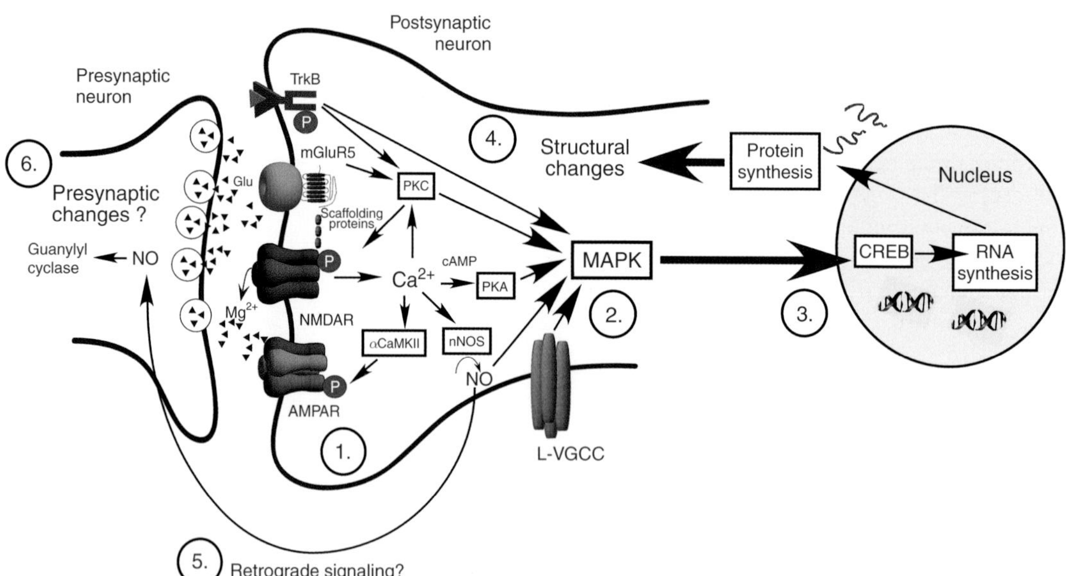

Figure 8 A model of fear memory consolidation in the amygdala. See text for details. (1) Acquisition and STM formation of fear conditioning requires events at the postsynaptic density, including activation of NMDARs, mGluR5, αCaMKII, and possibly PKC. Both αCaMKII and PKC may contribute to STM by influencing the conductance of NMDARs and AMPARs. (2) LTM formation of fear conditioning requires the activation of TrkB receptors, L-type VGCCs, and the cAMP-PKA signaling pathway. These pathways are thought to converge on ERK, which is thought to promote LTM and synaptic plasticity by translocating to the nucleus to influence gene expression. (3) CREB and CRE-mediated transcription are both required for LTM of fear conditioning. (4) The translation of CRE-mediated genes into proteins may lead to structural changes at LA spines that contribute to the permanence of LTM formation. (5) The activation of nNOS in LA neurons may promote retrograde signaling by NO and structural and/or functional changes on the presynaptic side of the synapse (6).

(Schafe et al., 2005). Finally, recent findings emphasizing a distributed network of plasticity in the amygdala have suggested that attention to synaptic plasticity at one synapse, or even one amygdala nucleus, will not be sufficient for a full understanding of how fear memories are acquired or consolidated (Repa et al., 2001; Paré et al., 2004). Accordingly, future experiments will need to consider not only how intracellular signaling mechanisms contribute to fear learning, but also how plasticity across amygdala synapses might be involved in fear memory formation.

21.8 Beyond 'Simple' Fear Conditioning

While great strides have been made in identifying the neural and molecular mechanisms that underlie auditory fear conditioning, we have also begun to learn a great deal about more complex aspects of fear learning. In this section, we will explore what is known regarding contextual fear learning, fear extinction, 'reconsolidation' of fear, instrumental fear learning, and memory modulation by the brain's fear system.

21.8.1 Contextual Fear Conditioning

In a typical auditory fear conditioning experiment, the animal not only learns to fear the tone that is paired with the foot shock, but also the context in which conditioning occurs. Contextual fear may also be induced by the presentation of foot shocks alone within a novel environment. In the laboratory, fear to the context is measured by returning the rat to the conditioning chamber on the test day and measuring freezing behavior (Blanchard et al., 1969; Fanselow, 1980).

In comparison to auditory fear conditioning, much less is known about the neural system underlying contextual fear. Much of the work examining the neuroanatomical substrates of contextual fear has relied exclusively on lesion methods, and, as in auditory fear conditioning the amygdala appears to play an essential role. For example, lesions of the amygdala, including the LA and basal nucleus, have been shown to disrupt both acquisition and expression of contextual fear conditioning (Phillips and LeDoux, 1992; Kim et al., 1993; Maren, 1998), as has reversible functional inactivation targeted to the LA (Muller et al., 1997). Contextual fear conditioning is also impaired by infusion of antagonists to NMDARs, mGluR5, and CaMKII into the LA, as well as inhibitors of PKA/PKC, RNA, and protein synthesis (Kim et al., 1991; Bailey et al., 1999; Goosens et al., 2000; Rodrigues et al., 2001, 2002, 2004a). Further, a recent study showed that memory consolidation for contextual fear is impaired by infusion of antisense oligonucleotides directed against EGR-1 (Malkani et al., 2004). Collectively, these findings suggest that essential aspects of the memory are encoded and stored in the amygdala via alterations in some of the same intracellular signaling mechanisms that underlie acquisition and consolidation of auditory fear conditioning. At this time, however, there are few data that allow us to distinguish between the involvement of different amygdala subnuclei in contextual fear, although recent lesion evidence suggests that the LA and anterior basal nuclei are critical, but not the posterior basal nucleus (Goosens and Maren, 2001). The CE is, of course, essential for the expression of contextual fear, as it is for auditory fear conditioning (Goosens and Maren, 2001). It remains unknown, however, whether the CE is also required for the acquisition and/or consolidation of contextual fear, or whether distributed plasticity in the LA underlies contextual fear learning.

The hippocampus has also been implicated in contextual fear conditioning, although its exact role has been difficult to define. A number of studies have shown that electrolytic and neurotoxic lesions of the hippocampus disrupt contextual, but not auditory, fear conditioning (Kim and Fanselow, 1992; Phillips and LeDoux, 1992; Kim et al., 1993; Maren et al., 1997). Posttraining lesions appear to be the most effective; pretraining lesions of the hippocampus have occasionally been shown to be without effect (Maren et al., 1997). This is presumably because the animal uses a nonhippocampal strategy to acquire fear to the contextual cues of the environment in the absence of an intact hippocampus during training. Posttraining hippocampal lesions, however, are only effective at impairing contextual fear if given shortly after training. If rats are given hippocampal lesions 28 days after training, there is no memory impairment (Kim and Fanselow, 1992). This 'retrograde gradient' of recall suggests that hippocampal-dependent memories are gradually transferred, over time, to other regions of the brain for permanent storage, an idea that is consistent with the findings of hippocampal-dependent episodic memory research in humans (Milner et al., 1998). The exact mechanism whereby these 'remote' contextual fear memories are consolidated remains unknown, but is thought to involve LTP-like changes in signaling between the hippocampus and regions of the cortex that make up the individual elements of the contextual representation (Frankland et al., 2001).

What role does the hippocampus play in contextual fear? One prominent view is that it is necessary for forming a representation of the context in which conditioning occurs and for providing the amygdala with that information during training and CS-US integration (Phillips and LeDoux, 1992; Young et al., 1994; Frankland et al., 1998). In support of this view, the hippocampal formation has been shown to project to the basal nucleus of the amygdala (Canteras and Swanson, 1992). This pathway has been shown to exhibit LTP (Maren and Fanselow, 1995), thus providing a potential neuroanatomical substrate through which contextual fear associations can be formed (Maren and Fanselow, 1995). Further, it has recently been shown that intrahippocampal infusions of the protein synthesis inhibitor anisomycin impair the ability of the hippocampus to form a contextual representation, but not the ability of the animal to form a context-shock association (Barrientos et al., 2002). In these experiments, the 'immediate shock deficit' paradigm was used to tease apart the contribution of the hippocampus to learning about a context and learning to fear one. Normally, immediate shock (i.e., that which is given soon after introduction to the conditioning chamber) is not sufficient to support contextual fear conditioning, presumably because it takes time for the hippocampus to form a representation of the context in which the animal finds itself. However, if the animal is *preexposed* to the conditioning chamber briefly on the day before training, it can subsequently acquire contextual fear following immediate shock, presumably because the animal now enters the training situation with a contextual representation already intact (Fanselow, 1980). In the Barrientos et al. study (2002), rats were given an infusion of anisomycin or vehicle into the dorsal hippocampus immediately after exposure to a novel context on the day before they received immediate shock, or immediately after receiving immediate shock on the day after they received preexposure. The findings showed that intrahippocampal anisomycin resulted in impaired contextual learning only in the first group (Barrientos et al., 2002). This important finding suggests that the protein synthesis in the hippocampus is necessary for learning about contexts, but not for contextual fear conditioning. A similar finding has recently been reported by Frankland and colleagues using manipulations of NMDARs, CaMKII, and CREB in the hippocampus (Frankland et al., 2004).

It is clear, however, that the hippocampus undergoes plastic changes during fear conditioning, some of which may be necessary for memory formation of contextual fear. For example, intrahippocampal infusion of the NMDAR antagonist APV impairs contextual fear conditioning (Stiedl et al., 2000; Young and Wang, 2004), and contextual, but not auditory, fear conditioning is impaired in mice that lack the NR1 subunit of the NMDA receptor exclusively in area CA1 of the hippocampus (Rampon and Tsien, 2000). Further, fear conditioning leads to increases in the activation of αCaMKII, PKC, ERK/MAPK, and CRE-mediated gene expression in the hippocampus (Atkins et al., 1998; Impey et al., 1998b; Hall et al., 2000). These findings add support to the notion that NMDAR-dependent plastic changes in the hippocampus, in addition to the amygdala, are required for contextual fear conditioning. However, it should be emphasized that the exact contribution of this NMDAR-mediated signaling to contextual fear conditioning remains unclear. For example, most of these studies cannot distinguish between a role for NMDAR-mediated plasticity in formation of contextual representations as opposed to a role in fear memory acquisition and storage. Further, regulation of intracellular signaling cascades in the hippocampus by fear conditioning, while potentially indicative of some type of memory storage, does not necessarily indicate that these changes are related to the acquisition *fear* memories. They may be related to declarative or explicit memories of the training experience that are acquired at the same time as fearful memories (LeDoux, 2000). Indeed, a number of studies have shown that hippocampal cells undergo plastic changes during and after fear conditioning (Doyère et al., 1995; Moita et al., 2003), including auditory fear conditioning which is spared following hippocampal lesions (Kim and Fanselow, 1992). Clearly, more research is needed before a convincing picture of the role of the hippocampus in contextual fear conditioning emerges.

21.8.2 Fear Extinction

Extinction is a process whereby repeated presentations of the CS in the absence of the US leads to a weakening of the expression of conditioning responding. While extinction of conditioned fear has been well documented in the behavioral literature, until recently we learned comparatively little about its neurobiological substrates. Work in a number of laboratories has recently implicated a number of structures, including the prefrontal cortex, amygdala, and hippocampus.

The medial prefrontal cortex (mPFC), and in particular the ventral mPFC, appears to play an important role in fear extinction. Early studies, for example, showed that selective lesions of the ventral mPFC retard the extinction of fear to an auditory CS while having no effect on initial fear acquisition (Morgan et al., 1993; Morgan and LeDoux, 1995). Further, neurons in the mPFC alter their response properties as the result of extinction (Garcia et al., 1999; Herry et al., 1999). Interestingly, studies by Quirk and colleagues suggest that the mPFC may not be necessary for fear extinction *per se*, but rather for the long-term recall of extinguished fear. For example, rats with mPFC lesions are able to extinguish within a session, but show impaired extinction between sessions (Quirk et al., 2000). Further, neurons in the mPFC fire strongly to a tone CS after behavioral extinction has occurred, and artificial stimulation of the mPFC that resembles responding in an extinguished rat is sufficient to inhibit behavioral expression of fear in nonextinguished rats (Milad and Quirk, 2002). Thus, it appears clear that the mPFC plays an essential role in long-term retention and/or expression of fear extinction. The question of whether the mPFC is a 'site of storage' of extinction or rather simply a region that is necessary for the long-term expression of extinguished memories has only begun to be explored. Recent studies, however, have shown that extinction training regulates the expression of the IEG cFos in regions of the mPFC (Santini et al., 2004). Further, intra-mPFC infusion of inhibitors to MEK or protein synthesis impairs long-term recall of fear extinction (Santini et al., 2004; Hugues et al., 2006), suggesting that essential aspects of the plasticity underlying extinction memory are localized in the mPFC.

The amygdala has also been shown to be an essential site of plasticity underlying fear extinction. Infusions of NMDAR antagonists or inhibitors of ERK/MAPK into the amygdala have been shown to impair fear extinction (Falls et al., 1992; Lu et al., 2001; Davis, 2002; Herry et al., 2006). Conversely, both systemic and intra-amygdala infusions of partial agonists of the NMDA receptor facilitate fear extinction (Walker et al., 2002). More recently, Ressler and colleagues showed that BDNF signaling in the amygdala was critical to the consolidation of fear extinction (Chhatwal et al., 2006). They showed, for example, that fear conditioning leads to an increase in BDNF expression in the LA and basal amygdala. Further, infusion of a viral vector encoding a dominant negative TrkB receptor into the amygdala impaired between-session, but not within-session, retention of fear extinction. These experiments suggest that some type of activity-dependent synaptic plasticity must take place in the amygdala during extinction learning, as it does during initial learning. After the memory of extinction is formed, the amygdala may then signal the mPFC to inhibit ongoing fear responses. Indeed, McDonald and colleagues have shown that the mPFC projects to GABAergic (GABA: gamma-aminobutyric acid) intercalated cells that are situated between the lateral and basal amygdala and the CE (McDonald et al., 1996), which may be important for regulating fear responses (Paré and Smith, 1993; Quirk and Gehlert, 2003; Quirk et al., 2003; Paré et al., 2004). In agreement with this hypothesis, a recent study has confirmed that stimulation of the mPFC neurons blunts the activity of CE neurons that are critical for the expression of fear responses (Quirk et al., 2003). Additional experiments will be necessary to define the exact contribution of connections between the mPFC and the amygdala in extinction processes, as well as the detailed biochemical mechanisms responsible for promoting fear extinction.

One of the more interesting facts about memories that have undergone extinction is that they are context specific. That is, an extinguished memory remains extinguished only in the context in which extinction has taken place, and responding returns or is subject to 'renewal' in a different context (Bouton and Bolles, 1979; Bouton and Ricker, 1994). This fact, along with the finding that fully extinguished memories are capable of 'reinstating' upon presentation of the US (Rescorla and Heth, 1975), has led to the long-held view that extinction does not result in the erasure of the original memory trace but is rather a new kind of learning that serves to inhibit expression of the old memory (Pavlov, 1927). Not surprisingly, recent studies have indicated that the hippocampus plays an important role in the contextual modulation of fear extinction. Maren and colleagues, for example, have shown that training-induced neurophysiological responses in the LA readily extinguish within a fear extinction session, but that this neural representation of extinction, like the behavior itself, is specific to the context in which extinction has taken place (Hobin et al., 2003). Further, functional inactivation of the hippocampus using the $GABA_A$ agonist muscimol can impair the context-specific expression of fear extinction (Corcoran and Maren, 2001). While it remains unclear how the hippocampus might inhibit the expression of LA spike firing and fear behavior in a context-specific manner, it has been proposed that projections from the hippocampus to the mPFC may be critical (Hobin et al., 2003).

21.8.3 Retrieval and 'Reconsolidation' of Fear Memories

Fear extinction is not the only way to turn a fear memory off. Another, perhaps more clinically efficacious way, is to interfere with that fear memory's *reconsolidation*. The idea that memory undergoes a second phase of consolidation, or 'reconsolidation,' upon retrieval has been the subject of speculation for decades (Sara, 2000). Early studies showed that amnesic manipulations at or around the time of memory retrieval, rather than at the time of initial learning, resulted in loss of the memory on subsequent recall tests (Misanin et al., 1968; Lewis et al., 1972). These early findings suggested that the retrieval process could render a memory susceptible to disruption in a manner very similar to a newly formed memory.

Interest in the reconsolidation process has been rekindled in recent years, due in part to the progress that has been made in identifying the cellular and molecular mechanisms underlying long-term synaptic plasticity and the initial phases of memory consolidation (Milner et al., 1998). Accordingly, this has provided researchers with a set of tools and learning paradigms with which to study the reconsolidation process. Several years ago, for example, Nader and colleagues showed that infusion of the protein synthesis inhibitor anisomycin into the amygdala immediately after retrieval of auditory fear conditioning impaired memory recall on subsequent tests (Nader et al., 2000). This effect was clearly dependent on retrieval of the memory; that is, no memory deficit was observed if exposure to the CS was omitted. Further, the effect was observed not only when the initial recall test and drug infusion were given shortly after training (i.e., 1 day), but also if given 14 days later, suggesting that the effect could not be attributable to disruption of the late phases of protein synthesis necessary for the initial training episode. Thus, following active recall of a fear memory, that memory appears to undergo a second wave of consolidation that requires protein synthesis in the amygdala. More recent work has shown that this process does not appear to be attributable to rapid extinction of fear during the recall test, since fear memories that have failed to reconsolidate after intra-amygdala infusion of anisomycin fail to renew in a different context (Duvarci and Nader, 2004). Further, memories that fail to reconsolidate do not appear to be subject to reinstatement (Duvarci and Nader, 2004), a finding which suggests that manipulations of a fear memory at or around the time of retrieval may result in permanent impairment of the memory.

Reconsolidation does not appear to be unique to the amygdala; hippocampal-dependent contextual memories also appear to be sensitive to manipulation at the time of retrieval. In a recent study, Debiec et al. (2002) gave rats intrahippocampal infusions of anisomycin following recall of contextual fear conditioning and found that memory retrieval was impaired on subsequent tests. Interestingly, reconsolidation of contextual fear was impaired even when memory reactivation and intrahippocampal anisomycin treatment were given 45 days after the initial training session, a time when lesion studies have shown that contextual memories should no longer depend on the hippocampus (Kim and Fanselow, 1992). The initial experiments by Kim and Fanselow, however, used only a single recall test after training and hippocampal lesions; the ability of the animal to recall contextual fear on subsequent tests was not examined. Surprisingly, when Debiec et al. *reactivated* the contextual memory prior to making a lesion of the hippocampus, even as long as 45 days after training, subsequent recall was impaired (Debiec et al., 2002). Thus, hippocampal-dependent contextual memories appear to undergo both a cellular and a systems-level reconsolidation following memory retrieval. That is, recall of an older, hippocampal-independent contextual memory must return to the hippocampus during retrieval and undergo a protein synthesis–dependent process of reconsolidation to be maintained. As in most hippocampal studies, however, it remains unclear what information is being reconsolidated – the memory of the context or the contextual fear memory.

How might the reconsolidation process be accomplished at the cellular and molecular levels? Recent studies have shown that fear reconsolidation, like the initial phases of consolidation, requires both PKA and ERK/MAPK in the amygdala (Duvarci et al., 2005; Tronson et al., 2006). Further, transient overexpression of a dominant negative isoform of CREB in the forebrain at the time of memory retrieval impairs reconsolidation of auditory and contextual fear conditioning (Kida et al., 2002). However, the reconsolidation process does not appear to be a mere recapitulation of the initial consolidation process; there have also been numerous reports of biochemical dissociations between consolidation and reconsolidation. These have included studies that have failed to find impairments in fear reconsolidation following inhibition of RNA synthesis (Parsons et al., 2006) or NO signaling (Schafe et al., 2005) in the amygdala. Further, reactivation of a contextual fear memory induces only a subset of genes in the hippocampus that are activated during the initial phases of memory consolidation (von Hertzen and Giese, 2005), and hippocampal-dependent reconsolidation of a contextual fear memory appears to be characterized by different classes of immediate early genes (Lee et al., 2004). Finally, a recent study has shown that blockade of β-adrenergic receptors in the LA impairs reconsolidation, but not consolidation, of fear conditioning (Debiec and Ledoux, 2004). Clearly, additional studies will be required for a full appreciation of how reconsolidation is accomplished at the cellular level.

21.8.4 Instrumental Fear Learning

In addition to its role in the rapid, reflexive learning that characterizes Pavlovian fear conditioning, the amygdala contributes to other fear-related aspects of behavior. Pavlovian fear conditioning, for example, is useful for learning to detect a dangerous object or situation, but the animal must also be able to use this information to guide ongoing behavior that is instrumental in avoiding that danger. In some experimental situations, the animal must learn to make a response (i.e., move away, press a bar, turn a wheel, etc.) that will allow it to avoid presentation of a shock or danger signal, a form of learning known as *active avoidance.* In other situations, the animal must learn *not* to respond, also known as *passive avoidance.* Both of these are examples of instrumental conditioning, and the amygdala plays a vital role in each.

Previously, we mentioned that only the LA and CE were critical for Pavlovian fear conditioning. However, we have recently begun to appreciate the significance of projections from the LA to the basal nucleus of the amygdala from studies that employ fear learning tasks that involve both classical and instrumental components (Killcross et al., 1997; Amorapanth et al., 2000). Amorapanth et al. (2000), for example, first trained rats to associate a tone with foot shock (the Pavlovian component). Next, rats learned to move from one side of a two-compartment box to the other to avoid presentation of the tone (the instrumental component), a so-called 'escape-from-fear' task. Findings showed that, while lesions of the LA impaired both types of learning, lesions of the CE impair only the Pavlovian component (i.e., the tone-shock association; **Figure 9(a)**). Conversely, lesions of the basal nucleus impaired only the instrumental component (learning to move to the second compartment; **Figure 9(b)**). Thus, different outputs of the LA appear to mediate Pavlovian and instrumental behaviors elicited by a fear-arousing stimulus (Amorapanth et al., 2000; **Figure 9(c)**). It is important to note, however, that these findings do not indicate that the basal nucleus is a site of motor control or a locus of memory storage for instrumental learning. Rather, the basal amygdala likely guides fear-related behavior and reinforcement learning via its projections to nearby striatal regions that are known to be necessary for instrumental learning and reward processes (Everitt et al., 1989, 1999; Robbins et al., 1989).

21.8.5 Memory Modulation by the Amygdala

Pavlovian fear conditioning is an implicit form of learning and memory. However, during most emotional experiences, including fear conditioning, explicit or declarative memories are also formed (LeDoux, 2000). These occur through the operation of the medial temporal lobe memory system involving the hippocampus and related cortical areas (Milner et al., 1998; Eichenbaum, 2000). The role of the hippocampus in the explicit memory of an emotional experience is much the same as its role in other kinds of experiences, with one important exception. During fearful or emotionally arousing experiences, the amygdala activates neuromodulatory systems in the brain and hormonal systems in the body via its projections to the hypothalamus, which can drive the hypothalamic-pituitary-adrenal (HPA) axis. Neurohormones released by these systems can, in turn, feed back to modulate the function of forebrain structures such as the hippocampus and serve to enhance the storage of the memory in these regions (McGaugh, 2000). The primary support for this model in animals comes from studies of *inhibitory avoidance learning,* a type of passive avoidance learning where the animal must learn not to enter a chamber in which it has previously received shock. In this paradigm, various pharmacological manipulations of the amygdala that affect neurotransmitter or

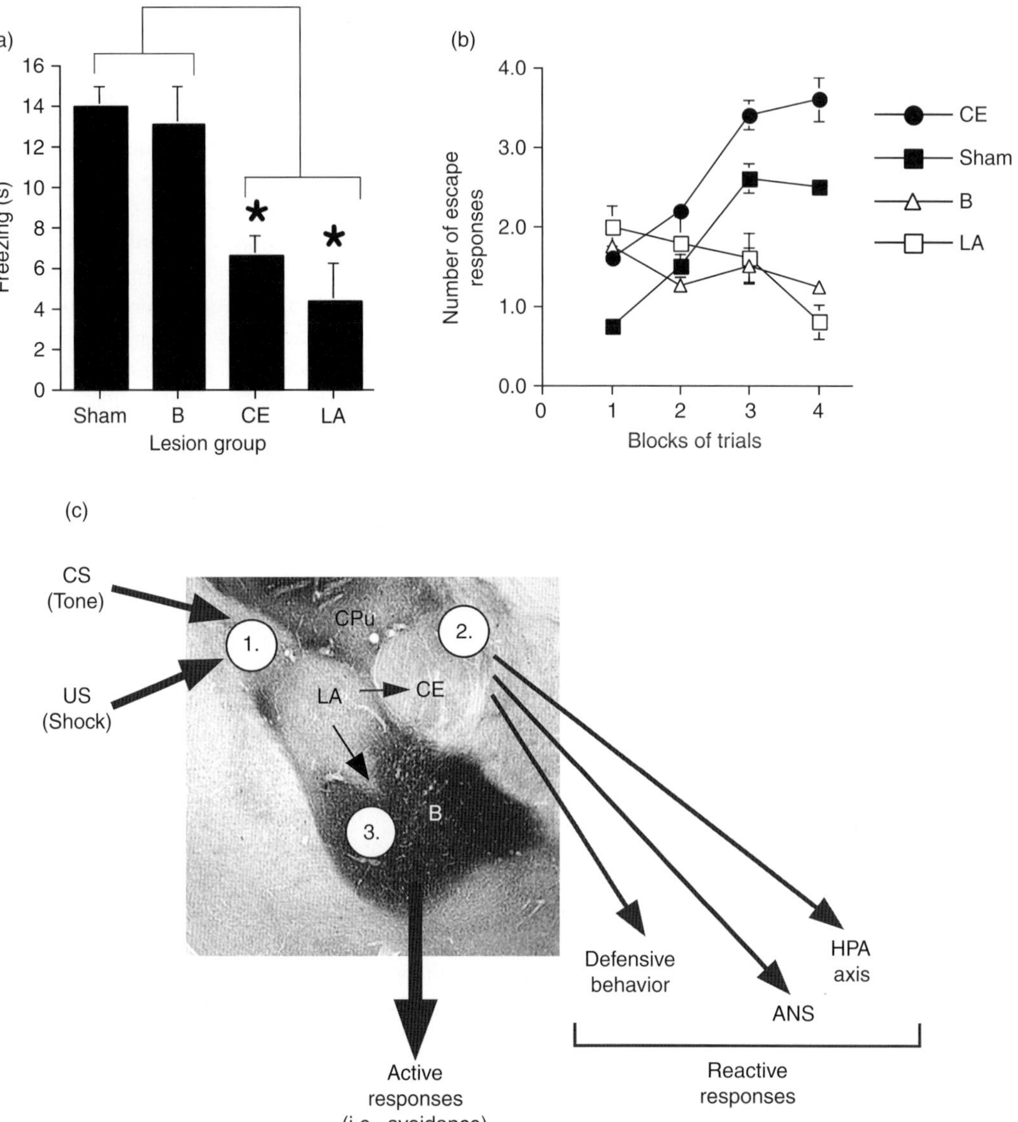

Figure 9 Active versus reactive fear. (a) Percent freezing in rats given auditory fear conditioning after receiving selective amygdala lesions. Auditory fear conditioning is impaired by lesions of the CE and LA, but spared by basal nucleus of the amygdala (B) lesions. (b) Number of escape responses across blocks of five trials during training in a one-way active avoidance task. Lesions of both LA and B impair this task, while lesions of CE do not. (c) The data are consistent with a model in which projections between LA and CE are sufficient for Pavlovian fear conditioning (reactive responses), while projections between LA and B are necessary for instrumental avoidance learning (active responses). HPA, hypothalamic-pituitary-adrenal; ANS, autonomic nervous system. Adapted from Amorapanth P, LeDoux JE, Nader K (2000) Different lateral amygdala outputs mediate reactions and actions elicited by a fear-arousing stimulus. *Nat Neurosci* 3: 74–79, with permission from Nature Publishing Group.

neurohormonal systems modulate the strength of the memory. For example, immediate posttraining blockade of adrenergic or glucocorticoid receptors in the amygdala impairs memory retention of inhibitory avoidance, while facilitation of these systems in the amygdala enhances acquisition and memory storage (McGaugh et al., 1993; McGaugh, 2000). The exact subnuclei in the amygdala that are critical for memory modulation remain unknown, as are the areas of the brain where these amygdala projections influence memory storage. Candidate areas include the hippocampus and entorhinal and parietal cortices (Izquierdo et al., 1997). Indeed, it would be interesting to know whether the changes in unit activity or the activation of intracellular signaling cascades in the hippocampus during and after fear conditioning, as discussed earlier, might be related to formation of such explicit memories, and how regulation of these signals depends on the integrity of the amygdala and its neuromodulators. Interestingly, a recent study has shown that stimulation of the basal nucleus of the amygdala can modulate the persistence of LTP in the hippocampus (Frey et al., 2001), which provides a potential mechanism whereby the amygdala can modulate hippocampal-dependent memories.

21.9 Fear Learning in Humans

Within the last 10 years, considerable progress has been made in understanding how the human fear learning system is organized and what features it shares with the fear learning system of lower vertebrates. In this final section, we will briefly summarize these findings. For a more comprehensive look at this topic, see Phelps and LeDoux (2005).

21.9.1 The Human Fear Learning System – Lesion and fMRI Studies

It has long been known that amygdala damage in humans confers deficits in fear conditioning (Bechara et al., 1995; LaBar et al., 1995). In these studies, fear conditioning is typically accomplished by pairing the presentation of visual stimuli with either mild electric shock to the skin or an aversive high-amplitude (i.e., 100 dB or more) tone. Conditioned fear is then measured by changes in skin conductance upon presentation of the CS. Damage to the amygdala in humans produces deficits in conditioned emotional responding to a CS even though the knowledge of the CS-US contingency remains intact (Bechara et al., 1995). That is, a patient with amygdala damage will not respond fearfully to the CS after it has been paired with an aversive US, but is capable of stating that the CS was previously presented and followed by the US. Interestingly, patients with selective hippocampal damage exhibit the converse effect; they will respond fearfully to the CS but cannot tell you why (Bechara et al., 1995).

Fear conditioning in humans also leads to increases in amygdala activity, as measured by functional magnetic resonance imaging (fMRI) (Buchel et al., 1998; LaBar et al., 1998). These changes largely mirror what has been seen in neurophysiological studies of amygdala activity in rodents, namely, increases in CS-elicited amygdala activity during and after fear conditioning, a corresponding attenuation of CS-elicited amygdala activity, and an increase in CS-elicited activity in the mPFC with extinction of the behavioral response (LaBar et al., 1998; Phelps et al., 2004). Further, as suggested by the animal work, the human fear learning system appears preferentially suited to use subcortical 'low-road' information during fear learning. In a study by Morris and colleagues, CS-elicited increases in amygdala activity were observed even if the CS was presented too fast to be perceived consciously, a so-called 'unseen CS' (Morris et al., 1999). When the activity of the amygdala during fear conditioning is cross-correlated with the activity in other regions of the brain, the strongest correlations are seen with subcortical (thalamic and collicular) rather than cortical areas, further emphasizing the importance of the direct thalamo-amygdala pathway in the human brain (Morris et al., 1999).

21.9.2 Instructed Fear – Using the High Road

In humans, direct experience with an aversive US does not appear necessary for fear learning to occur. In a series of experiments, Phelps and colleagues have demonstrated that simply telling a human subject that presentation of a CS *might* lead to an aversive outcome is sufficient to induce a learned fear state, a phenomenon known as 'instructed fear' (Phelps et al., 2001).

Like fears that are learned from direct experience, instructed fears require the amygdala (Funayama et al., 2001). Interestingly, however, it is the left amygdala that appears to be the most critical in this type of fear learning. In fMRI studies, the left amygdala is preferentially active in a paradigm utilizing instructed fear (Phelps et al., 2001), and amygdala lesions confined to the left hemisphere are most effective at impairing this type of fear learning (Phelps et al., 2001). In general, this stands in contrast to studies that have examined amygdala activation to fears that have been acquired through experience, especially those involving an 'unseen' CS. In those studies, amygdala activity is typically observed to be lateralized to the right amygdala (Morris et al., 1999). It has been hypothesized that this left lateralization in the instructed fear paradigm is the result of a linguistic/cognitive fear representation acquired through language, which, like other verbally mediated tasks, is mediated in the majority of individuals in the left hemisphere (Funayama et al., 2001).

21.9.3 Declarative Memory Formation and the Amygdala

It has long been recognized that memories formed during emotionally arousing situations are more vividly remembered than those formed under neutral circumstances. Earlier in this chapter, we reviewed evidence from the animal literature which provides a potential neural mechanism for this phenomenon, namely, that the amygdala and its various neurotransmitter systems modulate the strength of explicit or declarative memory formation by influencing the longevity of cellular processes such as LTP in the hippocampus (Frey et al., 2001). Does the human amygdala play a similar role in declarative memory formation? Evidence suggests that it does. For example, administration of the β-adrenergic antagonist propranolol to human subjects impairs long-term recall of an emotionally arousing short story (Cahill et al., 1994), while administration of the $\alpha 2$-adrenergic antagonist yohimbine, which is known to be anxiogenic, enhances recall (O'Carroll et al., 1999). A similar picture emerges in patients with bilateral amygdala damage; they cannot recall the details of an emotionally charged story to the extent that intact controls can (Cahill et al., 1995). Further, amygdala activity appears to correlate with the extent to which an emotionally arousing story is remembered. In one study, subjects in a positron emission tomography scanner were shown either emotionally arousing or emotionally neutral stories and tested for recall at a later time. The findings revealed that right amygdala blood flow during the emotionally arousing, but not neutral, stories correlated highly with the extent to which details of that story could be recalled at later test (Cahill et al., 1996). More recently, Dolan and colleagues studied amygdala-hippocampal activations and recall of emotionally arousing and neutral words in patients with varying degrees of hippocampal and amygdala damage. The findings revealed that left amygdala damage was inversely correlated with memory for the emotional words and also activity in the left hippocampus. Memory for neutral words, in contrast, was only related to the degree of hippocampal damage (Richardson et al., 2004). These findings parallel those found in the animal literature and suggest that interactions between the amygdala and hippocampal formation influence the strength of declarative memory in the human brain.

21.10 Conclusions

In this chapter, we have provided a comprehensive view of the neural system underlying fear learning, including the key synaptic events and downstream cellular cascades that are responsible for the acquisition and consolidation of fear memories in the amygdala. These findings provide a foundation for the continued study of the neural basis of emotional learning and memory at the cellular level, and also for bridging the gap between studies of memory formation and synaptic plasticity in the mammalian brain. These studies also provide us with a set of tools to continue our analysis of more complex and clinically relevant aspects of fear learning, including contextual control of learned fear, fear extinction, and reconsolidation. Finally, recent studies translating and extending what we have learned from laboratory rats to the human brain suggest that similar mechanisms and neural pathways are conserved across species.

Acknowledgments

This work was supported in part by National Institutes of Health grants MH 46516, MH 00956, MH 39774, and MH 11902 to J. E. L. and NSF grant 0444632 to G. E. S.

References

Abel T, Martin KC, Bartsch D, and Kandel ER (1998) Memory suppressor genes: Inhibitory constraints on the storage of long-term memory. *Science* 279: 338–341.
Abel T, Nguyen PV, Barad M, Deuel TA, Kandel ER, and Bourtchouladze R (1997) Genetic demonstration of a role for PKA in the late phase of LTP and in hippocampus-based long-term memory. *Cell* 88: 615–626.
Abraham WC, Mason SE, Demmer J, et al. (1993) Correlations between immediate early gene induction and the persistence of long-term potentiation. *Neuroscience* 56: 717–727.
Adams JP and Sweatt JD (2002) Molecular psychology: Roles for the ERK MAP kinase cascade in memory. *Annu. Rev. Pharmacol. Toxicol.* 42: 135–163.
Ali DW and Salter MW (2001) NMDA receptor regulation by Src kinase signalling in excitatory synaptic transmission and plasticity. *Curr. Opin. Neurobiol.* 11: 336–342.
Amorapanth P, LeDoux JE, and Nader K (2000) Different lateral amygdala outputs mediate reactions and actions elicited by a fear-arousing stimulus. *Nat. Neurosci.* 3: 74–79.

Anwyl R (1999) Metabotropic glutamate receptors: Electrophysiological properties and role in plasticity. *Brain Res. Brain Res. Rev.* 29: 83–120.

Arancio O, Antonova I, Gambaryan S, et al. (2001) Presynaptic role of cGMP-dependent protein kinase during long-lasting potentiation. *J. Neurosci.* 21: 143–149.

Arancio O, Kiebler M, Lee CJ, et al. (1996) Nitric oxide acts directly in the presynaptic neuron to produce long-term potentiation in cultured hippocampal neurons. *Cell* 87: 1025–1035.

Atkins CM, Selcher JC, Petraitis JJ, Trzaskos JM, and Sweatt JD (1998) The MAPK cascade is required for mammalian associative learning. *Nat. Neurosci.* 1: 602–609.

Bailey CH, Alberini C, Ghirardi M, and Kandel ER (1994) Molecular and structural changes underlying long-term memory storage in *Aplysia*. *Adv. Second Messenger Phosphoprotein Res.* 29: 529–544.

Bailey CH and Kandel ER (1993) Structural changes accompanying memory storage. *Annu. Rev. Physiol.* 55: 397–426.

Bailey CH, Montarolo P, Chen M, Kandel ER, and Schacher S (1992) Inhibitors of protein and RNA synthesis block structural changes that accompany long-term heterosynaptic plasticity in *Aplysia*. *Neuron* 9: 749–758.

Bailey DJ, Kim JJ, Sun W, Thompson RF, and Helmstetter FJ (1999) Acquisition of fear conditioning in rats requires the synthesis of mRNA in the amygdala. *Behav. Neurosci.* 113: 276–282.

Bakin JS and Weinberger NM (1990) Classical conditioning induces CS-specific receptive field plasticity in the auditory cortex of the guinea pig. *Brain Res.* 536: 271–286.

Barria A, Muller D, Derkach V, Griffith LC, and Soderling TR (1997) Regulatory phosphorylation of AMPA-type glutamate receptors by CaM-KII during long-term potentiation. *Science* 276: 2042–2045.

Barrientos RM, O'Reilly RC, and Rudy JW (2002) Memory for context is impaired by injecting anisomycin into dorsal hippocampus following context exploration. *Behav. Brain Res.* 134: 299–306.

Bartsch D, Ghirardi M, Skehel PA, et al. (1995) *Aplysia* CREB2 represses long-term facilitation: Relief of repression converts transient facilitation into long-term functional and structural change. *Cell* 83: 979–992.

Bauer EP, Schafe GE, and LeDoux JE (2002) NMDA receptors and L-type voltage-gated calcium channels contribute to long-term potentiation and different components of fear memory formation in the lateral amygdala. *J. Neurosci.* 22: 5239–5249.

Bechara A, Tranel D, Damasio H, Adolphs R, Rockland C, and Damasio AR (1995) Double dissociation of conditioning and declarative knowledge relative to the amygdala and hippocampus in humans. *Science* 269: 1115–1118.

Beck CH and Fibiger HC (1995) Conditioned fear-induced changes in behavior and in the expression of the immediate early gene c-fos: With and without diazepam pretreatment. *J. Neurosci.* 15: 709–720.

Ben-Ari Y, Aniksztejn L, and Bregestovski P (1992) Protein kinase C modulation of NMDA currents: An important link for LTP induction. *Trends Neurosci.* 15: 333–339.

Benke TA, Luthi A, Isaac JT, and Collingridge GL (1998) Modulation of AMPA receptor unitary conductance by synaptic activity. *Nature* 393: 793–797.

Bernabeu R, de Stein ML, Fin C, Izquierdo I, and Medina JH (1995) Role of hippocampal NO in the acquisition and consolidation of inhibitory avoidance learning. *Neuroreport* 6: 1498–1500.

Bernard JF and Besson JM (1990) The spino(trigemino)-pontoamygdaloid pathway: Electrophysiological evidence for an involvement in pain processes. *J. Neurophysiol.* 63: 473–490.

Blair HT, Tinkelman A, Moita MA, and LeDoux JE (2003) Associative plasticity in neurons of the lateral amygdala during auditory fear conditioning. *Ann. N.Y. Acad. Sci.* 985: 485–487.

Blair HT, Schafe GE, Bauer EP, Rodrigues SM, and LeDoux JE (2001) Synaptic plasticity in the lateral amygdala: A cellular hypothesis of fear conditioning. *Learn. Mem.* 8(5): 229–242.

Blanchard RJ and Blanchard DC (1969) Crouching as an index of fear. *J. Comp. Physiol. Psychol.* 67: 370–375.

Bliss TV and Collingridge GL (1993) A synaptic model of memory: Long-term potentiation in the hippocampus. *Nature* 361: 31–39.

Bliss TV and Lømo T (1973) Long-lasting potentiation of synaptic transmission in the dentate area of the anaesthetized rabbit following stimulation of the perforant path. *J. Physiol. (Lond.)* 232: 331–356.

Bohme GA, Bon C, Lemaire M, et al. (1993) Altered synaptic plasticity and memory formation in nitric oxide synthase inhibitor-treated rats. *Proc. Natl. Acad. Sci. USA* 90: 9191–9194.

Bordi F and LeDoux J (1992) Sensory tuning beyond the sensory system: An initial analysis of auditory response properties of neurons in the lateral amygdaloid nucleus and overlying areas of the striatum. *J. Neurosci.* 12: 2493–2503.

Bourtchuladze R, Frenguelli B, Blendy J, Cioffi D, Schutz G, and Silva AJ (1994) Deficient long-term memory in mice with a targeted mutation of the cAMP-responsive element-binding protein. *Cell* 79: 59–68.

Bouton ME and Bolles RC (1979) Contextual control of the extinction of conditioned fear. *Learn. Motiv.* 10: 445–466.

Bouton ME and Ricker ST (1994) Renewal of extinguished responding in a second context. *Anim. Learn. Behav.* 22: 317–324.

Brambilla R, Gnesutta N, Minichiello L, et al. (1997) A role for the Ras signalling pathway in synaptic transmission and long-term memory. *Nature* 390: 281–286.

Bredt DS and Snyder SH (1992) Nitric oxide, a novel neuronal messenger. *Neuron* 8: 3–11.

Buchel C, Morris J, Dolan RJ, and Friston KJ (1998) Brain systems mediating aversive conditioning: An event-related fMRI study. *Neuron* 20: 947–957.

Cahill L, Babinsky R, Markowitsch HJ, and McGaugh JL (1995) The amygdala and emotional memory. *Nature* 377: 295–296.

Cahill L, Haier RJ, Fallon J, et al. (1996) Amygdala activity at encoding correlated with long-term, free recall of emotional information. *Proc. Natl. Acad. Sci. USA* 93: 8016–8021.

Cahill L, McGaugh JL, and Weinberger NM (2001) The neurobiology of learning and memory: Some reminders to remember. *Trends Neurosci.* 24: 578–581.

Cahill L, Prins B, Weber M, and McGaugh JL (1994) Beta-adrenergic activation and memory for emotional events. *Nature* 371: 702–704.

Cahill L, Weinberger NM, Roozendaal B, and McGaugh JL (1999) Is the amygdala a locus of "conditioned fear"? Some questions and caveats. *Neuron* 23: 227–228.

Campeau S and Davis M (1995) Involvement of the central nucleus and basolateral complex of the amygdala in fear conditioning measured with fear-potentiated startle in rats trained concurrently with auditory and visual conditioned stimuli. *J. Neurosci.* 15: 2301–2311.

Campeau S, Miserendino MJ, and Davis M (1992) Intra-amygdala infusion of the N-methyl-D-aspartate receptor antagonist AP5 blocks acquisition but not expression of fear-potentiated startle to an auditory conditioned stimulus. *Behav. Neurosci.* 106: 569–574.

Canteras NS and Swanson LW (1992) Projections of the ventral subiculum to the amygdala, septum, and hypothalamus: A PHAL anterograde tract-tracing study in the rat. *J. Comp. Neurol.* 324: 180–194.

Cavus I and Teyler T (1996) Two forms of long-term potentiation in area CA1 activate different signal transduction cascades. *J. Neurophysiol.* 76: 3038–3047.

Chapman PF, Atkins CM, Allen MT, Haley JE, and Steinmetz JE (1992) Inhibition of nitric oxide synthesis impairs two different forms of learning. *Neuroreport* 3: 567–570.

Chapman PF, Kairiss EW, Keenan CL, and Brown TH (1990) Long-term synaptic potentiation in the amygdala. *Synapse* 6: 271–278.

Chhatwal JP, Stanek-Rattiner L, Davis M, and Ressler KJ (2006) Amygdala BDNF signaling is required for consolidation but not encoding of extinction. *Nat. Neurosci.* 9: 870–872.

Clugnet MC and LeDoux JE (1990) Synaptic plasticity in fear conditioning circuits: Induction of LTP in the lateral nucleus of the amygdala by stimulation of the medial geniculate body. *J. Neurosci.* 10: 2818–2824.

Corcoran KA and Maren S (2001) Hippocampal inactivation disrupts contextual retrieval of fear memory after extinction. *J. Neurosci.* 21: 1720–1726.

Davis HP and Squire LR (1984) Protein synthesis and memory: A review. *Psychol. Bull.* 96: 518–559.

Davis M (1992) The role of the amygdala in fear-potentiated startle: Implications for animal models of anxiety. *Trends Pharmacol. Sci.* 13: 35–41.

Davis M (1997) Neurobiology of fear responses: The role of the amygdala. *J. Neuropsychiatry Clin. Neurosci.* 9: 382–402.

Davis M (2002) Role of NMDA receptors and MAP kinase in the amygdala in extinction of fear: Clinical implications for exposure therapy. *Eur. J. Neurosci.* 16: 395–398.

De Oca BM, DeCola JP, Maren S, and Fanselow MS (1998) Distinct regions of the periaqueductal gray are involved in the acquisition and expression of defensive responses. *J. Neurosci.* 18: 3426–3432.

Debiec J and LeDoux JE (2004) Disruption of reconsolidation but not consolidation of auditory fear conditioning by noradrenergic blockade in the amygdala. *Neuroscience* 129: 267–272.

Debiec J, LeDoux JE, and Nader K (2002) Cellular and systems reconsolidation in the hippocampus. *Neuron* 36: 527–538.

Denninger JW and Marletta MA (1999) Guanylate cyclase and the NO/cGMP signaling pathway. *Biochim. Biophys. Acta* 1411: 334–350.

Derkach V, Barria A, and Soderling TR (1999) Ca2+/calmodulin-kinase II enhances channel conductance of alpha-amino-3-hydroxy-5-methyl-4-isoxazolepropionate type glutamate receptors. *Proc. Natl. Acad. Sci. USA* 96: 3269–3274.

Doherty AJ, Palmer MJ, Henley JM, Collingridge GL, and Jane DE (1997) (RS)-2-chloro-5-hydroxyphenylglycine (CHPG) activates mGlu5, but no mGlu1, receptors expressed in CHO cells and potentiates NMDA responses in the hippocampus. *Neuropharmacology* 36: 265–267.

Dolmetsch RE, Pajvani U, Fife K, Spotts JM, and Greenberg ME (2001) Signaling to the nucleus by an L-type calcium channel-calmodulin complex through the MAP kinase pathway. *Science* 294: 333–339.

Doron NN and LeDoux JE (1999) Organization of projections to the lateral amygdala from auditory and visual areas of the thalamus in the rat [published erratum appears in *J. Comp. Neurol*. 2000 Feb 14; 417(3): 385–386]. *J. Comp. Neurol.* 412: 383–409.

Doyère V, Redini-Del Negro C, Dutrieux G, Le Floch G, Davis S, and Laroche S (1995) Potentiation or depression of synaptic efficacy in the dentate gyrus is determined by the relationship between the conditioned and unconditioned stimulus in a classical conditioning paradigm in rats. *Behav. Brain Res.* 70: 15–29.

Doyle C, Holscher C, Rowan MJ, and Anwyl R (1996) The selective neuronal NO synthase inhibitor 7-nitro-indazole blocks both long-term potentiation and depotentiation of field EPSPs in rat hippocampal CA1 *in vivo*. *J. Neurosci.* 16: 418–424.

Duvarci S and Nader K (2004) Characterization of fear memory reconsolidation. *J. Neurosci.* 24: 9269–9275.

Duvarci S, Nader K, and LeDoux JE (2005) Activation of extracellular signal-regulated kinase-mitogen-activated protein kinase cascade in the amygdala is required for memory reconsolidation of auditory fear conditioning. *Eur. J. Neurosci.* 21: 283–289.

Edeline JM and Weinberger NM (1993) Receptive field plasticity in the auditory cortex during frequency discrimination training: Selective retuning independent of task difficulty. *Behav. Neurosci.* 107: 82–103.

Eichenbaum H (2000) A cortical-hippocampal system for declarative memory. *Nat. Rev. Neurosci.* 1: 41–50.

Engert F and Bonhoeffer T (1999) Dendritic spine changes associated with hippocampal long-term synaptic plasticity. *Nature* 399: 66–70.

Everitt BJ, Cador M and Robbins TW (1989) Interactions between the amygdala and ventral striatum in stimulus-reward associations: Studies using a second-order schedule of sexual reinforcement. *Neuroscience* 30: 63–75.

Everitt BJ, Parkinson JA, Olmstead MC, Arroyo M, Robledo P, and Robbins TW (1999) Associative processes in addiction and reward. The role of amygdala-ventral striatal subsystems. *Ann. N.Y. Acad. Sci.* 877: 412–438.

Falls WA, Miserendino MJ, and Davis M (1992) Extinction of fear-potentiated startle: Blockade by infusion of an NMDA antagonist into the amygdala. *J. Neurosci.* 12: 854–863.

Fanselow MS (1980) Conditioned and unconditional components of post-shock freezing. *Pavlov. J. Biol. Sci.* 15: 177–182.

Fanselow MS and LeDoux JE (1999) Why we think plasticity underlying Pavlovian fear conditioning occurs in the basolateral amygdala. *Neuron* 23: 229–232.

Fendt M and Schmid S (2002) Metabotropic glutamate receptors are involved in amygdaloid plasticity. *Eur. J. Neurosci.* 15: 1535–1541.

Fifkova E and Anderson CL (1981) Stimulation-induced changes in dimensions of stalks of dendritic spines in the dentate molecular layer. *Exp. Neurol.* 74: 621–627.

Fifkova E and Van Harreveld A (1977) Long-lasting morphological changes in dendritic spines of dentate granular cells following stimulation of the entorhinal area. *J. Neurocytol.* 6: 211–230.

Figurov A, Pozzo-Miller LD, Olafsson P, Wang T, and Lu B (1996) Regulation of synaptic responses to high-frequency stimulation and LTP by neurotrophins in the hippocampus. *Nature* 381: 706–709.

Fink CC and Meyer T (2002) Molecular mechanisms of CaMKII activation in neuronal plasticity. *Curr. Opin. Neurobiol.* 12: 293–299.

Frank DA and Greenberg ME (1994) CREB: A mediator of long-term memory from mollusks to mammals. *Cell* 79: 5–8.

Frankland PW, Cestari V, Filipkowski RK, McDonald RJ, and Silva AJ (1998) The dorsal hippocampus is essential for context discrimination but not for contextual conditioning. *Behav. Neurosci.* 112: 863–874.

Frankland PW, Josselyn SA, Anagnostaras SG, Kogan JH, Takahashi E, and Silva AJ (2004) Consolidation of CS and US representations in associative fear conditioning. *Hippocampus* 14: 557–569.

Frankland PW, O'Brien C, Ohno M, Kirkwood A, and Silva AJ (2001) Alpha-CaMKII-dependent plasticity in the cortex is required for permanent memory. *Nature* 411: 309–313.

Frey S, Bergado-Rosado J, Seidenbecher T, Pape HC, and Frey JU (2001) Reinforcement of early long-term potentiation (early-LTP) in dentate gyrus by stimulation of the basolateral amygdala: Heterosynaptic induction mechanisms of late-LTP. *J. Neurosci.* 21: 3697–3703.

Fu XZ, Zhang QG, Meng FJ, and Zhang GY (2004) NMDA receptor-mediated immediate Ser831 phosphorylation of GluR1 through CaMKIIalpha in rat hippocampus during early global ischemia. *Neurosci. Res.* 48: 85–91.

Fukunaga K and Miyamoto E (1999) Current studies on a working model of CaM kinase II in hippocampal long-term potentiation and memory. *Jpn. J. Pharmacol.* 79: 7–15.

Funayama ES, Grillon C, Davis M, and Phelps EA (2001) A double dissociation in the affective modulation of startle in humans: Effects of unilateral temporal lobectomy. *J. Cogn. Neurosci.* 13: 721–729.

Gabriel M, Saltwick SE, and Miller JD (1975) Conditioning and reversal of short-latency multiple-unit responses in the rabbit medial geniculate nucleus. *Science* 189: 1108–1109.

Gale GD, Anagnostaras SG, Godsil BP, et al. (2004) Role of the basolateral amygdala in the storage of fear memories across the adult lifetime of rats. *J. Neurosci.* 24: 3810–3815.

Garcia R, Vouimba RM, Baudry M, and Thompson RF (1999) The amygdala modulates prefrontal cortex activity relative to conditioned fear. *Nature* 402: 294–296.

Goosens KA, Holt W, and Maren S (2000) A role for amygdaloid PKA and PKC in the acquisition of long-term conditional fear memories in rats. *Behav. Brain Res.* 114: 145–152.

Goosens KA and Maren S (2001) Contextual and auditory fear conditioning are mediated by the lateral, basal, and central amygdaloid nuclei in rats. *Learn. Mem.* 8: 148–155.

Grant SG, O'Dell TJ, Karl KA, Stein PL, Soriano P, and Kandel ER (1992) Impaired long-term potentiation, spatial learning, and hippocampal development in fyn mutant mice. *Science* 258: 1903–1910.

Grosshans DR, Clayton DA, Coultrap SJ, and Browning MD (2002) LTP leads to rapid surface expression of NMDA but not AMPA receptors in adult rat CA1. *Nat. Neurosci.* 5: 27–33.

Grover LM and Teyler TJ (1990) Two components of long-term potentiation induced by different patterns of afferent activation. *Nature* 347: 477–479.

Guzowski JF, Lyford GL, Stevenson GD, et al. (2000) Inhibition of activity-dependent arc protein expression in the rat hippocampus impairs the maintenance of long-term potentiation and the consolidation of long-term memory. *J. Neurosci.* 20: 3993–4001.

Hall J, Thomas KL, and Everitt BJ (2000) Rapid and selective induction of BDNF expression in the hippocampus during contextual learning. *Nat. Neurosci.* 3: 533–535.

Hawkins RD, Kandel ER, and Siegelbaum SA (1993) Learning to modulate transmitter release: Themes and variations in synaptic plasticity. *Annu. Rev. Neurosci.* 16: 625–665.

Hawkins RD, Son H, and Arancio O (1998) Nitric oxide as a retrograde messenger during long-term potentiation in hippocampus. *Prog. Brain Res.* 118: 155–172.

Hayashi Y, Shi SH, Esteban JA, Piccini A, Poncer JC, and Malinow R (2000) Driving AMPA receptors into synapses by LTP and CaMKII: Requirement for GluR1 and PDZ domain interaction. *Science* 287: 2262–2267.

Helmstetter FJ and Bellgowan PS (1994) Effects of muscimol applied to the basolateral amygdala on acquisition and expression of contextual fear conditioning in rats. *Behav. Neurosci.* 108: 1005–1009.

Helmstetter FJ and Landeira-Fernandez J (1990) Conditional hypoalgesia is attenuated by naltrexone applied to the periaqueductal gray. *Brain Res.* 537: 88–92.

Helmstetter FJ and Tershner SA (1994) Lesions of the periaqueductal gray and rostral ventromedial medulla disrupt antinociceptive but not cardiovascular aversive conditional responses. *J. Neurosci.* 14: 7099–7108.

Herry C, Vouimba RM, and Garcia R (1999) Plasticity in the mediodorsal thalamo-prefrontal cortical transmission in behaving mice. *J. Neurophysiol.* 82: 2827–2832.

Herry C, Trifilieff P, Micheau J, Luthi A, and Mons N (2006) Extinction of auditory fear conditioning requires MAPK/ERK activation in the basolateral amygdala. *Eur. J. Neurosci.* 24: 261–269.

Hobin JA, Goosens KA, and Maren S (2003) Context-dependent neuronal activity in the lateral amygdala represents fear memories after extinction. *J. Neurosci.* 23: 8410–8416.

Holscher C, McGlinchey L, Anwyl R, and Rowan MJ (1996) 7-Nitro indazole, a selective neuronal nitric oxide synthase inhibitor *in vivo*, impairs spatial learning in the rat. *Learn. Mem.* 2: 267–278.

Holt W and Maren S (1999) Muscimol inactivation of the dorsal hippocampus impairs contextual retrieval of fear memory. *J. Neurosci.* 19: 9054–9062.

Huang YY and Kandel ER (1998) Postsynaptic induction and PKA-dependent expression of LTP in the lateral amygdala. *Neuron* 21: 169–178.

Huang YY, Martin KC, and Kandel ER (2000) Both protein kinase A and mitogen-activated protein kinase are required in the amygdala for the macromolecular synthesis-dependent late phase of long-term potentiation. *J. Neurosci.* 20: 6317–6325.

Hugues S, Chessel A, Lena I, Marsault R, and Garcia R (2006) Prefrontal infusion of PD098059 immediately after fear extinction training blocks extinction-associated prefrontal synaptic plasticity and decreases prefrontal ERK2 phosphorylation. *Synapse* 60: 280–287.

Impey S, Mark M, Villacres EC, Poser S, Chavkin C, and Storm DR (1996) Induction of CRE-mediated gene expression by stimuli that generate long-lasting LTP in area CA1 of the hippocampus. *Neuron* 16: 973–982.

Impey S, Obrietan K, Wong ST, et al. (1998a) Cross talk between ERK and PKA is required for Ca2+ stimulation of CREB-dependent transcription and ERK nuclear translocation. *Neuron* 21: 869–883.

Impey S, Smith DM, Obrietan K, Donahue R, Wade C, and Storm DR (1998b) Stimulation of cAMP response element (CRE)-mediated transcription during contextual learning [see comments]. *Nat. Neurosci.* 1: 595–601.

Ito I, Hidaka H, and Sugiyama H (1991) Effects of KN-62, a specific inhibitor of calcium/calmodulin-dependent protein kinase II, on long-term potentiation in the rat hippocampus. *Neurosci. Lett.* 121: 119–121.

Iwata J, LeDoux JE, and Reis DJ (1986) Destruction of intrinsic neurons in the lateral hypothalamus disrupts the classical conditioning of autonomic but not behavioral emotional responses in the rat. *Brain Res.* 368: 161–166.

Izquierdo I, Quillfeldt JA, Zanatta MS, et al. (1997) Sequential role of hippocampus and amygdala, entorhinal cortex and parietal cortex in formation and retrieval of memory for inhibitory avoidance in rats. *Eur. J. Neurosci.* 9: 786–793.

Jarrell TW, Gentile CG, Romanski LM, McCabe PM, and Schneiderman N (1987) Involvement of cortical and thalamic auditory regions in retention of differential bradycardiac conditioning to acoustic conditioned stimuli in rabbits. *Brain Res.* 412: 285–294.

Jasmin L, Burkey AR, Card JP, and Basbaum AI (1997) Transneuronal labeling of a nociceptive pathway, the spino-(trigemino-)parabrachio-amygdaloid, in the rat. *J. Neurosci.* 17: 3751–3765.

Jia Z, Lu Y, Henderson J, et al. (1998) Selective abolition of the NMDA component of long-term potentiation in mice lacking mGluR5. *Learn. Mem.* 5: 331–343.

Johnston D, Hoffman DA, Colbert CM, and Magee JC (1999) Regulation of back-propagating action potentials in hippocampal neurons. *Curr. Opin. Neurobiol.* 9: 288–292.

Jones MW, Errington ML, French PJ, et al. (2001) A requirement for the immediate early gene Zif268 in the expression of late LTP and long-term memories. *Nat. Neurosci.* 4: 289–296.

Josselyn SA, Shi C, Carlezon WA, Jr., Neve RL, Nestler EJ, and Davis M (2001) Long-term memory is facilitated by cAMP response element-binding protein overexpression in the amygdala. *J. Neurosci.* 21: 2404–2412.

Kang H and Schuman EM (1995) Long-lasting neurotrophin-induced enhancement of synaptic transmission in the adult hippocampus. *Science* 267: 1658–1662.

Kapp BS, Frysinger RC, Gallagher M, and Haselton JR (1979) Amygdala central nucleus lesions: Effect on heart rate conditioning in the rabbit. *Physiol. Behav.* 23: 1109–1117.

Kasai H, Matsuzaki M, Noguchi J, Yasumatsu N, and Nakahara H (2003) Structure-stability-function relationships of dendritic spines. *Trends Neurosci.* 26: 360–368.

Kelso SR, Nelson TE, and Leonard JP (1992) Protein kinase C-mediated enhancement of NMDA currents by metabotropic glutamate receptors in *Xenopus* oocytes. *J. Physiol.* 449: 705–718.

Kida S, Josselyn SA, de Ortiz SP, et al. (2002) CREB required for the stability of new and reactivated fear memories. *Nat. Neurosci.* 5: 348–355.

Killcross S, Robbins TW, and Everitt BJ (1997) Different types of fear-conditioned behaviour mediated by separate nuclei within amygdala. *Nature* 388: 377–380.

Kim JJ, DeCola JP, Landeira-Fernandez J, and Fanselow MS (1991) N-methyl-D-aspartate receptor antagonist APV blocks acquisition but not expression of fear conditioning. *Behav. Neurosci.* 105: 126–133.

Kim JJ and Fanselow MS (1992) Modality-specific retrograde amnesia of fear. *Science* 256: 675–677.

Kim JJ, Rison RA, and Fanselow MS (1993) Effects of amygdala, hippocampus, and periaqueductal gray lesions on short- and long-term contextual fear. *Behav. Neurosci.* 107: 1093–1098.

Ko GY and Kelly PT (1999) Nitric oxide acts as a postsynaptic signaling molecule in calcium/calmodulin-induced synaptic potentiation in hippocampal CA1 pyramidal neurons. *J. Neurosci.* 19: 6784–6794.

Korte M, Kang H, Bonhoeffer T, and Schuman E (1998) A role for BDNF in the late-phase of hippocampal long-term potentiation. *Neuropharmacology* 37: 553–559.

LaBar KS, Gatenby JC, Gore JC, LeDoux JE, and Phelps EA (1998) Human amygdala activation during conditioned fear acquisition and extinction: A mixed-trial fMRI study. *Neuron* 20: 937–945.

LaBar KS, LeDoux JE, Spencer DD, and Phelps EA (1995) Impaired fear conditioning following unilateral temporal lobectomy in humans. *J. Neurosci.* 15: 6846–6855.

Lamprecht R, Farb CR, and LeDoux JE (2002) Fear memory formation involves p190 RhoGAP and ROCK proteins through a GRB2-mediated complex. *Neuron* 36: 727–738.

Lamprecht R, Farb CR, Rodrigues SM, and LeDoux JE (2006) Fear conditioning drives profilin into amygdala dendritic spines. *Nat. Neurosci.* 9: 481–483.

LeDoux JE (2000) Emotion circuits in the brain. *Annu. Rev. Neurosci.* 23: 155–184.

LeDoux JE, Cicchetti P, Xagoraris A, and Romanski LM (1990) The lateral amygdaloid nucleus: Sensory interface of the amygdala in fear conditioning. *J. Neurosci.* 10: 1062–1069.

LeDoux JE and Farb CR (1991) Neurons of the acoustic thalamus that project to the amygdala contain glutamate. *Neurosci. Lett.* 134: 145–149.

LeDoux JE, Iwata J, Cicchetti P, and Reis DJ (1988) Different projections of the central amygdaloid nucleus mediate autonomic and behavioral correlates of conditioned fear. *J. Neurosci.* 8: 2517–2529.

LeDoux JE, Ruggiero DA, and Reis DJ (1985) Projections to the subcortical forebrain from anatomically defined regions of the medial geniculate body in the rat. *J. Comp. Neurol.* 242: 182–213.

LeDoux JE, Ruggiero DA, Forest R, Stornetta R, and Reis DJ (1987) Topographic organization of convergent projections to the thalamus from the inferior colliculus and spinal cord in the rat. *J. Comp. Neurol.* 264: 123–146.

LeDoux JE, Sakaguchi A, Iwata J, and Reis DJ (1986) Interruption of projections from the medial geniculate body to an archi-neostriatal field disrupts the classical conditioning of emotional responses to acoustic stimuli. *Neuroscience* 17: 615–627.

LeDoux JE, Sakaguchi A, and Reis DJ (1984) Subcortical efferent projections of the medial geniculate nucleus mediate emotional responses conditioned to acoustic stimuli. *J. Neurosci.* 4: 683–698.

Lee HK, Barbarosie M, Kameyama K, Bear MF, and Huganir RL (2000) Regulation of distinct AMPA receptor phosphorylation sites during bidirectional synaptic plasticity. *Nature* 405: 955–959.

Lee HK, Takamiya K, Han JS, et al. (2003) Phosphorylation of the AMPA receptor GluR1 subunit is required for synaptic plasticity and retention of spatial memory. *Cell* 112: 631–643.

Lee JL, Everitt BJ, and Thomas KL (2004) Independent cellular processes for hippocampal memory consolidation and reconsolidation. *Science* 304: 839–843.

Leuner B, Falduto J, and Shors TJ (2003) Associative memory formation increases the observation of dendritic spines in the hippocampus. *J. Neurosci.* 23: 659–665.

Lewis DJ, Bregman NJ, and Mahan JJ, Jr. (1972) Cue-dependent amnesia in rats. *J. Comp. Physiol. Psychol.* 81: 243–247.

Li XF, Stutzmann GE, and LeDoux JE (1996) Convergent but temporally separated inputs to lateral amygdala neurons from the auditory thalamus and auditory cortex use different postsynaptic receptors: *In vivo* intracellular and extracellular recordings in fear conditioning pathways. *Learn. Mem.* 3: 229–242.

Liao GY, Wagner DA, Hsu MH, and Leonard JP (2001) Evidence for direct protein kinase-C mediated modulation of N-methyl-D-aspartate receptor current. *Mol. Pharmacol.* 59: 960–964.

Lindquist DH, Jarrard LE, and Brown TH (2004) Perirhinal cortex supports delay fear conditioning to rat ultrasonic social signals. *J. Neurosci.* 24: 3610–3617.

Link W, Konietzko U, Kauselmann G, et al. (1995) Somatodendritic expression of an immediate early gene is regulated by synaptic activity. *Proc. Natl. Acad. Sci. USA* 92: 5734–5738.

Linke R, Braune G, and Schwegler H (2000) Differential projection of the posterior paralaminar thalamic nuclei to the amygdaloid complex in the rat. *Exp. Brain Res.* 134: 520–532.

Lisman J, Schulman H, and Cline H (2002) The molecular basis of CaMKII function in synaptic and behavioural memory. *Nat. Rev. Neurosci.* 3: 175–190.

Lu KT, Walker DL, and Davis M (2001) Mitogen-activated protein kinase cascade in the basolateral nucleus of amygdala is involved in extinction of fear-potentiated startle. *J. Neurosci.* 21: RC162.

Lu YF and Hawkins RD (2002) Ryanodine receptors contribute to cGMP-induced late-phase LTP and CREB phosphorylation in the hippocampus. *J. Neurophysiol.* 88: 1270–1278.

Lu YF, Kandel ER, and Hawkins RD (1999) Nitric oxide signaling contributes to late-phase LTP and CREB phosphorylation in the hippocampus. *J. Neurosci.* 19: 10250–10261.

Lu YM, Jia Z, Janus C, et al. (1997) Mice lacking metabotropic glutamate receptor 5 show impaired learning and reduced

CA1 long-term potentiation (LTP) but normal CA3 LTP. *J. Neurosci.* 17: 5196–5205.
MacDonald JF, Kotecha SA, Lu WY, and Jackson MF (2001) Convergence of PKC-dependent kinase signal cascades on NMDA receptors. *Curr. Drug Targets* 2: 299–312.
Magee JC and Johnston D (1997) A synaptically controlled, associative signal for Hebbian plasticity in hippocampal neurons [see comments]. *Science* 275: 209–213.
Malenka RC (2003) Synaptic plasticity and AMPA receptor trafficking. *Ann. N.Y. Acad. Sci.* 1003: 1–11.
Malenka RC and Nicoll RA (1993) NMDA-receptor-dependent synaptic plasticity: Multiple forms and mechanisms. *Trends Neurosci.* 16: 521–527.
Malenka RC and Nicoll RA (1999) Long-term potentiation – A decade of progress? *Science* 285: 1870–1874.
Malinow R (2003) AMPA receptor trafficking and long-term potentiation. *Philos. Trans. R. Soc. Lond. B Biol. Sci.* 358: 707–714.
Malkani S and Rosen JB (2000) Specific induction of early growth response gene 1 in the lateral nucleus of the amygdala following contextual fear conditioning in rats. *Neuroscience* 97: 693–702.
Malkani S, Wallace KJ, Donley MP, and Rosen JB (2004) An egr-1 (zif268) antisense oligodeoxynucleotide infused into the amygdala disrupts fear conditioning. *Learn. Mem.* 11: 617–624.
Mammen AL, Kameyama K, Roche KW, and Huganir RL (1997) Phosphorylation of the alpha-amino-3-hydroxy-5-methylisoxazole4-propionic acid receptor GluR1 subunit by calcium/calmodulin-dependent kinase II. *J. Biol. Chem.* 272: 32528–32533.
Maren S (1998) Overtraining does not mitigate contextual fear conditioning deficits produced by neurotoxic lesions of the basolateral amygdala. *J. Neurosci.* 18: 3088–3097.
Maren S (1999) Long-term potentiation in the amygdala: A mechanism for emotional learning and memory. *Trends Neurosci.* 22: 561–567.
Maren S (2000) Auditory fear conditioning increases CS-elicited spike firing in lateral amygdala neurons even after extensive overtraining. *Eur. J. Neurosci.* 12: 4047–4054.
Maren S (2001) Neurobiology of Pavlovian fear conditioning. *Annu. Rev. Neurosci.* 24: 897–931.
Maren S, Aharonov G, and Fanselow MS (1997) Neurotoxic lesions of the dorsal hippocampus and Pavlovian fear conditioning in rats. *Behav. Brain Res.* 88: 261–274.
Maren S, Aharonov G, Stote DL, and Fanselow MS (1996) N-methyl-D-aspartate receptors in the basolateral amygdala are required for both acquisition and expression of conditional fear in rats. *Behav. Neurosci.* 110: 1365–1374.
Maren S and Fanselow MS (1995) Synaptic plasticity in the basolateral amygdala induced by hippocampal formation stimulation *in vivo*. *J. Neurosci.* 15: 7548–7564.
Maren S, Yap SA, and Goosens KA (2001) The amygdala is essential for the development of neuronal plasticity in the medial geniculate nucleus during auditory fear conditioning in rats. *J. Neurosci.* 21: RC135.
Markram H, Lubke J, Frotscher M, and Sakmann B (1997) Regulation of synaptic efficacy by coincidence of postsynaptic APs and EPSPs [see comments]. *Science* 275: 213–215.
Matus A (2000) Actin-based plasticity in dendritic spines. *Science* 290: 754–758.
Mayford M, Bach ME, Huang YY, Wang L, Hawkins RD, and Kandel ER (1996) Control of memory formation through regulated expression of a CaMKII transgene. *Science* 274: 1678–1683.
McDonald AJ (1998) Cortical pathways to the mammalian amygdala. *Prog. Neurobiol.* 55: 257–332.
McDonald AJ, Mascagni F, and Guo L (1996) Projections of the medial and lateral prefrontal cortices to the amygdala: A Phaseolus vulgaris leucoagglutinin study in the rat. *Neuroscience* 71: 55–75.
McDonald AJ, Muller JF, and Mascagni F (2002) GABAergic innervation of alpha type II calcium/calmodulin-dependent protein kinase immunoreactive pyramidal neurons in the rat basolateral amygdala. *J. Comp. Neurol.* 446: 199–218.
McGaugh JL (2000) Memory – A century of consolidation. *Science* 287: 248–251.
McGaugh JL, Introini-Collison IB, Cahill LF, et al. (1993) Neuromodulatory systems and memory storage: Role of the amygdala. *Behav. Brain Res.* 58: 81–90.
McKernan MG and Shinnick-Gallagher P (1997) Fear conditioning induces a lasting potentiation of synaptic currents *in vitro*. *Nature* 390: 607–611.
Medina JF, Christopher Repa J, Mauk MD, and LeDoux JE (2002) Parallels between cerebellum- and amygdala-dependent conditioning. *Nat. Rev. Neurosci.* 3: 122–131.
Milad MR and Quirk GJ (2002) Neurons in medial prefrontal cortex signal memory for fear extinction. *Nature* 420: 70–74.
Milner B, Squire LR, and Kandel ER (1998) Cognitive neuroscience and the study of memory. *Neuron* 20: 445–468.
Misanin JR, Miller RR, and Lewis DJ (1968) Retrograde amnesia produced by electroconvulsive shock after reactivation of a consolidated memory trace. *Science* 160: 554–555.
Miserendino MJ, Sananes CB, Melia KR, and Davis M (1990) Blocking of acquisition but not expression of conditioned fear-potentiated startle by NMDA antagonists in the amygdala. *Nature* 345: 716–718.
Moita MA, Lamprecht R, Nader K, and LeDoux JE (2002) A-kinase anchoring proteins in amygdala are involved in auditory fear memory. *Nat. Neurosci.* 5: 837–838.
Moita MA, Rosis S, Zhou Y, LeDoux JE, and Blair HT (2003) Hippocampal place cells acquire location-specific responses to the conditioned stimulus during auditory fear conditioning. *Neuron* 37: 485–497.
Monfort P, Munoz MD, Kosenko E, and Felipo V (2002) Long-term potentiation in hippocampus involves sequential activation of soluble guanylate cyclase, cGMP-dependent protein kinase, and cGMP- degrading phosphodiesterase. *J. Neurosci.* 22: 10116–10122.
Monyer H, Sprengel R, Schoepfer R, et al. (1992) Heteromeric NMDA receptors: Molecular and functional distinction of subtypes. *Science* 256: 1217–1221.
Morgan MA and LeDoux JE (1995) Differential contribution of dorsal and ventral medial prefrontal cortex to the acquisition and extinction of conditioned fear in rats. *Behav. Neurosci.* 109: 681–688.
Morgan MA, Romanski LM, and LeDoux JE (1993) Extinction of emotional learning: Contribution of medial prefrontal cortex. *Neurosci. Lett.* 163: 109–113.
Morris JS, Ohman A, and Dolan RJ (1999) A subcortical pathway to the right amygdala mediating "unseen" fear. *Proc. Natl. Acad. Sci. USA* 96: 1680–1685.
Muller J, Corodimas KP, Fridel Z, and LeDoux JE (1997) Functional inactivation of the lateral and basal nuclei of the amygdala by muscimol infusion prevents fear conditioning to an explicit conditioned stimulus and to contextual stimuli. *Behav. Neurosci.* 111: 683–691.
Nader K, Schafe GE, and Le Doux JE (2000) Fear memories require protein synthesis in the amygdala for reconsolidation after retrieval. *Nature* 406: 722–726.
Nakanishi S (1992) Molecular diversity of glutamate receptors and implications for brain function. *Science* 258: 597–603.
Nakazawa T, Komai S, Tezuka T, et al. (2001) Characterization of Fyn-mediated tyrosine phosphorylation sites on GluR epsilon 2 (NR2B) subunit of the N-methyl-D-aspartate receptor. *J. Biol. Chem.* 276: 693–699.
Nakazawa T, Tezuka T, and Yamamoto T (2002) [Regulation of NMDA receptor function by Fyn-mediated tyrosine

phosphorylation]. *Nihon Shinkei Seishin Yakurigaku Zasshi* 22: 165–167.
Nguyen PV, Abel T, and Kandel ER (1994) Requirement of a critical period of transcription for induction of a late phase of LTP. *Science* 265: 1104–1107.
Nguyen PV and Kandel ER (1996) A macromolecular synthesis-dependent late phase of long-term potentiation requiring cAMP in the medial perforant pathway of rat hippocampal slices. *J. Neurosci.* 16: 3189–3198.
O'Carroll RE, Drysdale E, Cahill L, Shajahan P, and Ebmeier KP (1999) Stimulation of the noradrenergic system enhances and blockade reduces memory for emotional material in man. *Psychol. Med.* 29: 1083–1088.
Paré D, Quirk GJ, and Ledoux JE (2004) New vistas on amygdala networks in conditioned fear. *J. Neurophysiol.* 92: 1–9.
Paré D and Smith Y (1993) The intercalated cell masses project to the central and medial nuclei of the amygdala in cats. *Neuroscience* 57: 1077–1090.
Parsons RG, Gafford GM, Baruch DE, Riedner BA, and Helmstetter FJ (2006) Long-term stability of fear memory depends on the synthesis of protein but not mRNA in the amygdala. *Eur. J. Neurosci.* 23: 1853–1859.
Patterson SL, Abel T, Deuel TA, Martin KC, Rose JC, and Kandel ER (1996) Recombinant BDNF rescues deficits in basal synaptic transmission and hippocampal LTP in BDNF knockout mice. *Neuron* 16: 1137–1145.
Patterson SL, Pittenger C, Morozov A, et al. (2001) Some forms of cAMP-mediated long-lasting potentiation are associated with release of BDNF and nuclear translocation of phospho-MAP kinase. *Neuron* 32: 123–140.
Pavlov IP (1927) *Conditioned Reflexes.* London: Oxford University Press.
Phelps EA, Delgado MR, Nearing KI, and LeDoux JE (2004) Extinction learning in humans: Role of the amygdala and vmPFC. *Neuron* 43: 897–905.
Phelps EA and LeDoux JE (2005) Contributions of the amygdala to emotion processing: From animal models to human behavior. *Neuron* 48: 175–187.
Phelps EA, O'Connor KJ, Gatenby JC, Gore JC, Grillon C, and Davis M (2001) Activation of the left amygdala to a cognitive representation of fear. *Nat. Neurosci.* 4: 437–441.
Phillips RG and LeDoux JE (1992) Differential contribution of amygdala and hippocampus to cued and contextual fear conditioning. *Behav. Neurosci.* 106: 274–285.
Poremba A and Gabriel M (2001) Amygdalar efferents initiate auditory thalamic discriminative training-induced neuronal activity. *J. Neurosci.* 21: 270–278.
Quirk GJ, Armony JL, and LeDoux JE (1997) Fear conditioning enhances different temporal components of tone-evoked spike trains in auditory cortex and lateral amygdala. *Neuron* 19: 613–624.
Quirk GJ and Gehlert DR (2003) Inhibition of the amygdala: Key to pathological states? *Ann. N.Y. Acad. Sci.* 985: 263–272.
Quirk GJ, Likhtik E, Pelletier JG, and Pare D (2003) Stimulation of medial prefrontal cortex decreases the responsiveness of central amygdala output neurons. *J. Neurosci.* 23: 8800–8807.
Quirk GJ, Repa C, and LeDoux JE (1995) Fear conditioning enhances short-latency auditory responses of lateral amygdala neurons: Parallel recordings in the freely behaving rat. *Neuron* 15: 1029–1039.
Quirk GJ, Russo GK, Barron JL, and Lebron K (2000) The role of ventromedial prefrontal cortex in the recovery of extinguished fear. *J. Neurosci.* 20: 6225–6231.
Radley JJ, Johnson LR, Janssen WG, et al. (2006) Associative Pavlovian conditioning leads to an increase in spinophilin-immunoreactive dendritic spines in the lateral amygdala. *Eur. J. Neurosci.* 24: 876–884.
Rampon C, Tang YP, Goodhouse J, Shimizu E, Kyin M, and Tsien JZ (2000) Enrichment induces structural changes and recovery from nonspatial memory deficits in CA1 NMDAR1-knockout mice [see comments]. *Nat. Neurosci.* 3: 238–244.
Rampon C and Tsien JZ (2000) Genetic analysis of learning behavior-induced structural plasticity. *Hippocampus* 10: 605–609.
Rattiner LM, Davis M, French CT, and Ressler KJ (2004) Brain-derived neurotrophic factor and tyrosine kinase receptor B involvement in amygdala-dependent fear conditioning. *J. Neurosci.* 24: 4796–4806.
Rattiner LM, Davis M, and Ressler KJ (2005) Brain-derived neurotrophic factor in amygdala-dependent learning. *Neuroscientist* 11: 323–333.
Repa JC, Muller J, Apergis J, Desrochers TM, Zhou Y, and LeDoux JE (2001) Two different lateral amygdala cell populations contribute to the initiation and storage of memory. *Nat. Neurosci.* 4: 724–731.
Rescorla RA and Heth CD (1975) Reinstatement of fear to an extinguished conditioned stimulus. *J. Exp. Psychol. Anim. Behav. Process* 1: 88–96.
Ressler KJ, Paschall G, Zhou XL, and Davis M (2002) Regulation of synaptic plasticity genes during consolidation of fear conditioning. *J. Neurosci.* 22: 7892–7902.
Richardson CL, Tate WP, Mason SE, Lawlor PA, Dragunow M, and Abraham WC (1992) Correlation between the induction of an immediate early gene, zif/268, and long-term potentiation in the dentate gyrus. *Brain Res.* 580: 147–154.
Richardson MP, Strange BA, and Dolan RJ (2004) Encoding of emotional memories depends on amygdala and hippocampus and their interactions. *Nat. Neurosci.* 7: 278–285.
Robbins TW, Cador M, Taylor JR, and Everitt BJ (1989) Limbic-striatal interactions in reward-related processes. *Neurosci. Biobehav. Rev.* 13: 155–162.
Roberson ED, English JD, Adams JP, Selcher JC, Kondratick C, and Sweatt JD (1999) The mitogen-activated protein kinase cascade couples PKA and PKC to cAMP response element binding protein phosphorylation in area CA1 of hippocampus. *J. Neurosci.* 19: 4337–4348.
Rodrigues SM, Bauer EP, Farb CR, Schafe GE, and LeDoux JE (2002) The group I metabotropic glutamate receptor mGluR5 is required for fear memory formation and long-term potentiation in the lateral amygdala. *J. Neurosci.* 22: 5219–5229.
Rodrigues SM, Farb CR, Bauer EP, LeDoux JE, and Schafe GE (2004a) Pavlovian fear conditioning regulates Thr286 autophosphorylation of Ca2+/calmodulin-dependent protein kinase II at lateral amygdala synapses. *J. Neurosci.* 24: 3281–3288.
Rodrigues SM, Schafe GE, and LeDoux JE (2001) Intraamygdala blockade of the NR2B subunit of the NMDA receptor disrupts the acquisition but not the expression of fear conditioning. *J. Neurosci.* 21(17): 6889–6896.
Rodrigues SM, Schafe GE, and LeDoux JE (2004b) Molecular mechanisms underlying emotional learning and memory in the lateral amygdala. *Neuron* 44: 75–91.
Rogan MT and LeDoux JE (1995) LTP is accompanied by commensurate enhancement of auditory-evoked responses in a fear conditioning circuit. *Neuron* 15: 127–136.
Rogan MT, Staubli UV, and LeDoux JE (1997) Fear conditioning induces associative long-term potentiation in the amygdala. *Nature* 390: 604–607.
Romanski LM, Clugnet MC, Bordi F, and LeDoux JE (1993) Somatosensory and auditory convergence in the lateral nucleus of the amygdala. *Behav. Neurosci.* 107: 444–450.
Romanski LM and LeDoux JE (1992a) Equipotentiality of thalamo-amygdala and thalamo-cortico-amygdala circuits in auditory fear conditioning. *J. Neurosci.* 12: 4501–4509.

Romanski LM and LeDoux JE (1992b) Bilateral destruction of neocortical and perirhinal projection targets of the acoustic thalamus does not disrupt auditory fear conditioning. *Neurosci. Lett.* 142: 228–232.
Romanski LM and LeDoux JE (1993) Information cascade from primary auditory cortex to the amygdala: Corticocortical and corticoamygdaloid projections of temporal cortex in the rat. *Cereb. Cortex* 3: 515–532.
Roozendaal B, Koolhaas JM, and Bohus B (1991) Attenuated cardiovascular, neuroendocrine, and behavioral responses after a single footshock in central amygdaloid lesioned male rats. *Physiol. Behav.* 50: 771–775.
Rosen JB, Fanselow MS, Young SL, Sitcoske M, and Maren S (1998) Immediate-early gene expression in the amygdala following footshock stress and contextual fear conditioning. *Brain Res.* 796: 132–142.
Royer S, Martina M, and Pare D (1999) An inhibitory interface gates impulse traffic between the input and output stations of the amygdala. *J. Neurosci.* 19: 10575–10583.
Rumpel S, LeDoux J, Zador A, and Malinow R (2005) Postsynaptic receptor trafficking underlying a form of associative learning. *Science* 308: 83–88.
Samson RD and Paré D (2005) Activity-dependent synaptic plasticity in the central nucleus of the amygdala. *J. Neurosci.* 25: 1847–1855.
Santini E, Ge H, Ren K, Pena de Ortiz S, and Quirk GJ (2004) Consolidation of fear extinction requires protein synthesis in the medial prefrontal cortex. *J. Neurosci.* 24: 5704–5710.
Sara SJ (2000) Retrieval and reconsolidation: Toward a neurobiology of remembering. *Learn. Mem.* 7: 73–84.
Schafe GE, Atkins CM, Swank MW, Bauer EP, Sweatt JD, and LeDoux JE (2000) Activation of ERK/MAP kinase in the amygdala is required for memory consolidation of pavlovian fear conditioning. *J. Neurosci.* 20: 8177–8187.
Schafe GE, Bauer EP, Rosis S, Farb CR, Rodrigues SM, and LeDoux JE (2005a) Memory consolidation of Pavlovian fear conditioning requires nitric oxide signaling in the lateral amygdala. *Eur. J. Neurosci.* 22: 201–211.
Schafe GE, Doyère V, and LeDoux JE (2005b) Tracking the fear engram: The lateral amygdala is an essential locus of fear memory storage. *J. Neurosci.* 25: 10010–10015.
Schafe GE and LeDoux JE (2000) Memory consolidation of auditory Pavlovian fear conditioning requires protein synthesis and protein kinase A in the amygdala. *J. Neurosci.* 20: RC96.
Schafe GE, Nader K, Blair HT, and LeDoux JE (2001) Memory consolidation of Pavlovian fear conditioning: A cellular and molecular perspective. *Trends Neurosci.* 24: 540–546.
Schuman EM and Madison DV (1991) A requirement for the intercellular messenger nitric oxide in long-term potentiation. *Science* 254: 1503–1506.
Scicli AP, Petrovich GD, Swanson LW, and Thompson RF (2004) Contextual fear conditioning is associated with lateralized expression of the immediate early gene c-fos in the central and basolateral amygdalar nuclei. *Behav. Neurosci.* 118: 5–14.
Shen K and Meyer T (1999) Dynamic control of CaMKII translocation and localization in hippocampal neurons by NMDA receptor stimulation. *Science* 284: 162–166.
Silva AJ, Kogan JH, Frankland PW, and Kida S (1998) CREB and memory. *Annu. Rev. Neurosci.* 21: 127–148.
Silva AJ, Paylor R, Wehner JM, and Tonegawa S (1992a) Impaired spatial learning in alpha-calcium-calmodulin kinase II mutant mice. *Science* 257: 206–211.
Silva AJ, Stevens CF, Tonegawa S, and Wang Y (1992b) Deficient hippocampal long-term potentiation in alpha-calcium-calmodulin kinase II mutant mice [see comments]. *Science* 257: 201–206.
Soderling TR and Derkach VA (2000) Postsynaptic protein phosphorylation and LTP. *Trends Neurosci.* 23: 75–80.
Son H, Lu YF, Zhuo M, Arancio O, Kandel ER, and Hawkins RD (1998) The specific role of cGMP in hippocampal LTP. *Learn. Mem.* 5: 231–245.
Stanton PK and Gage AT (1996) Distinct synaptic loci of Ca2+/calmodulin-dependent protein kinase II necessary for long-term potentiation and depression. *J. Neurophysiol.* 76: 2097–2101.
Stevens CF (1998) A million dollar question: Does LTP = memory? *Neuron* 20: 1–2.
Stiedl O, Birkenfeld K, Palve M, and Spiess J (2000) Impairment of conditioned contextual fear of C57BL/6J mice by intracerebral injections of the NMDA receptor antagonist APV. *Behav. Brain Res.* 116: 157–168.
Stork O, Stork S, Pape HC, and Obata K (2001) Identification of genes expressed in the amygdala during the formation of fear memory. *Learn. Mem.* 8: 209–219.
Stuart GJ and Hausser M (2001) Dendritic coincidence detection of EPSPs and action potentials. *Nat. Neurosci.* 4: 63–71.
Suzuki Y, Ikari H, Hayashi T, and Iguchi A (1996) Central administration of a nitric oxide synthase inhibitor impairs spatial memory in spontaneous hypertensive rats. *Neurosci. Lett.* 207: 105–108.
Sweatt JD (2004) Mitogen-activated protein kinases in synaptic plasticity and memory. *Curr. Opin. Neurobiol.* 14: 311–317.
Tan SE and Liang KC (1996) Spatial learning alters hippocampal calcium/calmodulin-dependent protein kinase II activity in rats. *Brain Res.* 711: 234–240.
Tang YP, Shimizu E, Dube GR, et al. (1999) Genetic enhancement of learning and memory in mice. *Nature* 401: 63–69.
Toni N, Buchs PA, Nikonenko I, Bron CR, and Muller D (1999) LTP promotes formation of multiple spine synapses between a single axon terminal and a dendrite. *Nature* 402: 421–425.
Tronson NC, Wiseman SL, Olausson P, and Taylor JR (2006) Bidirectional behavioral plasticity of memory reconsolidation depends on amygdalar protein kinase A. *Nat. Neurosci.* 9: 167–169.
Tsien JZ (2000) Building a brainier mouse. *Sci. Am.* 282: 62–68.
Tsvetkov E, Carlezon WA, Benes FM, Kandel ER, and Bolshakov VY (2002) Fear conditioning occludes LTP-induced presynaptic enhancement of synaptic transmission in the cortical pathway to the lateral amygdala. *Neuron* 34: 289–300.
Turner BH and Herkenham M (1991) Thalamoamygdaloid projections in the rat: A test of the amygdala's role in sensory processing. *J. Comp. Neurol.* 313: 295–325.
Van Harreveld A and Fifkova E (1975) Swelling of dendritic spines in the fascia dentata after stimulation of the perforant fibers as a mechanism of post-tetanic potentiation. *Exp. Neurol.* 49: 736–749.
van Rossum D and Hanisch UK (1999) Cytoskeletal dynamics in dendritic spines: Direct modulation by glutamate receptors? *Trends Neurosci.* 22: 290–295.
von Hertzen LS and Giese KP (2005) Memory reconsolidation engages only a subset of immediate-early genes induced during consolidation. *J. Neurosci.* 25: 1935–1942.
Walker DL and Davis M (2000) Involvement of NMDA receptors within the amygdala in short- versus long- term memory for fear conditioning as assessed with fear-potentiated startle. *Behav. Neurosci.* 114: 1019–1033.
Walker DL, Ressler KJ, Lu KT, and Davis M (2002) Facilitation of conditioned fear extinction by systemic administration or intra-amygdala infusions of D-cycloserine as assessed with fear-potentiated startle in rats. *J. Neurosci.* 22: 2343–2351.
Watson JB and Rayner R (2000) Conditioned emotional reactions. 1920. *Am. Psychol.* 55: 313–317.

Weeber EJ, Atkins CM, Selcher JC, et al. (2000) A role for the beta isoform of protein kinase C in fear conditioning. *J. Neurosci.* 20: 5906–5914.
Weinberger NM (1993) Learning-induced changes of auditory receptive fields. *Curr. Opin. Neurobiol.* 3: 570–577.
Weisskopf MG, Bauer EP, and LeDoux JE (1999) L-type voltage-gated calcium channels mediate NMDA-independent associative long-term potentiation at thalamic input synapses to the amygdala. *J. Neurosci.* 19: 10512–10519.
Weisskopf MG and LeDoux JE (1999) Distinct populations of NMDA receptors at subcortical and cortical inputs to principal cells of the lateral amygdala. *J. Neurophysiol.* 81: 930–934.
Wilensky AE, Schafe GE, and LeDoux JE (2000) The amygdala modulates memory consolidation of fear-motivated inhibitory avoidance learning but not classical fear conditioning. *J. Neurosci.* 20: 7059–7066.
Wilensky AE, Schafe GE, Kristensen MP, and LeDoux JE (2006) Rethinking the fear circuit: The central nucleus of the amygdala is required for the acquisition, consolidation, and expression of pavlovian fear conditioning. *J. Neurosci.* 26: 12387–12396.
Woolf NJ (1998) A structural basis for memory storage in mammals. *Prog. Neurobiol.* 55: 59–77.
Worley PF, Bhat RV, Baraban JM, Erickson CA, McNaughton BL, and Barnes CA (1993) Thresholds for synaptic activation of transcription factors in hippocampus: Correlation with long-term enhancement. *J. Neurosci.* 13: 4776–4786.
Xing J, Ginty DD, and Greenberg ME (1996) Coupling of the RAS-MAPK pathway to gene activation by RSK2, a growth factor-regulated CREB kinase. *Science* 273: 959–963.
Yin JC, Del Vecchio M, Zhou H, and Tully T (1995) CREB as a memory modulator: Induced expression of a dCREB2 activator isoform enhances long-term memory in *Drosophila*. *Cell* 81: 107–115.
Yin JC and Tully T (1996) CREB and the formation of long-term memory. *Curr. Opin. Neurobiol.* 6: 264–268.
Yin JC, Wallach JS, Del Vecchio M, et al. (1994) Induction of a dominant negative CREB transgene specifically blocks long-term memory. *Cell* 79: 49–58.
Ying SW, Futter M, Rosenblum K, et al. (2002) Brain-derived neurotrophic factor induces long-term potentiation in intact adult hippocampus: Requirement for ERK activation coupled to CREB and upregulation of Arc synthesis. *J. Neurosci.* 22: 1532–1540.
Young LJ and Wang Z (2004) The neurobiology of pair bonding. *Nat. Neurosci.* 7: 1048–1054.
Young SL, Bohenek DL, and Fanselow MS (1994) NMDA processes mediate anterograde amnesia of contextual fear conditioning induced by hippocampal damage: Immunization against amnesia by context preexposure. *Behav. Neurosci.* 108: 19–29.
Zheng X, Zhang L, Wang AP, Bennett MV, and Zukin RS (1999) Protein kinase C potentiation of N-methyl-D-aspartate receptor activity is not mediated by phosphorylation of N-methyl-D-aspartate receptor subunits. *Proc. Natl. Acad. Sci. USA* 96: 15262–15267.
Zhuo M, Hu Y, Schultz C, Kandel ER, and Hawkins RD (1994) Role of guanylyl cyclase and cGMP-dependent protein kinase in long-term potentiation. *Nature* 368: 635–639.
Zou LB, Yamada K, Tanaka T, Kameyama T, and Nabeshima T (1998) Nitric oxide synthase inhibitors impair reference memory formation in a radial arm maze task in rats. *Neuropharmacology* 37: 323–330.

22 Conditioned Taste Aversion and Taste Learning: Molecular Mechanisms

K. Rosenblum, Department of Neurobiology and Ethology, Mount Carmel, University of Haifa, Haifa, Israel

22.1 Introduction

The sense of taste, together with that of odor, belongs to the family of chemical senses, and it is an important defensive sense, evolved to guide food intake and to aid in avoiding poisons. Moreover, the very existence of an organism is dependent on its ability to maintain intrinsic homeostasis in a continuously changing world. The guarding gate, both for the intake of energy and other metabolites necessary for the organism's survival and for the avoidance of poisonous substrates, is the sense of taste. In order to maintain homeostasis, the organism must recognize its bodily needs, identify the relevant substances that contain the means to satisfy these needs, and ensure that the process of ingestion maintains the balance between the needs and the intake. In addition and in parallel, the organism must avoid substances that will make it sick.

In order to consume the necessary and beneficial substances and to avoid the damaging ones that may cause malaise, the organism mainly uses taste and tags the substances as pleasant, indifferent, or unpleasant. However, the reaction of the organism to a specific substance is determined by a combination of automatic responses that developed during evolution and learning mechanisms that are plastic and can modify the perceived food value according to individual experience. An ethological view may account for the predisposition for different tastes according to the theory that the animals are well adapted to conditions that may occur with high probability and/or have critical survival value.

Learning the value of new tastes may be in line with or in contrast to this evolution-dependent genetic programming. There are just five different taste categories: Sweet, salt, bitter, sour, and the less well known umami (manifested in monosodium glutamate). However, combinations of different concentrations within these five categories and the additional information related to texture and temperature enable the characterization and identification of thousands of different tastes. Animals, including humans, can react to the various tastes by using two main strategies: Genetic programming (like sweet, dislike bitter), and complex learning mechanisms that involve the participation of several forebrain structures.

Taste learning has been found and studied in vertebrates and invertebrates and seems to be universal throughout the animal kingdom. However, most of the research into the biological mechanisms underlying taste learning has involved mice and rats, and the present chapter deals mainly with these studies. A simple sense stimulus such as taste can be very well defined in terms of a number of molecules (e.g., known molarities in a known volume). However, even simple unimodal taste input includes not only the chemical properties of a substance, but also other physical dimensions, such as temperature and texture, and association with other cues and modalities.

This chapter does not address taste recognition on the receptor level, nor taste reactivity as it is defined genetically. The aim of this chapter is first to describe taste behavior in the context of laboratory attempts to identify molecular and cellular mechanisms of learning and memory, to present the various learning paradigms used in the laboratory, and the relevant neuroanatomy. Later, I will review and discuss in detail the molecular and cellular mechanisms of taste learning in the gustatory cortex, which reside in the insular cortex. I focus this chapter on recent publications, because the earlier development of the subject is covered in a seminal book by Jan Bures, Federico Bermudez-Rattoni, and Takashi Yamamoto (Bures et al., 1998). Finally, I present the current working model of taste memory formation, consolidation, and retention and suggest future research directions.

22.2 Measuring Taste Learning, Memory, and Consolidation: The Behavioral Paradigms

Learning is conventionally classified from the behavioral point of view into nonassociative (habituation and sensitization), associative (relationships between amounts and events), and incidental learning (learning in the absence of an explicit external reinforcer). In addition, memory can be classified according to the temporal phases of short- and long-term memories. The use of several different behavioral paradigms enables the different classification and temporal phases to be analyzed. Taste learning and conditioned taste aversion are considered to be implicit learning paradigms and they can result in short-term memory (hours) or lifelong memory (Bures et al., 1998; Houpt and Berlin, 1999). In animals, as in humans, a subject can prefer one taste over another without recognizing either (Adolphs et al., 2005).

The most familiar taste-learning paradigm is an association between taste and malaise: The process of conditioned taste aversion (CTA). In CTA learning, an animal learns to avoid a novel food associated with delayed poisoning (Garcia et al., 1955; Bures et al., 1988). CTA can be explained as an associative learning paradigm: The novel taste is the conditioned stimulus (CS), the malaise-inducing agent is the unconditioned stimulus (UCS), and the learned avoidance of the taste is the conditioned response (CR). However, it was clear from the first time that CTA was reported scientifically (Garcia et al., 1955) that CTA has very special and unique features.

The most prominent characteristic of CTA learning is the long delay between the novel food that serves as the CS and the toxic substance that serves as the UCS. This time frame of association is measured in hours (1–12 h) (Bures et al., 1998), which is in strong contrast to other forms of association, which tolerate time frames of a few seconds. The long delay between the CS and the UCS can be explained on the sensory level or in terms of the slow release of a substance from the stomach. Moreover, short time frames or backward conditioning do not yield good association and learning (Schafe et al., 1995). Thus, the long delay between the CS and the UCS in CTA should be explained in terms of the neuronal system subserving the CTA learning. Theoretically, the internal representation of the novel taste is kept in an on-hold position for many hours, ready for the UCS to produce the association. It is not clear how the internal representation of taste is stored, but it is hypothesized that it underlies ongoing activity that is dependent in part on the gustatory cortex (Katz et al., 2002; Bahar et al., 2003; Berman et al., 2003). CTA has other special features such as one-trial learning that produces strong and stable long-term memory; it can produce aversion to odor by odor potentiation taste aversion (Schneider and Pinnow, 1994), and, in contrast to the strong association between taste and malaise, there is no or very weak association between other sensory stimuli (e.g., sound, light) and malaise or discomfort. Similarly, there is hardly any association between taste and noninternal stresses, such as pain.

CTA can be affected if the CS is experienced either before the CTA, i.e., latent inhibition of CTA (LI-CTA), or after it, i.e., CTA extinction, as can other learning paradigms, but with specific characteristics for taste learning. In LI-CTA, if a taste stimulus was learned with no negative consequence there will be decreased aversion for the same taste following CTA (Rosenblum et al., 1993). This modulation in behavior can be attributed either to reduced strength of the association at the time of the CTA or to competition during the retrieval phase (Lubow, 1989). LI-CTA can be used successfully in a method to study incidental taste learning, i.e., learning with no external reinforcer or association. One exposure to the novel taste has a significant effect on reducing the aversion elicited by CTA. However, a critical parameter is the amount of the novel taste consumed at the preexposure (Belelovsky et al., 2005), e.g., consuming 5 ml or less of a novel taste will produce no significant latent inhibition (LI) in rats (Belelovsky et al., 2005).

Experiencing a given taste after its association with malaise will reduce the aversion responses, i.e., the experience will cause an extinction of the learned CTA. The extinction of the association is dependent on the strength of the association, the number of extinction trials, and the amount of novel taste consumed during the session (Dudai, 2006). Extinction can be viewed as imparting an evolutionary advantage when the food supply is restricted and there is a constant need to test the negative or positive effects of a given food.

Two other behavioral phenomena that are important with respect to taste learning are attenuation of neophobia and taste interference. Neophobia to food, as to other stimuli, is manifested in the careful consumption of a novel food/taste. If a few exposures to the novel taste lead to no gastric consequences, consumption of the given food will increase and thus will reduce the primary neophobic response. In a similar way to extinction, attenuation of neophobia will mark a given taste as safe and will increase its consumption in response to other needs of the animal.

An interaction between different familiar and unfamiliar tastes can lead to overshadowing or blocking. However, in interference one taste can interfere with the learning of another taste (Merhav et al., 2006). Specifically, it was shown that when two novel tastes are given before an associated malaise, only the second taste will acquire the association (Best and Meachum, 1986), Moreover, by using the latent inhibition paradigm, it was shown that consumption of a novel taste after another taste will eliminate completely the effect of the first taste (Merhav et al., 2006). This interference was inversely correlated with the time between the two tastes, and could be established only if the second taste was novel but not if it was familiar.

The above behavioral paradigms were established mainly with rats and mice. In all methods, mild water restriction is needed to stimulate the animals to consume the taste in a specific time. However, harsh water deprivation can modulate the behavior, and the behavioral method itself determines the biological mechanisms underlying taste learning (Berkowitz et al., 1988; Bernstein et al., 1996a,b; El-Gabalawy et al., 1997; Koh et al., 2003; Wilkins and Bernstein, 2006). The following are the main methods used in these experiments.

1. Single pipette: Animals are presented with single pipette with a given taste. The amount of intake can be compared with the amount of water consumed on the previous day, following one of the behavioral manipulations described.
2. Multiple pipettes: A main problem with the single bottle setup is conflict between the animal's urges to drink, because it is water-deprived, and not to drink, because it underwent CTA. The most common behavioral test is to allow the animals to choose, during the retention phase, from a series of pipettes containing water or the taste that is under investigation. Usually, an aversion index is calculated (water/water + studied taste). The more aversive the animal is to the conditioned taste, the higher the aversion index will be.
3. Taste reactivity test: The amount of drinking measured in session with one or multiple pipettes does not necessarily mirror the attractiveness of a given taste. This can be measured directly according to several characteristic responses to palatable or unpalatable tastes, in a taste reactivity test (Grill and Norgren, 1978), or via the licking behavior (Halpern and Tapper, 1971).
4. Learning without ingestion: In some behavioral studies, it is possible or necessary, sometimes because of limitations of the experimental setup, e.g., when studying electrophysiology in the anesthetized animal, to test taste learning without ingestion or consumption of the novel food. In such cases, the test is performed by intraoral infusion of the food/taste onto the tongue to elicit the response of the taste buds. CTA and other taste learning can be acquired through this passive experience. However, it seems that learning with or without ingestion could involve different learning mechanisms (Bernstein et al., 1996a).

22.3 Neuroanatomy of Taste and Conditioned Taste Aversion Learning

The sensation of taste involves, similarly in principle to the other senses, chemical recognition but, in addition, the physical features are always associated with hedonic aspects of the sensory input. Indeed, functional analysis of the taste neuroanatomic pathway reveals a strong association with the reward and feeding centers in the brain, including the ventral tegmental area (VTA), the nucleus accumbens (NAcb), the ventral palladium (VP), and the lateral hypothalamus (LH). The central gustatory pathway has been studied extensively in humans, monkeys, and rodents. **Figure 1** shows a schematic depiction of the rat's main taste pathway. Following activation of the taste buds, three cranial nerves (VII, IX, X) convey the taste input to the rostral part of the nucleus of the solitary tract (NTS), the first relay nucleus. In addition, the NTS receives input both from the area postrema (AP), which is sensitive to blood-transported toxins, and from the vestibular system, which is sensitive to nausea caused by motion. Lesioning this part of the NTS induces severe impairment of taste preference, but CTA can be still learned (Shimura et al., 1997). Taste information is that transduced from the NTS to the parabrachial nucleus (PBN) in the pons. The main taste-responsive neurons in the NTS project to medial subnuclei of the PBN, and the PBN projects both to the parvocellular part of the ventralis postmedial thalamic nucleus (VPMpc) and to other forebrain structures, including the amygdala, the lateral hypothalamus, the substati innominata, and the bed nucleus of the stria terminalis.

Yamamoto et al. (1995) studied the effects of lesions to various forebrain structures including the PBN, the hippocampus, the VPMpc, the gustatory

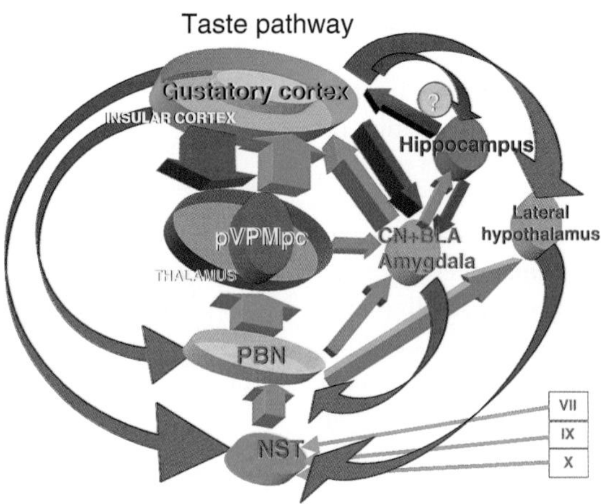

Figure 1 The neuroanatomy of the taste system. The processing of gustatory information begins with transduction of chemical stimuli which reach the oral cavity. Taste can be divided among five primary sensations: salty, sour, sweet, bitter, and umami. Typically, taste cells are broadly tuned and respond to several taste stimuli. The sensitivity to taste quality is not uniformly distributed throughout the oral cavity, and the same chemotopic arrangement is preserved to some degree at the gustatory relay. CN, central nucleus; BLA, basolateral amygdala.

Taste cells are innervated by cranial nerves VII, IX, X, which project to the primary gustatory nucleus in the brainstem (nucleus of solitary tract, NST). The NST sends information to three different systems:

1. The reflex system. This comprises medullary and reticular formation neurons which innervate the cranial motor nuclei (trigeminal, facial, hypoglossal).
2. The lemniscal system. The gustatory portion of the NST projects to the secondary nucleus situated in the dorsal pons (parabrachial nucleus, PBN). The PBN sends axons to the parvocellular part of the ventralis postmedial thalamic nucleus of the thalamus (VPMpc), which, in turn, relays gustatory information to the anterior part of the insular cortex (gustatory cortex, GC). The transition from the somatosensory lingual representation to the gustatory representation corresponds to the transition from the granular to the agranular insular cortex. The GC is thus situated dorsally to the intersection of middle cerebral artery and the rhinal sulcus and can be identified easily using these two markers. Although rodents have only a primary taste cortex, humans also have a second one.
3. The visceral-limbic system. The central gustatory pathway involves a collateral network of connections to the hypothalamus and limbic areas in the forebrain. The PBN is connected to the amygdala, the hypothalamus, and the bed-nucleus of the stria terminalis. All the limbic gustatory targets are interconnected with each other as well as with the PBN and the gustatory cortex. The GC and the thalamocortical system are required for acquisition and retention of taste information. The amygdala is required for learning the negative and possibly positive values of a taste. The prefrontal cortex is involved in CTA extinction. It is not clear what is the specific role of the hippocampus in taste learning, though it is hypothesized that it takes part in novel taste learning.

and enthorinal cortices, the amygdala, and the lateral and ventromedial hypothalamic nuclei, and reported that lesions to the PBN impaired both acquisition and retention of CTA. Other studies suggested that basic integration between taste and visceral inputs indeed took place at the level of the PBN.

The PBN projects to the VPMpc (Hamilton and Norgren, 1984), and from the relay station in the thalamus the taste information is transuded to the gustatory cortex (GC), which resides within the anterior portion of the insular cortex. Small lesions to the VPMpc did not affect CTA learning nor retrieval (Reilly and Pritchard, 1996), but a combination of lesions to the VPMpc and the GC eliminated CTA learning (Yamamoto, 1995).

Humans and monkeys have an additional, secondary area of taste, and it has been suggested that subdivisions within the insular cortex might serve as a secondary taste area in the rat brain. Similarly to the way the subcortical areas convert taste information, as described, the insular cortex also processes both taste information (in its anterior part) and visceral information (caudodorsally to the GC).

The first indication of the role of the GC in processing taste information was provided by Braun et al. (1972). Later, many experimental techniques, based on lesions, electrophysiology, imaging, correlative biochemistry, pharmacology, and, recently, direct imaging studies, were proven to be useful in analyzing the role of the GC in taste learning. It is clear that the GC plays a pivotal role in CTA acquisition and retention. Reversible inactivation of the amygdala and the insular cortex by microinjection of tetrodotoxin (TTX) to these two brain structures at different intervals before taste learning suggested that the insular cortex is pivotal for taste learning, whereas the amygdala is crucial for CTA formation (Gallo et al., 1992). The insular cortex and its gustatory portion can be anatomically divided into granular (normal neocortex), dysgranular, and agranular cortices (i.e., the gradual disappearance of the fourth layer). In rodents, most of the neurons that are responsive to taste stimuli reside within the dysgranular insular cortex. However, the input from the VPMpc terminates in both the granular and the dysgranular insular cortices. A topographical spatial organization of the GC in relation to the various taste stimuli was suggested recently by means of direct imaging of the GC *in vivo* (Accolla et al., 2007).

The experience of taste has other dimensions than the chemical input itself, including temperature and structure. These dimensions were hypothesized to be processed by the adjacent cortex, but also by the granular insular cortex itself (Simon et al., 2006).

The hippocampus, a forebrain structure known to be involved in many forms of learning, has been investigated also in relation to its role in taste learning. The role of the hippocampus in CTA is controversial; however, its involvement in neophobic responses to taste has been reported in several experiments. A temporal correlative response was found in the hippocampus and the GC. However, different molecular pathways were activated in the hippocampus and in the insular cortex (Yefet et al., 2006).

22.4 Long-Term Potentiation in the Insular Cortex

Long-term potentiation (LTP) is an attractive model for learning and memory: Activity-dependent, sustained increases in synaptic efficacy have been suggested to be the cellular manifestation of the learning process (Bliss and Collingridge, 1993; *See* Chapter 11). LTP was first described in the hippocampus but has been investigated in other brain structures, including the cortex; recently it was studied in the pathway from the basolateral amygdala to the insular cortex (Escobar et al., 1998) and in correlation with taste learning. High-frequency stimulation to the basolateral amygdala induced *N*-methyl-D-aspartate (NMDA)-dependent but metabotropic glutamate receptor (mGluR)-independent LTP in the insular cortex (Escobar et al., 1998, 2002). A pharmacological administration of the neurotrophin brain-derived neurotrophic factor (BDNF) locally to the insular cortex induced LTP that inclined slowly in a similar way to BDNF-induced LTP in the hippocampus (Escobar et al., 2003). Analysis of the molecular mechanisms of basolateral amygdala-insular cortex (IC) LTP identified correlative induction of extracellular signal-regulated protein kinase (ERK) activation and muscarine-dependent induction of several immediate early genes, including Zif268, Fos, Arc, and Homer (Jones et al., 1999). In a similar way to novel taste learning and to LTP in other brain structures, ERK was both correlative and necessary for LTP expression in the IC (Jones et al., 1999). It is clear from other studies that LTP and taste learning share molecular mechanisms in the IC. However, very little is known about the hypothesized possibility that LTP-like mechanisms in the IC subserve taste learning. A study that examined the possible interaction between the two found that LTP in the insular cortex enhanced CTA retention (Escobar and Bermudez Rattoni, 2000). However, much more investigation is needed to achieve better identification of the relevant circuit within the IC, and to prove that LTP-like processes underlie taste learning in the GC.

22.5 Processing of Taste in the Gustatory Cortex

Neuronal responses in the GC are driven by somatosensory and chemosensory inputs received from the oral cavity (Yamamoto et al., 1989; Ogawa et al., 1992a,b). Neurons in the GC are responsive to both the quality of a given taste, i.e., chemical identification, and its hedonic value, i.e., attractive, palatable, or repulsive (Yamamoto et al., 1989), and it is difficult to dissociate the two from one another. This may represent a unique feature of the taste sensory information, whereby a given stimulus is always tagged as pleasant, indifferent, or repulsive, i.e., this value represents one of the dimensions of gustatory processing, including the chemical and physical dimensions. Relatively very few cells (<10%) are responsive to a specific taste (Yasoshima and Yamamoto, 1998; Bahar et al., 2003), and most of the others are broadly tuned. Recently, however, direct imaging of the insular cortex was used to reveal some spatial distribution of the various taste stimuli within the GC (Accolla et al., 2007). An interesting correlation between neuronal activity in the GC and novel taste input is that the increased response to a novel taste was not detected until 1 day following learning (Bahar et al., 2003). Currently, there are no good models of taste coding in the taste system. The two main models of taste coding in the neuronal system are labeled line and cross-fiber patterns. Both models are static and noninteractive and are insufficient to describe taste learning (Katz et al., 2002). Another hypothesis is that the anatomical divisions of the insular cortex, i.e., granular, dysgranular, and agranular, serve as primary, secondary, and tertiary sensory cortices, respectively.

A recent review on the subject suggested that the gustatory pathways, including the GC, use distributed, ensemble codes of the various dimension of taste stimuli, i.e., chemical, thermal, and tactile, to produce an internal representation of a given taste (Simon et al., 2006). Other reviews summarized a vast amount of seminal research on taste, olfactory, food texture, and control of food intake (Rolls, 2004, 2006), but that research is not within the scope of the current chapter and mainly addressed monkeys.

22.6 Molecular Mechanisms of Taste Learning in the Taste Cortex

The previous sections introduced the behavioral, neuroanatomical, and cellular levels of analysis. The sections below discuss aspects of molecular mechanisms that subserve taste learning in the taste cortex, within the frameworks of the behavior and the neuroanatomy, in more detail. The working hypothesis underlying the research in the field is that during learning, physical or chemical information about the world is depicted in part by the organism's sensory system, i.e., in the present case, the taste system. This information is transformed into neuronal activity that uses neurotransmitters to create an internal representation of the received sensory information in the central nervous system (CNS). This neuronal creation or modification of an internal representation, i.e., sensory learning, comprises several different temporal phases: Acquisition, which immediately follows experiencing the sensory input, the imprinting of the internal representation in the CNS, a consolidation phase that is divided into two major processes: molecular consolidation, which is dependent on functional protein synthesis in the relevant brain area and is limited to several hours following learning; and system consolidation, which involves the transfer of information between brain areas and which has a temporal domain ranging from many days to months. The consolidation phase is defined in negative terms; it is the time window during which the memory trace is still fragile and can be disrupted by various interventions: behavioral (e.g., Merahv et al., 2006), pharmacological (Rosenblum et al., 1993), or others (Bures et al., 1998). In addition, it is highly likely that the consolidation phase contains subdivisions. For a given internal representation, the last phase is retrieval. However, any retrieval may have the dimension of relearning, as discussed in detail elsewhere (*See* Chapter 31).

Taste learning and CTA are highly suitable learning paradigms for studying the molecular mechanisms of learning and memory. Their relevant features include one-trial learning; strong incidental learning; clear and short learning time; minimal behavioral manipulation, since the animals can learn in their home cage with very little interference from other modalities; clear definition of the sensory input, which can be quantified in molecular terms; and clearly defined cortical area(s) subserving the learning. Within the framework of the present chapter, we will specifically discuss molecular mechanisms taking place in the GC which underlie the various phases of taste learning. It is important to note that two basic means of acquiring information are studies of the correlations between taste behavior and molecular modifications/processes and causality experiments, which show that a given biochemical pathway is necessary for a given phase in taste learning. In addition, it is highly likely that one signal transduction cascade can operate in one brain area and not another. For example, protein kinase B (PKB)/Akt phosphorylation is correlated with taste learning in the hippocampus but not in the GC (Yefet et al., 2006); also, ERK is activated in the GC but not in the hippocampus after the same length of time after learning (Yefet et al., 2006). These examples suggest that from the neuroanatomical point of view, positive correlation between molecular changes and learning is informative, whereas negative correlation can teach us very little. A summary of recent molecular observation related to taste learning and mainly to the taste cortex is presented in the following sections.

22.7 The Neurotransmitters in the Gustatory Cortex Involved in Taste Learning

Information on the physical and chemical properties of a given taste and also on its prominence reaches the GC via different neurotransmitters. Several different neurotransmitter systems are released in the GC, and the relevant receptors for these neurotransmitters are expressed in the GC. These include acetylcholine (ACh), dopamine, noradrenaline, gamma-aminobutyric acid (GABA), glutamate, and various neuropeptides. However, only the muscarinic and NMDA receptors have been studied extensively for their role in taste memory acquisition, consolidation, and retention. I will, therefore, focus mainly on these two neurotransmitter systems and their possible role in taste memory formation. The physical and chemical taste information is transferred from the oral cavity to the cortex via fast neurotransmission mediated by the neurotransmitter glutamate. This is consistent with other known modalities. Glutamate is the main excitatory neurotransmitter in the mammalian CNS, and it acts via both ionotropic and metabotropic effects. However, the prominence of a given taste is hypothesized to be mediated via activation of the neuromodulatory system (e.g., Kaphzan et al., 2006). It is thus conceivable that the interaction between the two systems produces a long-term taste memory trace and that it coincides on specific neurons and probably molecules that can serve as coincidence detectors of the sensory input and its meaning (Kaphzan et al., 2006). Glutamate can affect four types of receptors – alpha-amino-3-hydroxy-5-methyl-4-isoxazole propionic acid (AMPA), NMDA, kainate, and mGluRs – that can produce complex fast (ion influx) and slow (second messenger) changes in the neuron. These receptors are structurally and functionally multifaceted molecules. Microdialysis studies of the amygdala and the IC demonstrated enhanced glutamate release in both the amygdala and the IC, following induction of malaise (Miranda et al., 2002).

Application of the AMPA/kainate antagonist, NBQX, specifically to the insular cortex impaired both acquisition and retrieval of taste memory, which suggests that, in agreement with the general understanding, the AMPA receptor plays a major role in mediating the physical properties of the taste (Berman et al., 2000) and that normal activity of the AMPA receptor is needed to mediate taste properties in either learning or recognition. In contrast to the effects on the AMPA receptor antagonist, microinjection of the NMDA antagonist aminophosphonovaleric (APV) into the GC induced severe impairment of CTA and taste memory acquisition, but not of retrieval (Rosenblum et al., 1997; Berman et al., 2000). Thus, taste learning and CTA are dependent on the NMDA receptor in the insular cortex similarly to many other learning paradigms. Moreover, LTP in the insular cortex is NMDA-dependent, which suggests that similar molecular mechanisms subserve learning and LTP (Jones et al., 1999).

Application of the NMDA antagonist specifically to the insular cortex blocked taste memory formation and reduced the correlative activation of ERK (Rosenblum et al., 1997; Berman et al., 2000). It did not, however, reduce the basal level of ERK phosphorylation (Berman et al., 2000) as it did in hippocampal slices (Kaphzan et al., 2006). In addition, the NMDA antagonist, APV, did not affect the correlative increase in tyrosine phosphorylation of the NMDA receptor, suggesting that this increased phosphorylation is dependent on neuromodulatory neurotransmitters, most probably ACh (Rosenblum et al., 1997). Interestingly, APV microinjection to the insular cortex impaired long-term memory but did not affect short-term memory (Ferreira et al., 2002). These results are in contrast to the dogma that the NMDA receptor is crucial for memory formation but not for its consolidation, and may hint at the existence of unique molecular mechanisms that subserve the CS in the CTA case and that remain active for many hours.

Posttranslation modification and, especially, phosphorylation of the glutamate receptors, was hypothesized to play a major role in learning and LTP induction. The dogma suggests that changes in the steady state of the phosphorylation site of a specific receptor, e.g., the AMPA receptor, caused by modulation of the activity of kinases or phosphatases, alter the function of the receptor so as to increase or decrease synapse efficacy and thus to imprint a new cellular structure in the brain, which is manifested in the formation of an internal representation. However, on the assumption that the kinase/phosphatase modulation of activity is reversible, the memory of such a change is limited to the time span of the receptor that underwent phosphorylation. Different proteins are known to have different half-lives but, in any case, this cannot account for structural stability lasting more than a few days. In addition, the very rapid turnover of the receptors between different subcellular compartments shortens the time during which the receptor is expressed in the brain. Phosphorylation occurs on serine, threonine and, to a much smaller extent, tyrosine residues. However, tyrosine phosphorylation events have been found to be crucial in many cellular functions (Huang and Reichardt, 2003).

In the forebrain of mature animals, the NMDA receptor is composed of the NR1 subunits and a combination of NR2A and B subunits. The main tyrosine phosphorylated protein in the synapse is the 2B subunit of the NMDA receptor (Moon et al., 1994). However, it is clear that the 2A subunit is phosphorylated on tyrosine also, and in response to physiological inputs (Thornton et al., 2003). Tyrosine phosphorylation of both subunits induces modulation in the receptor function (Kalia et al., 2004), and it can be measured for a specific residue of a given protein, e.g., 1472 of the NR2B subunit, or as total tyrosine phosphorylation of a given protein after immunoprecipitation, or of a population of proteins. This measurement can be taken using antiphosphotyrosine antibodies for a population of proteins. Measuring tyrosine phosphorylation using general antiphosphotyrosine revealed that, compared with other tissues, the brain is highly phosphorylated on tyrosine residues in the absence of stimulation. In addition, following CTA or novel taste learning, tyrosine phosphorylation of a set of proteins was increased, but a familiar taste did not induce this correlative effect (Rosenblum et al., 1995). Following taste learning, the main molecular weights to be modulated in the insular cortex were 100, 115, and 180 kDa. At the same time, other proteins were unaffected by learning (Rosenblum et al., 1995). With regard to the findings of many other studies that identified correlations between posttranslation modifications and learning, the following questions can be raised in attempting to understand mechanistically the role of tyrosine phosphorylation in the GC during the formation of the internal representation of a taste:

- What is the identity of the tyrosine-phosphorylated proteins?
- What is the identity of the specific residue that is phosphorylated in a given protein?
- Is this phosphorylation event a mere correlation or a necessary step in memory formation?
- Can similar modifications be found in other learning paradigms or learning models?
- What is the time window and what is the physiological function of such phosphorylation?
- What are the upstream events that induce this phosphorylation in correlation with learning, and which neurotransmitters induce the modifications?
- What, and in which cortical layer, are the cells that are involved in these modifications? What is the localization, i.e., subcellular compartment, of such modification within the cells?

There are answers to some of these questions, whereas others are still subjects of ongoing research. It is clear that the NR2B is tyrosine phosphorylated in correlation with taste learning in the taste cortex (Rosenblum et al., 1997); a similar increase in NR2B tyrosine phosphorylation was detected in the hippocampus following LTP (Rosenblum et al., 1996; Rostas et al., 1996). As for the specific residue, the main tyrosine to be phosphorylated in the sequence of the NR2B is residue 1472. Indeed, a clear increase in pY1472 was correlated with taste learning in the GC. A recent study of genetic replacement of pY1472 in the mouse forebrain identified malfunction in amygdala-dependent learning, and suggested that the localization of the NR was defective in these transgenic mice (Nakazawa et al., 2006). In any case, mapping of the phosphorylation sites specifically on the NR and generally in synaptic proteins, which might explain synaptic plasticity, is currently the subject of proteomic investigation (Schrattenholz and Soskic, 2006).

In order to test the hypothesis that induced tyrosine phosphorylation is necessary for taste learning, the general tyrosine kinase inhibitor, genistein, was injected locally into the GC during taste learning; it inhibited the induced tyrosine phosphorylation of the NR2B and attenuated taste learning, which suggests that tyrosine phosphorylation during learning is crucial for memory formation.

What might be the identity of the neurotransmitter that induces tyrosine phosphorylation of the NR2B? Surprisingly, local blocking of the NMDA receptor itself by microinjection of APV into the GC blocked taste learning but did not affect the induced level of its tyrosine phosphorylation correlated with learning (Rosenblum et al., 1997). Thus, it seems that the process is not Ca^{2+} dependent and is involved in cross-talking with other receptors. Indeed, pharmacological activation of the muscarinic ACh receptor (AChR) in the GC induced tyrosine phosphorylation of the NR2B (Rosenlum et al., 1996). This cross talk between the two receptors may partly account for the important role played by muscarinic AChRs in novel taste learning. An interesting point is that the time window of increased tyrosine phosphorylation correlated with taste learning. The induction was still clear several hours following learning, in clear contrast to the behavior of other phosphorylation events that can be monitored only within minutes following learning. It is therefore suggested that the synaptic tyrosine phosphorylation represents an intermediate phase of molecular mechanisms and that it is not involved in the acquisition phase but rather in the consolidation phase. Another possibility is that this prolonged increase in tyrosine phosphorylation following learning is unique to taste learning and plays a role in the ability of the taste to be on hold, ready for association with malaise.

The involvement of muscarinic AChRs in taste and CTA learning was studied mainly through the administration of antagonists during the various phases of taste learning, followed by microdialysis measurements of ACh in the GC. Indeed, local application of atropine or scopolamine to the GC disrupted both taste learning and CTA (Naor and Dudai, 1996; Gutierrez et al., 2003; Berman et al., 2000). It was suggested that microinjection of scopolamine but not APV to the insular cortex attenuates the acquisition of familiarity of a novel taste (Gutierrez et al., 2003), though APV clearly affected latent inhibition of CTA (Rosenblum et al., 1997). Another study suggested that APV treatment impaired only long-term but not short-term taste memory (Ferreria et al., 2002). In a similar way to the prolonged duration of NR2B tyrosine phosphorylation, this result implies that the NR is more involved in the consolidation than in the acquisition processes. Microdialysis experiments have shown that ACh is released in the GC following consumption of novel but not of familiar tastes (Shimura et al., 1995; Miranda et al., 2000) in a similar way to other modalities. It is yet to be determined whether the prolonged endogenous release of ACh is the physiological reason for tyrosine phosphorylation of the NR; what is the exact function of such interaction? Other biochemical interactions between these two receptors may occur and await further analysis.

The glutamatergic and cholinergic systems were studied in detailed in the GC following novel taste aversion. Fascinatingly, the correlated expression of different immediate early genes in the GC that followed LTP induction was dependent both on NMDA and muscarinic AChR activation. However, the involvement of other neurotransmitters is well documented. Local microinjection of antagonists for the $GABA_AR$, dopamine (D1, 5), mGluR, and β-adrenergic neurotransmitters into the GC impaired both novel taste learning and CTA acquisition. However, only application of the AMPA/kainate antagonist and the $GABA_AR$ impaired CTA retrieval (Berman et al., 2000). A recent report suggests that metabotropic GABA receptors are differentially involved in CTA learning. The $GABA_{B(1a)}$ receptor was found necessary for CTA learning, whereas the $GABA_{B(1b)}$ receptor was involved in extinction of CTA (Jacobson et al., 2006), but the brain locus involved in these manipulations could not be identified. Various pharmacological tools have been used to assay the correlative induction of ERK with taste learning. It was found that antagonists for AMPA/kainate, dopamine (D1, 5), mGluR, and agonist of the $GABA_AR$ reduced the basal level of ERK activation, whereas $GABA_AR$ antagonist induced the levels of ERK activation in the GC (Berman et al., 2000). However, antagonists of the muscarinic AChR, NMDAR, AMPA/kainate, dopamine (D1, 5), and mGluR inhibited the induced expression of ERK with learning (Berman et al., 2000). It is clear from these experiments that cortical excitation is positively correlated with ERK activation and that antagonizing the muscarinic and the NMDA receptors is correlative with both taste and CTA learning, and with the correlative induction of ERK.

22.8 The Role of the MAPK/ERK Pathway in the Gustatory Cortex

ERK1 and ERK2 belong to the mitogen-activated protein kinase (MAPK) family of signal cascades. ERK is activated in and is necessary for the development of several forms of memory, such as fear conditioning, CTA memory, spatial memory, step-down inhibitory avoidance, and object recognition memory. Inhibition of MAP/ERK (MEK), the upstream kinase of ERK, affected both early and late phases of LTP in the hippocampus (Rosenblum et al., 2002). The role of ERK activation in the GC was first studied by means of radioactive kinase assays and, indeed, increased ERK activity was found in the GC, in correlation with novel taste learning. Later, most of the experiments in the field used phospho-specific antibodies that recognized the phosphorylated state of ERK as well as the activated state of these proteins in this unique case.

ERK activation was correlated with novel taste learning, whereas the actual amount of ERK protein was unchanged (Berman et al., 1998; Belelovsky et al., 2005). The time scale of the induced activation was a few minutes following consumption of a novel taste, and it could not be detected after more than 1 h. Microinjection of the MEK inhibitor into the GC prior to learning attenuated CTA memory; examination of other members of the MAPK family revealed that Jun N-terminal kinase 1/2 (JuNK1/2) was activated 1 h following novel taste learning, whereas p38 was not modified at any of the examined time points (Berman et al., 1998). A similar study in mice identified different temporal activation of ERK following novel taste learning (Swank and Sweatt, 2000). Further examination of the phosphorylation of the ERK substrate ELK-1 found a similar time scale for the relation between ERK activation and ELK-1 phosphorylation following novel taste learning as well as similarity in the neurotransmitters that induce ELK-1 phosphorylation in the GC in response to taste learning (Berman et al., 2003). Interestingly, the expression of LTP in the GC was found to be ERK dependent, and ERK was activated in correlation with LTP induction in the GC (Jones et al., 1999).

Similarly to other brain areas, ERK activation is correlated with learning, and possibly mainly with the consolidation phase of learning. Moreover, as discussed, the upstream mechanisms for ERK activation have been studied extensively in the GC and elsewhere. However, we know very little about the downstream targets of ERK or about the mechanisms in neurons that affect learning and synaptic plasticity. Much more proteomic research is needed to identify ERK substrates and to understand the effects of ERK on various neuronal processes, including trafficking, membrane properties, and nuclear targeting. One major role attributed to the ERK pathway is regulation of gene expression and, recently, translation regulation (Govindarajan et al., 2006).

22.9 The Role of Translation Regulation in Taste Memory Consolidation

Memory consolidation is defined biochemically by its dependence on functional protein synthesis within the relevant brain structures (Davis and Squire, 1984). Indeed, local application of the protein synthesis inhibitor anisomycin to the GC attenuated CTA and taste learning, as measured in the latent inhibition paradigm (Rosenblum et al., 1993). However, another study found that the same treatment had no effect on short-term memory, which suggests that short-term taste memory is independent of protein synthesis (Houpt and Berlin, 1999). Local application of anisomycin had a dose-dependent effect on CTA learning: Whereas 50- and 75-μg doses had no effect, 100- and 150-μg doses abolished CTA. This study (Rosenblum et al., 1993) is one of very few that measured the effect of anisomycin on protein synthesis *in vivo*. Local application of anisomycin inhibited more then 90% of protein synthesis in the GC for hours, but not in the hippocampus. Application of the same amount of anisomycin to the lateral ventricles did not affect either taste learning or CTA, and had a weaker and much faster effect on protein synthesis in the GC (Rosenblum et al., 1993; Meiri and Rosenblum, 1998). Usually, in order to achieve an effect on memory and LTP consolidation, one should apply the protein synthesis inhibitor(s) just before or immediately after learning, though some studies have suggested the existence of two or more sensitive periods for application of protein synthesis inhibitors. A recent study determined the temporal phase of sensitivity for protein synthesis inhibitors, and found that up to 100 min following novel taste learning, local application of anisomycin attenuated taste learning, which suggests that the short period after learning, i.e., the beginning of consolidation, is not the only sensitive period, but so, also, is a more advanced phase of consolidation.

As discussed, sensitivity for protein synthesis is a negative definition of memory consolidation. One may assume that following learning there is increased expression of proteins in the relevant brain areas, but it was only recently that scientists began to explore directly the possibility that the translation machinery is regulated during memory consolidation (Govindarajan et al., 2006). Translation comprises initiation, elongation, and termination phases. The initiation phase is the most highly regulated step and it is modulated via phosphorylation of initiation factors and ribosomal proteins (Proud, 2000). Analysis of taste learning in mice that lacked the translation repressor eukaryotic initiation factor 4E-binding protein (4E-BP2) revealed no difference in taste recognition but enhanced CTA learning (Banko et al., 2007). Similarly, mice with reduced phosphorylation of eukaryotic initiation factor 2 (eIF2α) exhibited enhanced taste learning, with no effect on taste recognition (Costa-Matiolli et al., 2006). In addition, it is clear that in these mice other forms of learning and plasticity are enhanced during the consolidation phase. Both the 4E-BP2 and eIF2α mice represent genetic modifications that enhanced translation initiation and thus induced better taste learning and memory. In contrast, knockout mice for both S6K1 and S6K2, which are characterized by reduced initiation rates, exhibited impaired taste learning.

Analysis of the initiation phase suggests a simple image: More initiation, better taste learning. However, the picture is more complex when the elongation phase of translation is analyzed.

The elongation phase requires activity of eukaryotic elongation factors (eEFs). Eukaryotic elongation factor 2 (eEF2) mediates ribosomal translocation (Ryazanov and Davydova, 1989) and is phosphorylated on Thr56 by a specific Ca^{+2}/calmodulin-dependent kinase. Phosphorylation of the kinase inhibits its activity and leads to general inhibition of protein synthesis (Nairn and Palfrey, 1987). Analysis of eEF2 phosphorylation in the GC, following novel taste learning, revealed that, in contrast to the simple hypothesis, the phosphorylation of eEF2 was increased and not decreased, which indicates an attenuation in translation elongation (Belelovsky et al., 2005). At the same time and among the same samples, the phosphorylation levels of S6K1 and ERK were increased, which suggests that the initiation levels were indeed increased (Belelovsky et al., 2005). On the assumption that the increased initiation and decreased elongation were taking place in the same neurons in the GC, one may suggest that this situation might lead to increased expression of mRNAs that are poorly initiated (see **Figure 2** for the proposed model). The suggested mechanisms could serve as a switch-like mechanism to express a specific set of mRNAs for a restricted time in a cellular microdomain such as the synapse.

It is clear that in the near future much more research will be aimed at understanding how regulation of the various phases of translation subserves consolidation processes. Other important proteins such as mammalian target of rapamycin (mTOR) and ERK are thought to be molecules that integrate the information delivered by the various neurotransmitters, in time and space, and translate it into a cellular decision that enables the consolidation of memories. In the near future, these very same molecules could serve as targets for possible cognitive enhancers in the consolidation phase.

22.10 Modulation of Specific Protein/mRNA Expression During Taste Learning and Consolidation

In many studies, a positive correlation was identified between enhanced expression of protein and/or mRNA, on the one hand, and learning in the relevant brain area(s), on the other hand (e.g., Guzowski, 2002). This correlation was assumed to be the positive aspect of the dependence of memory and synaptic plasticity on protein and mRNA inhibitors. As shown in **Figure 3** and discussed in detail earlier, many phosphorylation events are correlated with both novel taste learning and CTA learning. However, two conceptual observations can be derived from these findings. First, the posttranslation modulation that is correlated with novel taste learning is attributed to the meaning/prominence/novelty dimension and not to the physical/chemical dimension of the taste information (**Figure 3**); a familiar taste does not induce these correlations. One may suggest that the synaptic and neuronal activities underlying the formation of the taste memory *per se* are so small compared with the ongoing activity in the cortex that the biochemical methods used in these studies are not sensitive enough

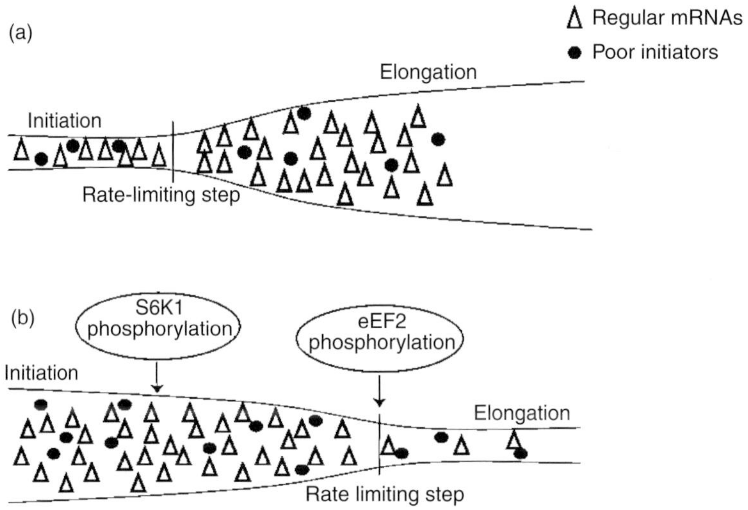

Figure 2 A proposal for the role of translation regulation underlying memory consolidation. (a) In a normal situation the rate-limiting step of protein synthesis is the initiation phase. The amount of protein synthesis is dependent on mRNA availability and the initiation rate as determined by ribosomal proteins and initiation factors. For a given amount of mRNA, regular mRNAs (triangles) are translated more than poor initiators (circles). A component of the intracellular signaling can alter the initiation rate, e.g., as in MAPK activation. (b) Taste memory consolidation is correlated with an increased initiation rate, which can be measured as increased ERK2 activation and decreased eIF2α phosphorylation and S6K1 phosphorylation. Within the same time frame, and possibly within the same cellular compartment, there is also a decrease in translation elongation, which can be detected in the increase in eEF2 phosphorylation. The end result of increasing initiation and decreasing elongation may be a shift in the rate-limiting step to the elongation phase. Together with the decrease in total protein synthesis, the synthesis of poorly initiated proteins such as α-Ca^{2+}/calmodulin-dependent protein kinase II (α-CaMKII) is probably increased. The mechanism described here can perform a switch-like function for various biological processes that shift protein expression patterns within a restricted time scale. In the cortex the mechanisms described can serve as molecular mechanisms that consolidate changes in synaptic strength over time. Adapted from Belelovsky K, Elkobi A, Kaphzan H, Nairn AC, and Rosenblum K (2005) A molecular switch for translational control in taste memory consolidation. *Eur. J. Neurosci.* 22: 2560–2568 with permission.

to detect the biochemical alterations subserving the physical properties of the taste. However, it is clear that some of the observed correlations (Rosenblum et al., 1997; Belelovsky et al., 2005) can be detected in the synaptosomal fraction. Another possibility lies in the strong link between taste and its perceived quality that is less inherent in other modalities. Taste is always perceived as good, bad, or indifferent, and thus the qualitative value of the physical input is a major building block in the memory of any taste.

The second observation is the difficulty of distinguishing between the biochemical correlations with the CTA or with the UCS itself, the malaise. In many experiments, the correlation between CTA and biochemical alterations can be detected following the UCS itself. In addition, the feeling of sickness is a strong input that can modulate several different parts of the brain.

What about mRNA or protein expression in the insular cortex that is correlated with taste learning or CTA?

The most common immediate early gene to be studied in correlation with learning is c-fos. Indeed, acute suppression, but not chronic genetic deficiency, of c-fos attenuated CTA learning (Yasoshima et al., 2006). Correlative studies for c-fos expression were carried out in Ilen Bernstein's laboratory (Wilkins and Bernstein, 2006; Koh et al., 2003; Koh and Bernstein, 2005) and elsewhere (Houpt et al., 1996; Ferriera et al., 2006). Exposure to a novel but not to a familiar taste induced c-fos expression in the central amygdala and the GC. The injection of the malaise-inducing agent LiCl induces c-fos in several brain structures, including the central amygdala and the IC. It is important to note that the posterior part of the IC processes visceral information and, therefore, it is possible that c-fos expression is not located in the same brain loci. The peak in c-fos expression can be detected about 1 h following novel taste learning and the malaise induced by the LiCl injection, and is degraded thereafter similarly to the processes in other brain areas subserving other learning paradigms (Wilkins and Bernstein, 2006).

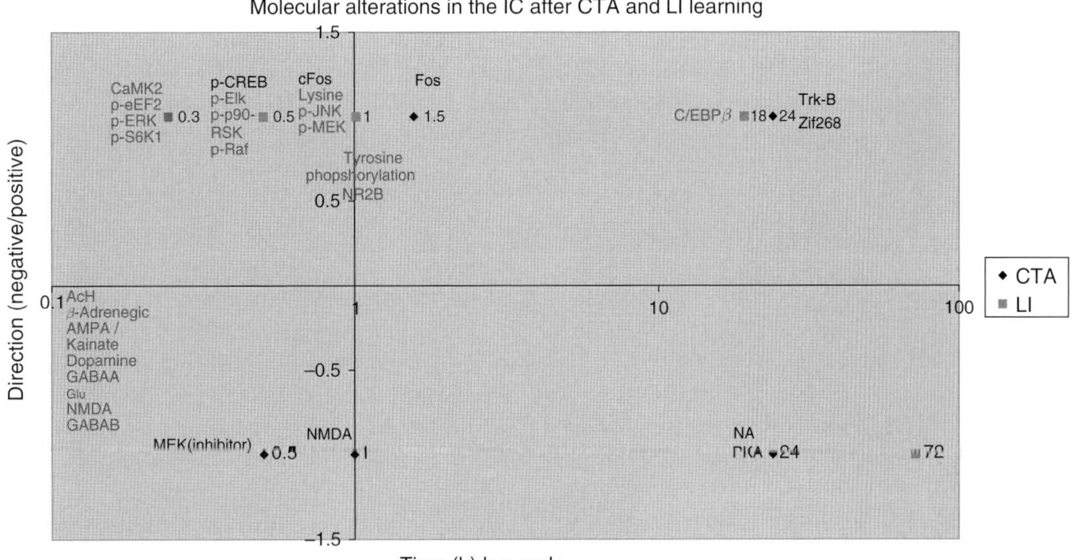

Figure 3 Summary of recent molecular analysis of taste learning in the rodent brain. The figure summarizes recent publications that examine the molecular mechanisms of taste learning; it shows whether the changes are correlative or are necessary for memory formation, and the direction of the changes. In addition, the figure indicates the method that was used and the temporal window of the changes. As can be seen, the research by Swank and Sweatt (2001) that used solid food with high metabolic value revealed a different time scale from that revealed by the other studies, which used liquid. In addition, the data in the figure can be divided into those related to CTA or novel taste learning; gene expression modulation, e.g., c-fos, or posttranslation regulation, e.g., MAPK activation; and manipulation affecting acquiring, retention, or both.

Another protein to be induced in correlation with taste learning in the GC is CCAAT enhancer binding protein β (C/EBPβ). However, the striking difference lies in the temporal phase of its induced expression. C/EBPβ is induced in both the hippocampus and the GC 18 h after taste learning (Yefet et al., 2006). Such late expression can be found following other learning paradigms (Taubenfeld et al., 2001). The correlative temporal increase in C/EBPβ 18 h following novel taste learning suggests that in a simple implicit learning task such as taste learning, both the hippocampus and the cortex are engaged in memory consolidation many hours after the acquisition phase. Moreover, another study demonstrated that this correlative induction of C/EBPβ can be deleted if another novel taste is consumed after the studied taste. A second novel taste induces memory interference that can be measured in behavior. However, at the same time, the second taste interferes with the correlative expression of C/EBPβ. Both the biochemical and behavioral interference suggest that a very long process of consolidation of taste information takes place, at least in part, in the GC (Merhav et al., 2006).

Careful analysis of the literature reveals very few correlations between mRNA-induced expression and taste learning. There are a few reports that identified induced expression of various mRNAs following CTA or LiCl injection (Lamprecht and Dudai, 1995, 1996). These investigations did not observe any modulation in mRNA expression in the insular cortex, following novel taste learning *per se.* Interestingly, LTP induced strong elevation in the expression of various mRNAs in the GC. These induced expressions were dependent on NMDA and muscarinic AChR (Jones et al., 1999). It is yet to be determined whether the major process that induces protein in the GC, in correlation with taste learning, is indeed translation and not transcription. Another possibility is that the temporal window for mRNA induction is prolonged and different from those in other learning paradigms, which would be consistent with the ability of the CS (novel taste) to maintain an on-hold position and to be associated with malaise hours later.

22.11 Temporal Phases in Taste Learning

The main feature of CTA learning is the long delay between the taste-related CS and the aversive internal symptoms (UCS). As a matter of fact, when first published in the scientific community, this long delay put the behavioral results into question (e.g., Garcia et al., 1955). The delayed CS–UCS association cannot be explained as a phenomenon related to transfer of the taste input but as one related to the processing machinery itself within the CNS. In a way that is not clear, a better association is created with a time interval in the range of many minutes than with shorter time intervals (Sachfe et al., 1995). Thus, the system is well suited for prolonged delay between the CS and the UCS. It may be assumed that taste sampling creates a taste memory that remains ready for association, for many minutes. This taste memory trace is both short-lived for an association (usually a few hours) and also long-lived (weeks or more), as can be measured in the latent inhibition paradigm. The creation of taste memory is dependent on the functional taste cortex. One way to study the stability of the taste memory trace, which is dependent on GC activity, is to examine the interactions between taste inputs. Indeed, it was shown recently that taste memory is fragile and can be disrupted for hours by learning another novel taste input (Merhav et al., 2006). This intrinsic limitation of the taste system may be related to its capacity for prolonged association. Interestingly, the interference interaction is only for a second taste over the first one. The inverse interaction of the first novel taste on the second one induces a facilitation effect for the second taste. This facilitation effect has a time window of a few hours; it is shorter than the interference effect and it may be attributed to molecular interactions within the same neuron, i.e., a similar phenomenon to that in the tagging hypothesis model in LTP or to interactions among neuromodulators released within vast GC areas over a long period.

In any case, the unique ability of the taste system to form an association in such a delayed manner presents the researcher with the possibility of studying associative learning in a time frame that allows biochemical/molecular experiments, and not only electrophysiological manipulations and measurements.

22.12 Summary and New Directions

It was clear from the first scientific report of CTA that some of its features do not suit the mainstream learning models (Garcia et al., 1955). The two main differences, which may in fact be linked to one another, are the long delay between the CS (taste) and the malaise, and the built-in meaning of a given taste input. Thus, the chemical internal representation of a given taste always has a value: good, bad, or indifferent. It is indeed possible that any taste input is remembered by its association with its value. Definitely, the biochemical correlates of taste learning in the taste cortex – those that have been identified so far – are always correlated with the novelty of the taste input, which is a major factor in the saliency of any input. This means that, according to the current synaptic-Hebbian view of memory formation, the biochemical correlates cannot be attributed to encoding of the physical properties of the taste input. It is possible that these biochemical and cellular modifications are too small to be detected with the currently available technology.

One may argue that any long-term memory trace is associated with a value; however, it is clear that incidental taste learning (i.e., with no known external associations) is genetically strongly associated with the implication of the input for the animal, and it is clear that food consumption is a major factor in animal survival. Whereas the various senses can report to the brain regarding the potential of a given food for the animal (e.g., sound, color, smell, texture, and shape), the taste conveys the essence of the food for the animal. It is interesting that in Hebrew the word 'taste' is synonymous with meaning or reasoning, while 'vision' (I see) is analogous to understanding in English.

In any case, the perceived value of a given taste can be changed rapidly. The association with malaise is strong (CTA), but past experience (the behavioral paradigm of LI-CTA) and future experience (the behavioral paradigm of CTA extinction) can modify the taste value, and all three learning modes are dependent, at least in part, on the GC.

Taste learning offers unique opportunities to study the biological mechanisms underlying learning and memory. In the last decade, a number of laboratories have contributed to vast progress in this field. The development of new research tools (e.g., multi-electrode arrays, genetic and molecular tools, and imaging techniques) enables us to ask new questions and to propose new hypotheses. Here are some of the major questions that will be addressed in the near future.

1. A major question in the neurobiology of learning and memory is whether the diverse experiences that create the internal representations are

modifications of a major internal representation or represent competition between different internal representations. It seems that the current knowledge of the taste system favors competition between different internal representations. However, further research is needed to obtain better evidence for one or the other of the options.

2. CTA learning is a hybrid between conscious learning, i.e., learning the taste information, and unconscious learning, i.e., visceral information. A major question concerns where this association takes place within the brain and neuronal circuit. The data so far indicate that the mainly subcortical structures, most probably the PBN, subserve the association. New tools and further analysis may enable us to answer this question.

3. Taste information is encoded, at least in part, by the GC, which resides within the insular cortex. However, very little is known about the circuit within the GC, and there are no good models that encompass the correlation between the electrophysiological and molecular information, on the one hand, and taste learning, on the other hand. A major line of research involves dissecting out the functional organization of the insular cortex on the circuit level, in order to better understand the encoding, consolidation, and retrieval processes, and it includes a number of questions. What types of cells produce the plasticity? Are they inhibitory interneurons, or excitatory cells? In which layer within the cortex do the correlative biochemical alterations take place? Does a given neuron contribute to the encoding of different tastes? Where within a given neuron do the modifications take place? The current experimental tools, which provide good spatial and temporal resolution, should provide answers to these basic questions in the near future.

4. Taste information can be kept on hold for many hours, waiting for an association, in contrast to other associations that have time windows measured in seconds. It is not clear if this unique ability represents distinct biological hardware, or if it is a prolongation of similar biological processes that underlie conventional association processes. A major question is how this associative potential is retained for many hours. If the mechanisms are similar to those in other learning paradigms, this unique ability of CS, which derives from processing mechanisms within the CNS, could be exploited to study association mechanisms by means of research tools with resolution times of minutes to hours, which could not be used in other learning paradigms, i.e., most molecular/biochemical tools.

5. The time frame of molecular modifications in the GC that are correlated with taste learning (see **Figure 2**) opens with posttranslation modifications within minutes after learning (e.g., ERK, eEF2; see **Figure 2** for more details), proceeds with other posttranslation modifications to synaptic proteins on a time scale of hours (e.g., tyrosine phosphorylation of the NR2B), and continues with protein expression on a time scale of hours to days following learning (e.g., the inductions of postsynaptic density 95 and C/EBPβ, which occur 3 and 18 h following learning, respectively). A major task will be to organize a temporal and spatial chart of these correlations in order to understand the stream of molecular and cellular events underlying taste memory formation.

In addition, the known identities of molecular events, and their time windows, are in accord with other brain structures that subserve other learning paradigms, for example, the expression of C/EBPβ in the relevant brain structure 18 h after learning. However, some of the events are different. For example, there are several indications that functional NMDA receptor in the GC is necessary for the consolidation phase, in contrast to other learning and LTP protocols, whereas the NMDA receptor is necessary mainly for the acquisition/induction phase. One possibility is that this is a unique feature of taste learning and that it is related to the ability of the taste memory trace to be associated after such a long delay. However, further analysis is needed to understand the role of NMDA receptor activity, localization, and posttranslation modification within the GC during taste memory formation.

6. In the last few years, the role of translation regulation in taste learning consolidation has been studied extensively. The results demonstrate intrinsic regulation of both the initiation and the elongation phases during taste memory formation. Moreover, it is clear that those genetic and pharmacological modifications that enhance the initiation phase also enhance performance. Much more research is needed to achieve understanding of translation regulation in memory consolidation to answer such questions as: What are the upstream neurotransmitters and signal transduction cascades? What are the targets and what are the mRNA populations and their localizations? However, the taste system can serve as a platform from which to study new targets for drugs, to be used as cognitive enhancers.

References

Accolla R, Bathellier B, Petersen CC, and Carleton A (2007) Differential spatial representation of taste modalities in the rat gustatory cortex. *J. Neurosci.* 27: 1396–1404.

Adolphs R, Tranel D, Koenigs M, and Damasio AR (2005) Preferring one taste over another without recognizing either. *Nat. Neurosci.* 8: 860–861.

Bahar A, Samuel A, Hazvi S, and Dudai Y (2003) The amygdalar circuit that acquires taste aversion memory differs from the circuit that extinguishes it. *Eur. J. Neurosci.* 17: 1527–1530.

Banko J, Merhav M, Stern E, Sonenberg N, Rosenblum K, and Klann E (2007) Behavioral alterations in mice lacking the translation repressor 4E-BP2. *Neurobiol. Learn. Mem.* 87(2): 248–256.

Belelovsky K, Elkobi A, Kaphzan H, Nairn AC, and Rosenblum K (2005) A molecular switch for translational control in taste memory consolidation. *Eur. J. Neurosci.* 22: 2560–2568.

Berkowitz RL, Chitkara U, Wilkins IA, Lynch L, Plosker H, and Bernstein HH (1988) Intravascular monitoring and management of erythroblastosis fetalis. *Am. J. Obstet. Gynecol.* 158: 783–795.

Berman DE, Hazvi S, Rosenblum K, Seger R, and Dudai Y (1998) Specific and differential activation of mitogen-activated protein kinase cascades by unfamiliar taste in the insular cortex of the behaving rat. *J. Neurosci.* 18(23): 10037–10044.

Berman DE, Hazvi S, Neduva V, and Dudai Y (2000) The role of identified neurotransmitter systems in the response of insular cortex to unfamiliar taste: Activation of ERK1-2 and formation of a memory trace. *J. Neurosci.* 20: 7017–7023.

Berman DE, Hazvi S, Stehberg J, Bahar A, and Dudai Y (2003) Conflicting processes in the extinction of conditioned taste aversion: Behavioral and molecular aspects of latency, apparent stagnation, and spontaneous recovery. *Learn. Mem.* 10: 16–25.

Bernstein CN, Pettigrew NM, el-Gabalawy HS, Sargent M, Meu Y, and Wilkins J (1996a) The differential expression of a novel intestinal epithelial glycoprotein in various forms of inflammatory bowel disease. *Am. J. Clin. Pathol.* 106: 42–51.

Bernstein CN, Sargent M, Gallatin WM, and Wilkins J (1996b) Beta 2-integrin/intercellular adhesion molecule (ICAM) expression in the normal human intestine. *Clin. Exp. Immunol.* 106: 160–169.

Best MR and Meachum CL (1986) The effect of stimulus preexposure on taste mediated enviromental conditioning: Potentiation and overshadowing. *Anim. Learn. Behav.* 14: 1–5.

Bliss TV and Collingridge GL (1993) A synaptic model of memory: Long-term potentiation in the hippocampus. *Nature* 361(6407): 31–39.

Braun JJ, Slick TB, and Lorden JF (1972) Involvement of the gustatory neocortex in the learning of taste aversions. *Physiol. Behav.* 9: 637–641.

Bures J, Bermudez-Rattoni F, and Yamamoto Y (1998) *Conditioned Taste Aversion: Memory of a Special Kind.* Oxford, New York: Oxford University Press.

Costa-Mattioli M, Gobert D, Stern E, et al. (2006) eIF2α phosphorylation regulates the switch from short- to long-term synaptic plasticity and memory. *Cell* 129(1): 195–206.

Davis HP and Squire LR (1984) Protein synthesis and memory: A review. *Psychol. Bull.* 96: 518–559.

Dudai Y (2006) Reconsolidation: The advantage of being refocused. *Curr. Opin. Neurobiol.* 16: 174–178.

El-Gabalawy H, King R, Bernstein C, et al. (1997) Expression of N-acetyl-D-galactosamine associated epitope in synovium: A potential marker of glycoprotein production. *J. Rheumatol.* 24: 1355–1363.

Escobar ML and Bermudez-Rattoni F (2000) Long-term potentiation in the insular cortex enhances conditioned taste aversion retention. *Brain Res.* 852(1): 208–212.

Escobar ML, Chao V, and Bermudez-Rattoni F (1998) In vivo long-term potentiation in the insular cortex: NMDA receptor dependence. *Brain Res.* 779(1–2): 314–319.

Escobar ML, Alcocer I, and Bermudez-Rattoni F (2002) In vivo effects of intracortical administration of NMDA and metabotropic glutamate receptors antagonists on neocortical long-term potentiation and conditioned taste aversion. *Behav. Brain Res.* 129: 101–106.

Escobar ML, Figueroa-Guzman Y, and Gomez-Palacio-Schjetnan A (2003) In vivo insular cortex LTP induced by brain-derived neurotrophic factor. *Brain Res.* 991(1–2): 274–279.

Ferreira G, Gutierrez R, De La Cruz V, and Bermudez-Rattoni F (2002) Differential involvement of cortical muscarinic and NMDA receptors in short- and long-term taste aversion memory. *Eur. J. Neurosci.* 16: 1139–1145.

Ferreira G, Miranda MI, De la Cruz V, Rodriguez-Ortiz CJ, and Bermudez-Rattoni F (2005) Basolateral amygdala glutamatergic activation enhances taste aversion through NMDA receptor activation in the insular cortex. *Eur. J. Neurosci.* 22: 2596–2604.

Ferreira G, Ferry B, Meurisse M, et al. (2006). Forebrain structures specifically activated by conditioned taste aversion. *Behav. Neurosci.* 120(4): 952–962.

Gallo M, Roldan G, and Bures J (1992) Differential involvement of gustatory insular cortex and amygdala in the acquisition and retrieval of conditioned taste aversion in rats. *Behav. Brain Res.* 52(1): 91–97.

Garcia J, Kimeldorf DJ, and Koelling RA (1955) Conditioned aversion to saccharin resulting from exposure to gamma radiation. *Science* 122: 157–158.

Govindarajan A, Kelleher RJ, and Tonegawa S (2006) A clustered plasticity model of long-term memory engrams. *Nat. Rev. Neurosci.* 7: 575–583.

Grill HJ and Norgren R (1978) The taste reactivity test. 1. Mimetic responses to gustatory stimuli in neurological normal rats. *Brain Res.* 143: 263–279.

Gutierrez R, Tellez LA, and Bermudez-Rattoni F (2003) Blockade of cortical muscarinic but not NMDA receptors prevents a novel taste from becoming familiar. *Eur. J. Neurosci.* 17: 1556–1562.

Guzowski JF (2002) Insights into immediate-early gene function in hippocampal memory consolidation using antisense oligonucleotide and fluorescent imaging approaches. *Hippocampus* 12: 86–104.

Halpern BP and Tapper DN (1971) Taste stimuli: Quality coding time. *Science* 171: 1256–1258.

Hamilton RB and Norgren R (1984) Central projections of gustatory nerves in the rat. *J. Comp. Neurol.* 222(4): 560–577.

Houpt TA and Berlin R (1999) Rapid, labile, and protein synthesis-independent short-term memory in conditioned taste aversion. *Learn. Mem.* 6: 37–46.

Houpt TA, Philopena JM, Joh TH, and Smith GP (1996) c-Fos induction in the rat nucleus of the solitary tract correlates with the retention and forgetting of a conditioned taste aversion. *Learn. Mem.* 3(1): 25–30.

Huang EJ and Reichardt LF (2003) Trk receptors: Roles in neuronal signal transduction. *Annu. Rev. Biochem.* 72: 609–642.

Jacobson LH, Kelly PH, Bettler B, Kaupmann K, and Cryan JF (2006) GABA(B(1)) receptor isoforms differentially mediate the acquisition and extinction of aversive taste memories. *J. Neurosci.* 26(34): 8800–8803.

Jones MW, French PJ, Bliss TV, and Rosenblum K (1999) Molecular mechanisms of long-term potentiation in the insular cortex in vivo. *J. Neurosci.* 19: RC36.

Kalia LV, Gingrich JR, and Salter MW (2004) Src in synaptic transmission and plasticity. *Oncogene* 23: 8007–8016.

Kaphzan H, O'Riordan KJ, Kile K, Levenson JM, and Rosenblum K (2006) NMDA and dopamine converge on the NMDA-receptor to induce ERK activation and synaptic depression in mature hippocampus. *PLoS ONE* 1(1): e138. doi:10.1371/journal.pone.0000138.

Katz DB, Nicolelis MA, and Simon SA (2002) Gustatory processing is dynamic and distributed. *Curr. Opin. Neurobiol.* 12: 448–454.

Koh MT and Bernstein IL (2005) Mapping conditioned taste aversion associations using c-Fos reveals a dynamic role for insular cortex. *Behav. Neurosci.* 119: 388–398.

Koh MT, Wilkins EE, and Bernstein IL (2003) Novel tastes elevate c-fos expression in the central amygdala and insular cortex: Implication for taste aversion learning. *Behav. Neurosci.* 117: 1416–1422.

Lamprecht R and Dudai Y (1995) Differential modulation of brain immediate early genes by intraperitoneal LiCl. *Neuroreport* 7: 289–293.

Lamprecht R and Dudai Y (1996) Transient expression of c-Fos in rat amygdala during training is required for encoding conditioned taste aversion memory. *Learn. Mem.* 3: 31–41.

Lubow RE (1989) *Latent Inhibition and Conditioned Attention Theory*. Cambridge: Cambridge University Press.

Meiri N and Rosenblum K (1998) Lateral ventricle injection of the protein synthesis inhibitor anisomycine impairs long-term memory in a spatial memory task. *Brain Res.* 789(1): 48–55.

Merhav M, Kuulmann-Vander S, Elkobi A, Jacobson-Pick S, Karni A, and Rosenblum K (2006) Behavioral interference and C/EBPbeta expression in the insular-cortex reveal a prolonged time period for taste memory consolidation. *Learn. Mem.* 13: 571–574.

Miranda MI, Ramirez-Lugo L, and Bermudez-Rattoni F (2000) Cortical cholinergic activity is related to the novelty of the stimulus. *Brain Res.* 882(1–2): 230–235.

Miranda MI, Ferreira G, Ramirez-Lugo L, et al. (2002). Glutamatergic activity in the amygdala signals visceral input during taste memory formation. *Proc. Natl. Acad. Sci. USA* 99(17): 11417–11422.

Moon IS, Apperson ML, and Kennedy MB (1994) The major tyrosine-phosphorylated protein in the postsynaptic density fraction is N-methyl-D-aspartate receptor subunit 2B. *Proc. Natl. Acad. Sci. USA* 91: 3954–3958.

Nairn AC and Palfrey HC (1987) Identification of the major Mr 100,000 substrate for calmodulin-dependent protein kinase III in mammalian cells as elongation factor-2. *J. Biol. Chem.* 262: 17299–17303.

Nakazawa T, Komai S, Watabe AM, et al. (2006) NR2B tyrosine phosphorylation modulates fear learning as well as amygdaloid synaptic plasticity. *EMBO J.* 25: 2867–2877.

Naor C and Dudai Y (1996) Transient impairment of cholinergic function in the rat insular cortex disrupts the encoding of taste in conditioned taste aversion. *Behav. Brain Res.* 79: 61–67.

Ogawa H, Hasegawa K, and Murayama N (1992a) Difference in taste quality coding between two cortical taste areas, granular and dysgranular insular areas, in rats. *Exp. Brain Res.* 91: 415–424.

Ogawa H, Murayama N, and Hasegawa K (1992b) Difference in receptive field features of taste neurons in rat granular and dysgranular insular cortices. *Exp. Brain Res.* 91: 408–414.

Proud CG (2000) Control of the elongation phase of protein synthesis. In: Sonenberg N, Hershy J, and Mathews M (eds.) *Translational Control of Gene Expression*, pp. 719–739. Cold Spring Harbor, NY: Cold Spring Harbor Laboratory Press.

Reilly S and Pritchard TC (1996) Gustatory thalamus lesions in the rat: Aversive and appetitive taste conditioning. *Behav. Neurosci.* 110: 746–759.

Rolls ET (2004) The functions of the orbitofrontal cortex. *Brain Cogn.* 55(1): 11–29.

Rolls ET (2006) Brain mechanisms underlying flavour and appetite. *Philos. Trans. R. Soc. Lond. B Biol. Sci.* 361: 1123–1136.

Rosenblum K, Meiri N, and Dudai Y (1993) Taste memory: The role of protein synthesis in gustatory cortex. *Behav. Neural Biol.* 59: 49–56.

Rosenblum K, Schul R, Meiri N, et al. (1995) Modulation of protein tyrosine phosphorylation in rat insular cortex after conditioned taste aversion training. *Proc. Natl. Acad. Sci. USA* 92(4): 1157–1161.

Rosenblum K, Dudai Y, and Richter-Levin G (1996) Long-term potentiation increases tyrosine phosphorylation of the N-methyl-D-aspartate receptor subunit 2B in rat dentate gyrus in vivo. *Proc. Natl. Acad. Sci. USA* 93: 10457–10460.

Rosenblum K, Berman DE, Hazvi S, Lamprecht R, and Dudai Y (1997) NMDA receptor and the tyrosine phosphorylation of its 2B subunit in taste learning in the rat insular cortex. *J. Neurosci.* 17: 5129–5135.

Rosenblum K, Futter M, Jones M, Hulme ED, and Bliss TVP (2000) ERKI/II regulation by the muscarinic acetylcholine receptors in neurones. *J. Neurosci.* 20(3): 977–985.

Rosenblum K, Futter M, Voss K, et al. (2002) The role of ERKI/II in late phase LTP. *J. Neurosci.* 22(13): 5432–5441.

Rostas JA, Brent VA, Voss K, Errington ML, Bliss TV, and Gurd JW (1996) Enhanced tyrosine phosphorylation of the 2B subunit of the N-methyl-D-aspartate receptor in long-term potentiation. *Proc. Natl. Acad. Sci. USA* 93: 10452–10456.

Ryazanov AG and Davydova EK (1989) Mechanism of elongation factor 2 (EF-2) inactivation upon phosphorylation. Phosphorylated EF-2 is unable to catalyze translocation. *FEBS Lett.* 251: 187–190.

Schafe GE, Sollars SI, and Bernstein IL (1995) The CS-US interval and taste aversion learning: A brief look. *Behav. Neurosci.* 109: 799–802.

Schneider K and Pinnow M (1994) Olfactory and gustatory stimuli in food-aversion learning of rats. *J. Gen. Psychol.* 121: 169–183.

Schrattenholz A and Soskic V (2006) NMDA receptors are not alone: Dynamic regulation of NMDA receptor structure and function by neuregulins and transient cholesterol-rich membrane domains leads to disease-specific nuances of glutamate-signalling. *Curr. Top. Med. Chem.* 6: 663–686.

Shimura T, Suzuki M, and Yamamoto T (1995) Aversive taste stimuli facilitate extracellular acetylcholine release in the insular gustatory cortex of the rat: A microdialysis study. *Brain Res.* 679: 221–226.

Shimura T, Tanaka H, and Yamamoto T (1997) Salient responsiveness of PBN neurons to conditioned stimulus after acquisition of taste aversionlearning in rats. *Neuroscience* 81: 239–247.

Simon SA, de Araujo IE, Gutierrez R, and Nicolelis MA (2006) The neural mechanisms of gustation: A distributed processing code. *Nat. Rev. Neurosci.* 7: 890–901.

Swank MW and Sweatt JD (2000) Increased histone acetyltransferase and lysine acetyltransferase activity and biphasic activation of the ERK/RSK cascade in insular cortex during novel taste learning. *J. Neurosci.* 21(10): 3383–3391.

Taubenfeld SM, Wiig KA, Monti B, Dolan B, Pollonini G, and Alberini CM (2001) Fornix-dependent induction of hippocampal CCAAT enhancer-binding protein [beta] and [delta] co-localizes with phosphorylated cAMP response element-binding protein and accompanies long-term memory consolidation. *J. Neurosci.* 21: 84–91.

Thornton C, Yaka R, Dinh S, and Ron D (2003) H-Ras modulates N-methyl-D-aspartate receptor function via inhibition of Src tyrosine kinase activity. *J. Biol. Chem.* 278: 23823–23829.

Wilkins EE and Bernstein IL (2006) Conditioning method determines patterns of c-fos expression following novel taste-illness pairing. *Behav. Brain Res.* 169: 93–97.
Yamamoto T, Matsuo R, Kiyomitsu Y, and Kitamura R (1989) Taste responses of cortical neurons in freely ingesting rats. *J. Neurophysiol.* 61: 1244–1258.
Yamamoto T, Fujimoto Y, Shimura Y, and Sakai N (1995) CTA in rats with excitoxic brain lesions. *Neurosci. Res.* 22: 31–49.
Yasoshima Y and Yamamoto T (1998) Short-term and long-term excitability changes of the insular cortical neurons after the acquisition of taste aversion learning in behaving rats. *Neuroscience* 84: 1–5.
Yasoshima Y, Sako N, Senba E, et al. (2006) Acute suppression, but not chronic genetic deficiency, of c-fos gene expression impairs long-term memory in aversive taste learning. *Proc. Natl. Acad. Sci. USA* 103: 7106–7111.
Yefet K, Merhav M, Kuulmann-Vander S, et al. (2006) Different signal transduction cascades are activated simultaneously in the rat insular cortex and hippocampus following novel taste learning. *Eur. J. Neurosci.* 24(5): 1434–1442.

23 Theory of Reward Systems

S. B. Ostlund, N. E. Winterbauer, and B. W. Balleine, University of California, Los Angeles, CA, USA

23.1 Introduction

Except, perhaps, for the unabashed moralist, knowledge alone does not determine choice of action, i.e., knowing that "action A leads to X and action B leads to Y" does not 'entail' choosing A or B. What enables choice, given this information, is some nonarbitrary means of establishing the relative merits of achieving X or Y. We argue that it is the reward system that provides this means. From this perspective, although the reward system is an extension of the general motivational processes of animals, its function is limited to actions over which animals can exert control and that are instrumental to achieving some goal or other, i.e., to goal-directed instrumental actions. Of course, although most aspects of an animal's behavioral repertoire can be described in goal-directed terms, many of these activities are not goal-directed at all and are reflexive responses elicited by stimuli or relations between stimuli. Establishing criteria for discerning goal-directed and non-goal-directed actions is a necessary step, therefore, in limiting our discussion of the reward system. In this chapter, we consider first the criteria for defining an action as goal-directed and then use that definition to describe the nature and function of the reward system in establishing primary rewarding events, like foods and fluids, both with respect to encoding reward value and to retrieving that value in order to choose between competing courses of action.

This research has established that the value of reward is determined by the quality of the emotional response associated with an event, the latter dependent on current motivational state, i.e., value essentially maps onto the relationship between the specific sensory features of an event and the particular, pleasant or unpleasant, emotional feedback generated when that event is contacted. This issue is taken up in more detail in the section titled 'Reward processes,' where we examine one of the main predictions of this account, that, in the context of secondary rewards, any event associated with a pleasant emotional reaction will support the performance of goal-directed actions. These are sensory events that acquire reward value through association with primary rewards (commonly mislabeled conditioned reinforcers). The procedures used to establish secondary rewards are identical to those commonly used to establish Pavlovian conditioned responses to a stimulus, raising the possibility that the functioning of the reward system can be reduced to the motivational processes that support Pavlovian conditioning. In the section titled 'Secondary reward' we examine this possibility and conclude, based on the extensive evidence standing against this claim, that Pavlovian conditioned responses (CRs) and goal-directed actions are controlled by fundamentally distinct incentive processes.

23.2 Reward Processes

23.2.1 Goal-Directed Actions and Behavioral Control

The critical distinction between reflexive and goal-directed actions is that the latter are controlled by a causal relationship to their consequences, whereas the former are not. There are many illustrations of this distinction but perhaps the most apposite is Sheffield's (1965) analysis based on the salivary response of dogs. Salivation was the conditioned and unconditioned reflex studied by Pavlov (1927). Nevertheless, from a goal-directed perspective, it is possible that dogs control this response in order to facilitate digestion or to improve the taste of food. Sheffield arranged a standard pairing between conditioned and unconditioned stimuli, in this case presentation of a tone followed by food delivery, but with a twist: If the dog salivated during the tone the food was not delivered on that trial. This arrangement maintains a Pavlovian relationship between the tone and food but abolishes any instrumental contingency between salivation and food. He reasoned that, if the salivation was goal-directed then this omission contingency should ensure that they stop salivating; indeed having never had the opportunity to learn that salivating improved the rewarding impact of the food by enhancing its flavor or improving its ingestion, they should never acquire salivation to the tone in the first place. Sheffield found that it was clearly the Pavlovian relationship controlling performance; during the course of over 800 tone-food pairings the dogs acquired and maintained salivation to the tone even though this resulted in them losing most of the food they could otherwise have obtained.

Salivation may be the exception of course, but in numerous studies over the last 40 years it has been established in a range of species that Pavlovian conditioned responses do not adjust to this kind of contingency, i.e., one in which performance of the conditioned response leads to the omission of the unconditioned stimulus. Rats acquire conditioned approach responses during a conditioned stimulus (CS) when doing so omits the food (Holland, 1979), pigeons peck at keys (Williams and Williams, 1969), chicks chase food away (Hershberger, 1986), and so on. In all of these studies, the evidence confirms that the performance of the Pavlovian CR does not depend on the relationship between the CR and the US.

In contrast, experiments assessing the performance of actions acquired during instrumental conditioning have found evidence that these responses do indeed depend on the contingency between action and outcome. Take, for example, instrumental lever pressing. Rats will acquire lever pressing for food quickly and without explicit shaping. Putting this response on an omission contingency, in which responding leads to the omission of an otherwise freely delivered food, rapidly reduces the performance of that response, more rapidly than simply delivering the outcome in an unpaired manner (Davis and Bitterman, 1971; Dickinson et al., 1998). Furthermore, numerous studies have demonstrated the exquisite sensitivity of the performance of instrumental lever pressing to changes in the net probability of outcome delivery given the action (i.e., the difference between probability of an outcome given a response and the probability of the outcome given no response). These changes can be highly selective; degrading one action–outcome contingency by delivering the outcome associated with that action noncontingently often has no effect on the performance of other actions (Colwill and Rescorla, 1986; Dickinson and Mulatero, 1989; Balleine and Dickinson, 1998a).

23.2.2 The Effect of Changes in Reward Value

Generally, therefore, goal-directed actions are those that, unlike Pavlovian CRs, are sensitive to the causal relation between the performance of the action and its specific outcome. It is important to note, however, that lever press responses can be controlled by two kinds of association. The first is the relationship between action and outcome described earlier. After extensive instrumental training, however, performance of an action can become habitual, elicited by various situational cues connected with the action through a process of sensorimotor association (Adams, 1981; Dickinson, 1985, 1994). Although the formation of these associations diminishes sensitivity to omission (Dickinson et al., 1998), it does not necessarily abolish it and, although this test distinguishes actions from Pavlovian conditioned reflexes, it does not provide an adequate assessment in itself to distinguish goal-directed actions from habits. Fortunately, there is a clear distinction between the functions of the instrumental outcome in the two forms of learning. Whereas the outcome serves as the second term of the action–outcome association that supports the acquisition and performance of goal-directed actions, it serves merely to strengthen or to reinforce the stimulus–response (S–R) associations that form habits. As such, the outcome forms no part of the associative structure that supports habitual performance. Based on this analysis, therefore, and combined with an assessment of sensitivity to changes in the instrumental contingency, the standard test of whether an action is goal-directed or not involves an assessment of the sensitivity of performance to a posttraining change in the reward value of the outcome. From an S–R perspective, when conducted posttraining, i.e., after a substantial S–R association has been established, a change in outcome value should be expected to have little if any effect on the subsequent tendency to perform the action. If an action is goal-directed, however, the change in value should potently alter performance.

Consider the case in which a hungry rat is trained to press a lever for a particular type of food pellet. According to a goal-directed account, it is the reward value of the food pellets that motivates performance. Consequently, if having trained the rat to perform this action, the reward value of the food pellets is reduced in some way, we should expect this devaluation to affect performance, i.e., the rat should be less inclined to press the lever after the devaluation. Given this scenario, the question at issue is whether the devaluation affects performance via the animal's knowledge of the contingency between lever pressing and the food pellets. In the first appropriately controlled study along these lines, Adams and Dickinson (1981) assessed this by training rats with two types of food pellets, sugar and grain, with only one type being delivered by lever pressing. The other type of pellet was presented independently of any instrumental action. Thus, any particular rat might have to work for sugar pellets by lever pressing, while receiving free deliveries of grain pellets every so often. The issue was whether the animals would reduce lever pressing more after the devaluation of the response-contingent pellets, the sugar pellets in our example, than after devaluation of the free pellets, the grain ones. Such an outcome could only occur if the effect of the devaluation was mediated by the instrumental contingency between lever pressing and the sugar pellets.

In this study, the pellets were devalued using conditioned taste aversion procedures; it is well established that a food aversion can be conditioned by inducing gastric illness, for example by the injection of lithium chloride (LiCl), shortly after the animal has consumed the food (Bernstein, 1999). In the Adams and Dickinson study, having trained the rats to lever press, half had a taste aversion conditioned to the sugar and half to the grain pellets. During aversion conditioning, the levers were withdrawn and the animals were given a series of sessions in each of which they were allowed to eat one type of pellet. The animals in the devaluation group received a LiCl injection after sessions in which they received the pellets that had been contingent on lever pressing during training but not following sessions with the free pellets. The control group, by contrast, had the aversion conditioned to the free pellets rather than the response-contingent ones. Although such food aversions can be established with a single pairing of consumption with illness when the food is novel, the treatment had to be repeated a number of times to suppress consumption in the present study. This is because the pellets were already familiar to the rats, having been presented during instrumental training.

After inducing these aversions, Adams and Dickinson were now in a position to ask whether devaluing the pellets that acted as the reward for lever pressing during training had a greater impact on performance than devaluing the freely delivered pellets. This result would be expected if the motivational properties of rewards are mediated by their instrumental relation to the action. In fact, this is just what Adams and Dickinson found: When subsequently given access to the lever again, the devaluation group pressed significantly less than the control group. Note that this test was conducted in extinction, during which neither type of pellet was presented, for if the pellets had been presented during testing, the reluctance of the devaluation group to press the lever could be explained simply in terms of the direct suppressive effect of presenting this aversive consequence. By testing in extinction, however, different performance in the two groups must have reflected integration of knowledge of the consequences of lever pressing acquired during training with the current reward value of the pellets. This suggestion was further confirmed by Colwill and Rescorla (1986) using a choice test. They trained hungry rats to perform two instrumental actions, lever pressing and chain pulling, with one action earning access to food pellets and the other earning access to a sucrose solution. The rats were then given several trials in which they were allowed to consume one of the outcomes with the levers and chains withdrawn and were then made ill by an injection of LiCl. All animals were then given a choice extinction test on the levers and chains again conducted in extinction, i.e., in the absence of either of the outcomes. Although S–R accounts should predict no effect of this treatment, Colwill and Rescorla found that animals performed less of the action whose training outcome was subsequently paired with LiCl than the other action, indicating that the rats had indeed encoded the consequences of their actions.

The importance of these demonstrations of the outcome devaluation effect lies in the fact that, together, they provide strong evidence that animals encode the specific features of the consequences or outcome of their instrumental actions. Furthermore, these studies show that instrumental performance is not only determined by the encoding of the action–outcome relation but also by the current reward value of the outcome. In recent years, considerable attention has been paid to the processes that contribute to the encoding of reward value, and the advances that have been made have come largely from asking how outcome devaluation works to change instrumental performance: How does taste aversion work to modify the rats' evaluation of the outcome and so change the course of its instrumental performance?

23.2.3 Incentive Learning and the Encoding of Reward Value

Perhaps the simplest account of the way taste aversion learning works to devalue the instrumental outcome can be derived from accounts of aversive conditioning generally according to which pairing the instrumental outcome with illness changes the evaluation of the outcome through the formation of a predictive association between the food or fluid and the aversive state induced by illness. The result of an effective pairing of the outcome with illness is, therefore, that the animal learns that the outcome now signals that aversive consequence. From this perspective, the outcome devaluation effect is the product of a practical inference process through which a previously encoded action–outcome relation is combined with learning that the outcome signals an aversive consequence to reduce subsequent performance of the action.

In contrast, Garcia (1989) introduced a more complex account according to which the change in the evaluation of the outcome induced by taste aversion learning is not due to changing what the outcome predicts but due to changes in how it tastes. Garcia related the change in taste to negative feedback from a system sensitive to illness that he identified as inducing a disgust or distaste reaction. It is important to see that this view implies that taste aversion learning involves not one learning process but two: (1) an effective pairing of the outcome with illness initially enables a connection between the sensory properties of the outcome and processes sensitive to illness; (2) this association is activated when the outcome is subsequently contacted to generate a distaste reaction and allow the animal to associate the outcome representation with disgust or distaste. This account predicts that, to induce outcome devaluation, it is not sufficient merely to pair the outcome with an injection of LiCl. Rather, a change in value is not induced until the second process is engaged when the outcome is again contacted.

The procedures employed to induce instrumental outcome devaluation, such as that described by Adams and Dickinson (1981), do not differentiate between these two accounts of taste aversion learning because the conditioning of an aversion to the outcome is usually conducted using multiple pairings of the outcome with illness. Clearly the pairings themselves would be sufficient to establish a signaling relation between the outcome and an aversive consequence. But the fact that the animals were allowed to contact the outcome on subsequent pairings could have provided the opportunity for the animals to associate the outcome representation with distaste. If a substantial aversion to the outcome could be conditioned with a single pairing of the outcome with illness, however, then these accounts of outcome devaluation make divergent predictions: On the signaling account, a devaluation effect should emerge, providing that an effective pairing between the taste and illness was produced; on Garcia's (1989) account it should not emerge until the rats have been reexposed to the devalued outcome. In a test of these divergent predictions, Balleine and Dickinson (1991) trained thirsty rats to lever press for water. After acquisition, the outcome was switched to sugar solution for a single session, after which the rats were given an injection of LiCl either immediately or after a delay (the latter treatment, as an unpaired control, should have induced relatively little aversion to the sucrose on either account). The critical question was whether, in the absence of further contact with the sucrose, the rats in the immediately poisoned group would display reduced performance on the lever relative to the delayed group.

To assess the influence of reexposure to the sucrose, half of each of the immediate and delayed groups were allowed merely to taste the sucrose, whereas the remainder were given water before two tests were conducted on the levers. The first test was conducted in extinction to assess the effects of devaluation and reexposure on the tendency to press. A second, punishment test was then conducted in which responding on the lever again delivered the sucrose, which allowed us to assess the strength of the aversion to sucrose. If a substantial aversion to the sucrose was conditioned in the immediately poisoned groups, then not only should a reliable punishment effect have emerged in the second test, but, on the signaling account, responding should also have been reduced in the extinction test in all of the immediately poisoned rats. In contrast, in Garcia's account, responding in the extinction test should be reduced in those immediately poisoned rats given reexposure to the sucrose. In fact, in this and in several other experiments along similar lines, Balleine and Dickinson (1991) and Balleine (1992) found consistent evidence for Garcia's account; although a single pairing between sucrose and illness invariably produced a reliable punishment effect in immediately poisoned rats, a devaluation effect only emerged in the critical extinction test if reexposure to the sucrose was given prior to the test.

These results suggest that outcome devaluation depends upon the interaction of two learning processes. The first process involves the conditioning of an association between the outcome and processes that are activated by the induction of illness by LiCl. The failure of this learning process to directly affect instrumental performance suggests that it is not, alone, sufficient to induce outcome devaluation. Rather, it appears to be necessary for feedback from this first learning process to become explicitly associated with the specific sensory features of the outcome itself for a change in the reward value of the instrumental outcome to occur and for performance to change. Indeed, considerable evidence now suggests that this second learning process critically determines the encoding of the rewarding properties of the instrumental outcome, a process referred to as incentive learning (Dickinson and Balleine, 1994, 1995).

The reason for emphasizing the role of incentive learning in instrumental outcome-devaluation effects is that it also appears to be the process by which other primary motivational states, such as hunger and thirst, encode the reward value of other goals such as foods and fluids. It is well established that the motivational state of rats is a major determinant of their instrumental performance; not surprisingly, hungry animals work more vigorously for a food reward than sated ones. But what current evidence suggests is that this is because a food-deprived state induces an animal to assign a higher incentive value to nutritive outcomes when they are contacted in that state and that this high rating of the incentive value of the outcome is then reflected in a more vigorous rate of performance. Although this suggestion stands contrary to general drive theories of motivation that suppose that increments in motivation elicit their effects on performance by increases in general activation (Hull, 1943), there are good empirical grounds for arguing that motivational states do not directly control performance (Dickinson and Balleine, 1994, 2002; Balleine, 2001). Balleine (1992) trained groups of undeprived rats to lever press for a food reward. After training, half of the rats were shifted to a food deprivation schedule, whereas the remainder were maintained undeprived before both groups were given an extinction test on the levers. Balleine found that performance of the groups on test did not differ even though the shift in motivational state was clearly effective. In a subsequent test where the animals could again earn the food pellets, the food-deprived rats pressed at a substantially higher rate than the undeprived rats. Although motivational state clearly did not exert any direct control over performance, as was found in taste aversion conditioning, the motivational state could control performance if the rats were given the opportunity for incentive learning by allowing them consummatory contact with the instrumental outcome in the test motivational state prior to the test. To demonstrate this, Balleine (1992) trained two further groups of rats to lever press when undeprived. Both groups were given prior exposure to the instrumental outcome when food-deprived before the test in which one group was tested undeprived and the other food-deprived. Now a clear difference in performance was found in that the rats tested when food-deprived and allowed to consume the instrumental outcome when food-deprived prior to test pressed at a higher rate than the other three groups that in turn did not differ. Balleine (1992) was able to confirm that this incentive learning effect depended upon the instrumental contingency. He trained undeprived rats to perform two actions, lever pressing and chain pulling, with one action earning access to food pellets and the other to a maltodextrin solution. All rats were then given a choice extinction test on the levers and chains. Prior to the test, however, the animals were given six sessions in which they were allowed to consume one instrumental outcome when food deprived and, on alternate days, the other outcome in the training, i.e., undeprived, state. On test, Balleine found that animals performed more of the action that, in training, had delivered the outcome reexposed in the food-deprived state prior to the test than the other action.

It should be noted that this role for incentive learning in instrumental performance following a shift in motivational state is not confined to posttraining increases in food deprivation. The same pattern of results was also found for the opposite shift, i.e., where rats were trained to lever press for food pellets when food-deprived and then tested when undeprived. In this case, rats only reduced their performance when food deprivation was reduced if they were allowed to consume the instrumental outcome when undeprived prior to the test (Balleine, 1992; Balleine and Dickinson, 1994). Finally, the generality of this role of incentive learning in instrumental performance has been confirmed for a number of different motivational systems and in a number of devaluation paradigms. For example, in addition to taste aversion learning, incentive learning has been found to mediate (1) specific satiety-induced outcome devaluation effects (Balleine and Dickinson, 1998b); (2) shifts from water deprivation to satiety (Lopez et al., 1992); (3) changes in outcome value mediated by drug states (Balleine et al., 1994, 1995a); and changes in the value of (4) thermoregulatory rewards (Hendersen and Graham, 1979) and (5) sexual rewards (Everitt and Stacey, 1987; Woodson and Balleine, 2002) (see Dickinson and Balleine, 1994, 2002; Balleine, 2001, for reviews). In all of these cases, it is clear that animals have to learn about changes in the incentive value of an instrumental outcome through consummatory contact with that outcome before this change will affect performance.

23.2.4 Incentive Learning as an Emotional Process

Traditional neobehaviorist learning theories argued that CRs, what were called fractional anticipatory goal responses, could exert a motivating effect on instrumental performance (Hull, 1943, 1952; Spence, 1956). Largely due to the subsequent work of Konorski (1967) and Mowrer (1960), however, it is now widely accepted that these effects reflect the conditioning of an affective state that can exert a direct modulatory influence over consummatory responses and, through a change in the emotional responses elicited during ingestion, on instrumental performance (Rescorla and Solomon, 1967; Dickinson, 1989). Recent research investigating the microstructure of orofacial taste reactivity responses in rats to various tastes has provided evidence, not only of specific ingestion and rejection responses to sweet and bitter tastes, but also that the ingestive taste reactivity responses are increased in hungry rats to tastes previously paired with nutrients (Myers and Sclafani, 2001). Likewise, rejection-related taste reactivity responses are increased to tastes previously paired with illness (Berridge et al., 1981). With respect to incentive learning, this approach suggests that, during this form of consummatory exposure, activation of the outcome representation activates its associated motivational system, which, through activation of attendant affective processes, generates feedback in the form of an emotional response. This process is illustrated in **Figure 1**. On this account, incentive learning depends on two processes: a feedback process: (**Figure 1 (a), (b)**) and a feedforward process (**Figure 1 (c)**). Presenting the instrumental outcome in some motivational state or other provides the opportunity for the formation of an association between the outcome representation and the motivation system (**Figure 1(a)**) that acts to open a feedback loop (**Figure 1(b)**). When the outcome is subsequently contacted, activation of the outcome representation acts to produce specific motivational activity that results directly in activity in affective structures productive of an emotional response. Incentive learning

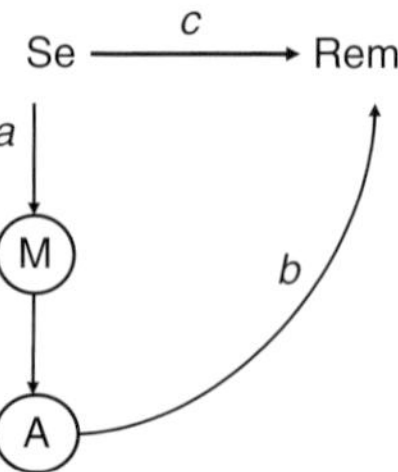

Figure 1 The structure of incentive learning. (a) Sensory features of the instrumental outcome (Se) are associated with a motivational process (M). (b) Through connections with affective structures (A) this connection provides feedback in the form of an emotional response (Rem). (c) Incentive learning reflects the association between Se and Rem based on their contiguous activity.

(**Figure 1(c)**), then, is the formation of a feedforward association between the outcome representation and an emotional response.

Taste aversion-induced outcome devaluation effects provide a good example of this process. In this case, this perspective argues that a taste is first associated with activation of a disgust system induced by LiCl. After this pairing, reexposure to the taste can drive the disgust system to activate the aversive affective system to generate an aversive emotional response. It is the contiguous pairing of the taste and the emotional response that, from this perspective, drives the reduction in reward value induced by reexposure. Notice that, if pairing a taste with illness conditions an association between the taste and disgust, then blocking the activity of the disgust system at the time of conditioning using an antiemetic, i.e., a drug that prevents or relieves illness or nausea, should be predicted to attenuate the formation of that association with the effect that, in the test sessions, rats should prefer a taste poisoned under the antiemetic to some other poisoned taste. But furthermore, if the expression of a previously conditioned aversion, and the consequent change in reward value, depends upon the ability of the taste representation to access the disgust system via an established connection, blocking the activity of the disgust system with an antiemetic during reexposure should be predicted to block the incentive learning effect; see **Figure 2**.

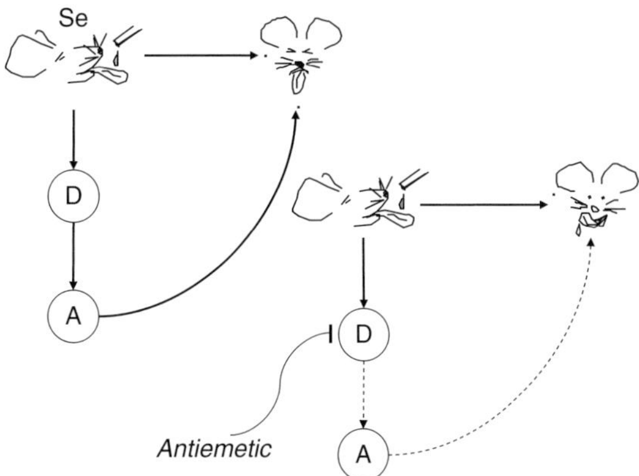

Figure 2 Incentive learning and taste aversion-induced outcome devaluation. The left panel shows the effect of reexposure to a poisoned outcome; the association between the taste (Se) and disgust (D) induced by pairing the taste with illness provokes feedback in the form of a disgust response, allowing the rat to learn about the change in value of the outcome. The right panel shows the predicted effect of an antiemetic on incentive learning. By blocking activity in the disgust system, the antiemetic should reduce the unpleasant emotional feedback and hence the change in value produced during reexposure to the taste. A, affective structures.

In accord with this suggestion, Limebeer and Parker (2000) reported that the antiemetic ondansetron blocked the expression of the aversive taste reactivity responses induced by a taste previously paired with illness. Furthermore, we have assessed this prediction by assessing the influence of ondansetron on reexposure to a poisoned taste on instrumental choice performance (Balleine et al., 1995b). In this experiment, thirsty rats were trained in a single session to perform two actions, lever pressing and chain pulling, with one action delivering a sucrose solution and the other a saline solution on a concurrent schedule. Immediately after this training session, all of the rats were given an injection of LiCl. Over the next 2 days the rats were given brief periods of reexposure to both the sucrose and the saline solutions. Prior to one reexposure session, rats were injected with ondansetron in an attempt to block the emotional effects of reexposure, whereas prior to the other session they were injected with vehicle. The next day, the rats were given a choice extinction test on the lever and chain. If reexposure devalues the instrumental outcome via the ability of the outcome representation to access the disgust system, blocking the activity of that system with ondansetron should attenuate the effects of reexposure such that, on test, the action that, in training, delivered the outcome subsequently reexposed under ondansetron should be performed more than the other action. This is, in fact, exactly what was found (Balleine et al., 1995a). The attenuation of incentive learning by ondansetron provides, therefore, strong confirmation of the suggestion that incentive learning depends critically upon negative feedback generated by an association between the outcome representation and a disgust system.

23.2.5 Retrieving Reward Value

Given the role of incentive learning in the encoding of reward, it is interesting to consider how the value conferred by this process is retrieved to determine choice performance. Because the choice tests are often conducted many days after incentive learning, in extinction the rat is forced to rely on their memory of specific action–outcome associations and the current relative value of the instrumental outcomes. So how is value encoded for retrieval during this test?

A currently influential theory, the somatic marker hypothesis (Damasio, 1994), proposes that value is retrieved through the operation of the same processes through which it was encoded. According to this view, decisions based on the value of specific goals are determined by reexperiencing the emotional effects associated with contact with that goal. With regard to outcome devaluation effects, for example, the theory could not be more explicit:

> When a bad outcome connected with a given response option comes to mind, however fleetingly, you experience an unpleasant gut feeling... that forces attention on the negative outcome to which the given action may lead, and functions as an automated alarm signal which says: Beware of danger ahead if you choose the option that leads to this outcome. The signal may lead you to reject, *immediately*, the negative course of action and thus make you choose between other alternatives (Damasio, 1994: 173).

An alternative theory proposes that reward values, once determined through incentive learning, are encoded abstractly (e.g., X is good or Y is bad and so on) and, as such, from this perspective they are not dependent on the original emotional effects induced by contact with the goal during the encoding of incentive value for their retrieval (see Balleine and Dickinson, 1998a; Balleine, 2005, for further discussion).

We have conducted several distinct series of experiments to test these two hypotheses and, in all of these, the data suggest that after incentive learning, incentive values are encoded abstractly and do not involve the original emotional processes that established those values during their retrieval (Balleine and Dickinson, 1994; Balleine et al., 1994, 1995a,b). One test of these two accounts was derived from consideration of the role of associations between the outcome representation and the disgust system in outcome devaluation described in the previous section. If the impact of outcome devaluation on performance is carried by emotional feedback induced by activation of the disgust system by the outcome representation, then, according to the somatic marker hypothesis, reducing the ability of the outcome representation to activate the disgust system during retrieval of incentive value on test by administering ondansetron prior to the test should be predicted to attenuate the effects of outcome devaluation on performance. This experiment replicated the procedures used in the experiment described earlier (Balleine et al., 1995b) except that, prior to the choice extinction test, half of the animals were injected with ondansetron, whereas the remainder were injected with vehicle. Based on the previous study, it was anticipated that the group given the injection of vehicle prior to the test would perform more of the action that, in training, had delivered the outcome reexposed under ondansetron. More importantly, if activation of the disgust system critically mediates the retrieval of incentive value during the test, as the somatic marker hypothesis suggests, then any difference found in the vehicle group should be attenuated in the group injected with ondansetron on test.

The results of this experiment were very clear; contrary to predictions of the somatic marker hypothesis, the injection of ondansetron on test had no impact whatsoever on performance in the choice extinction test. Whether injected with vehicle or ondansetron prior to the test, the action that, in training, delivered the outcome reexposed under ondansetron was performed more than the other action and to a similar degree. This finding suggests that, although activity in the disgust system determines the effects of incentive learning, the disgust system does not play a role once incentive learning has occurred, i.e., the retrieval of incentive value is not based on the same process through which it was encoded. In line with the proposal that reward value is encoded abstractly or symbolically and in contradiction to predictions from the somatic marker hypothesis position, in this and other similar studies we have found that the processes that determine the encoding of reward value are not required during the retrieval of that value during free choice tests in order for animals to select a course of action.

23.3 Secondary Reward

The suggestion that the reward process supporting instrumental conditioning is derived from an association between the sensory features of an event and an emotional response, together with the evidence for the abstract encoding of reward value, provides an immediate explanation as to how events not directly associated with primary motivational systems can serve as the goals of instrumental actions; from this perspective, any stimulus associated with an emotional response should be able to serve as a goal and so support the performance of goal-directed actions. In the past, the seemingly arbitrary nature of goals has been explained in terms of a process called conditioned reinforcement (Skinner, 1938). Within that literature, this process was proposed as the means by which arbitrary things, like colored pieces of paper, could serve as reinforcers supporting the development of new response tendencies through the acquisition of various stimulus-response associations. It is our view that the term conditioned reinforcement is a misnomer; it implies that the actions that they support are no more than habits. Of course, most human actions are acquired and maintained by goals that are associated with primary rewards and so have only an indirect connection to primary motivational systems and as such are more likely to be goal-directed actions than habits. We propose that the process that determines the acquisition of these goals be referred to, therefore, as secondary reward (SdR). Nevertheless, it is clear that the goal-directed status of these actions is something that stands in need of direct assessment.

There is, in addition, a further implication of this account. Although one should anticipate that secondary rewards will be the more potent, what this account of incentive learning portends is that, if the emotional response associated with an event determines whether it can serve as a goal, essentially any event can serve as the goal of an action providing it induces a positive change in emotional tone. In this section we describe research indicating that both stimuli associated with already established rewards and salient sensory events can serve as goals, allowing animals to acquire new responses based on the relationship of actions to these, sometimes weakly but nevertheless apparently rewarding, consequences.

23.3.1 Sensory Versus Secondary Reward

As mentioned, the older literature dealing with the phenomenon of conditioned reinforcement proposed that when neutral stimuli were associated with reinforcing ones, they could become conditioned reinforcers. A problem widely neglected within this literature, however, is the fact that apparently neutral stimuli turn out to be very difficult to come by. Indeed, the vast majority of experimentally utilized stimuli are demonstrably not neutral with respect to their ability to support instrumental responding even prior to any pairing with primary reward (Kish, 1966). The capacity of environmental stimuli, or more correctly, of change in the state of environmental stimuli to support instrumental behavior can, however, be well enough handled by the current claim that reward value is controlled by the emotional response associated with that event providing it is accepted that change in environmental stimuli provides a sufficiently positive change in that response. From this perspective, therefore, events that are sufficiently mild to induce a positive change provide a source of sensory reward (SeR), whether it is derived from generalization or perhaps by another source of motivation, such as a form of preparatory state produced by general affective arousal (Konorski, 1967) or perhaps, as has occasionally been proposed in the past, by a primary motivational process such as curiosity (Berlyne, 1960).

In order to use secondary reward as a tool to establish the way apparently arbitrary events can become the goals of instrumental action, it is important first to compare the influence of secondary and sensory rewards on the performance of actions. The question is, which secondary reward procedure should one employ to do so? The central position of this notion in Hull's conception of learning (Hull, 1943) and Skinner's utilization of it to explain the origin of human actions without apparent reinforcement (Skinner, 1938) drove considerable research during the middle part of the last century intended to establish or to disprove its applicability to the conditioning process. The most commonly used procedure to analyze SdR has been in chain schedules of instrumental reinforcement, where both instrumental training with the SdR and the pairing of the event with reward presumed to support that conditioned reinforcer occurred within a common sequence of behavior. Zimmerman (1969), for instance, gave rats the opportunity to press one lever in order to obtain the presentation of a stimulus light on a fixed interval. Once that stimulus was presented, a response on a second lever would result in the delivery of food. The stimulus light, via its forward pairings with the food, should have accrued associative strength over the course of performance. Because, however, responding on the first component of the chain also activated the second manipulandum in the chain, it is difficult to assert that the animal was responding for the stimulus rather than the opportunity to respond on that second manipulandum. Chain schedules, therefore, typically require some further intervention in order to partition the sources of support for instrumental responding. In this case, Zimmerman took advantage of the fact that the pattern of responding on fixed interval and variable interval schedules differs to assess whether the light was controlling performance on the first lever as a secondary reward.

To do this, he put the rewarding impacts of the light and food into competition with each other on the first lever. In a test phase, the light was presented as a result of responding on the first lever on a variable interval schedule, whereas the food was presented on the fixed interval schedule that had previously delivered the light and the second lever was shifted to an extinction schedule. Zimmerman found that the pattern of responding on the first lever shifted from that typical of a fixed interval schedule to that typical of a variable interval schedule, a finding consistent with the development of conditioned reinforcing properties by the stimulus light.

Although commonly employed, the difficulty of ruling out alternative interpretations of the source of instrumental performance on chain schedules leaves something to be desired. Since the second response, as in Zimmerman's study (1969), often becomes superfluous in the critical phase testing for the presence of SdR, it follows that it may not be necessary at all. Extinction studies of SdR reify this possibility, by utilizing a training phase where an instrumental action is paired with a stimulus that is immediately followed by the delivery of a reward. Because of the presence of the reward during training, the second, third, and higher components of the instrumental chain used to provide further conditioned stimuli and eventual primary reinforcement in chain studies of SdR are eliminated from the outset. A test phase is again required to detect the role of the SdR in the maintenance of that instrumental behavior. If the SdR plays no role in the maintenance of instrumental responding, then with or without its presence at an extinction test phase, animals should extinguish at the same rate. Instead, researchers usually find that animals extinguish much more slowly when the instrumental response leads to the delivery of the putative conditioned reinforcer than when it leads to no stimulus consequences (Bugelski, 1938).

Although these studies appear to confirm the basic effect, the most direct way to demonstrate and compare the secondary or sensory reward value of some event or other is to assess its ability to serve as the goal during the acquisition of a new action. If stimuli acquire the ability to reward instrumental actions in the course of pairing them with a primary reward, then it follows that one should be able to demonstrate the acquisition of instrumental actions that have as their sole outcome the delivery of a stimulus with a history of this pairing. This logic has been frequently employed in the detection of SdR, and procedures employing it have generally been referred to as acquisition of a new response, or simply, acquisition tests of SdR. Especially attractive is the absence of confounding effects of primary reward during training that could interfere with SdR interpretations of instrumental behaviors (Wike, 1966). Numerous experiments along these lines have been conducted by giving prior stimulus–outcome associations followed by training on a lever that delivers that stimulus. Work by Trevor Robbins and colleagues has demonstrated particularly clear acquisition of lever-press performance when that lever delivered a stimulus that was previously associated with food relative to an inactive lever that the rats could press but that had no scheduled consequences (Taylor and Robbins, 1984; Robbins et al., 1989).

We have conducted a similar experiment to those of Robbins using two different versions of their procedure, firstly to replicate their basic result but also to examine the effects of using a different control condition in which one lever delivered a stimulus that had previously been paired with food and the other lever delivered a familiar stimulus but that had not been paired with any rewarding consequence; a sensory reinforcement control (SeR). The results of this study are presented in **Figure 3**. As is clear from this figure, a good conditioned reinforcement effect was observed in both conditions: responding on the lever delivering the SdR was greater than on the inactive lever (left panel) and greater on the lever delivering the SdR than on the lever delivering the SeR. It is also clear, however, that the net size of the SdR effect is really much smaller than one might be led to believe from the difference between the active and inactive levers.

23.3.2 Do Secondary Rewards Reward, Reinstate, or Reinforce?

Describing events associated with primary reward as SdRs suggests that the responses that animals learn to gain access to SdRs are goal-directed. This is, however, a matter of dispute. It has often been argued in the past that, rather than developing reward value, the stimulus acquires the ability to drive instrumental responding in an S–R fashion, i.e., rather than acting as a goal in and of itself, it acts to reinforce the connection between situational cues and the response. That the conditioned reinforcing stimulus itself might not be the object of an instrumental action, but rather an elicitor of that action, is an explanation that has seen some theoretical and experimental exploration. Bugelski (1956), for instance, reinterpreted his

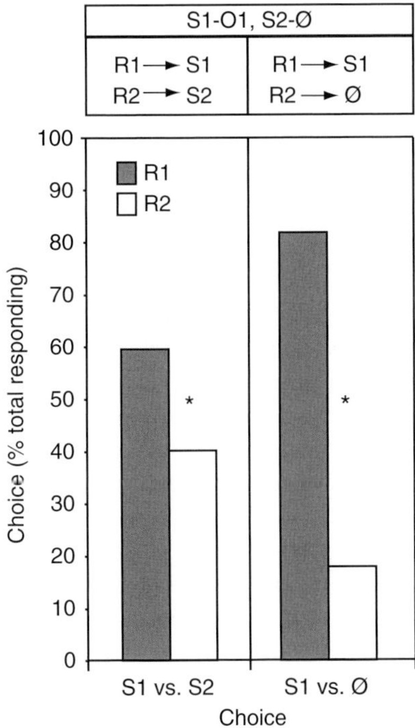

Figure 3 An assessment of secondary reward conducted in a choice test on two levers. Rats were first given pairings between one stimulus (S1) and a rewarding outcome (O1), whereas another stimulus was presented unpaired (S2). Some rats were then allowed to press two levers. In one group, one lever delivered S1 and the other S2 (left panel) in the other group, one lever delivered S1 and the other nothing (Ø). It is clear that both tasks revealed a secondary rewarding effect of S1 on performance. However, the effect is somewhat exaggerated by the choice between S1 and Ø. When sensory reward is taken into consideration, as it is in the choice between S1 and S2, the net secondary reward effect is significantly smaller.

earlier extinction test-conditioned reinforcement data (Bugelski, 1938) using this framework and found that it provided a satisfactory account of the results. During acquisition training, the SdR not only follows the instrumental response as a consequence, but on all trials except the first bears a forward predictive relationship with later occurrences of that response. It is at least possible that during acquisition the instrumental action is reinforced solely by the primary reinforcer, whereas the SdR becomes associated with the response itself. In extinction, it is argued, the conditioned reinforcer then acts, following the first response, to delay extinction through this conditioned ability to evoke or reinstate subsequent instrumental responses.

Wyckoff (1959) attempted to produce a quantitative model of SdR effects emphasizing the eliciting function, or cue properties, of the conditioned reinforcer. This model was based on the results of an experiment reported by Wyckoff et al. (1958) in which rats were given conditioning trials where a buzzer was followed by the delivery of water. Following this training, experimental rats were given the opportunity to press a lever in order to secure the delivery of the buzzer without water, and control rats were placed on an omission schedule, where the buzzer was delivered if they refrained from pressing the lever. Performance between the two groups was not reliably different, which led Wyckoff et al. to conclude that the buzzer functioned primarily not to reward lever pressing, in which case the experimental group should have pressed significantly more than the control animals, but to elicit lever pressing. This result, however, has not been replicated, suggesting that some feature of the experimental design, or a simple lack of power, prevented Wyckoff et al. from observing cue-independent conditioned reinforcing effects. Indeed, Ward (1960) conducted a formally very similar experiment, substituting food reward for water and the random delivery of the cue in the control group for the omission schedule, and demonstrated a reliably greater level of responding in experimental animals than in control animals.

An important source of evidence against the response elicitation account of SdR effects comes from an experimental series performed by Crowder and his colleagues. They employed a yoked control procedure in several different paradigms to demonstrate the existence of secondary reward above and beyond the effects of stimulus-based response elicitation. In all experiments, the experimental animals performed an instrumental action that was followed by the delivery of SdR. At the same time as that delivery, the yoked controls received noncontingent presentation of that same stimulus. If the stimulus elicited or reinstated further responding, it should have done so equally in both groups. Instead, in the extinction test paradigm (Crowder et al., 1959a), the acquisition of a new response paradigm (Crowder et al., 1959b), and in reacquisition (Crowder et al., 1959c) and retention SdR paradigms (Crowder et al., 1959d), they found superior performance in the experimental subjects whose actions were correlated with the delivery of the SdR. Although these results are not completely immune to criticism derived from the analysis of systematic sources of error in the yoked group (Church, 1964), they indicate the relatively small degree of support that elicitation or reinstatement accounts provide for instrumental responding in SdR paradigms.

One published study has attempted to assess whether lever pressing for the SdR is goal-directed by devaluing the primary reward previously associated with the SdR (Parkinson et al., 2005). In this study rats were given pairings of a light stimulus paired with sugar after which the sugar was paired with illness. Although this reduced responding to the sucrose, it did not affect the ability of the light to serve as a secondary reward for lever pressing; lever pressing was acquired and maintained to a comparable degree whether the sucrose had been devalued or not. The authors concluded that, as the lever pressing appeared to be independent of the value of the primary reward, performance acquired through SdR should be considered habitual. But what was not confirmed in this study, however, was whether the devaluation of the sucrose was successful in modifying the reward value of the light. Indeed, as the SdR value depends on the association of the light with the emotional response elicited by the sucrose, rather than by the sucrose itself (see **Figure 4**), it seems unlikely that SdR could be undermined in this way. Rather, what this account predicts is that devaluation of the SdR could only be induced by counterconditioning, i.e., pairing the light previously paired with sucrose with a noxious consequence, such as foot shock. Would lever pressing still have been maintained after this treatment? To date no studies along these lines have been conducted, although there is plenty of evidence from studies of conditioned punishment to conclude that at least the sensory rewarding component of stimuli is abolished by this means of devaluation (Killcross et al., 1997).

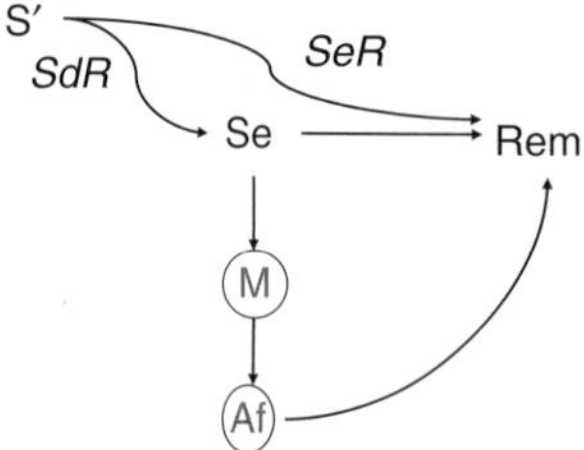

Figure 4 Sensory reward (SeR) is derived from the emotional effects (Rem) of stimulus change that can be produced by the presentation of even quite neutral stimuli (such as S′). Secondary reward (SdR) is derived from the pairing of S′ with an excitatory sensory event (Se in this diagram) previously established as a primary reward and through its association with an emotional response generated by its connection with both motivational (M) and affective (Af) processes (see **Figure 1**).

Other studies from our laboratory have, however, confirmed that actions acquired for a secondary reward are essentially goal-directed. As discussed with respect to primary reward, one of the criteria for defining an action as goal-directed is that it is sensitive to the causal relationship between the action and reward. In this experiment, rats were first given pairings between two distinct visual cues with one cue paired with sucrose and the other with food pellets. After this training, the rats were trained to press two levers, each associated with a different visual cue. In these sessions, one of the visual cues was also presented noncontingently; as such the noncontingent cue was the same as that presented contingent on pressing one lever but different from that presented for pressing the other lever. As such the specific R-SdR contingency was maintained on one lever but was degraded on the other. The results of this study are presented in **Figure 5**. As is clear from this figure, the rats were sensitive to the specific lever press–SdR contingency, reducing performance on the action delivering the same SdR as that delivered noncontingently relative to the other action. This result is not consistent with either the reinforcing or reinstating functions of SdRs (Winterbauer, 2006).

An important aspect of the establishment of a secondary reward is its pairing with primary reward. The procedures that establish SdRs are, in fact, identical to those used to establish Pavlovian CRs to a stimulus. The possibility that stimuli require something more than Pavlovian conditioning to become conditioned reinforcers has been entertained; Skinner (1938) proposed, for example, in a thesis later considered in detail in the work of Keller and Schoenfeld (1950), that only stimuli that act to set the occasion for responding to other Pavlovian stimuli could serve as SdRs. Again, as Wike (1966) suggested, although occasion setters may make better SdRs, there seems to be no requirement that all conditioned reinforcers be occasion setters. Work in our laboratory has largely confirmed this view, in that we show perfectly reasonable SdR effects without special modifications to the Pavlovian conditioning phase (Winterbauer, 2006). But this raises an important issue: If SdR can be established using Pavlovian procedures, are the processes underlying reward and those underlying Pavlovian incentive motivation all one and the same? Or is this no more than a superficial, procedural similarity?

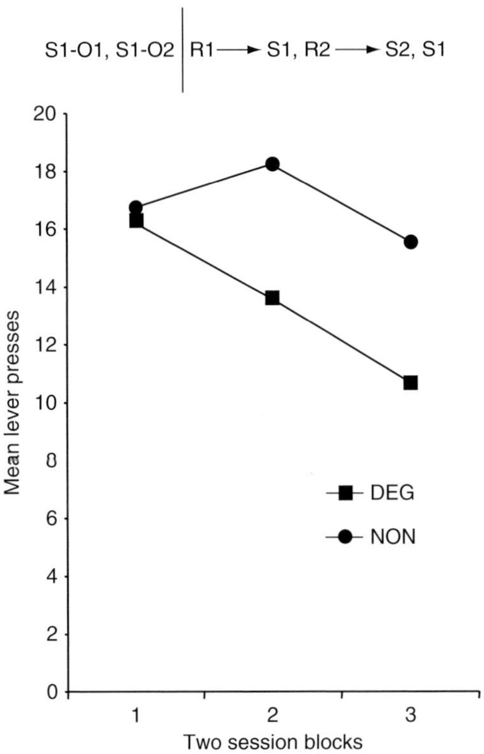

Figure 5 Contingency degradation in instrumental conditioning using secondary rewards. After establishing two stimuli (S1 and S2) as secondary rewards by pairing them with primary rewards, rats were trained to perform two lever-press responses (R1 and R2) with one earning S1 and the other S2. Noncontiguous presentations of one secondary reward (e.g., S1) degraded the response–outcome contingency (DEG) and caused a significant reduction in responding on the lever delivering S1 (DEG) relative to that delivering S2 (NON).

23.4 Reward and the Anticipation of Reward

The preceding sections have reviewed the considerable evidence suggesting that the influence of changes in reward value on goal-directed instrumental actions is an important determinant of action selection and of instrumental performance generally. Other factors can clearly influence performance, however. One of the most obvious, and perhaps best-documented, influences on action selection is that produced by stimuli 'associated' with reward. Advertising has a clear influence on action selection; if it did not the advertising industry would be a vacuous waste of time and of advertisers' money. Of course, advertisers are hoping that the stimuli that they associate with a particular product will provide the basis for quite specific changes in choice performance and, of course, by and large they do. It is important to recognize, however, that, despite a superficial similarity in some of the procedures used to establish the reward value of particular events, notably SdRs, there is substantial evidence suggesting that the influence of cues associated with reward on goal-directed instrumental actions is not mediated by the reward system. In this section, we describe this evidence as it has emerged from analyses of the relationship between Pavlovian and instrumental conditioning, particularly those proposing that the motivational processes engaged by reward and by the anticipation of reward are the same or, at the very least, interact with one another.

23.4.1 Pavlovian-Instrumental Interactions

In fact, some of the earliest evidence that the representation of the instrumental outcome takes part in action selection was found by studying how Pavlovian and instrumental learning processes interact. For instance, Trapold (1970) trained rats on a biconditional discrimination in which, on any given trial, subjects were allowed to choose between two actions (left and right lever press). Trials were initiated by the presentation of one of two discriminative stimuli (tone and clicker), signaling which of the actions would be rewarded (e.g., S1 → R1 and S2 → R2). The novel feature of this experiment, however, was that these cues also signaled the identity of the outcome that could be earned on that trial. Whereas the control groups earned either food pellets (food control) or sucrose solution (sucrose control) on both actions (e.g., S1 → R1 → O1 and S2 → R1 → O1), the experimental group was rewarded with one outcome (O1; e.g., pellets) for performing one action and a different outcome (O2; e.g., sucrose) for performing the other action (e.g., S1 → R1 → O1 and S2 → R2 → O2). Consequently, the experimental group differed from the control groups in that, for the former, each discriminative stimulus signaled not only a different response but also a different outcome. Interestingly, Trapold (1970) found that the experimental group acquired more rapidly than either control group despite the fact that the S–R arrangements needed to solve the discrimination were the same across conditions.

This phenomenon, known as the differential outcomes effect, provides clear evidence that reward expectations can be used to guide action selection.

Moreover, the representation mediating this effect appears to consist of richly detailed information about the sensory properties of the reward. In Trapold's (1970) study, the sucrose solution and grain-based pellets used to differentially reward the two actions were both nutritive outcomes and so should have held a similar incentive value for hungry rats. Since this motivational variable does not appear to have been used to discriminate between actions, rats probably relied instead on the sensory features (e.g., texture, odor, taste) of the anticipated outcome. There is even evidence that this effect can be obtained using outcomes that differ in one motivationally irrelevant sensory feature. Fedorchak and Bolles (1986) trained thirsty rats on a biconditional lever press discrimination task in which each correct response was rewarded with water. For two groups, the delivery of water was occasionally paired with a flashing light; whereas the light exclusively followed just one of the two S–R arrangements in the differential outcomes group, it followed both responses with an equal probability in the nondifferential control group. For a third group, the light was never paired with water. Once again, the group that received differential outcomes acquired more rapidly than the other two groups, demonstrating that the expectancy of a sensory event extraneous to outcome itself could be used to guide action selection.

How does differential outcomes training provide an advantage in discriminating between two actions? Clearly, it must have something to do with the Pavlovian contingencies embedded in the task (see **Figure 6**, top panel). It has long been argued that Pavlovian learning plays an important role in the control of instrumental performance (Rescorla and Solomon, 1967). Although we will discuss alternative accounts shortly, let us first consider the model Trapold and Overmier (1972) devised to explain the differential outcomes effect and similar findings (see **Figure 6**, middle panel). Their model was built within the general framework of traditional S–R theory (Hull, 1943), and so instrumental learning was assumed to involve the gradual recruitment of S–R associations through a conventional reinforcement process. However, Trapold and Overmier (1972) proposed that reward deliveries engage a second, Pavlovian learning process capable of supporting the acquisition of stimulus–reward associations. It was argued that through such learning, stimuli acquired the capacity to elicit a reward expectancy comprising the sensory features of that event. The final step in their argument was in allowing this reward

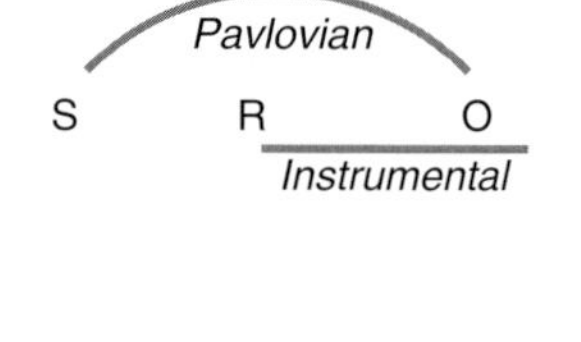

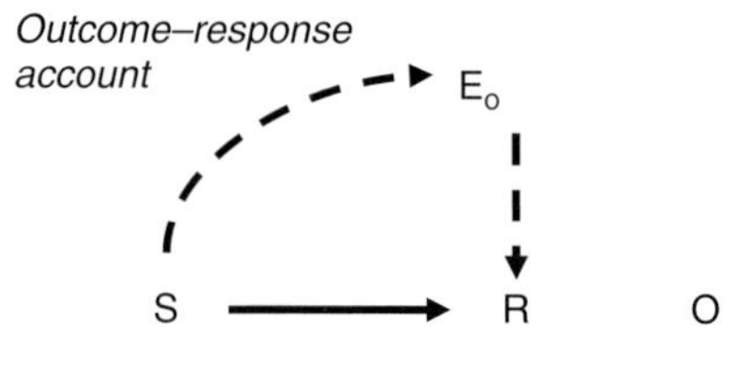

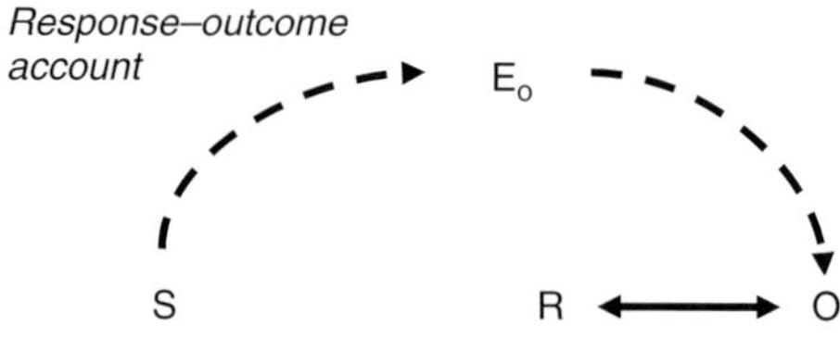

Figure 6 Schematic diagrams illustrating the associative structure proposed to underlie instrumental conditioning on various accounts. As shown in the top panel, the introduction of an instrumental (R–O) contingency is typically accompanied by an imbedded Pavlovian (S–O) contingency, arising from incidental pairings between contextual cues and reward. Two-process accounts of action selection have proposed that Pavlovian learning results in the generation of an outcome expectancy (E_o), which may guide performance by entering into association with the instrumental response (middle panel), or by retrieving any response that had earned the expected outcome (bottom panel).

expectancy to enter into S–R associations like any other sensorial event in the training environment, i.e., the expectation of reward was assumed to acquire discriminative control over performance. According to this analysis, the experimental group in Trapold's (1970) study was provided with an additional source of stimulus support for action selection; the correct choice was signaled by both an auditory cue and an expectation of the reward that could be earned on that trial.

The differential outcomes effect provides strong evidence that the Pavlovian learning can influence instrumental performance through a highly specific representation of the mediating outcome. Further evidence for this claim comes from studies of the so-called Pavlovian-instrumental transfer effect. For instance, Kruse et al. (1983) first trained rats using a biconditional procedure quite similar to that used in differential outcomes studies (e.g., Trapold, 1970;

Fedorchak and Bolles, 1986), such that each stimulus (clicker and tone) signaled both the response (left or right lever) that would be rewarded and the identity of its outcome (pellets or sucrose solution). During a separate Pavlovian training phase, the group of interest to our current discussion received pairings between a stimulus (pause in the background white noise) and one of the two outcomes (either pellets or sucrose). In a subsequent test phase, Kruse et al. (1983) found that presentations of this stimulus facilitated instrumental performance in an outcome-dependent manner; rats preferentially increased their performance of the action that had shared a common outcome with that cue, relative to the other action. Importantly, this test was conducted in extinction, indicating that this effect relied entirely on information acquired during earlier training phases.

Following Kruse et al. (1983), there have been numerous demonstrations of outcome-specific transfer (Colwill and Rescorla, 1988), even using actions that had been acquired through free operant training (Colwill and Motzkin, 1994; Delamater, 1995; Holland, 2004). The latter finding is important because it reveals that Pavlovian learning can influence action selection even under conditions in which anticipating reward provides no obvious advantage in obtaining reward. According to Trapold and Overmier (1972), the transfer effect emerges because the Pavlovian outcome expectancy selectively retrieves the response it signaled during training through the activation of an outcome–response association (see **Figure 6**, top panel). This account applies equally well to the free operant situation. Note that in any instrumental conditioning study there exists an embedded Pavlovian relationship between contextual cues and the reward delivery. In this case, cues that best predict reward should come to elicit an expectancy of reward capable of entering into association with the response.

Of course, the two-process account of Trapold and Overmier (1972) does not provide the only explanation for the influence of Pavlovian reward expectancies over instrumental performance. For instance, several two-process theories have been proposed that assume instrumental learning involves encoding some approximation of the action–outcome contingency arranged by the experimenter (Bolles, 1972; Asratyan, 1974). According to this view, Pavlovian outcome expectancies guide action selection by retrieving the action that had actually earned that outcome during training (see **Figure 6**, bottom panel).

23.4.2 The Two-Process Account of Reward Value

How is Pavlovian-instrumental transfer relevant to our interpretation of instrumental performance as an instance of goal-directed action? Recall that in order to be considered goal-directed, a behavior must be performed because of its expected consequences; performance should depend on the subject's capacity to (1) anticipate the outcome of the action (i.e., action–outcome learning) and (2) evaluate the incentive properties of that outcome (i.e., incentive learning). Two-process theories, however, tend to attribute incentive effects, such as the sensitivity of instrumental performance to outcome devaluation, to the Pavlovian process (Rescorla and Solomon, 1967). These accounts typically assume that Pavlovian learning provides the motivational support for instrumental performance. Even Trapold and Overmier (1972), who took an expressly associative approach, entertained the possibility that incentive manipulations have their effect by disrupting the capacity of the Pavlovian outcome expectancy to mediate response selection (e.g., through generalization decrement). Others have taken a more explicitly motivational position. Bolles (1972), for instance, proposed that Pavlovian and instrumental processes interact based on their shared outcome expectancies, but that this interaction is gated by the incentive value of mediating outcome. The two-process approach, therefore, provides a compelling explanation for the influence of reward value over performance. According to this account, instrumental responding is depressed following outcome devaluation, not because of a reduction in the reward value of the outcome and knowledge of the underlying response–outcome contingency, but because this treatment diminishes the Pavlovian support for performance.

The claim that Pavlovian learning plays a part in action selection is beyond doubt. The critical question, however, is whether these processes are responsible for the influence of reward value over performance. If so, it would be necessary to abandon the goal-directed interpretation of instrumental performance altogether. Note that since the two-process account uses the Pavlovian–instrumental interaction responsible for transfer to explain the sensitivity of performance to outcome devaluation, it predicts that these two apparently distinct forms of action selection should share a common associative structure. One way to evaluate this prediction, therefore, is to assess whether the associations guiding transfer and outcome devaluation are acquired at roughly the same rate. For instance, it has been repeatedly shown that, while sensitivity to outcome devaluation emerges with rather limited training (Holland, 2004; Yin et al., 2005), depending on training parameters used (e.g., number of action–outcome contingencies), this effect is either maintained (Colwill and Rescorla, 1985a) or attenuated (Adams, 1981; Holland, 2004) with training that is more extensive. Alternatively, recent evidence suggests that Pavlovian-instrumental transfer increases in magnitude with more extensive instrumental training (Holland, 2004).

It should also be possible to evaluate the two-process account by analyzing the content of the associations that mediate transfer and outcome devaluation. However, it is important to remember that individual two-process theories do not agree on what that content should be. Trapold and Overmier (1972), for instance, argued that the response becomes associated with an expectancy of reward generated by prevailing stimuli, resulting in an outcome–response association. As we have mentioned, others (e.g., Asratyan, 1974; Bolles, 1972) have proposed that the response becomes associated with the outcome it actually produces during training, in the form of a response–outcome association. Two-process theories, therefore, can be distinguished by determining whether the association responsible for action selection reflects the actual response–outcome contingency, or whether it is, instead, the product of the incidental stimulus–outcome contingency present during training. However, investigating the relative contribution of these two contingencies to instrumental learning is no trivial task. In any typical instrumental conditioning study, the outcome earned by the response is also predicted by the prevailing situational cues (i.e., the anticipated and earned outcomes are the same). Thus, one approach to the problem is to create a training situation in which this in not the case.

Several studies have used this basic strategy to assess the associative structure underlying transfer and outcome devaluation. For instance, Colwill (1994) reported evidence of outcome selective transfer with responses that had been concurrently trained on distinct action–outcome contingencies. Similarly, Colwill and Rescorla (1985b) reported that rats display an outcome-specific devaluation effect after concurrent training of this kind. Since rats given concurrent training are allowed to alternate freely between responses, the context should be associated equally with both outcomes, thereby preventing the development of specific outcome–response associations. The specificity of transfer and outcome devaluation despite this treatment, therefore, seems to suggest that both effects can be supported by response–outcome learning.

Rescorla and Colwill (1989) and Rescorla (1992) have attempted more directly to compare the relative contribution of outcome–response and response–outcome associations to these effects. For instance, Rescorla and Colwill (1989) investigated this issue by first pretraining rats on a common nose-poke response with four distinct stimuli; two stimuli (S1 and S3) signaled a pellet reward and two others (S2 and S4) signaled a sucrose solution. Next, they were given discrimination training on two responses (R1 and R2), such that one response, say R1, earned pellets and the other response, R2, earned sucrose. However, each response was also signaled by a stimulus that had previously been paired with the alternative outcome (i.e., S2 → R1 → O1 and S1 → R2 → O2). According to Trapold and Overmier's (1972) two-process account, this should have resulted in the formation of, for example, a sucrose–R1 association, even though R1 had actually been followed by pellets. During the transfer test, rats were allowed to perform each response in extinction while S3 and S4 were occasionally presented. In contrast to the predictions of the outcome–response view, it was found that stimulus presentations selectively facilitated performance based on the identity of the outcome that 'followed' a response during training (e.g., S3 increased R1 relative to R2). Furthermore, in a separate experiment, Rescorla and Colwill (1989) used the same strategy to investigate the structure underlying outcome devaluation performance. They found that, as with transfer, the sensitivity of instrumental performance to reward value was dominated by response–outcome learning; performance was suppressed by devaluing the outcome that the action had actually earned during training, not the outcome that was signaled by the discriminative stimulus (e.g., devaluing O1 decreased R1 relative to R2).

There is, however, reason to question whether these experiments provide a fair test of the outcome–response account. This basic approach, of course, depends entirely on the experimenter's capacity to create a situation in which the expectation of reward differs from the reward that is obtained by responding. In Rescorla and Colwill's (1989) study, for instance, each discriminative stimulus was pretrained so that it would signal a different outcome from the one that would be earned on that trial. Since this phase of the experiment was conducted over 4 days, however, it is possible that rats were able to learn the new stimulus–outcome relationships (e.g., S1 → O2), nullifying the effects of pretraining. Rescorla (1992) addressed this issue in an experiment otherwise quite similar to the first (Rescorla and Colwill, 1989), except that, during the discrimination phase, each stimulus continued to be paired with the outcome that it predicted during initial pretraining, while at the same time signaling that responding could earn the opposite outcome. These additional Pavlovian trials were added to encourage the persistence of the initial stimulus–outcome learning, thereby providing greater opportunity for any potential outcome–response associations to form during the instrumental discrimination training. Using this new procedure, Rescorla (1992) once again found no evidence that outcome–response associations play a part in outcome devaluation performance. However, the results of transfer testing were less straightforward. He observed that stimulus presentations tended to increase the performance of both responses, although this effect was larger for the response that had 'earned' the outcome signaled by the transfer stimulus than it was for the response that had been trained in 'anticipation' of that outcome. Thus, while these findings suggest that both outcome devaluation and transfer are dominated by response–outcome learning, they also indicate that outcome–response associations may play some, albeit limited, role in the latter.

This conclusion does not help the two-process account of reward value. According to this account, the processes underlying transfer and outcome devaluation should be identical. Perhaps more importantly, however, these studies illustrate the difficulty in attempting to dissociate the contributions of Pavlovian and instrumental learning to performance. Indeed, even in these studies it is possible that the subjects were able to confound the experimenter's intentions and acquire appropriate stimulus–outcome associations during instrumental training based on the relationship between the features of the individual response manipulanda and the outcome earned by those responses. For instance, rats trained to press a lever for pellets and pull a chain for sucrose solution may come to associate the lever itself with pellets and the chain with sucrose. Such learning would ensure that the rat anticipated the reward that they would actually obtain for performing the response, even in the presence of a context that signaled both rewards (e.g., Colwill and Rescorla, 1985b; Colwill, 1994) or a Pavlovian cue that signaled a different reward (e.g., Rescorla and Colwill, 1989; Rescorla, 1992).

This problem can be avoided, however, by training distinct action–outcome contingencies on a common response manipulandum. For instance, Dickinson et al. (1996) trained rats to push a vertically positioned pole to the left and right for different outcomes; for half the rats, left pushes earned food pellets and right pushes earned a maltodextrin solution, whereas the other half was trained with the opposite arrangement. Rats were then sated on one of the two outcomes in order to selectively reduce its reward value. Immediately after this treatment, they were given an extinction test in which the pole was available and could be pushed freely in either direction without consequence. Dickinson et al. (1996) found that, despite having both actions trained on a common manipulandum, the rats were able to use response–outcome training relationships to guide their action selection according to outcome value; rats were less likely to push the pole in the direction that had earned the now devalued outcome, relative to the other direction. This finding is incompatible with the two-process account, which predicts that outcome-selective devaluation should never emerge in the absence of differential stimulus–outcome contingencies. Instead, it provides strong support for the view that instrumental performance is goal-directed and that its sensitivity to reward value depends on response–outcome learning.

One final method for evaluation of the two-process account of reward value involves assessing the interaction between transfer and outcome devaluation. If these phenomena rely on the same underlying structure, then the capacity of a Pavlovian cue to facilitate performance should depend on the value of the mediating outcome representation. Colwill and Rescorla (1990) directly investigated the role of incentive value in outcome selective transfer. Rats were initially given biconditional discrimination training using differential outcomes, such that one stimulus (S1) signaled that pellets could be earned on one response (R1) and the other stimulus (S2) signaled that sucrose could be earned on a different response (R2). Subsequently, they were given free operant training on two new responses (R3 and R4), such that each earned a unique outcome (either pellets or sucrose). One outcome was then devalued through conditioned taste aversion and then a transfer test was conducted in extinction, with both R3 and R4 available. Although rats were, in general, less likely to perform the response that had earned the devalued outcome than the other response, both responses were selectively facilitated by presentations of the stimulus with which they shared a common outcome. Moreover, the magnitude of this transfer effect, measured in the difference from baseline performance, was comparable across responses. This basic finding, that devaluing an outcome fails to diminish its capacity to mediate Pavlovian-instrumental transfer, has since been replicated in a number of studies (Rescorla, 1994; Holland, 2004).

Altogether, there appears to be scant support for the two-process account of reward value. The associative processes supporting outcome devaluation and transfer appear to be acquired at different rates and encode somewhat different content. Furthermore, instrumental responses remain sensitive to outcome devaluation under conditions that cannot support differential stimulus–outcome learning. Finally, the Pavlovian-instrumental interaction responsible for transfer does not appear to depend on the reward value of the retrieved outcome. Instead, these findings strengthen the goal-directed view of instrumental action and, while demonstrating that reward anticipation influences action selection, it is also clear that this effect is not mediated by the reward system.

23.5 Summary and Conclusions

We have argued that the reward system is a specialization that developed in the service of goal-directed action allowing animals to encode the relative values of specific environmental events. These values provide the basis for choice, allowing animals to decide on a course of action based not only on knowledge or information as to the consequences of an action but on the basis of the value of those consequences.

Encoding the reward value of a particular event involves the formation of an association between the specific sensory representation of that event and an emotional response. In the case of primary rewards, the emotional response is directly determined by the activity of specific motivational and affective processes engaged during consummatory contact with the outcome. Thus, by virtue of their biologically active properties (e.g., nutrient, fluidic, pheromonal), rewarding events (food, fluid, sex objects, and so on) are readily able to activate these underlying systems that modify emotional responses as one of the consequences of that activation. Basing the evaluation of primary rewards on emotional responses is adaptive if those responses are determined by the operation of these basic motivational and affective systems, which is essential if the animal's choice between alternative courses of action is to remain, by and large, adaptive too. In the case of secondary rewards, the emotional response is, of course, determined by the primary reward with which it is paired. By basing the transfer of value from primary to secondary rewards on an emotional response, the selection of actions, even when they are directed toward achieving apparently quite arbitrary goals, can be understood as being constrained by primary motivational processes through their influence on emotional responses.

Finally, we addressed the distinction between the role the reward system plays in assigning reward value and the processes controlling the anticipation of reward. These are quite distinct aspects of behavioral control; although cues that signal forthcoming rewards can provide information that can be used by the goal-directed system, they do not depend, ultimately, on the reward system to play that role. As such, the influence of reward-related cues on action selection does not replace or explain away the functions of the reward system in this regard. Rather, the distinct processes mediating the effects of reward and of the anticipation of reward provides the basis for understanding the role that cognitive processes generally play in goal-directed action. Because it constrains the event relations to which an animal is exposed, there has been a long tradition of using Pavlovian conditioning to model the cognitive control of behavior. The fact that, ultimately, this system is concerned with the production of reflexive responses would, however, appear to render this approach perhaps a little too abstract. It makes more sense to study the role of cognition in a behavioral system within which information can act to influence performance. Based on the evidence reviewed here that animals are able to exert control over their instrumental actions, choose between actions based on the relative value of their consequences, and use predictive information to influence action selection, we suggest that instrumental conditioning provides the more precise model of this capacity.

Acknowledgments

The preparation of this chapter was supported by the National Institute of Mental Health, grant #56446.

References

Adams CD (1981) Variations in the sensitivity of instrumental responding to reinforcer devalaution. *Q. J. Exp. Psychol. B* 34: 77–98.

Adams CD and Dickinson A (1981) Instrumental responding following reinforcer devaluation. *Q. J. Exp. Psychol. B* 33: 109–121.

Asratyan EA (1974) Conditioned reflex theory and motivational behavior. *Acta Neurobiol. Exp.* 34: 15–31.

Balleine B (1992) Instrumental performance following a shift in primary motivation depends on incentive learning. *J Exp Psychol Anim Behav Process* 18: 236–250.

Balleine BW (2001) Incentive processes in instrumental conditioning. In: Klein RMS (ed.) *Handbook of Contemporary Learning Theories*, pp. 307–366. Hillsdale, NJ: Lawrence Erlbaum Associates.

Balleine B and Dickinson A (1991) Instrumental performance following reinforcer devaluation depends upon incentive learning. *Q. J. Exp. Psychol. B* 43: 279–296.

Balleine BW and Dickinson A (1994) The role of cholecystokinin in the motivational control of instrumental action. *Behav. Neurosci.* 108: 590–605.

Balleine BW and Dickinson A (1998a) Goal-directed instrumental action: Contingency and incentive learning and their cortical substrates. *Neuropharmacology* 37: 407–419.

Balleine BW and Dickinson A (1998b) The role of incentive learning in instrumental outcome revaluation by specific satiety. *Anim. Learn. Behav.* 26: 46–59.

Balleine B, Ball J, and Dickinson A (1994) Benzodiazepine-induced outcome revaluation and the motivational control of instrumental action in rats. *Behav. Neurosci.* 108: 573–589.

Balleine B, Davies A, and Dickinson A (1995a) Cholecystokinin attenuates incentive learning in rats. *Behav. Neurosci.* 109: 312–319.

Balleine B, Garner C, and Dickinson A (1995b) Instrumental outcome devaluation is attenuated by the anti-emetic ondansetron. *Q. J. Exp. Psychol.* B 48: 235–251.

Berlyne DEC (1960) *Contact, Arousal and Curiosity*. New York: McGraw-Hill.

Bernstein IL (1999) Taste aversion learning: A contemporary perspective. *Nutrition* 15: 229–234.

Berridge K, Grill HJ, and Norgren R (1981) Relation of consummatory responses and preabsorptive insulin release to palatability and learned taste aversions. *J. Comp. Physiol. Psychol.* 95: 363–382.

Bolles RC (1972) Reinforcement, expectancy, and learning. *Psychol. Rev.* 79: 394–409.

Bugelski BR (1956) *The Psychology of Learning*. New York: Holt.

Bugelski R (1938) Extinction with and without sub-goal reinforcement. *J. Comp. Psychol.* 26: 121–134.

Church RM (1964) Systematic effect of random error in the yoked control design. *Psychol. Bull.* 62.

Colwill RM (1994) Associative representations of instrumental contingencies. In: Medin DL (ed.) *The Psychology of Learning and Motivation*, pp. 1–72. New York: Academic Press.

Colwill RM and Motzkin DK (1994) Encoding of the unconditioned stimulus in Pavlovian conditioning. *Anim. Learn. Behav.* 22: 384–394.

Colwill RM and Rescorla RA (1985a) Instrumental responding remains sensitive to reinforcer devaluation after extensive training. *J. Exp. Psychol. Anim. Behav. Process.* 11: 520–536.

Colwill RM and Rescorla RA (1985b) Postconditioning devaluation of a reinforcer affects instrumental responding. *J. Exp. Psychol. Anim. Behav. Process.* 11: 120–132.

Colwill RM and Rescorla RA (1986) Associative structures in instrumental learning. In: *The Psychology of Learning and Motivation*, pp. 55–104 Orlando: Academic Press.

Colwill RM and Rescorla RA (1988) Associations between the discriminative stimulus and the reinforcer in instrumental learning. *J. Exp. Psychol. Anim. Behav. Process.* 14: 155–164.

Colwill RM and Rescorla RA (1990) Effect of reinforcer devaluation on discriminative control of instrumental behavior. *J. Exp. Psychol. Anim. Behav. Process.* 16: 40–47.

Crowder WF, Morris JB, and McDaniel MH (1959a) Secondary reinforcement or response facilitation? I. Resistance to extinction. *J. Psychol.* 48: 299–302.

Crowder WF, Gill K Jr, Hodge CC, and Nash FA Jr (1959b) Secondary reinforcement or response facilitation? II. Response acquisition. *J. Psychol.* 48: 303–306.

Crowder WF, Gay BR, Bright MG, and Lee MF (1959c) Secondary reinforcement or response facilitation? III. Reconditioning. *J. Psychol.* 48: 307–310.

Crowder WF, Gay BR, Fleming WC, and Hurst RW (1959d) Secondary reinforcement or response facilitation? IV. The retention method. *J. Psychol.* 48: 311–314.

Damasio A (1994) *Descartes' Error*. New York: G.P. Putnam's Sons.

Davis J and Bitterman ME (1971) Differential reinforcement of other behavior (DRO): A yoked-control comparison. *J. Exp. Anal. Behav.* 15: 237–241.

Delamater AR (1995) Outcome-selective effects of intertrial reinforcement in Pavlovian appetitive conditioning with rats. *Anim. Learn. Behav.* 23: 31–39.

Dickinson A (1985) Actions and habits: The development of behavioural autonomy. *Philos. Trans. R. Soc. Lond. B* 308: 67–78.

Dickinson A (1989) Expectancy theory in animal conditioning. In: Klein SB and Mowrer RR (eds.) *Contemporary Learning Theories: Pavlovian Conditioning and the Status of Traditional Learning Theories*, pp. 279–308. Hillsdale, NJ: Lawrence Erlbaum Associates.

Dickinson A (1994) Instrumental conditioning. In: Mackintosh NJ (ed.) *Animal Cognition and Learning*, pp. 4–79. London: Academic Press.

Dickinson A and Balleine BW (1994) Motivational control of goal-directed action. *Anim. Learn. Behav.* 22: 1–18.

Dickinson AB and Balleine B (1995) Motivational control of instrumental action. *Curr. Dir. Psychol. Sci.* 4: 162–167.

Dickinson A and Balleine BW (2002) The role of learning in the operation of motivational systems. In: Gallistel CR (ed.) *Learning, Motivation and Emotion, Vol. 3: Stevens' Handbook of Experimental Psychology,* 3rd edn., pp. 497–533. New York: John Wiley.

Dickinson A, Campos J, Varga Z, and Balleine BW (1996) Bidirectional control of instrumental conditioning. *Q. J. Exp. Psychol.* 49B: 289–306.

Dickinson A and Mulatero CW (1989) Reinforcer specificity of the suppression of instrumental performance on a non-contingent schedule. *Behav. Process.* 19: 167–180.

Dickinson A, Squire S, Varga Z, and Smith JW (1998) Omission learning after instrumental pretraining. *Q. J. Exp. Psychol.* 51B: 271–286.

Everitt BJ and Stacey P (1987) Studies of instrumental behavior with sexual reinforcement in male rats (*Rattus norvegicus*): II. Effects of preoptic area lesions, castration and testosterone. *J. Comp. Psychol.* 101: 407–419.

Fedorchak PM and Bolles RC (1986) Differential outcome effect using a biologically neutral outcome difference. *J. Exp. Psychol. Anim. Behav. Process.* 12: 125–130.

Garcia J (1989) Food for Tolman: Cognition and cathexis in concert. In: Archer T and Nilsson L-G (eds.) *Aversion, Avoidance and Anxiety*, pp. 45–85. Hillsdale, NJ: Lawrence Erlbaum Associates.

Hendersen RW and Graham J (1979) Avoidance of heat by rats: Effects of thermal context on the rapidity of extinction. *Learn. Motiv.* 10: 351–363.

Hershberger WA (1986) An approach through the looking-glass. *Anim. Learn. Behav.* 14: 443–451.

Holland PC (1979) Differential effects of omission contingencies on various components of Pavlovian appetitive conditioned responding in rats. *J. Exp. Psychol. Anim. Behav. Process.* 5: 178–193.

Holland PC (2004) Relations between Pavlovian-instrumental transfer and reinforcer devaluation. *J. Exp. Psychol. Anim. Behav. Process.* 30: 104–117.

Hull CL (1943) *Principles of Behavior*. New York: Appleton.

Hull CL (1952) *A Behavior System*. New York: Wiley.

Keller FS and Schoenfeld WN (1950) *Principles of Psychology: A Systematic Text in the Science of Behavior*. East Norwalk, CT: Appleton-Century-Crofts.

Killcross AS, Everitt BJ, and Robins TW (1997) Symmetrical effects of amphetamine and alpha-flupenthixol on conditioned punishment and conditioned reinforcement: Contrasts with midazolam. *Psychopharmacology (Berl)* 129: 141–152.

Kish GB (1966) Studies of sensory reinforcement. In: Honig WK (ed.) *Operant Behavior: Areas of Research and Application*, pp. 109–159. New York: Appleton-Century-Crofts.

Konorski J (1967) *Integrative Activity of the Brain*. Chicago: University of Chicago Press.

Kruse JM, Overmier JB, Konz WA, and Rokke E (1983) Pavlovian conditioned stimulus effects upon instrumental choice behavior are reinforcer specific. *Learn. Motiv.* 14: 165–181.

Limebeer CL and Parker LA (2000) The antiemetic drug ondansetron interferes with lithium-induced conditioned rejection reactions, but not lithium-induced taste avoidance in rats. *J. Exp. Psychol. Anim. Behav. Process.* 26: 371–384.

Lopez M, Balleine BW, and Dickinson A (1992) Incentive learning and the motivational control of instrumental performance by thirst. *Anim. Learn. Behav.* 20: 322–328.

Mowrer OH (1960) *Learning Theory and the Symbolic Processes*. New York: Wiley.

Myers KP and Sclafani A (2001) Conditioned enhancement of flavor evaluation reinforced by intragastric glucose. II. Taste reactivity analysis. *Physiol. Behav.* 74: 495–505.

Parkinson JA, Roberts AC, Everitt BJ, and Di Ciano P (2005) Acquisition of instrumental conditioned reinforcement is resistant to the devaluation of the unconditioned stimulus. *Q. J. Exp. Psychol. B* 58: 19–30.

Pavlov IP (1927) *Conditioned Reflexes: An Investigation of the Physiological Activity of the Cerebral Cortex*, Anrep GV (trans.). London: Oxford University Press.

Rescorla RA (1992) Response-outcome versus outcome-response associations in instrumental learning. *Anim. Learn. Behav.* 20: 223–232.

Rescorla RA (1994) Transfer of instrumental control mediated by a devalued outcome. *Anim. Learn. Behav.* 22: 27–33.

Rescorla RA and Colwill RM (1989) Associations with anticipated and obtained outcomes in instrumental learning. *Anim. Learn. Behav.* 17: 291–303.

Rescorla RA and Solomon RL (1967) Two-process learning theory: Relationships between Pavlovian conditioning and instrumental learning. *Psychol. Rev.* 74: 151–182.

Robbins TW, Cador M, Taylor JR, and Everitt BJ (1989) Limbic-striatal interactions in reward-related processes. *Neurosci. Biobehav. Rev.* 13: 155–162.

Sheffield FD (1965) Relation between classical and instrumental conditioning. In: Prokasy WF (ed.) *Classical Conditioning*, pp. 302–322. New York: Appleton-Century-Crofts.

Skinner BF (1938) *The Behavior of Organisms: An Experimental Analysis*. New York, London: D. Appleton-Century.

Spence KW (1956) *Behavior Theory and Conditioning*. New Haven: Yale University Press.

Taylor JR and Robbins TW (1984) Enhanced behavioural control by conditioned reinforcers following microinjections of d-amphetamine into the nucleus accumbens. *Psychopharmacology (Berl.)* 84: 405–412.

Trapold MA (1970) Are expectancies based upon different positive reinforcing events discriminably different? *Learn. Motiv.* 1: 129–140.

Trapold MA and Overmier JB (1972) The second learning process in instrumental conditioning. In: Black AA and Prokasy WF (eds.) *Classical Conditioning: II. Current Research and Theory*, pp. 427–452. New York: Appleton-Century-Crofts.

Ward GI (1960) Secondary reinforcement with cue stimulus effects reduced. *Proc. WV Acad. Sci.* 32: 205–208.

Wike EL (1966) *Secondary Reinforcement: Selected Experiments*. New York: Harper and Row.

Williams DR and Williams H (1969) Auto-maintenance in the pigeon: Sustained pecking despite contingent non-reinforcement. *J. Exp. Anal. Behav.* 12: 511–520.

Winterbauer NE (2006) *Conditioned Reinforcement.* PhD Thesis, University of California at Los Angeles.

Woodson JC and Balleine BW (2002) An assessment of factors contributing to instrumental performance for sexual reward in the rat. *Q. J. Exp. Psychol. B* 55: 75–88.

Wyckoff LB (1959) Toward a quantitative theory of secondary reinforcement. *Psychol. Rev.* 66: 68–78.

Wyckoff LB, Sidowski J, and Chambliss DJ (1958) An experimental study of the relationship between secondary reinforcing and cue effects of a stimulus. *J. Comp. Physiol. Psychol.* 51: 103–109.

Yin HH, Knowlton BJ, and Balleine BW (2005) Blockade of NMDA receptors in the dorsomedial striatum prevents action-outcome learning in instrumental conditioning. *Eur. J. Neurosci.* 22: 505–512.

Zimmerman DW (1969) Patterns of responding in a chained schedule altered by conditioned reinforcement. *Psychonom. Sci.* 16: 120–126.

24 The Molecular Mechanisms of Reward

C. A. Winstanley, University of British Columbia, Vancouver, Canada

E. J. Nestler, The University of Texas Southwestern Medical Center, Dallas, TX, USA

24.1 Introduction

This article considers the molecular mechanisms which have been implicated in aspects of reward processing and reward-related learning. A brief description of the nature of reward and the animal learning theory associated with its assessment is provided. The neural circuitry involved in implicating these psychological processes is then described, with emphasis placed on the nucleus accumbens (NAc), amygdala, and frontal cortex. Dopaminergic regulation of these structures has been shown to play a pivotal role in mediating reward-related behavior, and the intracellular signaling cascades affected by dopamine release have provided us with novel insight into the molecular basis of reward processing. In particular, data are considered from research into both drug addiction and depression, with a focus on the transcription factors cyclic adenosine monophosphate response element binding protein (CREB) and ΔFosB as well as some of their downstream targets. Dissociable roles are identified for different molecules in the regulation of reward. Furthermore, in parallel to data from neurochemical investigations, the behavioral effects of manipulating molecular pathways depend on both the region targeted and the time course of action. Greater understanding of reward processing at the molecular level is being achieved through combining expertise developed within the fields of psychology and molecular biology. Such an approach can further our knowledge of the detrimental changes in brain function which are inherent within addiction and affective disorders and which are associated with maladaptive assessment of reward and motivation.

24.2 Researching Reward Processes: What Do We Mean by Reward and How Do We Measure It?

Before we consider its molecular basis, we need to establish the nature of the psychological processes covered by the term 'reward.' This topic is dealt with in more detail elsewhere in this reference work (*See* Chapter 23); therefore, only a brief summary will be included here to enable discussion of subsequent experimental work. In its most simple terms, a reward is a positive stimulus, that is, something which the individual values and enjoys. Rewards carry emotional significance, and individuals are motivated to expend effort to attain them. The study of how reward and reward-related stimuli inform behavior contributes a significant amount to our knowledge of learning and memory processes.

In terms of animal learning theory, an innately rewarding stimulus, such as food, is known as an unconditioned stimulus (US). This elicits an unconditioned, automatic response (UR), for example, salivation. If the US is repeatedly paired with a previously neutral stimulus, such as a light, an association will be learned between presentation of the light and food reward, such that illumination of the light alone will cause the animal to salivate. The light is now regarded as a conditioned stimulus (CS), and the response it elicits is termed a conditioned response (CR). This process is known as Pavlovian conditioning and forms the basis of associative learning. Although conceptually quite simple, the effects that a CS can exert over behavior are far-reaching and can influence goal-directed behavior. For example, a rat can learn to press a lever to earn a food pellet through instrumental conditioning processes (see **Figure 1**). If delivery of that food pellet is repeatedly paired with presentation of a light CS, the CS will acquire some of the appetitive value of the food and become rewarding in its own right such that the rat will press the lever to turn the light on. The CS is then called a conditioned reinforcer (CRf).

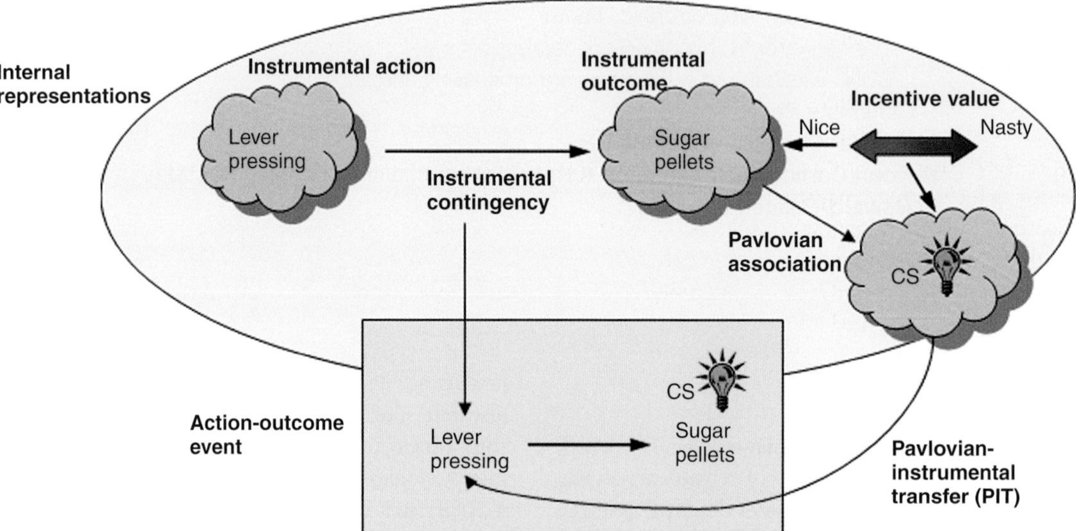

Figure 1 A schematic of some factors which affect instrumental learning. An action such as pressing a lever leads to the delivery of sugar pellets, accompanied by the onset of a stimulus light (the conditioned stimulus: CS). This action-outcome event (contained within the tan box) is detected and represented internally. Degrading the encoding of this contingency will have a direct effect on instrumental performance. The value of the outcome is determined by incentive learning (i.e., how nice the sugar pellets are). This can be affected by the motivational state of the animal. The attribution of incentive value affects the representation of the instrumental outcome, such that changing this value has an impact upon truly goal-directed instrumental behavior (see the section titled 'The prelimbic cortex'). The CS is also associated with the incentive value of the instrumental outcome through Pavlovian conditioning. Presentation of the CS can invigorate responding for the outcome through Pavlovian to instrumental transfer (PIT). Based on Cardinal RN, Parkinson JA, Hall J, and Everitt BJ (2002) Emotion and motivation: The role of the amygdala, ventral striatum, and prefrontal cortex. *Neurosci. Biobehav. Rev.* 26: 321–352; figure 2, p. 327; used with permission from Elsevier Science.

The noncontingent presentation of a CS can also influence ongoing instrumental responding in a process known as Pavlovian to instrumental transfer (PIT). For example, presentation of a tone associated with sucrose delivery will increase lever-pressing for sucrose (conditioned motivation). Conversely, if a light has been paired with a painful stimulus such as footshock, presentation of the light CS will decrease lever-pressing for reward (conditioned suppression).

These concepts inform more than just animal learning theory: experiments designed using these psychological constructs provide valuable insight into the processing of reward in psychopathology. The inability to find stimuli rewarding, as well as an excessive desire for certain rewards, are symptoms of several mental disorders, including depression, attention-deficit/hyperactivity disorder and drug addiction, among others. Research into the mechanisms of reward-related learning has therefore contributed to our understanding of these conditions. Just as a CS paired with food stimulates lever-pressing for reward in rats, stimuli paired with drug reward can lead to craving for drug and relapse to drug-seeking in both rats and human addicts (de Wit and Stewart, 1981; Childress et al., 1988). Failure to alter behavior when the incentive value of a reward changes also has obvious implications for substance abuse disorders, where addicts continue to use drugs despite increasingly negative consequences and reductions in the reward experienced. In rats, food reward can be devalued by pairing food delivery with an injection of lithium chloride, which induces nausea, or by feeding animals to satiation. Such devaluation procedures subsequently alter the way in which animals respond to food presentation or to a CS paired with that reward, making it possible to investigate the biological basis of this aspect of reward processing.

24.3 The Neural Circuitry of Reward

Considerable evidence has been amassed concerning the neural circuitry underpinning reward-related learning (see Cardinal, 2001, for review). The processing of reward occurs in a distributed network of structures comprising both cortical and subcortical areas, the majority of which are connected within the limbic or affective corticostriatal loop (**Figure 2**) (Alexander et al., 1986). Within this framework, structures involved in higher-order cognitive function such as the prefrontal cortex (PFC) interact with areas of the limbic system heavily implicated in emotional processing and memory, such as the amygdala and hippocampal formation. These structures are interconnected with the NAc, often described as the reward center of the brain. This circuit influences motor output and motivation via the ventral pallidum and mediodorsal thalamus, which also project back to the PFC. We will focus on three of the most studied areas: the NAc, the amygdala, and regions of the PFC. Given that the focus of this chapter is to discuss the molecular basis of reward, the majority of research of which has been undertaken in rodents, we will focus on data supporting a role for these regions in the reward system of the rat, although these areas and their homologues have been heavily implicated in reward processing in both monkeys and humans.

24.3.1 The Nucleus Accumbens

The NAc is probably the most widely studied region in terms of regulating reward-related learning. This region has been labeled the 'limbic-motor interface' due to its extensive connections with limbic structures, such as the amygdala, hippocampus, and PFC, in addition to its projections to motor output areas. The NAc is therefore thought to be a key node in the limbic corticostriatal loop, wherein diverse types of information from both cortical and subcortical structures are integrated and key signals generated to enable the implementation of behavioral change relevant to goal-seeking. The NAc can be divided into the core (NAc-C) and shell (NAc-Sh) subregions, which differ in both structure and function (Groenewegen et al., 1987; Voorn et al., 1989; Berendse et al., 1992). Whereas the NAc-C projects predominantly to the ventral pallidum, the shell also projects to subcortical structures, including the lateral hypothalamus and periaqueductal grey. Damage to the NAc does not prevent animals from making a response to earn food reward, or from adjusting their responding when the value of that reward changes, that is, animals are still capable of goal-directed behavior (see the section titled 'The prefrontal cortex'). However, the ability of a CS to regulate behavior is profoundly affected by NAc lesions. Damage to the NAc-C disrupts PIT and the acquisition of autoshaping, a Pavlovian conditioning paradigm where presentation of a CS with food delivery leads animals to approach the CS (Parkinson et al., 1999; Hall et al., 2001). Damage to the NAc also impairs conditioned place preference, where animals learn to associate a specific context or place with reward delivery and therefore spend more time in this location. Neither

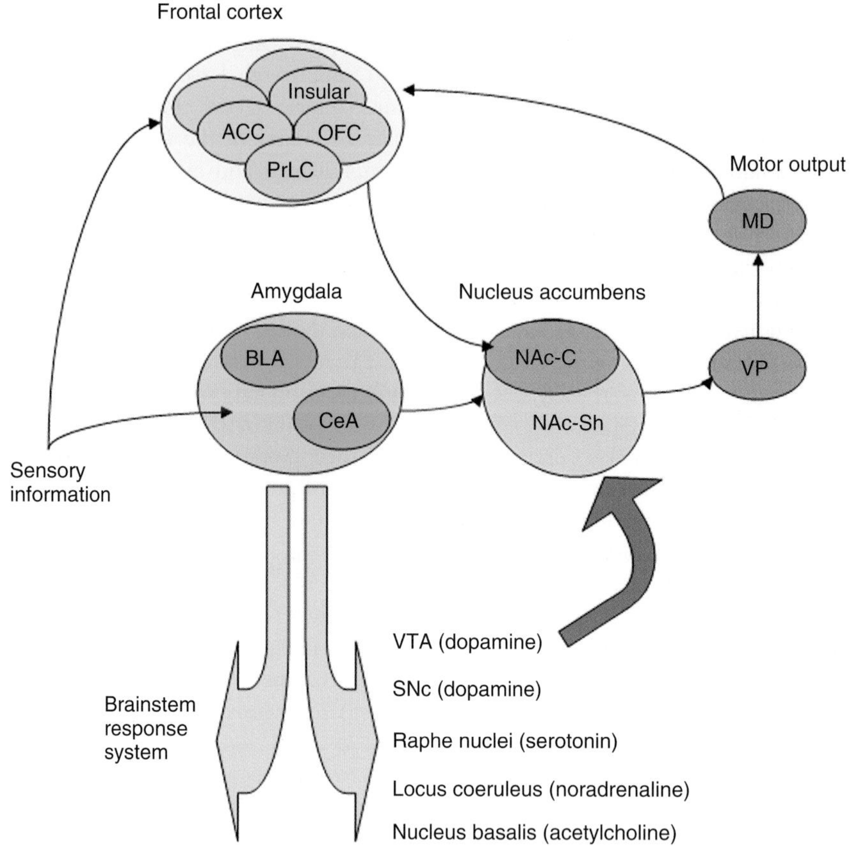

Figure 2 Simplified diagram of the limbic corticostriatal loop. (Abbreviations: ACC, anterior cingulate cortex, OFC, orbitofrontal cortex; PrLC, prelimbic cortex; BLA, basolateral amygdala; CeA, central amygdala; VTA, ventral tegmental area; SNc, substantia nigra pars compacta; NAc-C, nucleus accumbens core; NAc-Sh, nucleus accumbens shell; VP, ventral pallidum; MD, mediodorsal thalamus.) The frontal cortex is functionally heterogeneous, and several frontal regions are involved in different aspects of instrumental responding. As discussed in the text, the PrLC, part of the medial prefrontal cortex, is involved in detecting the instrumental action-outcome contingency and is essential for the maintenance of goal-directed behavior. The functions of the ACC are complex and are not described in detail here, but involve resolving response conflict and error detection, whereas the insular cortex, containing the primary gustatory cortex, encodes the primary sensory qualities of specific foods. The OFC plays a role in integrating changes in the incentive value of a reward with representations of the expected outcome, a function which is thought to depend on its connections with the BLA. The BLA is one of the primary structures involved in encoding CS-US associations and is necessary for the presentation of a CS to trigger retrieval of the motivational value of its associated US. It can work in concert with the CeA to influence brainstem function, arousal, and neurotransmitter release. As the 'limbic-motor interface,' the NAc combines information from both frontal and amygdalar systems, as well as from other inputs, to generate motivational drive. The NAc-Sh signals the motivational properties of unconditioned (primary) reinforcers, whereas the NAc-C has a more pronounced role in mediating the motivational impact which Pavlovian conditioned stimuli have on behavior. Adapted from Cardinal RN, Parkinson JA, Hall J, and Everitt BJ (2002) Emotion and motivation: The role of the amygdala, ventral striatum, and prefrontal cortex. *Neurosci. Biobehav. Rev.* 26: 321–352; figure 3, p. 329; used with permission from Elsevier Science.

damage to the core or shell abolishes CRf *per se*, but manipulations of the dopaminergic innervation of the NAc can alter responding for CRf (see the section titled 'Dopamine and reward'). As well, damage to the NAc results in decreased tolerance to the delay of reward, such that animals will choose a small immediate reward over a larger but more delayed one, a concept which has direct relevance to models of impulsive behavior (Cardinal et al., 2001). In contrast, selective lesions of the NAc-Sh do not appear to have such a pronounced effect on the conditioned responses to rewards, that is, reward-related learning, but this region plays an important role in the unconditioned response to primary reinforcers. In particular, the NAc-Sh appears to alter the motivational impact of rewards, such that inhibition of NAc-Sh activity induces overeating, an effect attributable to its connections with the lateral hypothalamus (Stratford and Kelley, 1999). Inhibition of neuronal firing is also observed when animals engage in a sequence of reward-seeking and consumption (Taha and Fields, 2006), which results in disinhibition of activity in target brain regions such as the hypothalamus. Activity within the NAc may therefore act to gate appetitive behavior through its influence over reward-related brain circuitry.

24.3.2 The Amygdala

The first indication that the amygdala was one of the most important brain regions for the processing of affective stimuli was the discovery that damage localized to this area produced marked deficits in emotional display and apparent fearlessness in monkeys (Kluver and Bucy, 1939). Humans with damage to the amygdala show a variety of impairments in emotional perception and expression, and can unwittingly endanger themselves through failing to process danger or risk. The amygdala can be divided into multiple nuclei based on cytoarchitectonic distinctions (Pitkanen, 2000). Functional dissociations have also been observed between the different units. In particular, the central nucleus (CeA) and basolateral nucleus (BLA) of the amygdala have been implicated in divergent forms of affective processing (Everitt et al., 2000). Both the BLA and CeA receive sensory input, yet the BLA has more prominent connections with the frontal cortices and ventral striatum, while the CeA shares more numerous connections with areas within the hypothalamus and brainstem.

It is generally thought that the BLA plays an integral role in Pavlovian conditioning involving both appetitive and aversive stimuli (*See* Chapter 21) (Davis, 1998; LeDoux, 2000). One of the most commonly used paradigms to measure emotional learning is fear conditioning, in which animals form an association between a painful footshock and a particular stimulus such as a light or tone. Animals rapidly learn this association and freeze during subsequent presentations of the CS, indicative of a state of fear, yet this freezing is much less evident following BLA or CeA lesions. More sophisticated analysis of Pavlovian conditioning procedures suggests that the BLA is necessary in order for presentation of the CS to trigger retrieval of the value of the US with which it was paired. Although BLA-lesioned animals show evidence of learning simple CS-US associations, changing the value of a reward does not alter the way in which the animal responds to the associated CS. For example, BLA-lesioned rats show aversion to a devalued food, but still approach the food magazine when the CS paired with the devalued food is presented (Hatfield et al., 1996). Likewise, although BLA-lesioned monkeys show preference for different foods (i.e., can still make value judgments), they are unable to alter their choice preference when the value of a particular food has been changed through devaluation. This idea that the BLA is involved in processing the incentive value of rewards and reward-related stimuli associated with them has been very influential and is thought to depend on its connections with the orbitofrontal cortex (OFC) (Baxter et al., 2000; see the section titled 'The orbitofrontal cortex'). Given its proximity to the hippocampus and other limbic structures heavily implicated in memory processing and storage, the BLA is ideally positioned to mediate the effect of emotional arousal on memory.

24.3.3 The Prefrontal Cortex

The PFC is involved in numerous higher-order cognitive functions, such as decision-making, attention, problem solving, strategy development, and working memory (*See* Chapter 9). Such processes exert powerful control over goal-directed behavior. The PFC is both structurally and functionally heterogeneous, and a discussion of the role of each subregion is beyond the scope of this article. We will focus on two areas which appear to be particularly important in reward processing: the medial PFC (mPFC) as exemplified by the prelimbic and anterior cingulate regions, and the ventral PFC encompassing the orbitofrontal and agranular insular cortices.

24.3.3.1 The prelimbic cortex

This region of the rat mPFC is involved in the acquisition of goal-directed behavior. In order for action to be considered goal-directed, it must fulfill two criteria: (1) the animal must be aware of the *causal* link between the instrumental action and its outcome (i.e., a rat pressing a lever for food knows that pressing the lever results in delivery of food reward) and (2) the outcome for which the animal is responding must be considered a goal by the animal (i.e., the rat *wants* the food). Instrumental responding ceases to be goal-directed once it becomes habitual, that is, the animal is insensitive to changes in the incentive value of the reward or to the presence of an instrumental contingency. Behavior is instead controlled by simple stimulus-response (S-R) associations in which stimuli or outcomes become directly associated with a motor response, so that the rat responds on the lever regardless of its motivational state. Damage to the prelimbic cortex (PrLC) not only retards acquisition of instrumental responding, but also disrupts the detection of instrumental contingencies (Balleine and Dickinson, 1998; Corbit and Balleine, 2003). These data indicate that rats with PrLC damage may acquire instrumental responses based on S-R associations and are no longer truly capable of goal-directed learning. The transition from goal-directed to habitual S-R responding can also happen naturally over time with repeated training and has some advantage in that it is thought to use fewer cognitive resources. However, habits are less flexible than goal-directed actions and can lead to maladaptive behavior, such as that commonly associated with addiction, where environmental stimuli trigger engagement in drug-taking even though drug intake itself is no longer rewarding.

In keeping with these data indicating that the mPFC is involved in maintaining cognitive flexibility, the PrLC is also thought to play an important role in extinction processes. Extinction refers to the decline in responding when that response no longer leads to the associated outcome. The role of the PrLC has been extensively studied in the extinction of conditioned fear (see Sotres-Bayon et al., 2004, for review). Repeated presentation of the CS in the absence of the associated shock reduces the ability of the CS to elicit fear-related responses such as freezing as the animal learns that the CS is no longer a reliable predictor of the US. This ability to update knowledge about what is, and what is not, an accurate predictor of a dangerous event is clearly important for adaptation and survival. Lesions to the mPFC encompassing the PrLC impair extinction of conditioned fear. The deficits in extinction observed in the absence of the PrLC may relate to the well-documented role of the frontal cortex in mediating behavioral inhibition and perseveration. Disconnection of the mPFC and the BLA also attenuates extinction of conditioned fear, suggesting that activity within the mPFC may act to inhibit the representations of the emotional value of the CS generated by the amygdala, highlighting the importance of prefrontal regulation of amygdala function in reward-related learning.

24.3.3.2 The orbitofrontal cortex

Perhaps more than any other region of the frontal cortex, the OFC has been heavily associated with the processing of rewarding or emotional stimuli and events. In humans, damage to the OFC produces a pattern of aberrant social behavior and maladaptive decision-making which is often described as impulsive. This behavior can be exemplified by performance of these patients on laboratory-based gambling tasks where subjects choose between different options to earn points. The optimal strategy is to choose options associated with small immediate gains but also low and infrequent losses, an approach which healthy volunteers learn. Persistent selection of options leading to large immediate gain but heavy losses in the long term is thought to reflect risky decision-making and is observed both in pathological gamblers (Cavedini et al., 2002) and substance abusers (Bechara et al., 2001) and in patients with damage to the OFC or BLA (Bechara et al., 1999). In the monkey, neurons within the OFC have been shown to fire preferentially to different food rewards and to decrease their firing rate specifically to a devalued reward (Critchley and Rolls, 1996). Similar to the BLA, the OFC therefore appears to be involved in creating representations of the incentive value of reward. The reciprocal connections between these two regions are well documented, and disconnection of the OFC and BLA prevents devaluation of reward from altering choice behavior in monkeys (Baxter et al., 2000). However, electrophysiology recordings in the rat suggest that the OFC may have a more sophisticated role to play in using this information. In a series of elegant studies, Schoenbaum and colleagues have developed the hypothesis that the OFC supports representations of outcome expectancy, that is, how rewarding the outcome of a certain action is anticipated as being (Schoenbaum et al., 2006). The BLA generates important information about the incentive value of reward-associated stimuli, which the OFC then uses to generate representations of the anticipated outcome predicted by those CS. Such outcome expectancy is then used to inform choice behavior.

Lesions to the OFC also affect aspects of impulsive and compulsive behavior in animals. As in humans, damage to the rodent or monkey OFC increases perseverative behavior and decreases cognitive flexibility. For example, in reversal learning paradigms, OFC-lesioned rats perseverate in responding to the previously rewarded stimulus (Schoenbaum et al., 2002; Chudasama and Robbins, 2003). In delay-to-reinforcement paradigms where rats choose between a small immediate versus a larger increasingly delayed reward, OFC-lesioned rats do not show such a strong aversion to the delay compared to their sham controls (Winstanley et al.,

2004). This deficit may arise from both perseverative tendencies as well as an inability to integrate the consequences of making a response with the incentive value of the reward, that is, the delay does not sufficiently devalue the reward.

24.4 Dopamine and Reward

Converging evidence from numerous studies has implicated dopamine as the single most important neurotransmitter involved in the signaling of reward. Using intracranial self-stimulation techniques, where animals respond for electrical stimulation into a particular region of the brain, it has been shown repeatedly that animals will work for stimulation of their dopamine system (Wise and Rompre, 1989). Likewise, the addictive properties of drugs of abuse can be attributed in part to their ability to potentiate dopaminergic transmission. In particular, dopaminergic regulation of the NAc is critically involved in this process. The ventral tegmental area (VTA) sends dopaminergic projections to numerous regions within the brain including the NAc, PFC, and other parts of the limbic system. Both natural and drug rewards increase dopamine efflux in the NAc-Sh, whereas CS associated with such reward increase dopamine efflux in the NAc-C. Although animals are still capable of finding things rewarding or pleasurable in the absence of dopamine, they are no longer motivated to earn reward (Salamone et al., 2003), that is, they are no longer capable of goal-directed behavior. Dopaminergic depletion of the NAc significantly decreases the amount of effort rats are willing to expend to earn reward, whereas manipulations which increase NAc dopamine function enhance goal-seeking.

Several groups have recorded from dopaminergic cells within the VTA in monkeys during Pavlovian conditioning paradigms. Using this methodology, it has been found that the firing of dopamine neurons may signal error prediction, that is, they are particularly active when an unexpected reward is delivered, and firing is suppressed when an expected reward does not appear (Montague et al., 2004; Schultz, 2006). The potentiation of dopamine function caused by drugs of abuse may therefore generate a powerful signal that the reward was larger or better than expected regardless of the actual experience created by the drug (Hyman et al., 2006). Not only are psychostimulant drugs like amphetamine rewarding in their own right, they also enhance the effects of conditioned reinforcers, an effect which can be induced by direct application of amphetamine or dopamine agonists into the NAc, and which is blocked by dopaminergic lesions of the NAc and by ablation of the NAc-Sh (see Cardinal et al., 2002). Similarly, PIT can be enhanced by intra-NAc amphetamine and is abolished by dopamine receptor antagonists. This general potentiation of reward-related learning and reward-seeking likely plays an important role in the generation and maintenance of addiction.

Dopamine also regulates reward-related processing within the PFC. Data from both *in vivo* observations and computational modeling has led to the suggestion that phasic dopamine release acts as a gating mechanism, signaling when internal representations of reward and related stimuli need to be updated (Cohen et al., 2002). Damage to dopaminergic innervation of the PFC alters reward-related learning in a manner consistent with this theory. For example, lesions to dopaminergic inputs to the mPFC cause a deficit in fear extinction (Morrow et al., 1999), and ablation of dopaminergic terminals within the OFC leads to persistent choice of a larger but delayed reward, similar to excitotoxic lesions of these structures. Pharmacological manipulations also suggest that there is an optimum level of dopamine function within the PFC, and that too much as well as too little can have a negative impact on a range of cognitive behaviors (Arnsten, 1997). Long-term drug use leads to cognitive deficits that have been largely attributed to dysfunction of the frontal cortex (Rogers and Robbins, 2001), and hypofunction of the OFC has been observed in recently abstinent cocaine abusers (Volkow and Fowler, 2000). In rats, repeated exposure to addictive drugs has been shown to alter reward-related learning in tasks known to be dependent on the integrity of the OFC (Schoenbaum et al., 2004). Given the importance of the dopamine system in facilitating reward-related learning and the ability of addictive drugs to modulate this system, it seems likely that dysregulation of the dopaminergic input to frontal regions is responsible for these cognitive impairments.

24.5 Cellular and Molecular Targets of the Dopamine-Reward System: Insights from Drug Addiction

Given that the dopaminergic system has been heavily implicated in mediating the highly rewarding nature of addictive drugs, and that addictive behavior appears to arise from the hijacking of normal reward systems, a significant proportion of the data concerning the molecular basis of reward have been obtained through studying the effects of drugs of abuse. The intracellular changes that occur following acute administration of an appetitive substance like cocaine can provide valuable information about the signaling cascades activated by such rewarding substances. However, the changes seen after repeated administration are of more relevance in determining the molecular basis of the alterations in reward-related learning underpinning the addicted state. Drug addiction is a chronic and often relapsing disorder, with human addicts remaining at risk of relapse even after years of abstinence. The fact that chronic drug intake produces such durable changes in brain function and behavior has led to the suggestion that long-lasting changes in gene transcription may play a prominent role (Nestler et al., 1993). This has led to a search for relatively stable markers of altered transcriptional regulation whose persistence matches the time course of aspects of addictive behavior. The contrasting effects of acute versus chronic administration of addictive drugs on intracellular signaling pathways can therefore provide information about different aspects of reward processing. The role played by these molecular mechanisms in the processing of natural rewards has also been studied in learning and memory paradigms, and also in animal models of depression.

The binding of dopamine, or any neurotransmitter or signaling molecule, by its membrane-bound receptors triggers the initiation of several intracellular signaling cascades which often culminate in the regulation of transcription factors (TFs), including those encoded by immediate early genes (**Figure 3**). In terms of our understanding of reward processing and addiction, a considerable amount of data is now available concerning the particular TF families activated by dopaminergic agents. In this section, we will focus on some specific examples of this aspect of gene regulation and consider the role of these different TFs in the development of addiction as well as in the response to natural rewards. In terms of reward-related learning, we will largely restrict our discussion to key areas within the affective corticostriatal loop highlighted in the previous section. However, it should be noted that many of these intracellular signaling pathways have been implicated in the emotional memory processes

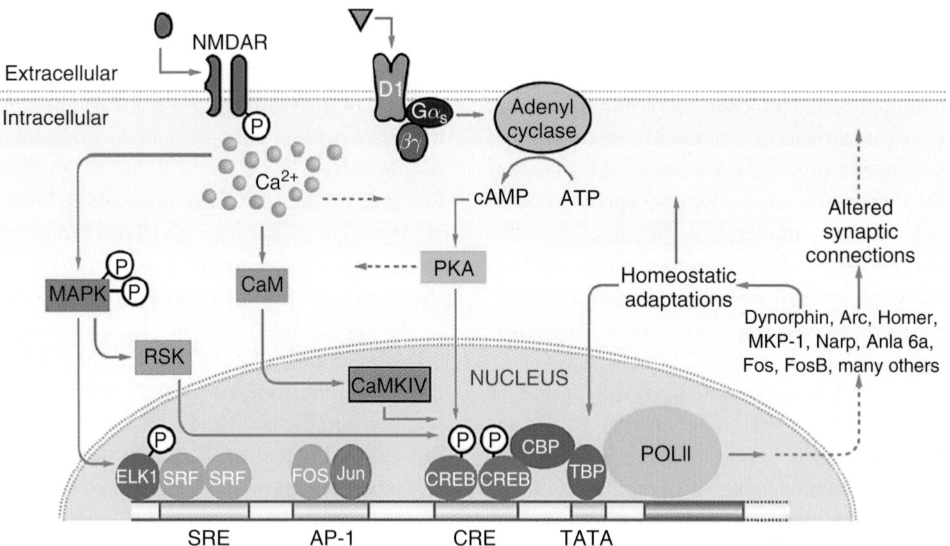

Figure 3 Regulation of gene expression within the striatum by dopamine and glutamate. Stimulation of dopaminergic D_1 receptors and glutamate receptors activates intracellular second messenger signaling cascades which result in changes in gene expression within the cell nucleus. Shown here are examples of DNA binding sites within the cFos promoter, including a serum response element (SRE), an activator protein-1 element (AP-1), and a cyclic adenosine monophosphate (cAMP) response element (CRE). Numerous other genes are also activated, including Homer, Arc, FosB, etc. Abbreviations: CBP, CREB binding protein; CREB, cAMP response element binding protein; MAPK, mitogen-activated protein kinase; NMDAR, *N*-methyl-D-aspartate glutamate receptor; PKA, protein kinase A; TBP, TATA binding protein; RSK, ribosomal S6 kinase; CaMKIV, Ca^{2+}/calmodulin-dependent kinase IV; ELK1, Ets-like transcription factor; SRF, serum response factor; POLII, RNA polymerase II; TATA describes a short sequence of base pairs that is rich in adenine (A) and thymidine (T) residues. Reprinted from Hyman SE, Malenka RC, and Nestler EJ (2006) Neural mechanisms of addiction: The role of reward-related learning and memory. *Annu. Rev. Neurosci.* 29: 565–598; used with permission from the Annual Reviews Permission Department.

involved in fear conditioning through their actions in the hippocampus (HPC).

Several techniques have been combined to determine whether these changes in TF regulation alter addiction-related behavior. Mice lacking these TFs have been developed, as have transgenic mice which either overexpress certain TFs or express mutant or dominant negative proteins which inhibit their effects. Reporter lines have also been developed, where the promoters regulated by a particular TF (e.g., cAMP response elements (CREs)) drive expression of a reporter gene expressing an easily visualized marker, such as β-galactosidase or green fluorescent protein (GFP). Such mice enable the consequences of different environmental manipulations on that TF to be determined. As well, viral vectors designed to express these proteins can be infused into specific regions using standard stereotaxic surgical techniques, which localizes the effects of changes in gene transcription to particular areas of interest. A small number of studies have infused antisense oligonucleotides into a certain brain area, although concerns remain about the toxicity and specificity of this approach. In addition to monitoring changes in cellular excitability and synaptic plasticity caused by these manipulations, development of these tools has made it possible to investigate the role these TFs play in reward-related learning. The majority of these studies have used conditioned place preference to assess the hedonic impact of substances of abuse given the relatively high throughput of this method. Instrumental responding for drug reward can also be assessed using self-administration paradigms, where animals learn to press a lever to obtain a drug infusion delivered into an indwelling intravenous catheter.

As mentioned before, one of the factors central to understanding addiction is the changes in behavior and brain function which occur following repeated rather than acute administration. In terms of behavioral output, one of the most widely studied phenomena is that of locomotor sensitization, whereby repeated administration of virtually any abused drug leads to a potentiation of the hyperlocomotor response seen after an acute drug injection in rodents. This increased sensitivity to the motor stimulating properties of addictive drugs is long-lasting, indicating that it could be mediated by some of the long-term changes in gene transcription and brain function which characterize the persistent nature of addiction. However, human addicts do not show sensitization to the arousing effects of drugs like cocaine following repeated use, with most users reporting tolerance of the drugs' stimulant effects. Nevertheless, it is hoped that understanding the changes in neuronal activity that accompany the development of locomotor sensitization may provide valuable insight into the changes in brain function caused by long-term drug use. The behavioral phenotype is very robust and easy to study, thereby facilitating the investigation of its underlying neurobiology. Furthermore, there is evidence to suggest that sensitization to psychostimulants enhances their ability to potentiate the impact of CS on behavior (Taylor and Horger, 1999). Some of the mechanisms underlying behavioral sensitization could also be involved in mediating the powerful ability of addictive drugs to influence goal-directed behavior and stimulate drug-seeking.

Given that addictive drugs heavily stimulate the dopamine system to cause long-term behavioral changes, it is likely that the regulatory mechanisms controlling neuronal plasticity within reward circuitry are targets of drugs of abuse. Repeated activation of neurotransmitter receptors leads to a change in the physiological state of neurons, rendering them more or less sensitive to subsequent stimulation. This could be mediated via changes in the effective strength of synaptic connections (referred to as synaptic plasticity), or via changes in the overall excitability of the affected neurons (referred to as whole-cell plasticity). The former in particular have been implicated in learning and memory processes. In keeping with this hypothesis, chronic administration of several, but not all, addictive drugs increases dendritic spine formation within the NAc (Robinson and Kolb, 2004). This increase in synaptic plasticity is proposed to underlie the locomotor sensitization discussed earlier. Considering the importance of the NAc in mediating the rewarding properties of addictive drugs, the majority of molecular studies have focused on manipulating gene transcription in this region.

24.5.1 The CREB and Fos Families of TFs

Ligand-binding at the dopamine D_1 receptor activates the cAMP second messenger signaling cascade, leading to the phosphorylation of protein kinase A (PKA) which can in turn phosphorylate downstream protein targets. Among the prominent targets of this signaling cascade is CREB. This transcription factor is constitutively expressed at fairly high levels throughout the brain, but needs to be phosphorylated for full transcriptional activity. In addition to PKA, CaM kinases such as Ca^{2+}/calmodulin kinase type IV (CaMKIV) and growth factor-associated kinases are all capable of performing this phosphorylation event, indicating that CREB activation is a point of functional convergence for several signaling pathways. Dimers of CREB bind to CRE sites located within the promoter regions of certain genes and alter the rate at which they are transcribed.

Acute administration of psychostimulant drugs stimulates phosphorylation of CREB through D_1 receptor-dependent mechanisms at several nodes within the reward circuitry, including the VTA, amygdala, PFC, and NAc. Increased expression of cFos, a product of an immediate early gene, is observed in similar locations, and its induction may be partly dependent on CREB activation, at least for amphetamine (Konradi et al., 1994). This occurs through CRE sites present in the promoter region of the cFos gene. cFos expression is also induced by several other intracellular signaling cascades, in particular, serum response factor (SRF) acting on serum response elements (SREs) within the cFos promoter. cFos is a member of the Fos family of transcription factors, which includes FosB, Fra1, and Fra2. These proteins heterodimerize with members of the Jun protein family to form the activator protein 1 (AP-1) transcription factor complex, which then binds to AP-1 sites within gene promoter regions. Increases in the activation of both cFos and CREB are rapid and transient, returning to basal levels within hours of the acute stimulus. In fact, repeated administration of drug causes the induction of cFos to desensitize, so that subsequent drug exposure no longer induces the robust elevation seen following first administration (Nestler et al., 2001). A similar pattern is observed in the expression of FosB. In contrast, the activation of CREB appears to become greater and more persistent with repeated drug exposures, an effect most firmly established within the NAc (Shaw-Lutchman et al., 2003). This pattern of expression suggests a more pronounced role for CREB-mediated gene transcription in aspects of addiction.

However, in contrast to all the TFs mentioned so far, isoforms of a truncated splice variant of FosB, known as ΔFosB, is only induced at high levels within the same reward-related areas following chronic, *but not acute*, administration of addictive drugs (**Figure 4**) (Nestler et al., 2001). The 35–37 kDa isoforms of ΔFosB dimerize predominantly with JunD to form an active AP-1 complex. These isoforms of ΔFosB also have an unusually long half-life due to their resistance to degradation by the proteosome, a property conferred at least in part by its truncated C-terminus and by a casein kinase 2–mediated phosphorylation (McClung et al., 2004). Once induced, levels of ΔFosB have been detected up to 2 months after cessation of drug treatment. Such accumulation has been observed following treatment with virtually any addictive substance, including cocaine, *d*-amphetamine, morphine, nicotine, alcohol, and phencyclidine (PCP). This relatively unique pattern of induction and stability has lead to the suggestion that ΔFosB may be a particularly important mediator of long-term changes in gene regulation associated with addiction.

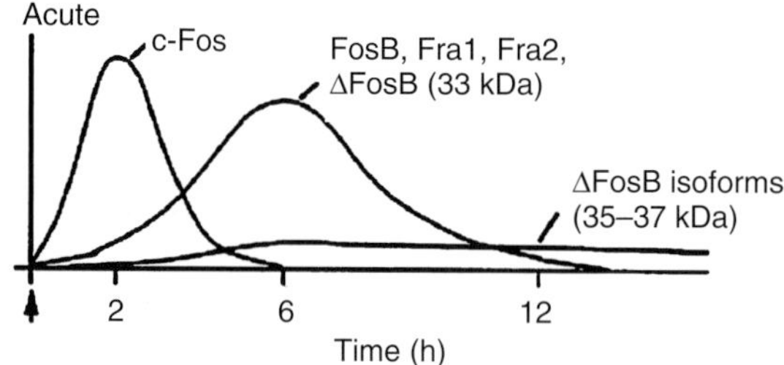

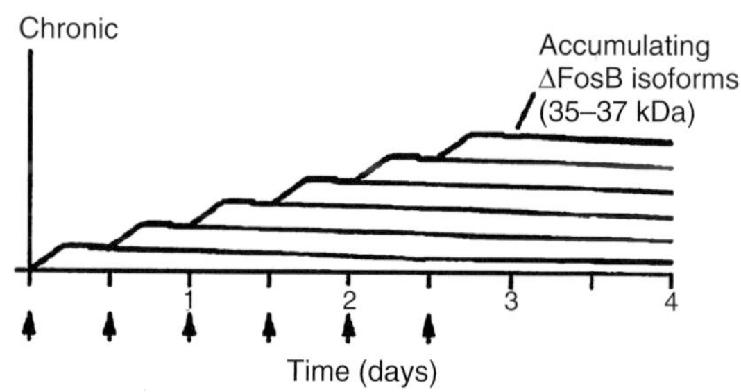

Figure 4 Diagrammatic representation of the induction of the Fos family of transcription factors (TFs) by acute and chronic drugs of abuse. The top panel charts the response to acute stimulation. cFos is rapidly induced, followed by FosB, Fra-1, and Fra-2. Levels of these TFs return to baseline between 6 and 12 hours poststimulation. Only a small increase is observed in levels of stabilized isoforms of ΔFosB. As shown in the bottom panel, this induction persists in the brain for a much longer time course and accumulates with chronic drug administration. Taken from Nestler EJ, Barrott M, and Self DW (2001) ΔFosB: A molecular switch for addiction. *Proc. Natl. Acad. Sci. USA* 98: 11042–11046; used with permission from National Academy of Sciences, USA.

Activation of PKA within the NAc reduces the rewarding effects of cocaine in self-administration and relapse assays, whereas inhibition of PKA has the opposite effect (Self et al., 1998). Likewise, overexpression of CREB in the NAc, through viral mediated gene transfer, decreases place conditioning to cocaine and to morphine, whereas overexpression of a dominant negative mutant form of CREB (mCREB), which cannot be phosphorylated due to a point mutation (Ser133 to Ala), potentiates the rewarding effects of both drugs (Carlezon et al., 1998; Barrot et al., 2002). Similar results are seen in transgenic mice that inducibly overexpress CREB or mCREB in the NAc and dorsal striatum. These data suggest that inhibition of CREB in the NAc enhances the hedonic value of cocaine and morphine; thereby animals 'like' the drug more, or alternatively could be facilitating the formation of the Pavlovian CS-US association between context and drug exposure. The viral infusions targeted the NAc-Sh, which is associated with encoding the rewarding properties of primary reinforcers rather than Pavlovian conditioning processes linking those rewards to environmental stimuli (see earlier). Therefore, it is likely that the behavioral changes observed arise from enhancing the rewarding effects of the drug. This interpretation is consistent with preliminary findings that mCREB decreases brain stimulation reward thresholds, while CREB has the opposite effect (Carlezon et al., 2005). Nevertheless, analysis of tissue from animals killed shortly after completion of the place conditioning test demonstrated increases in the phosphorylated form of CREB in the NAc core but not shell. Blocking this induction disrupted both the retrieval and consolidation of the CS-US association, indicating that CREB in the NAc-C is critically involved in this aspect of reward-related learning (Miller and Marshall, 2005). Thus, activation of CREB may play distinct roles in these two subregions of the NAc. CREB has been heavily implicated in multiple memory processes, particularly those underpinning long-term memory, which may reflect the known role for CREB in mediating certain changes in synaptic plasticity.

Transgenic mice have been developed which selectively overexpress ΔFosB within the NAc and dorsal striatum (Kelz et al., 1999). Furthermore, this overexpression is inducible (it occurs in adult animals) and is cell-type specific in that it is only observed in medium spiny neurons containing dynorphin/substance P (as opposed to those which contain enkephalin). The behavioral phenotype of these mice resembles animals treated chronically with drugs in several ways. The mice are more responsive to cocaine-induced hyperactivity, both acutely and after repeated administration, suggesting that ΔFosB expression may be involved in the development of locomotor sensitization. They also show enhanced place conditioning for cocaine and morphine, indicative of increased sensitivity to the rewarding properties of drugs or (as discussed earlier for CREB) of potential enhancement of the ability to form CS-US associations (Kelz et al., 1999; Zachariou et al., 2006b). Mice overexpressing ΔFosB self-administer lower doses of cocaine than wild-type controls and are more motivated to work for cocaine reward, as indicated by their elevated breakpoints in progressive ratio schedules (Colby et al., 2003). In contrast, mice overexpressing ΔcJun, a truncated form of cJun which acts as a dominant negative antagonist of all AP-1 mediated transcription, show reduced place conditioning to cocaine and morphine (Peakman et al., 2003). Together, these data may reflect more generalized increases in incentive motivation for reward.

One important molecular target of the dopamine system is dopamine and adenosine 3′5′-monophosphate-regulated phosphoprotein (32 kDa), or DARPP-32 as it is commonly known (Fienberg et al., 1998). DARPP-32 has been shown to be a potent modulator of both CREB and ΔFosB as well as many other facets of dopaminergic transmission. As with CREB, D_1-receptor-mediated activation of PKA induces the phosphorylation of DARPP-32 at threonine 34 (Thr34), which then acts as a potent inhibitor of protein phosphatase-1 (PP-1). In contrast, dopaminergic activation through D_2 receptors inhibits PKA signaling, through G-protein-coupled inhibition of adenylyl cyclase, leading to a decrease in phosphorylation of DARPP-32. Through its inhibition of PP-1, DARPP-32 regulates the phosphorylation of numerous proteins. With respect to TFs, mice lacking DARPP-32 show reduced phosphorylation of CREB in response to stimulant drugs of abuse, as well as reduced induction of cFos, in striatal regions (Fienberg et al., 1998). The mice also show reduced induction of ΔFosB after chronic stimulant administration. Consistent with these deficits in biochemical responses to drugs of abuse, DARPP-32 mutant mice show reduced responses to acute drug administration, including reduced locomotor activation and place conditioning (Zachariou et al., 2002). However, paradoxically, the mice show enhanced locomotor sensitization to chronic cocaine. The molecular basis of this latter abnormality is hard to explain on the basis of available data and requires more investigation (Hiroi et al., 1999). Mice in which Thr34 of DARPP-32 is mutated to Ala exhibit virtually the same biochemical and behavioral phenotype as DARPP-32 knockout mice, which demonstrates the importance of DARPP-32's phosphorylation by PKA in regulating its function (Zachariou et al., 2006a).

24.5.2 Clock

TFs traditionally associated with other roles of the dopamine system have also been recently implicated in reward-processing and the response to addictive drugs. For example, the dopaminergic system exerts an important influence over the entrainment of circadian rhythms during fetal development and in response to food and other stimuli, and disruption of the sleep cycle is observed in patients treated with dopaminergic drugs, such as *d*-amphetamine and L-DOPA. Abnormal circadian rhythms are also commonly found in substance abuse disorders. The most studied focus of circadian rhythms in brain is the suprachiasmatic nucleus (SCN) of the hypothalamus. This nucleus is particularly important for entraining the body's circadian rhythms to environmental lighting. The molecular basis of the circadian clock is now well established. The transcription factor Clock dimerizes with Bmal1 to form a transcription factor complex essential for accurate circadian rhythmicity (Vitaterna et al., 1994). The complex activates expression of Period and other proteins, which feed back and suppress their own expression in addition to regulating many other cellular targets. Increasing evidence indicates that this molecular clock operates in all tissues, which raises the interesting notion that many circadian rhythms are driven outside the SCN. For example, recent findings have shown that Clock is highly expressed within dopaminergic neurons of the VTA (McClung et al., 2005). Mice lacking functional Clock protein are hyperactive under baseline conditions, an effect which is most pronounced during the transition from the light to dark phases of their diurnal light cycle. Despite this hyperactivity, these mice show still greater activity following administration of cocaine as compared to littermate controls, and also show increased place conditioning to cocaine as well as decreased brain stimulation reward thresholds. These findings suggest that Clock, at the level of the VTA, may serve to dampen dopaminergic function and suppress reward, and that this may contribute to circadian rhythms in reward and motivation that have been well documented over the years.

24.6 The Role of CREB and ΔFosB in Response to Natural Rewards and Stress

Understanding the response to natural rewards has implications for research into depression due to the obvious relationship between value judgments and anhedonia. Pharmacologically, most currently used antidepressant treatments inhibit the reuptake of the monoamines serotonin and noradrenaline, or inhibit monoamine oxidase (a major catabolic enzyme for monoamine neurotransmitters). Although the dopamine system is critically associated with reward judgments, it is less well studied in the context of depressive etiology. However, changes in some of the same intracellular signaling mechanisms identified in drug addiction research are also affected in animal models of depression and within areas associated with reward-related learning such as the NAc, PFC, and BLA, as well as in areas more strongly associated with memory storage and retrieval such as the HPC (Nestler and Carlezon, 2006). Animal models of depression have generally focused on the response to stress, such as the forced swim test (FST), where antidepressants have been shown to increase the latency to immobility and decrease the total time rodents spend immobile when confined to a water-filled container. Similarly, antidepressants increase the time an animal struggles when suspended by its tail. A lack of struggling in these models is regarded as indicative of a state of behavioral despair. Likewise, animals exposed repeatedly to inescapable stressors, such as shocks, show an increased latency to escape when subsequently given the opportunity.

CREB activity in the NAc appears to play an important role in gating an individual's response to both rewarding and aversive stimuli (Barrot et al., 2002). Increased CRE-mediated transcription in the NAc has been observed following several stressors, including inescapable foot shocks, restraint stress, and the more natural stress of introducing an animal into a novel social group. Increased CREB expression reduces both the nociceptive reaction to painful stimuli and conditioned place aversion to naloxone withdrawal in morphine-dependent rats, whereas mCREB potentiates the response to these aversive stimuli. A similar pattern is observed in anxiety tests, where intra-NAc infusion of herpes simplex virus (HSV)-CREB appears to be anxiolytic and HSV-mCREB anxiogenic. In addition to modulating place conditioning for drug rewards, CREB in the NAc also alters preference for sucrose as assessed by a simple two-bottle choice test. Overexpression of CREB decreases sucrose preference, whereas mCREB increases sucrose preference. Conversely, levels of CRE-mediated transcription in the NAc decrease following protracted social isolation, a manipulation which increases anxiety and impairs initiation of sexual behavior. This phenotype can be rescued by overexpressing CREB within the NAc using viral-mediated gene transfer. Likewise, overexpressing mCREB in this region mimics these effects of isolation in nonisolated rats, an effect that can be reversed with the anxiolytic diazepam (Barrot et al., 2005).

In summary, CREB appears to reduce the impact of emotionally significant stimuli, whereas inhibition of CRE-mediated transcription enhances emotional responsivity. Although mCREB is not a naturally occurring protein, the endogenous inhibitor of CREB function, inducible cAMP early repressor (ICER), is capable of mediating the same functions as mCREB *in vivo* and is induced by both stress and amphetamine (Green et al., 2006). In keeping with this hypothesis that CREB in the NAc numbs the emotional response to stimuli, overexpression of CREB in the NAc induces depressive-like behavior in the FST and learned helplessness test, whereas inhibition of CREB function in this region, through overexpression of either mCREB and ICER, induces antidepressant-like behavior in these tests (Pliakas et al., 2001; Green et al., 2006).

The proposal that CREB gates the response to emotional stimuli within the NAc is consistent with recent elecrophysiological findings, where CREB was shown to increase the electrical excitability of NAc neurons and mCREB to cause the opposite effect (Dong et al., 2006). Moreover, direct inhibition of NAc neurons, via viral-mediated overexpression of a K^+ channel, which would mimic the mCREB effect, increased an animal's behavioral response to cocaine. These findings are interesting in light of work, cited earlier, where inhibition of NAc neurons has been linked with increases in goal-directed behavior.

The effect of CREB in the NAc contrasts with its established role in the HPC where, as noted earlier, CREB is thought to mediate long-term memory formation. Virally mediated overexpression of CREB in the HPC also produces antidepressant-like behavior in rats, an effect potentially mediated in part by CREB-induced elevations of brain-derived neurotrophic factor (BDNF; see section 'Brain-derived neurotrophic factor'). Changing CRE-mediated gene transcription within different brain areas, therefore, has very different effects (Carlezon et al., 2005). Such functional dissociations are not uncommon when considering the effects of neurotransmitters such as dopamine or serotonin. Therefore, it is not surprising that the same intracellular signaling mechanisms activated by these neurotransmitters likewise produce region-specific changes in behavior.

In comparison to CREB, less is known regarding the role of ΔFosB in regulating the response to natural rewards or stressors. ΔFosB upregulation is seen after chronic wheel-running behavior, an activity which rodents are thought to find pleasurable but potentially compulsive or 'addictive,' and mice overexpressing ΔFosB in striatal regions exhibit greater compulsive wheel-running than their wild-type littermates (Werme et al., 2002). Moreover, overexpression of ΔFosB in striatal regions, either by viral vectors or in inducible transgenic mice, increases motivation for food in progressive ratio and instrumental learning tests (Olausson et al., 2006). These findings support the hypothesis, mentioned earlier, that ΔFosB in this neural pathway promotes reward.

24.7 Target Genes of CREB and ΔFosB

This section will primarily focus on examples of the downstream targets of CREB and ΔFosB associated with reward processing, addiction, and depression-like behavior at the level of the brain's reward pathways. A broad survey of CREB and ΔFosB targets in the NAc has been published recently (McClung and Nestler, 2003). However, changes in targets upstream of the TFs considered here have also been associated with the response to rewarding stimuli, including the enzymes responsible for the synthesis and degradation of cAMP, namely adenylyl cyclase and cyclic nucleotide phosphodiesterases, respectively. Kinases such as PKA and extracellular signaling kinases (ERKs) have been implicated in the effects of addictive drugs as well as in numerous facets of learning and memory.

24.7.1 Dynorphin in the VTA-NAc Pathway

One of the primary mechanisms by which CREB is thought to affect reward-related learning and addiction is through induction of dynorphin within the NAc (**Figure 5**). Dopaminergic neurons in the VTA innervate GABAergic neurons in the NAc, which express dynorphin and in which activation of CREB has been observed after chronic treatment with addictive drugs. Dynorphin acts on κ opioid receptors expressed on the terminals of these

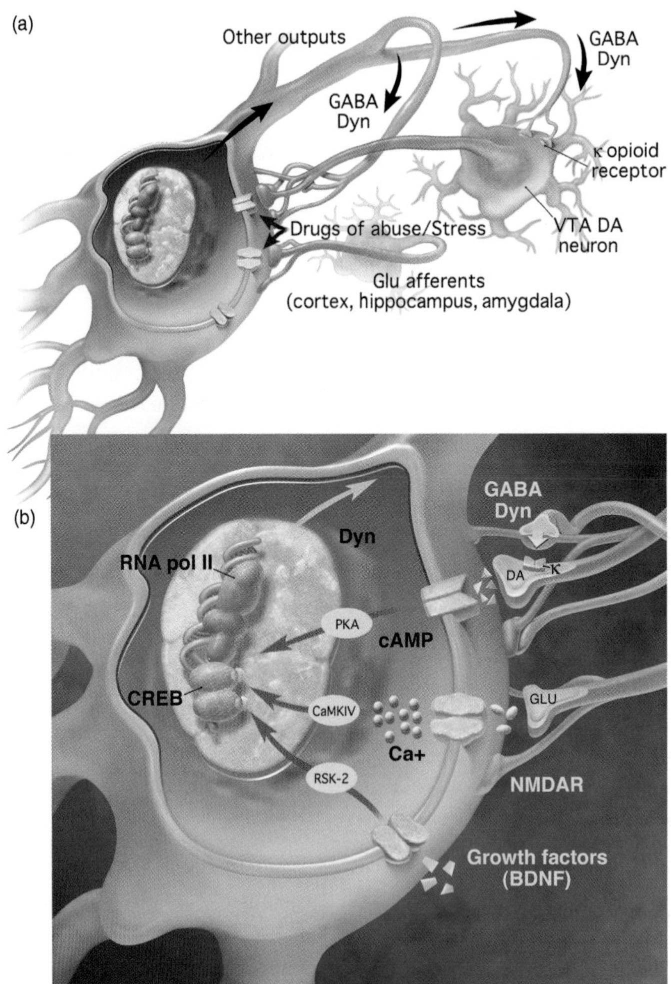

Figure 5 Regulation of NAc function by CREB and dynorphin (Dyn). The figure shows a dopaminergic neuron from the VTA innervating a medium spiny neuron within the NAc which expresses dynorphin. Glutamatergic input from other areas such as the PFC and amygdala, as well as BDNF (released from glutamatergic or dopaminergic projections) are also shown. Dynorphin acts as a negative feedback signal: when released, it binds to κ opioid receptors on dopaminergic neurons and inhibits their function. Drugs of abuse and stress increase CREB activity and induce dynorphin expression, upregulating this feedback loop. Activation of CREB could be caused by some of the mechanisms shown in the figure, all of which lead to its phosphorylation at Ser 133. Abbreviations: GABA, gamma-aminobutyric acid; NMDAR, *N*-methyl-D-aspartate receptor; PKA, protein kinase A; CaMKIV, Ca^{2+}/calmodulin-dependent protein kinase type IV; RSK-2, ribosomal S6 kinase-type 2; RNA pol II, RNA polymerase II complex. Taken from Nestler EJ, Barrot M, DiLeone RJ, Eisch AJ, Gold SJ, and Monteggia LM (2002) Neurobiology of depression. *Neuron* 34: 13–25; used with permission from Cell Press.

dopaminergic projections and inhibits their function, thereby forming a negative feedback loop to minimize the effects of dopaminergic stimulation. This dampening of the dopamine signal could contribute to the depressant-like effects of overexpressing CREB within the NAc and the reduction in place conditioning to addictive drugs (Carlezon et al., 2005). Increased ΔFosB is also primarily observed in dynorphin-containing cells within the NAc, but acts to decrease expression of dynorphin (Zachariou et al., 2006b) and to thereby potentiate dopaminergic signaling. Such reciprocal regulation of dynorphin by CREB and ΔFosB could explain some of the reciprocal behavioral changes observed following upregulation of these TFs. It could also account for the changes in reward processing that occur during different timepoints of withdrawal from addictive drugs. Drug-induced activation of CREB is relatively short-lived, yet increasing drug use potentiates CREB expression. The anhedonia and negative emotional symptoms which predominate during acute withdrawal could therefore arise partly from the ability of

CREB to downregulate dopaminergic signaling. In contrast, the sensitization to the rewarding effects of addictive drugs and the incubation of craving which predominate at later timepoints could be mediated in part by the prolonged expression of ΔFosB.

24.7.2 Cyclin-Dependent Kinase 5

Cyclin-dependent kinase 5 (Cdk5) was identified as a downstream target of ΔFosB within the NAc through microarray analysis (Bibb et al., 2001). Activation of Cdk5 alters dopaminergic signaling through phosphorylation of DARPP-32 at a different site from PKA, namely threonine 75 (Thr75) (see Benavides and Bibb, 2004). This converts DARPP-32 from an inhibitor of PP-1 to an inhibitor of PKA. The fact that DARPP-32 can function as either a protein phosphatase inhibitor or a protein kinase inhibitor, depending on the site at which it is phosphorylated, may be unique, and this high level of phosphorylation-site-specific regulation further highlights the importance of this molecule in intracellular signaling cascades. Furthermore, PKA activation can decrease phospho-Thr75 DARPP-32 through activation of protein phosphatase 2A (PP-2A). Acute administration of cocaine can increase phosphorylation of DARPP-32 at Thr34 and reduce it at Thr75 via activation of PKA and inhibition of the PP-2A pathway, respectively. However, chronic cocaine administration has the opposite effect, increasing phosphorylation of Thr75, and reducing the ability of D_1 receptor stimulation to activate PKA. Cdk5 is upregulated by chronic cocaine administration, and this effect appears to be mediated by ΔFosB: overexpression of ΔFosB induces Cdk5 expression, while expression of the dominant negative ΔcJun prevents the ability of cocaine to induce the enzyme (Bibb et al., 2001; Peakman et al., 2003).

The behavioral contribution of Cdk5 induction is complex. Intra-NAc infusion of the Cdk5 inhibitor roscovitine has been shown to potentiate the hyperlocomotor response to cocaine seen following chronic drug administration (Bibb et al., 2001). These behavioral data suggest that cocaine-induced upregulation of Cdk5 activity may be an attempt to compensate for overstimulation of the dopaminergic system. However, intra-NAc infusions of roscovitine also block the increase in dendritic spine proliferation seen in this region with chronic cocaine administration, which is correlated with the development of locomotor sensitization (Norrholm et al., 2003). As discussed earlier, these neuroplastic changes are one potential mechanism by which repeated drug administration perpetuates changes in learning and memory processes integral to the sensitized and addicted state. Chronic cocaine exposure, via ΔFosB, may therefore trigger an adaptive homeostatic response involving increased Cdk5 activity that ultimately commits the affected neurons to a maladaptive process of cytoarchitectural changes.

24.7.3 Nuclear Factor Kappa B

Nuclear factor kappa B (NFκB) is a transcription factor induced in many tissues by inflammation and immune responsiveness (see Chen and Greene, 2004). It is composed of two subunits, most commonly p50 and p65. Under basal conditions, it remains sequestered in the cytoplasm by inhibitory kappa B (IKB) protein. Upon phosphorylation by I kappa kinase (IKK), IKB releases an inactive dimer of p50 and p65, which can then be phosphorylated and transported to the nucleus where it can initiate gene transcription. This TF is more commonly associated with the field of immunology than neuroscience. However, in parallel to Cdk5, both ΔFosB overexpression and chronic cocaine treatment upregulate NFκB-related proteins such as p65, the precursor of p50 (p103), and IKB within the NAc (Ang et al., 2001). NFκB has been implicated in regulating cell survival and neuroplasticity and has been associated with long-term potentiation (LTP) and long-term depression (LTD), responses implicated in learning and memory processes. In terms of reward processing, intra-amygdala infusions of κB decoy DNA impaired fear-potentiated startle responses, suggesting that this molecule may play a role in the intracellular signaling pathway underpinning emotional CS-US learning (Yeh et al., 2002). Preliminary data also indicate that potentiating NFκB signaling within the NAc through overexpression of a constitutively active form of IKK increases place conditioning to cocaine and also increases local dendritic spine formation.

24.7.4 Brain-Derived Neurotrophic Factor

Neurotrophic factors facilitate neural growth and differentiation during development and also have a critical role to play in mediating neuronal survival and plasticity in adulthood. BDNF has been identified as an important downstream target of CREB and is implicated in numerous processes related to learning and memory, particularly within the HPC.

BDNF also modulates emotional learning within the amygdala, where increases in BDNF mRNA have been reported following fear conditioning. In addition, overexpression of a mutated dominant negative form of the tyrosine kinase B (TrkB) receptor within the amygdala blocks the acquisition of fear conditioning (Rattiner et al., 2004), indicating that the ability of BDNF to mediate changes in synaptic plasticity could be of particular import in the encoding of emotionally significant events in this region.

24.7.4.1 The neurotrophic hypothesis of depression

The neurotrophic hypothesis of depression suggests that a deficiency in neurotrophic support may contribute to the observed hippocampal pathology associated with depression (e.g., reduced hippocampal volume in depressed patients, decreases in dendritic arborization, decreased adult hippocampal neurogenesis), and that antidepressants relieve the symptoms of depression through increasing neurotrophic action. BDNF has been widely studied within the context of this hypothesis. Chronic administration of numerous antidepressant drugs increases expression of BDNF within the HPC despite their diverse pharmacological actions (Nibuya et al., 1995). Both acute and chronic stress decreases BDNF expression in hippocampal regions, effects which may contribute to the etiology of depression and which can be blocked by antidepressant treatment. Direct infusion of BDNF into the hippocampus also produces antidepressant-like effects on the FST and learned helplessness paradigms (Shirayama et al., 2002), while mice lacking BDNF do not show antidepressant behavioral responses (Monteggia et al., 2004, 2007), further indicating that BDNF may be important in mediating depressive symptoms.

Observations that both intra-cerebral infusions of BDNF (Pencea et al., 2001) and chronic administration of antidepressants (Malberg et al., 2000) increase adult neurogenesis has led to the suggestion that this may be one mechanism underlying the therapeutic action of antidepressants. However, a direct, causal relationship between neurogenesis, BDNF, and antidepressant action has proved difficult to demonstrate conclusively. Although X-ray irradiation of the brain blocks cell proliferation and also prevented the chronic effects of antidepressants in a novelty-suppressed feeding assay (Santarelli et al., 2003), irradiation also disrupts numerous intracellular signaling cascades, which may confound interpretation of these findings (Silasi et al., 2004).

Although it is clear that antidepressants can increase CREB and that CREB activity can increase BDNF expression, it is currently unclear as to whether CREB-mediated activation of BDNF is the critical pathway for the antidepressant actions of BDNF. Thus, the increase in BDNF caused by antidepressant administration is blocked in CREB-deficient mice (Conti et al., 2002), yet these mice still respond to antidepressant drugs in tests such as the FST. Although CREB phosphorylation is thought to have pro-survival properties in newly formed hippocampal neurons, the atypical antidepressant tianeptine increases hippocampal neurogenesis but does not activate the cAMP signaling cascade (Czeh et al., 2001). The role of CREB in the antidepressant effects of BDNF clearly merits further study (Malberg and Blendy, 2005).

24.7.4.2 BDNF within the VTA-NAc: Reward processing and addiction

In addition to its roles in neuroplastic responses, BDNF is critically involved in the regulation of dopaminergic neurotransmission. Through binding at TrkB receptors on dopaminergic terminals within the NAc, BDNF is capable of potentiating dopamine release in this region. In addition, BDNF acts directly on TrkB receptors expressed by NAc neurons. Hence, it is not surprising that this molecule has been implicated in addiction and reward-related learning. Direct administration of BDNF into the NAc or VTA increases cocaine-induced hyperactivity, whereas BDNF heterozygous knockout mice show reduced locomotor activity and reduced place conditioning to cocaine (Hall et al., 2003). Intra-NAc BDNF also increases responding for CRf (Horger et al., 1999), suggesting that induction of BDNF may contribute to the increases in incentive motivation for drugs that are associated with addiction. In support of this hypothesis, increases in BDNF have been observed in the NAc, BLA, and VTA following withdrawal from cocaine, and these increases appear to track the incubation (potentiation over time) of craving for cocaine as measured by drug-seeking behavior following presentation of a drug-paired CS (Grimm et al., 2003). A direct infusion of BDNF into the VTA can also potentiate such drug-seeking behavior (Lu et al., 2004).

However, despite these increases in incentive motivation for drugs and the potentiation of local dopaminergic transmission, increases in BDNF within the NAc and VTA appear to induce a pro-depressant phenotype. Intra-VTA infusions of BDNF decreased the latency to immobility in the FST, whereas overexpression of a mutant TrkB receptor within the NAc (which inhibits BDNF signaling) produces an antidepressant-like effect in the same task (Eisch et al., 2003). Recent data using the social defeat model of stress in mice provide further insight into the role of BDNF in affective processing. In this paradigm, an animal is defeated by a larger, dominant, and aggressive mouse and is then housed in close confinement with the aggressor (although the animals can no longer fight). Animals defeated chronically in this way develop a behavioral syndrome characterized by numerous indices of anhedonia which may reflect aspects of human depression, such as decreased preference for natural rewards such as sucrose, sex, and social interaction, as well as a general decrease in locomotor activity. Some of these changes are particularly long-lasting and are reversed by chronic antidepressant treatment (Berton et al., 2006). Knocking out BDNF within the VTA selectively, by use of a viral vector expressing the Cre recombinase, prevents the development of this depressive-like syndrome following social defeat. These data suggest that BDNF within the VTA-NAc pathway plays an important role in reward-related learning, and that overstimulation of this signaling pathway by repeated drug intake or chronic stress could lead to potentiated and maladaptive learning, both to rewarding and aversive stimuli. As with CREB, the effects of BDNF in the HPC versus the VTA-NAc appear to be diametrically opposed. Indeed, the observation that stress decreases BDNF in the HPC, yet increases it in the VTA-NAc, indicates that these areas mediate very different aspects of an animal's behavioral repertoire in response to stress.

24.7.5 Glutamate Receptors

In addition to the changes observed in dopaminergic signaling, repeated administration of addictive drugs increases the expression of both alpha-amino-3-hydroxy-5-methyl-4-isoxazole propionic acid (AMPA) and *N*-methyl-D-aspartate (NMDA) glutamate receptor (GluR) subunits within the VTA. The GluR1 subunit of the AMPA receptor has received particular attention (Carlezon et al., 2002). Increases in the number of GluR1 subunits present in an AMPA receptor increase its overall conductance as well as its permeability to calcium (Ca^{2+}) ions. Ca^{2+} is involved in numerous intracellular signaling pathways, and changes in levels of intracellular Ca^{2+} can alter the regulation of gene expression. Given that sensitizing regimes of drug administration increase the electrophysiological responsiveness of dopaminergic cells within the VTA to AMPA receptor agonists (Thomas and Malenka, 2003), and that the increase in GluR1 subunits is most prominent in animals showing behavioral signs of sensitization (Churchill et al., 1999), it has been suggested that upregulation of the GluR1 subunit may be one molecular mechanism underlying the potentiated response to chronic drug treatment. In support of this hypothesis, increasing GluR1 expression within the VTA increases both conditioned place preference and hyperlocomotion caused by morphine (Carlezon et al., 1997). Recent evidence indicates that drug-induced upregulation of GluR1 in the VTA may be mediated via drug induction of CREB in this brain region (Olson et al., 2005).

In contrast, increases in GluR1 subunit expression within the NAc-Sh can facilitate the extinction of cocaine-seeking (Sutton et al., 2003), suggesting that increased glutamatergic action within this region can reverse some of the detrimental adaptations caused by chronic drug intake. Chronic cocaine treatment has been shown to reduce the electrophysiological sensitivity of NAc neurons to AMPA agonists (Thomas and Malenka, 2003). This effect may be accounted for by increased levels of GluR2 subunits within the NAc, which decrease the conductance of AMPA receptors and reduce their permeability to Ca^{2+}. Overexpression of ΔFosB increases GluR2 levels within the NAc, while ΔcJun prevents the ability of cocaine to induce the protein (Kelz et al., 1999; Peakman et al., 2003). Moreover, viral-mediated overexpression of GluR2 within the NAc mimics the effects of increased ΔFosB, in that both manipulations enhance place conditioning to cocaine (Kelz et al., 1999). Drug-induced adaptations in several postsynaptic density proteins, which modulate GluR function, have also been observed in the NAc (Yao et al., 2004). It would, therefore, appear that drug-induced changes in the expression of different GluR subunits within different reward-related regions may have opposing actions on cellular excitability, yet may both contribute to the addicted phenotype.

24.8 Molecular Changes within the PFC

The majority of work to date has focused on changes in transcriptional regulation within the subcortical regions of reward-related circuitry, with an understandable emphasis on the NAc and VTA. However, changes in gene expression within the PFC have also been observed in models of addiction and depression, although less is known about their functional consequences (Kalivas, 2004). For example, a recent study examined patterns of cFos expression within the PrLC, NAc, and BLA following reexposure to a cocaine-associated context, as assessed by place conditioning. The authors observed a selective increase in GABAergic cells expressing cFos within the PrLC (Miller and Marshall, 2004). Similarly, a decrease in protein kinase C (PKC) has been observed in this region during retrieval of a discrete CS paired with cocaine during self-administration training (Thomas and Everitt, 2001). These data suggest that output from this region is reduced in response to cue exposure, a finding which may be of relevance to cue-elicited drug craving.

Alterations in G-protein-coupled receptor signaling pathways within the mPFC have recently been identified which may underlie potentiated responding to drug versus natural rewards and relapse to drug-seeking (Kalivas et al., 2005). The activator of G-protein signaling 3 (AGS3) is increased in the mPFC following withdrawal from cocaine self-administration, and reinstatement of cocaine seeking can be blocked by decreasing levels of AGS3. AGS3 sequesters the alpha subunit of inhibitory G proteins (Giα) and reduces signaling through Giα-coupled receptors such as D_2 dopamine receptors. It is thought that this reduction in D_2 receptor signaling leads to increased inhibition of PFC output to the NAc which can only be overcome by relatively strong inputs, such as drug reward. This hypothesis needs further investigation, but potentially provides a molecular mechanism to explain the increased control over goal-directed behavior exerted by drugs of abuse.

Increases in ΔFosB have also been reported in regions of the frontal cortex following chronic exposure to both addictive drugs and stressful manipulations (Perrotti et al., 2004). Recent evidence suggests that increased expression of ΔFosB within this region increases preference for sucrose, potentially indicative of an increased sensitivity to rewarding stimuli. Increased ΔFosB in this region also appears to sensitize animals to the locomotor stimulant actions of cocaine, yet produces tolerance to the disruptive effects of the psychostimulant on operant behavioral measures of motivation and impulsivity. These changes closely parallel those observed after chronic cocaine treatment. Further work aimed at understanding the changes in cognition caused by long-term drug use, and their underlying molecular basis, is clearly warranted.

24.9 Beyond Corticolimbic Circuitry: A Role for Hypothalamic Feeding Peptides in Reward-Related Learning?

The hypothalamus is one of the most important regions of the brain in terms of regulating more physiological aspects of reward such as the homeostatic control of hunger and thirst. Animals will preferentially self-stimulate the lateral hypothalamus (LH), a finding partially explained by the fact that dopaminergic fibers from the VTA to the NAc pass through this structure. Intriguingly, the threshold for LH self-stimulation in the perifornical region increases with weight loss, suggesting a relationship between the physiological homeostatic drive for natural rewards and the sensitivity of the brain to rewarding stimuli in general (see Shizgal et al., 2001). Although this region has not been associated with the more cognitive process of mediating goal-directed behavior, modulation of hypothalamic activity forms a critical part of the output pathway of the corticolimbic circuitry discussed earlier. The maintenance of energy balance depends on the allocation of behavior between feeding and competing activities; therefore, the signals of hunger or satiety generated by the hypothalamus have significant impact on the motivation for food reward and, therefore, potentially on numerous models of goal-seeking discussed previously. Whether modulation of this signal is also involved in assessment of the rewarding properties of addictive drugs is currently under investigation. The hypothalamic–pituitary adrenal axis is also one of the most prominent mechanisms by which the brain reacts to stress. Neurons in the paraventricular nucleus of the hypothalamus secrete corticotropin-releasing factor, which stimulates the release of adrenocorticotropin from the anterior pituitary. This in turn leads to production of glucocorticoids (cortisol in humans and corticosterone in rodents) within the adrenal cortex, which can have profound effects on behavior and brain function in numerous regions, as well as affecting general metabolism. Given that stress contributes to the development of affective psychiatric disorders such as depression and can trigger relapse to drug-seeking, a growing number of studies are addressing the role of signaling peptides within this region in reward-related learning and emotional processing. Some examples are considered in the following, though this is by no means an exhaustive list.

Melanin-concentrating hormone (MCH) is an orexigenic (pro-appetite) protein expressed within the lateral hypothalamus. The MCH_1 receptor is highly expressed within the NAc, and intra-NAc infusions of MCH increase food intake, whereas antagonists of the MCH_1 receptor have the opposite effect. MCH_1 receptor antagonists acting within the NAc also exert antidepressant effects within the FST, an effect which is also observed in MCH knockout mice (Georgescu et al., 2005) and with systemic administration of MCH antagonists (Borowsky et al., 2002). These data suggest that molecules primarily thought to control the regulation of food intake can also have an effect on mood through their influence on NAc function.

Orexin (hypocretin) may have a similar role to play. Expressed within the lateral hypothalamus, orexin increases food intake by promoting a state of wakefulness and arousal, and deficits in orexin are known to cause the sleep disorder narcolepsy (Mignot, 2001). This debilitating condition, characterized by daytime sleepiness, cataplexy, and other sleep abnormalities, is frequently associated with depression, and some of the sleep-related symptoms are treated with antidepressants (Daniels et al., 2001). Narcolepsy and depression are both associated with alterations in circadian rhythms, and a dampening in the naturally occurring diurnal variation in orexin levels has been observed in depressed patients (e.g., Salomon et al., 2003). One mechanism by which hypothalamic peptides may influence reward processing may be via their modulation of the dopaminergic system. For example, orexin neurons project prominently to the dopaminergic cells of the VTA, where orexin binds to orexin 1 (OX_1) receptors to stimulate the neurons. Administration of an OX_1 receptor antagonist blocks the development of locomotor sensitization to cocaine (Borgland et al., 2006), whereas orexin precipitates relapse to drug-seeking in animals withdrawn from cocaine self-administration through induction of a stress-like state (Boutrel et al., 2005). Orexin knockout mice also show reduced physical dependence on morphine as indicated by a reduction in the physical signs of naloxone-precipitated withdrawal symptoms (Georgescu et al., 2003).

Functional interactions between the dopaminergic system and another hypothalamic peptide family, the melanocortins, have been reported and have likewise been implicated in mediating drug reward. Mice lacking the melanocortin-4 (MC_4) receptor, which is highly expressed within the NAc, fail to develop locomotor sensitization, and direct intra-NAc infusions of an MC_4 antagonist peptide, SHU-9119, reduces cocaine self-administration and place conditioning. As with BDNF, this peptide also prevents cocaine from potentiating the response to CRf (Hsu et al., 2005).

Neuropeptide Y (NPY) is perhaps best known for its ability to antagonize the behavioral consequences of stress within the central nervous system (CNS) (see Heilig, 2004). Administration of NPY is anxiolytic in numerous animal models, which is thought to result in part from its actions at Y_1 receptors within the amygdala. Acute stress decreases NPY expression, whereas chronic stress exposure, which leads to behavioral habituation, reverses this effect so that NPY is upregulated. The hypothesis that increased NPY expression could mediate coping responses is supported by the observation that NPY transgenic rats are less sensitive to stressful manipulations (Thorsell et al., 2000). In keeping with the view that stress promotes depression, at least in vulnerable individuals, antidepressant treatments also increase NPY within the frontal cortex, providing another mechanism by which antidepressant drugs may confer their therapeutic benefit. Dysregulation of NPY regulation has also been implicated in drug addiction, particularly in relation to alcoholism, where it is thought to mediate the anxiolytic properties of alcohol, thereby increasing motivation to consume the drug (see Valdez and Koob, 2004).

Whether induction of these hypothalamic feeding peptides is regulated by the same TFs as other proteins implicated in reward and addiction has yet to be determined. However, it is known that NPY is a downstream target of CREB, and whether the behavioral effects of NPY expression likewise vary depending on its locus of action remains a possibility.

24.10 Overview

Within this article, we have briefly considered the psychological processes involved in signaling rewarding events, and the roles played by different regions within the corticostriatal loop associated with reward-related learning. Through analysis of the intracellular signaling cascades affected by the dopaminergic system, specific molecules involved in mediating aspects of reward processing have been highlighted, and data pertaining to their influence over reward-related behavior have been discussed. In parallel to much of what is known regarding the neurochemical basis of reward signaling, it is clear that different molecules can have very different effects on behavior depending on their locus of action. Likewise, the time course of molecular changes, whether transient or long-term, can have a profound influence on their behavioral consequences. The molecular tools have now been developed to directly manipulate intracellular signaling pathways and gene transcription at the level of different transcription factors and their downstream targets within highly circumscribed brain nuclei. As these advances in molecular biological techniques become more accessible, a wider array of behavioral and genetic studies will become possible. Although significant progress has been made in determining the role of such molecular events in reward-related learning, further integration between the fields of psychology and molecular biology will enable greater understanding of the biological basis of goal-directed behavior.

References

Alexander GE, DeLong MR, and Strick PL (1986) Parallel organization of functionally segregrated circuits linking basal ganglia and cortex. *Annu. Rev. Neurosci.* 9: 357–381.

Ang E, Chen J, Zagouras P, et al. (2001) Induction of nuclear factor-kappaB in nucleus accumbens by chronic cocaine administration. *J. Neurochem.* 79: 221–224.

Arnsten AFT (1997) Catecholamine modulation of prefrontal cortical cognitive function. *Trends Cogn. Sci.* 2: 436–447.

Balleine BW and Dickinson A (1998) Goal-directed instrumental action: Contingency and incentive learning and their cortical substrates. *Neuropharmacology* 37: 407–419.

Barrot M, Wallace DL, Bolanos CA, et al. (2005) Regulation of anxiety and initiation of sexual behavior by CREB in the nucleus accumbens. *Proc. Natl. Acad. Sci. USA* 102: 8357–8362.

Barrot M, Olivier JDA, Perrotti LI, et al. (2002) CREB activity in the nucleus accumbens shell controls gating of behavioral responses to emotional stimuli. *Proc. Natl. Acad. Sci. USA* 99: 11435–11440.

Baxter MG, Parker A, Lindner CC, Izquierdo AD, and Murray EA (2000) Control of response selection by reinforcer value requires interaction of amygdala and orbital prefrontal cortex. *J. Neurosci.* 20: 4311–4319.

Bechara A, Damasio H, Damasio AR, and Lee GP (1999) Different contributions of the human amygdala and ventromedial prefrontal cortex to decision-making. *J. Neurosci.* 19: 5473–5481.

Bechara A, Dolan S, Denburg N, Hindes A, Anderson SW, and Nathan PE (2001) Decision-making deficits, linked to a dysfunctional ventromedial prefrontal cortex, revealed in alcohol and stimulant abusers. *Neuropsychologia* 39: 376–389.

Benavides DR and Bibb JA (2004) Role of Cdk5 in drug abuse and plasticity. *Ann. N.Y. Acad. Sci.* 1025: 335–344.

Berendse HW, Galis-de Graaf Y, and Groenewegen HJ (1992) Topographical organization and relationship with ventral striatal compartments of prefrontal corticostriatal projections in the rat. *J. Comp. Neurol.* 316: 314–347.

Berton O, McClung CA, Dileone RJ, et al. (2006) Essential role of BDNF in the mesolimbic dopamine pathway in social defeat stress. *Science* 311: 864–868.

Bibb JA, Chen J, Taylor JR, et al. (2001) Effects of chronic exposure to cocaine are regulated by the neuronal protein Cdk5. *Nature* 410: 376–380.

Borgland SL, Taha SA, Sarti F, Fields HL, and Bonci A (2006) Orexin A in the VTA is critical for the induction of synaptic plasticity and behavioral sensitization to cocaine. *Neuron* 49: 589–601.

Borowsky B, Durkin MM, Ogozalek K, et al. (2002) Antidepressant, anxiolytic and anorectic effects of a melanin-concentrating hormone-1 receptor antagonist. *Nat. Med.* 8: 825–830.

Boutrel B, Kenny PJ, Specio SE, et al. (2005) Role for hypocretin in mediating stress-induced reinstatement of cocaine-seeking behavior. *Proc. Natl. Acad. Sci. USA* 102: 19168–19173.

Cardinal RN (2001) Neuropsychology of reinforcement processes in the rat. In: *Experimental Psychology*, p. 276. PhD Thesis, University of Cambridge.

Cardinal RN, Parkinson JA, Hall J, and Everitt BJ (2002) Emotion and motivation: The role of the amygdala, ventral striatum, and prefrontal cortex. *Neurosci. Biobehav. Rev.* 26: 321–352.

Cardinal RN, Pennicott DR, Sugathapala CL, Robbins TW, and Everitt BJ (2001) Impulsive choice induced in rats by lesions of the nucleus accumbens core. *Science* 292: 2499–2501.

Carlezon WA, Jr., Boundy VA, Haile CN, et al. (1997) Sensitization to morphine induced by viral-mediated gene transfer. *Science* 277: 812–814.

Carlezon WA, Jr., Duman RS, and Nestler EJ (2005) The many faces of CREB. *Trends Neurosci.* 28(8): 436–445.

Carlezon WA, Jr., and Nestler EJ (2002) Elevated levels of GluR1 in the midbrain: A trigger for sensitization to drugs of abuse? *Trends Neurosci.* 25: 610–615.

Carlezon WA, Jr., Thome J, Olson VG, et al. (1998) Regulation of cocaine reward by CREB. *Science* 282: 2272–2275.

Cavedini P, Riboldi G, Keller R, D'Annucci A, and Bellodi L (2002) Frontal lobe dysfunction in pathological gambling patients. *Biol. Psychiatry* 51: 334–341.

Chen LF and Greene WC (2004) Shaping the nuclear action of NF-kappaB. *Nat. Rev. Mol. Cell. Biol.* 5: 392–401.

Childress AR, McLellan AT, Ehrman R, and O'Brien CP (1988) Classically conditioned responses in opioid and cocaine dependence: A role in relapse? *NIDA Res. Monogr.* 84: 25–43.

Chudasama Y and Robbins TW (2003) Dissociable contributions of the orbitofrontal and infralimbic cortex to pavlovian autoshaping and discrimination reversal learning: Further evidence for the functional heterogeneity of the rodent frontal cortex. *J. Neurosci.* 23: 8771–8780.

Churchill L, Swanson CJ, Urbina M, and Kalivas PW (1999) Repeated cocaine alters glutamate receptor subunit levels in the nucleus accumbens and ventral tegmental area of rats that develop behavioral sensitization. *J. Neurochem.* 72: 2397–2403.

Cohen JD, Braver TS, and Brown JW (2002) Computational perspectives on dopamine function in prefrontal cortex. *Curr. Opin. Neurobiol.* 12: 223–229.

Colby CR, Whisler K, Steffen C, Nestler EJ, and Self DW (2003) Striatal cell type-specific overexpression of DeltaFosB enhances incentive for cocaine. *J. Neurosci.* 23: 2488–2493.

Conti AC, Cryan JF, Dalvi A, Lucki I, and Blendy JA (2002) cAMP response element-binding protein is essential for the upregulation of brain-derived neurotrophic factor transcription, but not the behavioral or endocrine responses to antidepressant drugs. *J. Neurosci.* 22: 3262–3268.

Corbit LH and Balleine BW (2003) The role of prelimbic cortex in instrumental conditioning. *Behav. Brain Res.* 146: 145–157.

Critchley HD and Rolls ET (1996) Hunger and satiety modify the responses of olfactory and visual neurons in the primate orbitofrontal cortex. *J. Neurophysiol.* 75: 1673–1686.

Czeh B, Michaelis T, Watanabe T, et al. (2001) Stress-induced changes in cerebral metabolites, hippocampal volume, and cell proliferation are prevented by antidepressant treatment with tianeptine. *Proc. Natl. Acad. Sci. USA* 98: 12796–12801.

Daniels E, King MA, Smith IE, and Shneerson JM (2001) Health-related quality of life in narcolepsy. *J. Sleep Res*. 10: 75–81.

Davis M (1998) Are different parts of the extended amygdala involved in fear versus anxiety? *Biol. Psychiatry* 44: 1239–1247.

de Wit H and Stewart J (1981) Reinstatement of cocaine-reinforced responding in the rat. *Psychopharmacology (Berl.)* 75: 134–143.

Dong Y, Green T, Saal D, et al. (2006) CREB modulates excitability of nucleus accumbens neuron. *Nat. Neurosci*. 9: 475–477.

Eisch AJ, Bolanos CA, de Wit J, et al. (2003) Brain-derived neurotrophic factor in the ventral midbrain-nucleus accumbens pathway: A role in depression. *Biol. Psychiatry* 54: 994–1005.

Everitt BJ, Cardinal RN, Hall J, Parkinson JA, and Robbins TW (2000) Differential involvement of amygdala subsystems in appetitive conditioning and drug addiction. In: Aggleton J (ed.) *The Amygdala: A Functional Analysis,* 2nd edn., pp. 353–391. Oxford: Oxford University Press.

Fienberg AA, Hiroi N, Mermelstein PG, et al. (1998) DARPP-32: Regulator of the efficacy of dopaminergic neurotransmission. *Science* 281: 838–842.

Georgescu D, Zachariou V, Barrot M, et al. (2003) Involvement of the lateral hypothalamic peptide orexin in morphine dependence and withdrawal. *J. Neurosci*. 23: 3106–3111.

Georgescu D, Sears RM, Hommel JD, et al. (2005) The hypothalamic neuropeptide melanin-concentrating hormone acts in the nucleus accumbens to modulate feeding behavior and forced-swim performance. *J. Neurosci*. 25: 2933–2940.

Green TA, Alibhai IN, Hommel JD, et al. (2006) Induction of inducible cAMP early repressor expression in nucleus accumbens by stress or amphetamine increases behavioral responses to emotional stimuli. *J. Neurosci*. 26: 8235–8242.

Grimm JW, Lu L, Hayashi T, Hope BT, Su TP, and Shaham Y (2003) Time-dependent increases in brain-derived neurotrophic factor protein levels within the mesolimbic dopamine system after withdrawal from cocaine: Implications for incubation of cocaine craving. *J. Neurosci*. 23: 742–747.

Groenewegen HJ, Vermeulen-van der Zee E, Kortschot AT, and Witter MP (1987) Organization of the projections from the subiculum to the ventral striatum in the rat: A study using anterograde transport of Phaseolus vulgaris leucoagglutinin. *Neuroscience* 23: 103–120.

Hall FS, Drgonova J, Goeb M, and Uhl GR (2003) Reduced behavioral effects of cocaine in heterozygous brain-derived neurotrophic factor (BDNF) knockout mice. *Neuropsychopharmacology* 28: 1485–1490.

Hall J, Parkinson JA, Connor TM, Dickinson A, and Everitt BJ (2001) Involvement of the central nucleus of the amygdala and nucleus accumbens core in mediating Pavlovian influences on instrumental behaviour. *Eur. J. Neurosci*. 13: 1984–1992.

Hatfield T, Han JS, Conley M, Gallagher M, and Holland P (1996) Neurotoxic lesions of basolateral, but not central, amygdala interfere with Pavlovian second-order conditioning and reinforcer devaluation effects. *J. Neurosci.* 16: 5256–5265.

Heilig M (2004) The NPY system in stress, anxiety and depression. *Neuropeptides* 38: 213–224.

Hiroi N, Fienberg AA, Haile CN, et al. (1999) Neuronal and behavioural abnormalities in striatal function in DARPP-32-mutant mice. *Eur. J. Neurosci*. 11: 1114–1118.

Horger BA, Iyasere CA, Berhow MT, Messer CJ, Nestler EJ, and Taylor JR (1999) Enhancement of locomotor activity and conditioned reward to cocaine by brain-derived neurotrophic factor. *J. Neurosci*. 19: 4110–4122.

Hsu R, Taylor JR, Newton SS, et al. (2005) Blockade of melanocortin transmission inhibits cocaine reward. *Eur. J. Neurosci*. 21: 2233–2242.

Hyman SE, Malenka RC, and Nestler EJ (2006) Neural mechanisms of addiction: The role of reward-related learning and memory. *Annu. Rev. Neurosci*. 29: 565–598.

Kalivas PW (2004) Glutamate systems in cocaine addiction. *Curr. Opin. Pharmacol*. 4: 23–29.

Kalivas PW, Volkow N, and Seamans J (2005) Unmanageable motivation in addiction: A pathology in prefrontal-accumbens glutamate transmission. *Neuron* 45: 647–650.

Kelz MB, Chen J, Carlezon WA, Jr., et al. (1999) Expression of the transcription factor deltaFosB in the brain controls sensitivity to cocaine. *Nature*. 401: 272–276.

Kluver H and Bucy PC (1939) Preliminary analysis of functions of the temporal lobes in monkeys. *Arch. Neurol. Psychiatry* 42: 979–997.

Konradi C, Cole RL, Heckers S, and Hyman SE (1994) Amphetamine regulates gene expression in rat striatum via transcription factor CREB. *J. Neurosci*. 14: 5623–5634.

LeDoux JE (2000) Emotion circuits in the brain. *Annu. Rev. Neurosci*. 23: 155–184.

Lu L, Dempsey J, Liu SY, Bossert JM, and Shaham Y (2004) A single infusion of brain-derived neurotrophic factor into the ventral tegmental area induces long-lasting potentiation of cocaine seeking after withdrawal. *J. Neurosci*. 24: 1604–1611.

Malberg JE and Blendy JA (2005) Antidepressant action: To the nucleus and beyond. *Trends Pharmacol. Sci*. 26: 631–638.

Malberg JE, Eisch AJ, Nestler EJ, and Duman RS (2000) Chronic antidepressant treatment increases neurogenesis in adult rat hippocampus. *J. Neurosci*. 20: 9104–9110.

McClung CA and Nestler EJ (2003) Regulation of gene expression and cocaine reward by CREB and DeltaFosB. *Nat. Neurosci*. 6: 1208–1215.

McClung CA, Sidiropoulou K, Vitaterna M, et al. (2005) Regulation of dopaminergic transmission and cocaine reward by the Clock gene. *Proc. Natl. Acad. Sci. USA* 102: 9377–9381.

McClung CA, Ulery PG, Perrotti LI, Zachariou V, Berton O, and Nestler EJ (2004) ΔFosB: A molecular switch for long-term adaptation. *Mol. Brain Res*. 132: 146–154.

Mignot E (2001) A commentary on the neurobiology of the hypocretin/orexin system. *Neuropsychopharmacology* 25: S5–13.

Miller CA and Marshall JF (2004) Altered prelimbic cortex output during cue-elicited drug seeking. *J. Neurosci.* 24: 6889–6897.

Miller CA and Marshall JF (2005) Molecular substrates for retrieval and reconsolidation of cocaine-associated contextual memory. *Neuron* 47: 873–884.

Montague PR, Hyman SE, and Cohen JD (2004) Computational roles for dopamine in behavioural control. *Nature* 431: 760–767.

Monteggia LM, Barrot M, Powell CM, et al. (2004) Essential role of brain-derived neurotrophic factor in adult hippocampal function. *Proc. Natl. Acad. Sci. USA* 101(29): 10827–10832.

Monteggia LM, Luikart B, Barrot M, et al. (2007) Brain-derived neurotrophic factor conditional knockouts show gender differences in depression-related behaviors. *Biol. Psychiatry* 61(2): 187–197.

Morrow BA, Elsworth JD, Rasmusson AM, and Roth RH (1999) The role of mesoprefrontal dopamine neurons in the acquisition and expression of conditioned fear in the rat. *Neuroscience* 92: 553–564.

Nestler EJ, Barrot M, DiLeone RJ, Eisch AJ, Gold SJ, and Monteggia LM (2002) Neurobiology of depression. *Neuron* 34(1): 13–25.

Nestler EJ, Barrot M, and Self DW (2001) ΔFosB: A molecular switch for addiction. *Proc. Natl. Acad. Sci. USA* 98: 11042–11046.

Nestler EJ and Carlezon WA, Jr. (2006) The mesolimbic dopamine reward circuit in depression. *Biol. Psychiatry* 59: 1151–1159.

Nestler EJ, Hope BT, and Widnell KL (1993) Drug addiction: A model for the molecular basis of neural plasticity. *Neuron* 11: 995–1006.

Nibuya M, Morinobu S, and Duman RS (1995) Regulation of BDNF and trkB mRNA in rat brain by chronic electroconvulsive seizure and antidepressant drug treatments. *J. Neurosci.* 15: 7539–7547.

Norrholm SD, Bibb JA, Nestler EJ, Ouimet CC, Taylor JR, and Greengard P (2003) Cocaine-induced proliferation of dendritic spines in nucleus accumbens is dependent on the activity of the neuronal kinase Cdk5. *Neuroscience* 116: 19–22.

Olausson P, Jentsch JD, Tronson N, Neve RL, Nestler EJ, and Taylor JR (2006) ΔFosB in the nucleus accumbens regulates food-reinforced instrumental behavior and motivation. *J. Neurosci.* 26: 9196–9204.

Olson VG, Zabetian CP, Bolanos CA, et al. (2005) Regulation of drug reward by cAMP response element-binding protein: Evidence for two functionally distinct subregions of the ventral tegmental area. *J. Neurosci.* 25(23): 5553–5562.

Parkinson JA, Olmstead MC, Burns LH, Robbins TW, and Everitt BJ (1999) Dissociation in effects of lesions of the nucleus accumbens core and shell on appetitive pavlovian approach behavior and the potentiation of conditioned reinforcement and locomotor activity by d-amphetamine. *J. Neurosci.* 19: 2401–2411.

Peakman MC, Colby C, Perrotti LI, et al. (2003) Inducible, brain region-specific expression of a dominant negative mutant of c-Jun in transgenic mice decreases sensitivity to cocaine. *Brain Res.* 970: 73–86.

Pencea V, Bingaman KD, Wiegand SJ, and Luskin MB (2001) Infusion of brain-derived neurotrophic factor into the lateral ventricle of the adult rat leads to new neurons in the parenchyma of the striatum, septum, thalamus, and hypothalamus. *J. Neurosci.* 21: 6706–6717.

Perrotti LI, Hadeishi Y, Ulery P, et al. (2004) Induction of ΔFosB in reward-related brain regions after chronic stress. *J. Neurosci.* 24: 10594–10602.

Pitkanen A (2000) Connectivity of the rat amygdaloid complex. In: Aggleton J (ed.) *The Amygdala: A Functional Analysis,* 2nd edn., pp. 31–117. Oxford: Oxford University Press.

Pliakas AM, Carlson RR, Neve RL, Konradi C, Nestler EJ, and Carlezon WA, Jr. (2001) Altered responsiveness to cocaine and increased immobility in the forced swim test associated with elevated cAMP response element-binding protein expression in nucleus accumbens. *J. Neurosci.* 21: 7397–7403.

Rattiner LM, Davis M, French CT, and Ressler KJ (2004) Brain-derived neurotrophic factor and tyrosine kinase receptor B involvement in amygdala-dependent fear conditioning. *J. Neurosci.* 24: 4796–4806.

Robinson TE and Kolb B (2004) Structural plasticity associated with exposure to drugs of abuse. *Neuropharmacology* 47(supplement 1): 33–46.

Rogers RD and Robbins TW (2001) Investigating the neurocognitive deficits associated with chronic drug misuse. *Curr. Opin. Neurobiol.* 11: 250–257.

Salamone JD, Correa M, Mingote S, and Weber SM (2003) Nucleus accumbens dopamine and the regulation of effort in food-seeking behavior: Implications for studies of natural motivation, psychiatry, and drug abuse. *J. Pharmacol. Exp. Ther.* 305: 1–8.

Salomon RM, Ripley B, Kennedy JS, et al. (2003) Diurnal variation of cerebrospinal fluid hypocretin-1 (Orexin-A) levels in control and depressed subjects. *Biol. Psychiatry* 54: 96–104.

Santarelli L, Saxe M, Gross C, et al. (2003) Requirement of hippocampal neurogenesis for the behavioral effects of antidepressants. *Science* 301: 805–809.

Schoenbaum G, Roesch MR, and Stalnaker TA (2006) Orbitofrontal cortex, decision-making and drug addiction. *Trends Neurosci.* 29: 116–124.

Schoenbaum G, Nugent S, Saddoris MP, and Setlow B (2002) Orbitofrontal lesions in rats impair reversal but not acquisition of go, no-go odor discriminations. *Neuroreport* 13: 885–890.

Schoenbaum G, Saddoris MP, Ramus SJ, Shaham Y, and Setlow B (2004) Cocaine-experienced rats exhibit learning deficits in a task sensitive to orbitofrontal cortex lesions. *Eur. J. Neurosci.* 19: 1997–2002.

Schultz W (2006) Behavioral theories and the neurophysiology of reward. *Annu. Rev. Psychol.* 57: 87–115.

Self DW, Genova LM, Hope BT, Barnhart WJ, Spencer JJ, and Nestler EJ (1998) Involvement of cAMP-dependent protein kinase in the nucleus accumbens in cocaine self-administration and relapse of cocaine-seeking behavior. *J. Neurosci.* 18: 1848–1859.

Shaw-Lutchman TZ, Impey S, Storm D, and Nestler EJ (2003) Regulation of CRE-mediated transcription in mouse brain by amphetamine. *Synapse* 48: 10–17.

Shirayama Y, Chen AC, Nakagawa S, Russell DS, and Duman RS (2002) Brain-derived neurotrophic factor produces antidepressant effects in behavioral models of depression. *J. Neurosci.* 22: 3251–3261.

Shizgal P, Fulton S, and Woodside B (2001) Brain reward circuitry and the regulation of energy balance. *Int. J. Obes. Relat. Metab. Disord.* 25(supplement 5): S17–S21.

Silasi G, Diaz-Heijtz R, Besplug J, et al. (2004) Selective brain responses to acute and chronic low-dose x-ray irradiation in males and females. *Biochem. Biophys. Res. Commun.* 325: 1223–1235.

Sotres-Bayon F, Bush DE, and LeDoux JE (2004) Emotional perseveration: An update on prefrontal-amygdala interactions in fear extinction. *Learn. Mem.* 11: 525–535.

Stratford TR and Kelley AE (1999) Evidence of a functional relationship between the nucleus accumbens shell and lateral hypothalamus subserving the control of feeding behavior. *J. Neurosci.* 19: 11040–11048.

Sutton MA, Schmidt EF, Choi KH, et al. (2003) Extinction-induced upregulation in AMPA receptors reduces cocaine-seeking behaviour. *Nature* 421: 70–75.

Taha SA and Fields HL (2006) Inhibitions of nucleus accumbens neurons encode a gating signal for reward-directed behavior. *J. Neurosci.* 26: 217–222.

Taylor JR and Horger BA (1999) Enhanced responding for conditioned reward produced by intra-accumbens amphetamine is potentiated after cocaine sensitization. *Psychopharmacology (Berl.1)* 142: 31–40.

Thomas KL and Everitt BJ (2001) Limbic-cortical-ventral striatal activation during retrieval of a discrete cocaine-associated stimulus: A cellular imaging study with gamma protein kinase C expression. *J. Neurosci.* 21: 2526–2535.

Thomas MJ and Malenka RC (2003) Synaptic plasticity in the mesolimbic dopamine system. *Philos. Trans. R. Soc. Lond. B Biol. Sci.* 358: 815–819.

Thorsell A, Michalkiewicz M, Dumont Y, et al. (2000) Behavioral insensitivity to restraint stress, absent fear suppression of behavior and impaired spatial learning in transgenic rats with hippocampal neuropeptide Y overexpression. *Proc. Natl. Acad. Sci. USA* 97: 12852–12857.

Valdez GR and Koob GF (2004) Allostasis and dysregulation of corticotropin-releasing factor and neuropeptide Y systems: Implications for the development of alcoholism. *Pharmacol. Biochem. Behav.* 79: 671–689.

Vitaterna MH, King DP, Chang AM, et al. (1994) Mutagenesis and mapping of a mouse gene, Clock, essential for circadian behavior. *Science* 264: 719–725.

Volkow ND and Fowler SJ (2000) Addiction, a disease of compulsion and drive: Involvement of the orbitofrontal cortex. *Cereb. Cortex* 10: 318–325.

Voorn P, Gerfen CR, and Groenewegen HJ (1989) Compartmental organisation of the ventral striatum of the rat: Immunohistochemical distribution of enkephalin, substance-p, dopamine and calcium-binding protein. *J. Comp. Neurol.* 289: 189–201.

Werme M, Messer C, Olson L, et al. (2002) DeltaFosB regulates wheel running. *J. Neurosci.* 22: 8133–8136.

Winstanley CA, Theobald DE, Cardinal RN, and Robbins TW (2004) Contrasting roles for basolateral amygdala and orbitofrontal cortex in impulsive choice. *J. Neurosci.* 24: 4718–4722.

Wise RA and Rompre PP (1989) Brain dopamine and reward. *Annu. Rev. Psychol.* 40: 191–225.

Yao WD, Gainetdinov RR, Arbuckle MI, et al. (2004) Identification of PSD-95 as a regulator of dopamine-mediated synaptic and behavioral plasticity. *Neuron* 41: 625–638.

Yeh SH, Lin CH, Lee CF, and Gean PW (2002) A requirement of nuclear factor-kappaB activation in fear-potentiated startle. *J. Biol. Chem.* 277: 46720–46729.

Zachariou V, Benoit-Marand M, Allen PB, et al. (2002) Reduction of cocaine place preference in mice lacking the protein phosphatase 1 inhibitors DARPP 32 or Inhibitor 1. *Biol. Psychiatry* 51: 612–620.

Zachariou V, Sgambato-Faure V, Sasaki T, et al. (2006a) Phosphorylation of DARPP-32 at Threonine-34 is required for cocaine action. *Neuropsychopharmacology* 31: 555–562.

Zachariou V, Bolanos CA, Selley DE, et al. (2006b) An essential role for DeltaFosB in the nucleus accumbens in morphine action. *Nat. Neurosci.* 9: 205–211.

25 Neurophysiology of Motor Skill Learning

R. J. Nudo, University of Kansas Medical Center, Kansas City, KS, USA

25.1 Introduction

Motor performance improves with practice. Movements are initially slow, variable, uncoordinated, and fractionated. After numerous repetitions, movements become fast, stereotyped, coordinated, and smooth, so that individual joint contractions blend into a single, transitionless action. Several aspects of cognitive and motor processing must be refined in order for such high levels of motor performance to be attained. Over the past several years, neurophysiological studies in experimental animals, especially in nonhuman primates, as well as neuroimaging studies in humans, have provided a wealth of data, which has helped to clarify the neural processes and structures underlying the development of skilled motor behavior. It now appears that a broad network of structures in the cerebral cortex, striatum, and cerebellum coordinate their activity to enable skilled motor behavior. Each of these structures probably plays a different role in either motor planning or execution, and some of these structures are critical to the learning of new motor tasks. This is evident since activity patterns are correlated with specific phases of learning, and this activity is altered as tasks are practiced and become highly skilled. In this chapter, we review the evidence from neurophysiological, neuroanatomical, and neuroimaging studies that shed light on brain mechanisms underlying motor skill learning.

25.2 Definition of Motor Skill Learning

As used in this chapter, motor skill refers primarily to fine motor skill, such as might be required in picking up small objects, writing, typing, and so on, and not gross motor skill, such as might be required to sit upright, crawl, or walk. While the learning of gross motor skills is important during development, during activities of daily living, and during recovery from certain severe neurological disorders, the current chapter focuses on fine motor skill and its acquisition. Skill learning is sometimes referred to as habit learning, defined as the process of successive adaptation of behavioral responses to contingencies in environmental stimuli (Mishkin et al., 1984). Habit or skill learning is one of several forms of implicit learning thought to be mediated by neural networks in the cerebellum, frontal cortex, and basal ganglia. Implicit learning is contrasted with declarative learning, which involves the temporal lobe (Squire, 2004).

Although a general sense of what is meant by motor skill exists among researchers, there is no general agreement regarding what constitutes the acquisition of motor skill. In our view, motor skill learning is operationally defined as a change in motor behavior, specifically referring to the increased use of novel, task-specific joint sequences and combinations, resulting from practice and/or repetition. Others have argued that changes in the speed of movement, even if not accompanied by reciprocal changes in the accuracy of movement, indicate skill learning (Fitts, 1954; Hallett et al., 1996). However, it should be cautioned that speed as the sole criterion for evidence of skill learning may, at least in some situations, be confounded, as they may occur as a function of motivational state, also called dispositional learning (Amsel, 1992).

25.3 Central Nervous System Structures Involved in Motor Skill Learning

It is now clear that the motor cortex does not execute motor tasks in isolation. A broad network minimally involving the primary and secondary motor areas, the dorsolateral prefrontal cortex, the posterior parietal cortex, the striatum, and the cerebellum is involved in both skill acquisition and in motor execution. One goal of recent research has been to differentiate the role of various structures in the actual movement execution versus the role of the structure in learning the task (usually a movement sequence) or storage of the learned motor program. While both cortical and subcortical structures are clearly involved in motor learning, this chapter focuses on cortical motor areas and their role in skill learning.

Classically, motor skill was viewed as a serial process. Premotor areas were thought to be critical for the learning and storage of motor sequences. Premotor areas were thought to send information to the primary motor cortex for execution of motor behavior via descending pathways to the spinal cord. While certain neuroanatomical and neurophysiological features of premotor and primary motor areas support this concept, the more modern view recognizes that each of the cortical motor areas are, to some extent, involved in motor learning and the storage of motor commands, and that motor skill does not reside in any one place. However, these areas may differ in their degree of involvement in skilled motor behaviors, depending upon various task demands (e.g., role of visual or somatosensory guidance, cognitive demands, bimanual involvement, etc.). Here we review both the basic anatomy and physiology of these various motor areas and evidence for their differential roles in motor skill learning.

25.3.1 Cortical Motor Areas in Nonhuman Primates

It is generally accepted that no single feature is sufficient for characterizing an area as a distinct region. Features used to define cortical motor fields include cytoarchitectonics, patterns of afferent and efferent connections, features of intrinsic connectivity, chemoarchitectonics, behavioral effects of ablation, and, particularly for motor cortical areas, the ability to elicit movements upon electrical stimulation.

A differentiated motor field has a unique cytoarchitecture, traditionally defined by stains for Nissl bodies and myelin. Additionally, areas have been examined and characterized based on cytochrome oxidase staining, acetylcholinesterase staining, neurofilament antibody staining, and receptor binding. Unique characteristics of cell types, laminar organization, cell density, fiber density, and various staining densities are all used for characterization. Extensive tract tracing studies have been used to identify subareas of motor cortex based on differential afferent and efferent connections with the thalamus, basal ganglia, and other cortical areas, as well as their projections to the spinal cord. Physiological criteria have also been used for differentiation. Intracortical microstimulation mapping procedures have helped to define somatotopic organization within each motor area, with attention paid to minimal threshold requirements for initiation of movements, as well as the characterization of the movements themselves. The relationship of single-unit activity to behavioral aspects of motor tasks in awake, freely moving animals has also been an important approach to distinguishing motor fields. Finally, motor areas have been characterized based on functional differences in ablation-behavior studies in nonhuman primates and functional imaging studies in humans.

The nomenclature used for subdivisions of primate motor areas has varied across laboratories. The generalized current scheme includes M1 (or Brodmann's area 4); four subdivisions of the lateral premotor cortex (PMd-c, PMd-r, PMv-c, and PMv-r, or F2, F7, F4, and F5, respectively); two premotor subdivisions on the mesial surface of the hemisphere (SMA and pre-SMA, or F3 and F6), and three subdivisions of the cingulate motor area within regions lining the cingulate sulcus (CMAr, CMAd, and CMAv, or area 24c, area 6c, and area 23c). M1 is the most easily recognizable area in histological stains, as it contains very large pyramidal neurons in layer V, the so-called Betz cells. Also, it contains a greatly reduced layer IV, compared with sensory cortex that contains a thick layer IV with substantial numbers of granule cells. For this reason, M1 is sometimes referred to as agranular cortex. **Figure 1** illustrates the location of the main cortical motor areas.

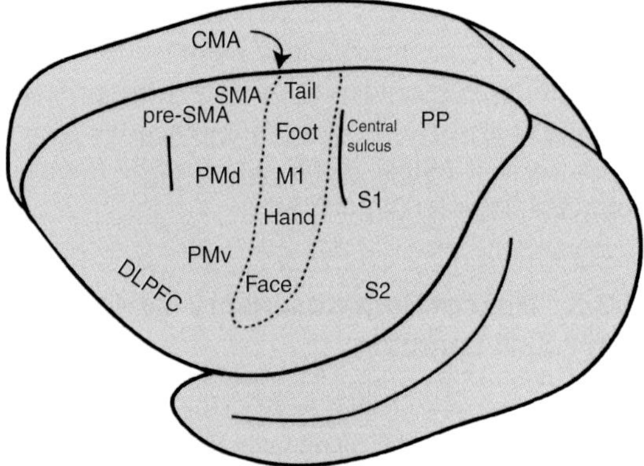

Figure 1 Location of cortical areas involved in motor skill learning and execution. Cortical areas are depicted on the brain of a squirrel monkey, a primate with few convolutions in its cortex. The areas depicted can be subdivided further on the basis of anatomical and physiological criteria. For example, SMA can be divided into a caudal component (SMA proper) and a rostral component (pre-SMA). CMA, cingulate motor areas; SMA, supplementary motor area; PMd, dorsal premotor cortex; PMv, ventral premotor cortex; DLPFC, dorsolateral prefrontal cortex; M1, primary motor cortex; PP, posterior parietal cortex; S1, primary somatosensory cortex; S2, second somatosensory area.

25.3.2 Cortical Motor Areas in Rodents

Because rodents are often used to study the role of motor cortex in motor skill learning, a brief comparative account of cortical motor areas in rodents is instructive. (While motor cortex in cats is also frequently a focus of motor learning experiments, this species will not be discussed in this review.) Intracortical microstimulation studies of sensorimotor cortex in the rat have shown a complete motor representation that is cytoarchitectonically defined as agranular cortex (Hall and Lindholm, 1974; Donoghue and Wise, 1982) and commonly called M1 based on its similarities to primate M1. In rodents, the portion of the agranular cortex in caudal portions of frontal cortex that is devoted to forelimb movements is referred to as the caudal forelimb area (CFA). In addition, a second motor representation of the forelimb has been identified in more rostral portions of the frontal cortex. This second forelimb representation, referred to as the rostral forelimb area (RFA), is smaller than the CFA (Neafsey et al., 1986). The RFA is separated from the CFA by a zone where intracortical microstimulation elicits vibrissa or neck movements.

Because the presence of a secondary motor area in rats would appear to parallel the differentiation of motor areas in primates, suggestions have been made that the RFA is a homolog of one of the primate secondary motor areas. Tract tracing studies of motor cortical connections in rat have shown differences in the thalamic, striatal, and cortical connections of CFA and RFA (Rouiller et al., 1993). Comparison of these connections to the pattern of connections of primate motor areas suggests that RFA has some similarities to primate premotor areas. Overall, based on its connections, CFA is more similar to the M1 forelimb area in primates, and RFA in some ways appears to be more similar to nonprimary motor cortex in primates. It is not currently possible to decide whether RFA is a homolog of primate premotor cortex, supplementary motor areas, or a combination of secondary motor areas in primates (Rouiller et al., 1993). A more comprehensive review of primate and rodent motor areas can be found in Nudo and Frost (2006).

25.3.3 Role of Somatosensory Cortex in Motor Skill Learning

While the present chapter focuses on motor output structures, it should be recognized that sensory information plays a critical role in the learning of new motor skills. For example, the somatosensory system is critical for skilled motor behavior. Various somatosensory regions in the parietal lobe of the cerebral cortex are intimately interconnected with motor cortical regions in the frontal lobe. Somatosensory information can be recorded from neurons in M1, and this information is segregated by submodality. Cutaneous inputs arrive in the more caudal aspects of M1, while proprioceptive inputs arrive in the more rostral aspects. Focal experimental lesions in rostral or caudal M1 result in distinct sensory-related deficits in skilled use of the hands. Lesions in either primary somatosensory cortex or M1 in nonhuman primates result in similar deficits. Thus, while there are clear structural and functional distinctions between M1 and S1, they are functionally codependent with regard to skilled motor behaviors.

25.4 Organization of Primary Motor Cortex and Its Role in Motor Skill Learning

The vast majority of studies examining the neurophysiological bases for motor skill learning have been performed in the primary motor cortex, or M1. The reasons for this bias are numerous: M1 is very accessible because of its location in the precentral gyrus. The portion of M1 that is most often examined, the M1 hand representation, is located on the dorsolateral surface. In most primates, however, a large portion of the M1 hand representation is buried in the anterior banks of the central sulcus, rendering accurate reconstruction of two-dimensional topographic maps more challenging. Nevertheless, neuronal population studies, especially from cells within the more rostral portions of M1, and to a lesser extent, the caudal portions of M1 within the depths of the central sulcus, are numerous. Thus, from the first functional localization studies in the 1800s to cellular responsivity studies of the present day, M1 is the primary focus of most cortical studies of motor control.

In primates at least, M1 is equivalent to Brodmann's area 4, based on cytoarchitectonic criteria. M1 contains a complete representation of skeletal and orofacial musculature organized in a topographic fashion, but with an exaggerated representation of the hands and face. This organization has been known since the late 1800s, primarily because of muscular contractions evoked from electrical stimulation of the cortical surface and, more recently, by more direct stimulation of the output neurons located in layer V, demonstrated by intracortical microstimulation. The most direct access to motor neurons in the spinal cord is via the corticospinal tract, originating in layer V pyramidal cells and terminating in intermediate and deep laminae of the spinal cord. In many primate species (and possibly other mammalian species), a subset of corticospinal neurons, so-called corticomotoneuronal cells, terminate monosynaptically onto spinal motor neurons. It is now known that corticomotoneuronal cells diverge to innervate multiple (on average, about four or five) motor neuron pools (**Figure 2**). Furthermore, corticomotoneuronal cells with different projection patterns intermingle within each local zone within M1 (Rathelot and Strick, 2006). Thus, the highly organized topographic arrangement inferred from electrical stimulation studies is valid only on a macroscopic scale. Substantial divergence and convergence exist in the connections between M1 and spinal cord motor neurons at a more focal level. It is possible that this anatomical arrangement confers on M1 a certain capacity for functional plasticity, since, depending upon the subset of neurons in a given zone that is activated, a different motor output might result.

M1 can access motor neurons in the spinal cord via more indirect routes also. For example, corticofugal neurons project monosynaptically to the red nucleus, which in turn projects monosynaptically and disynaptically to spinal cord motor neurons. These pathways are topographically organized on a macroscopic scale, much like the direct corticomotoneuronal pathway. Somewhat more diffuse access can be accomplished via M1 projections to the pontine and medullary reticular formation, which in turn projects to the spinal cord.

M1 also contains a rich array of intracortical connections that are thought to modulate the output of corticofugal cells. The role of local corticocortical fibers in shaping responses in the execution of skilled motor tasks is not well known. However, this

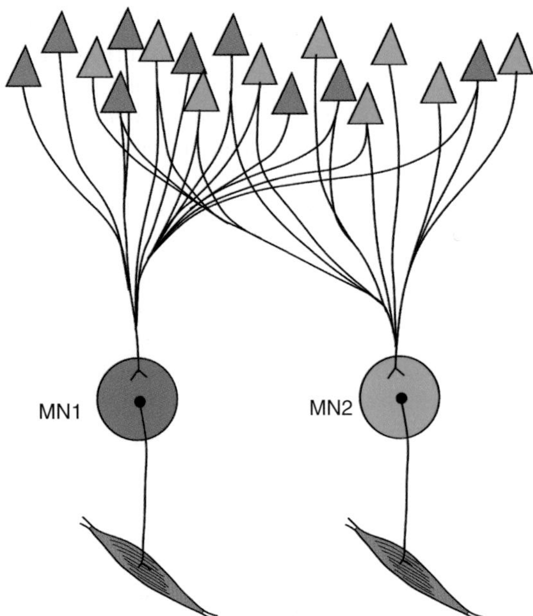

Figure 2 Divergence and convergence of corticospinal neurons in M1. Corticospinal neurons diverge to form monosynaptic connections with up to four or five motor neuron pools. Two such pools, MN1 and MN2, are shown in the figure. Corticospinal neurons projecting to a single motor neuron pool are represented over a large territory within M1. Thus, different corticospinal neuron populations (red and green triangles) are intermixed across the spatial domain of M1.

modulatory influence may provide another important substrate for plasticity in the output properties of motor cortex.

Virtually all mammalian species contain a cortical structure analogous (if not homologous) to primary motor cortex. Corticospinal neurons originating in layer V exist in every mammalian species studied to date, including primates, carnivores, rodents, insectivores, and marsupials. However, the number of corticospinal neurons, their penetration into the cord, their trajectory in the cord, and the proximity of their terminals to motor neuron cell bodies vary widely across species. A motor cortex, as defined by an area of the cerebral cortex whose stimulation results in movements of muscles of the body, seems to be universal among mammals.

25.4.1 Neurophysiological Changes in M1 Associated with Motor Skill Learning

Historically, it has been thought that since M1 is so intimately connected to motor neurons in the spinal cord, its role in motor behavior was concerned primarily with low-level execution of muscular contractions. However, several lines of evidence now suggest that it plays a very important role in skill acquisition and motor learning.

Neurophysiological studies in animal models, especially nonhuman primates, provide unique insight into the role of various cortical and subcortical networks in motor skill learning, since the activity of neuronal populations can be tracked over time in the same animals, as they perform a specific task. However, until recently, the most common paradigm was to examine neuronal activity in relation to movement only after an animal had been highly trained for several weeks to months. While this paradigm allows examination of the relationship of neuronal activity to control of movements, it does not provide much insight into the actual learning of the task. This is important since the acquisition of various aspects of motor skill might be mediated by different neuronal structures and processes.

Several human studies using transcranial magnetic stimulation have demonstrated that increased use of muscles expands their motor representations (Pascual-Leone and Torres, 1993; Tyc et al., 2005). Even simple movements repeated over a short period of time are effective in inducing cortical representational changes (Classen et al., 1998). Recent experiments in nonhuman primates have demonstrated that motor representations of hand movements expand in concert with the acquisition of new motor skills (Nudo et al., 1996). In these studies, monkeys were trained on an operant task requiring retrieval of food pellets from small wells. Behavioral performance was initially poor based on timing of retrievals and numbers of digit flexions required per retrieval. Behavioral performance increased asymptotically and reached plateau in about 10 days. At the end of the training period, both individual joint movements and specific joint movement combinations and sequences used by individual animals became represented over larger cortical territories (**Figure 3**). As digit skills were acquired, very little expansion of the total hand representation occurred. Instead, digit and wrist representations became redistributed. These effects were reversible, to some extent, though not completely. This suggests that once a novel motor task is learned, certain aspects of cortical topography are altered for an extremely long period of time. Changes in face motor cortex have also been

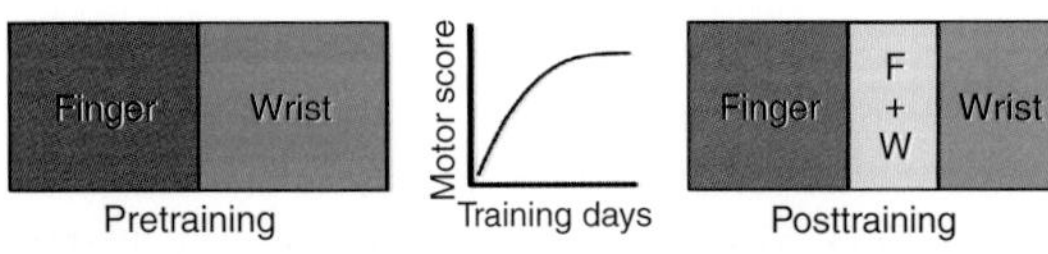

Figure 3 Alterations in motor representations in M1 as a result of motor skill training. After several days of practice at a novel motor task (pellet retrievals from small wells), monkeys display larger representations of the fingers and wrist. In addition, representations of multijoint movements (fingers + wrist) emerge. Current thresholds required for activating movements at multijoint sites are particularly low compared with at single-joint sites. From Nudo RJ, Milliken GW, Jenkins WM, and Merzenich MM (1996) Use-dependent alterations of movement representations in primary motor cortex of adult squirrel monkeys. *J. Neurosci.* 16: 785–807.

demonstrated after learning a novel tongue protrusion task (Sessle et al., 2007).

One of the more interesting aspects of these results is that movement combinations that were used in the task became represented over a larger cortical territory. This suggests that temporal correlation of movements (and presumably muscles) drives changes in cortical motor organization. It is possible that local intracortical connections couple various separate modules together to form muscle or movement synergies. After training, at sites where multiple joints are represented (as defined by similar thresholds for activation), the current levels required for evoking the multijoint movements are significantly lower than those required to evoke single-joint movements. Recently, analogous results have been demonstrated using functional magnetic resonance imaging after motor training in humans (McNamara et al., 2007). Thus, training may in some way prime specific intracortical connections to enhance the excitability of subsets of corticomotoneuronal cells that must fire concurrently for skilled tasks to be completed.

Subsequent microelectrode stimulation studies in monkeys and rats confirmed these initial findings and further suggested that skill acquisition was a necessary feature of the behavioral experience for neurophysiological map plasticity to occur, rather than simple movement execution alone. Monkeys that retrieve food pellets from larger wells than those used in the study described do not exhibit the slowly developing asymptotic learning curve compared with monkeys trained on the small-well task. Even though they execute the same number of digit movements, these animals demonstrate no systematic change in motor map topography in M1 (Plautz et al., 2000). Similar findings have been found in rodents. Rats trained in a novel task to retrieve food pellets from a rotating platform demonstrate expansions of distal forelimb representations in M1. However, rats trained to press a bar repeatedly with their distal forelimb show no map changes (Kleim et al., 1998). Presumably, the large-well pellet retrieval task in the monkey and the bar pressing task in the rat are skills that had already been acquired in the normal behavior of the animal. Only when novel tasks are taught that require the acquisition of new joint movement combinations is the motor cortex topography altered significantly.

Another paradigm for motor training, strength training, also does not appear to alter motor maps in M1. In comparison to nontrained control animals, rats that are trained to repetitively grasp and break a strand of dried pasta show expanded representations of the distal forelimb, presumably due to the novel skill required by the task. However, if rats are trained to break progressively larger bundles of pasta strands, a similar task that simply requires more force, the same expansions occur. That is, no further reorganization in distal forelimb representations occurs with strength training (Remple et al., 2001).

At the cellular level, both long-term potentiation (LTP) and long-term depression (LTD) can be generated in somatosensory and motor cortex of rats under specific conditions (Castro-Alamancos et al., 1995; Rioult-Pedotti et al., 2000). It has been suggested that extensive intracortical connections in superficial layers of motor cortex might undergo changes in synaptic efficacy that underlie neurophysiological changes in motor cortex during motor learning. In rats, when one limb is trained on a motor task, the amplitude of field potentials contralateral to the trained limb is significantly increased relative to the cortex opposite the untrained limb. Further, the trained cortex is less amenable to subsequent LTP induction (Rioult-Pedotti et al., 1998; Hodgson et al., 2005). However, others have argued that learning motor skill acquisition produces bidirectional changes in synaptic strength distributed throughout the intracortical networks of motor cortex. Unidirectional changes in the population of neural elements are suggested to occur during certain behavioral states not directly related to the learning process (i.e., stress; Cohen and Castro-Alamancos, 2005).

25.4.2 Neuroanatomical Correlates of Motor Skill Training in M1

Skill training is also associated with changes in the microanatomy within motor cortex, including dendritic reorganization, synaptogenesis, and changes in synapse morphology. Training rats on an acrobatic task that requires them to traverse a series of obstacles (horizontal ladder, grid platform, rope, barriers) results in increases in synapse to neuron ratios and dendritic processes in motor cortex (Jones et al., 1999; Bury and Jones, 2002). Similar synaptic and dendritic changes occur with reach training in rats (Withers and Greenough, 1989; Kleim et al., 2002). Training-induced structural reorganization is limited to the motor cortex region that undergoes neurophysiological reorganization (Kleim et al., 2002). More recent immunohistochemical studies have attempted to determine the proteins that are involved in these morphological changes. In rats, synaptophysin and GAP-43 expression appear to be correlated with the first 5 days of motor skill learning. However, microtubule-associated protein 2 (MAP-2) was not influenced by learning (Derksen et al., 2006). Brain-derived neurotrophic factor (BDNF) appears to be involved in learning-related plasticity in motor cortex. If BDNF is inhibited by injection of antisense oligodeoxynucleotides, receptor antagonists, or BDNF receptor antibodies, motor skill is impaired and neurophysiological organization is disrupted (Kleim et al., 2003; Adkins et al., 2006).

While studies at the genetic and molecular level of analysis are still few in number, recent studies suggest a time-dependent change in corticostriatal expression patterns of immediate early genes during motor training (Hernandez et al., 2006).

25.5 Secondary Motor Areas and Their Role in Motor Skill Learning

In addition to M1, there are several secondary motor areas (SMAs) recognized in the primate cortex (**Figure 1**). These areas have been defined as having direct connections to both M1 and the spinal cord. The premotor cortex, the SMA, and the cingulate motor cortex have been identified in all primate species examined, including prosimian primates. Each of these secondary areas has been divided into subareas based on differences in cortical architecture that are related to hodological and functional differences. The lateral premotor area is divided into ventral and dorsal areas (PMv and PMd, respectively), the SMA into SMA proper and pre-SMA, and the cingulate motor cortex into rostral (CMAr) and caudal (CMAc) divisions. As many as ten motor fields emerged early in primate evolution (Wu et al., 2000).

The premotor and supplementary motor areas appear to be involved in different aspects of movement compared to M1. This has been suggested simply from the timing of activity in the various cortical motor regions. Using time-resolved fMRI during a delayed cued finger movement task, activity in M1 was substantially weaker during movement preparation compared with during movement execution. However, activity in PM and SMA was equally high during both phases of the task (Richter et al., 1997).

25.5.1 Role of the SMA in Motor Skill Learning

A significant role in the planning, preparation, and initiation of voluntary movement has been ascribed to the secondary motor areas on the medial wall of the hemispheres, especially the supplementary motor area. Early stimulation studies demonstrating complex movements evoked at higher currents from stimulation of SMA first suggested that the medial motor areas are involved in more complex aspects of motor behavior (Thickbroom et al., 2000). Later, neuroimaging studies implicated the role of SMA in higher-order processes. In one very influential study examining cerebral blood flow, for example, the SMA was the only area activated when subjects mentally rehearsed a finger tapping sequence without actually executing it (Roland et al., 1980).

Based on these early results, the focus for SMA studies has been on its role in complex aspects of motor behavior, such as movement planning and sequencing. In daily activities, discrete movements must be coordinated in the proper sequence, and transitions from one movement to the next must be accomplished smoothly and rapidly. As movement sequences are practiced, the individual movements become more stereotyped (i.e., with decreased variability in kinematics and kinetics), and the time between different movements decreases. Eventually, one movement component blends into the next, and a smooth, coordinated action results. The SMA is thought to participate in this sequencing function. But it should be recognized that sequence learning requires several neural systems that are involved in cognitive, perceptual, motoric, and temporal aspects of learning (Grafton et al., 1998). Motor behaviors are controlled by a distributed network, and it may be too simplistic to think in terms of compartmentalized units that have mutually exclusive functions. For example, a recent 2-deoxyglucose study in nonhuman primates showed substantial metabolic activity in both SMA and pre-SMA associated with visually guided reaching movements. The intensity of activation was comparable to that of M1 in the same animals (Picard and Strick, 2003). Most neurons in SMA are active in relation to effector-related variables. However, a modest number appear to represent target direction independent of reach direction. Further, the largest number of neurons in SMA appears to be context-dependent, that is, activity is directional in one visuomotor mapping condition, but not others (Crutcher et al., 2004). While it is now clear that these areas are involved in diverse aspects of movement control, planning and timing are the major focus of investigations.

Many studies in nonhuman primates have demonstrated that the supplementary motor area is important in the control of sequential movements. Early studies demonstrated that SMA neurons are active during movements of either extremity (Brinkman and Porter, 1983), and SMA lesions result in deficits in bimanual coordination (Brinkman, 1981). More recent studies demonstrated that removal of SMA in monkeys does not cause paralysis or akinesia. However, monkeys were impaired at performance of a simple learned task in which they were required to raise their arm to obtain a food reward below (Thaler et al., 1995). They were less impaired if the task was paced by an external cue (tone). These deficits are similar to those observed in humans with damage to SMA. Patients with lesions involving the SMA, but sparing the lateral hemispheric surface, demonstrated difficulties in producing rhythmic motion unless the task was guided by auditory pacing (Halsband et al., 1993). These data have been cited as evidence for the role of SMA in self-initiated actions.

SMA is thought to play a role in modulating motor output based on kinesthetic inputs. A large percentage of neurons in SMA respond differentially to different instructions during a preparatory state (Tanji et al., 1980; Passingham, 1987). Also, neuronal discharge within SMA typically precedes activity in M1 (Deecke et al., 1985), but SMA response properties differ from those in M1 in that SMA activity is related to factors other than the execution of movement to a greater extent than neurons in M1 (Kurata and Tanji, 1985).

Neuronal activity in SMA is also thought to reflect internal models of movement dynamics, or the forces exerted by contracting muscles. Dynamic related signals are nearly comparable in SMA and M1 (Crutcher and Alexander, 1990). Movement dynamics are significantly represented in SMA during both motor planning and execution. This property is likely to play a particularly important role in motor learning, as SMA neurons shift their preferred direction in the direction of an external force when monkeys adapt to a perturbing force field, and back in the other direction when the monkeys readapt to the nonperturbed direction. This shift occurs during the instructed delay and during the movement-related time window (Padoa-Schioppa et al., 2004).

25.5.2 Two SMAs: Different Roles for SMA and Pre-SMA

Two SMA representations can be differentiated in primate species based on distinct cytoarchitecture, intracortical microstimulation, neuronal response properties, and connection patterns. These two areas, located on the mesial aspect of the frontal cortex, are referred to as SMA proper (or simply SMA; also called F3) and the pre-SMA (also called F6), situated more rostrally (Wu et al., 2000). Typically, in human neuroimaging studies, the SMA is differentiated from pre-SMA based their location relative to the anterior commissure, with the SMA proper lying caudal to the level of the commissure, and the pre-SMA lying rostral to the commissure. However, diffusion tensor imaging studies have revealed different patterns of connections in SMA and pre-SMA, and thus, more refined identification methods in humans are now available (Lehericy et al., 2004).

25.5.2.1 Basic differences in physiology and anatomy of SMA/pre-SMA

SMA contains a complete motor representation with the face-arm-leg regions arranged rostrocaudally (Luppino et al., 1991). Movements are elicited at low current thresholds. Arm movements can be elicited from pre-SMA, though larger currents are required (Matsuzaka et al., 1992). Compared to SMA, pre-SMA has only sparse spinal projections but connects more heavily with prefrontal cortex. For this reason, some investigators consider pre-SMA (as well as pre-PMd) to be a prefrontal cortical region rather than a premotor area. In general, SMA proper is thought to be involved primarily in simple tasks, while pre-SMA is activated during relatively complex tasks (Picard and Strick, 2001).

25.5.2.2 Role of SMA/pre-SMA in learning of motor sequences

Many cells in SMA and pre-SMA fire preferentially during the performance of new sequences (Nakamura et al., 1998). Studies of the role of SMA and pre-SMA in sequence learning have focused primarily on either movement sequences with the upper extremity or sequences of saccades (Muri et al., 1994). Neuronal responses to visual stimuli predominate in pre-SMA, while responses to somatosensory stimuli predominate in SMA proper (Matsuzaka et al., 1992). However, the current review focuses exclusively on movements of the upper extremity, and not on saccades.

Neurons in SMA/pre-SMA that are related to sequence learning start discharging after the illumination of the stimuli for each set; the discharge rate increases until the monkey presses the first button. As learning proceeds, these neurons discharge progressively less, so that in highly learned sequences, almost no activity is evident. Such neurons that preferentially are activated during new sequences are more common in pre-SMA. This role has often been referred to as reprogramming. In fact, neurophysiological studies in monkeys demonstrate that many pre-SMA cells are preferentially active only during the single trials where the animals are required to update to a new movement sequence (Shima et al., 1996). The activity is not related to a new association, since the sensory stimuli and the associations with different movements are already well learned. This suggests that pre-SMA is involved in updating motor plans or reprogramming.

Many SMA neurons display a gradual change in activity related to experience with a particular movement sequence. This suggests that activity in SMA is dynamically reorganized by experience (Lee and Quessy, 2003). It is possible for learning about motor tasks to occur in the absence of motor performance changes, for example, as measured by reaction time. This might occur during the observation of a motor task. The subject later demonstrates more rapid improvements in performance since some perceptual/cognitive aspect of the task was learned during the observation. It has been argued that SMA may play a role in sequence learning independent of the relationship with performance changes (Lee and Quessy, 2003).

One behavioral paradigm that is popular for studying motor sequence learning in nonhuman primates is the sequential button task, in which monkeys are required to press pairs of buttons in the proper sequence. This task has been used extensively by Hikosaka and colleagues, who generally train monkeys in sets of five consecutive pairs of button presses. Using a similar task in a PET study of cerebral blood flow in humans, SMA was more active (more blood flow) during the performance of a prelearned sequence compared with a new sequence (Jenkins et al., 1994). In contrast, pre-SMA is active during the process of learning the sequence (Hikosaka et al., 1996).

These results may explain the earlier lesion results. If SMA is more active after a motor sequence is learned (and thus, after external cues are no longer necessary to pace the task), damage to SMA would then result in deficits in performing the learned sequence. However, if external cues are then provided, the lateral premotor areas are engaged and can compensate for the deficit.

But many brain regions are active during new learning, such as dorsolateral prefrontal cortex, parietal cortex, lateral premotor area, cerebellum, and basal ganglia (Nakamura et al., 1999). Are either SMA or pre-SMA necessary for learning new sequences? In monkey studies, these areas can be differentially and temporarily inactivated using muscimol, a GABA agonist. Inactivation of either area increases reaction time of button presses for both novel and learned sequences. However, inactivation of pre-SMA, but not SMA, increases errors for novel sequences, but not learned sequences (Nakamura et al., 1999). These data provide further support that pre-SMA is more involved in the learning of new motor sequences. What specific factors related to new learning are disrupted by the inactivation (novelty detection, selective attention, decision making, error correction, switching motor plan, memory coding, retrieval, etc.) are not completely known.

Cells have also been found in SMA that appear to be responsive to a particular order of forthcoming movements (Tanji and Shima, 1994), supporting the view that SMA is particularly important in the relational order of sequence components (i.e., neurons fire during movement A only if movement A is preceded or followed by movement B). In addition, both SMA and pre-SMA neurons show selectivity for the numerical order of sequence components, although the incidence of such neurons is higher in pre-SMA. That is, these neurons may fire during movement A only if movement A is the second movement in the sequence (Clower and Alexander, 1998).

Before leaving this discussion of motor sequence learning, it should be emphasized that SMA and pre-SMA are probably not the only cortical motor areas involved in coding movement sequences. Recent data from monkeys have demonstrated that after long-term training on a sequence task, a large proportion of neurons in M1 were differentially active during a repeating sequence versus a random sequence (Matsuzaka et al., 2007). A large number of M1 neurons are active during the instruction period, similar to findings in premotor areas. When cells were sought that showed an interaction between movement direction and serial order (sequence-related cells), such cells were the most common type (40%). Only 17% of these cells were related to movement direction alone (Lu and Ashe, 2005). This suggests that M1 may represent sequential movements, as has been suggested for SMA and pre-SMA. It would appear that M1 participates in motor skill learning beyond the simple kinematic level, and thus, the neural network participating in more cognitive aspects of motor tasks may be broadly distributed.

A model for a more global network view of sequence learning has been proposed by Ashe and colleagues (2006). The basic principle of this model is that motor sequences involve both implicit and explicit learning depending upon the stage of the learning process (**Figure 4**). These two forms of learning are thought to employ somewhat different neural structures. Much of motor sequence learning is implicit, as elements of the movements are made in sequential order without specific awareness about the sequence. Ashe's model suggests that in these conditions, implicit processes originate in M1 and propagate to premotor areas. With repeated practice, learning may become explicit, as the subject is aware of the instructional set. In this case, explicit processes originate in prefrontal cortex and then propagate to premotor areas. In reality, both implicit and explicit processes probably interact, and thus neural correlates can be found across broad neuronal networks.

25.5.2.3 Role of SMA/pre-SMA in self-initiated versus externally guided movements

One of the central issues concerning the role of SMA/ pre-SMA in movement is its role in self-initiated movements as opposed to movements triggered by external stimuli, or externally guided movements. While a large percentage of neurons in SMA are active during IG movements, approximately 90% of task-related neurons are active before or during EG movements (Mushiake et al., 1991).

Both self-initiated and externally guided movements activate a common network of cortical areas including SMA, pre-SMA, cingulate cortex, M1, superior parietal cortex, and insular cortex. Neurophysiological data in animals seem to indicate that the mesial motor areas are more involved in self-initiated movements, while lateral premotor areas are involved in externally guided movements (Romo and Schultz, 1987; Thaler et al., 1988; Mushiake et al., 1991; Cunnington et al., 2002). Motor preparatory activity appears to arise primarily from mesial motor areas, supporting this view. Neuroimaging studies have demonstrated that mesial motor areas show greater activation with self-initiated compared with externally triggered movement (Rao et al., 1993; Wessel et al., 1997; Deiber et al., 1999; Jenkins et al., 2000; Hoshi and Tanji, 2006), and greater activation of lateral premotor areas for externally triggered (EG) movements.

Activity increases in both mesial motor areas and lateral premotor areas during a movement preparation period (Richter et al., 1997). M1 shows weak activation

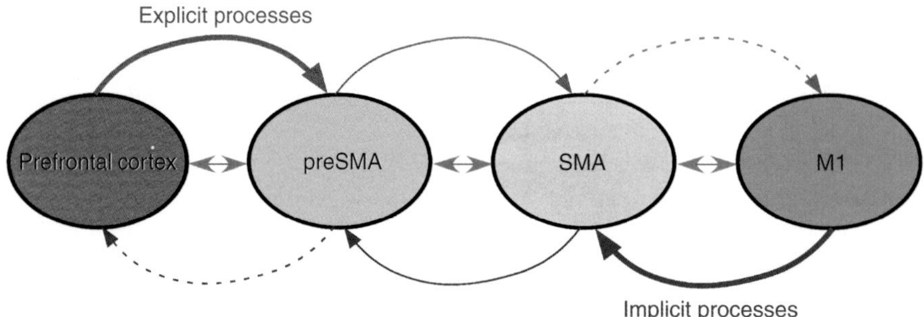

Figure 4 Cortical structures involved in the control of motor sequences. In this model, both explicit and implicit processes operate in the learning and execution of movement sequences. The degree of involvement of the two processes, and the underlying neural structures participating in the behavior, are a function of the stage of the learning process. Adapted from Ashe J, Lungu OV, Basford AT, and Lu X (2006) Cortical control of motor sequences. *Curr. Opin. Neurobiol.* 16: 213–221.

during this preparation period, and follows that of premotor areas in time (Wildgruber et al., 1997). Using rapid event-related functional magnetic resonance imaging that allows the timing of different motor cortical areas to be examined, activity has been examined using a finger sequence movement task. Using this approach, activity in SMA does not differ between self-initiated and externally guided sequences during movement, or between self-initiated premovement and movement. Both self-initiated movements and externally cued movements show strong activation in mesial motor areas. However, the timing of the activity in pre-SMA was significantly earlier for self-initiated compared with externally triggered movements. (Cunnington et al., 2002). Sequence complexity had a greater effect on SMA before rather than during movement, suggesting that SMA is more involved in preparatory processes (Elsinger et al., 2006).

Pre-SMA appears to be preferentially involved in self-initiated movements. Pre-SMA also appears to be activated when a mental representation of a movement is engaged, in the absence of actual movement (Koski et al., 2003). However, imagined movements are also correlated with activation in SMA, but the SMA was more active during movement execution (Cunnington et al., 2006).

Whether the SMA is involved in self-initiated movements is subject to debate (see discussion in Deiber et al., 1999), but other variables may modulate activity of SMA, in addition to the mode of movement initiation. Pre-SMA (as well as PMd) and not SMA was activated preferentially during an auditory conditional motor task, in which two different tones triggered different movements (Kurata et al., 2000). Pre-SMA activity appears to be rate dependent, with more extensive activation with faster movements. SMA is preferential for sequential rather than fixed movements, that is, the type of movement (Deiber et al., 1999).

One interesting aspect of the timing of movements focuses on whether motor areas are concerned with ordinal or interval properties of the timed movements. Timing control appears to be independent of sequence representation. That is, timing can be changed without changing the sequential order. During a sequential movement task, subjects had to attend to either the interval or the ordinal information of a sequence of visually presented stimuli. While the same motor areas were activated in both conditions, pre-SMA, lateral PMC, frontal opercular areas, basal ganglia, and left lateral cerebellar cortex were activated more strongly by interval information, while SMA, frontal eye field, M1 and S1, cuneus, and medial cerebellar cortex were more active for ordinal information. (Schubotz and von Cramon, 2001). Thus, different aspects of impending movement sequences may be processed by different areas.

25.5.2.4 Shift-related cells in pre-SMA

In monkeys, activity in response to visual cue signals during a preparatory phase that indicates the direction of an upcoming arm movement is abundant in pre-SMA. Also, pre-SMA contains an abundance of shift-related cells that respond when monkeys are instructed to shift the target of a future reach from a previous target to a new target (Matsuzaka and Tanji, 1996). Relatively few shift-related cells are found in SMA. The majority of SMA neurons are time-locked to movements.

25.5.2.5 Role of SMA in kinetics and dynamics of movement

Two aspects of reaching movements have been described based on kinematics versus dynamics of the action (Padoa-Schioppa et al., 2002). Kinematics refers to the evolution in time of the joint angles and hand position. Dynamics refers to the set of forces exerted by the muscles. The accomplishment of skilled reaching can be defined from a neural perspective as the generation of appropriate forces (dynamics) for a desired hand trajectory (kinematics). Thus the role that the central motor structures plays in the transformation of desired kinematics into dynamics is critical to our understanding of motor skill learning. Dynamics-related neural activity has been found in several motor structures including dentate and interpositus nuclei in the cerebellum, M1, SMA, PMd, PMv, and putamen. Neurophysiological studies suggest that dynamics-related activity in SMA occur during the motor planning phase. Thus, SMA is likely to participate in this kinetics-to-dynamics transformation (Padoa-Schioppa et al., 2002).

25.5.3 Lateral Premotor Cortical Areas and Their Role in Motor Skill Learning

25.5.3.1 Comparative aspects of lateral premotor areas

Recent studies indicate that premotor areas play an important role in sensory guidance of movement and some aspects of motor preparation. Premotor areas probably first appeared with the divergence of prosimian primates, as evidenced by lateral premotor representations coincident with distinct cytoarchitectonics rostral to the M1 representation. Two major subdivisions, PMd and PMv, have been identified in the prosimian Galago (Wu et al., 2000). PMd has been further subdivided in Galago into rostral and caudal components (PMd-r and PMd-c, respectively). These two PMd areas appear to be functionally distinct, as saccades are evoked from stimulation of PMd-r, and forelimb and body movements are evoked from PMd-c (Fujii et al., 2000). To the extent that Galagos represent a primordial state of primate motor cortex, it is likely that PMd-r, PMd-c, and PMv are homologs in all extant primates. Intracortical microstimulation studies have also identified PMv and PMd in New World and Old World monkeys (Gould et al., 1986; Stepniewska et al., 1993; Preuss et al., 1996; Frost et al., 2003; Hoshi and Tanji, 2004). The PMd has been shown to consist of representations of both hindlimb and forelimb (He et al., 1993; Ghosh and Gattera, 1995; Preuss et al., 1996; Raos et al., 2003), while PMv contains representations of the forelimb and orofacial muscles (Stepniewska et al., 1993; Preuss et al., 1996).

In addition to the areas noted that have been identified in prosimian primates and New World monkeys, the PMv is further differentiated in Old World monkeys. A total of four subareas of lateral premotor cortex are identifiable in macaques: PMd-c, PMd-r, PMv-c, and PMv-r (or F2, F7, F4, and F5, respectively) based on cytoarchitectonics and intracortical microstimulation results and connections (Rizzolatti and Fadiga, 1998; Rouiller et al., 1998; Morel et al., 2005).

Unlike macaque monkeys, there have been no delineations of subareas F4 and F5 (Pmv-c and Pmv-r) in PMv of prosimian primates or New World monkeys. In macaques, PMv is subdivided into caudal and rostral divisions based on cytoarchitectonic, connectional, histochemical, and physiological distinctions (Matelli et al., 1985, 1991; Luppino et al., 1999; Rizzolatti and Luppino, 2001; Rizzolatti et al., 2002; Morel et al., 2005).

Since direct corticospinal projections originate from dorsal and ventral premotor areas (as from M1, SMA, and CMA), it is possible that all frontal cortical areas may participate in movement dynamics.

25.5.3.2 Role of the ventral premotor cortex in motor control

The ventral premotor cortex was first characterized functionally by its involvement in visually guided motor behavior as its neurons discharge during preparation and execution of movements under visual guidance (Godschalk et al., 1981). PMv neurons also respond to tactile and proprioceptive stimulation (Graziano et al., 1997; Graziano, 1999). Thus, PMv has been implicated in the initiation and control of limb movements based on visual and somatosensory information (Kurata and Tanji, 1986; Gentilucci et al., 1988; Rizzolatti et al., 1988; Mushiake et al., 1991, 1997). PMv is important for the integration of visual information derived from extrapersonal three-dimensional space and involved in the spatial guidance of limb movements (Kakei et al., 2001). PMv neurons respond to somatosensory stimuli applied to either face or arm and to visual stimuli corresponding to peripersonal space (Gallese et al., 1996; Graziano et al., 1997). PMv neurons are selective for the three-dimensional shape of objects to be grasped (Murata et al., 1997), the direction or movement trajectory in visual/extrinsic space (Kakei et al., 2001; Schwartz et al., 2004), the attention to visuospatial stimuli (Boussaoud et al., 1993), and decisions making based on somatosensory signals (Romo et al., 2004).

Specific lesions of PMv in the area responding to visual object presentation (F5) result in deficits in visually guided grasping movements. Hand preshaping preceding grasping is markedly impaired. Monkeys were able to grasp objects, but only after compensation based on tactile correction (Fogassi et al., 2001). Animals show a reluctance to use the affected hand (Rizzolatti et al., 1983; Schieber, 2000), though the ability to make a precision grip appears unaffected (Schieber, 2000). During conditional visuomotor association tasks, movements have smaller amplitudes and slower velocities, but few direction errors are made (Kurata and Hoffman, 1994). Monkeys appear to lose the ability to perform a prism adaptation task after muscimol injection in PMv (Kurata and Hoshi, 1999). Lesions of the periarcuate region of frontal cortex (premotor cortex, probably primarily PMv) result in deficits in selecting the proper response to a conditional cue (Petrides, 1986).

In macaques, F4 appears to code goal-directed actions mediated by spatial locations (Rizzolatti et al., 2002), while F5 has been shown to be involved in motor-action recognition (Umilta et al., 2001). Human area 44 has been shown to be involved in sensorimotor transformations for grasping and manipulation (Binkofski et al., 1999) and is thought to be homologous to F5 in macaques (Rizzolatti et al., 2002).

Neurons in PMv reflect processes in extrinsic coordinates more often than neurons in M1 (Kakei et al., 2001). Effector-independent activity is more frequent in PMv than in PMd (Hoshi and Tanji, 2002). Premovement activity is less frequent in PMv than PMd (Boudreau et al., 2001). Activity of neurons in PMv co-varies with external force in a precision grip task (Hepp-Reymond et al., 1994, 1999). Dynamics of movement appear to be coded in both PMd and PMv (Xiao et al., 2006).

25.5.3.3 Role of dorsal premotor cortex in motor control

PMd is involved in movement parameters (Fu et al., 1993; Kurata, 1993; Crammond and Kalaska, 2000) and in the integration of internal body representation and target information for the preparation of motor actions (Kurata, 1994; Hoshi and Tanji, 2004). PMd neurons are active during a preparatory motor-set period (Weinrich and Wise, 1982) and in relation to visuomotor-association tasks (Kurata and Wise, 1988; Mitz et al., 1991). Neurons in PMd are active before expected visual signals (Mauritz and Wise, 1986) and during motor preparation (Wise and Mauritz, 1985; Kurata and Wise, 1988). Target-related activity prior to and during movement is more abundant in PMd than in M1 (Shen and Alexander, 1997). However, there is considerable overlap in function (Riehle and Requin, 1989; Kalaska et al., 1997).

Like SMA, neurons in PMd appear to reflect dynamics during motor planning, or the dynamics of upcoming movement. PMd may also be involved in the kinetics-to-dynamics transformation, though not to the degree that SMA is. During the premovement period, neurons in PMv are mostly not directionally tuned, which is more like M1.

Monkeys with PMd lesions exhibit increased direction errors during conditional visuomotor association tasks. However, movement amplitude and velocity are normal (Kurata and Hoffman, 1994). This contrasts with effects of PMv lesions.

25.5.3.4 Direct comparison of ventral and dorsal premotor cortex response properties

In a few studies, direct comparisons have been made between these two premotor areas. The results show that set-related activity is mainly found in PMd, while movement-related activity is found in both PMd and PMv (Kurata, 1993). PMv neurons mainly respond to visual target location, while PMd neurons respond to target location and arm direction (Hoshi and Tanji, 2004). PMv neurons predominantly reflect locations of visuospatial signals (Hoshi and Tanji, 2002, 2006). About half of PMd neurons reflect motor instructions about the cue (arm or target to be selected) (Hoshi and Tanji, 2006).

25.5.3.5 Role of dorsal and ventral premotor cortex in motor skill learning

Based on the response properties of premotor neurons and the effects of lesions to PMd and PMv, it would appear that premotor cortex plays a role in retrieval of movements from memory based on environmental context (Mitz et al., 1991). This would suggest an important role for premotor cortex in learning conditional associations between sensory stimuli and appropriate motor actions. When monkeys were trained to learn new conditional motor associations, over half the neurons tested in PMd changed their activity during the learning of the association (Mitz et al., 1991). As learning progressed, the activity of novel associations began to resemble familiar ones (Buch et al., 2006). Interestingly, after the response choice had been made, but prior to any feedback, activity increased in the putamen, but not in PMd (Buch et al., 2006). In an auditory conditional association task in humans, PMd and pre-SMA exclusively showed preferential activation, suggesting that these are sites where general sensorimotor integration for learning new associations takes place (Kurata et al., 2000).

In another popular paradigm for motor learning, neuronal activity is recorded in motor areas as animals learn to adapt to a novel force field. In this task, premotor neurons display plasticity related to learning of kinematic, dynamic, or memory properties (Xiao, 2005). A progressive change in movement-related representations have been reported in PMd in an instructed-delay paradigm (Messier and Kalaska, 2000).

25.5.3.6 Learning through observation: role of premotor cortex

There is now considerable interest in the role of motor cortical areas in learning new motor skills through observation. While motor skills are typically learned through physical practice, it is well known that motor performance can be improved simply by observing a skilled motor task (Vogt, 1995; Mattar and Gribble, 2005). It has been suggested that observing the movements of another individual is not simply the observation of visual patterns but the generation of an image of oneself for performing the action (Petrosini et al., 2003). Thus, it is likely that the same structures that are involved in motor execution are active during the observation.

The neural basis of imitation is becoming increasingly clear. In macaque monkeys, so-called mirror neurons located in the ventral premotor cortex (area F5) and posterior parietal cortex (area PF) fire not only when the monkey performs a particular motor action but also when the monkey observes someone else performing the same action (Rizzolatti et al., 1996). This phenomenon has been implicated in the human ability to imitate. Functional magnetic resonance imaging studies in humans confirm that similar regions may be active during both observed and executed actions (Koski et al., 2003). Further, these regions appear to be more active during specular imitation (i.e., the actor moves the left hand and the imitator moves the right hand, as if looking in a mirror), more so than during anatomic imitation (i.e., the actor and imitator move the right hand) (Koski et al., 2003).

25.5.4 CMAs and Their Role in Motor Behavior

The primate cingulate cortex, buried in the cingulate sulcus, has traditionally been divided into rostral and caudal architectonic subdivisions (areas 24 and 23). More recently, in the macaque, the caudal CMA has been further differentiated into three distinct areas – rostral (CMAr), dorsal (CMAd), and ventral (CMAv) – based on cytoarchitectonics and neuronal response properties (Walsh and Ebner, 1970; Vogt et al., 1987; Takada et al., 2001; Hatanaka et al., 2003). Because the CMAs are in close proximity to SMA and pre-SMA, it is likely that in many older studies in both nonhuman primates and humans, neuronal activation anywhere on the medial wall was attributed to SMA. Thus, caution should be taken when interpretating findings in which this distinction is not made clear. In general, the rostral cingulate zone is activated by complex tasks, while the caudal cingulated zone is activated during simple tasks (Picard and Strick, 1996).

CMAv receives proprioceptive input from the arm and hand (Cadoret and Smith, 1995). As with other secondary motor areas, the CMA areas send somatotopic projections directly to M1 and the spinal cord (Muakkassa and Strick, 1979; Dum and Strick, 1991, 1996; Luppino et al., 1993; He et al., 1995; Wang et al., 2001). The somatotopy of CMA has been examined using intracortical microstimulation, demonstrating at least a forelimb representation in each of the three subareas (Mitz and Wise, 1987; Luppino et al., 1991, 1994; Takada et al., 2001; Wang et al., 2001; Hatanaka et al., 2003). CMA also receives prominent afferent input from limbic structures and the prefrontal cortex, conveying information regarding motivation. Functional studies examining CMAs suggest that CMAr plays a unique role in the cognitive control of voluntary movements, while the caudal CMA (CMAd and CMAv) is directly involved in the execution of voluntary movement (Devinsky et al., 1995; Picard and Strick, 1996, 2001; Carter et al., 1999; Tanji et al., 2002).

Both the rostral and caudal cingulate areas are more active for self-initiated as opposed to externally triggered movements. In the caudal cingulate zone, activation is greater for sequential rather than for fixed movements, much like SMA proper (Deiber et al., 1999).

On the basis of deoxyglucose labeling techniques in monkeys, it has been suggested that CMAd is highly active during the preparation for and/or execution of a highly rehearsed, remembered movement sequence but is less active if the movement sequence is performed under visual guidance (Picard and Strick, 1997). In the same remembered movement sequence task, the CMAr and CMAv were not active. Instead, these areas are active during simple motor tasks (Shima et al., 1991).

CMAs are likely to play a role in motor learning. A learning paradigm that is popular in rabbits is trace eyeblink conditioning. Lesions of the caudal anterior cingulate cortex in rabbits prevent trace eyeblink conditioning (Weible et al., 2000). However, based on inputs from limbic and prefrontal structures, the role of cingulate areas in motor learning is likely to be related to transmitting information regarding motivation and memory of previous events, rather than simple sensorimotor transformations.

25.6 Phases of Motor Learning and Differential Activation of Motor Structures

Significant improvements in reaching accuracy occur in rats after less than one week of training. However, significant expansion of movement representations does not occur for at least ten days after training is initiated (Kleim et al., 2004). This mismatch between behavioral and neurophysiological endpoints suggests that plasticity in cortical maps reflects only certain aspects of the motor learning experience. Therefore, it is important to differentiate the various phases of motor learning.

Memory has often been described in terms of a short-term memory that is labile and susceptible to interference and a long-term memory that is more stable. The process of transferring information from short-term to long-term memory is referred to as consolidation. It has been argued that motor learning proceeds through similar stages and that different neural mechanisms may account for the two distinct functional stages (Shadmehr and Brashers-Krug, 1997). Stages of motor skill learning have also been described as consisting of a fast, within-session phase that occurs on a time scale of minutes and a second, slowly evolving phase that takes hours to occur. Whether these stages of motor learning that have been proposed based on human experiments have any relationship to neurophysiological and neuroanatomical findings from experimental animal models is still unclear. While the human studies are typically conducted over the course of several hours or a few days, the cortical plasticity demonstrated in animals takes place over one week or more. It is possible that the stages of motor learning described in human studies are the initial events in a much more protracted process.

Early and late phases of motor learning have been associated with different neuronal networks. In motor sequence learning, the early phase is thought to involve the corticostriatal and corticocerebellar networks, while the late phase is attributed to the corticostriatal network (see Doyon and Benali, 2005). In a pursuit rotor task requiring human subjects to track a moving target with a stylus, positron emission tomography studies have shown increased blood flow involving a large distributed network in cortex, striatum, and cerebellum during the execution of the task (Grafton et al., 1992). These included motor areas (M1, SMA, putamen, substantia nigra, anterior lobe, and inferior vermis of the cerebellum) and visual association areas (fusiform gyrus and extrastriate area 18). However, sequential positron emission tomography scans over the course of learning the pursuit task demonstrated increased cerebral blood flow in a smaller subset of motor structures including contralateral SMA, M1, and pulvinar thalamus. Thus, procedural motor learning is accomplished by a subregion of the larger network that is critical to the movement execution.

25.7 Summary

Significant advances have been made in the past several years in understanding the role of the various cortical motor areas in motor learning. It is clear that motor skill acquisition is associated with alterations in topographic maps of motor representations, structural changes in neuronal elements (synapses, dendrites, etc.), and differential expression of growth-related proteins. We now recognize that motor learning is a distributed process. While differentiation in the response properties of various cortical areas demonstrates their unique functions, there is considerable overlap. Primary motor cortex is most associated with movement-related aspects of learning motor tasks. The mesial areas are more related to learning motor sequences, especially when they are self-initiated. The lateral motor areas are more related to externally guided movements and the integration of sensory cues with motor commands, especially in forming conditional motor associations. Finally, the CMAs are involved in more cognitive and motivational aspects of motor learning.

References

Adkins DL, Boychuk J, Remple MS, and Kleim JA (2006) Motor training induces experience-specific patterns of plasticity across motor cortex and spinal cord. *J. Appl. Physiol.* 101: 1776–1782.

Amsel A (1992) *Frustration Theory: An Analysis of Dispositional Learning and Memory*. New York: Cambridge University Press.

Ashe J, Lungu OV, Basford AT, and Lu X (2006) Cortical control of motor sequences. *Curr. Opin. Neurobiol.* 16: 213–221.

Binkofski F, Buccino G, Posse S, Seitz RJ, Rizzolatti G, and Freund H (1999) A fronto-parietal circuit for object manipulation in man: Evidence from an fMRI-study. *Eur. J. Neurosci.* 11: 3276–3286.

Boudreau MJ, Brochier T, Pare M, and Smith AM (2001) Activity in ventral and dorsal premotor cortex in response to predictable force-pulse perturbations in a precision grip task. *J. Neurophysiol.* 86: 1067–1078.

Boussaoud D, Barth TM, and Wise SP (1993) Effects of gaze on apparent visual responses of frontal cortex neurons. *Exp. Brain Res.* 93: 423–434.

Brinkman C (1981) Lesions in supplementary motor area interfere with a monkey's performance of a bimanual coordination task. *Neurosci. Lett.* 27: 267–270.

Brinkman C and Porter R (1983) Supplementary motor area and premotor area of monkey cerebral cortex: Functional organization and activities of single neurons during performance of a learned movement. *Adv. Neurol.* 39: 393–420.

Buch ER, Brasted PJ, and Wise SP (2006) Comparison of population activity in the dorsal premotor cortex and putamen during the learning of arbitrary visuomotor mappings. *Exp. Brain Res.* 169: 69–84.

Bury SD and Jones TA (2002) Unilateral sensorimotor cortex lesions in adult rats facilitate motor skill learning with the "unaffected" forelimb and training-induced dendritic structural plasticity in the motor cortex. *J. Neurosci.* 22: 8597–8606.

Cadoret G and Smith AM (1995) Input-output properties of hand-related cells in the ventral cingulate cortex in the monkey. *J. Neurophysiol.* 73: 2584–2590.

Carter CS, Botvinick MM, and Cohen JD (1999) The contribution of the anterior cingulate cortex to executive processes in cognition. *Rev. Neurosci.* 10: 49–57.

Castro-Alamancos MA, Donoghue JP, and Connors BW (1995) Different forms of synaptic plasticity in somatosensory and motor areas of the neocortex. *J. Neurosci.* 15: 5324–5333.

Classen J, Liepert J, Wise SP, Hallett M, and Cohen LG (1998) Rapid plasticity of human cortical movement representation induced by practice. *J. Neurophysiol.* 79: 1117–1123.

Clower WT and Alexander GE (1998) Movement sequence-related activity reflecting numerical order of components in supplementary and presupplementary motor areas. *J. Neurophysiol.* 80: 1562–1566.

Cohen JD and Castro-Alamancos MA (2005) Skilled motor learning does not enhance long-term depression in the motor cortex in vivo. *J. Neurophysiol.* 93: 1486–1497.

Crammond DJ and Kalaska JF (2000) Prior information in motor and premotor cortex: Activity during the delay period and effect on pre-movement activity. *J. Neurophysiol.* 84: 986–1005.

Crutcher MD and Alexander GE (1990) Movement-related neuronal activity selectively coding either direction or muscle pattern in three motor areas of the monkey. *J. Neurophysiol.* 64: 151–163.

Crutcher MD, Russo GS, Ye S, and Backus DA (2004) Target-, limb-, and context-dependent neural activity in the cingulate and supplementary motor areas of the monkey. *Exp. Brain Res.* 158: 278–288.

Cunnington R, Windischberger C, Deecke L, and Moser E (2002) The preparation and execution of self-initiated and externally-triggered movement: A study of event-related fMRI. *Neuroimage* 15: 373–385.

Cunnington R, Windischberger C, Robinson S, and Moser E (2006) The selection of intended actions and the observation of others' actions: A time-resolved fMRI study. *Neuroimage* 29: 1294–1302.

Deecke L, Kornhuber HH, Lang W, Lang M, and Schreiber H (1985) Timing function of the frontal cortex in sequential motor and learning tasks. *Hum. Neurobiol.* 4: 143–154.

Deiber MP, Honda M, Ibanez V, Sadato N, and Hallett M (1999) Mesial motor areas in self-initiated versus externally triggered movements examined with fMRI: Effect of movement type and rate. *J. Neurophysiol.* 81: 3065–3077.

Derksen MJ, Ward NL, Hartle KD, and Ivanco TL (2006) MAP2 and synaptophysin protein expression following motor learning suggests dynamic regulation and distinct alterations coinciding with synaptogenesis. *Neurobiol. Learn. Mem.* 87: 404–415.

Devinsky O, Morrell MJ, and Vogt BA (1995) Contributions of anterior cingulate cortex to behaviour. *Brain* 118: 279–306.

Donoghue JP and Wise SP (1982) The motor cortex of the rat: cytoarchitecture and microstimulation mapping. *J. Comp. Neurol.* 212: 76–88.

Doyon J and Benali H (2005) Reorganization and plasticity in the adult brain during learning of motor tasks. *Curr. Opin. Neurobiol.* 15: 161–167.

Dum RP and Strick PL (1991) The origin of corticospinal projections from the premotor areas in the frontal lobe. *J. Neurosci.* 11: 667–689.

Dum RP and Strick PL (1996) Spinal cord terminations of the medial wall motor areas in macaque monkeys. *J. Neurosci.* 16: 6513–6525.

Elsinger CL, Harrington DL, and Rao SM (2006) From preparation to online control: Reappraisal of neural circuitry mediating internally generated and externally guided actions. *Neuroimage* 31: 1177–1187.

Fitts PM (1954) The information capacity of the human motor system in controlling the amplitude of movement. *J. Exp. Psychol.* 47: 381–391.

Fogassi L, Gallese V, Buccino G, Craighero L, Fadiga L, and Rizzolatti G (2001) Cortical mechanism for the visual guidance of hand grasping movements in the monkey: A reversible inactivation study. *Brain* 124: 571–586.

Frost SB, Barbay S, Friel KM, Plautz EJ, and Nudo RJ (2003) Reorganization of remote cortical regions after ischemic brain injury: A potential substrate for stroke recovery. *J. Neurophysiol.* 89: 3205–3214.

Fu QG, Suarez JI, and Ebner TJ (1993) Neuronal specification of direction and distance during reaching movements in the superior precentral premotor area and primary motor cortex of monkeys. *J. Neurophysiol.* 70: 2097–2116.

Fujii N, Mushiake H, and Tanji J (2000) Rostrocaudal distinction of the dorsal premotor area based on oculomotor involvement. *J. Neurophysiol.* 83: 1764–1769.

Gallese V, Fadiga L, Fogassi L, and Rizzolatti G (1996) Action recognition in the premotor cortex. *Brain* 119: 593–609.

Gentilucci M, Fogassi L, Luppino G, Matelli M, Camarda R, and Rizzolatti G (1988) Functional organization of inferior area 6 in the macaque monkey. I. Somatotopy and the control of proximal movements. *Exp. Brain Res.* 71: 475–490.

Ghosh S and Gattera R (1995) A comparison of the ipsilateral cortical projections to the dorsal and ventral subdivisions of the macaque premotor cortex. *Somatosens. Mot. Res.* 12: 359–378.

Godschalk M, Lemon RN, Nijs HG, and Kuypers HG (1981) Behaviour of neurons in monkey peri-arcuate and precentral cortex before and during visually guided arm and hand movements. *Exp. Brain Res.* 44: 113–116.

Gould HJ 3rd, Cusick CG, Pons TP, and Kaas JH (1986) The relationship of corpus callosum connections to electrical stimulation maps of motor, supplementary motor, and the frontal eye fields in owl monkeys. *J. Comp. Neurol.* 247: 297–325.

Grafton ST, Hazeltine E, and Ivry RB (1998) Abstract and effector-specific representations of motor sequences identified with PET. *J. Neurosci.* 18: 9420–9428.

Grafton ST, Mazziotta JC, Presty S, Friston KJ, Frackowiak RS, and Phelps ME (1992) Functional anatomy of human procedural learning determined with regional cerebral blood flow and PET. *J. Neurosci.* 12: 2542–2548.

Graziano MS (1999) Where is my arm? The relative role of vision and proprioception in the neuronal representation of limb position. *Proc. Natl. Acad. Sci. USA* 96: 10418–10421.

Graziano MS, Hu XT, and Gross CG (1997) Visuospatial properties of ventral premotor cortex. *J. Neurophysiol.* 77: 2268–2292.

Hall RD and Lindholm EP (1974) Organization of motor and somatosensory neocortex in the albino rat. *Brain Res.* 66: 23–38.

Hallett M, Pascual-Leone A, and Topka H (1996) Adaptation and skill-learning: Evidence for different neural substrates. In: Bloedel JR, Ebner TJ, Wise SP (eds.) *The Acquisition of Motor Behavior in Vertebrates*. Cambridge, MA: MIT Press.

Halsband U, Ito N, Tanji J, and Freund HJ (1993) The role of premotor cortex and the supplementary motor area in the temporal control of movement in man. *Brain* 116: 243–266.

Hatanaka N, Tokuno H, Hamada I, et al. (2003) Thalamocortical and intracortical connections of monkey cingulate motor areas. *J. Comp. Neurol.* 462: 121–138.

He SQ, Dum RP, and Strick PL (1993) Topographic organization of corticospinal projections from the frontal lobe: Motor areas on the lateral surface of the hemisphere. *J. Neurosci.* 13: 952–980.

He SQ, Dum RP, and Strick PL (1995) Topographic organization of corticospinal projections from the frontal lobe: Motor areas on the medial surface of the hemisphere. *J. Neurosci.* 15: 3284–3306.

Hepp-Reymond MC, Husler EJ, Maier MA, and QI HX (1994) Force-related neuronal activity in two regions of the primate ventral premotor cortex. *Can. J. Physiol. Pharmacol.* 72: 571–579.

Hepp-Reymond M, Kirkpatrick-Tanner M, Gabernet L, Qi HX, and Weber B (1999) Context-dependent force coding in motor and premotor cortical areas. *Exp. Brain Res.* 128: 123–133.

Hernandez PJ, Schiltz CA, and Kelley AE (2006) Dynamic shifts in corticostriatal expression patterns of the immediate early genes Homer 1a and Zif268 during early and late phases of instrumental training. *Learn. Mem.* 13: 599–608.

Hikosaka O, Sakai K, Miyauchi S, Takino R, Sasaki Y, and Putz B (1996) Activation of human presupplementary motor area in learning of sequential procedures: A functional MRI study. *J. Neurophysiol.* 76: 617–621.

Hodgson RA, Ji Z, Standish S, Boyd-Hodgson TE, Henderson AK, and Racine RJ (2005) Training-induced and electrically induced potentiation in the neocortex. *Neurobiol. Learn. Mem.* 83: 22–32.

Hoshi E and Tanji J (2002) Contrasting neuronal activity in the dorsal and ventral premotor areas during preparation to reach. *J. Neurophysiol.* 87: 1123–1128.

Hoshi E and Tanji J (2004) Functional specialization in dorsal and ventral premotor areas. *Prog. Brain Res.* 143: 507–511.

Hoshi E and Tanji J (2006) Differential involvement of neurons in the dorsal and ventral premotor cortex during processing of visual signals for action planning. *J. Neurophysiol.* 95: 3596–3616.

Jenkins IH, Brooks DJ, Nixon PD, Frackowiak RS, and Passingham RE (1994) Motor sequence learning: A study with positron emission tomography. *J. Neurosci.* 14: 3775–3790.

Jenkins IH, Jahanshahi M, Jueptner M, Passingham RE, and Brooks DJ (2000) Self-initiated versus externally triggered movements. II. The effect of movement predictability on regional cerebral blood flow. *Brain* 123: 1216–1228.

Jones TA, Chu CJ, Grande LA, and Gregory AD (1999) Motor skills training enhances lesion-induced structural plasticity in the motor cortex of adult rats. *J. Neurosci.* 19: 10153–10163.

Kakei S, Hoffman DS, and Strick PL (2001) Direction of action is represented in the ventral premotor cortex. *Nat. Neurosci.* 4: 1020–1025.

Kalaska JF, Scott SH, Cisek P, and Sergio LE (1997) Cortical control of reaching movements. *Curr. Opin. Neurobiol.* 7: 849–859.

Kleim JA, Barbay S, Cooper NR et al. (2002) Motor lering-ependentsynaptogenesis is localized to functionally reorganized motor cortex. *Neurobiol. Learn. Mem.* 77: 63–77.

Kleim JA, Barbay S, and Nudo RJ (1998) Functional reorganization of the rat motor cortex following motor skill learning. *J. Neurophysiol.* 80: 3321–3325.

Kleim JA, Bruneau R, Calder K, et al. (2003) Functional organization of adult motor cortex is dependent upon continued protein synthesis. *Neuron* 40: 167–176.

Kleim JA, Hogg TM, VandenBerg PM, Cooper NR, Bruneau R, and Remple M (2004) Cortical synaptogenesis and motor map reorganization occur during late, but not early, phase of motor skill learning. *J. Neurosci.* 24: 628–633.

Koski L, Iacoboni M, Dubeau MC, Woods RP, and Mazziotta JC (2003) Modulation of cortical activity during different imitative behaviors. *J. Neurophysiol.* 89: 460–471.

Kurata K (1993) Premotor cortex of monkeys: Set- and movement-related activity reflecting amplitude and direction of wrist movements. *J. Neurophysiol.* 69: 187–200.

Kurata K (1994) Information processing for motor control in primate premotor cortex. *Behav. Brain Res.* 61: 135–142.

Kurata K and Hoffman DS (1994) Differential effects of muscimol microinjection into dorsal and ventral aspects of the premotor cortex of monkeys. *J. Neurophysiol.* 71: 1151–1164.

Kurata K and Hoshi E (1999) Reacquisition deficits in prism adaptation after muscimol microinjection into the ventral premotor cortex of monkeys. *J. Neurophysiol.* 81: 1927–1938.

Kurata K and Tanji J (1985) Contrasting neuronal activity in supplementary and precentral motor cortex of monkeys. II. Responses to movement triggering vs. nontriggering sensory signals. *J. Neurophysiol.* 53: 142–152.

Kurata K and Tanji J (1986) Premotor cortex neurons in macaques: Activity before distal and proximal forelimb movements. *J. Neurosci.* 6: 403–411.

Kurata K, Tsuji T, Naraki S, Seino M, and Abe Y (2000) Activation of the dorsal premotor cortex and pre-supplementary motor area of humans during an auditory conditional motor task. *J. Neurophysiol.* 84: 1667–1672.

Kurata K and Wise SP (1988) Premotor cortex of rhesus monkeys: Set-related activity during two conditional motor tasks. *Exp. Brain Res.* 69: 327–343.

Lee D and Quessy S (2003) Activity in the supplementary motor area related to learning and performance during a sequential visuomotor task. *J. Neurophysiol.* 89: 1039–1056.

Lehericy S, Ducros M, Krainik A, et al. (2004) 3-D diffusion tensor axonal tracking shows distinct SMA and pre-SMA projections to the human striatum. *Cereb. Cortex* 14: 1302–1309.

Lu X and Ashe J (2005) Anticipatory activity in primary motor cortex codes memorized movement sequences. *Neuron* 45: 967–973.

Luppino G, Matelli M, Camarda RM, Gallese V, and Rizzolatti G (1991) Multiple representations of body movements in mesial area 6 and the adjacent cingulate cortex: An intracortical microstimulation study in the macaque monkey. *J. Comp. Neurol.* 311: 463–482.

Luppino G, Matelli M, Camarda R, and Rizzolatti G (1993) Corticocortical connections of area F3 (SMA-proper) and area F6 (pre-SMA) in the macaque monkey. *J. Comp. Neurol.* 338: 114–140.

Luppino G, Matelli M, Camarda R, and Rizzolatti G (1994) Corticospinal projections from mesial frontal and cingulate areas in the monkey. *Neuroreport* 5: 2545–2548.

Luppino G, Murata A, Govoni P, and Matelli M (1999) Largely segregated parietofrontal connections linking rostral intraparietal cortex (areas AIP and VIP) and the ventral premotor cortex (areas F5 and F4). *Exp. Brain Res.* 128: 181–187.

Matelli M, Luppino G, and Rizzolatti G (1985) Patterns of cytochrome oxidase activity in the frontal agranular cortex of the macaque monkey. *Behav. Brain Res.* 18: 125–136.

Matelli M, Luppino G, and Rizzolatti G (1991) Architecture of superior and mesial area 6 and the adjacent cingulate cortex in the macaque monkey. *J. Comp. Neurol.* 311: 445–462.

Matsuzaka Y, Aizawa H, and Tanji J (1992) A motor area rostral to the supplementary motor area (presupplementary motor area) in the monkey: Neuronal activity during a learned motor task. *J. Neurophysiol.* 68: 653–662.

Matsuzaka Y, Picard N, and Strick PL (2007) Skill representation in the primary motor cortex after long-term practice. *J. Neurophysiol.* 97: 1819–1832.

Matsuzaka Y and Tanji J (1996) Changing directions of forthcoming arm movements: Neuronal activity in the presupplementary and supplementary motor area of monkey cerebral cortex. *J. Neurophysiol.* 76: 2327–2342.

Mattar AA and Gribble PL (2005) Motor learning by observing. *Neuron* 46: 153–160.

Mauritz KH and Wise SP (1986) Premotor cortex of the rhesus monkey: Neuronal activity in anticipation of predictable environmental events. *Exp. Brain Res.* 61: 229–244.

McNamara A, Tegenthoff M, Dinse H, Buchel C, Binkofski F, and Ragert P (2007) Increased functional connectivity is crucial for learning novel muscle synergies. *Neuroimage* 35: 1211–1218.

Messier J and Kalaska JF (2000) Covariation of primate dorsal premotor cell activity with direction and amplitude during a memorized-delay reaching task. *J. Neurophysiol.* 84: 152–165.

Mishkin M, Malamut B, and Bachevalier J (1984) Memories and habits: Two neural systems. In: Lynch G, McGaugh JL, Weinberger NM (eds.) *Neurobiology of Learning and Memory*, pp. 65–77. New York: Guilford.

Mitz AR, Godschalk M, and Wise SP (1991) Learning-dependent neuronal activity in the premotor cortex: Activity during the acquisition of conditional motor associations. *J. Neurosci.* 11: 1855–1872.

Mitz AR and Wise SP (1987) The somatotopic organization of the supplementary motor area: Intracortical microstimulation mapping. *J. Neurosci.* 7: 1010–1021.

Morel A, Liu J, Wannier T, Jeanmonod D, and Rouiller EM (2005) Divergence and convergence of thalamocortical projections to premotor and supplementary motor cortex: A multiple tracing study in the macaque monkey. *Eur. J. Neurosci.* 21: 1007–1029.

Muakkassa KF and Strick PL (1979) Frontal lobe inputs to primate motor cortex: Evidence for four somatotopically organized "premotor" areas. *Brain Res.* 177: 176–182.

Murata A, Fadiga L, Fogassi L, Gallese V, Raos V, and Rizzolatti G (1997) Object representation in the ventral premotor cortex (area F5) of the monkey. *J. Neurophysiol.* 78: 2226–2230.

Muri RM, Rosler KM, and Hess CW (1994) Influence of transcranial magnetic stimulation on the execution of memorised sequences of saccades in man. *Exp. Brain Res.* 101: 521–524.

Mushiake H, Inase M, and Tanji J (1991) Neuronal activity in the primate premotor, supplementary, and precentral motor cortex during visually guided and internally determined sequential movements. *J. Neurophysiol.* 66: 705–718.

Mushiake H, Tanatsugu Y, and Tanji J (1997) Neuronal activity in the ventral part of premotor cortex during target-reach movement is modulated by direction of gaze. *J. Neurophysiol.* 78: 567–571.

Nakamura K, Sakai K, and Hikosaka O (1998) Neuronal activity in medial frontal cortex during learning of sequential procedures. *J. Neurophysiol.* 80: 2671–2687.

Nakamura K, Sakai K, and Hikosaka O (1999) Effects of local inactivation of monkey medial frontal cortex in learning of sequential procedures. *J. Neurophysiol.* 82: 1063–1068.

Neafsey EJ, Bold EL, Haas G, et al. (1986) The organization of the rat motor cortex: A microstimulation mapping study. *Brain Res.* 396: 77–96.

Nudo RJ and Frost SB (2006) The evolution of motor cortex and motor systems. In: Kaas JH (ed.) *Evolution of Nervous Systems*, pp. 373–396. Oxford: Academic Press.

Nudo RJ, Milliken GW, Jenkins WM, and Merzenich MM (1996) Use-dependent alterations of movement representations in primary motor cortex of adult squirrel monkeys. *J. Neurosci.* 16: 785–807.

Padoa-Schioppa C, Li CS, and Bizzi E (2002) Neuronal correlates of kinematics-to-dynamics transformation in the supplementary motor area. *Neuron* 36: 751–765.

Padoa-Schioppa C, Li CS, and Bizzi E (2004) Neuronal activity in the supplementary motor area of monkeys adapting to a new dynamic environment. *J. Neurophysiol.* 91: 449–473.

Pascual-Leone A and Torres F (1993) Plasticity of the sensorimotor cortex representation of the reading finger in Braille readers. *Brain* 116: 39–52.

Passingham RE (1987) Two cortical systems for directing movement. *Ciba Found. Symp.* 132: 151–164.

Petrides M (1986) The effect of periarcuate lesions in the monkey on the performance of symmetrically and asymmetrically reinforced visual and auditory go, no-go tasks. *J. Neurosci.* 6: 2054–2063.

Petrosini L, Graziano A, Mandolesi L, Neri P, Molinari M, and Leggio MG (2003) Watch how to do it! New advances in learning by observation. *Brain Res. Brain Res. Rev.* 42: 252–264.

Picard N and Strick PL (1996) Motor areas of the medial wall: A review of their location and functional activation. *Cereb. Cortex* 6: 342–353.

Picard N and Strick PL (1997) Activation on the medial wall during remembered sequences of reaching movements in monkeys. *J. Neurophysiol.* 77: 2197–2201.

Picard N and Strick PL (2001) Imaging the premotor areas. *Curr. Opin. Neurobiol.* 11: 663–672.

Picard N and Strick PL (2003) Activation of the supplementary motor area (SMA) during performance of visually guided movements. *Cereb. Cortex* 13: 977–986.

Plautz EJ, Milliken GW, and Nudo RJ (2000) Effects of repetitive motor training on movement representations in adult squirrel monkeys: Role of use versus learning. *Neurobiol. Learn. Mem.* 74: 27–55.

Preuss TM, Stepniewska I, and Kaas JH (1996) Movement representation in the dorsal and ventral premotor areas of owl monkeys: A microstimulation study. *J. Comp. Neurol.* 371: 649–676.

Rao SM, Binder JR, Bandettini PA, et al. (1993) Functional magnetic resonance imaging of complex human movements. *Neurology* 43: 2311–2318.

Raos V, Franchi G, Gallese V, and Fogassi L (2003) Somatotopic organization of the lateral part of area F2 (dorsal premotor cortex) of the macaque monkey. *J. Neurophysiol.* 89: 1503–1518.

Rathelot JA and Strick PL (2006) Muscle representation in the macaque motor cortex: An anatomical perspective. *Proc. Natl. Acad. Sci. USA* 103: 8257–8262.

Remple MS, Bruneau RM, VandenBerg PM, Goertzen C, and Kleim JA (2001) Sensitivity of cortical movement representations to motor experience: Evidence that skill learning but not strength training induces cortical reorganization. *Behav. Brain Res.* 123: 133–141.

Richter W, Andersen PM, Georgopoulos AP, and Kim SG (1997) Sequential activity in human motor areas during a delayed cued finger movement task studied by time-resolved fMRI. *Neuroreport* 8: 1257–1261.

Riehle A and Requin J (1989) Monkey primary motor and premotor cortex: Single-cell activity related to prior information about direction and extent of an intended movement. *J. Neurophysiol.* 61: 534–549.

Rioult-Pedotti MS, Friedman D, and Donoghue JP (2000) Learning-induced LTP in neocortex. *Science* 290: 533–536.

Rioult-Pedotti MS, Friedman D, Hess G, and Donoghue JP (1998) Strengthening of horizontal cortical connections following skill learning. *Nat. Neurosci.* 1: 230–234.

Rizzolatti G, Camarda R, Fogassi L, Gentilucci M, Luppino G, and Matelli M (1988) Functional organization of inferior area 6 in the macaque monkey. II. Area F5 and the control of distal movements. *Exp. Brain Res.* 71: 491–507.

Rizzolatti G and Fadiga L (1998) Grasping objects and grasping action meanings: The dual role of monkey rostroventral

premotor cortex (area F5). *Novartis Found. Symp.* 218: 81–95; discussion 95–103.
Rizzolatti G, Fadiga L, Gallese V, and Fogassi L (1996) Premotor cortex and the recognition of motor actions. *Brain Res. Cogn. Brain Res.* 3: 131–141.
Rizzolatti G, Fogassi L, and Gallese V (2002) Motor and cognitive functions of the ventral premotor cortex. *Curr. Opin. Neurobiol.* 12: 149–154.
Rizzolatti G and Luppino G (2001) The cortical motor system. *Neuron* 31: 889–901.
Rizzolatti G, Matelli M, and Pavesi G (1983) Deficits in attention and movement following the removal of postarcuate (area 6) and prearcuate (area 8) cortex in macaque monkeys. *Brain* 106: 655–673.
Roland PE, Larsen B, Lassen NA, and Skinhoj E (1980) Supplementary motor area and other cortical areas in organization of voluntary movements in man. *J. Neurophysiol.* 43: 118–136.
Romo R, Hernandez A, and Zainos A (2004) Neuronal correlates of a perceptual decision in ventral premotor cortex. *Neuron* 41: 165–173.
Romo R and Schultz W (1987) Neuronal activity preceding self-initiated or externally timed arm movements in area 6 of monkey cortex. *Exp. Brain Res.* 67: 656–662.
Rouiller EM, Moret V, and Liang F (1993) Comparison of the connectional properties of the two forelimb areas of the rat sensorimotor cortex: Support for the presence of a premotor or supplementary motor cortical area. *Somatosens. Mot. Res.* 10: 269–289.
Rouiller EM, Tanne J, Moret V, Kermadi I, Boussaoud D, and Welker E (1998) Dual morphology and topography of the corticothalamic terminals originating from the primary, supplementary motor, and dorsal premotor cortical areas in macaque monkeys. *J. Comp. Neurol.* 396: 169–185.
Schieber MH (2000) Inactivation of the ventral premotor cortex biases the laterality of motoric choices. *Exp. Brain Res.* 130: 497–507.
Schubotz RI and von Cramon DY (2001) Interval and ordinal properties of sequences are associated with distinct premotor areas. *Cereb. Cortex* 11: 210–222.
Schwartz AB, Moran DW, and Reina GA (2004) Differential representation of perception and action in the frontal cortex. *Science* 303: 380–383.
Sessle BJ, Adachi K, Avivi-Arber L, et al. (2007) Neuroplasticity of face primary motor cortex control of orofacial movements. *Arch. Oral Biol.* 52: 334–337.
Shadmehr R and Brashers-Krug T (1997) Functional stages in the formation of human long-term motor memory. *J. Neurosci.* 17: 409–419.
Shen L and Alexander GE (1997) Preferential representation of instructed target location versus limb trajectory in dorsal premotor area. *J. Neurophysiol.* 77: 1195–1212.
Shima K, Aya K, Mushiake H, Inase M, Aizawa H, and Tanji J (1991) Two movement-related foci in the primate cingulate cortex observed in signal-triggered and self-paced forelimb movements. *J. Neurophysiol.* 65: 188–202.
Shima K, Mushiake H, Saito N, and Tanji J (1996) Role for cells in the presupplementary motor area in updating motor plans. *Proc. Natl. Acad. Sci. USA* 93: 8694–8698.
Squire LR (2004) Memory systems of the brain: A brief history and current perspective. *Neurobiol. Learn. Mem.* 82: 171–177.
Stepniewska I, Preuss TM, and Kaas JH (1993) Architectonics, somatotopic organization, and ipsilateral cortical connections of the primary motor area (M1) of owl monkeys. *J. Comp. Neurol.* 330: 238–271.
Takada M, Tokuno H, Hamada I, et al. (2001) Organization of inputs from cingulate motor areas to basal ganglia in macaque monkey. *Eur. J. Neurosci.* 14: 1633–1650.
Tanji J, Shima K, and Matsuzaka Y (2002) Reward-based planning of motor selection in the rostral cingulate motor area. *Adv. Exp. Med. Biol.* 508: 417–423.
Tanji J, Taniguchi K, and Saga T (1980) Supplementary motor area: Neuronal response to motor instructions. *J. Neurophysiol.* 43: 60–68.
Tanji M and Shima K (1994) Role for supplementary motor area cells in planning several movements ahead. *Nature* 371: 413–416.
Thaler D, Chen YC, Nixon PD, Stern CE, and Passingham RE (1995) The functions of the medial premotor cortex. I. Simple learned movements. *Exp. Brain Res.* 102: 445–460.
Thaler DE, Rolls ET, and Passingham RE (1988) Neuronal activity of the supplementary motor area (SMA) during internally and externally triggered wrist movements. *Neurosci. Lett.* 93: 264–269.
Thickbroom GW, Byrnes ML, Sacco P, Ghosh S, Morris IT, and Mastaglia FL (2000) The role of the supplementary motor area in externally timed movement: The influence of predictability of movement timing. *Brain Res.* 874: 233–241.
Tyc F, Boyadjian A, and Devanne H (2005) Motor cortex plasticity induced by extensive training revealed by transcranial magnetic stimulation in human. *Eur. J. Neurosci.* 21: 259–266.
Umilta MA, Kohler E, Gallese V, et al. (2001) I know what you are doing. A neurophysiological study. *Neuron* 31: 155–165.
Vogt BA, Pandya DN, and Rosene DL (1987) Cingulate cortex of the rhesus monkey: I. Cytoarchitecture and thalamic afferents. *J. Comp. Neurol.* 262: 256–270.
Vogt S (1995) On relations between perceiving, imagining and performing in the learning of cyclical movement sequences. *Br. J. Psychol.* 86: 191–216.
Walsh TM and Ebner FF (1970) The cytoarchitecture of somatic sensory-motor cortex in the opossum (*Didelphis marsupialis virginiana*): A Golgi study. *J. Anat.* 107: 1–18.
Wang Y, Shima K, Sawamura H, and Tanji J (2001) Spatial distribution of cingulate cells projecting to the primary, supplementary, and pre-supplementary motor areas: A retrograde multiple labeling study in the macaque monkey. *Neurosci. Res.* 39: 39–49.
Weible AP, McEchron MD, and Disterhoft JF (2000) Cortical involvement in acquisition and extinction of trace eyeblink conditioning. *Behav. Neurosci.* 114: 1058–1067.
Weinrich M and Wise SP (1982) The premotor cortex of the monkey. *J. Neurosci.* 2: 1329–1345.
Wessel K, Zeffiro T, Toro C, and Hallett M (1997) Self-paced versus metronome-paced finger movements. A positron emission tomography study. *J. Neuroimaging* 7: 145–151.
Wildgruber D, Erb M, Klose U, and Grodd W (1997) Sequential activation of supplementary motor area and primary motor cortex during self-paced finger movement in human evaluated by functional MRI. *Neurosci. Lett.* 227: 161–164.
Wise SP and Mauritz KH (1985) Set-related neuronal activity in the premotor cortex of rhesus monkeys: Effects of changes in motor set. *Proc. R. Soc. Lond. B Biol. Sci.* 223: 331–354.
Withers GS and Greenough WT (1989) Reach training selectively alters dendritic branching in subpopulations of layer II-III pyramids in rat motor-somatosensory forelimb cortex. *Neuropsychologia* 27: 61–69.
Wu CW, Bichot NP, and Kaas JH (2000) Converging evidence from microstimulation, architecture, and connections for multiple motor areas in the frontal and cingulate cortex of prosimian primates. *J. Comp. Neurol.* 423: 140–177.
Xiao J (2005) Premotor neuronal plasticity in monkeys adapting to a new dynamic environment. *Eur. J. Neurosci.* 22: 3266–3280.
Xiao J, Padoa-Schioppa C, and Bizzi E (2006) Neuronal correlates of movement dynamics in the dorsal and ventral premotor area in the monkey. *Exp. Brain Res.* 168: 106–119.

26 The Role of Sleep in Memory Consolidation

J. D. Payne, Beth Israel Deaconess Medical Center, Harvard Medical School, Harvard University, Boston, MA, USA

J. M. Ellenbogen, Beth Israel Deaconess Medical Center, Brigham and Women's Hospital, Harvard Medical School, Boston, MA, USA

M. P. Walker and R. Stickgold, Beth Israel Deaconess Medical Center, Harvard Medical School, Boston, MA, USA

26.1 The Role of Sleep in Memory Consolidation

We spend about a third of our lives sleeping, yet in spite of decades of scientific inquiry, the function of sleep remains an enigma. This is not to say that progress has not been made. From antiquity until the 1950s, sleep was generally believed to be a state of inactivity where the brain was turned off and the body rested, but we now know that the sleeping brain can be equally, and sometimes more, active than the brain in its awake state. Even during deep or slow wave sleep, when the brain is relatively quiescent compared to rapid eye movement sleep or wakefulness, it is still roughly 80% activated and thus capable of elaborate information processing (Steriade, 1999; Hobson, 2005).

Numerous hypotheses have been put forward to explain the functions of sleep, including energy conservation, brain detoxification, immune regulation, tissue restoration, and predator avoidance. More recently, the hypothesis that sleep plays a key role in the consolidation of memories has gained considerable attention (Smith, 1985; Maquet, 2001; Smith, 2001; Stickgold et al., 2001). Following two seminal papers in 1994 (Karni et al., 1994; Wilson and McNaughton, 1994), the publication rate on this topic increased fivefold over the next 10 years (Stickgold and Walker, 2005).

Despite this resurgence of attention, the question of how sleep contributes to memory consolidation is actually quite old. In the first century AD, the Roman rhetorician Quintilian, commenting on the benefits of sleep, noted that "what could not be repeated at first is readily put together on the following day; and the very time which is generally thought to cause forgetfulness is found to strengthen the memory."

In this chapter, we review the accumulating evidence supporting a sleep–memory connection, which converges from studies at the molecular, cellular, physiological, and behavioral levels of analysis (Maquet, 2001; Smith, 2001; McNaughton et al., 2003; see also Gais and Born, 2004a; Stickgold, 2005; but see Vertes and Siegel, 2005). We begin with a précis of the field's history before turning to a review of its present status. We attempt to operationally define the terms sleep and memory, and offer our opinions on the field's strengths and shortcomings. In the first half of this chapter, we examine sleep's role in the strengthening of perceptual and procedural skills, and in the second half, we devote our attention to sleep's role in the consolidation of episodic memories. Our primary intention is to alert memory researchers to the growing field of sleep and memory, as well as to spark enthusiasm for a new way of researching memory systems that holds much promise for understanding both sleep and memory.

Although our review covers mainly behavioral and physiological evidence in humans, we point the interested reader to a growing animal literature on this topic. Numerous studies have examined the reactivation of neuronal patterns during post-training sleep, which show that neuronal activation sequences associated with various memory tasks are replayed during subsequent sleep. We touch briefly upon these studies toward the end of the chapter, but we refer the reader to the following articles for a deeper understanding of this fascinating topic (Wilson and McNaughton, 1994; Qin et al., 1997; McNaughton et al., 2003; Sirota et al., 2003; Ribeiro and Nicolelis, 2004). Other studies have begun to illuminate the molecular aspects of sleep-dependent memory consolidation, which we will not discuss here, but which certainly deserve attention as well (Smith et al., 1991; Nakanishi et al., 1997; Ribeiro et al., 1999; Graves et al., 2001; Benington and Frank, 2003).

26.2 Definitions of Sleep and Memory

Before turning to a discussion of the relationship between sleep and memory, we will first attempt to define both terms, as confusion has often arisen due to oversimplifications of one or both. We thus begin the chapter with a brief overview of the neurobiological characteristics associated with the various stages of sleep, and the different types of memory.

26.3 Stages of Sleep

Sleep progresses through a series of stages, which can be divided broadly into rapid eye movement or REM sleep (also called paradoxical sleep, due to the many wake-like features seen in this sleep stage), and non-rapid eye movement or NREM sleep. NREM sleep can be further subdivided into four NREM stages (1–4) corresponding, in that order, to increasing depth of sleep (Rechtschaffen and Kales, 1968). Slow wave sleep (stages 3 and 4) is the deepest of the NREM phases, and is the phase from which people have the most difficulty awakening.

In healthy adults, NREM and REM sleep alternate in approximately 90-min cycles throughout the night (so-called ultradian cycles). However, the relative contributions of NREM and REM sleep to these cycles varies across the night, with more of NREM stages 3 and 4 (slow wave sleep, SWS) early in the night, and more REM sleep late in the night. Thus, more than 80% of a night's SWS is concentrated in the first half of the night, while the second half of the night contains roughly twice as much REM sleep as the first half. This distribution of sleep stages has implications for some of the research paradigms described later in this chapter.

As NREM sleep progresses from stage 1 through stages 3 and 4 (SWS), electroencephalographic (EEG) activity steadily slows. In stage 1 sleep (drowsiness) there is an attenuation of the normally occurring alpha rhythm (8–13 Hz). In its place, a mixture of frequencies with a slower theta frequency (4–7 Hz) begin to emerge. Stage 2 NREM sleep is characterized by a continued reduction in EEG frequencies combined with two signature waveforms: large electrical sharp waves called K complexes and short synchronized bursts of 11- to 16-Hz oscillations called sleep spindles. Slow wave sleep is characterized by high-voltage, low-frequency (<4 Hz) EEG oscillations, which are an expression of underlying synchrony between the thalamus and cerebral cortex (Amzica and Steriade, 1995).

REM sleep, on the other hand, is characterized by low-amplitude, mixed-frequency EEG oscillations that are similar to the EEG patterns seen in wake. Periodic bursts of rapid eye movement also occur, along with a nearly complete loss of muscle tone.

As the brain passes through these sleep stages, it undergoes marked neurochemical alterations. In NREM sleep, acetylcholine neurons in the brainstem and forebrain become strikingly less active (Hobson et al., 1975) and serotonergic and noradrenergic neurons also reduce their firing rates relative to waking levels. In REM sleep, both of these aminergic systems are strongly inhibited, while acetylcholine neurons become intensely active, in some cases more active than in wake (Marrosu et al., 1995). The brain in REM sleep is thus largely devoid of aminergic modulation and dominated by acetylcholine. Thus, sleep consists of myriad physiological states and many neurochemical and neurohormonal mechanisms. When considering the role of sleep in memory consolidation, one must take this dynamic model of sleep into account (Payne and Nadel, 2004; Walker and Stickgold, 2004).

26.4 Types of Memory

Like sleep, memory can be subdivided into different types. In contrast to earlier perspectives, in which memory was viewed as a single system subserved by a restricted part of the brain, most modern views posit several types of memory, each obeying different rules of operation, and each drawing on distinct neural systems that interact to produce the subjective sense of remembering. This insight is critical if we are to understand the role of sleep in human memory consolidation because it raises the possibility of many complex interactions among the dynamic processes of sleep and memory, where the neurochemistry associated with distinct sleep/brain states differentially influences the various types of memory.

Various taxonomies are used to classify the different memory systems (Schacter and Tulving, 1994), most of which agree on a distinction between two broad classes of memory. First, there are memories of the events in our lives and the knowledge of the world that we obtain from these events. Typically, this class of memories can be explicitly retrieved, and for this reason it is often referred to as explicit or declarative (i.e., that which can be declared). Second, there are memories for the various skills, procedures, and habits we acquire through experience – so-called 'how-to' memories. These memories are not so easily made explicit and are usually only evident through performance improvements in various behaviors. Thus, this class of memories is referred to as procedural or implicit. The neural mechanisms that support these memory systems appear to be partially dissociable; however, it is important to remember that they interact as well.

Explicit memory can be further subdivided into episodic and semantic memories (Tulving, 1972). Episodic memory concerns those aspects of explicit remembering that incorporate the specific context of an experienced event, including the time and place of its occurrence. Semantic memory, on the other hand, is concerned with the knowledge one acquires during events, but is itself separated from the specific event in question. Thus, our knowledge about the meaning of words and facts about the world, though acquired in the context of some specific experience, appears to be stored in a form that is context-independent (e.g., not bound to the originating context).

Beyond these, there is also evidence for an emotional memory system that mediates the encoding and consolidation of emotionally charged events (McGaugh et al., 1993; Cahill and McGaugh, 1996; McGaugh et al., 1996; Cahill, 2000; Packard and Cahill, 2001). This system is particularly concerned with learning about fearful and unpleasant stimuli, although growing evidence suggests it plays a role in memory for pleasant information as well (Hamann et al., 1999; Hamann et al., 2002; Hamann, 2003; Kensinger, 2004).

The explicit memory system is governed by the hippocampus and surrounding medial temporal areas, while procedural and implicit memory are thought to be independent of the hippocampal complex, relying instead on various subcortical and neocortical structures (Squire, 1992; Schacter and Tulving, 1994). The emotional memory system is critically modulated by the amygdala, a limbic structure located deep in the subcortical brain and richly connected to the hippocampus. It is important to note that because each of these memory systems is subserved by different brain areas, information dependent on each is open to differential processing during sleep. Thus, when attempting to answer the seemingly straightforward question – how does sleep influence memory? – we find that it quickly branches into numerous questions, depending on what kind of sleep and what kind of memory we are talking about.

Although memory consolidation is a complex, multistep process, we define it here as a slow process that converts a still-labile memory trace into a more stable or enhanced form (e.g., Dudai, 2004). As such, the benefits of sleep are sometimes seen as a reduction in the normal decay of a memory (assessed via performance on a memory task), while other times they are seen as actual enhancements in performance.

26.5 Procedural and Implicit Memory

Sleep appears to benefit both procedural/implicit and explicit memory. Since most of the recent work has focused on sleep and procedural memory, we begin our review here. A wide range of perceptual, motor, and cognitive abilities are gradually acquired through continuous interactions with the environment, and in many cases this occurs in the absence of conscious awareness. Converging data suggest that these abilities are acquired slowly and are not attained solely during the learning episode. While some learning certainly develops quickly, performance on various tasks improves further, and without additional practice, simply through the passage of time (so-called off-line improvement), suggesting that memory traces continue to be processed over long periods of time. Importantly for our purposes, these longer periods often contain sleep, and the consolidation occurring during them may be dependent on this sleep.

26.5.1 Visual Discrimination Learning

Early work investigating the effect of sleep on implicit learning used a visual texture discrimination task (VDT) that was originally developed by Karni and Sagi (1991). The task requires participants to determine the orientation (vertical or horizontal) of an array of diagonal bars that is embedded in one visual quadrant against a background of exclusively horizontal bars (**Figure 1**). At the center of the screen is the fixation target, which is either the letter T or L. This target screen is succeeded first by a blank screen for a variable interstimulus interval (ISI), and then by a mask (a screen covered with randomly oriented V letters, with a superimposed V and L in the center). Subjects must determine the orientation of the array, and the performance is estimated by the ISI corresponding to 80% correct responses (Karni and Sagi, 1993; Karni et al., 1994).

Amnesic patients with damage to the hippocampal complex, who cannot acquire knowledge explicitly, show normal performance improvements on the VDT. This was shown using a group of five densely amnesic patients. All five had extensive medial temporal lobe damage, including damage to the hippocampal formation. These patients were trained on the task on day 1 and retested on days 2 and 5. In spite of having no conscious recollection of having taken the test before, they showed substantially improved performance (Stickgold, 2003).

In neurologically normal subjects, improvement on the VDT develops slowly after training (Karni and Sagi, 1993; Stickgold et al., 2000a), with no improvement when retesting occurs on the same day as training (**Figure 2(a)**, open circles). Instead, improvement is only observed after a night of sleep (**Figure 2(a)**, filled circles).

This was true even for a group of subjects that were retested only 9 h after training. Importantly, there was not even a trend to greater improvement when the training–retest interval was increased from 9 to 22.5 h, suggesting that additional wake time after the night of sleep provided no additional benefit. While further wake time provided no benefit, additional nights of sleep did produce incremental improvement. When subjects were retested 2–7 days after training, 50% greater improvement was observed than after a single night of sleep (**Figure 2(b)**, green bars). Critically, another group of subjects was sleep-deprived on the first night after training. These subjects were allowed two full nights of recovery sleep before being retested 3 days later. They failed to show any residual learning, suggesting that performance enhancements are dependent on a normal first night of sleep (**Figure 2(b)**, red bar). Time alone is clearly not enough to produce

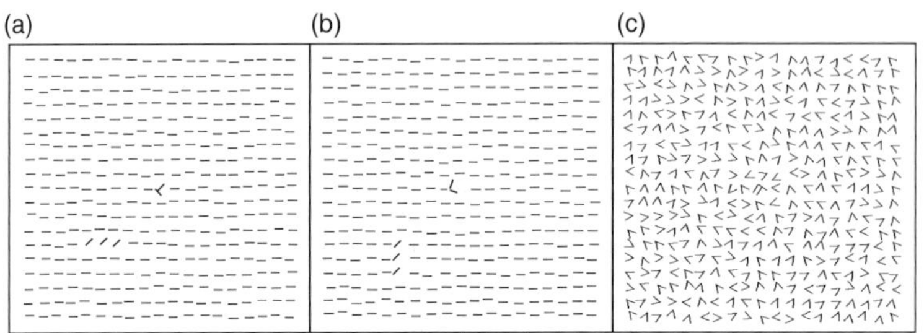

Figure 1 Sample screens from the visual texture discrimination task (VDT). See text for explanation.

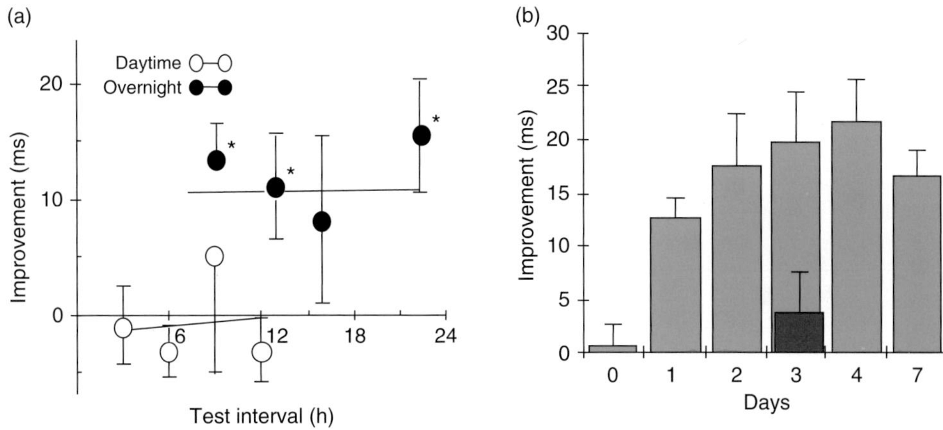

Figure 2 Sleep-dependent improvement on the VDT. All subjects were trained and then retested only a single time. Each point in (a) and each bar in (b) represents a separate group of subjects. Error bars in (a) and (b) are S.E.M.s. From Stickgold R, James L, and Hobson A (2000a) Visual discrimination learning requires post-training sleep. *Nat. Neurosci.* 2(12): 1237–1238; Stickgold R, Whidbee D, et al. (2000b) Visual discrimination task improvement: A multi-step process occurring during sleep. *J. Cogn. Neurosci.* 12: 246–254.

long-term benefits from VDT training. It appears that sleep is also required (Stickgold et al., 2000a).

Initially, improvement on this task appeared to depend solely on REM sleep, because subjects who underwent selective deprivation of REM sleep showed no improvement on the task (Karni et al., 1994). Later studies, however, showed that optimal performance on this task requires both SWS and REM sleep (Stickgold et al., 2000b).

When subjects were trained and their subsequent sleep monitored in the sleep laboratory, the amount of improvement was proportional to the amount of SWS during the first quarter of the night (**Figure 3(a)**), as well as to the amount of REM sleep in the last quarter (**Figure 3(b)**). Indeed, the product of these two sleep parameters explained more than 80% of the intersubject variance (**Figure 3(d)**). No significant correlations were found for sleep stages during other parts of the night (**Figure 3(c)**) or for the amount of Stage 2 sleep at any time during the night.

Gais et al. (2000) came to a similar conclusion by examining improvement after 3 h of sleep either early or late in the night. They found that 3 h of early night sleep, which was rich in SWS, produced an 8-ms improvement; but after a full night of sleep, which added REM-rich sleep late in the night, a 26-ms improvement was observed, three times that seen with early sleep alone. Interestingly, however, 3 h of REM-rich, late-night sleep actually produced deterioration in performance (Gais et al., 2000).

Daytime naps also lead to performance benefits on the VDT. To lay the groundwork for the nap studies, Mednick et al. (2002) showed that VDT performance suffers from repeated, same-day testing. When subjects were trained on the task and then tested at numerous time points throughout the day, their performance deteriorated (i.e., their ISI threshold was higher). **Figure 4** depicts tests given at 9.00 a.m., 12.00 p.m., 4.00 p.m., and 7.00 p.m., with performance worsening significantly on each successive test. However, if subjects are allowed to take an afternoon nap after the second test, their performance improves. Interestingly, 30-min naps prevented the normal deterioration seen during sessions 3 and 4 (Mednick et al., 2002), and longer naps ranging from 60 to 90 min, and containing both SWS and REM sleep, actually enhance performance (Mednick et al., 2003). Taken together, these studies suggest that both SWS and REM sleep play roles in the sleep-dependent memory consolidation of this task.

At this point, sleep's role in visual discrimination learning (as measured by VDT performance) is clear. But the VDT represents a very specific type of sensory memory that may or may not share its sleep dependency with other procedural tasks. This raises the question of whether the sleep effects observed with the VDT generalize to other forms of procedural memory. Studies of sleep-dependent auditory and motor skill learning strongly suggest that they do.

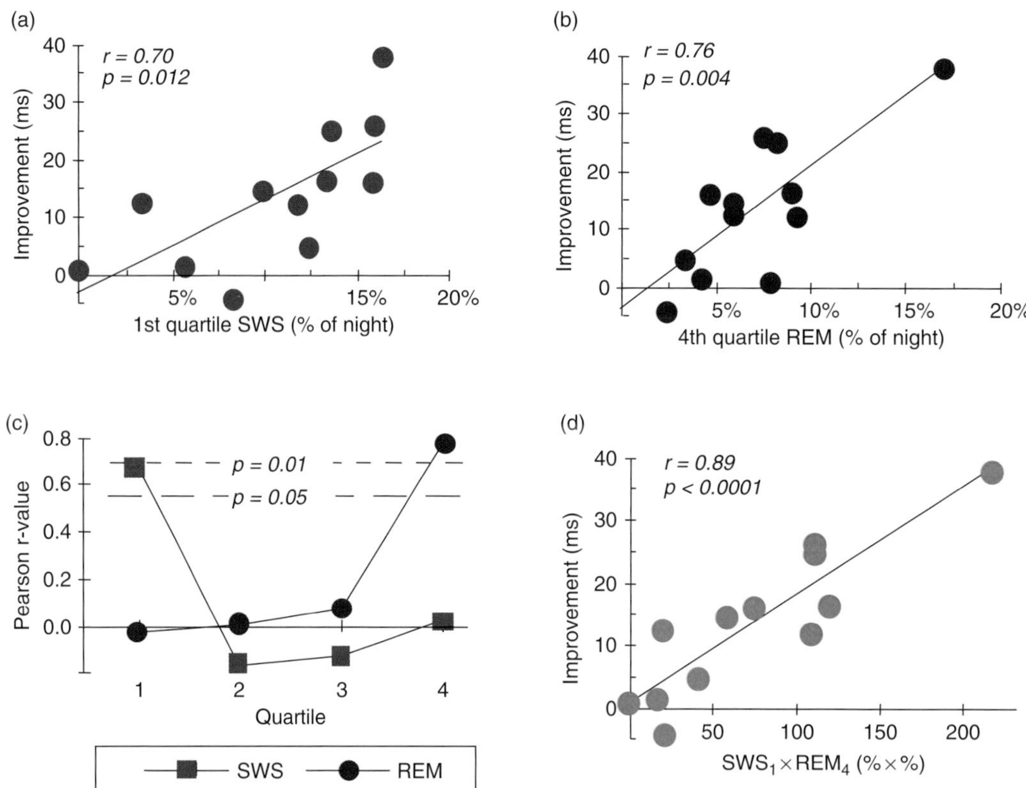

Figure 3 REM and SWS dependence of VDT learning. From Stickgold R, Whidbee D, Schirmer B, et al. (2000b) Visual discrimination task improvement: A multi-step process occurring during sleep. *J. Cogn. Neurosci.* 12: 246–254.

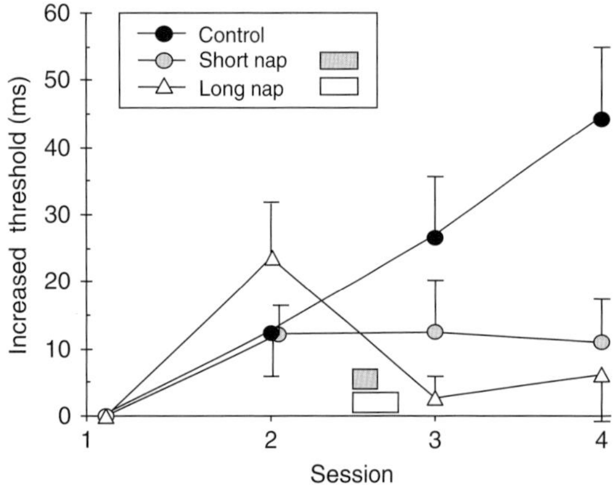

Figure 4 Deterioration in VDT performance with repeated same-day testing and recovery following napping. Note that the ordinate reflects changes in ISI threshold and, as such, higher values indicate worse performance. From Mednick SC, Nakayama K, Cantero JL, et al. (2002) The restorative effect of naps on perceptual deterioration. *Nat. Neurosci.* 5: 677–681.

26.5.2 Auditory Learning

Gaab et al. (2004) have shown that delayed performance improvements in memory for pitch develop only across periods of sleep and not across similar periods spent awake. Atienza and colleagues (Atienza et al., 2002, 2004) have also presented evidence of both time- and sleep-dependent auditory memory consolidation, including sleep-dependent changes in brain-evoked response potentials (ERPs). Although post-training sleep deprivation did not prevent continued behavioral improvements, ERP changes associated with the automatic shift of attention to relevant stimuli, which normally develop in the 24–72 h after training, failed to develop following a posttraining night of sleep deprivation. These findings highlight the danger of presuming that a lack of behavioral improvement is equivalent to an absence of beneficial plastic changes in the brain, and they demonstrate the importance of using combined behavioral and physiological analyses (Gaab et al., 2004; Walker and Stickgold, 2006).

Finally, Fenn et al. (2003) have demonstrated that sleep benefits learning on a synthetic speech-recognition task. Training on a small set of words improved performance on novel words that used the same phoneme but a different acoustic pattern.

Importantly, sleep benefited this ability to generalize phonological categories across different acoustic patterns. Time spent awake after initial training resulted in a degradation of performance on this task, but a subsequent night of sleep restored it. This suggests a process of sleep-dependent consolidation capable of reestablishing previously learned complex auditory skill memory, as well as a form of sleep-dependent generalization of learning, which is a hallmark of flexible learning in humans (Fenn et al., 2003). These studies suggest that, as with visual discrimination learning, sleep provides an important benefit to auditory skill learning. In the next section, we show that motor memory benefits from sleep as well.

26.5.3 Motor Memory

Numerous studies have demonstrated a relationship between sleep and various types of motor memory (Smith and MacNeill, 1994; Fischer et al., 2002; Walker et al., 2002; Maquet et al., 2003). As an example, Walker et al. (2002) have demonstrated sleep-dependent improvements on a finger-tapping task. The task requires subjects to type the numeric sequence 4-1-3-2-4 as quickly and accurately as possible. Training consisted of twelve 30-s trials, separated by 30-s rest periods. All subjects show considerable improvement during the 12 trials of the training session (a fast learning component), but 12 h later, subjects performed very differently depending on whether the 12-h interval was filled with time spent sleeping or time spent awake. When trained in the morning and retested 12 h later, only an additional nonsignificant 4% improvement was seen in performance, but when tested again the next morning, a large and robust (14%) improvement was seen (**Figure 5(a)**). The failure to improve during the daytime could not be due to interference from related motor activity because subjects who were required to wear mittens and refrain from fine motor activities during this time showed a similar pattern of wake/sleep improvement (**Figure 5(b)**).

In contrast, when subjects were trained in the evening, improvement was observed the following morning (after sleep), but not across an additional 12 h of wake (**Figure 5(c)**). Thus, improved performance resulted specifically from a night of sleep, as opposed to the simple passage of time. Curiously, unlike the findings for the VDT, overnight improvement on this task correlated with the amount of stage 2 NREM during the night, especially during the last quarter of the night. These findings are in agreement with those of Smith and colleagues (Smith and MacNeill, 1994; Tweed et al., 1999; Fogel et al., 2001), who have also shown that stage 2 sleep, and possibly the sleep spindles which reach peak density

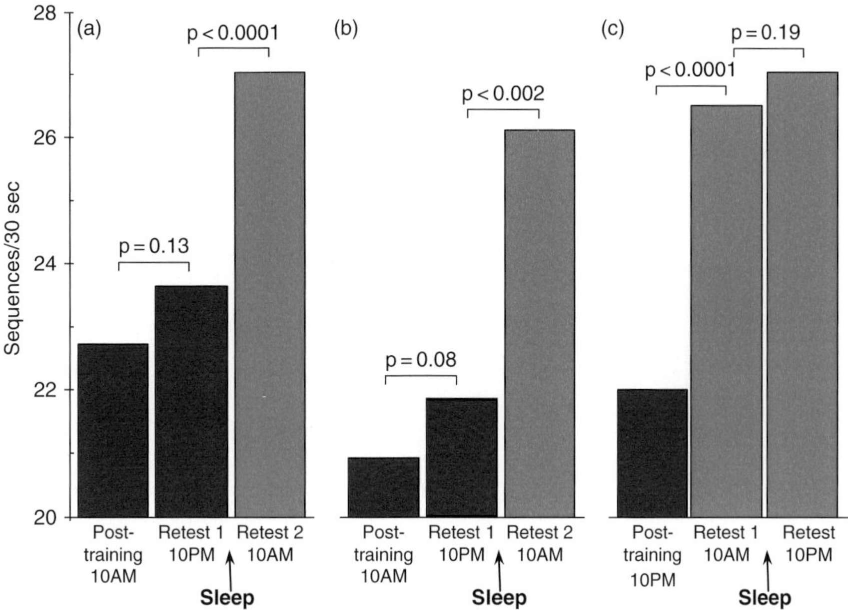

Figure 5 Sleep-dependent motor learning. Improvement in speed was seen in all three groups over a night of sleep, but not over 12 h of daytime wake. From Walker MP, Brakefield T, Hobson JA, and Stickgold R (2002) Practice with sleep makes perfect: Sleep dependent motor skill learning. *Neuron* 35(1): 205–211.

during late night stage 2 sleep, are critical for simple motor memory consolidation. This seems plausible, as sleep spindles have been proposed to trigger intracellular mechanisms that are required for synaptic plasticity (Sejnowski and Destexhe, 2000).

It is important to note that this sleep-based improvement was not due to a speed/accuracy trade-off. When the number of errors per 30-s trial was compared between evening and morning, the number of errors actually decreased, although not significantly (Walker et al., 2002). However, when error rates (i.e., errors per sequence) were calculated, a highly significant 43% decrease in the error rate was seen overnight (**Figure 6**), while a 20% increase in the error rate was found across 12 h spent awake (Walker et al., 2003).

At least for a simple motor task then, sleep appears to benefit both speed and accuracy. More recent studies have shown that these sleep-dependent benefits appear to be specific to both the motor sequence learned and the hand used to perform the task (Fischer et al., 2002; Korman et al., 2003).

This motor sequence task has been examined to determine where precisely in the motor program the sleep-dependent improvement occurs (Kuriyama et al., 2004). In the sequence mentioned above (4-1-3-2-4), there are four unique key-press transitions; 4 to 1, 1 to 3, 3 to 2, and 2 to 4. When the speed between transitions was analyzed for individual subjects prior to sleep, sticking points emerged. While some transitions were easy (i.e., fast), others were problematic (i.e., slow), as if the sequence was being parsed or chunked into smaller bits during pre-sleep learning (Walker and Stickgold, 2006). After a night of sleep, these problematic points were preferentially improved, whereas transitions that had already been mastered prior to sleep did not change. Subjects who were trained and retested after a daytime wake interval showed no such improvements.

These findings suggest that the sleep-dependent consolidation process involves the unification of smaller motor memory units into a single motor memory representation, thereby improving problem points in the sequence. This overnight process would therefore offer a greater degree of performance automation, effectively optimizing speed across the motor program, and would explain the sleep-dependent improvements in speed and accuracy previously reported (Walker and Stickgold, 2006). But importantly, it suggests that the role of sleep is subtle and complex and does more than simply strengthen memories; sleep may encourage the restructuring and reorganization of memories – an important and often overlooked aspect of memory consolidation. We will return to this idea later in the chapter.

Fisher et al. (2002), using a different sequential finger-tapping task, which involves finger-to-thumb movements instead of keyboard typing, have shown

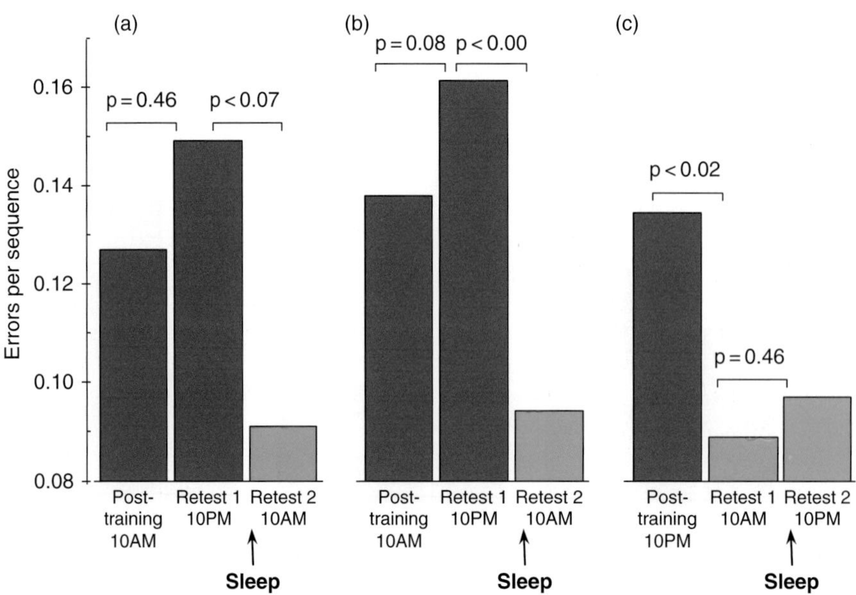

Figure 6 Sleep-dependent motor learning. Improvement in accuracy was seen in all three groups over a night of sleep, but not over 12 h of daytime wake. From Walker MP, Brakefield T, Hobson JA, and Stickgold R (2002) Practice with sleep makes perfect: Sleep dependent motor skill learning. *Neuron* 35(1): 205–211.

that sleep following training is critical for delayed performance improvements. However, they found this improvement to be most strongly correlated with REM sleep rather than stage 2 NREM sleep (see 'Stages of sleep' above).

This discrepancy in sleep stage correlations mirrors similar discrepancies in the declarative memory section below, and remains to be resolved. Nonetheless, it is possible that the more novel finger-to-thumb task requires REM sleep, whereas the keyboard typing task, so similar to the well-learned typing most of us do regularly, is consolidated during stage 2 NREM sleep. A similarly subtle distinction has been reported by Robertson et al. (2004), who found that sleep-dependent enhancement of performance on a perceptual-motor sequence task again correlated with NREM, but only when subjects were explicitly aware of the presence of a repeating sequence, and not when knowledge of the sequence was gained only implicitly (Robertson et al., 2004).

Moving to another type of motor memory – motor adaptation – Maquet et al. (2003) showed that sleep benefits performance on a pursuit task. Participants were trained on a task in which the target trajectory was only predictable on the horizontal axis. This meant that optimal performance could only be achieved by developing an implicit model of the motion characteristics of the learned trajectory. Half of the subjects were sleep deprived on the first post-training night, while the other half were allowed to sleep normally. Three days later, after 2 full days of recovery sleep, performance was superior in the sleep group compared to the sleep-deprived group, and fMRI revealed that the superior temporal sulcus (STS) was differentially more active for the learned trajectory in subjects who slept than in sleep-deprived subjects. Moreover, increased functional connectivity was observed between the STS and the cerebellum, and between the supplementary eye field and the frontal eye field, suggestive of sleep-related plastic changes during motor skill learning in areas involved in smooth pursuit and eye movements.

Similarly, Smith and MacNeill (1994) demonstrated that selective stage 2 NREM sleep deprivation impairs memory for a pursuit rotor task and Huber et al. (2004) demonstrated improved performance on a motor reaching-adaptation task across a night of sleep, but not across an equivalent period of time spent awake. Here, daytime motor skill practice was accompanied by a subsequent increase in NREM slow-wave EEG activity over parietal cortex. This increase was proportional to the amount of delayed learning that developed overnight. Subjects who showed the greatest increase in slow-wave activity in the parietal cortex during NREM sleep showed the largest benefit in motor skill performance the following day (Huber et al., 2004).

Taken together, these findings strongly suggest that sleep is fundamentally important for the development of motor skill memory. Initial daytime learning benefits are supplemented by a night of sleep, which triggers additional learning without the need for further training. Although the role of the various sleep stages in skill memory remains unclear, overnight memory improvements tend to exhibit a strong relationship to NREM sleep, and, in some cases, to specific NREM sleep stages at specific times of the night (Walker and Stickgold, 2006).

Admittedly, visual discrimination, finger tapping, and motor adaptation are all relatively basic, low-level procedural tasks that may become automated fairly quickly. What about more complex implicit and procedural tasks? Animal work clearly demonstrates that complex tasks (e.g., instrumental conditioning, avoidance or maze learning) benefit from sleep, with rats showing increases in REM sleep that continue until the tasks are mastered (Smith et al., 1980; Smith and Wong, 1991; Hennevin et al., 1995). For instance, Smith and Wong (1991) trained rats on a complex operant bar press task, on which only some rats demonstrated increases in REM sleep after training. This split successfully predicted which rats would improve on the task and which rats would fail. Furthermore, after training rats on an avoidance task, Datta (2000) observed an increase in PGO waves (waves of neural activity that are generated in the pons and activate the forebrain during REM sleep) during the first four post-training REM sleep episodes. Changes in REM density observed during the first three of these episodes were proportional to improvement in task performance. These data suggest that the activation of pontine cells that generate PGO waves during REM sleep lead in turn to the activation of forebrain and cortical structures involved in memory consolidation and perhaps to the initiation of these consolidation processes (Datta, 2000).

Recently, Datta and colleagues examined whether the activation of PGO waves could reverse the learning impairment seen after REM sleep deprivation. Rats were trained on a two-way avoidance-learning task and either slept normally or underwent REM sleep deprivation. In addition, they either received a saline injection (placebo) or a carbachol injection in the P-wave generator. The rats that received both saline and REM sleep deprivation showed learning deficits when compared with the saline-injected rats that slept. But a carbachol-induced activation of PGO waves prevented this learning impairment in the sleep-deprived rats, suggesting that the PGO waves mediated the normal sleep-based memory consolidation (Datta et al., 2004).

Depriving rats of REM sleep after training also leads to performance deficits in complex skills, particularly if the deprivation occurs during so-called critical periods or paradoxical sleep windows (Smith et al., 1995; Smith and Rose, 1996). Two such critical periods emerged in rats attempting to learn a shuttle avoidance task when 20 trials per day were given over a 5-day period. The first occurred 9–12 h after training and the second occurred 17–20 h after training. If the rats were deprived of REM sleep during these windows, their memory for the task was significantly impaired. However, with more intensive training, the window appears earlier. When rats were given 100 training trials in a single session, the critical period appeared at 1–4 h after the end of the shuttle avoidance training (Smith and Butler, 1982).

Critical periods thus appear to vary depending on the task and the intensity of training, and hint at the complexity of sleep–memory relationships that we discuss later. Nonetheless, critical periods are thought to mirror the time after acquisition when REM sleep would typically increase over normal levels. These REM windows may not be prevalent in humans, however, who appear to be sensitive to deprivation during any REM period when trying to learn new complex skills (Smith, 1995).

REM sleep has been implicated in complex procedural learning in humans as well. In a PET (positron emission tomography) study of visuomotor skill memory using the serial reaction time task (SRTT) (Maquet et al., 2000), six spatially permanent position markers were shown on a computer screen and subjects watched for stimuli to appear below these markers. When a stimulus appeared in a particular position, subjects reacted as quickly as possible by pressing a corresponding key on the keyboard. Because the stimuli were generated in an order defined by a probabilistic finite-state grammar, improvement on the task (compared to randomly generated sequences) reflects implicitly acquired knowledge of this grammar (Maquet et al., 2000).

Neuroimaging was performed on three groups of subjects. One group was scanned while they were awake, both at rest and during performance of the task, providing information about which brain regions are typically activated by the task. A second group of subjects was trained on the task during the afternoon and then scanned the night after training, both while awake and during various sleep stages. Thus, group 2 was included to determine if similar brain regions were reactivated during sleep. A post-sleep session was also conducted to verify that learning had indeed occurred. Finally, a third group, never trained on the task, was scanned while sleeping to ensure that the pattern of activation present in natural sleep was different from the pattern of activation present after training.

Results showed that in REM sleep, as compared to resting wakefulness, several brain areas used during task performance were more active in trained than in nontrained subjects. These included occipital, parietal, anterior cingulate, motor and premotor cortices, and the cerebellum – all of which are consistent with the component processes involved in the visual and motor functioning involved in this task. Behavioral data confirmed that trained subjects improved significantly more across the night.

More recently, Peigneux et al. (2003), using the same task, showed that the level of acquisition of probabilistic rules attained prior to sleep was correlated with the increase in activation of task-related cortical areas during posttraining REM sleep. This suggests that cerebral reactivation is modulated by the strength of the memory traces developed during the learning episode, and as such, these data provide the first experimental evidence linking behavioral performance to reactivation during REM sleep (Peigneux et al., 2003). As with previously described animal studies (Datta, 2000), these findings suggest that it is not simply experiencing the task that modifies sleep physiology, but the process of memory consolidation associated with successful learning of the task.

These results support the hypothesis that implicit/procedural memory traces in humans can be reactivated during REM sleep, and that this reactivation is linked to improved consolidation. Indeed, looking a bit more closely at the literature, human REM sleep has also been linked to memory for complex logic games, foreign language acquisition, and to intensive studying (Smith, 2001). It is interesting that these more complex conceptual–procedural tasks often show REM sleep relationships, while more basic procedural tasks benefit mainly from NREM sleep. In order to understand these differences in sleep stage correlations, it is helpful to draw on a proposal by Greenberg and Pearlman (1974), who suggested that habitual reactions may be REM sleep-independent, while activities involving the assimilation of unusual or unrelated information require REM sleep for optimal consolidation. Such a distinction would support Pearlman's suggestion that simpler tasks are learned without a REM sleep dependency, while the learning of more complex tasks is dependent on posttraining REM sleep (Pearlman, 1979; Greenberg and Pearlman, 1974).

The above findings provide encouraging evidence that sleep-based processes can aid in procedural memory consolidation, not only for basic forms of sensory and motor memory in humans, but for complex procedural and conceptual knowledge as well. Moreover, it argues that the consolidation of familiar skills, or those that are similar to other well-learned skills, may be reliant on NREM sleep stages (particularly stage 2 NREM sleep), whereas REM sleep may be required for the integration of new concepts or skills with pre-existing information that is already stored in memory. This is an important question that warrants future investigation.

Although much remains to be understood about the precise relationship of specific sleep stages to different procedural memory processes, we can say with confidence that sleep generally aids in the consolidation of implicit and procedural forms of memory. Evidence in support of this relationship is now so overwhelming that strong positions to the contrary will, at minimum, have to be revised (Vertes and Eastman, 2000; Siegel, 2001).

26.6 Episodic Memory

We turn next to the relationship between sleep and the consolidation of episodic memories. Interest in this relationship can be traced back to a landmark study by Jenkins and Dallenbach (1924), which showed that a period of sleep led to better retention of nonsense syllables than an equivalent period of wakefulness. They interpreted this work to mean that sleep, being an inactive state, transiently protected memory from interference, whereas reduction of recall during wakefulness was due to interference.

> "The results of our study as a whole indicate that forgetting is not so much a matter of the decay of old impressions and associations as it is a matter of interference, inhibition, or obliterations of the old by the new" (Jenkins and Dallenbach, 1924: p. 612).

This interpretation struck a serious blow to the then dominant trace decay theory of forgetting, which posited that the simple passage of time was responsible for forgetting.

Nonetheless, the fact that memories were protected during sleep led to increased interest in the topic (particularly among interference theorists), and Jenkins and Dallenbach's (1924) finding was quickly replicated in better-controlled studies (e.g. Lovatt and Warr, 1968; Benson and Feinberg, 1977). Researchers began to wonder if sleep was actively promoting memory formation, rather than simply reducing interference. Moreover, they began to hypothesize that some types of sleep played a bigger role in episodic memory consolidation than others (The relationship between sleep and the consolidation of semantic memory has received scant attention to date, although see Stickgold et al. (1999) and Brualla et al. (1998) for evidence of semantic memory processing during sleep.).

After the discovery of REM sleep by Aserinsky and Kleitman (1953), the prevailing hypothesis – inspired by psychoanalytic theory – was that memory content would show up in REM sleep, because this was the only stage of sleep in which dreams were thought to occur. (It is now clear that dreams and other types of mental content can occur in all sleep stages, including SWS (Foulkes, 1966; see also Payne and Nadel, 2004)). It made a great deal of intuitive sense that REM sleep should be the stage involved in the reprocessing and consolidation of episodic memories, because, as noted above, the brain during REM sleep is intensely active and looks like it is engaging in some sort of cognitive processing.

This hypothesis was initially supported by several REM sleep-deprivation studies, which showed that such deprivation interfered with memory for prose passages (Empson and Clarke, 1970) and increased the time interval over which memories remained fragile and susceptible to electroconvulsive shock (Fishbein et al., 1971). However, as summarized in Smith (2001), REM deprivation studies in humans provided mixed results on the whole (Chernik, 1972) (see Johnson et al., 1974; Lewin and Glaubman, 1975), which may not be surprising given that sleep deprivation suffers from many confounds, including disrupted natural sleep, decreased levels of arousal and motivation, and increased levels of stress (Maquet, 2001). The stress hormone cortisol, for example, often impairs memory at high levels but can facilitate some aspects of memory at low to moderate levels (Payne and Nadel, 2004; Payne et al., 2004).

Seeking to avoid the confounds inherent in sleep deprivation studies, Ekstrand and colleagues developed a procedure that attempted to isolate SWS, which is prevalent early in the night, from REM sleep, which is maximal late in the night (see 'Stages of sleep' section above). These researchers were thus the first to systematically investigate the impact of different sleep stages on memory performance while controlling for the unspecific effects of REM sleep deprivation. Their findings implicated NREM, particularly stage 4 SWS, as the most beneficial sleep stage for episodic memory consolidation. Yaroush et al. (1971) required subjects to study a paired-associates list just before bedtime. Half of the subjects were awakened after 4 h of early sleep (dense in SWS) and tested for recall. The other half were allowed to sleep for 4 h prior to awakening; they then studied the list and returned to sleep for another 4 h late in the night (REM-rich sleep) before being awakened to recall the word pairs. A third group of subjects were trained during the day and returned 4 h later for the recall test. The early night group remembered more of the words than either the late night or wake groups in several tests of memory (paced and unpaced tests, matching, and relearning tests), suggesting that early sleep, rich in SWS, benefited episodic memory (Yaroush et al., 1971).

In a follow up-study, Barrett and Ekstrand (1972) replicated this effect while attempting to control for circadian differences. Here, all subjects were required to learn and recall at the same time of day; the retention interval was always between 3.00 a.m. to 7.00 a.m. One group remained awake until training at 3.00 a.m., slept for 4 h, and then were awakened at 7.00 a.m. for testing. Another group arrived in the lab at 10.00 p.m., slept for 4 h prior to training, awakened at 2.50 a.m. to train, returned to sleep for another 4 h and then awakened for testing at 6.50 a.m.. As in the Yaroush et al. (1971) study, recall of word pairs was better in the first-half sleep condition than in either the second-half sleep or wake conditions, thus replicating the early sleep effect while controlling for time of day (Barrett and Ekstrand, 1972).

Fowler et al. (1973) replicated the early sleep effect, this time in the sleep laboratory, where they showed that SWS was indeed most prevalent early in the night (first-half of sleep), while REM was maximal late in the night (second-half of sleep) in spite of the experimental awakenings. The authors pointed out that their findings were not easy to reconcile with an interference theory of forgetting. Subjects in the first and second half of night conditions slept for equivalent amounts of time during the retention interval, so simple protection against interference should have been equal in both groups. Unless one wanted to argue that dreaming is as much an interfering factor as a waking mental activity (and this remains to be determined), it seemed that early-night SWS, and perhaps particularly stage 4 sleep, was most important for episodic memory consolidation (Fowler et al., 1973).

More than 20 years later, Born and colleagues revived this procedure (Plihal and Born, 1997; Plihal and Born 1999a,b). In the first of their studies (Plihal and Born, 1997), both episodic (recall of semantically related paired associates) and procedural (performance on a mirror tracing task) memory were assessed within the same subjects. Participants were trained to criterion on both tasks and then retested after 3-h retention intervals, containing either early or late nocturnal sleep. The results showed that memory improvements were greater after sleep than after a corresponding period of wake, but more importantly, the different periods of sleep seemed to support consolidation of different types of memory. Recall of paired associates improved more after 3 h of early sleep rich in SWS than after 3 h of late sleep rich in REM, or after a 3-h period of wake. Conversely, mirror tracing improved more after 3 h of late, REM-rich sleep than after 3 h spent either in early sleep or awake.

In a related study, Plihal and Born (1999a) examined different measures of episodic and implicit memory in order to separate the effects of type of material (verbal vs. nonverbal) from type of memory (episodic vs. procedural). Thus, a nonverbal episodic memory task (spatial rotation) and a verbal implicit task (word-stem priming) were used in the same early versus late night sleep procedure, and the findings mirrored the previous results. Compared to wake, recall of spatial memory was enhanced after early retention sleep but not late retention sleep, while priming was enhanced more after late than early retention sleep.

It is important to note that this early-/late-night sleep procedure suffers not only from confounds associated with sleep deprivation, but also from an incomplete separation of REM and NREM sleep. Early sleep is an imperfect proxy for SWS, and similarly, late sleep is an imperfect proxy for REM sleep. SWS does appear in the second half of the night, and REM appears in the first half of the night, and thus one cannot exclude the possibility that REM and SWS during these periods contributed to the noted consolidation effects. Moreover, the distribution of Stage 2 NREM sleep is not entirely equal in both halves of the night. Thus, one cannot examine early versus late sleep and make definitive conclusions about SWS versus REM sleep.

In addition, SWS is tested by training subjects before they go to sleep (at around 10.00 or 11.00 p.m.) and then awakening them 3 h later for memory testing. REM sleep, on the other hand, is tested by awakening subjects to train in the middle of the night. These subjects then return to sleep before being awakened 3 h later for memory testing. Training in the middle of the night may well be less effective than training that occurs before subjects have slept at all, which means that the lack of improvement seen after REM awakenings in some experiments may be confounded; what looks like a failure to consolidate may simply reflect a difference in the quality of encoding and degree of attentional resources available for the task after being awakened in the middle of the night as opposed to in the evening prior to sleep. Finally, control groups that are awake for similar periods in the night are acutely sleep deprived, limiting the validity of the comparisons. Therefore, while the value of this creative procedure is that it manipulates sleep stages experimentally, a number of problems limits the clear interpretation of these findings.

In spite of these problems, two neuroimaging investigations of episodic memory consolidation have also suggested an important role for SWS. The first of these investigated performance on a hippocampally dependent virtual maze task (Peigneux et al., 2004). Daytime learning of the task was associated with hippocampal activity. Then, during posttraining sleep, there was a reemergence of hippocampal activation, and it occurred specifically during SWS. The most compelling finding, however, is that the increase in hippocampal activation seen during posttraining SWS was proportional to the amount of improvement seen the next day (see also Peigneux et al., 2003 described above). This suggests that the re-expression of hippocampal activation during SWS reflects the off-line reprocessing of spatial episodic memory traces, which in turn leads to the plastic changes underlying the improvement in memory performance seen the next day.

The second study (Takashima et al., 2006) investigated the time course of episodic memory consolidation across 90 days. Subjects studied 360 photographs of landscapes and were then tested on subsets of the photographs either after a nap the same day, or after 2, 30, or 90 days. Prior to each test, subjects studied 80 new pictures, and then were tested on 80 of the original pictures and the 80 new ones, as well as 80 pictures they had never seen before. All memory retrieval sessions occurred during fMRI scanning.

Following the initial 90-min nap, stage 2 sleep was positively correlated with successful recall of both remote and recent items, indicating a nonspecific benefit of stage 2 NREM sleep on episodic memory. This is an intriguing finding, given that stage 2 is where sleep spindles are most prominent (see the section titled 'Electrophysiological signatures'). Slow-wave sleep, on the other hand, was correlated only with memory for remote (but not recent) items. Because performance on remote items increased with longer SWS duration, but performance for recent items did not, the effect on memory performance for remote items cannot be explained by a general effect of SWS on memory retrieval processes. The authors also point out that this brief period of SWS may have had an even longer-lasting effect on memory, because there was a linear relationship between the amount of SWS during the nap and recognition memory performance after both 2 and 30 days, whereas there continued to be no such correlation for recent items. This finding is striking, given that this was a nap rather than a full night of sleep, and that only 15 of the 24 subjects reached SWS. Finally, longer SWS durations led to decreases in hippocampal activation when remote items were successfully retrieved (it should be noted that while this finding appears to support traditional consolidation theory (Squire and Cohen, 1984), the hippocampus remained active during successful retrieval throughout the study (up to the last test at 90 days), suggesting that episodic memories may never become completely independent of the hippocampus (Nadel and Moscovitch, 1997; Moscovitch et al., 2006). These findings strongly suggest that episodic memories can undergo initial consolidation within a rather short time frame and that this consolidation is promoted by SWS.

In another nap study, Tucker et al. (2006) found that naps containing only NREM sleep enhanced declarative memory for word pairs. Performance on episodic (paired-associates) and procedural (mirror tracing) memory tasks were tested 6 h after training, either with or without an intervening nap. While there was no difference between nap and wake subjects on the procedural memory task, the nap subjects performed significantly better on the paired associate task relative to the subjects who remained awake

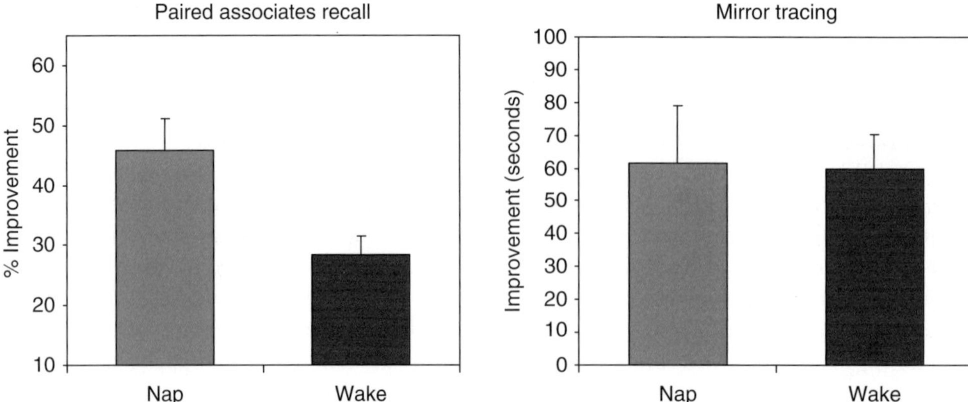

Figure 7 A brief daytime nap benefits episodic memory. Note that the nap (which did not contain REM sleep) benefited episodic, but not procedural, memory. From Tucker MA, Hirota Y, Wamsley EJ, et al. (2006) A daytime nap containing solely non-REM sleep enhances declarative but not procedural memory. *Neurobiol. Learn. Mem.* 86(2): 241–247.

(**Figure** 7). Subjects in the nap condition also showed a weak correlation between improved recall and the amount of SWS in the nap, further supporting the relationship between episodic memory and SWS (Tucker et al., 2006). It will be interesting to see a follow-up study in which the contribution of REM sleep physiology is assessed.

These results should not be taken to mean that REM sleep mediates the consolidation of procedural memories, whereas SWS mediates the consolidation of episodic memories. Matters are clearly not so simple. Recall that improvement on a visual discrimination task depended on SWS as well as REM (Gais et al., 2000), and improvement on a motor task correlated with stage 2 NREM sleep (Smith and MacNeill, 1994). Moreover, emotionally charged episodic memories may rely on REM sleep for their consolidation (see 'Emotional episodic memory' section below).

There are two possible interpretations of these apparent contradictions. First, the sleep stage dependency of these various memory tasks may depend on aspects of the task other than simply whether they are episodic or procedural, perhaps depending more on the intensity of training, the emotional salience of the task, or even the manner in which information is encoded (e.g., deep versus shallow encoding or implicit versus explicit). The second possibility involves an inherent oversimplification in correlating performance improvements with sleep stages as they are classically defined. Indeed, mounting evidence points to several electrophysiological, neurotransmitter, and neuroendocrine mechanisms that may underlie these effects and which do not necessarily correlate with any single sleep stage (see section below), and sleep staging, as it has been defined for 40 years, may not capture all of the key elements that lead to memory consolidation enhanced by sleep.

At an even more basic level, none of the verbal episodic memory studies described above demonstrated that a full night of sleep can produce the kinds of benefits seen following a half-night of sleep or an afternoon nap. The idea of early SWS-rich sleep, but not late REM-rich sleep, being linked to improvements in episodic memory performance, for example, loses much of its interest if these early-night benefits were lost across the second half of the night, such that they would not be available the following day.

Fortunately, several very recent reports dispel this concern (e.g., Ellenbogen et al., 2006a; Gais et al., 2006b). These studies demonstrate lasting benefits of a full night of sleep on episodic memory. For example, Ellenbogen et al. (2006a) showed that a full night of sleep not only strengthened memory for unrelated paired associates, but also made these memories more resistant to interference than an equivalent period of time spent awake.

Using a classic AB-AC interference paradigm (Barnes and Underwood, 1959), subjects first learned a list of paired associates, A_iB_i. After either a 12-h period including a night with 7–8 h of sleep, or an equivalent 12-h period of wakefulness during the day, half of the subjects in each group recalled the previously learned word pairs (cued recall). The other half learned a new list of paired associates, A_iC_i, before being tested for recall of the original list. To control for circadian effects and to demonstrate that the effects of sleep persist, an additional group of subjects was trained at the same circadian time as the sleep group (9.00 p.m.), and tested 24 rather than 12 h later.

While sleep provided modest protection against memory deterioration even in the absence of interference training, it provided a large and dramatic protection against post-sleep interference, and this benefit was sustained throughout the subsequent waking day (**Figure 8**). Thus, memories after sleep were highly resistant to interference and remained resistant across the subsequent day, demonstrating significantly better recall after 24 h than memories encoded in the morning and tested just 12 h later, without sleep. This study suggests that sleep does more than simply protect memories from interference while asleep: sleep stabilizes memories, making them resistant to future interference during the subsequent wake period.

A study by Gais et al. (2006b) provides additional evidence that sleep does more than protect memories against interference (see Wixted, 2004 for a full review of the interference argument). Subjects learned English–German vocabulary lists in the morning (8.00 a.m.) or in the evening (8.00 p.m.) and were tested immediately via cued recall to establish a baseline memory retention score. They were then retested after 24 or 36 h, either at the same circadian time or at a different circadian time (i.e., subjects trained at 8.00 a.m. and were retested at 8.00 p.m. or vice-versa). Subjects went to sleep either soon after training and initial testing (approximately 3 h in the 8.00 p.m. training condition) or after a significant delay (approximately 15 h in the 8.00 a.m. training condition).

Subjects who slept soon after training (and were retested either 24 or 36 h later) performed better on the retest session, suggesting that a night of sleep shortly after training benefited their performance on the task. In a second experiment, subjects were similarly trained in the evening either prior to sleep or to a night of sleep deprivation. Sleep-deprived subjects were allowed to sleep the following day, where they made up much of their lost sleep. However, the deprived subjects did not sleep until 10 h after training, whereas control subjects went to sleep a mere 3 h after training. In both conditions, recall testing took place 48 h after initial learning, again in the evening, to allow for recovery sleep in the deprivation condition. Although no differences emerged in the initial test on the first evening, there was a clear deficit after a night of sleep deprivation. Subjects remembered more words when they slept the night following training than when they remained awake, thus providing further evidence that sleep benefits memory consolidation. Importantly, both the 24 h groups (a.m. and p.m.

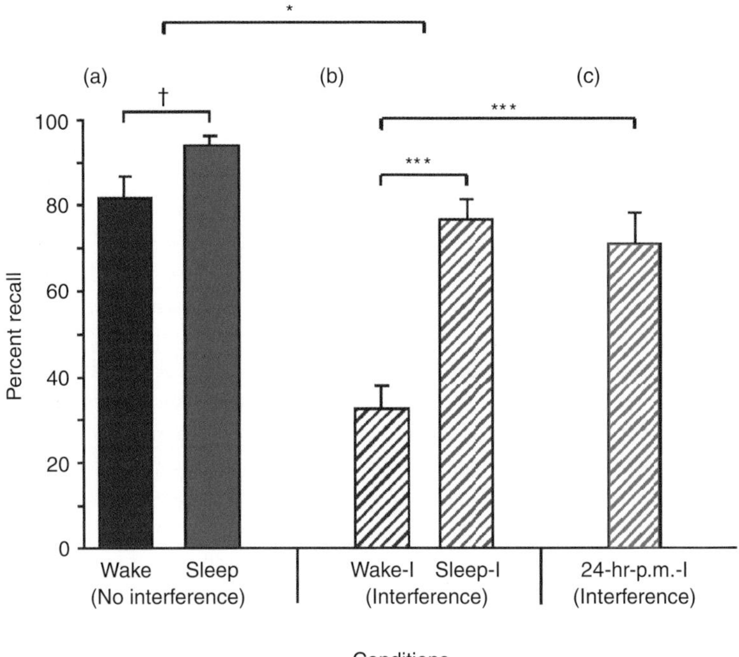

Figure 8 Sleep makes memory resistant to interference. Note that this beneficial effect of sleep was seen after 12 nighttime hours including sleep and remained 24 hours later. From Ellenbogen JM, Hulbert JC, Stickgold R, et al. (2006a) Interfering with theories of sleep and memory: Sleep, declarative memory, and associative interference. *Current Biology* 16(13): 1290–1294.

training) underwent identical amounts of waking interference, as did the two 48-h groups (controls and sleep-deprived), which strongly suggests that the sleep benefits cannot be explained by a decrease in waking interference.

Thus, it appears quite unlikely that sleep merely offers a permissive, interference-free environment for memory consolidation. It is plausible that sleep also activates unique neurobiological processes that play an active role in consolidation (for a recent review, see Ellenbogen et al., in press). This would suggest that there are sleep-specific neural processes that contribute to memory consolidation – an argument we review in the section titled 'Electrophysiological signatures'.

26.6.1 Emotional Episodic Memory

Sleep also appears to contribute to the consolidation of emotional episodic memories. This is interesting in light of the many early studies that demonstrated slow, time-dependent improvements in emotional memory, where memory for emotionally laden events, or emotional aspects of complex events, often continued to improve over days and even weeks (Kleinsmith and Kaplan, 1963; Kleinsmith et al., 1963; Kleinsmith and Kaplan, 1964). While it is well known that memories of emotional events are encoded and subsequently persist more strongly than memories for neutral events (McGaugh, 2000; Kensinger, 2004), only recently has sleep's contribution to this apparent consolidation effect been examined (Hu et al., 2006; Wagner et al., 2001).

Hu et al. (in press) examined the impact of a full night of sleep on both axes of emotional affect – valence (positive/negative) and arousal (high/low), across both remember and know measures of memory for pictures. Results showed that a night of sleep improved memory accuracy for emotionally arousing pictures relevant to an equivalent period of daytime wakefulness, but only for know judgments. No differences were observed for remember judgments. Moreover, memory bias changed across a night of sleep relative to wake, such that subjects became more conservative when making remember judgments, especially for emotionally arousing pictures. No bias differences were observed for know judgments between sleep and wake. These findings provide further evidence that the facilitation of memory for emotionally salient information may preferentially develop during sleep. Whether these effects emerge primarily after REM-rich, late night sleep, as in Wagner et al. (2001) (discussed in the section titled 'Neurohormones and neurotransmitters'), remains to be investigated. Nonetheless, the enhancing impact of sleep on the remembrance of emotional episodic information is becoming increasingly clear.

26.7 Electrophysiological Signatures

But what is it about sleep that leads to memory consolidation? Several electrophysiological signatures of sleep, recorded in animals with cortical electrodes as well as in the human EEG, reflect synchronized oscillatory patterns of neuronal activity in the cortex that may actively promote memory consolidation. There are still relatively few studies examining these proposed neurophysiological mechanisms. However, we expect the number to increase dramatically in the near future, and so we review what is currently known here.

26.7.1 Sleep Spindles

Sleep spindles are one example of such a mechanism. Sleep spindles are bursts of coherent brain activity visible on the EEG, which are most evident during stage 2 sleep. They consist of brief 11- to 16-Hz waves lasting 0.5–1.5 s. In animals, the initiation of cortical sleep spindles tends to occur with high-frequency ($\sim$200 Hz) ripples that ride on hippocampal sharp waves in NREM sleep (Siapas and Wilson, 1998). This co-occurrence of hippocampal sharp waves and cortical spindles may underlie the integration of information between the hippocampus and neocortex as memories are consolidated during sleep (Buzsáki, 1996).

In support of this hypothesis, several human studies have shown a correlation between hippocampally dependent episodic learning and cortical sleep spindles. In one such study (Gais et al., 2002), subjects studied a long list of unrelated word pairs 1 h prior to sleep, on two separate occasions, at least a week apart. In one case, they were instructed to imagine a relationship between the two nominally unrelated words, while in the other they were simply asked to count the number of letters containing curved lines in each word pair. Such instructions lead to deep, hippocampally mediated encoding and shallow, cortically mediated encoding, respectively. During the subsequent nights of sleep, subjects showed significantly higher spindle densities on the nights following deep encoding, averaging 34% more spindles in the first 90 min of sleep. Moreover, sleep spindle density was positively correlated both with immediate recall tested in the final stage of training and with recall the next morning, after sleep. Thus, those who learned better had more spindles the following night, and those with more spindles showed better performance the next morning.

These findings mirror previous observations by Meier-Koll et al. (1999), who reported a similar increase in spindles following learning of a hippocampally dependent maze task, and by Clemens et al. (2005) who found a correlation between spindle density and overnight verbal memory retention (although not between spindle density and memory for faces). Interestingly, Smith and colleagues have reported increased spindle density after intensive training on a pursuit rotor task, and after combined training on several simple procedural motor tasks (Fogel and Smith, 2006; Fogel et al., 2007). Thus, spindles might contribute to the consolidation of both explicit and implicit memories (Meier-Koll et al., 1999; Clemens et al., 2005; Fogel and Smith, 2006).

But sleep spindles also appears to correlate strongly with IQ (Bodizs et al., 2005; Schabus et al., 2006), and it can thus be difficult to discern whether high spindle content correlates with overnight improvement in memory *per se*, or whether both reflect correlations with IQ. While this is not problematic when repeated measures or factorial designs compare nights with and without preceding memory encoding, the correlation with IQ confounds correlational studies that show more posttraining spindles in subjects who subsequently show better recall.

26.7.2 Slow Waves

Given the evidence for early night facilitation of episodic memory recall (e.g., Plihal and Born, 1997, 1999a,b), it is not surprising that neurophysiologic markers associated with slow-wave sleep (SWS) have also been implicated in memory consolidation. Slow-wave rhythms, including both classical delta activity (1–4 Hz), and the more recently characterized cortical slow oscillations (<1 Hz) increase as humans pass into SWS. Indeed, these cortical slow oscillations are now considered a hallmark of SWS (Steriade and Timofeev, 2003). Such slow oscillatory activity in neuronal networks allows distant ensembles to become synchronized in rats and has been hypothesized to facilitate the binding and consolidation of memories that are dispersed across distant brain regions (Buzsáki and Draguhn, 2004).

Cortical slow oscillations have recently been observed in humans in conjunction with increased EEG coherence. EEG coherence is a large-scale measure of the coactivation of distant brain regions. Molle et al. (2004) recently showed that increased EEG coherence, which was strong during the memorization of word pairs, reappeared with cortical slow oscillations during subsequent slow wave sleep. Interestingly, while there were only marginal increases in coherence when measured over all NREM sleep, this coherence was dramatically increased when the analysis was time-locked to the occurrence of cortical slow oscillations (Molle et al., 2004).

This finding suggests that slow oscillations are important for the reprocessing of memories during sleep, a conclusion that is based on two assumptions. First, it assumes that high coherence between EEG signals from different sites on the scalp reflect an increased interplay between the underlying neuronal networks, and second, it assumes that efficient encoding of associations in episodic memory is facilitated by the large-scale synchrony of cortical neuronal activity measured by EEG coherence. Given these assumptions, the finding suggests that cortical slow oscillations may be of particular functional significance for the reprocessing of newly acquired associative memories during human SWS.

Slow oscillations also appear to exert a grouping influence over spindle activity. Molle et al. (2002) examined the temporal dynamics between spindle activity and slow oscillations in the human EEG during NREM stage 2 and SWS. They found that during human SWS, rhythmic activity in the spindle frequency range correlated with periods of slow oscillations. They also showed that discrete spindles identified during NREM stage 2 sleep coincided with the depolarizing portion of the cortical slow oscillations and were preceded by pronounced hyperpolarizing half-waves (Molle et al., 2002). These results suggest that slow rhythmic depolarizations and hyperpolarizations in cortical neurons might alternately drive and inhibit thalamically generated spindle activity, thereby contributing indirectly to memory consolidation through their regulation of spindles.

There are two distinct mechanisms by which spindles might provide the conditions necessary to induce long-term synaptic changes. Relevant cortical neural networks may be selectively activated during spindle activity as a result of previous learning, and, in turn, this activation may induce activity in, and thus modification of, related networks within the hippocampal complex. Alternatively, hippocampal activity driven by recent learning might selectively prime relevant cortical networks, which would then be activated and modified during subsequent sleep spindles (Siapas and Wilson, 1998). Either way, the spindles themselves may induce long-term synaptic changes in the neocortex.

Sleep spindles and slow oscillations represent promising candidate mechanisms for sleep-dependent memory consolidation, but it is important to note that a causal role for these electrophysiological signatures remains to be demonstrated. Nevertheless, they provide preliminary support, in humans, for the idea that the hippocampus and neocortex cooperate to integrate new information into long-term memory during sleep (Buzsáki, 1996).

26.7.3 Hippocampal and Cortical Replay

This hippocampal–neocortical communication paradigm is important, because it is intimately intertwined with theories of memory consolidation. New memories are at least initially dependent on connections between medial temporal and neocortical regions, and increased communication between these regions after training on a memory task may reflect consolidation of these recently acquired memories. A growing literature demonstrates precisely these effects in animals, where hippocampally dependent learning leads to post-training reactivations in brain areas involved in memory processing.

In the earliest studies, Pavlides and Winson (1989) demonstrated spontaneous neuronal replay of task-specific firing patterns during posttraining sleep, with individual hippocampal place cells that discharged during spatial exploration increasing their firing rates during subsequent sleep. Recording from large ensembles of place cells in the CA1 field of the hippocampus, Wilson and McNaughton (1994) showed that pairs of cells that fired together as rats passed through specific locations in an open field also fired together during subsequent SWS. This cellular activity during sleep mimicked the firing patterns seen when the task was performed, suggesting that information acquired during wake is re-expressed during sleep and that this reactivation forms a neurophysiological substrate of sleep-dependent memory consolidation (Pavlides and Winson, 1989; Wilson and McNaughton, 1994).

Since then, numerous studies have reported neuronal replay during both SWS (Skaggs and McNaughton, 1996; Kudrimoti et al., 1999; Lee and Wilson, 2002) and REM sleep (Poe et al., 2000; Louie and Wilson, 2001). Interestingly, the replay of temporal patterns of activity during SWS occurs on a time scale 20 times faster than the previous waking pattern (Lee and Wilson, 2002), while during REM it occurs in close to real time, averaging just 40% slower than in wake (Louie and Wilson, 2001).

The finding, discussed above (Siapas and Wilson, 1998), of temporal correlations during SWS between hippocampal sharp-wave/ripples and the initiation of individual prefrontal sleep spindles, along with similar correlations between the hippocampus and somatosensory cortex (Sirota et al., 2003) provides a mechanism by which such neuronal replay could lead to consolidation in both hippocampal and cortical networks.

26.7.4 Theta Rhythm

There is evidence in both humans and animals that theta frequency (4–7 Hz) oscillations are associated with enhanced learning and memory during the waking state (Bastiaansen and Hagoort, 2003), and it has been suggested that the integration of information within hippocampal and neocortical circuits may be mediated by theta activity. Although there is little theta activity during SWS, it is at waking levels during REM sleep, when hippocampal cell discharge is modulated at the theta frequency. This theta activity may aid memory reprocessing during REM sleep by enabling information to flow from the neocortex (through the superficial layers of the entorhinal cortex) into the hippocampus, where it can reverberate within hippocampal circuitry (i.e., replay). In contrast, during the sharp-wave and ripple activity of SWS, information may flow in the opposite direction, out of the hippocampus and back to the neocortex (through deep layers of the entorhinal cortex Buzsáki, 1996; Buzsáki, 1998), thus allowing information to flow throughout the complete neocortex–hippocampal circuit. Indeed, it has been proposed that high levels of the neurotransmitter acetylcholine and the neurohormone cortisol during REM sleep, and low levels during SWS, might modulate communication between hippocampus and neocortex as memories undergo consolidation (Payne and Nadel, 2004). In this view, as in others (Giuditta et al., 1995;Ficca et al., 2000), both SWS and REM sleep are thought to contribute to the consolidation of episodic memories. In addition, for emotional memory processing, cooperative theta oscillations between hippocampal and amygdala regions during REM sleep may play an important role as well (Pare et al., 2002).

26.8 Neurohormones and Neurotransmitters

Many modulatory neurotransmitters contribute to memory formation. Acetylcholine, however, has received the most attention by the sleep community to date, most likely because it is critically involved in control of the NREM/REM cycle, and because it is present at particularly high levels during REM sleep and low levels during SWS (Hobson et al., 1998).

Acetylcholine, although mainly involved in memory encoding, appears to also play a role in the flow of information between memory systems during different stages of sleep. According to a model by Hasselmo (1999), acetylcholine inhibits feedback loops both within the hippocampus and between the hippocampus and neocortex. As a result, the high cholinergic activity seen during wakefulness minimizes consolidation and promotes encoding of new episodic memories, whereas the low cholinergic activity in SWS blocks new input and supports the replay of recently encoded information in the hippocampus. This replay may then lead to integration of this information within hippocampal and neocortical memory stores (Buzsáki, 1996; Hasselmo, 1999; Payne and Nadel, 2004).

To investigate the role of acetylcholine in the consolidation of episodic memory during sleep, Gais and Born (2004b) trained subjects on a list of paired associates, as well as a mirror tracing task, before 3 h of SWS-rich nocturnal sleep or wakefulness during which they received a placebo or an infusion of the cholinesterase inhibitor physostigmine (which increases cholinergic tone). When tested after 3 h of sleep, recall on the paired-associates task was impaired in the physostigmine group, while procedural memory performance was unaffected (Gais and Born, 2004b). This provides initial support for Hasselmo's (1999) model and suggests that the inhibition of cholinergic activity during SWS is critical for sleep-based episodic memory consolidation.

As with neurotransmitters, hormonal fluctuations across the sleep cycle may also help to explain why different sleep stages contribute differentially to the consolidation of episodic memories. Activation of the neuroendocrine hypothalamic–pituitary–adrenocortical (HPA) system, for instance, results in the release of the stress hormone cortisol from the adrenal glands. Cortisol then feeds back onto the brain, where the hippocampus and frontal cortex, arguably two of the most critical memory regions, contain the highest number of cortisol receptors in humans (Lupien and Lepage, 2001). Several studies have demonstrated cortisol-induced memory impairments with episodic memory tasks during wake (Kim and Diamond, 2002; Payne et al., 2002; Payne et al., 2006). Intriguingly, cortisol levels are at their lowest during early nocturnal sleep, while achieving a diurnal maximum during late night sleep (Plihal and Born 1999b; Born and Wagner, 2004).

Plihal and Born (1997, 1999a) have thus argued that the circadian suppression of cortisol release early in the night makes this SWS-rich sleep an ideal physiological environment for episodic memory consolidation. Naturally low cortisol levels during early sleep promote more efficient consolidation of episodic memories than is seen during late, REM-rich sleep, when cortisol levels are high. In support of this view, Plihal and Born (1999b) showed that artificially elevating cortisol levels during early sleep eradicated the normal episodic memory benefit seen during this period, suggesting that the salubrious environment provided by early sleep is a result, at least in part, of the naturally low levels of cortisol during this time.

Cortisol levels in the Plihal and Born (1999b) study were elevated to levels similar to those typically seen in response to mild to moderate stressors, that are sufficient to disrupt episodic memory function during wakefulness (Kirschbaum et al., 1996; de Quervain et al., 2003; de Quervain, 2006).

In another study suggestive of a cortisol-related influence on memory consolidation (Wagner et al., 2001), memory for emotionally laden narrative material was facilitated after late night, REM-rich sleep periods. At first blush, this result seems to contradict the evidence reviewed in the section titled 'Emotional episodic memory', which demonstrated that late night REM sleep does not support episodic memory consolidation, perhaps due to high cortisol levels. Yet studies have consistently shown that cortisol facilitates memory for emotional episodic materials, while impairing closely matched neutral materials during wakefulness (Buchanan and Lovallo, 2001; Payne et al., 2006). Given the role of cortisol in enhancing emotional episodic information, the late-night enhancement of emotional memory in this study is not surprising.

In addition to cortisol, other hormones (e.g., growth hormone) are known to impact memory function in the waking state, and also vary across sleep, suggesting that they might contribute to sleep-based memory consolidation. Although initial studies of growth hormone have failed to find such an effect (Gais et al., 2006a), further investigation of the neurochemistry underlying the relationship between sleep and memory consolidation is a productive avenue for future research. Indeed, it seems especially important to forge ahead into precisely this neuromodulatory realm, where the chemical basis of the sleep/memory consolidation connection is examined.

26.9 Concluding Comments

Over the past 10 years, the field of sleep and memory has grown exponentially, with reports of sleep–memory interactions emerging from myriad disciplines, ranging form cellular and molecular studies in animals to behavioral and neuroimaging studies in humans. In our view, sleep undoubtedly mediates memory processes, but the way in which it does so remains largely unknown. This makes the future of the field truly exciting, but also challenging. Much remains to be done, from uncovering the mechanisms of brain plasticity that underlie sleep-based memory processing, to untangling the complex relationship between the various sleep stages and types of memory. In so doing, memory researchers may find a field in which some of the more recalcitrant problems of basic memory research can also be answered.

Acknowledgments

Supported in part by grants from the U.S. National Institutes of Health, MH 48832 and MH 65292 to R.S., MH 69935 to M.P.W., and from the Harvard University Mind Brain and Behavior Interfaculty Initiative to J.D.P.

References

Amzica F and Steriade M (1995) Disconnection of intracortical synaptic linkages disrupts synchronization of a slow oscillation. *J. Neurosci.* 15: 4658–4677.

Aserinsky E and Kleitman N (1953) Regularly occurring periods of ocular motility and concomitant phenomena during sleep. *Science* 118: 273–274.

Atienza M, Cantero JL, and Dominguez-Marin E (2002) The time course of neural changes underlying auditory perceptual learning. *Learn. Mem.* 9(3): 138–150.

Atienza M, Cantero JL, and Stickgold R (2004) Post-training sleep enhances automaticity in perceptual discrimination. *J. Cogn. Neurosci.* 16: 53–64.

Barnes JM and Underwood BJ (1959) Fate of first-list associations in transfer theory. *J. Exp. Psychol.* 58: 97–105.

Barrett TR and Ekstrand BR (1972) Effect of sleep on memory. 3. Controlling for time-of-day effects. *J. Exp. Psychol.* 96(2): 321–327.

Bastiaansen M and Hagoort P (2003) Event-induced theta responses as a window on the dynamics of memory. *Cortex* 39(4–5): 967–992.

Benington JH and Frank MG (2003) Cellular and molecular connections between sleep and synaptic plasticity. *Prog. Neurobiol.* 69(2): 71–101.

Benson K and Feinberg I (1977) The beneficial effect of sleep in an extended Jenkins and Dallenbach paradigm. *Psychophysiology* 14(4): 375–84.

Bodizs R, Kis T, Lázár AS, et al. (2005) Prediction of general mental ability based on neural oscillation measures of sleep. *J. Sleep Res.* 14(3): 285–292.

Born J and Wagner U (2004) Memory consolidation during sleep: Role of cortisol feedback. *Ann. N. Y. Acad. Sci.* 1032: 198–201.

Brualla J, Romero MF, Serrano M, and Valdizan JR (1998) Auditory event-related potentials to semantic priming during sleep. *Electroencephalogr: Clin. Neurophysiol.* 108(3): 283–290.

Buchanan TW and Lovallo WR (2001) Enhanced memory for emotional material following stress-level cortisol treatment in humans. *Psychoneuroendocrinology* 26(3): 307–317.

Buzsáki G (1996) The hippocampo-neocortical dialogue. *Cereb. Cortex* 6: 81–92.

Buzsáki G (1998) Memory consolidation during sleep: A neurophysiological perspective. *J. Sleep Res.* 7(Suppl 1): 17–23.

Buzsáki G and Draguhn A (2004) Neuronal oscillations in cortical networks. *Science* 304(5679): 1926–1929.

Cahill L (2000) Neurobiological mechanisms of emotionally influenced, long-term memory. *Prog. Brain Res.* 126: 29–37.

Cahill L and McGaugh JL (1996) Modulation of memory storage. *Curr. Opin. Neurobiol.* 6(2): 237–242.

Chernik D (1972) Effect of REM sleep deprivation on learning and recall by humans. *Percept. Motor Skills* 34: 283–294.

Clemens Z, Fabó D, and Halász P (2005) Overnight verbal memory retention correlates with the number of sleep spindles. *Neuroscience* 132(2): 529–535.

Datta S (2000) Avoidance task training potentiates phasic pontine-wave density in the rat: A mechanism for sleep-dependent plasticity. *J. Neurosci.* 20(22): 8607–8613.

Datta S, Mavanji V, Ulloor J, et al. (2004) Activation of phasic pontine-wave generator prevents rapid eye movement sleep deprivation-induced learning impairment in the rat: A mechanism for sleep-dependent plasticity. *J. Neurosci.* 24(6): 1416–1427.

de Quervain DJ (2006) Glucocorticoid-induced inhibition of memory retrieval: implications for posttraumatic stress disorder. *Ann. N. Y. Acad. Sci.* 1071: 216–220.

de Quervain DJ, Henke K, Aerni A, et al. (2003) Glucocorticoid-induced impairment of declarative memory retrieval is associated with reduced blood flow in the medial temporal lobe. *Eur. J. Neurosci.* 17(6): 1296–1302.

Dudai Y (2004) The neurobiology of consolidations, or, how stable is the engram? *Ann. Rev. Psychol.* 55: 51–86.

Ellenbogen JM, Hulbert JC, Stickgold R, et al. (2006a) Interfering with theories of sleep and memory: Sleep, declarative memory, and associative interference. *Curr. Biol.* 16(13): 1290–1294.

Ellenbogen JM, Payne JD, and Stickgold R (2006b) The role of sleep in declarative memory consolidation: Passive, permissive, active or none? *Curr. Opin. Neurobiol.* 16(6): 716–722.

Empson JA and Clarke PR (1970) Rapid eye movements and remembering. *Nature* 227(5255): 287–288.

Fenn KM, Nusbaum HC, and Margoliash D (2003) Consolidation during sleep of perceptual learning of spoken language. *Nature* 425(6958): 614–616.

Ficca G, Lombardo P, Rossi L, et al. (2000) Morning recall of verbal material depends on prior sleep organization. *Behav. Brain Res.* 112(1–2): 159–163.

Fischer S, Hallschmid M, Elsner AL, et al. (2002) Sleep forms memory for finger skills. *Proc. Natl. Acad. Sci. USA* 99(18): 11987–11991.

Fishbein W, McGaugh JL, and Swarz JR (1971) Retrograde amnesia: Electroconvulsive shock effects after termination of rapid eye movement sleep deprivation. 172(978): 80–82.

Fogel S, Jacob J, and Smith C (2001) Increased sleep spindle activity following simple motor procedural learning in humans. *Actas Fisiol.* 7: 123.

Fogel SM and Smith CT (2006) Learning-dependent changes in sleep spindles and stage 2 sleep. *J. Sleep Res.* 15(3): 250–255.

Fogel SM, Smith CT, and Cote KA (2007) Dissociable learning-dependent changes in REM and non-REM sleep in declarative and procedural memory systems. *Behav. Brain. Res.* 180: 48–61.

Fowler MJ, Sullivan MJ, and Ekstrand BR (1973) Sleep and memory. *Science* 179(70): 302–304.

Gaab N and Paetzold M, et al. (2004) The influence of sleep on auditory learning: A behavioral study. *Neuroreport* 15(4): 731–734.

Gais S and Born J (2004a) Declarative memory consolidation: Mechanisms acting during human sleep. *Learn. Mem.* 11(6): 679–685.

Gais S and Born J (2004b) Low acetylcholine during slow-wave sleep is critical for declarative memory consolidation. *Proc. Natl. Acad. Sci. USA* 101(7): 2140–2144.

Gais S, Plihal W, Wagner U, et al. (2000) Early sleep triggers memory for early visual discrimination skills. *Nat. Neurosci.* 3(12): 1335–1339.

Gais S, Molle M, Helms K, et al. (2002) Learning-dependent increases in sleep spindle density. *J. Neurosci.* 22(15): 6830–6844.

Gais S, Hullemann P, Hallschmid M, et al. (2006a) Sleep-dependent surges in growth hormone do not contribute to sleep-dependent memory consolidation. *Psychoneuroendocrinology* 31(6): 786–791.

Gais S, Lucas B, and Born J (2006b) Sleep after learning aids memory recall. *Learn. Mem.* 13(3): 259–262.

Giuditta A and Ambrosini MV, et al. (1995) The sequential hypothesis of the function of sleep. *Behav. Brain Res.* 69: 157–166.

Graves L, Pack A, and Abel T (2001) *Sleep and memory: a molecular perspective. A* 24: 237–243.

Greenberg R and Pearlman CA (1974) Cutting the REM nerve: an approach to the adaptive function of REM sleep. *Perspect. Biol. Med.* 17: 513–521.

Hamann S (2003) Nosing in on the emotional brain. *Nat. Neurosci.* 6(2): 106–108.

Hamann SB, Ely TD, Grafton ST, et al. (1999) Amygdala activity related to enhanced memory for pleasant and aversive stimuli. *Nat. Neurosci.* 2(3): 289–293.

Hamann SB, Ely TD, Hoffman JM, et al. (2002) Ecstasy and agony: Activation of the human amygdala in positive and negative emotion. *Psychol. Sci.* 13(2): 135–141.

Hasselmo ME (1999) Neuromodulation: Acetylcholine and memory consolidation. *Trends Cogn. Sci.* 3: 351–359.

Hennevin E, Hars B, Maho C, et al. (1995) Processing of learned information in paradoxical sleep: Relevance for memory. *Behav. Brain Res.* 69: 125–135.

Hobson JA (2005) Sleep is of the brain, by the brain and for the brain. *Nature* 437(7063): 1254–1256.

Hobson JA, McCarley RW, and Wyzinski PW (1975) Sleep cycle oscillation: Reciprocal discharge by two brainstem neuronal groups. *Science* 189: 55–58.

Hobson JA, Stickgold R, and Pace-Schott EF (1998) The neuropsychology of REM sleep dreaming. *Neuroreport* 9: R1–R14.

Huber R, Ghilardi MF, Massimini M, et al. (2004) Local sleep and learning. *Nature* 430(6995): 78–81.

Hu P, Stylos-Allan M, and Walker M (2006) Sleep facilitates consolidation of emotional declarative memory. *Psychol. Sci.* 17: 891–898.

Jenkins JG and Dallenbach KM (1924) LXXII. Obliviscence during sleep and waking. *Am. J. Psychol.* 35: 605–612.

Johnson LC, Naitoh P, Moses JM, et al. (1974) Interaction of REM deprivation and stage 4 deprivation with total sleep loss: experiment 2. *Psychophysiology* 11(2): 147–159.

Karni A and Sagi D (1991) Where practice makes perfect in texture discrimination: evidence for primary visual cortex plasticity. *Proceedings of the National Academy of Science of the United States of America* 88: 4966–4970.

Karni A and Sagi D (1993) The time course of learning a visual skill. *Nature* 365: 250–252.

Karni A, Tanne D, Rubenstein BS, et al. (1994) Dependence on REM sleep of overnight improvement of a perceptual skill. *Science* 265(5172): 679–682.

Kensinger EA (2004) Remembering emotional experiences: The contribution of valence and arousal. *Rev. Neurosci.* 15(4): 241–251.

Kim JJ and Diamond DM (2002) The stressed hippocampus, synaptic plasticity and lost memories. *Nat. Rev. Neurosci.* 3(6): 453–462.

Kirschbaum C, Wolf OT, May M, et al. (1996) Stress- and treatment-induced elevations of cortisol levels associated with impaired declarative memory in healthy adults. *Life Sci.* 58(17): 1475–1483.

Kleinsmith LJ and Kaplan S (1963) Paired-associate learning as a function of arousal and interpolated interval. *J. Exp. Psychol.* 65: 190–193.

Kleinsmith LJ and Kaplan S (1964) Interaction of arousal and recall interval in nonsense syllable paired-associate learning. *J. Exp. Psychol.* 67: 124–126.

Kleinsmith LJ, Kaplan S, Tarte RD, et al. (1963) The relationship of arousal to short- and longterm verbal recall. *Can. J. Psychol.* 17: 393–397.

Korman M, Raz N, Flash T, et al. (2003) Multiple shifts in the representation of a motor sequence during the acquisition of skilled performance. *Proc. Natl. Acad. Sci. USA* 100(21): 12492–12497.

Kudrimoti HS, Barnes CA, and McNaughton BL (1999) Reactivation of hippocampal cell assemblies: Effects of behavioral state, experience, and EEG dynamics. *J. Neurosci.* 19(10): 4090–4101.

Kuriyama K, Stickgold R, and Walker MP (2004) Sleep-dependent learning and motor-skill complexity. *Learn. Mem.* 11(6): 705–713.

Lee AK and Wilson MA (2002) Memory of sequential experience in the hippocampus during slow wave sleep. *Neuron* 36(6): 1183–1194.

Lewin I and Glaubman H (1975) The effect of REM deprivation: Is it detrimental, beneficial or neutral? *Psychophysiology* 12: 349–353.

Louie K and Wilson MA (2001) Temporally structured replay of awake hippocampal ensemble activity during rapid eye movement sleep. *Neuron* 29(1): 145–156.

Lovatt DJ and Warr PB (1968) Recall after sleep. *Am. J. Psychol.* 81(2): 253–257.

Lupien SJ and Lepage M (2001) Stress, memory, and the hippocampus: can't live with it, can't live without it. *Behav. Brain Res.* 127(1–2): 137–158.

Maquet P (2001) The role of sleep in learning and memory. *Science* 294(5544): 1048–1052.

Maquet P, Laureys S, Peigneux P, et al. (2000) Experience-dependent changes in cerebral activation during human REM sleep. *Nat. Neurosci.* 3(8): 831–836.

Maquet P, Laureys S, Perrin F, et al. (2003) Festina lente: evidence for fast and slow learning processes and a role for sleep in human motor skill learning. *Learn. Mem.* 10(4): 237–239.

Marrosu F, Portas C, Mascia MS, et al. (1995) Microdialysis measurement of cortical and hippocampal acetylcholine release during sleep-wake cycle in freely moving cats. *Brain Res.* 671: 329–332.

McGaugh JL (2000) Memory – a century of consolidation. *Science* 287(5451): 248–251.

McGaugh JL, Introini-Collison IB, Cahill LF, et al. (1993) Neuromodulatory systems and memory storage: Role of the amygdala. *Behav. Brain Res.* 58(1–2): 81–90.

McGaugh JL, Cahill L, and Roozendhaal B (1996) Involvement of the amygdala in memory storage: Interaction with other brain systems. *Proc. Natl. Acad. Sci. USA* 93(24): 13508–13514.

McNaughton BL and Barnes CA, et al. (2003) Off-line reprocessing of recent memory and its role in memory consolidation: A progress report. In: Maquet P, Smith C, and Stickgold R (eds.) *Sleep and Plasticity*, pp. 225–246. London: Oxford University Press.

Mednick SC, Nakayama K, and Cantero JL (2002) The restorative effect of naps on perceptual deterioration. *Nat. Neurosci.* 5: 677–681.

Mednick S, Nakayama K, and Stickgold R (2003) Sleep dependent learning: A nap is as good as a night. *Nat. Neurosci.* 6: 697–698.

Meier-Koll A, Bussmann B, Schmidt C, et al. (1999) Walking through a maze alters the architecture of sleep. *Percept. Mot. Skills* 88: 1141–1159.

Molle M, Marshall L, Gais S, et al. (2002) Grouping of spindle activity during slow oscillations in human non-rapid eye movement sleep. *J. Neurosci.* 22(24): 10941–10947.

Molle M, Marshall L, and Gais S (2004) Learning increases human electroencephalographic coherence during subsequent slow sleep oscillations. *Proc. Natl. Acad. Sci. USA* 10(38): 13963–13968.

Moscovitch M, Nadel L, Winocur G, et al. (2006) The cognitive neuroscience of remote episodic, semantic and spatial memory. *Curr. Opin. Neurobiol.* 16(2): 179–190.

Nadel L and Moscovitch M (1997) Memory consolidation, retrograde amnesia and the hippocampal complex. *Curr. Opin. Neurobiol.* 7(2): 217–227.

Nakanishi H, Sun Y, Nakamura RK, et al. (1997) Positive correlations between cerebral protein synthesis rates and deep sleep in *Macaca mulatta*. *Eur. J. Neurosci.* 9(2): 271–279.

Packard MG and Cahill L (2001) Affective modulation of multiple memory systems. *Curr. Opin. Neurobiol.* 11(6): 752–756.

Pare D, Collins DR, and Pelletier JG (2002) Amygdala oscillations and the consolidation of emotional memories. *Trends Cogn. Sci.* 6: 306–314.

Pavlides C and Winson J (1989) Influences of hippocampal place cell firing in the awake state on the activity of these cells during subsequent sleep episodes. *J. Neurosci.* 9: 2907–2918.

Payne JD and Nadel L (2004) Sleep, dreams, and memory consolidation: The role of the stress hormone cortisol. *Learn. Mem.* 11(6): 671–678.

Payne JD, Nadel L, Allen JJ, et al. (2002) The effects of experimentally induced stress on false recognition. *Memory* 10(1): 1–6.

Payne JD, Nadel L, Britton WB, et al. (2004) The biopsychology of trauma and memory. In: *Memory and Emotion*, pp. 76–128. Oxford University Press.

Payne JD, Jackson ED, Ryan L, et al. (2006) The impact of stress on neutral and emotional aspects of episodic memory. *Memory* 14(1): 1–16.

Pearlman C (1979) REM Sleep and information processing: Evidence from animal studies. *Neurosci. Biobehav. Rev.* 3: 57–68.

Peigneux P, Laureys S, Fuchs S, et al. (2003) Learned material content and acquisition level modulate cerebral reactivation during posttraining rapid-eye-movement sleep. *Neuroimage* 20(1): 125–134.

Peigneux P, Laureys S, Fuchs S, et al. (2004) Are spatial memories strengthened in the human hippocampus during slow wave sleep? *Neuron* 44: 535–545.

Plihal W and Born J (1997) Effects of early and late nocturnal sleep on declarative and procedural memory. *J. Cogn. Neurosci.* 9(4): 534–547.

Plihal W and Born J (1999a) Effects of early and late nocturnal sleep on priming and spatial memory. *Psychophysiology* 36: 571–582.

Plihal W and Born J (1999b) Memory consolidation in human sleep depends on inhibition of glucocorticoid release. *Neuroreport* 10(13): 2741–2747.

Poe GR, Nitz DA, McNaughton BL, et al. (2000) Experience-dependent phase-reversal of hippocampal neuron firing during REM sleep. *Brain Res.* 855(1): 176–180.

Qin YL, McNaughton BL, Skaggs WE, et al. (1997) Memory reprocessing in corticocortical and hippocampocortical neuronal ensembles. *Philos. Trans. R. Soc. Lond. B Biol. Sci.* 352(1360): 1525–1533.

Rechtschaffen A and Kales A (1968) *A Manual of Standardized Terminology Techniques and Scoring System for Sleep Stages of Human Subjects*. Los Angeles: University of California Los Angeles, Brain Information Service.

Ribeiro S, Goyal V, Mello CV, et al. (1999) Brain gene expression during REM sleep depends on prior waking experience. *Learn. Mem.* 6: 500–508.

Ribeiro S and Nicolelis MA (2004) Reverberation, storage, and postsynaptic propagation of memories during sleep. *Learn. Mem.* 11(6): 686–696.

Robertson EM, Pascual-Leone A, and Press DZ (2004) Awareness modifies the skill-learning benefits of sleep. *Curr. Biol.* 14(3): 208–212.

Schabus M, Hodlmoser K, Gruber G, et al. (2006) Sleep spindle-related activity in the human EEG and its relation to general cognitive and learning abilities. *Eur. J. Neurosci.* 23(7): 1738–1746.

Schacter DL and Tulving E (1994) *Memory Systems 1994*. Cambridge, MA: MIT Press.

Sejnowski TJ and Destexhe A (2000) Why do we sleep? *Brain Res.* 886(1–2): 208–223.

Siapas AG and Wilson MA (1998) Coordinated interactions between hippocampal ripples and cortical spindles during slow-wave sleep. *Neuron* 21(5): 1123–1128.

Siegel JM (2001) The REM sleep-memory consolidation hypothesis. *Science* 294(5544): 1058–1063.

Sirota A, Csicsvari J, Buhl D, et al. (2003) Communication between neocortex and hippocampus during sleep in rodents. *Proc. Natl. Acad. Sci. USA* 100(4): 2065–2069.

Skaggs WE and McNaughton BL (1996) Replay of neuronal firing sequences in rat hippocampus during sleep following spatial experience. *Science* 271(5257): 1870–1873.

Smith C (1985) Sleep states and learning: a review of the animal literature. *Neurosci. Biobehav. Rev.* 9(2): 157–168.

Smith C (1995) Sleep states and memory processes. *Behav. Brain Res.* 69(1–2): 137–145.
Smith C (2001) Sleep states and memory processes in humans: Procedural versus declarative memory systems. *Sleep Med. Rev.* 5(6): 491–506.
Smith C and Butler S (1982) Paradoxical sleep at selective times following training is necessary for learning. *Physiol. Behav.* 29(3): 469–473.
Smith C and MacNeill C (1994) Impaired motor memory for a pursuit rotor task following stage 2 sleep loss in college students. *J. Sleep Res.* 3: 206–213.
Smith C and Rose GM (1996) Evidence for a paradoxical sleep window for place learning in the Morris water maze. *Physiol. Behav.* 59(1): 93–97.
Smith C and Wong PT (1991) Paradoxical sleep increases predict successful learning in a complex operant task. *Behav. Neurosci.* 105(2): 282–288.
Smith C, Young J, and Young W (1980) Prolonged increases in paradoxical sleep during and after avoidance-task acquisition. *Sleep* 3(1): 67–81.
Smith C, Tenn C, and Annett R (1991) Some biochemical and behavioural aspects of the paradoxical sleep window. *Can. J. Psychol.* 45(2): 115–124.
Smith C, Conway J, and Rose C (1995) Paradoxical sleep deprivation impairs reference memory in the radial maze task. *Sleep Res.* 24: 456.
Squire LR (1992) Declarative and nondeclarative memory: Multiple brain systems supporting learning and memory. *J. Cogn. Neurosci.* 4: 231–243.
Squire LR, Cohen NJ, and Nadel L (1984) The medial temporal region and memory consolidation: A new hypothesis. In: Weingartner H and Parker E (eds.) *Memory Consolidation*, pp. 185–210. Hillsdale, NJ: Erlbaum.
Steriade M (1999) Coherent oscillations and short-term plasticity in corticothalamic networks. *Trends Neurosci.* 22: 337–345.
Steriade M and Timofeev I (2003) Neuronal plasticity in thalamocortical networks during sleep and waking oscillations. *Neuron* 37(4): 563–76.
Stickgold R (2003) Human studies of sleep and off-line memory reprocessing. In: Maquet P, Smith C, and Stickgold R (eds.) *Sleep and Plasticity*, London: Oxford University Press.
Stickgold R (2005) Sleep-dependent memory consolidation. *Nature* 437: 1272–1278.
Stickgold R and Walker MP (2005) Sleep and memory: The ongoing debate. *Sleep* 28: 1225–1227.
Stickgold R, James L, and Hobson A (2000a) Visual discrimination learning requires post-training sleep. *Nat. Neurosci.* 2(12): 1237–1238.
Stickgold R, Whidbee D, Schirmer B, et al. (2000b) Visual discrimination task improvement: A multi-step process occurring during sleep. *J. Cogn. Neurosci.* 12: 246–254.
Stickgold R, Hobson JA, Fosse R, et al. (2001) Sleep, learning and dreams: Off-line memory reprocessing. *Science* 294: 1052–1057.
Takashima A, Petersson KM, Rutters F, et al. (2006) Declarative memory consolidation in humans: A prospective functional magnetic resonance imaging study. *Proc. Natl. Acad. Sci. USA* 103(3): 756–761.
Tucker MA, Hirota Y, Wamsley EJ, et al. (2006) A daytime nap containing solely non-REM sleep enhances declarative but not procedural memory. *Neurobiol. Learn. Mem.* 86(2): 241–247.
Tulving E (1972) Episodic and semantic memory. In: Tulving E and Donaldson W (eds.) *Organization of Memory*, pp. 381–403. New York: Academic Press.
Tweed S, Aubrey JB, Nader R, et al. (1999) Deprivation of REM sleep or stage 2 sleep differentially affects cognitive procedural and motor procedural memory. *Sleep* 22: S241.
Vertes RP and Eastman KE (2000) The case against memory consolidation in REM sleep. *Behav. Brain Sci.* 23: 867–876.
Vertes RP and Siegel JM (2005) Time for the sleep community to take a critical look at the purported role of sleep in memory processing. *Sleep* 28: 1228–1229.
Wagner U, Gais S, and Born J (2001) Emotional memory formation is enhanced across sleep intervals with high amounts of rapid eye movement sleep. *Learn. Mem.* 8: 112–119.
Walker MP and Stickgold R (2004) Sleep-dependent learning and memory consolidation. *Neuron* 44(1): 121–133.
Walker MP and Stickgold R (2006) Sleep, memory, and plasticity. *Annu. Rev. Psychol.* 57: 139–166.
Walker MP, Brakefield T, Hobson JA, and Stickgold R (2002) Practice with sleep makes perfect: Sleep dependent motor skill learning. *Neuron* 35(1): 205–211.
Walker MP, Brakefield T, Seidman J, et al. (2003) Sleep and the time course of motor skill learning. *Learn. Mem.* 10: 275–284.
Wilson MA and McNaughton BL (1994) Reactivation of hippocampal ensemble memories during sleep. *Science* 265: 676–679.
Wixted JT (2004) The psychology and neuroscience of forgetting. *Annu. Rev. Psychol.* 55: 235–269.
Yaroush R, Sullivan MJ, and Ekstrand BR (1971) Effect of sleep on memory. II: Differential effect of first and second half of the night. *J. Exp. Psychol.* 88: 361–366.

27 Memory Modulation

J. L. McGaugh and B. Roozendaal, University of California at Irvine, Irvine, CA, USA

27.1 Introduction

Brain systems have many tasks to perform in enabling the formation of memories. New information must be encoded and stored in ways that enable the information subsequently to be retrieved and expressed in behavior. Understanding the cellular mechanisms and brain systems responsible for enabling and orchestrating these various complex tasks is the aim of research on the neurobiology of learning and memory. A key role in such orchestration is played by systems that modulate the consolidation of memories of recent experiences. Our memories are not all created equally strong: Some experiences are well remembered, while others are remembered poorly, if at all. Understanding the neurobiological processes and systems that contribute to such differences in the strength of our memories is a special quest of research on memory modulation. Not only do modulatory systems influence neurobiological processes underlying the consolidation of new information, but more recent evidence indicates that these systems also affect other mnemonic processes, including memory extinction, memory recall, and working memory.

Research on memory modulation was stimulated by findings reported a little over half a century ago that, in rats, retention of a recently learned response was impaired by administration of electroconvulsive shock (ECS) (Duncan, 1949; Gerard, 1949). These findings were the first to provide compelling evidence supporting the hypothesis proposed half a century earlier (Müller and Pilzecker, 1900) that neural memory traces activated by new experiences perseverate in a fragile state and gradually become consolidated. Subsequent studies using ECS and other treatments to impair brain functioning shortly after training provided extensive evidence that such treatments impair memory by interfering with time-dependent processes involved in memory consolidation (McGaugh, 1966; McGaugh and Herz, 1972). The findings of such studies also revealed that susceptibility to posttraining modulating influences is a common feature of animal memory: Posttraining treatments affect memory in mollusks, fish, insects, and birds, as well as rodents and primates (Cherkin, 1969; Agranoff, 1980; Menzel, 1983; Kandel, 2001).

In providing evidence that new memories remain fragile for a while before becoming consolidated, the findings of Duncan and Gerard suggested the possibility that memory consolidation might also be enhanced by stimulating brain functioning. In support of this implication, many studies subsequently reported that, in rats, retention is enhanced by injections of stimulant drugs, including strychnine, the GABAergic antagonists picrotoxin and bicuculline, pentylenetetrazole, and amphetamine, administered shortly after training, and that such treatments are generally ineffective when administered several hours after learning (Breen and McGaugh, 1961; McGaugh and Petrinovich, 1965; McGaugh, 1966, 1973; Doty and Doty, 1966; Evangelista and Izquierdo, 1971; McGaugh and Herz, 1972; Grecksch and Matthies, 1981; Carr and White, 1984; Brioni and McGaugh, 1988; Castellano and Pavone, 1988). Such a time-dependent susceptibility thus clearly suggests that the drugs affected memory by modulating the consolidation of recently acquired information.

In studies of the effects of treatments modulating learning and memory it is essential to distinguish the effects of the treatments on memory from the effects of the treatments on, e.g., attentional, motivational and motor processes that may directly affect the behavior used to make inferences about memory. The use of posttraining treatments to alter brain functioning shortly after training has provided an effective technique for excluding such performance effects in investigating the effects of modulatory treatments on memory consolidation (McGaugh, 1966, 1989; McGaugh and Herz, 1972).

27.2 Endogenous Modulation of Consolidation

Memory consolidation appears to be a highly adaptive function because, as noted above, evidence of consolidation is found in a wide variety of animal species. But why do our long-term memories and those of other animals consolidate slowly? There seems to be no *a priori* reason to assume that neurobiological mechanisms are not capable of consolidating memory quickly. Considerable evidence suggests that the slow consolidation of memories may serve a highly important adaptive function by enabling endogenous processes activated by an experience, and thus occurring shortly after the event, to modulate memory strength. In a paper published shortly after those reporting that posttraining drug administration can enhance memory consolidation (e.g., Breen and McGaugh, 1961; McGaugh, 1966), Livingston suggested that stimulation of the limbic system and brainstem reticular formation might promote the storage of recently activated brain events by initiating a "neurohormonal influence (favoring) future repetitions of the same neural activities" (Livingston, 1967, p. 576). Kety subsequently offered the more specific suggestion that adrenergic catecholamines released in emotional states may serve "to reinforce and consolidate new and significant sensory patterns in the neocortex" (Kety, 1972, p. 73). Although the specific details of current findings and theoretical interpretations differ in many ways from those early views offered by Livingston and Kety, recent findings are consistent with their general hypotheses.

27.3 Modulating Influences of Adrenal Stress Hormones

Emotionally arousing experiences are generally well remembered (Christianson, 1992; McGaugh, 2003). As William James (1890) noted, "An experience may be so exciting emotionally as to almost leave a scar on the cerebral tissue" (James, 1890, p. 670). The susceptibility of memory consolidation processes to modulating influences induced after learning provides the opportunity for neurobiological processes activated by emotional arousal to regulate the strength of memory traces representing important experiences (McGaugh, 1983; McGaugh and Gold, 1989). Extensive evidence indicates that stress hormones released by the adrenal glands, epinephrine and cortisol (corticosterone in rodents), by emotionally arousing experiences modulate memory consolidation (McGaugh and Roozendaal, 2002). It is well established that, in rats and mice, hormones of the adrenal medulla and adrenal cortex are released during and immediately after stressful stimulation of the kinds used in aversively motivated learning tasks (McCarty and Gold, 1981; McGaugh and Gold, 1989; Aguilar-Valles et al., 2005), and that removal of these stress hormones by adrenalectomy generally results in memory impairment (Borrell et al., 1983, 1984; Oitzl and de Kloet, 1992; Roozendaal et al., 1996b; Roozendaal, 2000).

27.3.1 Epinephrine

Gold and van Buskirk (1975, 1978) were the first to report that, in adrenally intact rats, systemic posttraining injections of the adrenomedullary hormone epinephrine enhance long-term retention of inhibitory avoidance. As found in previous studies of the memory-enhancing effects of stimulant drugs, the epinephrine effects were dose dependent and time dependent. Moderate doses of posttraining epinephrine enhanced retention performance, whereas lower doses or higher doses were less effective. Furthermore, as was found with stimulant drugs, memory enhancement was greatest when epinephrine was administered shortly after training (**Figure 1**). Comparable effects were obtained in subsequent experiments using many different types of training tasks commonly used in experiments with rats and mice, including inhibitory avoidance, active avoidance, discrimination learning, and appetitively motivated tasks (Izquierdo and Dias, 1985; Sternberg et al., 1985; Introini-Collison and McGaugh, 1986; Liang et al., 1986; Costa-Miserachs et al., 1994). Additionally, numerous studies have shown that peripherally administered amphetamine, which increases the release of epinephrine from the adrenal medulla, also enhances memory consolidation when given shortly after training (Martinez et al., 1980).

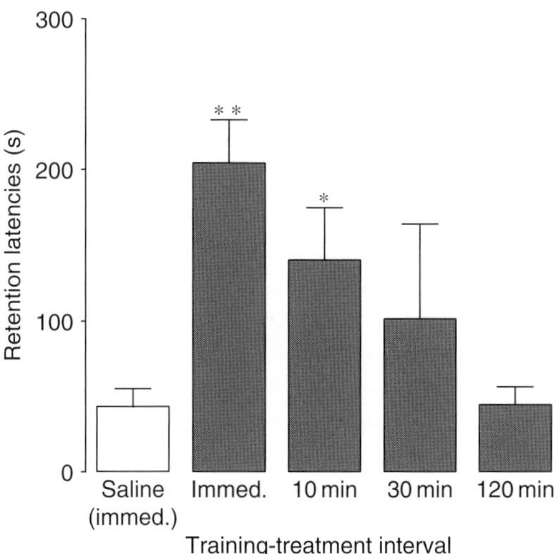

Figure 1 Posttraining systemic injection of epinephrine induces time-dependent memory enhancement. Epinephrine (0.1 mg/kg, ip) enhanced 24-h retention performance on an inhibitory avoidance task when injected either immediately or 10 min after training but was ineffective when given 30 or 120 min after training. Results represent retention latencies (mean + SEM) in seconds. *, $p < .05$; **, $p < .01$ as compared with the saline group. From Gold PE and van Buskirk R (1975) Facilitation of time-dependent memory processes with posttrial epinephrine injections. *Behav. Biol.* 13: 145–153.

Epinephrine effects on memory consolidation appear to be initiated, at least in part, by the activation of β-adrenoceptors located in the periphery, as this hormone does not readily cross the blood–brain barrier (Weil-Malherbe et al., 1959). Sotalol, a β-adrenoceptor antagonist that does not readily enter the brain, blocks the enhancing effects of peripherally administered epinephrine on memory for inhibitory avoidance training (Introini-Collison et al., 1992). Epinephrine effects are most likely mediated by activation of β adrenoceptors located on vagal afferents that project to the nucleus of the solitary tract (NTS) in the brain stem (Schreurs et al., 1986), which sends noradrenergic projections to forebrain regions involved in memory consolidation, including the amygdala (Ricardo and Koh, 1978). Furthermore, the NTS regulates noradrenergic activity of the forebrain via indirect projections to noradrenergic cell groups in the locus coeruleus (Williams and Clayton, 2001). Vagotomy attenuates the memory-enhancing effects induced by systemic administration of 4-OH-amphetamine, a peripherally acting derivative of amphetamine that induces epinephrine release (Williams and Jensen, 1991). The evidence that inactivation of the NTS with the sodium channel blocker lidocaine prevents epinephrine effects on memory consolidation, as well as the finding that the β-adrenoceptor agonist clenbuterol infused into the NTS posttraining enhances memory, very strongly suggests that epinephrine effects on memory consolidation are mediated via activation of the NTS (Williams and McGaugh, 1993). Additionally, the finding that, in rats as well as human subjects, posttraining electrical stimulation of vagal afferents enhances memory consolidation provides further evidence that projections mediated by the ascending vagus are involved in regulating memory consolidation (Clark et al., 1995, 1999; Ghacibeh et al., 2006).

Thus, the NTS appears to be an interface between peripheral adrenergic activation and brain processes regulating memory consolidation. However, posttraining peripheral administration of β-adrenoceptor agonists that are able to enter the brain, including dipivefrin and clenbuterol, also enhance memory consolidation. The memory enhancement induced by dipivefrin and clenbuterol is blocked by the β-adrenoceptor antagonist propranolol, which readily enters the brain, but not by the peripherally acting antagonist sotalol (Introini-Collison et al., 1992). Considered together, these findings indicate that the modulatory effects of epinephrine on memory consolidation are initiated by activation of peripheral β-adrenoceptors, but that memory consolidation is also modulated by direct activation of β-adrenoceptors within the brain. As discussed below, noradrenergic activation of the basolateral region of the amygdala (BLA), arising from noradrenergic cell groups in the NTS and locus coeruleus, is critically involved in mediating the effects of epinephrine, as well as those of many other neuromodulatory systems, on memory consolidation (Roozendaal, 2007).

Other findings suggest that epinephrine may also influence memory consolidation by enhancing glycogenolysis in the liver (Messier and White, 1984, 1987; Gold, 1995). Posttraining peripheral administration of glucose produces dose- and time-dependent effects on memory comparable to those produced by epinephrine (Gold, 1986). Additionally, doses of epinephrine and glucose that are optimal for enhancing retention induce comparable levels of plasma glucose (Hall and Gold, 1986). β-Adrenoceptor antagonists do not block glucose effects on memory (Gold et al., 1986). Glucose readily enters the brain and, thus, can directly influence brain glucoreceptors (Oomura et al., 1988). The finding that intracerebroventricular injections of glucose produce dose- and time-dependent enhancement of memory consolidation clearly suggests that peripherally administered glucose may affect memory by directly altering brain functioning (Lee et al., 1988). However, the finding that memory is also influenced by peripherally administered fructose, a sugar that has little influence on the brain, suggests that this sugar, as well as glucose, may also act, at least in part, at peripheral sites in influencing memory (Messier and White, 1987). In support of this view, Talley et al. (2002) showed that vagotomy blocks the memory-enhancing effects of peripherally administered L-glucose, an enantiomer of glucose that does not cross the blood–brain barrier.

27.3.2 Glucocorticoids

There is also extensive evidence that adrenocortical hormones are involved in modulating memory consolidation (for reviews, see de Kloet, 1991; Bohus, 1994; McEwen and Sapolsky, 1995; Lupien and McEwen, 1997; Roozendaal, 2000). As with epinephrine, posttraining injections of glucocorticoids produce dose- and time-dependent enhancement of memory (Cottrell and Nakajima, 1977; Sandi and Rose, 1994; Roozendaal and McGaugh, 1996a; Zorawski and Killcross, 2002; Okuda et al., 2004). However, in contrast to epinephrine, glucocorticoids are highly lipophylic and, thus, readily enter the brain and bind directly to mineralocorticoid receptors (MRs) and glucocorticoid receptors (GRs) (McEwen et al., 1968; de Kloet, 1991). These two receptor types differ in their affinity for corticosterone and synthetic ligands. MRs have a high affinity for the natural steroids corticosterone and aldosterone, whereas GRs have a high affinity for synthetic ligands such as dexamethasone and the GR agonist RU 28362 (Reul and de Kloet, 1985; Sutanto and de Kloet, 1987; Reul et al., 1990). As a consequence, MRs are mostly saturated during basal levels of corticosterone, whereas GRs become occupied by higher levels of corticosterone induced by stressful stimulation.

The memory-modulating effects of glucocorticoids released following arousing stimulation appear to involve the selective activation of the low-affinity GRs (Oitzl and de Kloet, 1992; Roozendaal et al., 1996b; Lupien and McEwen, 1997), as blockade of GRs, but not MRs, shortly before or immediately after training impairs long-term memory. Such findings provide strong support for the hypothesis that endogenously released glucocorticoids enhance memory consolidation. Glucocorticoids are known to act through intracellular and intranuclear receptors and can affect gene transcription either by direct binding of receptor homodimers to DNA (Beato et al., 1995; Datson et al., 2001) or via protein–protein interactions with other transcription factors such as Jun or Fos (Heck et al., 1994). However, as discussed later, glucocorticoids may also act more rapidly by interacting with membrane receptors and/or potentiating the efficacy of the norepinephrine signal cascade via an interaction with G-protein-mediated actions (Roozendaal et al., 2002b).

27.3.3 Adrenergic-Glucocorticoid Interactions

Evidence from several kinds of studies indicates that catecholamines and glucocorticoids released from the adrenal glands interact in influencing memory consolidation. Glucocorticoids alter the sensitivity of epinephrine in influencing memory consolidation in adrenalectomized rats (Borrell et al., 1983, 1984). Further, in adrenally intact rats, administration of meytrapone, a corticosterone-synthesis inhibitor that reduces the elevation of circulating corticosterone induced by aversive stimulation, attenuates the memory-enhancing effects of epinephrine administered posttraining (Roozendaal et al., 1996a). Such findings suggest that synergistic actions of epinephrine and corticosterone may be essential in mediating stress effects on memory enhancement.

The studies cited above used emotionally arousing footshock training, conditions that induce the release of both corticosterone and epinephrine. Studies using an object recognition task investigated whether adrenergic activation induced by emotional arousal is essential in enabling corticosterone effects on memory consolidation (Okuda et al., 2004). Rats were given either extensive habituation to an apparatus or no prior habituation and were then allowed to explore objects in the apparatus. Placing rats in a novel testing apparatus evokes novelty-induced arousal, and habituation of rats to the apparatus is known to reduce this arousal response (de Boer et al., 1990). Corticosterone administered immediately posttraining to nonhabituated (i.e., emotionally aroused) rats enhanced their 24-h retention performance. In contrast, posttraining corticosterone did not enhance retention of object recognition in habituated rats (Okuda et al., 2004), providing evidence that training-associated emotional arousal may be essential for enabling glucocorticoid effects on memory consolidation. Other findings indicated that training-induced adrenergic activation is a critical component of emotional arousal in enabling glucocorticoid effects on memory consolidation. As is shown in **Figure 2**, the β-adrenoceptor antagonist propranolol, coadministered with the corticosterone immediately after the object recognition training, blocked the corticosterone-induced memory enhancement (Roozendaal et al., 2006b). To investigate whether a pharmacologically induced increase in adrenergic activity enables glucocorticoid effects on memory consolidation, a low dose of the α_2-adrenoceptor antagonist yohimbine was administered to well-habituated (i.e., nonaroused) rats immediately after object recognition training. Corticosterone administered together with yohimbine induced dose-dependent enhancement of memory consolidation (Roozendaal et al., 2006b). Posttraining injections of corticosterone and yohimbine separated by a 4-h delay did not enhance memory consolidation. These findings are thus consistent with the hypothesis that adrenergic activation is essential in enabling glucocorticoid enhancement of memory consolidation. The nature of this interaction is discussed in more detail later.

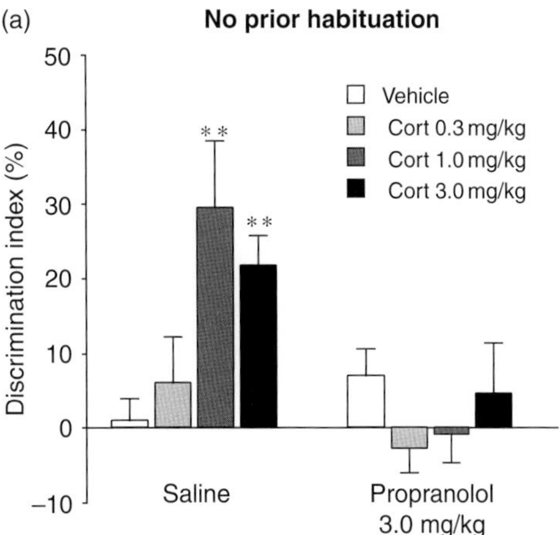

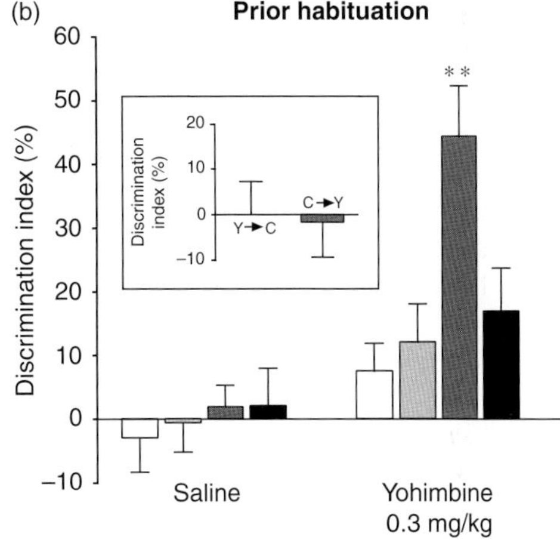

Figure 2 Glucocorticoid effects on memory consolidation for object recognition training require adrenergic activation. (a) Immediate posttraining administration of the β-adrenoceptor antagonist propranolol (3.0 mg/kg, sc) blocked the corticosterone-induced enhancement of object recognition memory in naïve rats. (b) The α_2-adrenoceptor antagonist yohimbine (0.3 mg/kg, sc) enabled a corticosterone effect on object recognition memory in habituated rats. Inset: Posttraining injections of yohimbine (0.3 mg/kg, sc) and corticosterone (1.0 mg/kg, sc) separated by a 4-h delay did not induce memory enhancement. Y → C; Yohimbine administered immediately after training and corticosterone 4 h later; C → Y; corticosterone administered immediately after training and yohimbine 4 h later. Results represent discrimination index (mean ± SEM) in percentage on a 24-h retention trial. $**$, $p < .01$, as compared with the corresponding vehicle group. From Roozendaal B, Okuda S, Van der Zee EA, and McGaugh JL (2006b) Glucocorticoid enhancement of memory requires arousal-induced noradrenergic activation in the basolateral amygdala. *Proc. Natl. Acad. Sci. USA* 103: 6741–6746.

27.3.4 Other Neuromodulatory Systems

As discussed earlier in this chapter, drugs affecting many other neuromodulatory and transmitter systems also influence memory consolidation. The dose- and time-dependent enhancement of memory induced by the stimulant drugs known to act via GABA (picrotoxin, bicuculline) and catecholamines (amphetamine, clenbuterol) has also been obtained in studies investigating the effects of opiate receptor antagonists (Messing et al., 1979; Introini and Baratti, 1984) and muscarinic cholinergic receptor agonists (Stratton and Petrinovich, 1963; Flood et al., 1981; Baratti et al., 1984; Introini-Collison and McGaugh, 1988; Power et al., 2003b), as well as drugs and hormones affecting several other systems, including corticotropin-releasing hormone (Roozendaal et al., 2002a), adrenocorticotropin (Gold and van Buskirk, 1976), vasopressin (de Wied, 1984), oxytocin (Bohus, 1980), substance P (Huston and Staubli, 1981; Schlesinger et al., 1986), histamine (Passani et al., 2001; da Silva et al., 2006), and cholecystokinin (Flood et al., 1987). Additionally, many studies have investigated interactions of these systems in modulating memory consolidation (McGaugh, 1989; McGaugh and Gold, 1989).

As is discussed below, the effects of many neuromodulatory systems are mediated by interactions with noradrenergic and muscarinic cholinergic systems within the amygdala. The initial research investigating such interactions investigated the effects of peripherally administered drugs and hormones (McGaugh and Cahill, 1997). Considerable evidence indicates that opiate and GABAergic influences on memory consolidation are mediated via adrenergic influences. The finding that the β-adrenoceptor antagonist propranolol blocks the memory-enhancing effects of the opiate receptor antagonist naloxone (Izquierdo and Graudenz, 1980) is consistent with evidence that opiates regulate the release of norepinephrine in the brain (Arbilla and Langer, 1978; Nakamura et al., 1982). Further, the β-adrenoceptor agonist clenbuterol blocks the memory impairment induced by the GABAergic agonist muscimol (Introini-Collison et al., 1994). As discussed below, such findings are consistent with the hypothesis that opioids and GABA impair memory by decreasing norepinephrine release in the brain (Quirarte et al., 1998; Hatfield et al., 1999). Thus, noradrenergic activation appears to be critical for opioid peptidergic and GABAergic influences on memory consolidation.

In contrast to the effects of opioid peptidergic and GABAergic drugs, cholinergic effects do not appear to be mediated by adrenergic activation. However, there is extensive evidence that muscarinic activity is a requirement for norepinephrine-induced memory enhancement. Systemic injections of the muscarinic cholinergic receptor antagonist atropine attenuate the memory-enhancing effects of the β-adrenoceptor agonist clenbuterol as well as that of epinephrine (Introini-Collison and McGaugh, 1988; Introini-Collison and Baratti, 1992). Thus, cholinergic activation appears to provide modulatory influences on memory consolidation that are downstream from adrenergic activation.

27.4 Involvement of the Amygdala in Modulating Memory Consolidation

Goddard's (1964) finding that electrical stimulation of the amygdala administered shortly after rats were trained on an aversively motivated task impaired their memory of the training was the first to suggest that the amygdala plays a role in influencing memory consolidation. The conclusion that the amygdala stimulation disrupted the consolidation of the memory of the training was confirmed by many subsequent findings from other laboratories (Kesner and Wilburn, 1974; McGaugh and Gold, 1976). One possible interpretation of these findings is that the stimulation disrupted the consolidation of memory processes occurring within the amygdala. However, many subsequent findings have indicated that amygdala stimulation modulates memory consolidation via influences mediated by amygdala efferent projections to other brain regions. The finding that posttraining electrical stimulation of the amygdala can either enhance or impair memory, depending on the stimulation intensity and the training conditions (Gold et al., 1975), clearly indicates that the effects are modulatory and not simply memory impairing. Further, the evidence that lesions of the stria terminalis (a major amygdala pathway) block the memory-impairing effects of posttraining electrical stimulation (Liang and McGaugh, 1983) strongly suggested that the modulation involves amygdala projections to other brain regions (see following).

27.4.1 Noradrenergic Influences in the BLA

Experiments by Kesner and Ellis (Ellis and Kesner, 1981; Kesner and Ellis, 1983) and Gallagher et al.

(1981) were the first to use posttraining drug infusions to investigate the involvement of neuromodulatory systems in the amygdala in memory consolidation. β-Adrenoceptor antagonists infused into the amygdala impaired rats' retention of inhibitory avoidance, and concurrent infusion of norepinephrine blocked the memory impairment (Gallagher et al., 1981). These investigators also found that, as is found with systemic administration (Messing et al., 1979; Izquierdo and Graudenz, 1980), posttraining intra-amygdala infusions of opioid peptidergic agonists and antagonists impaired and enhanced memory, respectively. The findings of more recent studies indicate that the BLA is selectively involved in such amygdala memory modulatory influences. The adjacent central nucleus does not appear to play a significant role, if any, in modulating memory consolidation (Tomaz et al., 1992; Parent and McGaugh, 1994; Roozendaal and McGaugh, 1996a, 1997a; DaCunha et al., 1999; McGaugh et al., 2000). Thus, the effects of relatively large intraamygdala drug infusion volumes typically used in most early studies as well as many recent studies are likely the result of selective influences on BLA activity. Moreover, findings of more recent studies indicating that posttraining intraamygdala infusions of drugs influence retention performance tested 24 h or longer after the training but do not affect performance tested within a few hours after training, provide strong evidence that the treatments selectively affect the consolidation of long-term memory (Bianchin et al., 1999; Schafe and LeDoux, 2000; Barros et al., 2002).

Other early findings also implicated the amygdala in adrenergic influences on memory consolidation. Adrenal demedullation or posttraining administration of epinephrine alter the memory-modulating effects of electrical stimulation of the amygdala (Liang et al., 1985), and lesions of either the amygdala or the stria terminalis block epinephrine effects on memory consolidation (Cahill and McGaugh, 1991; Liang and McGaugh, 1983). Although earlier studies reported evidence suggesting that epinephrine induces the release of norepinephrine in the brain (Gold and van Buskirk, 1978), the finding that posttraining intraamygdala infusions of the β-adrenoceptor antagonist propranolol block epinephrine effects on memory consolidation (Liang et al., 1986) provided the first evidence suggesting that epinephrine effects on memory are mediated by noradrenergic activation within the amygdala. In support of this implication, many subsequent studies reported that posttraining infusions of norepinephrine or the β-adrenoceptor agonist clenbuterol into the amygdala (or selectively into the BLA) produce dose-dependent enhancement of memory consolidation (Liang et al., 1986, 1990, 1995; Introini-Collison et al., 1991, 1996; Izquierdo et al., 1992; Bianchin et al., 1999; Ferry and McGaugh, 1999; Hatfield and McGaugh, 1999; LaLumiere et al., 2003, 2005; Huff et al., 2005). Furthermore, posttraining intra-amygdala infusions of β-adrenoceptor antagonists impair retention and block the memory-enhancing effects of norepinephrine coadministered (Liang et al., 1986, 1995; Salinas and McGaugh, 1995).

In addition to β-adrenoceptor influences, α-adrenoceptor activation in the BLA also modulates memory consolidation. Intra-BLA infusions of the α_1-adrenoceptor antagonist prazosin impair inhibitory avoidance memory, whereas infusions of the nonselective α-adrenoceptor agonist phenylephrine, administered together with yohimbine, an α_2-adrenoceptor antagonist, enhance retention (Ferry et al., 1999a). The α_1-adrenoceptor-induced memory enhancement most likely involves an interaction with β-adrenoceptors, as posttraining intra-BLA infusions of the β-adrenoceptor antagonist atenolol block the memory enhancement produced by activation of α_1-adrenoceptors. The finding that posttraining intraamygdala infusions of the synthetic cyclic adenosine monophosphate (cAMP) analog 8-bromo-cAMP enhance retention (Liang et al., 1995) is consistent with the hypothesis that activation of β-adrenoceptors modulates memory via a direct coupling to adenylate cyclase. Thus, the finding that intra-BLA infusions of the α_1-adrenoceptor antagonist prazosin do not prevent the memory enhancement induced by concurrently infused 8-bromo-cAMP suggests that the memory-enhancing effects of α_1-adrenoceptor activation are mediated by an interaction with β-adrenoceptors upstream from cAMP, probably at the G-protein level (Ferry et al., 1999b).

There is extensive evidence indicating that noradrenergic activity within the BLA also plays an important role in mediating the modulatory effects of other hormones and neurotransmitters on memory consolidation (Roozendaal, 2007). Many studies have reported that, as with peripherally administered drugs, intra-BLA infusions of the GABAergic receptor antagonists bicuculline and picrotoxin enhance memory consolidation and that GABAergic receptor agonists impair memory (e.g., Brioni et al., 1989; Izquierdo et al., 1992; Bianchin et al., 1999; Wilensky et al., 2000; Huff et al., 2005). Similarly, the opioid peptidergic antagonist naloxone enhances memory when infused into the amygdala posttraining, whereas opioid peptidergic agonists impair memory consolidation (McGaugh et al., 1988; Introini-Collison et al., 1989). Consistent with the evidence from studies using peripheral drug administration, β-adrenoceptor antagonists infused into the amygdala block the memory-enhancing effects of bicuculline or naloxone infused concurrently (McGaugh et al., 1988, 1990; Introini-Collison et al., 1989). In contrast, intraamygdala injections of α_1- or α_2-adrenoceptor antagonists do not block naloxone effects on memory consolidation (McGaugh et al., 1988). Thus, as was found with peripherally administered drugs, GABAergic and opioid peptidergic influences within the BLA appear to modulate memory consolidation by influencing β-adrenoceptor activation via influences on the release of norepinephrine. Ragozino and Gold (1994) reported that posttraining intraamygdala infusions of glucose block the memory impairment induced by the opiate drug morphine. However, such glucose infusions do not attenuate the memory impairment induced by propranolol (Lennartz et al., 1996; McNay and Gold, 1998). Thus, glucose effects do not appear to act via adrenergic activation within the amygdala.

Other recent studies reported that β-adrenoceptor activation within the BLA is also required for mediating the memory-modulatory effects of corticotropin-releasing hormone (CRH) and orphanin FQ/nociceptin (OFQ/N), a recently discovered opioid-like peptide. Retention is enhanced by posttraining intra-BLA infusions of CRH (Liang and Lee, 1988) and impaired by a CRH receptor antagonist (Roozendaal et al., 2002a). Unlike CRH, posttraining intra-BLA infusions of OFQ/N impair retention, and an OFQ/N receptor antagonist enhances retention (Roozendaal et al., 2007). Atenolol infused into the BLA blocks the memory-enhancing effect of CRH and the OFQ/N antagonist, whereas it potentiates the memory-impairing effect of OFQ/N administered concurrently (Roozendaal et al., 2007). These findings thus indicate that, as with many other neuromodulatory systems, endogenously released CRH and OFQ/N interact with noradrenergic activity within the BLA in modulating memory consolidation. Similar findings were obtained in studies of the effects of dopamine. Posttraining intra-BLA infusions of dopamine induce dose-dependent memory enhancement that is blocked by coinfusion of a β-adrenoceptor antagonist as well as D1 or D2 receptor antagonists (LaLumiere et al., 2004). However, noradrenergic activation within the BLA affecting memory also appears to require concurrent interaction with dopamine receptors, as dopamine receptor antagonists block the memory-enhancing effects of posttraining intra-BLA infusions of clenbuterol (LaLumiere et al., 2004).

The extensive evidence indicating that adrenoceptor activation within the amygdala is critical for the modulation of memory consolidation suggests that emotionally arousing learning experiences should induce the release of norepinephrine within the amygdala and that drugs and hormones that enhance memory consolidation should increase the release. Findings of studies using *in vivo* microdialysis and high-performance liquid chromatography to measure ongoing changes in norepinephrine levels in the amygdala strongly support these implications. As is shown in **Table 1**, footshock comparable to that typically used in inhibitory avoidance training significantly increases amygdala norepinephrine levels (Galvez et al., 1996; Quirarte et al., 1998). Moreover, drugs and hormones that enhance memory consolidation (e.g., epinephrine, picrotoxin, and naloxone) potentiate footshock-induced increases in norepinephrine levels in the

Table 1 Treatment effects on memory and amygdala norepinephrine levels

Treatment	*Effect on memory*	*Effect on amygdala norepinephrine levels*	*Reference*
Footshock	Varies directly with footshock intensity	Varies with footshock intensity	Quirarte et al. 1998
Epinephrine	Enhances	Increases	Williams et al. 1998
Corticosterone	Enhances	Increases	McIntyre et al. 2004
Muscimol	Impairs	Decreases	Hatfield et al. 1999
Picrotoxin	Enhances	Increases	Hatfield et al. 1999
β-endorphin	Impairs	Decreases	Quirarte et al. 1998
Naloxone	Enhances	Increases	Quirarte et al. 1998
Orphanin FQ/nociceptin	Impairs	Decreases	Kawahara et al. 2004

amygdala, and drugs that impair consolidation (e.g., muscimol, β-endorphin, and OFQ/N) decrease amygdala norepinephrine levels (Quirarte et al., 1998; Williams et al., 1998; Hatfield et al. 1999; Kawahara et al., 2004). Additionally, stimulation of the vagus nerve or the NTS increases norepinephrine levels in the amygdala and enhances memory consolidation (Clayton and Williams, 2000; Hassert et al., 2004). McIntyre et al. (2002) investigated norepinephrine levels in the amygdala induced by inhibitory avoidance training. Consistent with findings of previous studies using footshock (Galvez et al., 1996; Quirarte et al., 1998; Hatfield et al., 1999), norepinephrine levels increased following the training. However, the duration of the increased norepinephrine levels seen after training was greater than that previously found with footshock stimulation alone (i.e., without training). Additionally, and importantly, the increase in norepinephrine levels assessed in individual animals over an interval of 90 min after training correlated highly with their subsequent retention performance, tested the following day (**Figure 3**).

27.4.2 Glucocorticoid Influences in the BLA

There is extensive evidence that glucocorticoids affect memory consolidation through influences involving the BLA. The findings of studies of the effects of glucocorticoids on memory for inhibitory avoidance training are similar to those of studies of the effects of epinephrine. Lesions of the BLA or stria terminalis block the memory-enhancing effects of posttraining systemic injections of the synthetic glucocorticoid dexamethasone (Roozendaal and McGaugh, 1996a,b). Furthermore, memory is modulated by either systemic or intra-BLA infusions of glucocorticoids (Roozendaal and McGaugh, 1996a, 1997a), and like the effects of epinephrine, such modulation requires noradrenergic activation within the amygdala. Intra-BLA infusions of a β-adrenoceptor antagonist block the memory-enhancing effects of systemic injections of dexamethasone or corticosterone, as well as the effects of the GR agonist RU 28362 infused into the BLA concurrently (Quirarte et al., 1997; Roozendaal et al., 2002b, 2006a,b).

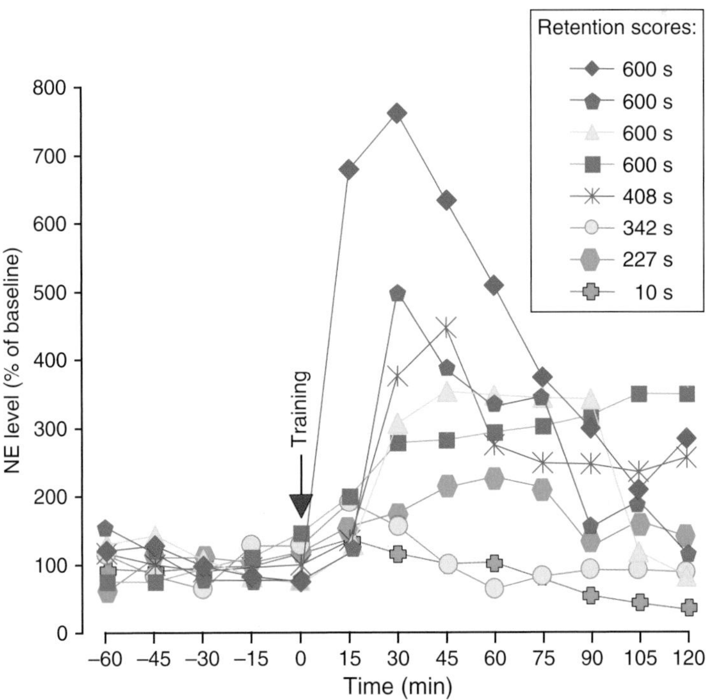

Figure 3 Norepinephrine levels in the amygdala in individual animals following inhibitory avoidance training. Percent of baseline norepinephrine following inhibitory avoidance training is graphed for each individual rat. The key notes retention score on the following day. Amygdala norepinephrine levels correlate with 24-h retention performance. Correlation values for the first five posttraining samples varied from +0.75 to +0.92. From McIntyre CK, Hatfield T, and McGaugh JL (2002) Amygdala norepinephrine levels after training predict inhibitory avoidance retention performance in rats. *Eur. J. Neurosci.* 16: 1223–1226.

As discussed above, studies investigating the effects of glucocorticoids administered systemically after object recognition training found that, in naïve (i.e., emotionally aroused) rats, propranolol blocked the memory enhancement induced by corticosterone and that, in habituated (i.e., emotionally less aroused) rats, corticosterone enhanced memory only when norepinephrine release was stimulated by yohimbine (Roozendaal et al., 2006b). A subsequent experiment (Roozendaal et al., 2006b) found that, in naive rats, intra-BLA infusions of a β-adrenoceptor antagonist blocked the effects of systemically administered corticosterone on object recognition memory. Further, in habituated rats, corticosterone activated BLA neurons, as assessed by phosphorylated cAMP response-element binding (pCREB) immunoreactivity levels, only in animals also given yohimbine. Considered together, these findings provide strong evidence that the BLA is a critical locus of the synergistic actions of glucocorticoids and emotional arousal-induced noradrenergic activation in influencing memory consolidation.

Findings of studies investigating the mechanism of glucocorticoid interactions with the noradrenergic system suggest that activation of GRs in the BLA may facilitate memory consolidation by potentiating the norepinephrine signaling cascade through an interaction with G-protein-mediated effects. The enhancement of memory for inhibitory avoidance training induced by posttraining intra-BLA infusions of the GR agonist RU 28362 is blocked by concurrent infusion of Rp-cAMPs, a drug that inhibits protein kinase A activity and thus blocks the norepinephrine signaling cascade (Roozendaal et al., 2002b). Moreover, intra-BLA infusions of the GR antagonist RU 38486 attenuate the memory-enhancing effects of the β-adrenoceptor agonist clenbuterol infused concurrently such that a much higher dose of clenbuterol (100 ng vs. 1 ng) is required to induce memory enhancement (Roozendaal et al., 2002b).

As was found with epinephrine, glucocorticoid effects on memory consolidation also appear to involve brain stem nuclei, including the NTS, that send noradrenergic projections to the BLA. A GR antagonist infused into the NTS attenuates the memory-enhancing effects of systemically administered dexamethasone (Roozendaal et al., 1999b). Moreover, the finding that posttraining infusions of RU 28362 into the NTS enhance inhibitory avoidance retention and that intra-BLA infusions of a β-adrenoceptor antagonist block the enhancement (Roozendaal et al., 1999b) provides additional evidence that the NTS influence on memory consolidation involves noradrenergic activation of the BLA (Williams et al., 1998, 2000; Clayton and Williams, 2000; Miyashita and Williams 2002).

27.4.3 Cholinergic Influences in the BLA

The finding that stria terminalis lesions block the memory-enhancing effect of systemically administered cholinergic drugs (Introini-Collison et al., 1989) provided the first evidence suggesting that muscarinic cholinergic influences within the amygdala may be involved in regulating memory consolidation. Subsequent studies have provided extensive evidence that posttraining intraamygdala infusions of muscarinic cholinergic receptor agonists and antagonists enhance and impair, respectively, memory for many kinds of training, including inhibitory avoidance, Pavlovian fear conditioning, conditioned place preference, and change in reward magnitude (Introini-Collison et al., 1996; Vazdarjanova and McGaugh, 1999; Salinas et al., 1997; Passani et al., 2001; Power and McGaugh, 2002; Schroeder and Packard, 2002; Power et al., 2003a,b; LaLumiere et al., 2004). Results of experiments using posttraining infusions of the muscarinic cholinergic receptor agonist oxotremorine administered together with selective antagonists indicate that both M1 and M2 muscarinic cholinergic receptor types are involved in the memory-enhancing effects of cholinergic activation (Power et al., 2003a). The finding that lesions of the nucleus basalis, the major source of cholinergic innervation of the BLA, impair inhibitory avoidance retention and that posttraining intra-BLA infusions of either oxotremorine or the acetylcholinesterase inhibitor physostigmine attenuate the memory impairment provided additional evidence that cholinergic activation within the BLA regulates memory consolidation (Power and McGaugh, 2002).

As noted above, in contrast to the effects of GABAergic and opioid peptidergic drugs, cholinergic effects on memory consolidation do not require concurrent noradrenergic activation. A β-adrenoceptor antagonist does not block the memory-enhancing effect of intraamygdala infusions of oxotremorine. However, a low and otherwise ineffective dose of the muscarinic cholinergic receptor antagonist atropine blocks the memory enhancement induced by intraamygdala infusions of clenbuterol (Dalmaz et al., 1993; Salinas et al., 1997). Thus, cholinergic activation in the BLA appears to act downstream from adrenergic activation in modulating memory consolidation. Other findings indicate that cholinergic activation within the BLA is critical for enabling glucocorticoid as well as dopamine enhancement of memory consolidation. Atropine infused into the BLA blocks the memory-enhancing effects of RU 28362 or dopamine infused concurrently as well as the effects of systemically administered dexamethasone (Power et al., 2000; LaLumiere et al., 2004). Conversely, cholinergic activation within the BLA affecting memory also appears to require concurrent interaction with dopamine, as dopamine receptor antagonists block the memory-enhancing effects of posttraining intra-BLA infusions of oxotremorine (LaLumiere et al., 2004).

Studies of the effects of histamine receptor antagonists and agonists infused into the BLA provide additional evidence of a role of acetylcholine in the BLA in modulating consolidation (Passini et al., 2001). H_3 receptor antagonists (ciproxifan, clobenprobit, or thioperamide) infused into the BLA decrease acetylcholine release, as assessed by *in vivo* microdialysis, and concurrent infusions of the H_2 receptor agonist cimetidine block the decreased acetylcholine release. Moreover, posttraining intra-BLA infusions of H_3 receptor antagonists, administered in doses found to decrease acetylcholine release, impair memory for contextual fear conditioning (Passani et al., 2001). As other studies have reported that posttraining systemically administered H_3 receptor antagonists enhance memory and block memory impairment induced by a muscarinic cholinergic antagonist (Bernaerts et al., 2004), it seems likely that the central and peripheral actions of H_3 receptor antagonists involve different actions. There is also evidence that acetylcholine is released within the amygdala during training. Studies using *in vivo* microdialysis have shown that acetylcholine levels in the amygdala increase while rats perform a spontaneous alternation task and that the increase is correlated with performance on the task (Gold, 2003; McIntyre et al., 2003). As this task is known to involve hippocampal functioning, these findings are consistent with other evidence, discussed below, suggesting that the amygdala influences memory processing that involves the hippocampus. **Figure 4** summarizes some of the neuromodulatory interactions within the BLA involved in regulating memory consolidation.

27.4.4 Other Neuromodulatory Influences in the BLA

The BLA is also involved in mediating the modulatory effects of other hormones and neurotransmitters on memory consolidation. For example, a recent study reported not only that the reproductive hormone relaxin binds to specific receptors in hypothalamic regions to regulate reproductive behaviors but also that posttraining intra-BLA infusions of relaxin also induce dose-dependent impairment of inhibitory avoidance memory (Ma et al., 2005). Other recent studies implicated the amygdala in the memory-modulatory effects of bombesin (gastrin-releasing peptide). Posttraining intra-BLA infusions of the bombesin receptor antagonist RC-3095 impair memory of inhibitory avoidance (Roesler et al., 2004b), whereas temporary inactivation of the BLA blocked the memory-modulatory effects of systemically administered bombesin or its antagonist (Rashidy Pour and Razvani, 1998; Roesler et al., 2004b). Furthermore, the finding that bombesin infused into the NTS also modulates memory consolidation (Williams and McGaugh, 1994) and that inactivation of the NTS blocks the effects of peripherally administered bombesin (Rashidy-Pour and Razvani, 1998) suggests that noradrenergic activity may be essential in mediating the effects of bombesin on memory consolidation. This suggestion is supported by the evidence that the bombesin receptor antagonist selectively impaired memory consolidation of aversively motivated inhibitory avoidance training and not that of emotionally less arousing object recognition training (Roesler et al., 2004a), which, as discussed above, induces less noradrenergic activation of the BLA.

27.5 Involvement of the Amygdala in Modulating Memory Extinction

Several studies have investigated whether extinction learning (i.e., learning that cues that previously predicted aversive or appetitive consequences no longer predict such consequences) is regulated by the same neuromodulatory systems that regulated the original learning. An early study found that posttraining peripheral administration of picrotoxin enhances the extinction of cued fear conditioning (McGaugh et al., 1990). Experiments using intra-BLA infusions have found that the GABAergic antagonist bicuculline and norepinephrine administered posttraining enhance extinction of contextual fear conditioning (Berlau and McGaugh, 2006). If such extinction involves the same processes engaged by fear conditioning, the effects of bicuculline would be expected to require β-adrenoceptor activation. Consistent with

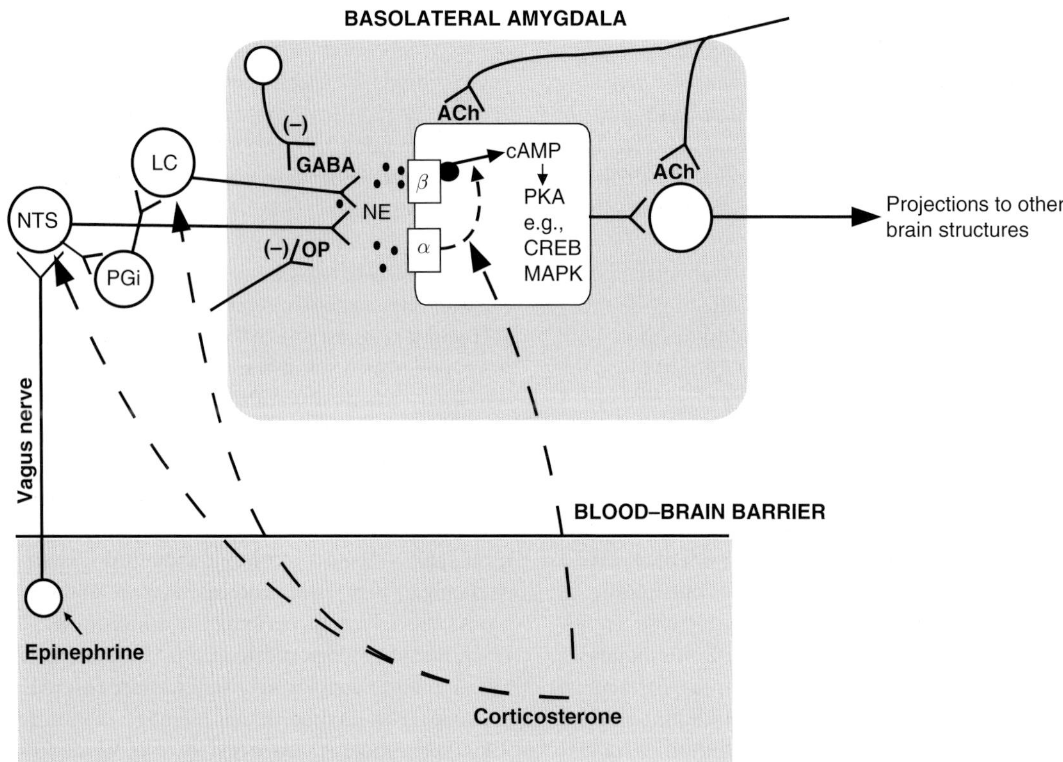

Figure 4 Schematic summarizing the role of the noradrenergic system of the basolateral amygdala in memory consolidation. Norepinephrine (NE) is released in the basolateral amygdala following training in aversively motivated tasks and binds to both β-adrenoceptors and α_1-adrenoceptors at postsynaptic sites. The β-adrenoceptor is coupled directly to adenylate cyclase to stimulate cAMP formation. The α_1-adrenoceptor modulates the response induced by β-adrenoceptor stimulation. Intracellular cAMP can initiate a cascade of molecular events in the basolateral amygdala. The memory-modulatory effects of several other neuromodulatory influences, including that of epinephrine, glucocorticoid, opioid peptidergic, and GABAergic systems, are mediated by converging influences on the noradrenergic system of the basolateral amygdala. Drug interactions with the noradrenergic system can occur at both presynaptic and postsynaptic loci. These noradrenergic effects in the basolateral amygdala are required for regulating memory consolidation in other brain regions. α, α_1-adrenoceptor; ACh, acetylcholine; β, β-adrenoceptor; cAMP, adenosine 3′,5′-cyclic monophosphate; CREB, cAMP-response element-binding protein; GABA, gamma-aminobutyric acid; LC, locus coeruleus; MAPK, mitogen-activated protein kinase, NTS, nucleus of the solitary tract; OP, opioid peptide; PGi, nucleus paragigantocellularis; PKA, protein kinase A. From McGaugh JL (2000) Memory: A century of consolidation. *Science* 287: 248–251, and Roozendaal B (2000) Glucocorticoids and the regulation of memory consolidation. *Psychoneuroendocrinology* 25: 213–238.

that implication, posttraining infusions of bicuculline did not enhance extinction memory consolidation when infused into the BLA together with a low and otherwise ineffective dose of propranolol. Additionally, the GABAergic agonist muscimol coinfused into the BLA with norepinephrine posttraining did not block the memory enhancement induced by norepinephrine. These findings are consistent with the evidence discussed above indicating that norepinephrine effects in the BLA act downstream from GABAergic influences (Introini-Collison et al., 1994; McGaugh and Cahill, 1997). Other studies have reported that extinction of fear conditioning is enhanced by pre- or postextinction infusions of the *N*-methyl-D-aspartate (NMDA) partial agonist d-cycloserine (Walker et al., 2002; Ledgerwood et al., 2003, 2005). Furthermore, intra-BLA infusions of d-cycloserine block the impairing effects of concurrent administration of the GABAergic agonist muscimol on the consolidation of extinction memory (Akirav, 2007). Consistent with extensive evidence of glucococorticoid enhancement of consolidation of memory of fear-based training, dexamethasone administered systemically after extinction training or intra-amygdally prior to extinction also enhanced extinction of fear-potentiated startle (Yang et al., 2006). Furthermore, corticosterone given systemically immediately after retention testing on a contextual fear conditioning task facilitated extinction of this memory (Cai et al., 2006). Other studies have reported that the BLA modulates the extinction of conditioned place preference. Glucose or oxotremorine infused into the BLA immediately after extinction training enhanced the extinction of amphetamine-induced place preference (Schroeder and Packard, 2003, 2004).

27.6 Amygdala Interactions with Other Brain Systems in Modulating Memory

Although many of the experiments investigating BLA involvement in memory consolidation have used inhibitory avoidance training and testing (Parent and McGaugh, 1994; Izquierdo et al., 1997; McGaugh et al., 2000; McGaugh and Izquierdo, 2000; Wilensky et al., 2000), comparable effects of posttraining amygdala treatments have been obtained in experiments using many different kinds of training tasks, including contextual fear conditioning (Sacchetti et al., 1999; Vazdarjanova and McGaugh, 1999; LaLumiere et al., 2003), cued fear conditioning (Sacchetti et al., 1999; Schafe and LeDoux, 2000; Roozendaal et al., 2006a), Y-maze discrimination training (McGaugh et al., 1988), change in reward magnitude (Salinas et al., 1997), conditioned place preference (Hsu et al., 2002; Schroeder and Packard, 2003, 2004), radial-arm maze appetitive training (Packard and Chen, 1999), water-maze spatial and cued training (Packard et al., 1994; Packard and Teather, 1998), conditioned taste aversion (Miranda et al., 2003), olfactory training (Kilpatrick and Cahill, 2003a), object recognition (Roozendaal et al., 2006b), extinction of contextual fear conditioning (Berlau and McGaugh, 2006), and extinction of conditioned reward (Schroeder and Packard, 2003). Thus, although there is abundant evidence that the BLA is involved in modulating memory of aversively motivated training, such as footshock training used in inhibitory avoidance and Pavlovian fear conditioning, the evidence also clearly indicates that the BLA modulates the consolidation of memory for many different kinds of training experiences (McGaugh, 2002; Packard and Cahill, 2001), and as these different training experiences are known to engage different brain systems both during training and during the consolidation occurring after training (Quillfeldt et al., 1996; Zanatta et al., 1996; Izquierdo et al., 1997; Packard and Knowlton, 2002; Gold, 2004), the BLA-induced modulation no doubt involves influences on processing occurring in these other brain regions.

As discussed above, there is considerable evidence that neuromodulatory interactions occurring within the amygdala influence memory consolidation. Such influences may be, at least in part, a result of influences on neuroplasticity within the amygdala. However, several kinds of evidence suggest that alterations in amygdala functioning affect memory consolidation through amygdala influences on other brain regions involved in memory consolidation. The BLA sends projections to many other brain regions, some via the stria terminalis (Young, 1993; Pitkänen, 2000; Petrovich et al., 2001; Price, 2003; Sah et al., 2003). The evidence, discussed above, that stria terminalis lesions block the memory-modulating effects of electrical stimulation and intraamygdala drug infusions strongly suggests that modulation within the amygdala is not sufficient to affect memory: efferent projections seem required. The evidence that posttraining BLA treatments affect memory for many kinds of training clearly suggests that processing in different brain regions is required. This implication is supported by the finding that training known to involve the amygdala (e.g., Pavlovian fear conditioning) induces the expression of several transcriptionally regulated genes implicated in synaptic plasticity in many brain areas, including the hippocampus, striatum, and cortex, as well as the amygdala (Ressler et al., 2002). These effects appear to be involved in memory consolidation and not simply a result of nonspecific effects of stress or arousal, as they were found only when the stimuli used in the training-induced learning. The findings of the many types of studies discussed later provide compelling evidence that the amygdala interacts with other brain regions in modulating the consolidation of memory for different kinds of training.

27.6.1 BLA Interactions with the Caudate Nucleus, Hippocampus, and Nucleus Accumbens

The amygdala projects directly to the caudate nucleus (via the stria terminalis) and both directly and indirectly to the hippocampus (Pitkänen, 2000; Petrovich et al., 2001). The evidence that stria terminalis lesions block the memory-enhancing effects of oxotremorine that was infused posttraining into the caudate nucleus suggests that efferents from the amygdala influence memory processing involving the caudate nucleus (Packard et al., 1996). There is considerable evidence that the caudate nucleus and hippocampus are involved in different kinds of learning (e.g., Packard and McGaugh, 1992, 1996; McDonald and White, 1993; Packard and Cahill, 2001). In studies of rats given water-maze training, Packard and colleagues (Packard et al., 1994; Packard and Teather, 1998) found that amphetamine that was infused posttraining into the caudate nucleus selectively enhanced memory of visually cued training, whereas infusions administered into the dorsal hippocampus selectively enhanced memory of spatial training. In contrast, amphetamine infused into the amygdala posttraining enhanced memory for both types of training. Additionally, inactivation of the hippocampus (with lidocaine) prior to testing blocked retention of the spatial training, and inactivation of the caudate nucleus blocked retention of the visually cued training. But importantly, inactivation of the amygdala prior to retention testing did not block memory of either kind of training. Thus, although the amygdala modulates the consolidation of both caudate nucleus-dependent and hippocampus-dependent tasks, such findings suggest that it is not a locus of memory for either type of training. Additionally, in rats trained in a radial-arm maze spatial task, lidocaine infused into the amygdala blocked the memory enhancement induced by posttraining intrahippocampal infusions of glutamate (Packard and Chen, 1999). Such findings are consistent with extensive evidence that the hippocampus is involved in the learning of contextual information (Hirsh, 1974; Rudy and Sutherland, 1989; Phillips and LeDoux, 1992; Eichenbaum et al., 1996; McNish et al., 1997; Matus-Amat et al., 2004).

In fear conditioning tasks, including inhibitory avoidance, that are typically used in memory modulation studies, the rats learn that footshock occurs in a specific context. Further, that information can be learned if rats are first exposed to the context and then, on a subsequent day, given a brief footshock. As is shown in **Figure 5**, infusions of oxotremorine administered into the hippocampus after context exposure enhanced the subsequent conditioning, but infusions administered after the footshock training were ineffective (Malin and McGaugh, 2006). In contrast, oxotremorine infused into the rostral anterior cingulate cortex selectively enhanced memory when administered after the footshock. Oxotremorine infused into the BLA enhanced retention when administered after either the context or footshock training, consistent with extensive evidence that BLA activity modulates memory for many different kinds of experiences. Other findings of studies of the effects of posttraining intraamygdala infusions of a GR agonist provide additional evidence of BLA–hippocampus interactions in memory consolidation. As is shown in **Figure 6**, unilateral posttraining intrahippocampal infusions of the specific GR agonist RU 28362 enhanced rats' retention of inhibitory avoidance training, and the retention enhancement was blocked selectively by ipsilateral infusions of a β-adrenoceptor antagonist into the BLA (Roozendaal et al., 1999a). The memory enhancement induced by GR activation in the hippocampus is also blocked by lesions of the BLA, stria terminalis, or nucleus accumbens (Roozendaal and McGaugh, 1997b; Roozendaal et al., 2001).

The BLA projects to the nucleus accumbens primarily via the stria terminalis (Kelley et al., 1982; Wright et al., 1996). The possible involvement of the BLA–stria terminalis–nucleus accumbens pathway in modulating memory consolidation was suggested by the finding that lesions of the nucleus accumbens, like lesions of the BLA, block the memory-enhancing effects of systemically administered dexamethasone (Roozendaal and McGaugh, 1996a; Setlow et al., 2000). Furthermore, the finding that unilateral lesions of the BLA combined with contralateral (unilateral) lesions of the nucleus accumbens also blocked the dexamethasone effect strongly indicates that these two structures interact via the stria terminalis in influencing memory consolidation (Setlow et al., 2000). Further evidence of BLA–nucleus accumbens interactions in modulating memory consolidation is provided by the finding (LaLumiere et al., 2005) that memory enhancement induced by intra-BLA infusions of dopamine is blocked by infusions of a dopamine receptor antagonist into the nucleus accumbens shell (but not the core). Conversely, a dopamine receptor antagonist infused into the BLA blocks the memory enhancement induced by infusions of dopamine infused into the nucleus accumbens shell posttraining (**Figure 7**).

As the hippocampus is known to project to the nucleus accumbens, that region may be a critical locus of converging BLA and hippocampal modulatory influences on memory consolidation (Mulder et al., 1998). The finding that inactivation of the nucleus accumbens with infusions of bupivacaine prior to training blocks the acquisition of contextual fear conditioning provides evidence consistent with this hypothesis (Haralambous and Westbrook, 1999). It is not known whether the BLA–nucleus accumbens

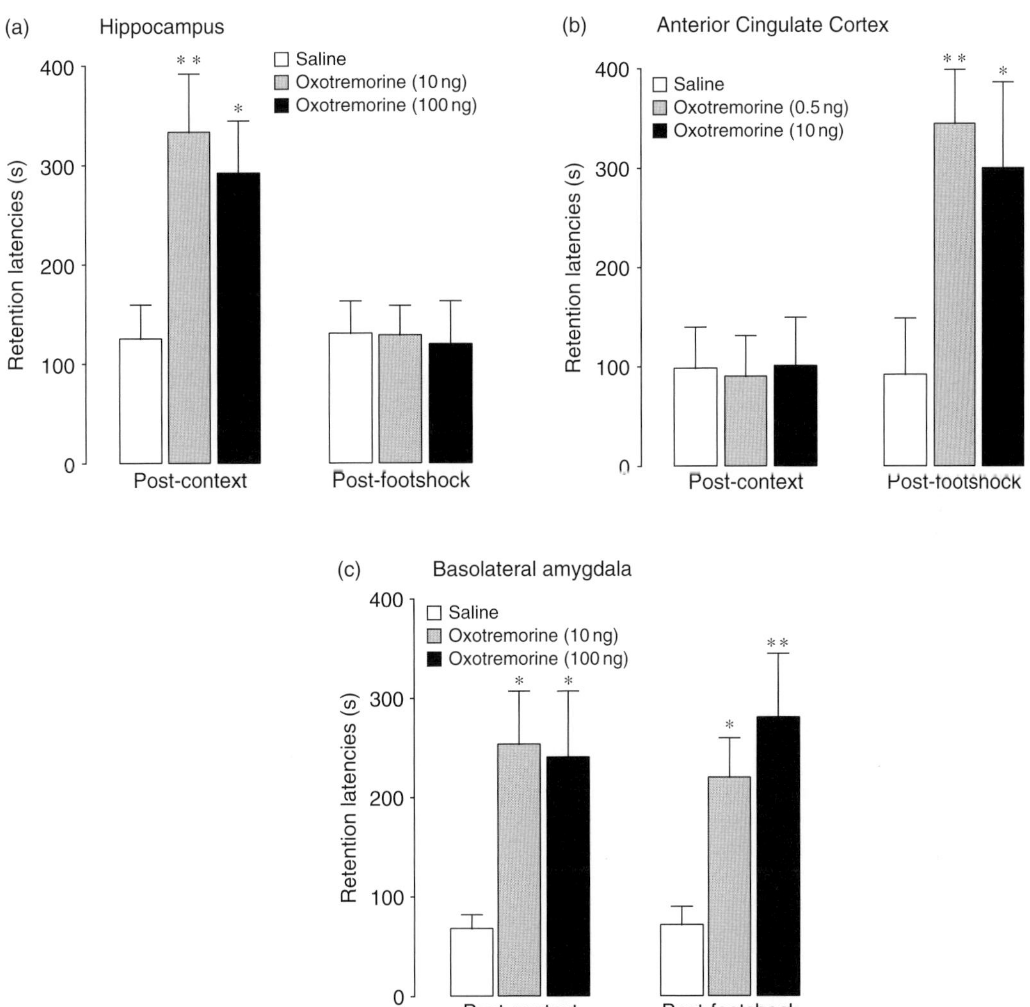

Figure 5 Differential involvement of the hippocampus, anterior cingulate cortex, and basolateral amygdala in memory for context and footshock. (a) Posttraining infusions of the muscarinic cholinergic receptor agonist oxotremorine (10 or 100 ng in 0.5 μl) into the dorsal hippocampus enhanced 48-h inhibitory avoidance retention latencies when administered after context exposure but not after the shock exposure given 24 h later. (b) Posttraining infusions of oxotremorine (0.5 or 10 ng in 0.5 μl) into the anterior cingulate cortex selectively enhanced 48-h inhibitory avoidance retention latencies when administered after the shock experience but not after the context exposure. (c) Posttraining infusions of oxotremorine (10 or 100 ng in 0.2 μl) into the basolateral amygdala enhanced 48-h inhibitory avoidance retention latencies when administered after either the context exposure or the shock experience. Results represent retention latencies (mean + SEM) in seconds. $*$, $p < .05$; $**$, $p < .01$ compared with the corresponding saline group. From Malin EL and McGaugh JL (2006) Differential involvement of the hippocampus, anterior cingulate cortex and basolateral amygdala in memory for context and footshock. *Proc. Natl. Acad. Sci. USA* 103: 1959–1963.

and hippocampus–nucleus accumbens pathways are also involved in mediating other BLA neuromodulatory influences on memory consolidation.

Other findings indicate that noradrenergic stimulation of the BLA that enhances memory consolidation also increases dorsal hippocampal levels of activity-regulated cytoskeletal protein (Arc) (McIntyre et al., 2005), an immediate-early gene implicated in hippocampal synaptic plasticity and memory consolidation processes (Guzowski et al., 2000). Additionally, inactivation of the BLA with infusions of lidocaine impairs memory consolidation and decreases Arc protein levels in the dorsal hippocampus (McIntyre et al., 2005). Further, the finding that intra-BLA infusions of muscimol attenuate the increase in Arc mRNA induced by contextual fear conditioning provides

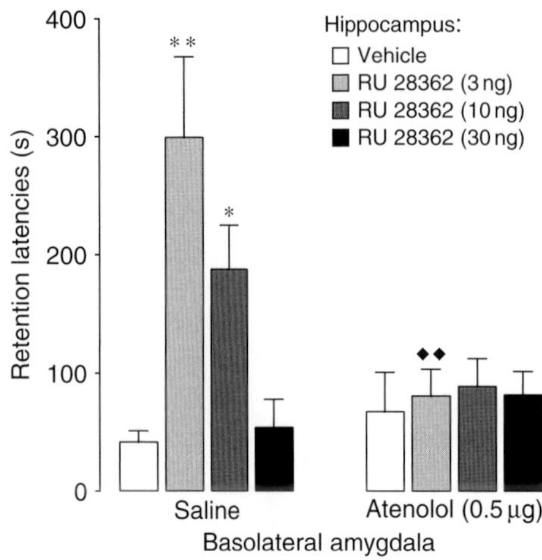

Figure 6 Glucocorticoid effects in the hippocampus on memory consolidation require noradrenergic activity of the basolateral amygdala. Immediate posttraining unilateral infusions of the glucocorticoid receptor agonist RU 28362 (3, 10, or 30 ng in 0.5 µl) induced dose-dependent enhancement of 48-h inhibitory avoidance retention latencies in rats given saline infusions into the basolateral amygdala concurrently. Ipsilateral infusions of the β-adrenoceptor antagonist atenolol (0.5 µg in 0.2 µl) into the basolateral blocked the memory enhancement induced by the glucocorticoid receptor agonist. Results represent retention latencies (mean + SEM) in seconds. $*$, $p < .05$; $**$, $p < .01$ compared with the corresponding vehicle group. ◆◆, $p < .01$ compared with the corresponding saline group. From Roozendaal B, Nguyen BT, Power A, and McGaugh JL (1999a) Basolateral amygdala noradrenergic influence enables enhancement of memory consolidation induced by hippocampal glucocorticoid receptor activation. *Proc. Natl. Acad. Sci. USA* 96: 11642–11647.

further evidence that the BLA modulates memory consolidation via regulation of Arc expression in the hippocampus (Huff et al., 2006).

Studies of BLA influences on hippocampal neuroplasticity provide additional important evidence of amygdala–hippocampal interactions (Abe, 2001). Electrical stimulation of the BLA enhances the induction of long-term potentiation (LTP) in the dentate gyrus of the hippocampus (Ikegaya et al., 1995b; Akirav and Richter-Levin, 1999; Frey et al., 2001; Almaguer-Melian et al., 2003). Also, selective lesions of the BLA or infusions of a β-adrenoceptor antagonist into the BLA block the induction of LTP in the dentate gyrus (Ikegaya et al., 1994, 1995a, 1997). Consistent with the findings of BLA modulation of memory, norepinephrine and corticosterone both influence the effects of BLA stimulation on dentate gyrus LTP (Akirav and Richter-Levin, 2002). Recent findings indicate that electrical stimulation of the BLA also enhances LTP at cortical synapses onto striatal neurons (Popescu et al., 2007). Such findings fit well with the evidence that posttraining amygdala activation enhances consolidation of striatal-dependent memory (Packard et al., 1994; Packard and Teather, 1998).

The recent findings that Pavlovian fear conditioning induces an increase in synchronization of theta-frequency activity in the lateral amygdala and CA1 region of the hippocampus strongly suggest that activation of an amygdala–hippocampus circuit is involved in fear-based learning (Pape et al., 2005). More generally, studies of synchronized oscillatory activity occurring within the BLA suggest that such activity may facilitate the temporal lobe as well as neocortical processes involved in consolidating explicit or declarative memory (Paré, 2003; Pelletier and Paré, 2004). Importantly, there is also evidence that the firing of cells in the BLA of cats is increased greatly by a single footshock and that the increased firing lasts for at least 2 h (Pelletier et al., 2005). Such increased firing may serve to modulate memory processing in efferent brain regions, including the entorhinal cortex and hippocampus (Paré et al., 2002; Pelletier and Paré, 2004; McGaugh, 2005). This view is supported by additional physiological evidence that, in cats, during the early stages of reward-based learning, training-induced BLA activity increases the impulse transmission from perirhinal to entorhinal cortical regions (Paz et al., 2006).

27.6.2 BLA–Cortical Interactions in Memory Consolidation

It is now well established that posttraining infusions of drugs into various cortical regions can impair or enhance the consolidation of memory for several kinds of training (Ardenghi et al., 1997; Izquierdo et al., 1997; Baldi et al., 1999; Sacchetti et al., 1999; Malin and McGaugh, 2006). The findings of several recent studies indicate that the BLA modulates cortical functioning involved in memory consolidation. Neurons within the BLA project directly to the entorhinal cortex (Paré et al., 1995; Paré and Gaudreau, 1996; Pikkarainen et al., 1999; Petrovich et al., 2001). The memory enhancement induced by posttraining drug infusions administered into the entorhinal cortex (Izquierdo and Medina, 1997) requires a functioning BLA, as lesions of the BLA prevent the memory enhancement induced by 8-bromo-cAMP infused posttraining into the

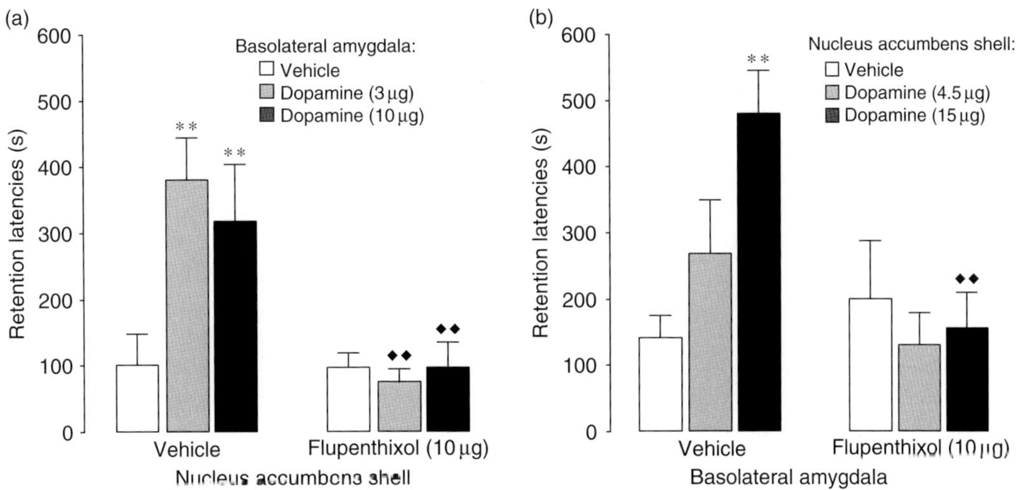

Figure 7 Modulation of memory consolidation by the basolateral amygdala or nucleus accumbens shell requires concurrent dopamine receptor activation in both brain regions. (a) Intrabasolateral amygdala infusions of dopamine (3 or 10 μg in 0.2 μl) immediately after inhibitory avoidance training produced enhancement of 48-h retention performance in rats receiving vehicle into the nucleus accumbens shell. Infusion of the general dopamine receptor antagonist *cis*-flupenthixol (10 μg in 0.3 μl) into the nucleus accumbens shell blocked the memory enhancement induced by dopamine infusions into the basolateral amygdala. (b) Intranucleus accumbens shell infusions of dopamine (4.5 or 15 μg in 0.3 μl) also induced memory enhancement, and this effect was blocked by concurrent infusions of *cis*-flupenthixol (10 μg in 0.2 μl) into the basolateral amygdala. Results represent retention latencies (mean + SEM) in seconds. ∗∗, $p < .01$ compared with the vehicle group; ◆◆, $p < .01$ compared with the corresponding vehicle group. From LaLumiere RT, Nawar EM, and McGaugh JL (2005) Modulation of memory consolidation by the basolateral amygdala or nucleus accumbens shell requires concurrent dopamine receptor activation in both brain regions. *Learn. Mem.* 12: 296–301.

entorhinal cortex (Roesler et al., 2002). Other recent studies have reported that BLA lesions or blocking of β-adrenoceptors in the BLA also block the memory-enhancing effects of 8-bromo-cAMP infused posttraining into the insular cortex (Miranda and McGaugh, 2004) and of oxotremorine infused into the rostral anterior cingulate cortex (Malin et al., 2007). Additionally, the finding that lesions of the rostral anterior cingular cortex block the memory-enhancing effects of oxotremorine infused posttraining into the BLA indicates that cortical functioning is essential for BLA memory-modulatory effects (Malin et al., 2007). However, other evidence indicates that the rostral anterior cingulate cortex and the BLA serve quite different functions in memory. As discussed earlier, the anterior cingulate cortex appears to play a somewhat selective role in memory for nociceptive information, whereas extensive evidence indicates that the BLA is not dedicated to the modulation of any specific kinds of information (Packard et al., 1994; Malin and McGaugh, 2006). The BLA appears to be promiscuous in its modulation of emotionally influenced memory consolidation (McGaugh, 2002).

Other recent studies reported evidence indicating interactions between the BLA and the medial prefrontal cortex in regulating memory consolidation. Inactivation of the medial prefrontal cortex with the AMPA-receptor antagonist CNQX impairs consolidation of inhibitory avoidance memory (Liang et al., 1996). In contrast, activation of noradrenergic and dopaminergic mechanisms in the medial prefrontal cortex enhances consolidation of inhibitory avoidance and trace fear conditioning (Liang, 2001; Runyan and Dash, 2004). A GR agonist infused into the medial prefrontal cortex induces similar memory enhancement. However, and importantly, lesions of the BLA block this GR agonist-induced memory enhancement. Furthermore, consistent with the evidence of reciprocal inhibitory influences between both brain regions (McDonald, 1991; Perez-Jaranay and Vives, 1991; Rosenkranz and Grace, 2002), infusions of RU 28362 into the medial prefrontal cortex after inhibitory avoidance training increases BLA activity, as assessed with phosphorylation of extracellular-regulated kinase (ERK), a member of the mitogen-activated protein kinase family (Roozendaal et al., unpublished findings). Further, blockade of this increase in phosphorylated ERK levels in the BLA with the MEK inhibitor PD98059 blocks the memory enhancement induced by medial prefrontal cortex GR agonist infusions. Interestingly, infusions of a GR agonist into the BLA induce a similar increase in phosphorylated ERK activity in the medial prefrontal cortex, suggesting mutual interactions between both brain regions in regulating memory consolidation.

It is likely that the BLA also influences cortical functioning, at least in part, via its projection through the stria terminalis (Price, 1981) to the nucleus basalis, which provides cholinergic activation of the cortex. Studies have reported findings suggesting that the nucleus basalis–cortical projections may be essential for learning-induced cortical plasticity (Miasnikov et al., 2001, 2006; Weinberger, 2003). Stimulation of the BLA activates the cortex, as indicated by EEG desynchronization, and potentiates nucleus basalis influences on cortical activation. Moreover, inactivation of the nucleus basalis with lidocaine blocks the BLA effects on cortical activation (Dringenberg and Vanderwolf, 1996; Dringenberg et al., 2001). Thus, the BLA may influence cortical functioning in memory consolidation, at least in part, through its effects on the nucleus basalis and consequent cholinergic activation of the cortex. In support of this suggestion, Power et al. (2002) reported that selective lesions of cortical nucleus basalis corticopetal cholinergic projections induced by 192-IgG saporin blocked the dose-dependent enhancement of inhibitory avoidance induced by posttraining intra-BLA infusions of norepinephrine (**Figure 8**). Thus, it is clear that cortical cholinergic activity is required for BLA influences on memory consolidation. **Figure 9** summarizes the interaction of the BLA with other systems in regulating memory consolidation.

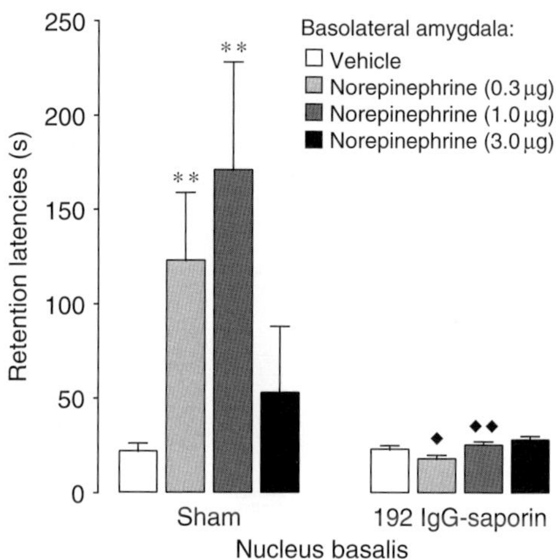

Figure 8 Lesions of nucleus basalis cholinergic neurons with 192 IgG-saporin block the memory enhancement induced by posttraining infusions of norepinephrine into the basolateral amygdala. Intrabasolateral amygdala infusions of norepinephrine (0.3, 1.0, or 3.0 ng in 0.2 μl) immediately after inhibitory avoidance training produced a dose-dependent enhancement of 48-h retention performance in sham-operated rats. Rats with 192 IgG-saporin lesions did not show memory enhancement with norepinephrine infusions. Results represent retention latencies (mean + SEM) in seconds. ∗∗, $p < .01$ compared with the saline group; ◆, $p < .05$; ◆◆, $p < .01$ compared with the corresponding sham-lesion group. From Power AE, Thal LJ, and McGaugh JL (2002) Lesions of the nucleus basalis magnocellularis induced by 192 IgG-saporin block memory enhancement with posttraining norepinephrine in the basolateral amygdala. *Proc. Natl. Acad. Sci. USA* 99: 2315–2319.

27.7 Amygdala Activity and Modulation of Human Memory Consolidation

As discussed above, the findings of animal experiments very clearly provide extensive evidence that stress hormones released by emotional experiences influence memory consolidation and that the influence is mediated by activation of the BLA. The findings of many human studies of effects of emotional arousal, stress hormones, and amygdala activation on memory are consistent with those of animal studies (Cahill and McGaugh, 1998, 2000; Cahill, 2000; Dolan, 2000; Buchanan and Adolphs, 2004; LaBar and Cabeza, 2006). Cortisol administered to subjects prior to presentations of words or pictures enhanced subsequent recall (Buchanan and Lovallo, 2001; Abercrombie et al., 2003, 2006; Kuhlmann and Wolf, 2006). Amphetamine administered to human subjects, either before or after they learned lists of words, also enhanced long-term memory (Soetens et al., 1993, 1995). Administration of propranolol to subjects prior to their viewing an emotionally arousing slide presentation blocked the enhancing effects of emotional arousal on long-term memory (Cahill et al., 1994). Propranolol also blocks the memory enhancement produced by stress-released epinephrine (Nielson and Jensen, 1994). Further, epinephrine or cold pressor stress (which stimulates the release of adrenal stress hormones) administered to subjects after they viewed emotionally arousing slides enhanced the subjects' long-term memory of the slides (Cahill and Alkire, 2003; Cahill et al., 2003). Similar effects were produced by

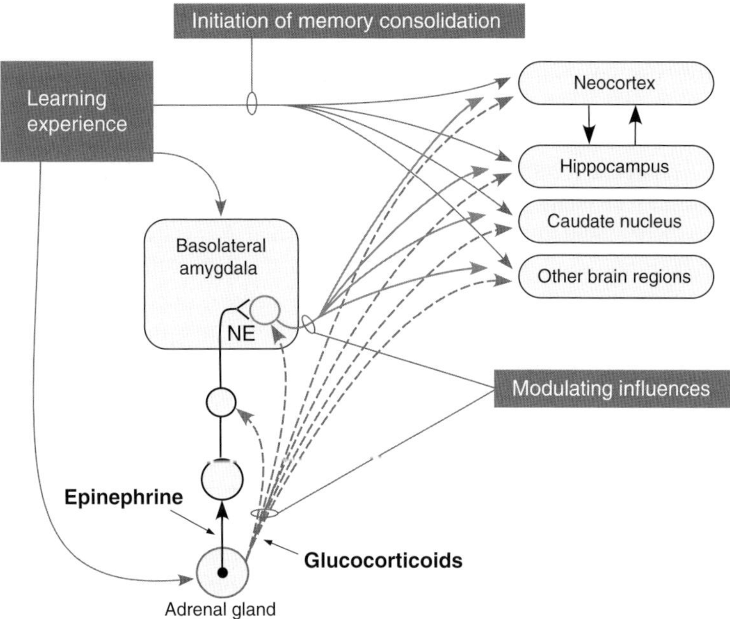

Figure 9 Schematic summarizing interactions of the basolateral amygdala with other brain regions in mediating emotional arousal-induced modulation of memory consolidation. Experiences initiate memory consolidation in many brain regions involved in the forms of memory represented. Emotionally arousing experiences also release adrenal epinephrine and glucocorticoids and activate the release of norepinephrine in the basolateral amygdala. The basolateral amygdala modulates memory consolidation by influencing neuroplasticity in other brain regions. From McGaugh JL (2000) Memory: A century of consolidation. *Science* 287: 248–251.

administration of the α_2-adrenoceptor antagonist yohimbine, which stimulates norepinephrine release (O'Carroll et al., 1999; Southwick et al., 2002). These findings of studies of memory in human subjects are, thus, consistent with those of the animal experiments discussed above in providing evidence of the central roles of emotional activation and stress hormones in modulating memory consolidation.

Recent human studies have also provided extensive evidence that amygdala activation is involved in enabling the enhanced memory induced by emotional arousal. Memory for emotionally arousing material is not enhanced in human subjects with selective bilateral lesions of the amygdala, as it is in normal subjects (Cahill et al., 1995; Adolphs et al., 1997). Studies using positron emission tomography (PET) and functional magnetic resonance imaging (fMRI) brain imaging have provided additional evidence that the influence of emotional arousal on human memory involves amygdala activation. In the first study of the relationship between amygdala activity during encoding and subsequent memory, Cahill et al. (1996) reported that amygdala activity assessed by PET imaging as subjects viewed emotionally arousing films correlated highly (+0.93) with the subjects' recall of the films assessed in a surprise memory test 3 weeks later. Importantly, the degree of emotional arousal rather than the valence of the emotionally arousing material appears to be critical in influencing memory. In a subsequent study using PET imaging, Hamann et al. (1999, 2002) reported that amygdala activity induced by viewing either pleasant or unpleasant slides correlated highly with memory for the slides assessed 1 month later. Studies using fMRI have obtained highly similar findings. Canli et al. (2000) found that subjects' memory for a series of scenes tested 3 weeks after brain scanning correlated highly with amygdala activity induced by viewing the scenes. Furthermore, and importantly, the relationship between amygdala activity during encoding and subsequent memory was greatest for the scenes that the subjects had rated as being the most emotionally intense.

Human memory studies have provided additional evidence of the importance of noradrenergic acti vation of the amygdala. When assessed during encoding, PET imaging of amygdala activity that is assessed over many minutes of arousal as well as event-related fMRI of amygdala activity induced by single items both predict long-term memory of the arousing stimuli (Cahill et al., 1996; Canli et al., 2000). And, importantly, β-adrenoceptor antagonists (e.g., propranolol) block the increase in amygdala activity and enhanced retention induced by emotional stimuli obtained in fMRI studies (Strange and Dolan, 2004; van Stegeren et al., 2005). Thus, β-adrenergic activation of the amygdala appears to be essential for the short-latency modulation induced by brief and mild emotional arousal used in fMRI studies as well as the effects found in human and animal studies, with longer intervals of time between learning and stress hormone activation or administration.

An additional finding of human brain imaging studies of memory studies is that, with both PET and fMRI experiments, activity of the right amygdala is related to enhanced memory in men, whereas activity of the left amygdala is correlated with enhanced memory in women (Cahill et al., 2001, 2004; Canli et al., 2001). Understanding the bases of such sex differences may provide further insights into mechanisms of emotional arousal underlying influences on memory consolidation.

Other findings based on an analysis of PET and fMRI scans provide evidence, consistent with that from many animal studies, indicating that amygdala activation influences memory processing in other brain regions. The activity of the amygdala and hippocampal/parahippocampal regions are correlated during emotional arousal (Hamann et al., 1999), and such activation is correlated with subsequent retention (Dolcos et al., 2004). The results of a 'path analysis' (structural equation modeling) study (Kilpatrick and Cahill, 2003b) of amygdala activity scanned, using PET, while subjects viewed neutral or emotionally arousing films (Cahill et al., 1996) suggest that emotional arousal increased amygdala influences on activity of the ipsilateral parahippocampal gyrus and ventrolateral prefrontal cortex. Such findings provide additional evidence that amygdala influences on activity of other brain regions are critical in creating lasting memories.

27.8 Involvement of the Amygdala in Modulating Memory Retrieval and Working Memory

Most studies investigating neuromodulatory influences on memory have focused on the neurobiological mechanisms underlying the consolidation of recent experiences. However, there is also much evidence that neuromodulatory systems influence memory retrieval and working memory. Most of such studies have investigated the effects of either peripherally administered hormones and neurotransmitters or the effects of direct infusions of a variety of drugs into the hippocampus and medial prefrontal cortex, brain regions that are critically involved in regulating memory retrieval and working memory. However, consistent with its role in memory consolidation, recent findings indicate that the BLA, via its projections to these brain regions, also plays an important modulatory role in regulating drug effects on these memory functions.

27.8.1 Memory Retrieval

Several studies investigated the effects of peripherally administered hormones and drugs on memory retrieval in rats. Stress exposure or the glucocorticoid corticosterone administered systemically shortly before testing for memory of training on inhibitory avoidance or water-maze spatial tasks (24 h earlier) produces temporary impairment of retention performance (Bohus, 1973; de Quervain et al., 1998; Yang et al., 2003; Roozendaal et al., 2004a; Pakdel and Rashidy-Pour, 2006; Sajadi et al., 2006). As the same treatments administered shortly before training do not affect either acquisition or retention performance assessed immediately after acquisition, such findings indicate that glucocorticoids impair retention by influencing memory retrieval. These findings are consistent with those indicating that stress exposure or glucocorticoids administered immediately after a learning session also impair retention performance tested 30–60 min after the session, that is, at a time when the memory trace has not yet been consolidated into long-term memory (Diamond et al., 1999; Woodson et al., 2003; Okuda et al., 2004). Similarly, as is found with memory consolidation, glucocorticoid effects on memory retrieval depend on concurrent activation of noradrenergic mechanisms. The β-adrenoceptor antagonist propranolol administered systemically 30 min before inhibitory avoidance retention testing blocks the memory retrieval impairment induced by concurrent injections of corticosterone (Roozendaal et al., 2004a). As stimulation of β_1-adrenoceptors with systemic injections of the selective agonist xamoterol induces a memory retrieval impairment comparable to that seen after corticosterone administration (Roozendaal et al., 2004b), the findings suggest that glucocorticoid effects on memory retrieval impairment involve activation of noradrenergic mechanisms. Norepinephrine effects on memory retrieval are most likely dose dependent, as other studies reported that under other conditions, norepinephrine or noradrenergic stimulation can also enhance memory retrieval (Sara and Devauges, 1989; Devauges and Sara, 1991; Barros et al., 2001; Murchison et al., 2004). Peripheral administration of the opioid peptidergic antagonist naloxone or D2, but not D1, dopamine receptor antagonists also block the impairing effect of concurrently administered corticosterone or dexamethasone on memory retrieval (Rashidy-Pour et al., 2004; Pakdel and Rashidy-Pour, 2006). Other studies have reported that memory retrieval is also influenced by systemic administration of drugs affecting several other modulatory systems, including epinephrine, adrenocorticotropin, β-endorphin, vasopressin, acetylcholine, and serotonin (e.g., Altman et al., 1987; Izquierdo et al., 2002; Sato et al., 2004). In investigating drug effects on learning and memory, including memory retrieval, it is critically important to distinguish the effects of the drugs on memory retrieval from those on other processes that may affect the behavior used to assess memory. Not all of the studies cited above adequately controlled for such performance effects.

Many studies have reported evidence indicating that the hippocampus is involved in memory retrieval (Hirsch, 1974; Squire et al., 2001). Inactivation of the hippocampus with local infusions of the glutamatergic AMPA/kainate receptor antagonist LY326325 or the GABAergic agonist muscimol impairs memory retrieval of water-maze spatial and contextual fear conditioning tasks (Holt and Maren, 1999; Riedel et al., 1999). As the GR agonist RU 28362 administered into the hippocampus shortly before retention testing also impairs retrieval of spatial memory (Roozendaal et al., 2003, 2004b), such findings indicate that glucocorticoid-induced memory retrieval impairment depends, in part, on GR activation in the hippocampus. Consistent with the findings of experiments of peripherally administered drugs, a β-adrenoceptor antagonist infused into the hippocampus prevents the retrieval-impairing effect of a GR agonist administered concurrently (Roozendaal et al., 2004b). Other studies have shown that the effect of novelty stress on memory retrieval is blocked by intrahippocampal infusions of the AMPA-receptor antagonist CNQX and the metabotropic glutamate receptor antagonist MCPG, as well as the cAMP blocker Rp-cAMPs (Izquierdo et al., 2000). In contrast, infusions of the protein synthesis inhibitor anisomycin do not block corticosterone effects on memory retrieval (Sajadi et al., 2006), suggesting that stress and corticosterone may influence memory retrieval through a rapid, protein synthesis-independent mechanism.

Retrieval of memory of emotionally arousing information also induces activation of the BLA (Hall et al., 2001; Boujabit et al., 2003). Furthermore, intra-BLA infusions of norepinephrine or CNQX affect memory retrieval of inhibitory avoidance training (Liang et al., 1996; Barros et al., 2001). In contrast, intra-BLA infusions of a GR agonist do not appear to affect memory retrieval (Roozendaal et al., 2003). However, the BLA interacts with the hippocampus in mediating glucocorticoid effects on memory retrieval. Lesions of the BLA or infusions of a β-adrenoceptor antagonist into the BLA block the impairing effect of a GR agonist infused into the hippocampus on memory retrieval (Roozendaal et al., 2003, 2004b). These findings are thus consistent with those described earlier on memory consolidation (e.g., Roozendaal and McGaugh, 1997b; Roozendaal et al., 1999a) and indicate that the BLA regulates memory retrieval via interactions with other brain regions.

The findings of studies examining stress hormone effects on memory retrieval in humans are consistent with those of animal experiments and indicate that glucocorticoids impair memory retrieval via an interaction with noradrenergic mechanisms. Stress-level cortisol or cortisone administration to human subjects impairs delayed, but not immediate, recall on episodic tasks (de Quervain et al., 2000; Wolf et al., 2001; Buchanan and Adolphs, 2004; Buss et al., 2004; Het et al., 2005; Kuhlmann et al., 2005a,b, 2006), and the β-adrenoceptor antagonist propranolol given orally blocks the impairing effect of glucocorticoids on memory retrieval (de Quervain et al., 2007). Recent findings from an $H_2^{15}O$-PET study indicate that glucocorticoid effects on memory retrieval in human subjects are also mediated, at least in part, by actions in the hippocampus (de Quervain et al., 2003). However, other findings of human imaging studies indicate that the amygdala is also activated during the retrieval of previously learned emotionally arousing material and that the effect is independent of the valence of the emotional material (Dolan, 2000). Further, recent findings of human brain imaging studies are consistent with findings of animal studies in indicating that the amygdala and hippocampus interact during the retrieval of emotionally arousing information (Dolcos et al., 2005; Greenberg et al., 2005; Smith et al., 2006).

27.8.2 Working Memory

Evidence from lesion, pharmacological, imaging, and clinical studies indicates that working memory, a dynamic process whereby information is updated continuously, depends on the integrity of the medial prefrontal cortex (Brito et al., 1982; Fuster, 1991; Taylor et al., 1999; Rowe et al., 2000; Levy and Fallow, 2001; Stern et al., 2001; Lee and Kesner, 2003). Decrements in prefrontal cortical function are induced by local depletion of norepinephrine and dopamine, suggesting that these monoamines regulate prefrontal cortical function (Brozoski et al., 1979; Bubser and Schmidt, 1990; Cai et al., 1993). The importance of endogenous norepinephrine and dopamine stimulation in the medial prefrontal cortex is indicated by studies in which local infusion of either noradrenergic α_2 (Li et al., 1999) or dopaminergic D1 antagonists (Sawaguchi and Goldman-Rakic, 1991; Seamans et al., 1998) administered into the medial prefrontal cortex impairs performance on working memory tasks. In contrast, activation of α_2-adrenoceptors with guanfacine improves working memory functions in rats and monkeys. Together, these data suggest that norepinephrine and dopamine are necessary for optimal medial prefrontal cortical function.

Excessive levels of norepinephrine or dopamine, however, impair working memory. The impairing effects of high doses of norepinephrine are mediated by activation of the α_1- and β-adrenoceptor (Arnsten and Jentsch, 1997; Arnsten et al., 1999; Birnbaum et al., 1999; Ramos et al., 2005). In contrast, α_2-adrenoceptor activation enhances working memory (Taylor et al., 1999). Electrophysiological studies have shown increased medial prefrontal cortical activity in the delay period during which the information needs to be retained (Fuster, 1991). Adrenergic agents that enhance working memory increase this neuronal activity during the delay period, whereas adrenergic drugs that impair working memory decrease such neuronal activity (Li et al., 1999). Dopaminergic D1 receptor agonists influence working memory following an inverted-U-shaped dose–response relationship. Too little or too much D1 receptor stimulation impairs prefrontal cortical activity and working memory in mice, rats, and monkeys (Cai and Arnsten, 1997; Zahrt et al., 1997; Li et al., 1999; Lidow et al., 2003).

Working memory deficits are also observed following exposure to stress (Arnsten and Goldman-Rakic, 1998). Mild uncontrollable stress impairs performance on a delayed alternation task but does not impair performance on nonmnemonic control tasks that have similar motivational and motor demands (Murphy et al., 1996). Mild stress, such as noise or exposure to the predator odor TMT, increases norepinephrine and dopamine turnover in the medial prefrontal cortex (Finlay et al., 1995; Morrow et al., 2000). The medial prefrontal cortex response to stress is blocked by anxiolytic benzodiazepine drugs and mimicked by the anxiogenic benzodiazepine inverse agonist FG7142 (Tam and Roth, 1985; Murphy et al., 1996; Birnbaum et al., 1999). Also, like stress, glucocorticoid administration impairs working memory. Basal levels of endogenous glucocorticoids are required to maintain prefrontal cortical function (Mizoguchi et al., 2004), but systemic injections of stress doses of corticosterone or intramedial prefrontal cortical administration of the GR agonist RU 28362 impair working memory, as assessed by delayed alternation performance, in rats (Roozendaal et al., 2004c). Additionally, stress-level cortisol treatment impairs prefrontal cortex-dependent inhibitory control of behaviors in squirrel monkeys (Lyons et al., 2000), as well as working memory performance in human subjects (Lupien et al., 1999; Young et al., 1999; Wolf et al., 2001). Glucocorticoids appear to interact with noradrenergic mechanisms in inducing working memory impairment, as systemic administration of the β-adrenoceptor antagonist propranolol blocks the working memory impairment of corticosterone administered concurrently (Roozendaal et al., 2004c). Such findings suggest that corticosterone effects on working memory impairment may involve a facilitation of noradrenergic mechanisms in the medial prefrontal cortex. This hypothesis is supported by findings of an *in vivo* microdialysis study indicating that systemic administration of corticosterone increases levels of norepinephrine in the medial prefrontal cortex (Thomas et al., 1994).

Glucocorticoid-induced working memory impairment also depends on interactions of the medial prefrontal cortex with the BLA. As discussed earlier, the BLA both sends projections to and receives projections from the medial prefrontal cortex (McDonald, 1991; Perez-Jaranay and Vives, 1991; Rosenkranz and Grace, 2002). The BLA itself does not appear to play a significant role in working memory (Wan et al., 1994; Bianchin et al., 1999; Roozendaal et al., 2004c), but lesions of the BLA block the impairment induced by either systemic administration of corticosterone or infusions of a GR agonist into the medial prefrontal cortex (Roozendaal et al., 2004c) (**Figure 10**). These findings thus indicate that the BLA interacts with the medial prefrontal cortex in regulating stress hormone effects on working memory.

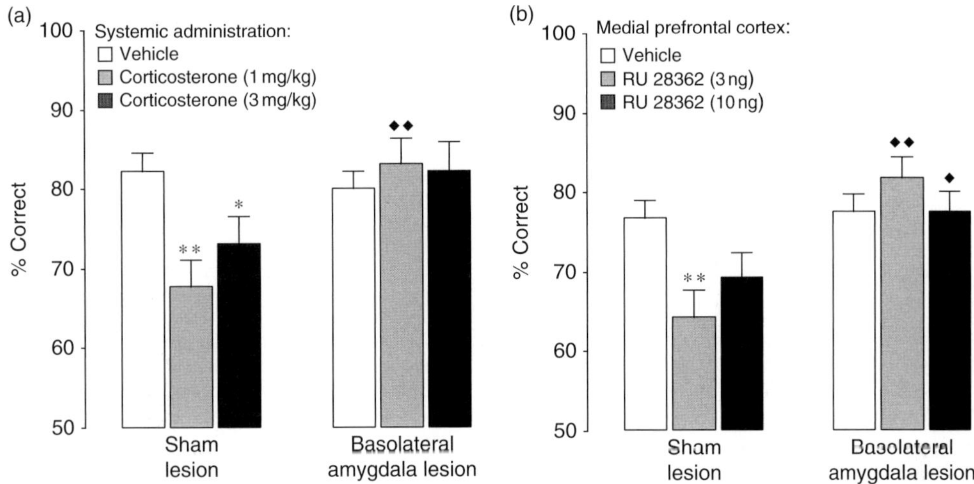

Figure 10 The basolateral amygdala interacts with the medial prefrontal cortex in mediating glucocorticoid effects on working memory. Systemic injections of corticosterone (1.0 or 3.0 mg/kg, ip) (a) or infusions of the specific glucocorticoid receptor agonist RU 28362 (3.0 or 10.0 ng in 0.5 μl) into the medial prefrontal cortex (b) impaired delayed alternation performance in sham-lesioned rats. Lesions of the basolateral amygdala blocked working memory impairment induced by either corticosterone or RU 28362. Results represent percent correct choices (mean + SEM). *, $p < .05$; **, $p < .01$ compared with the corresponding vehicle group; ◆, $p < .05$; ◆◆, $p < .01$ compared with the corresponding sham-lesion group. From Roozendaal B, McReynolds JR, and McGaugh JL (2004c) The basolateral amygdala interacts with the medial prefrontal cortex in regulating glucocorticoid effects on working memory impairment. *J. Neurosci.* 24: 1385–1392.

27.9 Concluding Comments

Research investigating memory modulation evolved from many sources. Key, of course, was Müller and Pilzecker's (1900) perseveration–consolidation hypothesis proposed over a century ago. The subsequent findings that treatments such as electroconvulsive shock administered after training-induced retrograde amnesia (Duncan, 1949; McGaugh and Herz, 1972) provided critical evidence supporting that hypothesis. Those findings also suggested the possibility that posttraining treatments that stimulate brain activity might enhance memory consolidation. This implication was confirmed by evidence that posttraining administration of stimulant drugs enhances long-term memory (Breen and McGaugh, 1961; McGaugh, 1966, 1973). Livingston's (1967) hypothesis that activation of the limbic system might promote the storage of recently activated brain events, as well as Kety's (1972) proposal that adrenergic catecholamines released by emotional states may serve to influence consolidation, suggested physiological processes that might mediate the posttraining modulation of memory consolidation induced by stimulant drugs. Although the findings obtained in studies of memory modulation fit perhaps in a general way with these early ideas, there are many more parts to this memory modulatory system, and they interact in complex ways that were not anticipated. The early studies of adrenal stress hormone influences on memory consolidation (e.g., Gold and van Buskirk, 1975, 1976; McGaugh, 1989; McGaugh and Gold, 1989; Roozendaal, 2007) provided compelling evidence that peripheral hormones released by emotional arousals play an important role. The findings (e.g., Liang et al., 1986) suggesting that stress hormones as well as drugs affect memory by noradrenergic activation of the amygdala (i.e., the BLA) provided strong evidence suggesting that the BLA is an essential part of a memory-modulatory system. This suggestion has now been confirmed by the extensive findings that the BLA interacts with many other brain regions in modulating memory consolidation (McGaugh, 2000, 2002, 2004). The findings indicating that stress hormones modulate memory retrieval and working memory via noradrenergic influences and the BLA provide yet other chapter to the story of memory modulation (Roozendaal, 2002; Roozendaal et al., 2003, 2004a). Of course, our understanding of memory-modulatory systems is incomplete. Much more needs to be discovered about how the BLA interacts with other brain systems and how it acts to influence neuroplasticity in other brain regions involved in consolidating newly acquired information of many different kinds. But in the past several decades, research on memory modulation has made significant progress in understanding how emotional arousal influences the consolidation and retrieval of significant experiences. Research findings have revealed at least some understanding of why it is, as William James (1890) noted, that emotional experiences may leave scars on the cerebral tissue.

References

Abe K (2001) Modulation of hippocampal long-term potentiation by the amygdala: A synaptic mechanism linking emotion and memory. *Jap. J. Pharmacol.* 86: 18–22.

Abercrombie HC, Kalin NH, Thurow ME, Rosenkranz MA, and Davidson RJ (2003) Cortisol variation in humans affects memory for emotionally laden and neutral information. *Behav. Neurosci.* 117: 506–516.

Abercrombie HC, Speck NS, and Monticelli RM (2006) Endogenous cortisol elevations are related to memory facilitation only in individuals who are emotionally aroused. *Psychoneuroendocrinology* 31: 187–196.

Adolphs R, Cahill L, Schul R, and Babinsky R (1997) Impaired declarative memory for emotional material following bilateral amygdala damage in humans. *Learn. Mem.* 4: 51–54.

Agranoff BW (1980) Biochemical events mediating the formation of short-term and long-term memory. In: Tsukada Y and Agranoff W (eds.) *Neurobiological Basis of Learning and Memory*, pp. 135–147. New York: Wiley.

Aguilar-Valles A, Sanchez E, de Gortari P, et al. (2005) Analysis of the stress response in rats trained in the water-maze: Differential expression of corticotropin-releasing hormone, CRH-R1, glucocorticoid receptors and brain-derived neurotrophic factor in limbic regions. *Neuroendocrinology* 82: 306–319.

Akirav I (2007) NMDA partial agonist reverses blocking of extinction of aversive memory by GABA(A) agonist in the amygdala. *Neuropsychopharmacology* 32: 542–550.

Akirav I and Richter-Levin G (1999) Biphasic modulation of hippocampal plasticity by behavioral stress and basolateral amygdala stimulation in the rat. *J. Neurosci.* 19: 10530–10535.

Akirav I and Richter-Levin G (2002) Mechanisms of amygdala modulation of hippocampal plasticity. *J. Neurosci.* 22: 9912–9921.

Almaguer-Melian W, Martinez-Marti L, Frey JU, and Bergado JA (2003) The amygdala is part of the behavioural reinforcement system modulating long-term potentiation in rat hippocampus. *Neuroscience* 119: 319–322.

Altman HJ, Stone WS, and Ogren SO (1987) Evidence for a possible functional interaction between serotonergic and cholinergic mechanisms in memory retrieval. *Behav. Neural Biol.* 48: 49–62.

Arbilla S and Langer SA (1978) Morphine and β-endorphin inhibit release of noradrenaline from cerebral cortex but not of dopamine from rat striatum. *Nature* 271: 559–561.

Ardenghi P, Barros D, Izquierdo LA, et al. (1997) Late and prolonged post-training memory modulation in entorhinal and parietal cortex by drugs acting on the cAMP/protein kinase A signalling pathway. *Behav. Pharm.* 8: 745–751.

Arnsten AFT and Goldman-Rakic PS (1998) Noise stress impairs prefrontal cortical cognitive function in monkeys: Evidence for a hyperdopaminergic mechanism. *Arch. Gen. Psychiatry* 55: 362–369.

Arnsten AFT and Jentsch JD (1997) The alpha-1 adrenergic agonist, cirazoline, impairs spatial working memory performance in aged monkeys. *Pharmacol. Biochem. Behav.* 58: 55–59.

Arnsten AFT, Mathew R, Ubriani R, Taylor JR, and Li BM (1999) Alpha-1 noradrenergic receptor stimulation impairs prefrontal cortical cognitive function. *Biol. Psychiatry* 45: 26–31.

Baldi E, Lorenzini C, Sacchetti B, Tassoni G, and Bucherelli C (1999) Effects of combined medial septal area, fimbria-fornix and entorhinal cortex tetrodotoxin inactivations on passive avoidance response consolidation in the rat. *Brain Res.* 821: 503–510.

Baratti CM, Introini IB, and Huygens P (1984) Possible interaction between central cholinergic muscarinic and opioid peptidergic systems during memory consolidation in mice. *Behav. Neural Biol.* 40: 155–169.

Barros DM, Mello e Souza T, De David T, et al. (2001) Simultaneous modulation of retrieval by dopaminergic D1, β-noradrenergic serotonergic-1_a and cholinergic muscarinic receptors in cortical structures of the rat. *Behav. Brain Res.* 124: 1–7.

Barros DM, Pereira P, Medina JH, and Izquierdo I (2002) Modulation of working memory and of long, but not short-term memory by cholinergic mechanisms in the basolateral amygdala. *Behav. Pharmacol.* 13: 163–167.

Beato M, Herrlich P, and Schutz G (1995) Steroid hormone receptors: Many actors in search of a plot. *Cell* 83: 851–857.

Berlau DJ and McGaugh JL (2006) Enhancement of extinction memory consolidation: The role of the noradrenergic and GABAergic systems within the basolateral amygdala. *Neurobiol. Learn. Mem.* 86: 123–132.

Bernaerts P, Lamberty Y, and Tirelli E (2004) Histamine H3 antagonist thioperamide dose-dependently enhances memory consolidation and reverses amnesia induced by dizocilpine or scopolamine in a one-trial inhibitory avoidance task in mice. *Behav. Brain Res.* 154: 211–219.

Bianchin M, Mello e Souza T, Medina JH, and Izquierdo I (1999) The amygdala is involved in the modulation of long-term memory, but not in working or short-term memory. *Neurobiol. Learn. Mem.* 71: 127–131.

Birnbaum S, Gobeske KT, Auerbach J, Taylor JR, and Arnsten AFT (1999) A role for norepinephrine in stress-induced cognitive deficits: Alpha-1-adrenoceptor mediation in the prefrontal cortex. *Biol. Psychiatry* 46: 1266–1274.

Bohus B (1973) Pituitary-adrenal influences on avoidance and approach behavior of the rat. In: Zimmerman E, Gispen WH, Marks BH, and de Wied D (eds.) *Progress in Brain Research. Drugs Effects on Neuroendocrine Regulations*, pp. 407–430. Amsterdam: Elsevier.

Bohus B (1980) Vasopressin, oxytocin and memory: Effects on consolidation and retrieval processes. *Acta. Psychiatr. Belg.* 80: 714–720.

Bohus B (1994) Humoral modulation of memory processes. Physiological significance of brain and peripheral mechanisms. In: Delacour J (ed.) *The Memory System of the Brain, vol. 4*, pp. 337–364. Advanced Series of Neuroscience., New Jersey: World Scientific.

Boujabit M, Bontempi B, Destrade C, and Gisquet-Verrier P (2003) Exposure to a retrieval cue in rats induces changes in regional brain glucose metabolism in the amygdala and other related brain structures. *Neurobiol. Learn. Mem.* 79: 57–71.

Borrell J, de Kloet ER, and Bohus B (1984) Corticosterone decreases the efficacy of adrenaline to affect passive avoidance retention of adrenalectomized rats. *Life Sci.* 34: 99–104.

Borrell J, de Kloet ER, Versteeg DH, and Bohus B (1983) Inhibitory avoidance deficit following short-term adrenalectomy in the rat: The role of adrenal catecholamines. *Behav. Neural Biol.* 39: 241–258.

Breen RA and McGaugh JL (1961) Facilitation of maze learning with posttrial injections of picrotoxin. *J. Comp. Physiol. Psychol.* 54: 498–501.

Brioni JD and McGaugh JL (1988) Post-training administration of GABAergic antagonists enhances retention of aversively motivated tasks. *Psychopharmacology* 96: 505–510.

Brioni JD, Nagahara AH, and McGaugh JL (1989) Involvement of the amygdala GABAergic system in the modulation of memory storage. *Brain Res.* 487: 105–112.

Brito GNO, Thomas GJ, Davis BJ, and Gingold SI (1982) Prelimbic cortex, mediodorsal thalamus, septum and delayed alternation in rats. *Exp. Brain Res.* 46: 52–58.

Brozoski T, Brown RM, Rosvold HE, and Goldman PS (1979) Cognitive deficit caused by regional depletion of dopamine in prefrontal cortex of rhesus monkey. *Science* 205: 929–931.

Bubser M and Schmidt W (1990) 6-OHDA lesion of the rat prefrontal cortex increases locomotor activity, impairs acquisition of delayed alternation tasks, but does not affect uninterrupted tasks in the radial maze. *Behav. Brain Res.* 37: 157–168.

Buchanan TW and Adolphs R (2004) The neuroanatomy of emotional memory in humans. In: Reisberg D and Hertel P (eds.) *Emotion and Memory*, pp. 42–75. Oxford: Oxford University Press.

Buchanan TW and Lovallo WR (2001) Enhanced memory for emotional material following stress-level cortisol treatment in humans. *Psychoneuroendocrinology* 26: 307–317.

Buss C, Wolf OT, Witt J, and Hellhammer DH (2004) Autobiographic memory impairment following acute cortisol administration. *Psychoneuroendocrinology* 29: 1093–1096.

Cahill L (2000) Modulation of long-term memory in humans by emotional arousal: Adrenergic activation and the amygdala. In: Aggleton JP (ed.) *The Amygdala*, pp. 425–446. London: Oxford University Press.

Cahill L and Alkire M (2003) Epinephrine enhancement of human memory consolidation: Interaction with arousal at encoding. *Neurobiol. Learn. Mem.* 79: 194–198.

Cahill L, Babinsky R, Markowitsch HJ, and McGaugh JL (1995) The amygdala and emotional memory. *Nature* 377: 295–296.

Cahill L, Gorski L, and Le K (2003) Enhanced human memory consolidation with post-learning stress: Interaction with the degree of arousal at encoding. *Learn. Mem.* 10: 270–274.

Cahill L, Haier RJ, Fallon J, et al. (1996) Amygdala activity at encoding correlated with long-term, free recall of emotional information. *Proc. Natl. Acad. Sci. USA* 93: 8016–8021.

Cahill L, Haier RJ, White NS, et al. (2001) Sex-related difference in amygdala activity during emotionally influenced memory storage. *Neurobiol. Learn. Mem.* 75: 1–9.

Cahill L and McGaugh JL (1991) NMDA-induced lesions of the amygdaloid complex block the retention enhancing effect of posttraining epinephrine. *Psychobiology* 19: 206–210.

Cahill L and McGaugh JL (1998) Mechanisms of emotional arousal and lasting declarative memory. *TINS* 21: 294–299.

Cahill L and McGaugh JL (2000) Emotional learning. In: Kazdin AE (ed.) *Encyclopedia of Psychology*, pp. 175–177. Washington, DC: American Psychological Association, and New York: Oxford University Press.

Cahill L, Prins B, Weber M, and McGaugh JL (1994) β-adrenergic activation and memory for emotional events. *Nature* 371: 702–704.

Cahill L, Uncapher M, Kilpatrick L, Alkire MT, and Turner J (2004) Sex-related hemispheric lateralization of amygdala function in emotionally influenced memory: An FMRI investigation. *Learn. Mem.* 11: 261–266.

Cai JX and Arnsten AFT (1997) Dose-dependent effects of the dopamine D1 receptor agonists A77636 or SKF81297 on spatial working memory in aged monkeys. *J. Pharm. Exp. Ther.* 283: 183–189.

Cai JX, Ma YY, Xu L, and Hu XT (1993) Reserpine impairs spatial working memory performance in monkeys: Reversal by the alpha-2 adrenergic agonist, clonidine. *Brain Res.* 614: 191–196.

Cai W-H, Blundell J, Han J, Greene RW, and Powell CM (2006) Postreactivation glucocorticoids impair recall of established fear memory. *J. Neurosci.* 26: 9560–9566.

Canli T, Zhao Z, Brewer J, Gabrieli JD, and Cahill L (2000) Event-related activation in the human amygdala associates with later memory for individual emotional experience. *J. Neurosci.* 20: RC99.

Canli T, Zhao Z, Desmond JE, Kang E, Gross J, and Gabrieli JD (2001) An fMRI study of personality influences on brain reactivity to emotional stimuli. *Behav. Neurosci.* 115: 33–42.

Carr GD and White NM (1984) The relationship between stereotypy and memory improvement produced by amphetamine. *Psychopharmacology* 82: 203–209.

Castellano C and Pavone F (1988) Effects of ethanol on passive avoidance behavior in the mouse: Involvement of GABAergic mechanisms. *Pharmacol. Biochem. Behav.* 29: 321–324.

Cherkin A (1969) Kinetics of memory consolidation: Role of amnesic treatment parameters. *Proc. Natl. Acad. Sci. USA* 63: 1094–1101.

Christianson SA (ed.) (1992) *The Handbook of Emotion and Memory: Research and Theory*. Hillsdale, NJ: Lawrence Erlbaum.

Clark KB, Krahl SE, Smith DC, and Jensen RA (1995) Post-training unilateral vagal stimulation enhances retention performance in the rat. *Neurobiol. Learn. Mem.* 63: 213–216.

Clark KB, Naritoku DK, Smith DC, Browning RA, and Jensen RA (1999) Enhanced recognition memory following vagus nerve stimulation in human subjects. *Nat. Neurosci.* 2: 94–98.

Clayton EC and Williams CL (2000) Adrenergic activation of the nucleus tractus solitarius potentiates amygdala norepinephrine release and enhances retention performance in emotionally arousing and spatial tasks. *Behav. Brain Res.* 112: 151–158.

Costa-Miserachs D, Portell-Cortes IK, Aldavert-Vera L, Torras-Garcia M, and Morgado-Bernal I (1994) Long-term memory facilitation in rats by posttraining epinephrine. *Behav. Neurosci.* 108: 469–474.

Cottrell GA and Nakajima S (1977) Effect of corticosteroids in the hippocampus on passive avoidance behavior in the rat. *Pharmacol. Biochem. Behav.* 7: 277–280.

Da Cunha C, Roozendaal B, Vazdarjanova A, and McGaugh JL (1999) Microinfusions of flumazenil into the basolateral but not the central nucleus of the amygdala enhance memory consolidation in rats. *Neurobiol. Learn. Mem.* 72: 1–7.

Dalmaz C, Introini-Collison IB, and McGaugh JL (1993) Noradrenergic and cholinergic interactions in the amygdala and the modulation of memory storage. *Behav. Brain Res.* 58: 167–174.

da Silva WC, Bonini JS, Bevilaqua LR, Izquierdo I, and Cammarota M (2006) Histamine enhances inhibitory avoidance memory consolidation through a H2 receptor-dependent mechanism. *Neurobiol. Learn. Mem.* 86: 100–106.

Datson NA, van der Perk J, de Kloet ER, and Vreugdenhil E (2001) Identification of corticosteroid-responsive genes in rat hippocampus using serial analysis of gene expression. *Eur. J. Neurosci.* 14: 675–689.

de Boer SF, Koopmans SJ, Slangen JL, and van der Gugten J (1990) Plasma catecholamine, corticosterone and glucose responses to repeated stress in rats: Effect of interstressor interval length. *Physiol. Behav.* 47: 1117–1124.

de Kloet ER (1991) Brain corticosteroid receptor balance and homeostatic control. *Fron. Neuroendocrin.* 12: 95–164.

de Quervain DJ-F, Aemi A, and Roozendaal B (2007) Preventive effect of β-adrenoceptor blockade on glucocorticoid-induced memory retrieval defecits. *Am. J. Psych.* 164: 967–969.

de Quervain DJ-F, Henke K, Aerni A, et al. (2003) Glucocorticoid-induced impairment of declarative memory retrieval is associated with reduced blood flow in the medial temporal lobe. *Eur. J. Neurosci.* 17: 1296–1302.

de Quervain DJ-F, Roozendaal B, and McGaugh JL (1998) Stress and glucocorticoids impair retrieval of long-term spatial memory. *Nature* 394: 787–790.

de Quervain DJ-F, Roozendaal B, Nitsch RM, McGaugh JL, and Hock C (2000) Acute cortisone administration impairs retrieval of long-term declarative memory in humans. *Nat. Neurosci.* 3: 313–314.

Devauges V and Sara SJ (1991) Memory retrieval enhancement by locus coeruleus stimulation: Evidence for mediation by beta-receptors. *Behav. Brain Res.* 43: 93–97.

de Wied D (1984) Neurohypophyseal hormone influences on learning and memory processes. In: Lynch G, McGaugh JL, and Weinberger NM (eds.) *Neurobiology of Learning and Memory*, pp. 289–312. New York: The Guilford Press.

Diamond DM, Park CR, Heman KL, and Rose GM (1999) Exposing rats to a predator impairs spatial working memory in a radial arm water maze. *Hippocampus* 9: 542–552.

Dolan RJ (2000) Functional neuroimaging of the amygdala during emotional processing and learning. In: Aggleton JP (ed.) *The Amygdala*, pp. 631–654. London: Oxford University Press.

Dolcos F, LaBar KS, and Cabeza R (2004) Interaction between the amygdala and the medial temporal lobe memory system predicts better memory for emotional events. *Neuron* 42: 855–863.

Dolcos F, LaBar KS, and Cabeza R (2005) Remembering one year later: Role of the amygdala and the medial temporal lobe memory system in retrieving emotional memories *Proc. Natl. Acad. Sci. USA* 102: 2626–2631.

Doty B and Doty L (1966) Facilitating effects of amphetamine on avoidance conditioning in relation to age and problem difficulty. *Psychopharmacology* 9: 234–241.

Dringenberg H and Vanderwolf C (1996) Cholinergic activation of the electrocorticogram: An amygdaloid activating system. *Exp. Brain Res.* 108: 285–296.

Dringenberg H, Saber AJ, and Cahill L (2001) Enhanced frontal cortex activation in rats by convergent amygdaloid and noxious sensory signals. *Neuroreport* 12: 1295–1298.

Duncan CP (1949) The retroactive effect of electroshock on learning. *J. Comp. Physiol. Psychol.* 42: 32–44.

Eichenbaum H, Schoenbaum G, Young B, and Bunsey M (1996) Functional organization of the hippocampal memory system. *Proc. Natl. Acad. Sci. USA* 93: 13500–13507.

Ellis ME and Kesner RP (1981) Physostigmine and norepinephrine: Effects of injection into the amygdala on taste associations. *Physiol. Behav.* 27: 203–209.

Evangelista AM and Izquierdo I (1971) The effect of pre- and post-trial amphetamine injections on avoidance responses of rats. *Psychopharmacologia* 20: 42–47.

Ferry B and McGaugh JL (1999) Clenbuterol administration into the basolateral amygdala post-training enhances retention in an inhibitory avoidance task. *Neurobiol. Learn. Mem.* 72: 8–12.

Ferry B, Roozendaal B, and McGaugh JL (1999a) Involvement of alpha$_1$-adrenergic receptors in the basolateral amygdala in modulation of memory storage. *Eur. J. Pharmacol.* 372: 9–16.

Ferry B, Roozendaal B, and McGaugh JL (1999b) Basolateral amygdala noradrenergic influences on memory storage are mediated by an interaction between beta- and alpha$_1$-receptors. *J. Neurosci.* 19: 5119–5123.

Finlay JM, Zigmond MJ, and Abercrombie ED (1995) Increased dopamine and norepinephrine release in the medial prefrontal cortex induced by acute and chronic stress: Effects of diazepam. *Neurosci.* 64: 619–628.

Flood JF, Landry DW, and Jarvik ME (1981) Cholinergic receptor interactions and their effects on long-term memory processing. *Brain Res.* 215: 177–185.

Flood JF, Smith GE, and Morley JE (1987) Modulation of memory processing by cholecystokinin: Dependence on the vague nerve. *Science* 236: 832–834.

Frey S, Bergado-Rosado J, Seidenbecher T, Pape H-C, and Frey JU (2001) Reinforcement of early long-term potentation (early-LTP) in dentate gyrus by stimulation of the basolateral amygdala: Heterosynaptic induction mechanisms of late-LTP. *J. Neurosci.* 21: 3697–3703.

Fuster JM (1991) The prefrontal cortex and its relation to behavior. *Prog. Brain Res.* 87: 201–211.

Gallagher M, Kapp BS, Pascoe JP, and Rapp PR (1981) A neuropharmacology of amygdaloid systems which contribute to learning and memory. In: Ben-Ari Y (ed.) *The Amygdaloid Complex*, pp. 343–354. Amsterdam: Elsevier/North-Holland.

Galvez R, Mesches M, and McGaugh JL (1996) Norepinephrine release in the amygdala in response to footshock stimulation. *Neurobiol. Learn. Mem.* 66: 253–257.

Gerard RW (1949) Physiology and psychology. *Am. J. Psychol.* 106: 161–173.

Ghacibeh GA, Shenker JI, Shenal B, Uthman BM, and Heilman KM (2006) The influence of vagus nerve stimulation on memory. *Cog. Behav. Neurol.* 19: 119–122.

Goddard GV (1964) Amygdaloid stimulation and learning in the rat. *J. Comp. Physiol. Psychol.* 58: 23–30.

Gold PE (1986) Glucose modulation of memory storage. *Behav. Neural Biol.* 45: 342–349.

Gold PE (1995) Role of glucose in regulating the brain and cognition. *Am. J. Clin. Nutr.* 61: 987S–995S.

Gold PE (2003) Acetylcholine modulation of neural systems involved in learning and memory. *Neurobiol. Learn. Mem.* 80: 194–210.

Gold PE (2004) Coordination of multiple memory systems. *Neurobiol. Learn. Mem.* 82: 230–242.

Gold PE, Hankins L, Edwards RM, Chester J, and McGaugh JL (1975) Memory interference and facilitation with posttrial amygdala stimulation: Effect on memory varies with footshock level. *Brain Res.* 86: 509–513.

Gold PE and van Buskirk R (1975) Facilitation of time-dependent memory processes with posttrial epinephrine injections. *Behav. Biol.* 13: 145–153.

Gold PE and van Buskirk R (1976) Enhancement and impairment of memory processes with post-trial injections of adrenocorticotrophic hormone. *Behav. Biol.* 16: 387–400.

Gold PE and van Buskirk R (1978) Post-training brain norepinephrine concentrations: Correlation with retention performance of avoidance training with peripheral epinephrine modulation of memory processing. *Behav. Biol.* 23: 509–520.

Gold PE, Vogt J, and Hall JL (1986) Post-training glucose effects on memory: Behavioral and pharmacological characteristics. *Behav. Neural Biol.* 46: 145–155.

Grecksch G and Matthies H (1981) Differential effects of intrahippocampally or systemically applied picrotoxin on memory consolidation in rats. *Pharmacol. Biochem. Behav.* 14: 613–616.

Greenberg DL, Rice HJ, Cooper JJ, Cabeza R, Rubin DC, and LaBar KS (2005) Co-activation of the amygdala hippocampus and inferior frontal gyrus during autobiographical memory retrieval. *Neuropsychologia* 43: 659–674.

Guzowski JF, Lyford GL, Stevenson GD, et al. (2000) Inhibition of activity-dependent arc protein expression in the rat hippocampus impairs the maintenance of long-term potentiation and consolidation of long-term memory. *J. Neurosci.* 20: 3993–4001.

Hall JL and Gold PE (1986) The effects of training, epinephrine, and glucose injections on plasma glucose levels in rats. *Behav. Neural Biol.* 46: 156–167.

Hall J, Thomas KL, and Everitt BJ (2001) Cellular imaging of zif 268 expression in the hippocampus and amygdala during contextual and cued fear memory retrieval: Selective activation of hippocampal CA1 neurons during recall of contextual memory. *J. Neurosci.* 21: 2186–2193.

Hamann SB, Eli TD, Grafton ST, and Kilts CD (1999) Amygdala activity related to enhanced memory for pleasant and aversive stimuli. *Nat. Neurosci.* 2: 289–303.

Hamann SB, Eli TD, Hoffman JM, and Kilts CD (2002) Ecstacy and agony: Activation of the human amygdala in positive and negative emotions. *Psychol. Sci.* 13: 135–141.

Haralambous T and Westbrook RF (1999) An infusion of bupivacaine into the nucleus accumbens disrupts the acquisition but not the expression of contextual fear conditioning. *Behav. Neurosci.* 113: 925–940.

Hassert DL, Miyashita T, and Williams CL (2004) The effects of peripheral vagal nerve stimulation at a memory-modulating intensity on norepinephrine output in the basolateral amygdala. *Behav. Neurosci.* 118: 79–88.

Hatfield T and McGaugh JL (1999) Norepinephrine infused into the basolateral amygdala posttraining enhances retention in a spatial water maze task. *Neurobiol. Learn. Mem.* 71: 232–239.

Hatfield T, Spanis C, and McGaugh JL (1999) Response of amygdalar norepinephrine to footshock and GABAergic drugs using *in vivo* microdialysis and HPLC. *Brain Res.* 835: 340–345.

Heck S, Kullmann M, Gast A, et al. (1994) A distinct modulating domain in glucocorticoid receptor monomers in the repression of activity of the transcription factor AP-1. *EMBO J.* 13: 4087–4095.

Het S, Ramlow G, and Wolf OT (2005) A meta-analytic review of the effects of acute cortisol administration on human memory. *Psychoneuroendocrinology* 30: 771–784.

Hirsh R (1974) The hippocampus and contextual retrieval of information from memory: A theory. *Behav. Biol.* 12: 421–444.

Holt W and Maren S (1999) Muscimol inactivation of the dorsal hippocampus impairs contextual retrieval of fear memory. *J. Neurosci.* 19: 9054–9062.

Huff NC, Frank M, Wright-Hardesty K, et al. (2006) Amygdala regulation of immediate-early gene expression in the hippocampus induced by contextual fear conditioning. *J. Neurosci.* 26: 1616–1623.

Huff NC, Wright-Hardesty KJ, Higgins EA, Matus-Amat P, and Rudy JW (2005) Context pre-exposure obscures amygdala modulation of contextual-fear conditioning. *Learn. Mem.* 12: 456–460.

Hsu EH, Schroeder JP, and Packard M (2002) The amygdala mediates memory consolidation for an amphetamine conditioned place preference. *Behav. Brain Res.* 129: 93–100.

Huston JP and Staubli U (1981) Substance P and its effects on learning and memory. In: Martine JL, Jr., Jensen RA, Messing RB, Rigter H, and McGaugh, JL (eds.) *Endogenous Peptides and Learning and Memory Processes*, pp. 521–540. New York: Academic Press.

Ikegaya Y, Saito H, and Abe K (1994) Attenuated hippocampal long-term potentiation in basolateral amygdala-lesioned rats. *Brain Res.* 656: 157–164.

Ikegaya Y, Saito H, and Abe K (1995a) Requirement of basolateral amygdala neuron activity for the induction of long-term potentiation in the dentate gyrus *in vivo*. *Brain Res.* 671: 351–354.

Ikegaya Y, Saito H, and Abe K (1995b) High-frequency stimulation of the basolateral amygdala facilitates the induction of long-term potentiation in the dentate gyrus *in vivo*. *Neurosci. Res.* 22: 203–207.

Ikegaya Y, Saito H, Abe K, and Nakanishi K (1997) Amygdala beta-noradrenergic influence on hippocampal long-term potentiation *in vivo*. *Neuroreport* 8: 3143–3146.

Introini IB and Baratti CM (1984) The impairment of retention induced by β-endorphin in mice may be mediated by reduction of central cholinergic activity. *Behav. Neural Biol.* 41: 152–163.

Introini-Collison IB, Arai Y, and McGaugh JL (1989) Stria terminalis lesions attenuate the effects of posttraining oxotremorine and atropine on retention. *Psychobiology* 17: 397–401.

Introini-Collison IB and Baratti CM (1992) Memory-modulatory effects of centrally acting noradrenergic drugs: Possible involvement of brain cholinergic mechanisms. *Behav. Neural Biol.* 57: 248–255.

Introini-Collison IB, Castellano C, and McGaugh JL (1994) Interaction of GABAergic and β-noradrenergic drugs in the regulation of memory storage. *Behav. Neural Biol.* 61: 150–155.

Introini-Collison IB, Dalmaz C, and McGaugh JL (1996) Amygdala β-noradrenergic influences on memory storage involve cholinergic activation. *Neurobiol. Learn. Mem.* 65: 57–64.

Introini-Collison IB and McGaugh JL (1986) Epinephrine modulates long-term retention of an aversively-motivated discrimination task. *Behav. Neural Biol.* 45: 358–365.

Introini-Collison IB and McGaugh JL (1988) Modulation of memory by posttraining epinephrine: Involvement of cholinergic mechanisms. *Psychopharmacology* 94: 379–385.

Introini-Collison IB, Miyazaki B, and McGaugh JL (1991) Involvement of the amygdala in the memory-enhancing effects of clenbuterol. *Psychopharmacology* 104: 541–544.

Introini-Collison IB, Saghafi D, Novack G, and McGaugh JL (1992) Memory-enhancing effects of posttraining dipivefrin and epinephrine: Involvement of peripheral and central adrenergic receptors. *Brain Res.* 572: 81–86.

Izquierdo I, daCunha C, Rosat R, Jerusalinsky D, Ferreira MBC, and Medina JH (1992) Neurotransmitter receptors involved in posttraining memory processing by the amygdala, medial septum and hippocampus of the rat. *Behav. Neural Biol.* 58: 16–26.

Izquierdo I and Dias RD (1985) Influence on memory of posttraining or pre-test injections of ACTH, vasopressin, epinephrine and β-endorphin, and their interaction with naloxone. *Psychoneuroendocrinology* 10: 165–172.

Izquierdo I and Graudenz M (1980) Memory facilitation by naloxone is due to release of dopaminergic and β-adrenergic systems from tonic inhibition. *Psychopharmacology* 67: 265–268.

Izquierdo I and Medina JH (1997) Memory formation: The sequence of biochemical events in the hippocampus and its connection to activity in other brain structures. *Neurobiol. Learn. Mem.* 68: 285–316.

Izquierdo I, Quillfeldt JA, Zanatta MS, et al. (1997) Sequential role of hippocampus and amygdala, entorhinal cortex and parietal cortex in formation and retrieval of memory for inhibitory avoidance in rats. *Eur. J. Neurosci.* 9: 786–793.

Izquierdo LA, Barros DM, Medina JH, and Izquierdo I (2000) Novelty enhances retrieval of one-trial avoidance learning in rats 1 or 31 days after training unless the hippocampus is inactivated by different receptor antagonists and enzyme inhibitors. *Behav. Brain Res.* 117: 215–220.

Izquierdo LA, Barros DM, Medina JH, and Izquierdo I (2002) Stress hormones enhance retrieval of fear conditioning acquired either one day or many months before. *Behav. Pharmacol.* 13: 203–213.

James W (1890) *Principles of Psychology,* New York: Henry Holt and Company.

Kandel ER (2001) The molecular biology of memory storage: A dialog between genes and synapses. *Biosci. Rep.* 21: 565–611.

Kawahara Y, Hesselink MB, van Scharrenburg G, and Westerink BHC (2004) Tonic inhibition by orphanin FQ/ nociceptin of noradrenaline neurotransmission in the amygdala. *Eur. J. Pharmacol.* 485: 197–200.

Kelley AE, Domesick VB, and Nauta WJ (1982) The amygdalostriatal projection in the rat – An anatomical study by anterograde and retrograde tracing methods. *Neuroscience* 7: 615–630.

Kesner RP and Ellis ME (1983) Memory consolidation: Brain region and neurotransmitter specificity. *Neurosci. Lett.* 39: 295–300.

Kesner RP and Wilburn MW (1974) A review of electrical stimulation of the brain in context of learning and retention. *Behav. Biol.* 10: 259–293.

Kety S (1972) Brain catecholamines affective states and memory. In: McGaugh JL (ed.) *The Chemistry of Mood, Motivation and Memory*, pp. 65–80. New York: Raven Press.

Kilpatrick L and Cahill L (2003a) Modulation of memory consolidation for olfactory learning by reversible inactivation of the basolateral amygdala. *Behav. Neurosci.* 117: 184–188.

Kilpatrick L and Cahill L (2003b) Amygdala modulation of parahippocampal and frontal regions during emotionally influenced memory storage. *Neuroimage* 20: 2091–2099.

Kuhlman S and Wolf OT (2006) Arousal and cortisol interact in modulating memory consolidation in healthy young men. *Behav. Neurosci.* 120: 217–223.

Kuhlman S, Kirschbaum C, and Wolf OT (2005a) Effects of oral cortisol treatment in healthy young women on memory retrieval of negative and neutral words. *Neurobiol. Learn. Mem.* 83: 158–162.

Kuhlman S, Piel M, and Wolf OT (2005b) Impaired memory retrieval after psychosocial stress in healthy young men. *J. Neurosci.* 25: 2977–2982.

LaBar KS and Cabezza R (2006) Cognitive neuroscience of emotional memory. *Nat. Rev. Neurosci.* 7: 54–64.

LaLumiere RT, Buen T-V, and McGaugh JL (2003) Posttraining intra-basolateral amygdala infusions of norepinephrine enhance consolidation of memory for contextual fear conditioning. *J. Neurosci.* 23: 6754–6758.

LaLumiere RT, Nawar EM, and McGaugh JL (2005) Modulation of memory consolidation by the basolateral amygdala or nucleus accumbens shell requires concurrent dopamine receptor activation in both brain regions. *Learn. Mem.* 12: 296–301.

LaLumiere RT, Nguyen L, and McGaugh JL (2004) Posttraining intra-basolateral amygdala infusions of dopamine modulate consolidation of inhibitory avoidance memory: Involvement of noradrenergic and cholinergic systems. *Eur. J. Neurosci.* 20: 2804–2810.

Ledgerwood L, Richardson R, and Cranney J (2003) Effects of D-cycloserine on extinction of conditioned freezing. *Behav. Neurosci.* 117: 341–349.

Ledgerwood L, Richardson R, and Cranney J (2005) D-cycloserine facilitates extinction of learned fear: Effects on reacquisition and generalized extinction. *Biol. Psychiat.* 57: 841–847.

Lee I and Kesner RP (2003) Time-dependent relationship between the dorsal hippocampus and the prefrontal cortex in spatial memory. *J. Neurosci.* 23: 1517–1523.

Lee MK, Graham S, and Gold PE (1988) Memory enhancement with posttraining central glucose injections. *Behav. Neurosci.* 102: 591–595.

Lennartz RC, Hellems KL, Mook ER, and Gold PE (1996) Inhibitory avoidance impairments induced by intra-amygdala propranolol are reversed by glutamate but not glucose. *Behav. Neurosci.* 110: 1033–1039.

Levy F and Farrow M (2001) Working memory in ADHD: Prefrontal/parietal connections. *Curr. Drug Targets* 2: 347–352.

Li B-M, Mao Z-M, Wang M, and Mei Z-T (1999) Alpha-2 adrenergic modulation of prefrontal cortical neuronal activity related to spatial working memory in monkeys. *Neuropyschopharmacology* 21: 601–610.

Liang KC (2001) Epinephrine modulation of memory: Amygdala activation and regulation of long-term memory storage. In: Gold PE and Greenough WT (eds.) *Memory Consolidation: Essays in Honor of James L. McGaugh*, pp. 165–183. Washington, DC: American Psychological Association.

Liang KC, Bennett C, and McGaugh JL (1985) Peripheral epinephrine modulates the effects of posttraining amygdala stimulation on memory. *Behav. Brain Res.* 15: 93–100.

Liang KC, Chen L, and Huang T-E (1995) The role of amygdala norepinephrine in memory formation: Involvement in the memory enhancing effect of peripheral epinephrine. *Chin. J. Physiol.* 38: 81–91.

Liang KC, Hu S-J, and Chang SH (1996) Formation and retrieval of inhibitory avoidance memory: Differential roles of glutamate receptors in the amygdala and medial prefrontal cortex. *Chin. J. Physiol.* 39: 155–166.

Liang KC, Juler RG, and McGaugh JL (1986) Modulating effects of post-training epinephrine on memory: Involvement of the amygdala noradrenergic system. *Brain Res.* 368: 125–133.

Liang KC and Lee EH (1988) Intra-amygdala injections of corticotropin releasing factor facilitate inhibitory avoidance learning and reduce exploratory behavior in rats. *Psychopharmacology* 96: 232–236.

Liang KC and McGaugh JL (1983) Lesions of the stria terminalis attenuate the enhancing effect of post-training epinephrine on retention of an inhibitory avoidance response. *Behav. Brain Res.* 9: 49–58.

Liang KC, McGaugh JL, and Yao H-Y (1990) Involvement of amygdala pathways in the influence of posttraining amygdala norepinephrine and peripheral epinephrine on memory storage. *Brain Res.* 508: 225–233.

Lidow MS, Koh P-O, and Arnsten AFT (2003) D1 dopamine receptors in the mouse prefrontal cortex: Immunocytochemical and cognitive neuropharmacological analyses. *Synapse* 47: 101–108.

Livingston RB (1967) Reinforcement. In: Quarton GC, Melnechuk T, and Schmitt FO (eds.) *The Neurosciences: A Study Program*, pp. 514–576. New York: Rockefeller University Press.

Lupien SJ, Gillin CJ, and Hauger RL (1999) Working memory is more sensitive than declarative memory to the acute effects of corticosteroids: A dose-response study in humans. *Behav. Neurosci.* 113: 420–430.

Lupien SJ and McEwen BS (1997) The acute effects of corticosteroids on cognition: Integration of animal and human model studies. *Brain Res. Rev.* 24: 1–27.

Lyons DM, Lopez JM, Yang C, and Schatzberg AF (2000) Stress-level cortisol treatment impairs inhibitory control of behavior in monkeys. *J. Neurosci.* 20: 7816–7821.

Ma S, Roozendaal B, Burazin TCD, Tregear GW, McGaugh JL, and Gundlach AL (2005) Relaxin receptor activation in the basolateral amygdala impairs memory consolidation. *Eur. J. Neurosci.* 22: 2117–2122.

Malin EL, Ibrahim DY, Tu JW, and McGaugh JL (2007) Involvement of the rostral anterior cingulate cortex in consolidation of inhibitory avoidance memory: Interaction with the basolateral amygdala. *Neurobiol. Learn. Mem.* 87: 295–302.

Malin EL and McGaugh JL (2006) Differential involvement of the hippocampus, anterior cingulate cortex and basolateral amygdala in memory for context and footshock. *Proc. Natl. Acad. Sci. USA* 103: 1959–1963.

Martinez JL, Jr., Vasquez BJ, Rigter H, et al. (1980) Attenuation of amphetamine-induced enhancement of learning by adrenal demedullation. *Brain Res.* 195: 433–443.

Matus-Amat P, Higgins EA, Barrientos RM, and Rudy JW (2004) The role of the dorsal hippocampus in the acquisition and retrieval of context memory representations. *J. Neurosci.* 24: 2431–2439.

McCarty R and Gold PE (1981) Plasma catecholamines: Effects of footshock level and hormonal modulators of memory storage. *Horm. Behav.* 15: 168–182.

McDonald AJ (1991) Organization of amygdaloid projections to the prefrontal cortex and associated striatum in the rat. *Neuroscience* 44: 1–14.

McDonald RJ and White NM (1993) A triple dissociation of memory systems: Hippocampus, amygdala and dorsal striatum. *Behav. Neurosci.* 107: 3–22.

McEwen BS and Sapolsky RM (1995) Stress and cognitive function. *Curr. Opin. Neurobiol.* 5: 205–216.

McEwen BS, Weiss JM, and Schwartz LS (1968) Selective retention of corticosterone by limbic structures in the rat brain. *Nature* 220: 911–912.

McGaugh JL (1966) Time-dependent processes in memory storage. *Science* 153: 1351–1358.

McGaugh JL (1973) Drug facilitation of learning and memory. *Annu. Rev. Pharmacol.* 13: 229–241.

McGaugh JL (1983) Hormonal influences on memory. *Annu. Rev. Psychol.* 34: 297–323.

McGaugh JL (1989) Involvement of hormonal and neuromodulatory systems in the regulation of memory storage. *Annu. Rev. Neurosci.* 12: 255–287.

McGaugh JL (2000) Memory: A century of consolidation. *Science* 287: 248–251.

McGaugh JL (2002) Memory consolidation and the amygdala: A systems perspective. *TINS* 25: 456–461.

McGaugh JL (2003) *Memory and Emotion: The Making of Lasting Memories.* London: Weidenfeld and Nicolson The Orion House Group Ltd., and New York: Columbia University Press.

McGaugh JL (2004) The amygdala modulates the consolidation of memories of emotionally arousing experiences. *Annu. Rev. Neurosci.* 27: 1–28.

McGaugh JL (2005) Emotional arousal and enhanced amygdala activity: New evidence for the old perseveration-consolidation hypothesis. *Learn. Mem.* 12: 77–79.

McGaugh JL and Cahill L (1997) Interaction of neuromodulatory systems in modulating memory storage. *Behav. Brain Res.* 83: 31–38.

McGaugh JL, Ferry B, Vazdarjanova A, and Roozendaal B (2000) Amygdala role in modulation of memory storage. In: Aggleton JP (ed.) *The Amygdala*, pp. 391–423. London: Oxford University Press.

McGaugh JL and Gold PE (1976) Modulation of memory by electrical stimulation of the brain. In: Rosenzweig MR and Bennett EL (eds.) *Neural Mechanisms of Learning and Memory*, pp. 549–560. Cambridge: MA: MIT Press.

McGaugh JL and Gold PE (1989) Hormonal modulation of memory. In: Brush RB and Levine S (eds.) *Psychoendocrinology*, pp. 305–339. New York: Academic Press.

McGaugh JL and Herz MJ (1972) *Memory Consolidation.* San Francisco: Albion Publishing Company.

McGaugh JL, Introini-Collison IB, and Nagahara AH (1988) Memory-enhancing effects of posttraining naloxone: Involvement of β-noradrenergic influences in the amygdaloid complex. *Brain Res.* 446: 37–49.

McGaugh JL, Introini-Collison IB, Nagahara AH, Cahill L, Brioni JD, and Castellano C (1990) Involvement of the amygdaloid complex in neuromodulatory influences on memory storage. *Neurosci. Biobehav. Rev.* 14: 425–431.

McGaugh JL and Izquierdo I (2000) The contribution of pharmacology to research on the mechanisms of memory formation. *TIPS* 21: 208–210.

McGaugh JL and Petrinovich LF (1965) Effects of drugs on learning and memory. *Internatl. Rev. Neurobiol.* 8: 139–196.

McGaugh JL and Roozendaal B (2002) Role of adrenal stress hormones in forming lasting memories in the brain. *Curr. Opin. Neurobiol.* 12: 205–210.

McIntyre CK, Hatfield T, and McGaugh JL (2002) Amygdala norepinephrine levels after training predict inhibitory avoidance retention performance in rats. *Eur. J. Neurosci.* 16: 1223–1226.

McIntyre CK, Marriott LK, and Gold PF (2003) Cooperation between memory systems: Acetylcholine release in the amygdala correlates positively with performance on a hippocampus-dependent task. *Behav. Neurosci.* 117. 320–326.

McIntyre CK, Miyashita T, Setlow B, et al. (2005) Memory-influencing intra-basolateral amygdala drug infusions modulate expression of Arc protein in the hippocampus. *Proc. Natl. Acad. Sci. USA* 102: 10718–10723.

McIntyre CK, Roozendall B, and McGaugh JL (2004) Glucocorticoid treatment enhances training-induced norepinephrine release in the amygdala. *Soc. Neurosci. Abstr.* 772: 12.

McNay EC and Gold PE (1998) Memory modulation across neural systems: Intra-amygdala glucose reverses deficits caused by intraseptal morphine on a spatial task but not on an aversive task. *J. Neurosci.* 18: 3853–3858.

McNish KA, Gewirtz JC, and Davis M (1997) Evidence of contextual fear after lesions of the hippocampus: A disruption of freezing but not fear-potentiated startle. *J. Neurosci.* 17: 9353–9360.

Menzel R (1983) Neurobiology of learning and memory: The honeybee as a model system. *Naturwissenschaften* 70: 504–511.

Messier C and White NM (1984) Contingent and non-contingent actions of sucrose and saccharin reinforcers: Effects on taste preference and memory. *Physiol. Behav.* 32: 195–203.

Messier C and White NM (1987) Memory improvement by glucose, fructose, and two glucose analogs: A possible effect on peripheral glucose transport. *Behav. Neural Biol.* 48: 104–127.

Messing RB, Jensen RA, Martinez JL, Jr., et al. (1979) Naloxone enhancement of memory. *Behav. Neural Biol.* 27: 266–275.

Miasnikov AA, Chen JC, and Weinberger NM (2006) Rapid induction of specific associative behavioral memory by stimulation of the nucleus basalis in the rat. *Neurobiol. Learn. Mem.* 86: 47–65.

Miasnikov AA, McLin D, 3rd, and Weinberger NM (2001) Muscarinic dependence of nucleus basalis induced conditioned receptive field plasticity. *Neuroreport* 12: 1537–1542.

Miranda MI, LaLumiere RT, Buen TV, Bermudez-Rattoni F, and McGaugh JL (2003) Blockade of noradrenergic receptors in the basolateral amygdala impairs taste memory. *Eur. J. Neurosci.* 18: 2605–2610.

Miranda MI and McGaugh JL (2004) Enhancement of inhibitory avoidance and conditioned taste aversion memory with insular cortex infusions of 8-Br-cAMP: Involvement of the basolateral amygdala. *Learn. Mem.* 11: 312–317.

Miyashita T and Williams CL (2002) Glutamatergic transmission in the nucleus of the solitary tract modulates memory through influences on amygdala noradrenergic systems. *Behav. Neurosci.* 116: 13–21.

Mizoguchi K, Ishige A, Takeda S, Aburada M, and Tabita T (2004) Endogenous glucocorticoids are essential for maintaining prefrontal cortical cognitive function. *J. Neurosci.* 24: 5492–5499.

Morrow BA, Roth RH, and Elsworth JD (2000) TMT, a predator odor, elevates mesoprefrontal dopamine metabolic activity and disrupts short-term working memory in the rat. *Brain Res. Bull.* 52: 519–523.

Müller GE and Pilzecker A (1900) Experimentelle Beitrage zur Lehre vom Gedachtniss. *Z. Psychol.* 1: 1–288.

Mulder AB, Hodenpijl MG, and Lopes da Silva FH (1998) Electrophysiology of the hippocampal and amygdaloid projections to the nucleus accumbens of the rat: Convergence, segregation, and interaction of inputs. *J. Neurosci.* 18: 5095–5102.

Murchison CF, Zhang XY, Zhang WP, Ouyang M, Lee A, and Thomas SA (2004) A distinct role for norepinephrine in memory retrieval. *Cell* 117: 131–143.

Murphy BL, Arnsten AFT, Goldman-Rakic PS, and Roth RH (1996) Increased dopamine turnover in the prefrontal cortex impairs spatial working memory performance in rats and monkeys. *Proc. Natl. Acad. Sci. USA* 93: 1325–1329.

Nakamura S, Tepper JM, Young SJ, Ling N, and Groves PM (1982) Noradrenergic terminal excitability: Effects of opioids. *Neurosci. Lett.* 30: 57–62.

Nielson KA and Jensen RA (1994) Beta-adrenergic receptor antagonist antihypertensive medications impair arousal-induced modulation of working memory in elderly humans. *Behav. Neural Biol.* 62: 190–200.

O'Carroll RE, Drysdale E, Cahill L, Shajahan P, and Ebmeier KP (1999) Stimulation of the noradrenergic system enhances and blockade reduces memory for emotional material in man. *Psychol. Med.* 29: 1083–1088.

Okuda S, Roozendaal B, and McGaugh JL (2004) Glucocorticoid effects on object recognition memory require training-associated emotional arousal. *Proc. Natl. Acad. Sci. USA* 101: 853–858.

Oitzl MS and de Kloet ER (1992) Selective corticosteroid antagonists modulate specific aspects of spatial orientation learning. *Behav. Neurosci.* 108: 62–71.

Oomura Y, Nakano Y, Lenard L, Nishino H, and Aou S (1988) Catecholaminergic and opioid mechanisms in conditioned food intake behavior of the monkey amygdala. In: Woody CD, Alkon DL, and McGaugh JL (eds.) *Cellular Mechanisms of Conditioning and Behavioral Plasticity*, pp. 109–118. New York: Plenum.

Packard MG and Cahill L (2001) Affective modulation of multiple memory systems. *Curr. Opin. Neurobiol.* 11: 752–756.

Packard MG, Cahill L, and McGaugh JL (1994) Amygdala modulation of hippocampal-dependent and caudate nucleus-dependent memory processes. *Proc. Natl. Acad. Sci. USA* 91: 8477–8481.

Packard MG and Chen SA (1999) The basolateral amygdala is a cofactor in memory enhancement produced by intrahippocampal glutamate injections. *Psychobiology* 27: 377–385.

Packard MG, Introini-Collison IB, and McGaugh JL (1996) Stria terminalis lesions attenuate memory enhancement produced by intra-caudate nucleus injections of oxotremorine. *Neurobiol. Learn. Mem.* 65: 278–282.

Packard MG and Knowlton BJ (2002) Learning and memory functions of the basal ganglia. *Annu. Rev. Neurosci.* 25: 563–593.

Packard MG and McGaugh JL (1992) Double dissociation of fornix and caudate nucleus lesions on acquisition of two water maze tasks: Further evidence for multiple memory systems. *Behav. Neurosci.* 106: 439–446.

Packard MG and McGaugh JL (1996) Inactivation of hippocampus or caudate nucleus with lidocaine differentially affects expression of place and response learning. *Neurobiol. Learn. Mem.* 65: 65–72.

Packard MG and Teather L (1998) Amygdala modulation of multiple memory systems: Hippocampus and caudate-putamen. *Neurobiol. Learn. Mem.* 69: 163–203.

Pakdel R and Rashidy-Pour A (2006) Glucocorticoid-induced impairment of long-term memory retrieval in rats: An interaction with dopamine D2 receptors. *Neurobiol. Learn. Mem.* 85: 300–306.

Pape H-C, Narayanan RT, Smid J, Store O, and Seidenbecher T (2005) Theta activity in neurons and networks of the amygdala related to long-term fear memory. *Hippocampus* 15: 874–880.

Paré D (2003) Role of the basolateral amygdala in memory consolidation. *Prog. Neurobiol.* 70: 409–420.

Paré D, Collins DR, and Pelletier JG (2002) Amygdala oscillations and the consolidation of emotional memories. *TICS* 6: 306–314.

Paré D, Dong J, and Gaudreau H (1995) Amygdalo-entorhinal relations and their reflection in the hippocampal formation: Generation of sharp potentials. *J. Neurosci.* 15: 2482–2503.

Paré D and Gaudreau H (1996) Projection cells and interneurons of the lateral and basolateral amygdala: Distinct firing patterns and differential relation to theta and delta rhythms in conscious cats. *J. Neurosci.* 16: 3334–3350.

Parent MB and McGaugh JL (1994) Posttraining infusion of lidocaine into the amygdala basolateral complex impairs retention of inhibitory avoidance training. *Brain Res.* 661: 97–103.

Passani MB, Cangioli I, Baldi E, Bucherelli C, Mannaioni PF, and Blandina P (2001) Histamine H_3 receptor-mediated impairment of contextual fear conditioning and *in vivo* inhibition of cholinergic transmission in the rat basolateral amygdala. *Eur. J. Neurosci.* 14: 1–13.

Paz R, Pelletier JG, Bauer EP, and Paré D (2006) Emotional enhancement of memory via amygdala-driven facilitation of rhinal interactions. *Nat. Neurosci.* 9: 1321–1329.

Pelletier JG and Paré D (2004) Role of amygdala oscillations in the consolidation of emotional memories. *Biol. Psychiat.* 55: 559–562.

Pelletier JG, Likhtik E, Filali M, and Paré D (2005) Lasting increases in basolateral amygdala activity after emotional arousal: Implications for facilitated consolidation of emotional memories. *Learn. Mem.* 12: 96–102.

Perez-Jaranay JM and Vives F (1991) Electrophysiological study of the response of medial prefrontal cortex neurons to stimulation of the basolateral nucleus of the amygdala in the rat. *Brain Res.* 564: 97–101.

Petrovich GD, Canteras NS, and Swanson LW (2001) Combinatorial amygdalar inputs to hippocampal domains and hypothalamic behavior systems. *Brain Res. Rev.* 38: 247–289.

Phillips RG and LeDoux JE (1992) Differential contribution of amygdala and hippocampus to cued and contextual fear conditioning. *Behav. Neurosci.* 106: 274–285.

Pikkarainen M, Ronko S, Savander V, Insausti R, and Pitkänen A (1999) Projections from the lateral, basal, and accessory basal nuclei of the amygdala to the hippocampal formation in rat. *J. Comp. Neurol.* 403: 229–260.

Pitkänen A (2000) Connectivity of the rat amygdaloid complex. In: Aggleton JP (ed.) *The Amgydala*, pp. 31–117. London: Oxford University Press.

Popescu AT, Saghyan AA, and Paré D (2007) NMDA-dependent facilitation of corticostriatal plasticity by the amygdala. *Proc. Natl. Acad. Sci. USA.* 104: 341–346.

Power AE and McGaugh JL (2002) Phthalic acid amygdalopetal lesion of the nucleus basalis magnocellularis induces reversible memory deficits in rats. *Neurobiol. Learn. Mem.* 77: 373–388.

Power AE, McIntyre CK, Litmanovich A, and McGaugh JL (2003a) Cholinergic modulation of memory in the basolateral amygdala involves activation of both m1 and m2 receptors. *Behav. Pharmacol.* 14: 207–213.

Power AE, Roozendaal B, and McGaugh JL (2000) Glucocorticoid enhancement of memory consolidation in the rat is blocked by muscarinic receptor antagonism in the basolateral amygdala. *Eur. J. Neurosci.* 12: 3481–3487.

Power AE, Thal LJ, and McGaugh JL (2002) Lesions of the nucleus basalis magnocellularis induced by 192 IgG-saporin block memory enhancement with posttraining norepinephrine in the basolateral amygdala. *Proc. Natl. Acad. Sci. USA* 99: 2315–2319.

Power AE, Vazdarjanova A, and McGaugh JL (2003b) Muscarinic cholinergic influences in memory consolidation. *Neurobiol. Learn. Mem.* 80: 178–183.

Price JL (1981) Toward a consistent terminology for the amygdaloid complex. In: Ben-Ari Y (ed.) *The Amygdaloid Complex*, pp. 13–18. North Holland: Elsevier.

Price JL (2003) Comparative aspects of amygdala connectivity. *Ann. N. Y. Acad. Sci.* 985: 50–58.

Quillfeldt JA, Zanatta MS, Schmitz PK, et al. (1996) Different brain areas are involved in memory expression at different times from training. *Neurobiol. Learn. Mem.* 66: 97–102.

Quirarte GL, Galvez R, Roozendaal B, and McGaugh JL (1998) Norepinephrine release in the amygdala in response to footshock and opioid peptidergic drugs. *Brain Res.* 808: 134–140.

Quirarte GL, Roozendaal B, and McGaugh JL (1997) Glucocorticoid enhancement of memory storage involves noradrenergic activation in the basolateral amygdala. *Proc. Natl. Acad. Sci. USA* 94: 14048–14053.

Ragozzino ME and Gold PE (1994) Task-dependent effects of intra-amygdala morphine injections: Attenuation by intra-amygdala glucose injections. *J. Neurosci.* 14: 7478–7485.

Ramos BP, Colgan L, Nou E, Ovadia S, Wilson SR, and Arnsten AFT (2005) The beta-1 adrenergic antagonist, betaxolol, improves working memory performance in rats and monkeys. *Biol Psychiat.* 58: 894–900.

Rashidy-Pour A and Razvani ME (1998) Unilateral reversible inactivations of the nucleus tractus solitarius and amygdala attenuate the effects of bombesin on memory storage. *Brain Res.* 814: 127–132.

Rashidy-Pour A, Sadeghi H, Taherain AA, Vafaei AA, and Fathollahi Y (2004) The effects of acute restraint stress and dexamethasone on retrieval of long-term memory in rats: An interaction with opiate system. *Behav. Brain Res.* 154: 193–198.

Ressler KJ, Paschall G, Zhou X-L, and Davis M (2002) Regulation of synaptic plasticity genes during consolidation of fear conditioning. *J. Neurosci.* 22: 7892–7902.

Ricardo JA and Koh ET (1978) Anatomical evidence of direct projections from the nucleus of the solitary tract to the hypothalamus, amygdala, and other forebrain structures in the rat. *Brain Res.* 153: 1–26.

Riedel G, Micheau J, Lam AG, et al. (1999) Reversible neural inactivation reveals hippocampal participation in several memory processes. *Nat. Neurosci.* 2: 898–905.

Reul JMHM and de Kloet ER (1985) Two receptor systems for corticosterone in rat brain: Microdistribution and differential occupation. *Endocrinology* 117: 2505–2511.

Reul JMHM, de Kloet ER, van Sluys FA, Rijnberk A, and Rothuizen J (1990) Binding characteristics of mineralocorticoid and glucocorticoid receptors in dog brain and pituitary. *Endocrinology* 127: 907–915.

Roesler R, Kopschina MI, Rosa RM, Henriques JA, Souza DO, and Schwartsmann G (2004a) RC-3095, a bombesin/gastrin-releasing peptide receptor antagonist, impairs aversive but not recognition memory in rats. *Eur. J. Pharmacol.* 486: 35–41.

Roesler R, Lessa D, Venturella R, et al. (2004b) Bombesin/gastrin-releasing peptide receptors in the basolateral amygdala regulate memory consolidation. *Eur. J. Neurosci.* 19: 1041–1045.

Roesler R, Roozendaal B, and McGaugh JL (2002) Basolateral amygdala lesions block the memory-enhancing effect of 8-Br-cAMP infused into the entorhinal cortex of rats after training. *Eur. J. Neurosci.* 15: 905–910.

Roozendaal B (2000) Glucocorticoids and the regulation of memory consolidation. *Psychoneuroendocrinology* 25: 213–238.

Roozendaal B (2002) Stress and memory: Opposing effects of glucocorticoids on memory consolidation and memory retrieval. *Neurobiol. Learn. Mem.* 78: 578–595.

Roozendaal B (2007) Norepinephrine and long-term memory function. In: Ordway GA, Schwartz MA, and Frazer A (eds.) *Brain Norepinephrine: Neurobiology and Therapeutics*, pp. 236–274. Cambridge: Cambridge University Press.

Roozendaal B, Carmi O, and McGaugh JL (1996a) Adrenocortical suppression blocks the memory-enhancing effects of amphetamine and epinephrine. *Proc. Natl. Acad. Sci. USA* 93: 1429–1433.

Roozendaal B, de Quervain DJ-F, Ferry B, Setlow B, and McGaugh JL (2001) Basolateral amygdala-nucleus accumbens interactions in mediating glucocorticoid effects on memory consolidation. *J. Neurosci.* 21: 2518–2525.

Roozendaal B, de Quervain DJ-F, Schelling G, and McGaugh JL (2004a) A systemically administered β-adrenoceptor antagonist blocks corticosterone-induced impairment of contextual memory retrieval in rats. *Neurobiol. Learn. Mem.* 81: 150–154.

Roozendaal B, Griffith QK, Buranday J, de Quervain DJ-F, and McGaugh JL (2003) The hippocampus mediates glucocorticoid-induced impairment of spatial memory retrieval: Dependence on the basolateral amygdala. *Proc. Natl. Acad. Sci. USA* 100: 1328–1333.

Roozendaal B, Hahn EL, Nathan SV, de Quervain DJ-F, and McGaugh JL (2004b) Glucocorticoid effects on memory retrieval require concurrent noradrenergic activity in the hippocampus and basolateral amygdala. *J. Neurosci.* 24: 8161–8169.

Roozendaal B, Holloway BL, Brunson KL, Baram TZ, and McGaugh JL (2002a) Involvement of stress-released corticotropin-releasing hormone in the basolateral amygdala in regulating memory consolidation. *Proc. Natl. Acad. Sci. USA* 99: 13908–13913.

Roozendaal B, Hui GK, Hui IR, Berlau DJ, McGaugh JL, and Weinberger NM (2006a) Basolateral amygdala noradrenergic activity mediates corticosterone-induced enhancement of auditory fear conditioning. *Neurobiol. Learn. Mem.* 86: 249–255.

Roozendaal B, Lengvilas R, McGaugh JL, Civelli O, and Reinscheid RK (2007) Orphanin FQ/nociceptin interactions with the basolateral amygdala noradrenergic system in memory consolidation. *Learn. Mem.* 14: 29–35.

Roozendaal B and McGaugh JL (1996a) Amygdaloid nuclei lesions differentially affect glucocorticoid-induced memory enhancement in an inhibitory avoidance task. *Neurobiol. Learn. Mem.* 65: 1–8.

Roozendaal B and McGaugh JL (1996b) The memory-modulatory effects of glucocorticoids depend on an intact stria terminalis. *Brain Res.* 709: 243–250.

Roozendaal B and McGaugh JL (1997a) Glucocorticoid receptor agonist and antagonist administration into the basolateral but not central amygdala modulates memory storage. *Neurobiol. Learn. Mem.* 67: 176–179.

Roozendaal B and McGaugh JL (1997b) Basolateral amygdala lesions block the memory-enhancing effect of glucocorticoid administration in the dorsal hippocampus of rats. *Eur. J. Neurosci.* 9: 76–83.

Roozendaal B, McReynolds JR, and McGaugh JL (2004c) The basolateral amygdala interacts with the medial prefrontal cortex in regulating glucocorticoid effects on working memory impairment. *J. Neurosci.* 24: 1385–1392.

Roozendaal B, Nguyen BT, Power A, and McGaugh JL (1999a) Basolateral amygdala noradrenergic influence enables enhancement of memory consolidation induced by hippocampal glucocorticoid receptor activation. *Proc. Natl. Acad. Sci. USA* 96: 11642–11647.

Roozendaal B, Okuda S, Van der Zee EA, and McGaugh JL (2006b) Glucocorticoid enhancement of memory requires arousal-induced noradrenergic activation in the basolateral amygdala. *Proc. Natl. Acad. Sci. USA* 103: 6741–6746.

Roozendaal B, Portillo-Marquez G, and McGaugh JL (1996b) Basolateral amygdala lesions block glucocorticoid-induced modulation of memory for spatial learning. *Behav. Neurosci.* 110: 1074–1083.

Roozendaal B, Quirarte GL, and McGaugh JL (2002b) Glucocorticoids interact with the basolateral amygdala β-adrenoceptor-cAMP/PKA system in influencing memory consolidation. *Eur. J. Neurosci.* 15: 553–560.

Roozendaal B, Williams CL, and McGaugh JL (1999b) Glucocorticoid receptor activation in the rat nucleus of the solitary tract facilitates memory consolidation: Involvement of the basolateral amygdala. *Eur. J. Neurosci.* 11: 1317–1323.

Rosenkranz JA and Grace AA (2002) Cellular mechanisms of infralimbic and prelimbic prefrontal cortical inhibition and dopaminergic modulation of basolateral amygdala neurons *in vivo*. *J. Neurosci.* 22: 324–337.

Rowe JB, Toni I, Josephs O, Frackowiak RS, and Passingham RE (2000) The prefrontal cortex: Response selection of maintenance within working memory? *Science* 288: 1656–1660.

Rudy JW and Sutherland RJ (1989) The hippocampal formation is necessary for rats to learn and remember configural discriminations. *Behav. Brain Res.* 34: 97–109.

Runyan JD and Dash PK (2004) Intra-medial prefrontal administration of SCH-23390 attenuates ERK phosphorylation and long-term memory for trace fear conditioning in rats. *Neurobiol. Learn. Mem.* 82: 65–70.

Sacchetti B, Lorenzini CA, Baldi E, Tassoni G, and Bucherelli C (1999) Auditory thalamus, dorsal hippocampus, basolateral amygdala, and perirhinal cortex role in the consolidation of conditioned freezing to context and to acoustic conditioned stimulus in the rat. *J. Neurosci.* 19: 9570–9578.

Sah P, Faber ES, Lopez De Armentia M, and Power J (2003) The amygdaloid complex: Anatomy and physiology. *Physiol. Rev.* 83: 803–834.

Sajadi AA, Samaei SA, and Rashidy-Pour A (2006) Intra-hippocampal microinjections of anisomycin did not block glucocorticoid-induced impairment of memory retrieval in rats: An evidence for non-genomic effects of glucocorticoids. *Behav. Brain Res.* 173: 158–162.

Salinas JA, Introini-Collison IB, Dalmaz C, and McGaugh JL (1997) Posttraining intra-amygdala infusions of oxotremorine and propranolol modulate storage of memory for reductions in reward magnitude. *Neurobiol. Learn. Mem.* 68: 51–59.

Salinas JA and McGaugh JL (1995) Muscimol induces retrograde amnesia for changes in reward magnitude. *Neurobiol. Learn. Mem.* 63: 277–285.

Sandi C and Rose SPR (1994) Corticosterone enhances long-term potentiation in one-day-old chicks trained in a weak passive avoidance learning paradigm. *Brain Res.* 647: 106–112.

Sara SJ and Devauges V (1989) Idazoxan, an α-2 antagonist, facilitates memory retrieval in the rat. *Behav. Neural Biol.* 51: 401–411.

Sato T, Tanaka K, Teramoto T, et al. (2004) Effect of pretraining administration of NC-1900, a vasopressin fragment analog, on memory performance in non- or CO2-amnesic mice. *Pharmacol. Biochem. Behav.* 78: 309–317.

Sawaguchi T and Goldman-Rakic PS (1991) D1 dopamine receptors in prefrontal cortex: Involvement in working memory. *Science* 251: 947–950.

Schafe GE and LeDoux JE (2000) Memory consolidation of auditory Pavlovian fear conditioning requires protein synthesis and protein kinase A in the amygdala. *J. Neurosci.* 20: RC96.

Schlesinger K, Pelleymounter MA, van de Kamp J, Bader DL, Stewart KM, and Chase TN (1986) Substance P facilitation of memory: Effects in an appetitively motivated learning task. *Behav. Neural Biol.* 45: 230–239.

Schreurs J, Seelig T, and Schulman H (1986) β2-adrenergic receptors on peripheral nerves. *J. Neurochem.* 46: 294–296.

Schroeder JP and Packard MG (2002) Posttraining intra-basolateral amygdala scopolamine impairs food- and amphetamine-induced conditioned place preferences. *Behav. Neurosci.* 116: 922–927.

Schroeder JP and Packard MG (2003) Systemic or intra-amygdala injections of glucose facilitate memory consolidation for extinction of drug-induced conditioned reward. *Eur. J. Neurosci.* 17: 1482–1488.

Schroeder JP and Packard MG (2004) Facilitation of memory for extinction of drug-induced conditioned reward: Role of amygdala and acetylcholine. *Learn. Mem.* 11: 641–647.

Seamans JK, Floresco SB, and Phillips AG (1998) D1 receptor modulation of hippocampal-prefrontal cortical circuits integrating spatial memory with executive functions in the rat. *J. Neurosci.* 18: 1613–1621.

Setlow B, Roozendaal B, and McGaugh JL (2000) Involvement of a basolateral amygdala complex – Nucleus accumbens pathway in glucocorticoid-induced modulation of memory storage. *Eur. J. Neurosci.* 12: 367–375.

Smith AP, Stephan KE, Rugg MD, and Dolan RJ (2006) Task and content modulate amygdala-hippocampal connectivity in emotional retrieval. *Neuron* 49: 631–638.

Soetens E, Casaer S, D'Hooge R, and Hueting JE (1995) Effect of amphetamine on long-term retention of verbal material. *Psychopharmacology* 119: 155–162.

Soetens E, D'Hooge R, and Hueting JE (1993) Amphetamine enhances human-memory consolidation. *Neurosci. Lett.* 161: 9–12.

Southwick S, Davis M, Horner B, et al. (2002) Relationship of enhanced norepinephrine activity during memory consolidation to enhanced long-term memory in humans. *Am. J. Psychiat.* 159: 1420–1422.

Squire LR, Clark RE, and Knowlton BJ (2001) Retrograde amnesia. *Hippocampus* 11: 50–56.

Stern CE, Sherman SJ, Kirchhoff BA, and Hasselmo ME (2001) Medial temporal and prefrontal contributions to working memory tasks with novel and familiar stimuli. *Hippocampus* 11: 337–346.

Sternberg DB, Isaacs K, Gold PE, and McGaugh JL (1985) Epinephrine facilitation of appetitive learning: Attenuation with adrenergic receptor antagonists. *Behav. Neural Biol.* 44: 447–453.

Strange BA and Dolan RJ (2004) β-adrenergic modulation of emotional memory-evoked human amygdala and hippocampal responses. *Proc. Natl. Acad. Sci. USA* 101: 11454–11458.

Stratton LO and Petrinovich LF (1963) Post-trial injections of an anticholinesterase drug and maze learning in two strains of rats. *Psychopharmacologia* 5: 47–54.

Sutanto W and de Kloet ER (1987) Species-specificity of corticosteroid receptors in hamster and rat. *Endocrinology* 121: 1405–1411.

Talley CP, Clayborn H, Jewel E, McCarty R, and Gold PE (2002) Vagotomy attenuates effects of L-glucose but not of D-glucose on spontaneous alternation performance. *Physiol. Behav.* 77: 243–249.

Tam S-Y and Roth RH (1985) Selective increase in dopamine metabolism in the prefrontal cortex by the anxiogenic beta-carboline FG 7142. *Biochem. Pharmacol.* 34: 1595–1598.

Taylor JR, Birnbaum S, Ubriani R, and Arnsten AFT (1999) Activation of cAMP-dependent protein kinase A in prefrontal cortex impairs working memory performance. *J. Neurosci.* 19: RC23.

Thomas DN, Post RM, and Pert A (1994) Central and systemic corticosterone differentially affect dopamine and norepinephrine in the frontal cortex of the awake and freely moving rat. *Ann. N.Y. Acad. Sci.* 764: 467–469.

Tomaz C, Dickinson-Anson H, and McGaugh JL (1992) Basolateral amygdala lesions block diazepam-induced anterograde amnesia in an inhibitory avoidance task. *Proc. Natl. Acad. Sci. USA* 89: 3615–3619.

van Stegeren AH, Goekoop R, Everaerd W, et al. (2005) Noradrenaline mediates amygdala activation in men and women during encoding of emotional material. *Neuroimage* 24: 898–909.

Vazdarjanova A and McGaugh JL (1999) Basolateral amygdala is involved in modulating consolidation of memory for classical fear conditioning. *J. Neurosci.* 19: 6615–6622.

Walker DL, Ressler KJ, Lu KT, and Davis M (2002) Facilitation of conditioned fear extinction by systemic administration or intra-amygdala infusions of D-cycloserine as assessed with fear-potentiated startle in rats. *J. Neurosci.* 22: 2343–2352.

Wan, R-Q, Pang K, and Olton DS (1994) Hippocampal and amygdaloid involvement in nonspatial and spatial working memory in rats: Effects of delay and interference. *Behav. Neurosci.* 108: 866–882.

Weil-Malherbe H, Axelrod J, and Tomchick R (1959) Blood-brain barrier for adrenalin. *Science* 129: 1226–1228.

Weinberger NM (2003) The nucleus basalis and memory codes: Auditory cortical plasticity and the induction of specific, associative behavioral memory. *Neurobiol. Learn. Mem.* 80: 268–284.

Wilensky AE, Schafe GE, and LeDoux JE (2000) The amygdala modulates memory consolidation of fear-motivated inhibitory avoidance learning but not classical fear conditioning. *J. Neurosci.* 20: 7059–7066.

Williams CL and Clayton EC (2001) Contribution of brainstem structures in modulating memory storage processes. In: Gold PE and Greenough WT (eds.) *Memory Consolidation: Essays in Honor of James L. McGaugh*, pp. 141–163. Washington, DC: American Psychological Association.

Williams CL and Jensen RA (1991) Vagal afferents: A possible mechanism for the modulation of peripherally acting agents. In: Frederickson RCA, McGaugh JL, and Felten DL (eds.) *Peripheral Signaling of the Brain: Role in Neural-Immune Interactions, Learning and Memory*, pp. 467–472. New York: Hogrefe and Huber.

Williams CL and McGaugh JL (1993) Reversible lesions of the nucleus of the solitary tract attenuate the memory-modulating effects of posttraining epinephrine, *Behav. Neurosci.* 107: 1–8.

Williams CL and McGaugh JL (1994) Enhancement of memory processing in an inhibitory avoidance and radial maze task by posttraining infusion of bombesin into the nucleus tractus solitarius. *Brain Res.* 654: 251–256.

Williams CL, Men D, and Clayton EC (2000) The effects of noradrenergic activation of the nucleus tractus solitarius on memory and in potentiating norepinephrine release in the amygdala. *Behav. Neurosci.* 114: 1131–1144.

Williams CL, Men D, Clayton EC, and Gold PE (1998) Norepinephrine release in the amygdala after systemic injections of epinephrine or inescapable footshock: Contribution of the nucleus of the solitary tract. *Behav. Neurosci.* 112: 1414–1422.

Wolf OT, Convit A, McHugh PF, et al. (2001) Cortisol differentially affects memory in young and elderly men. *Behav. Neurosci.* 115: 1002–1011.

Woodson JC, Macintosh D, Fleshner M, and Diamond DM (2003) Emotion-induced amnesia in rats: Working memory-specific impairment, corticosterone-memory correlation, and fear versus arousal effects on memory. *Learn. Mem.* 10: 326–336.

Wright CI, Beijer AVJ, and Groenewegen HJ (1996) Basal amygdaloid afferents to the rat nucleus accumbens are compartmentally organized. *J. Neurosci.* 16: 1877–1893.

Yang Y, Cao J, Xiong W, et al. (2003) Both stress experience and age determine the impairment or enhancement effect of stress on spatial memory retrieval. *J. Endocrinl.* 178: 45–54.

Yang YL, Chao PK, and Lu KT (2006) Systemic and intra-amygdala administration of glucocorticoid agonist and antagonist modulate extinction of conditioned fear. *Neuropsychopharmacology* 31: 912–924.

Young AH, Sahakian BJ, Robbins TW, and Cowen PJ (1999) The effects of chronic administration of cortisone in cognitive function in normal male volunteers. *Psychopharmacology* 145: 260–266.

Young MP (1993) The organization of neural systems in the primate cerebral cortex. *Proc. R. Soc. Lond. B Biol. Sci.* 252: 13–18.

Zahrt J, Taylor JR, Mathew RG, and Arnsten AF (1997) Supranormal stimulation of D1 dopamine receptors in the rodent prefrontal cortex impairs spatial working memory performance. *J. Neurosci.* 17: 8528–8535.

Zanatta MS, Schaeffer E, Schmitz PK, et al. (1996) Sequential involvement of NMDA receptor-dependent processes in hippocampus, amygdala, chlorhinal cortex and parietal cortex in memory processing. *Behav. Pharmacol.* 7: 341–345.

Zorawski M and Killcross S (2002) Posttraining glucocorticoid receptor agonist enhances memory in appetitive and aversive Pavlovian discrete-cue conditioning paradigms. *Neurobiol. Learn. Mem.* 78: 458–464.

28 Memory-Enhancing Drugs

P. E. Gold, University of Illinois at Urbana-Champaign, Champaign, IL, USA

28.1 Background

28.1.1 Introduction

The formation of new memories can be impaired in many ways, from lesioning brain regions to blocking neurotransmitter actions to interfering with activation of transcription factors. Thus, the ability to interfere with memory processing is readily demonstrated. Remarkably, there are also treatments that can enhance memory processing. Like studies that impair memory, evidence for enhancement of memory offers insights into possible mechanisms responsible for forming new memories. Development of drugs that enhance memory – cognitive enhancers, 'smart pills,' anti-aging drugs – also address a more romantic vision of ways to make us smarter and to keep us that way as we age. Descriptions of tests of drug enhancement of memory during aging will be included in the discussions of some of the drugs; a more complete and recent discussion of drug enhancement in aging and Alzheimer's disease can be found in Disterhoft and Oh (2006). The ability to enhance memory and other cognitive functions raises a host of ethical issues about whether and when we should use these treatments; these issues are also covered elsewhere (cf. Rose, 2002; Farah et al., 2004).

28.1.2 Early Studies of Drug Enhancement of Learning and Memory

Pharmacological treatments that produce amnesia receive much of the attention as tools with which to investigate the neurobiological bases of learning and memory. Many of these treatments impair memory when administered near the time of training. In particular, the findings that some treatments impair memory when given after training (i.e., the treatments produce retrograde amnesia) provide much of the evidence for memory consolidation, the view that memory formation takes time to reach completion.

There is also a significant literature showing that some drugs can enhance memory. What is perhaps the first demonstration that a drug could improve memory was provided about 90 years ago by Karl

Lashley (Lashley, 1917), who showed that injections of low doses of strychnine increased the rate of food-motivated maze learning. The current era of tests of drug enhancement of memory can be traced to McGaugh and Petrinovich (1959), who extended Lashley's findings and reported enhanced maze learning in rats that received strychnine 10 min prior to training on each of 5 days. Subsequent experiments showed that strychnine, and also pentylenetetrazol, enhanced memory in rats, mice, rabbits, and cats. Enhanced memory was evident for a wide range of tasks in addition to food-motivated mazes, including discrimination learning, avoidance learning, and classical conditioning (Kelemen and Bovet, 1961; McGaugh and Thomson, 1962; Hunt and Krivanek, 1966; Benevento and Kandel, 1967; Cholewiak et al., 1968).

28.1.3 The Posttraining Design

These early findings were very encouraging, but the designs of the experiments left open many interpretations of the effects beyond specific actions on learning and memory processing. For example, strychnine might alter exploration in a manner that fostered better learning (Whishaw and Cooper, 1970). This is just one of many performance variables – others include sensory acuity, motivation to find food, attention, and retrieval mechanisms – that could lead to more rapid learning by mechanisms other than effects on memory. Considerations such as these led to the use of an experimental design shared with studies of retrograde amnesia. These are demonstrations that treatments administered after training can retroactively impair or enhance memory (Duncan, 1949; McGaugh, 1966).

Retrograde effects on memory provide much of the support for studies of memory consolidation (McGaugh, 1966, 2000; Gold and McGaugh, 1975; Gold, 2006). In addition to addressing issues regarding memory consolidation, the use of the posttraining design is very important for distinguishing between drug enhancement of memory formation and modification of performance variables (Gold and McGaugh, 1978; Gold, 1986; McGaugh, 1989). With a posttraining design, all subjects – control and experimental alike – are trained in the absence of drug treatment. Because the drug is administered after training, there can be no differences in performance variables such as motivation or locomotor activity during training that can explain later improvements on tests of memory. The tests of memory are generally administered 24 h or more after training and drug treatment, at a time when the direct effects of the drug have dissipated. The additional demonstration of a retrograde enhancement gradient, in which the enhancement of memory decreases as the time between training and treatment increases, is an important procedure to ensure that the drug administered after training is not having residual effects on memory tests given later, typically 1 or more days after the training-treatment procedure. For example, consider findings that a drug enhances memory at 24 h after training if the drug is administered within a few minutes of training but not if administered 4 h later. Restated, the findings show that the drug-induced enhancement of memory is evident when the drug is administered 24 h before testing but not 20 h before testing. Findings such as these do not support interpretations of the enhanced memory as the result of lingering effects of the drug, but instead convincingly demonstrate the absence of a proactive effect on memory processing during testing.

28.1.4 Posttraining Drug Enhancement of Memory

The posttraining design has been used to great benefit in the era of drug enhancement of memory that began in the 1960s and continues now. McGaugh and colleagues led the studies that examined the efficacy of a wide range of drugs in enhancing memory for learning in many tasks in rodents (McGaugh, 1966, 1989, 2000). In most of these experiments, rats were trained daily and received the drug treatment at variable delays after training. The major overall findings were that (1) posttraining administration of any of several drugs could enhance memory, (2) the dose-response was an inverted-U or more complex function, and (3) the effects on memory decreased with time between training and testing. Most of the drugs found to enhance memory were stimulants, including strychnine, pentylenetetrazol, caffeine, and amphetamine, among others. There were also differences reported in the dose-response functions across rat and mouse strains, across ages, and across tasks. Some of these variables will be discussed again later in considering hormonal enhancement of memory. Of interest, memory enhancement was evident not only for appetitive and aversive tasks, but also for latent memory, for example, learning about a spatial maze on 'pretraining' trials administered without reward or punishment (McGaugh, 1989). In addition, the posttraining design has been used effectively in demonstrating enhancement of memory in humans with drugs and other treatments (Parker et al., 1980; Manning et al., 1992; Soetens et al., 1993; Nielson et al., 1996; Bruce et al., 1999; Scholey and Fowles, 2002; Cahill and Alkire, 2003).

28.1.5 Memory Consolidation versus Memory Modulation

One of the striking features that came from studies of enhancement of memory with drugs, as well as impairments of memory with many treatments, was that the time courses of retrograde enhancement and retrograde amnesia were very different in different experimental conditions (Gold and McGaugh, 1975; Gold, 2006). Across amnestic treatments, retrograde amnesia and enhancement gradients might be as short as 500 ms or as long as weeks. The variability in the time windows during which memory is susceptible to modification has important implications for the goals of studies of memory consolidation, whether using treatments that enhance or impair memory. One of the key goals of memory consolidation experiments has been the identification of the time needed to form new memories, a time often based on the temporal properties obtained in retrograde amnesia or enhancement studies. One set of temporal properties comes from retrograde amnesia and enhancement gradients. Because these are highly variable, it is difficult to use any one temporal gradient to discuss the time needed for memory formation. A second set of temporal properties is often identified through amnesia studies that test the time after training to the onset of amnesia. These studies also yield a wide range of time parameters, from minutes to many hours (cf. Gold, 2006). Thus, it seems very difficult to fit these times, with poor temporal constraints, into a framework of memory consolidation, a practice nonetheless prevalent even today in investigations into cellular and molecular mechanisms of memory.

If memory consolidation studies do not yield a time constant for the formation of memory, then the issue is why do memories remain susceptible to modification during the time soon after training? It was thinking such as this that led to the development of an alternative way to think about drugs that enhance memory. Perhaps if retrograde amnesia and enhancement gradients do not reflect the time needed for memory formation, the gradients reflect the ability of some endogenous responses to experience to modulate later memory for that experience. Simply put, events that lead to high arousal, and particularly the neurochemical and hormonal consequences of the arousal, will modulate later memory (Gold and McGaugh, 1975; Gold, 1987; Cahill and McGaugh, 1998). And it is clear in many contexts that experiences with high arousal and affect are those best remembered.

The special role of postexperiential modulation of memory is well illustrated for learning about events that are unexpected and rather quick. Two examples are experiencing a near-accident while driving through an intersection or receiving a footshock when entering a dark compartment. In both instances, the neuroendocrine responses to the incidents largely come after, not before, the experience. The idea of modulation of memory is that the formation of new memories retains the capacity to be regulated by the ensuing neurobiological components of emotion and arousal. In general terms, the implication is that organismic responses that evolved to respond physiologically to potentially dangerous situations, including both endocrine and brain responses, were adopted by brain processes involved in the formation of memory as mechanisms through which to select from all experiences those that should be best remembered.

A major implication of this view is that memory for a mild experience will be made stronger by administration of treatments that activate some of the biological responses associated with emotion and arousal. In particular, this thinking predicts that treatments that activate or mimic hormonal and neurochemical functions related to emotion and arousal will enhance memory. As described next, these are precisely the results obtained in more recent studies that examine drugs aimed at hormones and neuromodulators.

28.2 Peripheral Factors

28.2.1 Epinephrine

Epinephrine is perhaps the hormone best studied and best understood as an enhancer of memory formation processes. In early experiments (Gold and van Buskirk, 1975), rats were trained in a one-trial inhibitory avoidance task using a footshock of low intensity. Soon after training, the rats received an injection of epinephrine. When tested for memory 24 h later, those rats that received the epinephrine had higher avoidance latencies (**Figure 1**, left graph). The effects were time-dependent; enhancement of memory decreased as the time after training increased. In addition, the

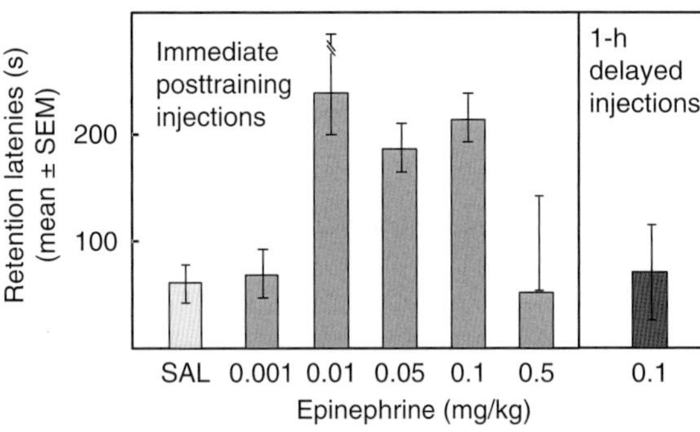

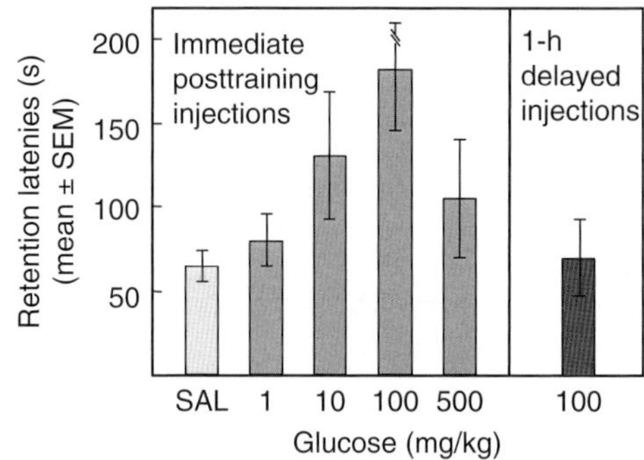

Figure 1 Dose-response function for epinephrine and glucose effects on memory in rats. Rats were trained in a one-trial inhibitory avoidance task; received injections of saline (SAL), epinephrine, or glucose immediately after training; and were tested 24 h later. Note the inverted-U dose-response curve for enhancement of memory seen on the test trial. Note also that injections of epinephrine or glucose 1 h after training did not significantly enhance memory on tests 24 h later. Left from Gold PE and van Buskirk RB (1975) Facilitation of time dependent memory processes with posttrial epinephrine injections. *Behav. Biol.* 13: 145–153; used with permission; right from Gold PE (1986) Glucose modulation of memory storage processing. *Behav. Neural Biol.* 45: 342–349; used with permission.

effects were dose-dependent, following an inverted-U dose-response curve. When circulating levels of epinephrine were measured after training and epinephrine injections, the findings indicated that the epinephrine dose optimal for enhancing memory resulted in peak circulating levels comparable to those seen after training with more intense footshock (Gold and McCarty, 1981; McCarty and Gold, 1981). Thus, epinephrine apparently mimicked an endogenous response to training, and the mimicry promoted the formation of new memory much as would a higher footshock level.

Later experiments showed that epinephrine, like strychnine and analeptics studied earlier, enhanced memory for a wide range of tasks, including not only avoidance tasks but also food- and water-motivated mazes, unrewarded spontaneous alternation measures of spatial working memory, and habituation and extinction (Gold, 1995). In humans, epinephrine enhances verbal memory for emotional information (Cahill and Alkire, 2003).

The proximal mechanisms by which epinephrine enhances memory have received considerable attention. Circulating epinephrine is largely excluded from the brain (Axelrod et al., 1959), indicating that it is likely that the hormone acts directly on peripheral targets in a manner that leads to regulation of brain functions. There are two main positions, which are not mutually exclusive, regarding the nature of the peripheral target. One position is that epinephrine acts on β-adrenergic receptors on the vagus nerve, with vagal afferents carrying to the brain information about the epinephrine signal (Williams and Clayton, 2003). The principal evidence for this view is that epinephrine effects on memory are blocked by inactivation of the vagus terminal field in the nucleus tractus solitarius (Clayton and Williams, 2000). Furthermore, posttraining vagal stimulation enhances memory in both rats and humans (Clark et al., 1998, 1999) and results in release of norepinephrine in the amygdala (Hassert et al., 2004). Together, the findings suggest that epinephrine may regulate brain memory processes via actions on vagal afferents. More direct tests (e.g., blockade of the effects of epinephrine on memory in vagotomized rats, neurophysiological measures of vagal activity, and neurochemical measures in the vagal terminal field, the nucleus tractus solitarius) have not yet been performed.

The effects of epinephrine on memory are also blocked by inactivation of the locus coeruleus or amygdala, as well as by blockade of β-adrenergic receptors in the amygdala, the latter presumably blocking central norepinephrine actions and not direct actions in the amygdala of circulating epinephrine. In addition, epinephrine injections result in release of central norepinephrine throughout the brain, including the amygdala (Gold and van Buskirk, 1978a,b; Williams et al., 1998). A second proximal mechanism proposed to mediate epinephrine enhancement of memory is based on a classic physiological response to epinephrine release from the adrenal medulla, an increase in blood glucose levels mediated in large part by liberation of hepatic glucose stores (McNay and Gold, 2002). These findings comprise the next section.

28.2.2 Glucose

Posttraining injections of glucose enhance memory in time- and dose-dependent manner similar to that of epinephrine (**Figure 1**, right graph). The dose-response function has an inverted-U form, with maximal enhancement of memory obtained at doses that lead to blood glucose levels similar to those attained after epinephrine doses that enhance memory (Gold, 1986; Hall and Gold, 1986). In addition, although enhancement of memory with epinephrine is blocked by peripheral coadministration of adrenergic receptor antagonists (Gold and van Buskirk, 1978b), enhancement of memory by glucose remains intact in the presence of adrenergic antagonists (Gold, 1986). In addition, modest food restriction, to deplete hepatic glucose stores, reduces the efficacy with which epinephrine but not glucose enhances memory (Talley et al., 2000); enhancement of memory with glucose is also intact after vagotomy (Talley et al., 2002) These findings suggest that increases in blood glucose levels subsequent to epinephrine release contribute importantly to the effects of the hormone on memory.

Like epinephrine, glucose enhances memory after training on a wide range of aversive tasks, including inhibitory avoidance (Gold, 1986; Kopf et al., 2001; Rashidy-Pour, 2001), conditioned emotional response (Messier and White, 1984), and swim (Oomura et al., 1993; Li et al., 1998) tasks. Although tests of glucose, like those of epinephrine, grew from considerations of stress and arousal responses and therefore initially involved aversive tasks, glucose also enhances memory for nonaversive tasks, including spatial memory in a radial arm maze and nonmatching to sample task (Winocur and Gagnon, 1998), spatial working memory in spontaneous alternation tasks (Ragozzino et al., 1996; McNay and Gold, 2002), operant bar pressing (Messier et al., 1990), and habituation of exploratory behavior (Kopf and Baratti, 1996). Moreover, glucose also enhances verbal memory in humans, including in healthy young adult and aged populations, as well as in individuals with Down syndrome and Alzheimer's disease (Manning et al., 1993; for reviews, see Korol, 2002; McNay and Gold, 2002; Messier, 2004; Gold, 2005). In individuals with Alzheimer's disease, the effects of glucose were particularly pronounced both in terms of percent improvement and breadth of cognitive domains (**Figure 2**). Of interest, the dose of glucose that enhances memory in humans results in increases in circulating levels comparable to those related to glucose and epinephrine enhancement of

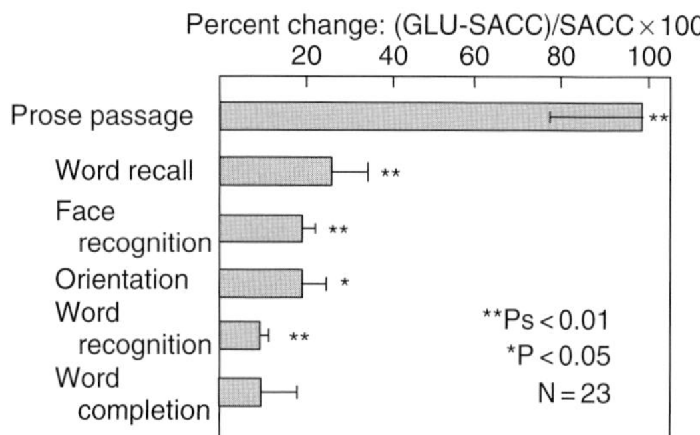

Figure 2 Glucose enhancement of cognitive functions in individuals with Alzheimer's disease. The patients were each tested on two occasions, once soon after ingesting a fruit drink sweetened with saccharin (SACC, control) and once after ingesting a fruit drink sweetened with glucose (GLU). On the glucose treatment day compared to the saccharin treatment day, the patients performed better when tested for memory of new information, on a narrative prose passage and word recall tests, as well as retrieval of old information included in the face recognition and orientation tests. From Manning CA, Ragozzino M, and Gold PE (1993) Glucose enhancement of memory in patients with Alzheimer's disease. *Neurobiol. Aging* 14: 523–528; used with permission.

memory in rodents. The pervasive enhancement of memory by glucose across multiple classes of memory and species suggests that glucose may play a key role in regulating neural plasticities involved in the formation of memory in multiple neural systems. Because of this, the mechanisms by which glucose mediates its effects on memory are important for understanding basic properties of memory formation. In addition, development of drugs targeting these mechanisms has the potential to enhance memory in human populations, particularly those with cognitive dysfunctions.

In contrast to circulating epinephrine, which is excluded from the brain, glucose has ready access to brain targets via a facilitated transport system (Choeiri et al., 2005; McNay and Gold, 2002). The direct access to the brain opens the possibility that glucose effects on memory are a result of direct brain actions. Consistent with this possibility, microinjections of glucose into the lateral ventricles (Lee et al., 1988) or into any of several neural sites also enhance memory. For example, glucose injections into the medial septum (Ragozzino et al., 1995; Stefani and Gold, 1998; Talley et al., 1999), hippocampus (Ragozzino et al., 1998; Krebs and Parent, 2005), and amygdala (Ragozzino et al., 1994; Lennartz et al., 1996; McNay and Gold, 1998) all enhance memory for some tasks, presumably by upregulating the contributions of these systems to memory.

During the past decade, it has become clear that different brain systems are especially important for processing different attributes of memory (cf. White and McDonald, 2002; Poldrack and Packard, 2003; Gold, 2004; Korol, 2004). Consistent with this view, microinjections of glucose into different brain regions are generally effective at enhancing memory in those tasks typically associated with each memory system. The roles of multiple memory systems are, however, more complex than just separation of functions. In many instances, damage to or inactivation of one system can enhance learning associated with a different system. These demonstrations are taken as evidence that memory systems at times compete for control over learning and memory functions. If damage of a brain region can enhance learning and memory for a task best associated with another neural system, then enhancement of processing in one brain area might impair learning and memory for a noncanonical task. Like hippocampal damage or inactivation, glucose injections into the striatum impaired learning of a spatial task, suggesting that glucose upregulated striatal processing in a manner that interfered with hippocampal functions (Pych et al., 2006). Related to these issues, glucose injections into the hippocampus or striatum alter the preference for selection of place and response strategies (Canal et al., 2005) in a T-maze that can be solved using either strategy (Tolman et al., 1946; Packard and McGaugh, 1996).

These findings raise significant issues important for developing drugs to enhance learning and memory. If multiple memory systems compete with each other for control over learning, systemically administered drugs might enhance the memory processing of brain systems that are positively and negatively associated with learning the task. Yet, the findings suggest otherwise. As noted earlier, most drugs that enhance memory do so for a wide range of tasks. Assessments of fluxes in extracellular glucose levels during learning as well as measures of glucose effects on neurotransmitter functions offer clues that might reconcile this apparent paradox. Glucose levels in the brain appear to respond to training in a region specific manner. Specifically, extracellular glucose levels are depleted in the hippocampus but not the striatum when rats are engaged in a spatial working memory task (McNay et al., 2001). Systemic injections of glucose block that depletion but, in the absence of depletion, do not appear to increase extracellular glucose levels. Thus, there may be regional specificity that links delivery of glucose to those brain areas that are engaged by the task.

Similar relationships appear in examinations of release of acetylcholine in the hippocampus while rats are tested on a spatial working memory task and receive glucose to enhance memory. In this experiment (Ragozzino et al., 1996), glucose augmented the testing-related increase in release of acetylcholine in the hippocampus. Importantly, however, glucose did not lead to an increase in acetylcholine release in control animals resting in a holding cage. Thus, the neurochemical effects of glucose were restricted to conditions under which the brain area was activated. In showing that glucose delivery and neurochemical consequences were sensitive to cognitive functions, the findings suggest that other systemic drug treatments might similarly be amenable to functional targeting of action. This possibility has important implications for development of memory-enhancing drug treatments and needs more experimental investigation.

At a mechanistic level, one promising candidate for glucose effects on memory is that glucose may act by modulating the conductance of central adenosine triphosphate-sensitive potassium (K-ATP) channels. These channels are best characterized for their significant contribution to the resting baseline membrane potential of pancreatic β-cells and thereby regulate of insulin secretion (Ashcroft, 2005; Hansen, 2006). When blood glucose levels rise, intracellular ATP levels increase. The high ATP levels inhibit the K-ATP channels and depolarize the cells, activating voltage-sensitive Ca^{++} channels with an influx of Ca^{++} triggering release of insulin. Because of the significance of these channels to regulation of blood glucose levels, including in patients with diabetes, there is a relatively large repertoire of drugs aimed at these channels, particularly including drugs that act at a sulfonylurea regulatory subunit of the K-ATP channels to open and close the channels. K-ATP channel conductance is decreased by increases in intracellular ATP levels and by sulfonylurea-class drugs such as glibenclamide and is increased by decreases in intracellular ATP concentration and by drugs such as lemakalim.

Of potential interest to understanding glucose effects on brain function, K-ATP channels exist in the brain and are widely distributed (cf. Liss and Roeper, 2001). In the ventromedial hypothalamus, the channels appear to be important in regulating food intake, apparently sensing extracellular glucose levels in manner much like that seen in pancreatic β-cells. The wide brain distribution of the channels points to other functions as well, in particular linking cellular excitability and metabolic states. With findings showing dynamic changes in extracellular glucose levels in the context of memory tests, fluctuations in extracellular glucose may modulate cell excitability. According to this view, decreases in K-ATP channel conductance would increase cellular sensitivity to depolarizing stimuli and increase the likelihood of stimulus-evoked neurotransmitter release, a possibility for which there is a good deal of evidence (e.g., Amoroso et al., 1990; Fellows et al., 1993; Panten et al., 1996). Additionally, there may be significant contributions of K-ATP channels to regulation of excessive glutamate release and subsequent excitotoxity after hypoxia and other brain insults, as well as involvement in neurodegenerative conditions like Alzheimer's disease and Parkinson's disease (Haddad and Jiang, 1994; Dirnagl et al., 1999; Yamada et al., 2001; cf. Liss and Roeper, 2001).

With respect to learning and memory, injections of glibenclamide, a drug that closes K-ATP channels, attenuated impairments of inhibitory (passive) avoidance memory produced by intraventricular injections of various K-ATP channel openers (Ghelardini et al., 1998). Several experiments have examined the effects on memory of direct brain injections of drugs that act at the K-ATP channel. The findings support the view that glucose may modulate learning and memory processes by acting on central K-ATP channels. Injections of glibenclamide into either the medial septum or the hippocampus result in enhanced memory (Stefani and Gold, 1998, 2001; Stefani et al., 1999). Conversely, injections of lemakalim or galanin, drugs that open the K-ATP channel, impair alternation performance; these impairments can be reversed by concomitant glucose administration (**Figure 3**). With systemic injections as well, drugs that open and close K-ATP channels block and potentiate, respectively, glucose enhancement of memory (Rashidy-Pour, 2001). Moreover, a recent paper suggests that the K-ATP channel blocker, glibenclamide, can override central nervous system deficits observed in humans under experimental hypoglycemia (Bingham et al., 2003). Subjects made hypoglycemic via glucose/insulin clamps exhibited impaired performance on a four-choice reaction time test. The impairments were reversed by pretreatment with glibenclamide. These findings add to the evidence that K-ATP channels may be a step subsequent to glucose actions in regulating brain and cognitive functions.

An elegant approach to understanding the mechanism by which glucose enhances memory is found in a recent paper that examined possible molecular

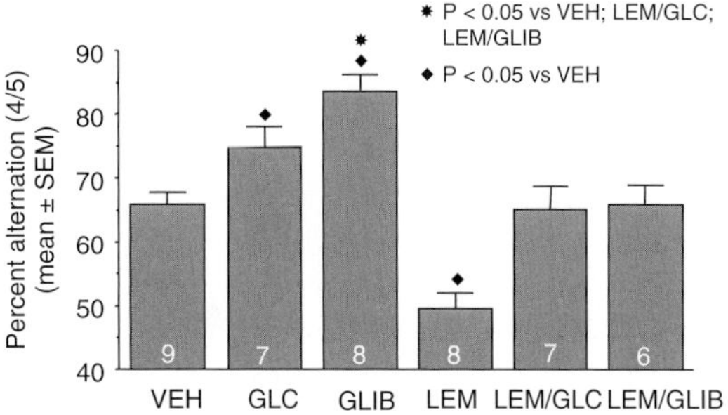

Figure 3 Effects of K^+-ATP channel modulators on memory in young rats. Drugs were injected into the hippocampus prior to spontaneous alternation testing on a 4-arm plus-shaped maze. Like glucose (GLC), the channel opening drug glibenclamide (GLIB) enhanced alternation scores, while the channel closing drug lemakalim (LEM) impaired alternation scores. Combination treatments were additive. VEH, vehicle. From Stefani MR and Gold PE (2001) Intra-hippocampal infusions of K-ATP channel modulators influence spontaneous alternation performance: Relationships to acetylcholine release in the hippocampus. *J. Neurosci.* 21: 609–614; used with permission.

pathways that might be regulated by glucose (Dash et al., 2006). The experiments examined possible glucose activation of the tuberous sclerosis complex-mammalian target of rapamycin (TSC-mTOR) pathway. The selection for investigation of the TSC-mTOR cascade was based on a convergence of signaling pathways important for mediating the effects of growth factors in promoting protein synthesis important for memory formation with the pathways involved in nutrient-mediated growth processes. Rats were weakly trained on the hidden platform version of the swim task. The rats received posttraining injections of glucose or of treatments that impair the TSC-mTOR pathway. The findings indicate that glucose activated the pathway and enhanced memory, whereas treatments that interfered with the pathway impaired memory (**Figure 4**). Moreover, glucose was unable to enhance memory in the presence of inhibition of the TSC-mTOR pathway. In addition to supporting a specific molecular basis for glucose enhancement of memory, this experiment also opens a new avenue of investigation in which drugs long known to enhance memory can be used to identify the molecular bases of memory formation. Moreover, the findings open the possibility of future drug development targeting, from a multitude of potential actions of glucose, to those cellular and molecular responses specifically related to memory formation.

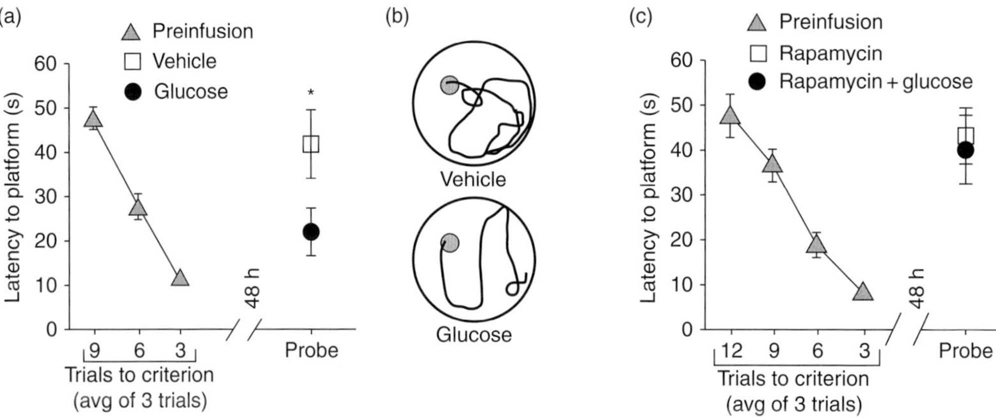

Figure 4 (a) Posttraining infusion of glucose augments long-term spatial memory. Animals were trained in the hidden platform version of the Morris water maze by using a soft criterion and then were infused with either vehicle ($n = 9$) or 20 μg/hippocampus glucose ($n = 10$). Training and probe trial performance (latency) are shown. (b) Representative probe trial traces of a vehicle-infused and a glucose-infused animal showing the path taken before the first platform crossing. Glucose-infused animals had a reduced mean distance traveled and an increased number of platform crossings when compared with vehicle-infused rats (not shown) (c) Posttraining administration of glucose did not enhance memory in the presence of the mTOR inhibitor rapamycin. Animals were infused with either 0.9 ng of rapamycin/hippocampus or 0.9 ng of rapamycin plus 20 μg of glucose/hippocampus. Error bars indicate SEM. From Dash PK, Orsi SA, and Moore AN (2006) Spatial memory formation and memory-enhancing effect of glucose involves activation of the tuberous sclerosis complex–mammalian target of rapamycin pathway. *J. Neurosci.* 26: 8048–8056; used with permission.

Pharmacological enhancement of memory by epinephrine and glucose has yielded interesting relationships with age-related impairments of memory (Gold, 2004, 2006). Aged rats and mice exhibit rapid forgetting across tasks, including inhibitory avoidance tasks. A hypothesis that decreases in release of epinephrine from the adrenals into blood during training might be diminished in aged rats was incorrect. Contrary to the hypothesis, epinephrine release after simple handling or after footshock was substantially greater in aged (2-year-old) rats than in young adult rats (Mabry et al., 1995a,c). Under conditions of greater stress such as immersion in cold water as in the swim task, aged rats produced extraordinarily high circulating levels of epinephrine as compared to young rats (Mabry et al., 1995b).

An explanation for the surprising result that aging was accompanied by increased rather than decreased release of a key memory-enhancing hormone comes from studies of differences in increases in blood glucose in young and old rats after stress. Aged rats exhibit increases in glucose levels that are absent at low levels of stress or doses of injected epinephrine and diminished at high levels of stress or epinephrine dose (Mabry et al., 1995a). Thus, the findings open the possibility that there is an impairment of the mechanisms by which epinephrine leads to glucose liberation from hepatic stores. Related to this view is evidence that glucose enhances memory in aged rats (McNay and Gold, 2001). Moreover, when engaged in a spatial working memory task sensitive to manipulations of the hippocampus, extracellular levels decline in both young and aged rats, but do so to much greater magnitude and duration in aged rats. Injections of glucose that enhance memory in aged rats block this considerable depletion of extracellular glucose levels in the hippocampus. Whether these endocrine, neurochemical, and behavior results are related to glucose effects on neurotransmitters like acetylcholine or are based on other actions of glucose requires additional attention.

28.2.3 ACTH and Glucocorticoids

In addition to enhancement of memory by epinephrine and glucose, there is extensive evidence showing that other humoral factors also enhance memory. A spate of papers in the 1970s and 1980s examined the effects of adrenocorticotropic hormone (ACTH) on memory (cf. de Wied, 1990). As with other drugs that enhance memory, ACTH did so with an inverted-U dose-response curve and in a retrograde time-dependent manner (Gold and van Buskirk, 1976). One of the most intriguing aspects of that work was the identification of the site on the ACTH molecule most important for enhancing memory (de Wied, 1999). The 39 amino acids that comprise ACTH are cleaved from the precursor protein proopiomelanocortin. Most of the memory-enhancing properties were retained with the small peptide $ACTH_{4-9}$. Importantly, although the small peptides had effects on memory formation, they did not lead to the release of corticosterone from the adrenal cortex. Thus, the peptides had actions on memory that did not depend on the classic hormonal response to ACTH. Perhaps because of limitations on the analytical and pharmacological methods of the time, these studies were not continued in parallel with those of epinephrine and glucose.

Of more intense current interest is the contribution of glucocorticoids to memory formation. Although not necessary for the effects on memory of the small ACTH-based peptides, corticosterone itself also enhances memory for many tasks, with characteristics again including inverted-U dose-response curves and retrograde temporal gradients (cf., McEwen, 2001; Luine, 2002; Roozendaal, 2002; Wolf, 2003; Diamond et al., 2004; Sandi, 2004; Korol and Gold, 2007). The inverted-U dose-response curve may result from differential binding at low and high concentrations to mineralocorticoid and glucocorticoid receptors (Oitzl and de Kloet, 1992; Pavlides et al., 1996; Ahmed et al., 2006).

As is true for many modulators, the amygdala appears to be important for mediating the effects of corticosterone on memory (Roozendaal, 2002, 2003). Lesions of the stria terminalis or injections of β-adrenergic antagonists into the amygdala block the memory enhancement produced by systemic corticosterone administration.

Glucocorticoid enhancement of memory may be accomplished by interactions with norepinephrine modulation of memory. In particular, enhancement of memory after intra-amygdala injections of a glucocorticoid agonist was blocked by coadministration of either a β-adrenergic receptor antagonist or a protein kinase A inhibitor (Roozendaal et al., 2002). In the converse experiment, a glucocorticoid antagonist attenuated memory enhancement produced by a β-adrenergic receptor agonist, but not by an analog of adenosine 3′,5′-cyclic monophosphate (cAMP), a presumed downstream product of norepinephrine actions important for the enhancement of memory. Thus, the interaction of glucocorticoids and norepinephrine to enhance memory may come at a cell

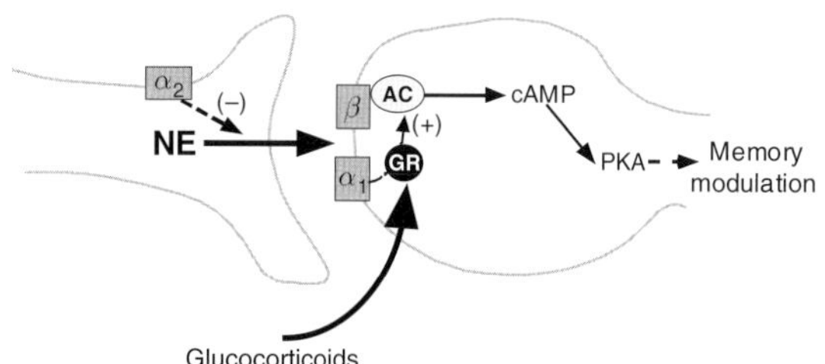

Figure 5 Schematic summarizing glucocorticoid effects on the β-adrenoceptor-AMP/protein kinase A (PKA) signaling pathway in the basolateral nucleus of the amygdala in influencing memory consolidation. Norepinephrine (NE) is released following training in aversively motivated tasks and binds to both β-adrenoceptors and α_1-adrenoceptors at postsynaptic sites. The β-adrenoceptor is coupled directly to adenylate cyclase to stimulate cAMP formation. The α_1-adrenoceptor modulates the response induced by β-adrenoceptor stimulation. Glucocorticoids may facilitate the β-adrenoceptor-cAMP system via a coupling with α_1-adrenoceptors. Other studies have demonstrated that cAMP may initiate a cascade of intracellular events involving activation of cAMP-dependent protein kinase (PKA). Our findings suggest that these effects in the basolateral amygdala are required for regulating memory consolidation in other brain regions. Abbreviations: α_1, α_1-adrenoceptor; α_2, α_2-adrenoceptor; AC, adenylate cyclase; β, β-adrenoceptor; GR, glucocorticoid receptor; cAMP, adenosine 3′,5′-cyclic monophosphate. From Roozendaal B, Quirarte GL, and McGaugh JL (2002) Glucocorticoids interact with the basolateral amygdala b-adrenoreceptor-cAMP/PKA system in influencing memory consolidation. *Eur. J. Neurosci.* 15: 553–560; used with permission.

locus between norepinephrine activation of postsynaptic β-receptors and the initiation of a molecular cascade through cAMP. A schematic of possible interactions of glucocorticoids with neurotransmitters and cAMP is shown in **Figure 5**.

28.2.4 Estrogen

Estrogen appears to act both to enhance memory and to regulate the cognitive strategy used to solve learning tasks (cf. Dohanich, 2002; Korol, 2004; Korol and Gold, 2007). Posttraining injections of estrogen enhance memory in rodents trained in the swim task (Packard and Teather, 1997a,b; Gresack and Frick, 2006), inhibitory and active avoidance tasks (Farr et al., 2000; Rhodes and Frye, 2006), and object recognition task (Gresack and Frick, 2006). Estrogen regulation of acetylcholine release at the time of training may contribute to the effects on memory (Marriott and Korol, 2003; Gibbs et al., 2004).

In contrast to other drugs noted earlier, estrogen appears to enhance learning and memory for some tasks and to impair learning and memory for others (Korol, 2004). The differences might be mediated by differential actions of estrogen on multiple memory systems (White and McDonald, 2002; Gold, 2004; Kesner and Rogers, 2004; White, 2004). Direct comparisons of estrogen effects across different versions of a food-motivated maze reveal that estrogen, administered for 2 days prior to training, enhances memory for hippocampus-sensitive place learning but impairs memory for striatum-sensitive response learning (**Figure 6**; Korol and Kolo, 2002). Estrogen status is also related to whether rats select place or response solutions to a T-maze that can be solved equally well using either strategy. Naturally cycling female rats preferentially exhibit place response at high estrogen and response strategies at low estrogen phases of their estrus cycle (Korol et al., 2004). Also, ovariectomized rats given estrogen choose place strategies, whereas those not given estrogen show response strategies. These findings suggest that estrogen can be viewed at once as a memory-enhancing and a memory-impairing treatment, depending on the specific task attributes. These differential effects seem likely to have their bases in actions of estrogen on different memory systems. Consistent with this view, estrogen administered directly to the hippocampus or striatum reveals enhanced memory for spatial tasks and for response tasks, respectively (Zurkovsky et al., 2007).

One aspect of the interest in estrogen and memory is that decreases in estrogen levels might lead to cognitive changes at the time of menopause. In addition to findings obtained in rodents, as earlier, support for this view came from several experiments that examined the effects of hormone replacement therapies on women, finding evidence for enhancement of memory in several experimental settings (for reviews see: Sherwin, 2006; Maki, 2006). In contrast, the findings of the large randomized controlled trials in the Women's Health Initiative Memory (WHIM) study failed to support the idea that hormone replacement therapy protected against cognitive decline in postmenopausal women (Espeland et al., 2004;

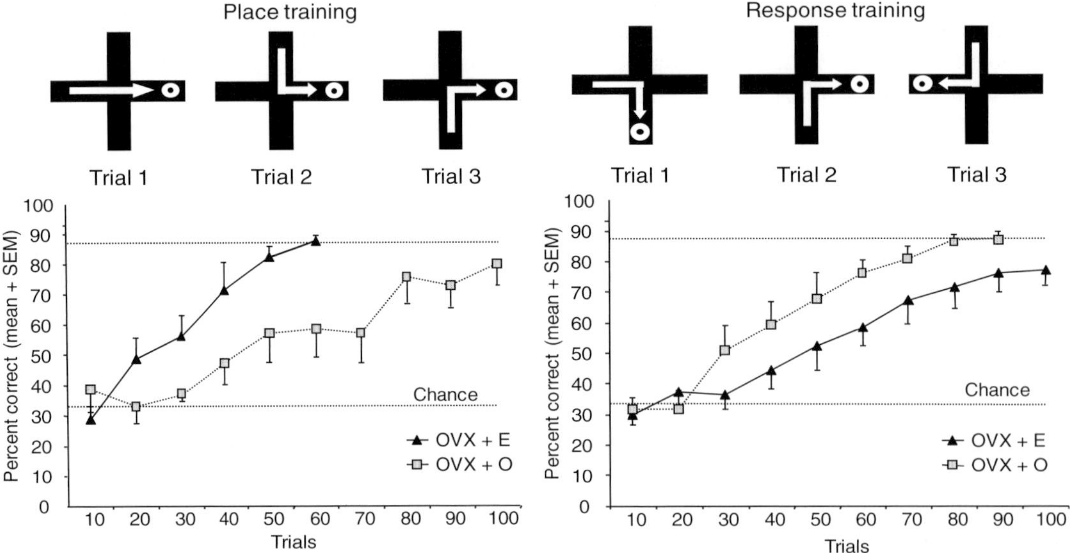

Figure 6 Effects of estrogen on maze learning in ovariectomized rats. Top figures show graphical representation of training protocols for place and response tasks in a plus-shaped maze. Place training required rats to locate food reward in an arm that maintained its position relative to the room cues throughout training. Start arms were randomly assigned across the other three arms. Response training required rats to locate food by making a right or left (not shown) turn. The goal arm was varied across training but maintained its position relative to the start arm with respect to the correct turn. Bottom graphs show learning curves, with trials groups into 10-trial blocks, in place and response versions of the maze for ovariectomized rats trained after treatment with oil (O) or estradiol (E). For place training, E-treated rats had steeper learning curves than did O-treated rats, suggesting faster learning. For response learning, E-treated rats were slower to acquire the task than were O-treated rats. Note that data reflect training until all rats reached criterion. OVX, ovariectomy. From Korol DL and Kolo LL (2002) Estrogen-induced changes in place and response learning in young adult female rats. *Behav. Neurosci.* 116: 411–420; used with permission.

Shumaker et al., 2004). Of several variables, it appears that time since menopause before the start of a hormone regimen may be especially important. In the WHIM experiments, hormone therapy began in women at approximately 72 years of age, whereas those in smaller prior studies had tested women at or close to the time of menopause. This difference has led to suggestions that there is a time window after decline in ovarian function during which the hormones are most effective at enhancing cognition (Gibbs and Gabor, 2003; Maki, 2006; Sherwin, 2006). The time window has direct support in studies of both rodents and nonhuman primates (e.g., Lacreuse et al., 2002; Daniel et al., 2006). There is also evidence that fitness and exercise may interact with hormone treatments in postmenopausal women, augmenting the positive effects and blunting negative effects of the hormones on both brain and cognitive measures (Erickson et al., 2007).

28.3 Neurotransmitters

28.3.1 Overview

Drugs targeting many neurotransmitters can enhance memory. For most neurotransmitters, or at least for specific receptors, the effects on memory of agonists and antagonists oppose each other. For example, systemic and central administration of norepinephrine and glutamate receptor agonists enhances memory, whereas administration of their antagonists impairs memory; gamma-aminobutyric acid (GABA) and opioid agonists impair memory, and antagonists enhance memory. With central injections, intrahippocampal injections of many drugs with these targets of action similarly enhance and impair memory (Izquierdo et al., 1992; Packard, 1999; Farr et al., 2000; Roesler et al., 2003). Particularly when injected systemically, these effects are often additive (Gold, 1995). Combined subthreshold doses of two memory-enhancing drugs often enhance memory, and coadministration of a memory-enhancing and -impairing drug often cancels their respective effects on memory.

However, injections into specific brain regions are not always additive across drugs, suggesting hierarchical arrangements that cannot always be explained by simple interactions across neurochemical systems and instead suggesting serial processing, at least in part, of neurotransmitter functions in modulation of memory. Additivity might explain findings that intra-amygdala injections of clenbuterol (β-noradrenergic agonist) enhance memory and that the enhancement is blocked by atropine (muscarinic antagonist) (Introini-Collison et al., 1996); injections of cholinergic antagonists can themselves impair memory (Izquierdo et al., 1993). However, memory enhancement with the cholinergic muscarinic receptor agonist, oxotremorine, injected into the amygdala is not blocked by propranolol (Introini-Collison et al., 1996). Studies examining the interactions between neurotransmitter-related drugs have provided insights into the organization of neurochemical substrates of memory modulation (McGaugh et al., 1993; Gold, 1995; McIntyre et al., 2003b; Power et al., 2003), although the full nature of these interactions awaits further clarification.

Nonetheless, the general pharmacological picture seems quite clear, especially for systemically administered drugs. When administered near the time of training on many tasks, drugs that activate or mimic norepinephrine, acetylcholine, or glutamate enhance memory, and drugs that activate or mimic GABA or opioids impair memory. The converse examples exist for drugs that interfere with the functions of the respective neurochemical systems.

The roles of many of these neurotransmitter systems are often characterized in different manners. The roles of acetylcholine and norepinephrine are described in terms of modulating memory formation (Gold, 2003; Power et al., 2003; McIntyre et al., 2003b). In contrast, the role ascribed to glutamate is generally one of being intrinsic to memory formation, a direct component of the processes that make memories rather than of processes that regulate or modulate memory formation (Riedle et al., 2003). Drugs that act at the *N*-methyl-D-aspartate (NMDA) receptor for glutamate are thought to be permissive in enabling permanent changes in synaptic efficacy, as seen in several forms of long-term potentiation. However, some of these functions are modulatory in nature (i.e., amplifying the main tetanus- or experience-induced changes in synaptic efficacy). The designations of modulator and mediator become quite murky as the pharmacological evidence grows.

28.3.2 Acetylcholine

Research in the early 1980s provided evidence that postmortem examinations of the brains of individuals with Alzheimer's disease revealed dramatic loss of forebrain cholinergic markers (Bartus et al., 1982; Whitehouse et al., 1982; Coyle et al., 1983; Winkler et al., 1998). These findings led to successful experiments in rats and mice revealing enhancement of memory and attention in young and aged rats and mice, as well as in rodent models of Alzheimer's disease, using drugs that augment cholinergic functions (Dutar et al., 1995; Everitt and Robbins, 1997; Iversen, 1998; Woolf, 1998; Disterhoft et al., 1999; Hasselmo, 1999; Sarter et al., 1999; van der Zee and Luiten, 1999; Sarter and Bruno, 2000). The promise of these agents led directly to the development of cholinesterase inhibitors that block the breakdown of acetylcholine to treat cognitive decline in Alzheimer's disease. Currently prescribed drugs include tacrine (Cognex), donepizil (Aricept), rivastigmine (Exelon), and galantamine (Reminyl) (cf. Disterhoft and Oh, 2006).

The drugs most often tested include agents that augment cholinergic functions indirectly or by direct receptor actions. Many studies examine the effects of acetylcholinesterase inhibitors, such as physostigmine, on memory in rodents. By inhibiting the degradation of acetylcholine after it is released from terminals, physostigmine increases the local concentration and the duration of the neurochemical actions of acetylcholine. Acetylcholinesterase inhibitors enhance learning and memory in rodents for tasks including inhibitory avoidance (Riekkinen et al., 1991), place and object recognition (Lamirault et al., 2003), and discrimination training (Marighetto et al., 2000). Acetylcholinesterase inhibitors are also very effective at reversing the impairing effects on memory of many drugs and brain lesions that impair memory (cf. Iversen, 1998; Gold and Stone, 1988). Drugs acting at either muscarinic or nicotinic cholinergic receptors also enhance learning, memory, and neural plasticity in rats and mice in many contexts and support the view that the neurotransmitter has important functions in regulating memory processing (e.g., Power et al., 2003; Gold, 2004; Hasselmo, 2006; Levin et al., 2006).

Acetylcholine appears to have many functions relevant to enhancement of memory. Release of acetylcholine may contribute to the memory-enhancing effects of glucose (**Figure** 7). Although neither peripheral nor intrahippocampal injections of glucose themselves increase the release of acetylcholine in the hippocampus, the injections augment acetylcholine release in the hippocampus while rats are engaged in a hippocampus-sensitive task (Ragozzino et al., 1996, 1998). In general, the magnitude of the increase in release is associated with enhancement of memory by glucose.

Another function of acetylcholine may be to balance the relative contributions of different memory systems to memory (Gold, 2003), perhaps regulating

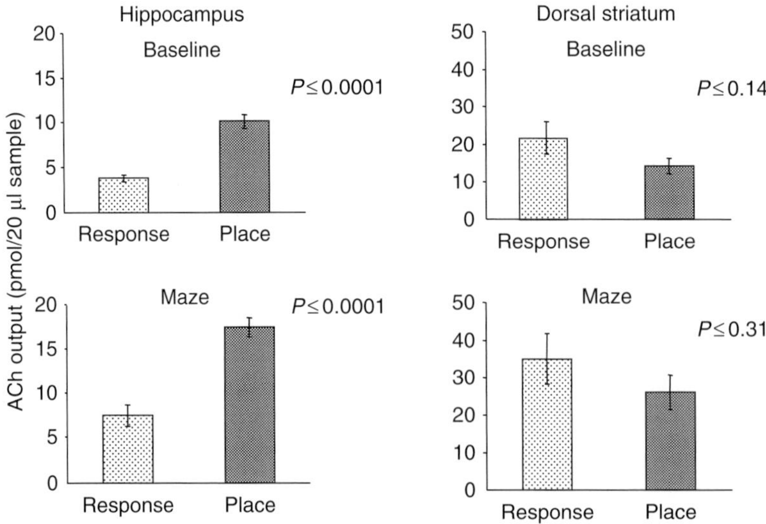

Figure 7 Acetylcholine (ACh) content in microdialysis samples collected concurrently from the hippocampus and dorsal striatum. Note the difference in *y*-axes for the two brain areas. Extracellular concentrations of ACh were greater in the striatum than in the hippocampus. Within the hippocampus, ACh release was significantly greater in rats that used a spatial strategy than in rats that used a response strategy. This was evident both prior to and during training. Although the scores were not significantly different at baseline or during training, the relationship between ACh release in the striatum of rats in the two groups was in the direction opposite that seen in the hippocampus. From McIntyre CK, Marriott LK, and Gold PE (2003a) Patterns of brain acetylcholine release predict individual differences in preferred learning strategies in rats. *Neurobiol. Learn. Mem.* 79: 177–183; used with permission.

the content of memory by modulating the level of activation of multiple memory systems. In one example, rats trained on a dual-solution T-maze solved equally well using either place (hippocampus-sensitive) or response (striatum-sensitive) solutions. The ratio of release of acetylcholine in the hippocampus versus dorsolateral striatum, measured just before training, predicted whether individual rats would show a preference for learning using a place or response solution (McIntyre et al., 2003b). These shifts may be related to evidence showing that acetylcholine shifts the cognitive function from attention at low levels of release to memory consolidation at higher levels of release (Hasselmo and McGaughy, 2004). These findings fit a broader context of evidence that acetylcholine regulates signal-to-noise ratios at the time of learning, regulates theta rhythms in the hippocampus, and modulates neuronal excitability (cf. Gold, 2003). More generally, the results suggest that acetylcholine enhances memory processing in multiple memory systems. By upregulating some systems more than others, the consequence would be that acetylcholine may alter the quality of memories as well as the strength of memories.

Acetylcholine also promotes neural plasticity assessed anatomically in the brains of honeybees (**Figure 8**; Ismail et al., 2006). New foragers exhibit substantial growth in the size of the mushroom body neuropil after extensive foraging experience. However, less experience is needed before neuropil growth is evident if a bee's foraging experience is coupled with administration of pilocarpine, a muscarinic agonist. Acetylcholine appears to promote neuroplasticity in somatosensory cortex (Dykes, 1997) and permit neurophysiological plasticity in auditory cortex during classical conditioning to tones (Weinberger, 2003, 2004).

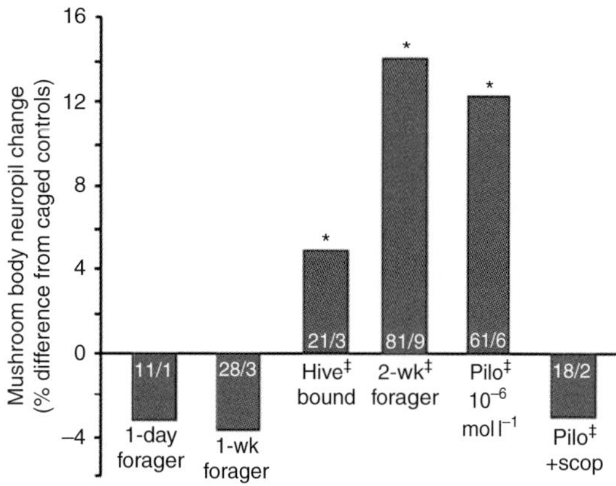

Figure 8 Effects of foraging experience with and without muscarinic agonist on the mushroom bodies. Estimates of the volume of the mushroom body neuropil were made for a total of 309 individuals, across nine experiments, conducted over three field seasons. To facilitate comparisons across all treatments, the % difference in neuropil volume relative to the caged control group in each experiment was calculated. Statistical analysis of these data used a mixed analysis of variance model ($F = 39.00$; $P < 0.0001$) and Dunnett *post hoc* tests (groups showing significant differences from the caged control group are indicated with the % difference). Key experimental groups are shown with the % difference indicated. Sample sizes are given in each bar (number of brains/number of trials). From Ismail N, Robinson GE, and Fahrbach SE (2006) Stimulation of muscarinic receptors mimics experience-dependent plasticity in the honey bee brain. *Proc. Natl. Acad. Sci. USA* 103: 207–211; used with permission.

28.3.3 Norepinephrine

Considerable evidence indicates that release of norepinephrine, particularly in the amygdala, may be a key brain component mediating enhancement of memory by a wide range of drugs (McIntyre et al., 2003; McGaugh, 2004). To some extent, interest in the role of norepinephrine in memory grew from the apparent involvement of the neurotransmitter in mediating the effects of epinephrine on memory. Indirect measures of norepinephrine release after epinephrine injections under conditions that enhance memory revealed release of norepinephrine throughout the brain (Gold and van Buskirk, 1978a,b); intermediate and high levels of release were associated with memory enhancement and impairment, respectively. More recent experiments, using *in vivo* microdialysis to study more directly release of norepinephrine, have found that peripheral epinephrine injections result in release of epinephrine within the amygdala (Williams et al., 1998). In addition, the magnitude of posttraining release of norepinephrine in the amygdala is positively correlated with later memory after inhibitory avoidance training. Posttraining injections of norepinephrine or β-adrenergic agonists directly into the amygdala enhance memory in an inverted-U dose-response manner (Liang et al., 1990; Hatfield and McGaugh, 1999).

The amygdala, and particularly the basolateral nucleus of the amygdala, may be a central mediator of many memory-enhancing treatments. For example, interference with noradrenergic functions in the amygdala, by lesions or by injections of β-adrenergic antagonists such as propranolol, block enhancement of memory by epinephrine, corticosterone, and GABA and opioid antagonists (McGaugh et al., 1988; Introini-Collison et al., 1989; Roozendaal et al., 1999). Moreover, there are considerable interactions between norepinephrine and acetylcholine within the amygdala. Often, the effects of cholinergic drugs on memory are not blocked by interference with β-noradrenergic receptors, in contrast to interactions of the β-noradrenergic receptors with other memory-enhancing treatments, results suggesting convergence of cholinergic and noradrenergic mechanisms within the amygdala to enhance memory (cf. McIntyre et al., 2003b).

Thus, neurochemical mechanisms in the amygdala may be a core mechanism common to the enhancement of memory with a wide range of treatments. Identifying the neurochemical bases of these effects may offer a plan for rational development of therapeutic agents targeted directly at mechanisms underlying memory enhancement by many treatments.

28.3.4 Glutamate

As the major excitatory neurotransmitter in the brain, it is not surprising that drugs that interfere with glutamate functions impair memory formation (cf. Riedel et al., 2003, for comprehensive review). A focus on memory-enhancing glutamatergic drugs yields far fewer examples, although there is clear evidence that glutamate itself enhances memory when injected directly into memory systems important for the learning task. Glutamate injections directly into the amygdala, administered immediately after presentation of a weak taste as the conditioned stimulus, enhance acquisition of a conditioned taste aversion to that taste (Miranda et al., 2002). In the same experiment, the investigators found that presentation of an unconditioned stimulus, lithium chloride, resulted in large increases in glutamate release measured with *in vivo* microdialysis. Other examples of glutamate enhancement of memory include enhancement of inhibitory avoidance training with posttraining injections of glutamate into the locus coeruleus (Clayton and Williams, 2000). Because the locus coeruleus is the site of cell bodies of neurons that distribute norepinephrine to the forebrain, the enhancement may be mediated by norepinephrine release at sites distal to the site of injection. Glutamate may also enhance memory processing at sites proximal to the injection. Using a dual-solution maze in which a rat could find food reward using either place or response solutions, glutamate infusions into the hippocampus or striatum differentially enhance place and response learning assessed on later probe trials (Packard, 1999).

Glutamate acts at several receptors with quite different functions, including both ligand-gated ion channels (ionotropic receptors) and G-protein-coupled (metabotropic) receptors. One receptor that has received attention is the metabotropic glutamate receptor subtype 5 (Simonyi et al., 2005). Posttraining injections of a drug, 3,3′-difluorobenzaldezine, that enhances these receptors facilitate later memory for spatial memory (Balschun et al., 2006). There is also evidence that ampakines, drugs that enhance alpha-amino-3-hydroxy-5-methyl-4-isoxazole propionic acid (AMPA)-type glutamate receptors, enhance learning and long-term potentiation (Lynch, 2006). AMPA receptors are responsible for fast excitatory neurotransmission mediated by glutamate, and the receptor modulation may reflect general increases in neural excitability as a mechanism of action. Enhancement of memory in a delayed matching to sample task has been seen in sleep-deprived monkeys (Porrino et al., 2005), although studies using post-training designs and unimpaired versus impaired memory have not been assessed. Of interest, parallel brain imaging studies show that the ampakines led to normalization of changes in metabolic activity in those brain areas where alterations were seen after sleep deprivation and not in other areas. These findings are reminiscent of the effects, described earlier, of glucose on acetylcholine release in the hippocampus when rats were engaged in training but not when rats were at rest (Ragozzino et al., 1996). The situational selectivity of such drug effects deserves considerable attention in developing drugs effective in enhancing multiple forms of memory.

28.4 Intracellular Factors

28.4.1 Calcium Channel Blockers

Considerable evidence suggests that dysfunctions of calcium regulation can impair memory and that such dysfunctions might contribute to those impairments during aging (cf. Disterhoft et al., 1996, 2004; Foster and Kumar, 2002; Foster, 2006). Disterhoft and colleagues have provided extensive evidence suggesting that drugs that attenuate age-related increases in calcium during activation of hippocampal (CA1) pyramidal neurons can enhance learning and memory in aged rabbits and rats. The task involves following the presentation of a tone with an air puff to the cornea, after a short delay, to establish an eyeblink classical conditioning response. Acquisition of this learned response is slowed or absent in aged rabbits and rats. Neurophysiological recordings from CA1 neurons reveal that there are age-related increases in the afterhyperpolarization (AHP) evident after a burst of action potentials. The AHP is characterized by an outward potassium current mediated by an influx of calcium that occurs with the action potential and serves to limit additional action potentials during its occurrence.

Of particular relevance to aging and memory, the AHPs are greatly enhanced in hippocampal pyramidal neurons of aged versus young animals, suggesting that the pyramidal neurons are less excitable and, perhaps, less able to participate in or to initiate mechanisms of learning and memory. Administration of nimodipine, an L-type calcium channel antagonist, reversed the age-related impairments in conditioning and in the AHPs (Deyo et al., 1989; Disterhoft et al., 1996; cf. Disterhoft et al., 2004). Of additional interest, drugs that augment cholinergic functions, including cholinesterase inhibitors and muscarinic receptor agonists, also enhanced learning and memory in this system and attenuated the AHP in aged animals (cf. Disterhoft and Oh, 2006). Findings such as these offer an excellent opportunity to address the mechanisms in common across treatment domains.

28.4.2 Intracellular Molecular Targets

As discussed earlier, considerable evidence quite consistently identifies classes of drugs, particularly those acting on specific neurotransmitters and receptors, that enhance memory. However, the cellular mechanisms by which the drugs act are less clear. Also unclear is whether deeper understanding of the most effective drugs to enhance memory will come from more specific identification of neurotransmitter receptors that mediate enhancement of memory, from examinations of combination drug protocols that act on multiple receptors (e.g., memory enhancing drug cocktails) or from drugs that act on putative intracellular mechanisms that might mediate memory enhancement by one or several neurotransmitters.

Of possible intracellular mechanisms that might contribute to enhancement of memory, cAMP response element-binding protein (CREB) has received considerable attention as an important regulator of memory formation (Silva et al., 1998; Izquierdo et al., 2002; Barco et al., 2003; Tully et al., 2003; Carlezon et al., 2005; Josselyn and Nguyen, 2005). In particular, CREB is often thought to facilitate the conversion of early to late stages of memory. Phosphorylation of CREB is correlated with memory formation (Izquierdo et al., 2002), and interference with CREB functions impairs memory formation (Guzowski and McGaugh, 1997). Although there have been significant attempts to identify pharmacological agents that might enhance CREB functions and thereby enhance memory (Barco et al., 2003; Tully et al., 2003), explicit tests of such drugs are not yet readily found. Also missing, for CREB as well as for many other putative components of the molecular biology of memory formation, are tests of whether these factors are the mediators of enhancement of memory by neurotransmitter actions or whether the factors elicit changes in neurotransmission related to modulation of memory. It seems unlikely that CREB is essential for memory. Epinephrine enhances memory in CREB-knockout mice (Frankland et al., 2004), and memory seems normalized by spaced versus massed training trials (Kogan et al., 1997). These findings suggest that activation of CREB is not necessary for memory formation or for modulation of memory, though it may be a step that precedes or interacts with the mechanisms by which systemic epinephrine injections modulate memory.

The absence of more information examining interrelationships between intracellular molecules implicated in memory processing and memory-enhancing treatments appears to be based on two elements. First, molecular cascades important to memory have primarily been identified with drugs that block specific components of these cascades. Complementary drugs that activate these cascades often do not exist or have not received sufficient attention in this regard. Second, the paucity of studies examining molecular cascades in memory enhancement may reflect the presumption in such studies that investigations are examining the mechanisms of memory formation rather than the mechanisms that modulate memory formation. At this point, either modulation or mechanism of memory formation seems to provide a plausible explanation of the findings obtained with studies of molecular cascades of memory, though the view that the molecules make new memories is dominant in research efforts.

A recent study explicitly related memory enhancement to an intracellular molecular target (McIntyre et al., 2005). Memory-enhancing injections of clenbuterol, a β-adrenergic agonist, were administered immediately after inhibitory avoidance training. Consistent with past findings, the treatment enhanced later memory. This treatment also resulted in increased expression of Arc protein. Arc is localized to dendritic regions near points of synaptic stimulation and appears to be associated with synaptic plasticity and memory (Guzowski et al., 2005). This is an early study in what promises to be a very useful approach of coupling memory-enhancing treatments to gene and protein responses important for the enhancement of memory.

28.5 Conclusions

Even over 50 years after the main demonstrations that drugs can enhance memory, the findings still seem quite remarkable in several respects. Although it is rather easy to imagine that interference with neural activity can impair memory, it is more surprising, at least to this writer, that drug perturbation of neural activity can also improve memory formation. Many of the drugs that enhance memory are related to neurotransmitters. For example, amphetamine augments catecholamine functions by blocking reuptake mechanisms. β-adrenergic, nicotinic, and glutamatergic receptor agonists act largely on postsynaptic receptors to mimic the action of the neurotransmitters norepinephrine, acetylcholine and glutamate, respectively. Although these neurotransmitters all appear to have a positive role in memory formation, the drugs that mimic them do not match the temporal and spatial patterning that appears to be a key element of neural processing generally, and in the formation of memory in particular. The apparent illogic may be addressed by findings that many neurotransmitters, notably including norepinephrine, acetylcholine, glutamate, and others, may have important extrasynaptic functions with release sites for neurotransmitters that are not always associated with close postsynaptic appositions (Descarries and Mechawar, 2000; Bach-y-rita, 2001; Descarries et al., 2004; Carmignoto and Fellin, 2006; Vizi and Mike, 2006). Findings such as these suggest that the temporal and spatial properties of neural activity may not apply to all neurotransmitters in all brain areas and may instead function much like local hormones, changing the functional state of the areas they bathe. One of those functional states may be readiness to alter connectivity in response to information flow, a function consistent with the idea of modulation of memory. Another explanation is based on the neurophysiological responses to some neurotransmitters involved in enhancement of memory. An example here is that the iontophoretic application of low levels of norepinephrine, serotonin, or acetylcholine can enhance both the postsynaptic excitation and inhibition produced by glutamate and GABA, respectively. In this way, the neuromodulators may enhance the impact of information flowing through traditional synapses, augmenting the signal-to-noise ratio and thereby enhancing memory formation.

It is also possible to move beyond these system-level views of how memory-enhancing drugs might work to the cellular and molecular bases by which they work. Mechanisms at this level might be the consequence of receptor binding leading to biochemical cascades important to memory or might be, similarly but less directly, the consequence of amplification of signals handled by other neurotransmitters, as discussed earlier. In contrast to the investigations of drugs that impair memory, far less attention has been given to the cellular and molecular bases by which well-studied drugs enhance memory. This is a research area ripe for future investigations.

Acknowledgments

Preparation of this chapter was supported by USPHS grants NIA AG07648 and DA 16951 from the National Institutes of Health.

References

Ahmed T, Frey JU, and Korz V (2006) Long-term effects of brief acute stress on cellular signaling and hippocampal LTP. *J. Neurosci.* 26: 3951–3958.

Amoroso S, Schmid-Antomarchi H, Fosset M, and Lazdunski M (1990) Glucose, sulfonylureas, and neurotransmitter release: Role of ATP-sensitive K^+ channels. *Science* 247: 852–854.

Ashcroft FM (2005) ATP-sensitive potassium channelopathies: Focus on insulin secretion. *J. Clin. Invest.* 115: 2047–2058.

Axelrod J, Weil-Malherbe H, and Tomchick R (1959) The physiological disposition of H3-epinephrine and its metabolite metanephrine. *J. Pharmacol. Exp. Ther.* 127: 251–256.

Bach-y-Rita P (2001) Nonsynaptic diffusion neurotransmission in the brain: Functional considerations. *Neurochem. Res.* 26: 871–873.

Balschun D, Zuschratter W, and Wetzel W (2006) Allosteric enhancement of metabotropic glutamate receptor 5 function promotes spatial memory. *Neuroscience* 142: 691–702.

Barco A, Pittenger C, and Kandel ER (2003) CREB, memory enhancement and the treatment of memory disorders: Promises, pitfalls and prospects. *Expert Opin. Ther. Targets* 7: 101–114.

Bartus RT, Dean RL III, Beer B, and Lippa AS (1982) The cholinergic hypothesis of geriatric memory dysfunction. *Science* 217: 408–417.

Benevento LA and Kandel GL (1967) Influence of strychnine on classically conditioned defensive reflexes in the cat. *J. Comp. Physiol. Psychol.* 63: 117–120.

Bingham E, Hopkins D, Pernet A, Reid H, Macdonald IA, and Amiel SA (2003) The effects of KATP channel modulators on counterregulatory responses and cognitive function during acute controlled hypoglycaemia in healthy men: A pilot study. *Diabet. Med.* 20: 231–237.

Bruce KR, Pihl RO, Mayerovitch JI, and Shestowsky JS (1999) Alcohol and retrograde memory effects: Role of individual differences. *J. Stud. Alcohol* 60: 130–136.

Cahill L and Alkire MT (2003) Epinephrine enhancement of human memory consolidation: Interaction with arousal at encoding. *Neurobiol. Learn. Mem.* 79: 194–198.

Cahill L and McGaugh JL (1998) Mechanisms of emotional arousal and lasting declarative memory. *Trends Neurosci.* 21: 294–299.

Canal C, Stutz SJ, and Gold PE (2005) Glucose injections into the hippocampus or striatum of rats prior to T-maze training: modulation of learning rates and strategy selection. *Learn. Mem.* 12: 367–374.

Carlezon WA Jr. Duman RS, and Nestler EJ (2005) The many faces of CREB. *Trends Neurosci.* 28: 436–445.

Carmignoto G and Fellin T (2006) Glutamate release from astrocytes as a non-synaptic mechanism for neuronal synchronization in the hippocampus. *J. Physiol. Paris* 99: 98–102.

Choeiri C, Staines W, Miki T, Seino S, and Messier C (2005) Glucose transporter plasticity during memory processing. *Neuroscience* 130: 591–600.

Cholewiak RW, Hammond R, Seigler IC, and Papsdorf JD (1968) Effects of strychnine sulphate on classically conditioned nictitating membrane responses of rabbits. *J. Comp. Physiol. Psychol.* 66: 77–81.

Clark KB, Smith DC, Hassert DL, Browning RA, Naritoku DK, and Jensen RA (1998) Posttraining electrical stimulation of vagal afferents with concomitant vagal efferent inactivation enhances memory storage processes in the rat. *Neurobiol. Learn. Mem.* 70: 364–373.

Clark KB, Naritoku DK, Smith DC, Browning RA, and Jensen RA (1999) Enhanced recognition memory following vagus nerve stimulation in human subjects. *Nat. Neurosci.* 2: 94–98.

Clayton EC and Williams CL (2000) Noradrenergic receptor blockade of the NTS attenuates the mnemonic effects of epinephrine in an appetitive light-dark discrimination learning task. *Neurobiol. Learn. Mem.* 74: 135–145.

Coyle JT, Price DL, and DeLong MR (1983) Alzheimer's disease: A disorder of the cortical cholinergic innervation. *Science* 219: 1184–1190.

Daniel JM, Hulst JL, and Berbling JL (2006) Estradiol replacement enhances working memory in middle-aged rats when initiated immediately after ovariectomy but not after a long-term period of ovarian hormone deprivation. *Endocrinology* 147: 607–614.

Dash PK, Orsi SA, and Moore AN (2006) Spatial memory formation and memory-enhancing effect of glucose involves activation of the tuberous sclerosis complex–mammalian target of rapamycin pathway. *J. Neurosci.* 26: 8048–8056.

de Wied D (1990) Neurotrophic effects of ACTH/MSH neuropeptides. *Acta Neurobiol. Exp.* 50: 353–366.

de Wied D (1999) Behavioral pharmacology of neuropeptides related to melanocortins and the neurohypophyseal hormones. *Eur. J. Pharmacol.* 375: 1–11.

Descarries L and Mechawar N (2000) Ultrastructural evidence for diffuse transmission by monoamine and acetylcholine neurons of the central nervous system. *Prog. Brain Res.* 125: 27–47.

Descarries L, Mechawar N, Aznavour N, and Watkins KC (2004) Structural determinants of the roles of acetylcholine in cerebral cortex. *Prog. Brain Res.* 145: 45–58.

Deyo RA, Strauble KT, and Disterhoft JF (1989) Nimodipene facilitates associative learning in aging rabbits. *Science* 243: 809–811.

Diamond DM, Park CR, and Woodson JC (2004) Stress generates emotional memories and retrograde amnesia by inducing an endogenous form of hippocampal LTP. *Hippocampus* 14: 281–291.

Dirnagl U, Iadecola C, and Moskowitz MA (1999) Pathobiology of ischaemic stroke: An integrated view. *Trends Neurosci.* 22: 391–397.

Disterhoft JF and Oh MM (2006) Pharmacological and molecular enhancement of learning in aging and Alzheimer's disease. *J. Physiol. Paris* 99: 180–192.

Disterhoft JF, Thompson LT, Moyer JR Jr. and Mogul DJ (1996) Calcium-dependent afterhyperpolarization and learning in young and aging hippocampus. *Life Sci.* 59: 413–420.

Disterhoft JF, Wu WW, and Ohno M (2004) Biophysical alterations of hippocampal pyramidal neurons in learning, ageing and Alzheimer's disease. *Ageing Res. Rev.* 3: 383–406.

Disterhoft JF, Kronforst-Collins M, Oh MM, Power JM, Preston AR, and Weiss C (1999) Cholinergic facilitation of trace eyeblink conditioning in aging rabbits. *Life Sci.* 64: 541–548.

Dohanich GP (2002) Gonadal steroids, learning and memory. In: Pfaff DW, Arnold AP, Etgen AM, Fahrbach SW, and Rubin RT (eds.) *Hormones, Brain and Behavior*, pp. 265–327. San Diego: Academic Press.

Duncan CP (1949) The retroactive effect of electroshock on learning. *J. Comp. Physiol. Psychol.* 42: 32–44.

Dutar P, Bassant MH, Senut MC, and Lamour Y (1995) The septohippocampal pathway: Structure and function of a central cholinergic system. *Physiol. Rev.* 75: 393–427.

Dykes RW (1997) Mechanisms controlling neuronal plasticity in somatosensory cortex. *Can. J. Physiol. Pharmacol.* 75: 535–545.

Erickson KI, Colcombe SJ, Elavsky S, et al. (2007) Interactive effects of fitness and hormone treatment on brain health in postmenopausal women. *Neurobiol. Aging* 28: 179–185.

Espeland MA, Rapp SR, Shumaker SA, et al., for the Women's Health Initiative (2004) Conjugated equine estrogens and global cognitive function in postmenopausal women. *JAMA* 291: 2959–2968.

Everitt BJ and Robbins TW (1997) Central cholinergic systems and cognition. *Annu. Rev. Psychol.* 48: 649–684.

Farah MJ, Illes J, Cook-Deegan R, et al. (2004) Neurocognitive enhancement: What can we do and what should we do? *Nat. Rev. Neurosci.* 5: 421–425.

Farr SA, Banks WA, and Morley JE (2000) Estradiol potentiates acetylcholine and glutamate-mediated post-trial memory processing in the hippocampus. *Brain Res.* 864: 263–269.

Fellows LK, Boutelle MG, and Fillenz M (1993) ATP-sensitive potassium channels and local energy demands in the rat hippocampus: An in vivo study. *J. Neurochem.* 61: 949–954.

Foster TC (2006) Biological markers of age-related memory deficits: Treatment of senescent physiology. *CNS Drugs* 20: 153–166.

Foster TC and Kumar A (2002) Calcium dysregulation in the aging brain. *Neuroscientist* 8: 297–301.

Frankland PW, Josselyn SA, Anagnostaras SG, Kogan JH, Takahashi E, and Silva AJ (2004) Consolidation of CS and US representations in associative fear conditioning. *Hippocampus* 14: 557–569.

Ghelardini C, Galeotti N, and Bartolini A (1998) Influence of potassium channel modulators on cognitive processes in mice. *Br. J. Pharmacol.* 123: 1079–1084.

Gibbs RB and Gabor R (2003) Estrogen and cognition: Applying preclinical findings to clinical perspectives. *J. Neurosci. Res.* 74: 637–643.

Gibbs RB, Gabor R, Cox T, and Johnson DA (2004) Effects of raloxifene and estradiol on hippocampal acetylcholine release and spatial learning in the rat. *Psychoneuroendocrinology* 29: 741–748.

Gold PE (1986) Glucose modulation of memory storage processing. *Behav. Neural Biol.* 45: 342–349.

Gold PE (1987) Sweet memories. *Am. Sci.* 75: 151–155.

Gold PE (1995) Modulation of emotional and non-emotional memories: Same pharmacological systems, different neuroanatomical systems. In: McGaugh JL, Weinberger NM, and Lynch GS (eds.) *Brain and Memory: Modulation and Mediation of Neural Plasticity*, pp. 41–74. New York: Oxford University Press.

Gold PE (2003) Acetylcholine modulation of neural systems involved in learning and memory. *Neurobiol. Learn. Mem.* 80: 194–210.

Gold PE (2004) Coordination of multiple memory systems. *Neurobiol. Learn. Mem.* 82: 230–242.

Gold PE (2005) Glucose and age-related changes in memory. *Neurobiol. Aging* 26S: S60–S64.

Gold PE (2006) The many faces of amnesia. *Learn. Mem.* 13: 506–514.

Gold PE and McCarty R (1981) Plasma catecholamines: Changes after footshock and seizure producing frontal cortex stimulation. *Behav. Neural Biol.* 31: 247–260.

Gold PE and McGaugh JL (1975) A single trace, two process view of memory storage processes. In: Deutsch D and Deutsch JA (eds.) *Short-Term Memory*, pp. 355–390. New York: Academic Press.

Gold PE and McGaugh JL (1978) Neurobiology and memory: Modulators, correlates and assumptions. In: Teyler T (ed.) *Brain and Learning*, pp. 93–103. Stamford, CT: Greylock Publishers.

Gold PE and Stone WS (1988) Neuroendocrine factors in age-related memory dysfunctions: Studies in animals and humans. *Neurobiol. Aging* 9: 709–717.

Gold PE and van Buskirk RB (1975) Facilitation of time dependent memory processes with posttrial epinephrine injections. *Behav. Biol.* 13: 145–153.

Gold PE and van Buskirk RB (1976) Enhancement and impairment of memory processes with posttrial injections of adrenocorticotrophic hormone. *Behav. Biol.* 16: 387–400.

Gold PE and van Buskirk RB (1978a) Posttraining brain norepinephrine concentrations: Correlation with retention performance of avoidance training and with peripheral epinephrine modulation of memory processing. *Behav. Biol.* 23: 509–520.

Gold PE and van Buskirk RB (1978b) Effects of α- and β-adrenergic receptor antagonists on post-trial epinephrine modulation of memory: Relationship to post-training brain norepinephrine concentrations. *Behav. Biol.* 24: 168–184. Gold et al., (1986).

Gresack JE and Frick KM (2006) Post-training estrogen enhances spatial and object memory consolidation in female mice. *Pharmacol. Biochem. Behav.* 84: 112–119.

Guzowski JF and McGaugh JL (1997) Antisense oligodeoxynucleotide-mediated disruption of hippocampal cAMP response element binding protein levels impairs consolidation of memory for water maze training. *Proc. Natl. Acad. Sci. USA* 94: 2693–2698.

Guzowski JF, Timlin JA, Roysam B, McNaughton BL, Worley PF, and Barnes CA (2005) Mapping behaviorally relevant neural circuits with immediate-early gene expression. *Curr. Opin. Neurobiol.* 15: 599–606.

Haddad GG and Jiang C (1994) Mechanisms of neuronal survival during hypoxia: ATP-sensitive K+ channels. *Biol. Neonate* 65: 160–165.

Hall JL and Gold PE (1986) The effects of training, epinephrine, and glucose injections on plasma glucose levels in rats. *Behav. Neural Biol.* 46: 156–176.

Hansen JB (2006) Towards selective Kir6.2/SUR1 potassium channel openers, medicinal chemistry and therapeutic perspectives. *Curr. Med. Chem.* 13: 361–376.

Hasselmo ME (1999) Neuromodulation: Acetylcholine and memory consolidation. *Trends Cogn. Sci.* 3: 351–359.

Hasselmo ME (2006) The role of acetylcholine in learning and memory. *Curr. Opin. Neurobiol.* 16: 710–715.

Hasselmo ME and McGaughy J (2004) High acetylcholine levels set circuit dynamics for attention and encoding and low acetylcholine levels set dynamics for consolidation. *Prog. Brain Res.* 145: 207–231.

Hassert DL, Miyashita T, and Williams CL (2004) The effects of peripheral vagal nerve stimulation at a memory-modulating intensity on norepinephrine output in the basolateral amygdala. *Behav. Neurosci.* 118: 79–88.

Hatfield T and McGaugh JL (1999) Norepinephrine infused into the basolateral amygdala posttraining enhances retention in a spatial water maze task. *Neurobiol. Learn. Mem.* 71: 232–239.

Hunt E and Krivanek J (1966) The effects of pentylenetetrazole and methylphenoxypropane on discrimination learning. *Psychopharmacologia* 9: 1–16.

Introini-Collison IB, Nagahara AH, and McGaugh JL (1989) Memory enhancement with intra-amygdala posttraining naloxone is blocked by concurrent administration of propranolol. *Brain Res.* 476: 94–101.

Introini-Collison IB, Dalmaz C, and McGaugh JL (1996) Amygdala β-noradrenergic influences on memory storage involve cholinergic activation. *Neurobiol. Learn. Mem.* 65: 57–64.

Ismail N, Robinson GE, and Fahrbach SE (2006) Stimulation of muscarinic receptors mimics experience-dependent plasticity in the honey bee brain. *Proc. Natl. Acad. Sci. USA* 103: 207–211.

Iversen SD (1998) The pharmacology of memory. *C R Acad. Sci. III* 321: 209–215.

Izquierdo I, da Cunha C, Rosat R, Jerusalinsky D, Ferreira MB, and Medina JH (1992) Neurotransmitter receptors involved in post-training memory processing by the amygdala, medial septum, and hippocampus of the rat. *Behav. Neural Biol.* 58: 16–26.

Izquierdo I, Bianchin M, Silva MB, et al. (1993) CNQX infused into rat hippocampus or amygdala disrupts the expression of memory of two different tasks. *Behav. Neural Biol.* 59: 1–4.

Izquierdo LA, Barros DM, Vianna MR, et al. (2002) Molecular pharmacological dissection of short- and long-term memory. *Cell Mol. Neurobiol.* 22: 269–287.

Josselyn SA and Nguyen PV (2005) CREB, synapses and memory disorders: Past progress and future challenges. *Curr. Drug Targets CNS Neurol. Disord.* 4: 481–497.

Kelemen K and Bovet D (1961) Effect of drugs upon the defensive behavior of rats. *Acta Physiol. Acad. Sci. Hung.* 19: 143–154.

Kesner RP and Rogers J (2004) An analysis of independence and interactions of brain substrates that subserve multiple attributes, memory systems and underlying processes. *Neurobiol. Learn. Mem.* 82: 199–215.

Kogan JH, Frankland PW, Blendy JA, et al. (1997) Spaced training induces normal long-term memory in CREB mutant mice. *Curr. Biol.* 7: 1–11.

Kopf SR and Baratti CM (1996) Effects of posttraining administration of glucose on retention of a habituation response in mice: Participation of a central cholinergic mechanism. *Neurobiol. Learn. Mem.* 65: 253–260.

Kopf SR, Buchholzer ML, Hilgert M, Loffelholz K, and Klein J (2001) Glucose plus choline improve passive avoidance behaviour and increase hippocampal acetylcholine release in mice. *Neuroscience* 103: 365–371.

Korol DL and Gold PE (2007) Modulation of learning and memory by adrenal and ovarian hormones. In: Kesner RP and Martinez JL (eds.) *Neurobiology of Learning and Memory*, pp. 243–267. Oxford: Elsevier Science.

Korol DL (2002) Enhancing cognitive function across the life span. *Ann. N. Y. Acad. Sci.* 959: 167–179.

Korol DL (2004) Role of estrogen in balancing contributions from multiple memory systems. *Neurobiol. Learn. Mem.* 82: 309–323.

Korol DL and Kolo LL (2002) Estrogen-induced changes in place and response learning in young adult female rats. *Behav. Neurosci.* 116: 411–420.

Korol DL, Malin EL, Borden KA, Busby RA, and Couper-Leo J (2004) Shifts in preferred learning strategy across the estrous cycle in female rats. *Horm. Behav.* 45: 330–338.

Krebs DL and Parent MB (2005) The enhancing effects of hippocampal infusions of glucose are not restricted to spatial working memory. *Neurobiol. Learn. Mem.* 83: 168–172.

Lacreuse A, Wilson ME, and Herndon JG (2002) Estradiol, but not raloxifene, improves aspects of spatial working memory in aged, ovariectomized rhesus monkeys. *Neurobiol. Aging* 23: 589–600.

Lamirault L, Guillou C, Thal C, and Simon H (2003) 9-Dehydrogalanthaminium bromide, a new cholinesterase inhibitor, enhances place and object recognition memory in young and old rats. *Neurobiol. Learn. Mem.* 80: 113–122.

Lashley KS (1917) The effects of strychnine and caffeine upon the rate of learning. *Psychobiology* 1: 141–170.

Lee MK, Graham S, and Gold PE (1988) Memory enhancement with posttraining intraventricular glucose injections in rats. *Behav. Neurosci.* 102: 591–595.

Lennartz RC, Hellems KL, Mook ER, and Gold PE (1996) Inhibitory avoidance impairments induced by intra-amygdala propranolol are reversed by glutamate but not glucose. *Behav. Neurosci.* 110: 1–7.

Levin ED, McClernon FJ, and Rezvani AH (2006) Nicotinic effects on cognitive function: Behavioral characterization, pharmacological specification, and anatomic localization. *Psychopharmacology* 184: 523–539.

Li AJ, Oomura Y, Sasaki K, et al. (1998) A single pre-training glucose injection induces memory facilitation in rodents performing various tasks: Contribution of acidic fibroblast growth factor. *Neuroscience* 85: 785–794.

Liang KC, McGaugh JL, and Yao HY (1990) Involvement of amygdala pathways in the influence of post-training intra-amygdala norepinephrine and peripheral epinephrine on memory storage. *Brain Res.* 508: 225–233.

Liss B and Roeper J (2001) Molecular physiology of neuronal K-ATP channels (review). *Mol. Membr. Biol.* 18: 117–127.

Luine V (2002) Sex differences in chronic stress effects on memory in rats. *Stress* 5: 205–216.

Lynch GS (2006) Glutamate-based therapeutic approaches: Ampakines. *Curr. Opin. Pharmacol.* 6: 82–88.

Mabry TR, Gold PE, and McCarty R (1995a) Age-related changes in plasma catecholamine and glucose responses of F-344 rats to footshock as in inhibitory avoidance training. *Neurobiol. Learn. Mem.* 64: 146–155.

Mabry TR, Gold PE, and McCarty R (1995b) Age-related changes in plasma catecholamine responses to acute swim stress. *Neurobiol. Learn. Mem.* 63: 260–268.

Mabry TR, Gold PE, and McCarty R (1995c) Age-related changes in plasma catecholamine responses to chronic intermittent stress. *Physiol. Behav.* 58: 49–56.

Maki PM (2006) Hormone therapy and cognitive function: Is there a critical period for benefit? *Neuroscience* 138: 1027–1030.

Manning CA, Parsons MW, and Gold PE (1992) Anterograde and retrograde enhancement of 24-hour memory by glucose in elderly humans. *Behav. Neural Biol.* 58: 125–130.

Manning CA, Ragozzino M, and Gold PE (1993) Glucose enhancement of memory in patients with Alzheimer's disease. *Neurobiol. Aging* 14: 523–528.

Marighetto A, Touzani K, Etchamenday N, et al. (2000) Further evidence for a dissociation between different forms of mnemonic expressions in a mouse model of age-related cognitive decline: Effects of tacrine and S 17092, a novel prolyl endopeptidase inhibitor. *Learn. Mem.* 7: 159–169.

Marriott LK and Korol DL (2003) Short-term estrogen treatment in ovariectomized rats augments hippocampal acetylcholine release during place learning. *Neurobiol. Learn. Mem.* 80: 315–322.

McCarty R and Gold PE (1981) Plasma catecholamines: Effects of footshock level and hormonal modulators of memory storage. *Horm. Behav.* 15: 168–182.

McEwen BS (2001) Plasticity of the hippocampus: Adaptation to chronic stress and allostatic load. *Ann. N. Y. Acad. Sci.* 933: 265–277.

McGaugh JL (1966) Time-dependent processes in memory storage. *Science* 153: 1351–1358.

McGaugh JL (1989) Dissociating learning and performance: Drug and hormone enhancement of memory storage. *Brain Res. Bull.* 23: 339–345.

McGaugh JL (2000) Memory: A century of consolidation. *Science* 287: 248–251.

McGaugh JL (2004) The amygdala modulates the consolidation of memories of emotionally arousing experiences. *Annu. Rev. Neurosci.* 27: 1–28.

McGaugh JL and Petrinovich LF (1959) The effect of strychnine sulphate on maze-learning. *Am. J. Psychol.* 72: 99–102.

McGaugh JL and Thomson CW (1962) Facilitation of simultaneous discriminate learning with strychnine sulphate. *Psychopharmacologia* 3: 166–172.

McGaugh JL, Introini-Collison IB, and Nagahara AH (1988) Memory-enhancing effects of posttraining naloxone: Involvement of β-noradrenergic influences in the amygdaloid complex. *Brain Res.* 446: 37–49.

McGaugh JL, Introini-Collison IB, Cahill LF, et al. (1993) Neuromodulatory systems and memory storage: Role of the amygdala. *Behav. Brain Res.* 58: 81–90.

McIntyre CK, Marriott LK, and Gold PE (2003a) Patterns of brain acetylcholine release predict individual differences in preferred learning strategies in rats. *Neurobiol. Learn. Mem.* 79: 177–183.

McIntyre CK, Power AE, Roozendaal B, and McGaugh JL (2003b) Role of the basolateral amygdala in memory consolidation. *Ann. N. Y. Acad. Sci.* 985: 273–293.

McIntyre CK, Miyashita T, Setlow B, et al. (2005) Memory-influencing intra-basolateral amygdala drug infusions modulate expression of Arc protein in the hippocampus. *Proc. Natl. Acad. Sci. USA* 102: 10718–10723.

McNay EC and Gold PE (1998) Memory modulation across neural systems: Intra-amygdala glucose reverses deficits caused by intra-septal morphine on a spatial task, but not on an aversive task. *J. Neurosci.* 18: 3853–3858.

McNay EC and Gold PE (2001) Age-related differences in hippocampal extracellular fluid glucose concentration during behavioral testing and following systemic glucose administration. *J. Gerontol. A Biol. Sci. Med. Sci.* 56A: B66–B71.

McNay EC and Gold PE (2002) Food for thought: Fluctuations in brain extracellular glucose provide insight into the mechanisms of memory modulation. *Behav. Cogn. Neurosci. Rev.* 1: 264–280.

McNay EC, McCarty RM, and Gold PE (2001) Fluctuations in glucose concentration during behavioral testing: Dissociations both between brain areas and between brain and blood. *Neurobiol. Learn. Mem.* 75: 325–337.

Messier C (2004) Glucose improvement of memory: A review. *Eur. J. Pharmacol.* 490: 33–57.

Messier C and White NM (1984) Contingent and non-contingent actions of sucrose and saccharin reinforcers: Effects on taste preference and memory. *Physiol. Behav.* 32: 195–203.

Messier C, Durkin T, Mrabet O, and Destrade C (1990) Memory-improving action of glucose: Indirect evidence for a facilitation of hippocampal acetylcholine synthesis. *Behav. Brain Res.* 39: 135–143.

Miranda MI, Ferreira G, Ramirez-Lugo L, and Bermudez-Rattoni F (2002) Glutamatergic activity in the amygdala signals visceral input during taste memory formation. *Proc. Natl. Acad. Sci. USA* 99: 11417–11422.

Nielson KA, Radtke RC, and Jensen RA (1996) Arousal-induced modulation of memory storage processes in humans. *Neurobiol. Learn. Mem.* 66: 133–142.

Oitzl MS and de Kloet ER (1992) Selective corticosteroid antagonists modulate specific aspects of spatial orientation learning. *Behav. Neurosci.* 106: 62–71.

Oomura Y, Sasaki K, and Li AJ (1993) Memory facilitation educed by food intake. *Physiol. Behav.* 54: 493–498.

Packard MG (1999) Glutamate infused posttraining into the hippocampus or caudate-putamen differentially strengthens place and response learning. *Proc. Natl. Acad. Sci. USA* 96: 12881–12886.

Packard MG and McGaugh JL (1996) Inactivation of the hippocampus or caudate nucleus with lidocaine differentially affects expression of place and response learning. *Neurobiol. Learn. Mem.* 65: 65–72.

Packard MG and Teather LA (1997a) Intra-hippocampal estradiol infusion enhances memory in ovariectomized rats. *Neuroreport* 8: 3009–3013.

Packard MG and Teather LA (1997b) Posttraining estradiol injections enhance memory in ovariectomized rats: Cholinergic blockade and synergism. *Neurobiol. Learn. Mem.* 68: 172–188.

Panten U, Schwanstecher M, and Schwanstecher C (1996) Sulfonylurea receptors and mechanism of sulfonylurea action. *Exp. Clin. Endocrinol.* 104: 1–9.

Parker ES, Birnbaum IM, Weingartner H, Hartley JT, Stillman RC, and Wyatt RJ (1980) Retrograde enhancement of human memory with alcohol. *Psychopharmacology* 69: 219–222.

Pavlides C, Ogawa S, Kimura A, and McEwen BS (1996) Role of adrenal steroid mineralocorticoid and glucocorticoid receptors in long-term potentiation in the CA1 field of hippocampal slices. *Brain Res.* 738: 229–235.

Poldrack RA and Packard MG (2003) Competition among multiple memory systems: Converging evidence from animal and human brain studies. *Neuropsychology* 41: 245–251.

Porrino LJ, Daunais JB, Rogers GA, Hampson RE, and Deadwyler SA (2005) Facilitation of task performance and removal of the effects of sleep deprivation by an ampakine (CX717) in nonhuman primates. *PLoS. Biol.* 3: e299.

Power AE, Vazdarjanova A, and McGaugh JL (2003) Muscarinic cholinergic influences in memory consolidation. *Neurobiol. Learn. Mem.* 80: 178–193.

Pych JC, Kim M, and Gold PE (2006) Effects of injections of glucose into the dorsal striatum on learning of place and response mazes. *Behav. Brain Res.* 167: 373–378.

Ragozzino ME, Wenk GL, and Gold PE (1994) Glucose attenuates morphine-induced decrease in hippocampal acetylcholine output: An in vivo microdialysis study in rats. *Brain Res.* 655: 77–82.

Ragozzino ME, Hellems K, Lennartz RC, and Gold PE (1995) Pyruvate infusions into the septal area attenuate spontaneous alternation impairments induced by intraseptal morphine injections. *Behav. Neurosci.* 109: 1074–1080.

Ragozzino ME, Unick KE, and Gold PE (1996) Hippocampal acetylcholine release during memory testing in rats: Augmentation by glucose. *Proc. Natl. Acad. Sci.* 93: 4693–4698.

Ragozzino ME, Pal SN, Unick K, Stefani MR, and Gold PE (1998) Modulation of hippocampal acetylcholine release and of memory by intrahippocampal glucose injections. *J. Neurosci.* 18: 1595–1601.

Rashidy-Pour A (2001) ATP-sensitive potassium channels mediate the effects of a peripheral injection of glucose on memory storage in an inhibitory avoidance task. *Behav. Brain Res.* 126: 43–48.

Rhodes ME and Frye CA (2006) ERbeta-selective SERMs produce mnemonic-enhancing effects in the inhibitory avoidance and water maze tasks. *Neurobiol. Learn. Mem.* 85: 183–191.

Riedel G, Platt B, and Micheau J (2003) Glutamate receptor function in learning and memory. *Behav. Brain Res.* 140: 1–47.

Riekkinen P Jr. Riekkenen M, Lahtinen H, Sirvio J, Valjakka A, and Riekkinen P (1991) Tetrahydroaminoacridine improves passive avoidance retention defects induced by aging and medial septal lesion but not by fimbria-fornix lesion. *Brain Res. Bull.* 27: 587–594.

Roesler R, Schroder N, Vianna MR, et al. (2003) Differential involvement of hippocampal and amygdalar NMDA receptors in contextual and aversive aspects of inhibitory avoidance memory in rats. *Brain Res.* 975: 207–213.

Roozendaal B (2002) Stress and memory: Opposing effects of glucocorticoids on memory consolidation and memory retrieval. *Neurobiol. Learn. Mem.* 78: 578–595.

Roozendaal B (2003) Systems mediating acute glucocorticoid effects on memory consolidation and retrieval. *Prog. Neuropsychopharmacol. Biol. Psychiatry* 27: 1213–1223.

Roozendaal B, Nguyen BT, Power AE, and McGaugh JL (1999) Basolateral amygdala noradrenergic influence enables enhancement of memory consolidation induced by hippocampal glucocorticoid receptor activation. *Proc. Natl. Acad. Sci. USA* 96: 11642–11647.

Roozendaal B, Quirarte GL, and McGaugh JL (2002) Glucocorticoids interact with the basolateral amygdala b-adrenoceptor-cAMP/PKA system in influencing memory consolidation. *Eur. J. Neurosci.* 15: 553–560.

Rose SPR (2002) 'Smart drugs': Do they work? Are they ethical? Will they be legal? *Nat. Rev. Neurosci.* 3: 975–979.

Sandi C (2004) Stress, cognitive impairment and cell adhesion molecules. *Nat. Rev. Neurosci.* 5: 917–930.

Sarter M and Bruno JP (2000) Cortical cholinergic inputs mediating arousal, attentional processing and dreaming: Differential afferent regulation of the basal forebrain by telencephalic and brainstem afferents. *Neuroscience* 95: 933–952.

Sarter M, Bruno JP, and Turchi J (1999) Basal forebrain afferent projections modulating cortical acetylcholine, attention and implications for neuropsychiatric disorders. *Ann. N. Y. Acad. Sci.* 877: 368–382.

Scholey AB and Fowles KA (2002) Retrograde enhancement of kinesthetic memory by alcohol and by glucose. *Neurobiol. Learn. Mem.* 78: 477–483.

Sherwin BB (2006) Estrogen and cognitive aging in women. *Neuroscience* 138: 1021–1026.

Shumaker SA, Legault C, Kuller L, et al. (2004) Conjugated equine estrogens and incidence of probable dementia and mild cognitive impairment in postmenopausal women. *JAMA* 291: 2947–2958.

Silva AJ, Kogan JH, Frankland PW, and Kida S (1998) CREB and memory. *Annu. Rev. Neurosci.* 21: 127–148.

Simonyi A, Schachtman TR, and Christoffersen GR (2005) The role of metabotropic glutamate receptor 5 in learning and memory processes. *Drug News Perspect.* 18: 353–361.

Soetens E, D'Hooge R, and Hueting JE (1993) Amphetamine enhances human-memory consolidation. *Neurosci. Lett.* 161: 9–12.

Stefani MR and Gold PE (1998) Intra-septal injections of glucose and glibenclamide attenuate galanin-induced spontaneous alternation performance deficits in the rat. *Brain Res.* 813: 50–56.

Stefani MR and Gold PE (2001) Intra-hippocampal infusions of K-ATP channel modulators influence spontaneous alternation performance: Relationships to acetylcholine release in the hippocampus. *J. Neurosci.* 21: 609–614.

Stefani MR, Nicholson GM, and Gold PE (1999) ATP-sensitive potassium channel blockade enhances spontaneous alternation performance in the rat: A potential mechanism for glucose-mediated memory enhancement. *Neuroscience* 93: 557–563.

Talley CP, Arankowsky-Sandoval G, McCarty R, and Gold PE (1999) Attenuation of morphine-induced behavioral changes in mice and rats by D- and L-glucose. *Neurobiol. Learn. Mem.* 71: 62–79.

Talley CEP, Kahn S, Alexander L, and Gold PE (2000) Epinephrine fails to enhance performance of food-deprived rats on a delayed spontaneous alternation task. *Neurobiol. Learn. Mem.* 73: 79–86.

Talley CP, Clayborn H, Jewel E, McCarty R, and Gold PE (2002) Vagotomy attenuates effects of L-glucose but not D-glucose on spontaneous alternation performance. *Physiol. Behav.* 77: 243–249.

Tolman EC, Ritchie BF, and Kalish D (1946) Studies in spatial learning, II: Place learning versus response learning. *J. Exp. Psychol.* 35: 221–229.

Tully T, Bourtchouladze R, Scott R, and Tallman J (2003) Targeting the CREB pathway for memory enhancers. *Nat. Rev. Drug. Discov.* 2: 267–277.

van der Zee EA and Luiten PG (1999) Muscarinic acetylcholine receptors in the hippocampus, neocortex and amygdala: A review of immunocytochemical localization in relation to learning and memory. *Prog. Neurobiol.* 58: 409–471.

Vizi ES and Mike A (2006) Nonsynaptic receptors for GABA and glutamate. *Curr. Top. Med. Chem.* 6: 941–948.

Weinberger NM (2003) The nucleus basalis and memory codes: Auditory cortical plasticity and the induction of specific, associative behavioral memory. *Neurobiol. Learn. Mem.* 80: 268–284.

Weinberger NM (2004) Specific long-term memory traces in primary auditory cortex. *Nat. Rev. Neurosci.* 5: 279–290.

Whishaw IQ and Cooper RM (1970) Strychnine and suppression of exploration. *Physiol. Behav.* 5: 647–649.

White NM and McDonald RJ (2002) Multiple parallel memory systems in the brain of the rat. *Neurobiol. Learn. Mem.* 77: 125–184.

White NM (2004) The role of stimulus ambiguity and movement in spatial navigation: A multiple memory systems analysis of location discrimination. *Neurobiol. Learn. Mem.* 82: 216–229.

Whitehouse PJ, Price DL, Struble RG, Clark AW, Coyle JT, and Delon MR (1982) Alzheimer's disease and senile dementia: Loss of neurons in the basal forebrain. *Science* 215: 1237–1239.

Williams CL, Men D, Clayton EC, and Gold PE (1998) Norepinephrine release in the amygdala following systemic injection of epinephrine or escapable footshock: Contribution of the nucleus of the solitary tract. *Behav. Neurosci.* 112: 1414–1422.

Williams CL and Clayton EC (2003) Contribution of brainstem structures in modulating memory storage processes. In: Gold PE and Greenough WT (eds.) *Memory Consolidation. Essays in Honor of James L. McGaugh – A Time to Remember*, pp. 141–164. Washington, DC: APA Press.

Winkler J, Thal LJ, Gage FH, and Fisher LJ (1998) Cholinergic strategies for Alzheimer's disease. *J. Mol. Med.* 76: 555–567.

Winocur G and Gagnon S (1998) Glucose treatment attenuates spatial learning and memory deficits of aged rats on tests of hippocampal functions. *Neurobiol. Aging* 19: 233–241.

Wolf OT (2003) HPA axis and memory. *Best Pract. Res. Clin. Endocrinol. Metab.* 17: 287–299.

Woolf NJ (1998) A structural basis for memory storage in mammals. *Prog. Neurobiol.* 55: 59–77.

Yamada K, Ji JJ, Yuan H, et al. (2001) Protective role of ATP-sensitive potassium channels in hypoxia-induced generalized seizure. *Science* 292: 1543–1546.

Zurkovsky L, Brown SL, Boyd SE, Fell JA, and Korol DL (2007) Estrogen modulates learning in female rats by acting directly at distinct memory systems. *Neuroscience* 144: 26–37.

29 Extinction: Behavioral Mechanisms and Their Implications

M. E. Bouton and A. M. Woods, University of Vermont, Burlington, VT, USA

Extinction is one of the best-known phenomena in all of learning theory. In Pavlovian learning, extinction occurs when the conditioned stimulus (CS) that has been associated with a biologically significant event (unconditioned stimulus, US) is now presented repeatedly without the US. In operant or instrumental learning, extinction occurs when an action or behavior that has been associated with a reinforcer is no longer reinforced. In either case, the learned performance declines. Extinction is important because it allows behavior to change and adapt as the environment also changes. Despite its fame and importance, however, it is not necessarily obvious how extinction works. One surprisingly common idea is that extinction involves the destruction of what was originally learned. Although this idea is built into several models of learning and memory (e.g., Rescorla and Wagner, 1972; McClelland and Rumelhart, 1985; see also McCloskey and Cohen, 1989), there is ample evidence that much of the original learning survives extinction (e.g., see Rescorla, 2001; Bouton, 2002, 2004; Myers and Davis, 2002; Delamater, 2004). This chapter selectively reviews results and theory from the behavioral literature in an effort to understand what is learned in extinction, what causes extinction, and how we can use our understanding of extinction to address certain clinical issues outside the laboratory.

There has been renewed interest in extinction in recent years. One reason is that as neuroscientists have made progress in understanding the brain mechanisms behind acquisition processes in learning (e.g., *See* Chapters 23, 21), they have naturally turned their attention to extinction and inhibition too. A detailed review of the biological work is beyond the scope of this chapter, although we consider some of its implications in the final sections. Another reason for renewed interest in extinction is that it is now clearly understood to be part of cognitive behavioral therapy. That is, in clinical settings, extinction is often the basis of treatment that is used to effectively eliminate maladaptive behaviors, thoughts, or emotions (e.g., Bouton, 1988; Conklin and Tiffany, 2002). However, as this chapter highlights, extinction does not result in a permanent removal of the behavior but instead leaves the organism vulnerable to relapse. This conclusion provides one illustration of how basic research on extinction provides information that is practically important.

The first part of this chapter introduces several extinction phenomena that any adequate theory of extinction will need to explain and accommodate. These phenomena suggest that extinction does not destroy the original learning, but instead involves new learning that is at least partly modulated by the context. They also potentially contribute to lapse and relapse effects that may occur after extinction therapies. The second part of the chapter then asks: if extinction is an example of new learning, what events reinforce or cause it? We come to the conclusion that extinction is mainly caused by generalization decrement and by new learning caused by the violation of an expectancy of reinforcement. The third part of the chapter takes knowledge from the first two sections and asks what can be done to optimize extinction learning in a way that eliminates the possibility of relapse. Our discussion in the first two sections expands and updates discussions in Bouton (2004); the last section updates a discussion in Bouton et al. (2006b).

29.1 Six Recovery Effects after Extinction

A number of experimental manipulations can be conducted after extinction that cause the extinguished response to return to performance. All of them are consistent with the idea that extinction involves new learning, and it therefore leaves the CS with two available meanings or associations with the US. As is true for an ambiguous word, the context is crucial in selecting between them.

29.1.1 Renewal

The renewal effect is perhaps the most fundamental postextinction phenomenon. In this effect (e.g., Bouton and Bolles, 1979a; Bouton and King, 1983), a change of context after extinction can cause a robust return of conditioned responding. Several versions of the renewal effect have been studied, but all cases of it support the idea that (1) extinction does not destroy the original learning and (2) the response triggered by the extinguished CS depends on the current context. In the most widely studied version, ABA renewal, conditioning is conducted in one context (Context A) and extinction is then conducted in a second one (Context B). (The contexts are typically separate and counterbalanced apparatuses housed in different rooms of the laboratory that differ in their tactile, olfactory, and visual respects.) When the CS is returned to the original conditioning context (Context A), responding to the CS returns (e.g., Bouton and Bolles, 1979a; Bouton and King, 1983; Bouton and Peck, 1989). In a second version, ABC renewal, conditioning is conducted in Context A, extinction is conducted in Context B, and then testing is conducted in a third, "neutral" context – Context C. Here again, a renewal of responding is observed (e.g., Bouton and Bolles, 1979a; Bouton and Brooks, 1993; Harris et al., 2000; Duvarci and Nader, 2004). In a final version, AAB renewal, conditioning and extinction are both conducted in the same context (Context A) and then the CS is tested in a second context (Context B). Here again, conditioned responding returns (e.g., Bouton and Ricker, 1994; Tamai and Nakajima, 2000), although there is currently less evidence of this type of renewal in operant than in Pavlovian conditioning (e.g., Nakajima et al., 2000; Crombag and Shaham, 2002).

Research on the renewal effect has helped us understand how contexts control behavior—in addition to understanding extinction itself. Several facts about the renewal effect are worth noting. First, it has been observed in virtually every conditioning preparation in which it has been investigated (see, e.g., Bouton, 2002, for a review). Second, it can occur after very extensive extinction training. In fear conditioning (conditioned suppression) in rats, Bouton and Swartzentruber (1989) observed it when 84 extinction trials followed eight conditioning trials. Other evidence suggests that it can occur after as many as 160 extinction trials (Gunther et al., 1998; Rauhut et al., 2001; Denniston et al., 2003), although at least one report suggests that it might not survive an especially massive extinction treatment (800 extinction trials after eight conditioning trials; Denniston et al., 2003). Third, the role of the context is different from the one anticipated by standard models of classical conditioning (e.g., Rescorla and Wagner, 1972; Pearce and Hall, 1980; Wagner, 1981; Wagner and Brandon, 1989, 2001). Those models accept the view that the context is merely another CS that is presented in compound with the target CS during reinforcement or nonreinforcement. It therefore enters into simple excitatory or inhibitory associations with the US. In the ABA renewal effect, for example, Context A might acquire excitatory associations with the US, and Context B might acquire inhibitory associations. Either kind of association would summate with the CS to produce the renewal effect (inhibition in B would reduce responding to the CS, whereas excitation in A would enhance it). However, a number of experiments have shown that the renewal effect can occur in the absence of demonstrable excitation in Context A or inhibition in Context B (e.g., Bouton and King, 1983; Bouton and Swartzentruber, 1986, 1989). These findings, coupled with others showing that strong excitation in a context does not influence performance to a CS unless the CS is under the influence of extinction (described later; Bouton, 1984; Bouton and King, 1986), suggest that direct associations in a context are neither necessary nor sufficient for a context to influence responding to a CS. The implication (e.g., Bouton, 1991b; Bouton and Swartzentruber, 1986) is that the contexts modulate or set the occasion for the current CS–US or CS–no US association (e.g., Holland, 1992; Swartzentruber, 1995; Schmajuk and Holland, 1998). Put another way, they activate or retrieve the CS's current relation with the US (*See* Chapter 31).

Another fact about renewal is that it appears to be supported by many kinds of contexts, including physical, temporal, emotional, and physiological ones (e.g., Bouton, 2000). For example, when fear extinction is conducted in the interoceptive context provided by benzodiazepine tranquilizers chlordiazepoxide and diazepam, renewed fear was observed when the rat was tested in the original nondrug state (Bouton et al., 1990). Cunningham (1979) had reported compatible evidence with alcohol, and we have recently collected similar observations with the benzodiazepine midazolam. State-dependent learning or retention can be conceptualized as the drug playing the role of context (e.g., Overton, 1985).

A further important characteristic of the renewal effect is that it implies that extinction learning is more context specific than original conditioning. This asymmetry in context dependence between conditioning and extinction must be true if one observes ABC and AAB renewal; in either case, conditioning transfers better to the final test context than extinction does. There is typically no measurable effect of switching the context after conditioning on responding to the CS in either fear or appetitive conditioning paradigms (e.g., Bouton and King, 1983; Bouton and Peck, 1989). This is also true of taste aversion learning (e.g., Rosas and Bouton, 1998) and human causal learning, in which humans are asked to judge the causal relationship between cues and outcomes presented over a series of trials (e.g., Rosas et al., 2001). The presence of the renewal effect indicates that extinction, on the other hand, is especially context specific. Some research suggests that both conditioning and extinction become somewhat context specific after extinction has occurred (Harris et al., 2000). However, there is little question that extinction comes under relatively more contextual control than original conditioning.

The reason for the difference in the context dependence of conditioning and extinction has been the subject of recent research. Given the similarities between extinction and inhibition, Bouton and Nelson (1994) and Nelson and Bouton (1997) asked whether pure inhibition (as acquired in the feature-negative paradigm, in which a CS is paired with the US when it is presented alone, but not when it is combined with an inhibitory CS) was context specific. Inhibition acquired by the inhibitory CS transferred without disruption to a new context; thus, extinction is not context specific merely because it is a form of inhibition. A second reason why extinction might be context specific is that it is the second thing the organism learns about the CS. Nelson (2002) confirmed that excitatory conditioning (tone–food pairings) transferred undisturbed across contexts, unless the tone had first been trained as a conditioned inhibitor, as discussed earlier, in the feature-negative paradigm. Conversely, inhibition to a conditioned inhibitor also transferred across contexts unless the CS had first been trained as a conditioned excitor (through tone–food pairings). Thus, regardless of whether the association was excitatory or inhibitory, the second thing learned was more context specific than the first (cf. Rescorla, 2005). Compatible data had been shown by Swartzentruber and Bouton (1992), who found that excitatory conditioning was context specific if it had been preceded by nonreinforced preexposure to the CS.

The evidence therefore suggests that the learning and memory system treats the first association as context free, but the second association as a kind of context-specific exception to the rule. (The main exception to the second-association rule is latent inhibition, in which the first phase can be shown to exert a context-dependent influence on the second phase (e.g., Hall and Channell, 1985), despite the fact that it is arguably the first thing learned. Latent inhibition is unique, however, in that the CS is not paired with anything significant in the first phase. One possibility, therefore, is that the CS is in part encoded as a feature of the context, making it difficult to extract it from that context when it is paired with the US in Phase 2 (cf. Gluck and Myers, 1993)).

There may be functional reasons for this (Bouton, 1994). A conditioning trial provides a sample from which an animal may make inferences about the state of the world (e.g., Staddon, 1988). Statistically, if the world is composed of two types of trials (CS–US and CS–no US), then the probability of sampling a particular type of trial will reflect its true prevalence in the world. Therefore, an early run of conditioning trials would reflect its high incidence in the population; a subsequent trial of another type might reflect an exception to the rule. Learning and memory may thus be designed to treat second-learned information as conditional and context-specific. At a more mechanistic level, recent research in human predictive learning (Rosas and Callejas-Aguilera, 2006) and in taste-aversion learning with rats (Rosas and Callejas-Aguilera, 2007) suggests that ambiguity introduced by conflicting information in Phase 2 leads the participants to pay attention to the context. The key finding is that after conflicting information about one CS or predictor is introduced, other subsequently learned associations are context dependent, even if they are entirely new or learned in a separate context. Thus, the introduction of a competing, conflicting association appears to encourage the participant to pay attention to all contexts.

It is worth concluding this section by noting the direct relevance of the renewal effect to exposure therapy in humans. Several studies have now shown that an exposure treatment that diminishes fear of spiders in one context (a room or a patio outdoors) can still allow a renewal of the fear when exposure to the spider was tested in the other context (Mystkowski et al., 2002; see also, e.g., Mineka et al., 1999; Vansteenwegen et al., 2005). Similar renewal has also been reported in the study of cue exposure therapy with both alcohol (Collins and Brandon, 2002) and cigarette users (Thewissen et al., 2006). Both types of participants reported a renewed urge to use the drug when tested in a context that was different from the one in which exposure to drug-related cues (e.g., visual and/or olfactory cues associated with the drug) had taken place; the alcohol participants also demonstrated renewal of a salivation response. All such results suggest limits to the effectiveness of cue exposure therapy (see also Conklin, 2006). However, renewal effects can be attenuated if the participant is reminded of extinction just prior to the renewal test. Collins and Brandon (2002) found that presenting explicit cues (a unique pencil, eraser, and clipboard) that had been a feature of the extinction context reduced renewal of the aforementioned reactivity to alcohol cues. Mystkowski et al. (2006) reported that renewal of spider fear could be decreased if human participants mentally reinstated (imagined) stimuli from the treatment context before being tested in a different context. Both studies extended earlier findings that the renewal effect can be reduced in rats if cues that were part of the extinction context were later presented before the test (Brooks and Bouton, 1994). Renewal can be viewed as due to a failure to retrieve extinction outside the extinction context (*See* Chapter 31). Retrieval cues can provide a "bridge" between the extinction context and possible relapse contexts which allows for the generalization of extinction learning between the contexts (see Bouton et al., 2006b).

29.1.2 Spontaneous Recovery

Pavlov (1927) first observed spontaneous recovery, another well-known postextinction effect that involves recovery of the conditioned response as time passes following extinction. There are several available explanations of spontaneous recovery (for a discussion, see Brooks and Bouton, 1993; Devenport et al., 1997; Robbins, 1990; Rescorla, 2004a), and it seems likely to be multiply determined. However, we have argued (e.g., Bouton, 1988, 1993) that just as extinction is relatively specific to its physical context, it may also be specific to its temporal context. The passage of time might also bring about changes in internal and external stimulation that provide a gradually changing context. Spontaneous recovery can be seen as the renewal effect that occurs when the CS is tested outside its temporal context. Both are due to a failure to retrieve memories of extinction outside the extinction context. Consistent with this perspective, a cue that is presented intermittently during the extinction session and again just before the final test (an 'extinction cue') can attenuate both spontaneous recovery and renewal by reminding the subjects of extinction (Brooks and Bouton, 1993, 1994; Brooks, 2000). Interestingly, changing the physical and temporal contexts together can have a bigger effect than changing either context alone, as if their combination creates an even larger context change (Rosas and Bouton, 1997, 1998).

A series of experiments in appetitive conditioning with rats further suggests that temporal context can include the intertrial interval (ITI), the time between successive extinction trials (Bouton and García-Gutiérrez, 2006). Previous experiments had shown that rats that received extinction trials spaced by either 4 or 16-min ITIs showed equivalent spontaneous recovery when tested 72 h later (Moody et al., 2006). However, when the retention interval was 16 min rather than 72 h (Bouton and García-Guiterrez, 2006), rats that had received extinction trials separated by the 4-min interval showed spontaneous recovery, whereas rats that had received the extinction trials separated by the 16-min interval did not. These results are consistent with the possibility that the ITI was coded as part of the extinction context. Thus, analogous to a renewal effect, conditioned responding returned when the animals were tested after an interval between trials that differed from the ITI that was used in extinction. However, a mismatch between the extinction ITI and the retention interval is not always sufficient to produce renewal; rats that received extinction trials spaced by 16 min and then received a short retention interval of 4 min failed to show spontaneous recovery. This anomaly is consistent with results that emerged in discrimination experiments in which the different ITIs were used as signals about whether or not the next CS presentation would be reinforced (see Bouton and García-Gutiérrez, 2006). Specifically, rats readily learned that a 16-min ITI signaled reinforcement of a CS, whereas a 4-min ITI did not. In contrast, they had considerably more difficulty learning that a 4-min ITI signaled reinforcement and a 16-min ITI did not. The results suggest that there are interesting constraints on how the interval between trials may be coded and/or used as a context.

29.1.3 Rapid Reacquisition

A third effect further indicates that conditioning is not destroyed in extinction. In rapid reacquisition, when CS–US pairings are reintroduced after extinction, the reacquisition of responding can be more rapid than initial acquisition with a novel CS (e.g., Napier et al., 1992; Ricker and Bouton, 1996; Weidemann and Kehoe, 2003). Although such an effect again suggests that the original learning has been 'saved' through extinction, the early literature was often difficult to interpret because many early designs were not equipped to rule out less interesting explanations (see Bouton, 1986, for a review). To add to the complexity, studies of fear conditioning (conditioned suppression) (Bouton, 1986; Bouton and Swartzentruber, 1989) and flavor aversion learning (Danguir and Nicolaidis, 1977; Hart et al., 1995) have shown that reacquisition can be slower than acquisition with a new CS. (It is more rapid than initial acquisition with a CS that has received the same number of nonreinforced trials without conditioning (Bouton and Swartzentruber, 1989).) In fear conditioning, slow reacquisition requires extensive extinction training; more limited extinction training yields reacquisition that is neither fast nor slow (Bouton, 1986). At least part of the reason these preparations support slow reacquisition is that both typically involve very few initial conditioning trials. In contrast, procedures in which rapid reacquisition has been shown (conditioning of the rabbit nictitating membrane response (NMR) and rat appetitive conditioning) have usually involved a relatively large number of initial conditioning trials. Consistent with a role for number of trials, Ricker and Bouton (1996) demonstrated that slow reacquisition occurred in an appetitive conditioning preparation when the procedure used the number of conditioning and extinction trials that had been used in previous fear conditioning experiments. In rabbit NMR and heart rate conditioning, extensive extinction training has abolished rapid reacquisition, although slow reacquisition has yet to be observed (Weidemann and Kehoe, 2003).

Ricker and Bouton (1996) suggested that rapid reacquisition may partly be an ABA renewal effect that occurs when the animal has learned that previous USs or conditioning trials are part of the original context of conditioning. That is, when CS–US pairings are resumed after extinction (a series of CS–no US trials), they return the animal to the original conditioning context. The hypothesis is compatible with Capaldi's (1967, 1994) sequential analysis of extinction, which has made excellent use of the idea that responding on a particular trial is determined by how the animal has learned to respond in the presence of similar memories of previous trials. Presumably, conditioning preparations that employ a relatively large number of conditioning trials (e.g., rabbit NMR) allow many opportunities for the animal to learn that previous reinforced trials are part of the context of conditioning. Furthermore, Ricker and Bouton (1996) reported evidence that high responding during the reacquisition phase was more likely after a reinforced than a nonreinforced trial, which had signaled conditioning and extinction, respectively.

Bouton et al. (2004) reasoned that if rapid reacquisition is caused by recent reinforced trials generating ABA renewal, then an extinction procedure that includes occasional reinforced trials among many nonreinforced trials should slow down rapid reacquisition by making recent reinforced trials part of the context of both conditioning and extinction. Consistent with this hypothesis, a very sparse partial reinforcement procedure in extinction slowed reacquisition compared to a group that had received simple extinction. Evidence of a similar slowed reacquisition effect has also been obtained in instrumental conditioning (Woods and Bouton, 2007) when a lever-press response was sparsely reinforced during extinction and then paired again more consistently with the reinforcer. Such a result is consistent with the idea that rapid reacquisition is at least partly an ABA renewal effect. Because the partial reinforcement treatment involved many more CS–US (or response–reinforcer) pairings than simple extinction, it is difficult to reconcile with the view that rapid reacquisition is a simple function of the strength of an association that remains after extinction (e.g., Kehoe, 1988; Kehoe and Macrae, 1997). Slowing rapid reacquisition of an instrumental response may be especially relevant from a clinical perspective, because instrumental learning is often involved in maladaptive behaviors such as substance abuse (e.g., Bouton, 2000). The evidence suggests that extinction (i.e., strict abstinence) might not be the most effective treatment to prevent relapse in all situations (cf. Alessi et al., 2004). A more successful technique might be one that permits occasional reinforcers during treatment (e.g., see Sobell and Sobell, 1973; Marlatt and Gordon, 1985) and therefore provides a bridge between the extinction and testing contexts (see also Bouton et al., 2006b).

29.1.4 Reinstatement

A fourth context-dependent postextinction phenomenon is reinstatement. In this effect, the extinguished response returns after extinction if the animal is merely reexposed to the US alone (e.g., Pavlov, 1927; Rescorla and Heth, 1975; Bouton and Bolles, 1979b). If testing of the CS is contemporaneous with US delivery, then the USs may cause a return of responding because they were encoded as part of the conditioning context (as earlier; see Reid, 1958; Baker et al., 1991; Bouton et al., 1993). On the other hand, in many studies of reinstatement, testing is conducted at an interval of at least 24 h after US reexposure; here one still observes reinstatement compared to controls that were not reexposed to the US (e.g., Rescorla and Heth, 1975; Bouton and Bolles, 1979b). In this case, evidence strongly suggests that the effect is due to conditioning of the context. When the US is presented after extinction, the organism associates it with the context; this contextual conditioning then creates reinstatement. For example, if the reinstating USs are presented in an irrelevant context, there is no reinstatement when the CS is tested again (e.g., Bouton and Bolles, 1979b; Bouton and King, 1983; Bouton, 1984; Baker et al., 1991; Wilson et al., 1995; Frohardt et al., 2000). Independent measures of contextual conditioning also correlate with the strength of reinstatement (Bouton and King, 1983; Bouton, 1984). Recent evidence that the effect in fear conditioning is abolished by excitotoxic lesions of the bed nucleus of the stria terminalis (Waddell et al., 2006), a brain area thought to control anxiety (e.g., Walker et al., 2003), suggests that in the fear-conditioning situation, at least, the effect may be mediated by anxiety conditioned in the context. Also, if the animal receives extensive extinction exposure to the context after the reinstatement shocks are presented, reinstatement is not observed (Bouton and Bolles, 1979b; Baker et al., 1991). These results indicate that mere reexposure to the US is not sufficient to generate reinstatement. It is necessary to test the CS in the context in which the US has been reexposed.

This effect of context conditioning is especially potent with an extinguished CS. For example, Bouton (1984) compared the effects of US exposure in the same or a different context on fear of a partially extinguished CS or another CS that had reached the same low level of fear through simple CS–US pairings (and no extinction). Although contextual conditioning enhanced fear of the extinguished CS, it had no impact on the nonextinguished CS (see also Bouton and King, 1986). This result is consistent with the effects of context switches mentioned earlier: An extinguished CS is especially sensitive to manipulations of the context. One reason is that contextual conditioning may be another feature of the conditioning context; its presence during a test may cause a return of responding after extinction because of another ABA renewal effect (Bouton et al., 1993).

29.1.5 Resurgence

Another recovery phenomenon has been studied exclusively in operant conditioning. In resurgence, a new behavior is reinforced at the same time the target behavior is extinguished. When reinforcement of the new behavior is discontinued, the original response can resurge. Resurgence can occur in two different forms. In one, a response (R1) is first trained and then extinguished. After R1 is extinguished, a new response (R2) is trained and subsequently extinguished. Recovery, or resurgence, of R1 happens during the extinction of R2 (Epstein, 1983; Lieving and Lattal, 2003, Experiment 1). The other version of the procedure, which can be called the ALT-R procedure (for reinforcement of an alternative response), involves first training R1 and then reinforcing R2 during the extinction of R1. When R2 then undergoes extinction, recovery of R1 occurs (Leitenberg et al., 1970, 1975; Rawson et al., 1977; Epstein, 1985; Lieving and Lattal, 2003). Like the other recovery phenomena described earlier, both forms of resurgence support the idea that extinction does not produce unlearning.

There has been little research designed to uncover the actual mechanisms behind resurgence. One possibility is that extinction of R2 could cause an increase in behavioral variability, or frustration, that might result in an increase in any alternative behavior, not just R1 (e.g., Neuringer et al., 2001). Few studies have included a control response to show that resurgence is unique to an extinguished response. The sole exception is a study by Epstein (1983), who reported that pigeons rarely pecked an alternative, previously nonreinforced response key. An explanation with specific regard to the ALT-R procedure is that reinforcement of R2 during extinction of R1 physically prevents the animal from emitting R1 and thus prevents exposure to the R1–no reinforcer contingency (Leitenberg et al., 1975; Rawson et al., 1977). It is also possible, however, that resurgence follows from the mechanisms implicated in the other recovery effects described earlier. In particular, resurgence observed in the ALT-R procedure could be due to the fact that extinction of R1 occurs in the context of R2 responding. Then, given that extinction is context-specific, R1 would return when extinction of R2 occurs and the frequency of R2 decreases. That is, little R2 responding would return the animal to the context in which R1 had been reinforced, and thus recovery of R1 in the ALT-R procedure would be analogous to an ABA renewal effect.

A somewhat different explanation would be required to explain the form of resurgence in which R1 is extinguished before R2 training begins. In this case, testing of R1 occurs after extinction of R2, and thus responding on R2 would be minimal in both the extinction and testing conditions and thus no renewal effect should result. For this scenario, we might suggest the following explanation. The reinforcer is consistently presented during training of R2, which occurs simultaneously with extinction of R1, and thus this would continuously reinstate responding to R1 (e.g., Rescorla and Skucy, 1969; Baker et al., 1991). Reinstatement of R1 is possible due to conditioning of background context or due to the fact that the reinforcer is a discriminative stimulus signaling to make the response (e.g., Baker et al., 1991). While R2 is being reinforced, the response will interfere with the reinstated performance of R1. However, when R2 then undergoes extinction, the reinstated R1 responding (i.e., resurgence) can then be revealed. In this case, then, resurgence may be an example of the basic reinstatement effect.

29.1.6 Concurrent Recovery

Concurrent recovery is another effect indicating that extinction does not destroy original learning. To date, the phenomenon has been studied exclusively in rabbit NMR conditioning: In that preparation, extinguished responding to a target CS can return if a completely different CS is separately paired with the US (e.g., Weidemann and Kehoe, 2004, 2005). One interesting fact about concurrent recovery is that the effect does not necessarily depend on extinction. Rather, similar to a "learning to learn" effect in which conditioning with one CS increases the subsequent rate of conditioning with other CSs (e.g., Kehoe and Holt, 1984), responding to a weakly conditioned target CS can be increased as a result of conditioning with a different CS (Schreurs and Kehoe, 1987). Kehoe (1988) has interpreted these phenomena from a connectionist perspective. He has suggested that the effects occur because inputs from different CSs might converge on a common hidden unit. When a nontarget CS is paired with the US, it strengthens the association of the common hidden unit with the US and thereby allows more responding when the target CS is again presented. This account suggests that extinction plays no special role in enabling concurrent recovery, although the effects that reinforcing one CS has on responding to extinguished and nonextinguished target CSs have not been compared.

A different account of concurrent recovery is that it might merely be a reinstatement effect that occurs due to presentation of the US (with another CS) after extinction of the target CS. Thus, rather than depending on new CS–US pairings, the mere presence of the US alone might be enough to produce concurrent recovery and would suggest that it is similar to a basic reinstatement effect. This possibility appears unlikely in the case of NMR conditioning, because exposure to the US on its own after extinction does not cause much reinstatement in that preparation (e.g., Napier et al., 1992). However, in the many other preparations where reinstatement does occur (e.g., fear conditioning or appetitive conditioning), a demonstration of concurrent recovery might merely be a reinstatement effect – exposure to CS–US pairings simply involves reexposure to the US (see Rescorla and Heth, 1975; Bouton and Bolles, 1979b, for evidence of reinstatement when the US is presented with or without a CS). Additional work on concurrent recovery is required to determine whether it differentially influences an extinguished CS and, importantly, whether it (like reinstatement) is context specific. Perhaps reinforcing a CS in the same context where a target CS was previously extinguished could remove the contextual inhibition that had accrued there or allow excitation to generalize to the target CS via common associations between the CSs and the context (cf. Honey and Hall, 1989).

29.1.7 Summary

A great deal of research thus indicates that responding to an extinguished CS is susceptible to any of a number of recovery effects, suggesting that extinction is not unlearning. Indeed, based on the results of a number of tests that allow a specific comparison of the strength of the CS–US association before and after extinction (e.g., Delamater, 1996; Rescorla, 1996a), Rescorla (2001) has suggested that extinction involves no unlearning whatsoever; the original CS–US association seems to survive essentially intact. Extinction must thus depend on other mechanisms. The renewal effect, and the fact that extinction leaves the CS so especially sensitive to manipulations of context, is consistent with the idea that extinction involves new learning that is especially context-dependent. We have therefore suggested that extinction leaves the CS under a contextually modulated form of inhibition (e.g., Bouton, 1993): The presence of the extinction context retrieves or sets the occasion for a CS–no US association.

29.2 What Causes Extinction?

A theoretically and clinically significant question in the field of learning and memory is what event or behavioral process actually causes the loss of responding during extinction? Several ideas have been examined and are discussed next.

29.2.1 Discrimination of Reinforcement Rate

One possibility is that the animal eventually learns that the rate of reinforcement in the CS is lower in extinction than it was during conditioning. Gallistel and Gibbon (2000) have argued that the animal continually decides whether or not to respond in extinction by comparing the current rate of reinforcement in the CS with its memory of the rate that prevailed in conditioning. Because rate is the reciprocal of time, the animal computes a ratio between the amount of time accumulated in the CS during extinction and the amount of time accumulated in the CS between USs during conditioning. When the ratio exceeds a threshold, the animal stops responding.

This approach has been tested in several experiments. Haselgrove and Pearce (2003) examined the impact of varying the duration of the CS during extinction; when longer CSs are used in extinction, time in the CS accumulates more quickly, and the animal should stop responding after fewer trials. In some experiments, rats were given appetitive conditioning with a 10-s CS and then given extinction exposures to a series of 10-s or 270-s presentations of the CS. When responding was examined at the start of each CS, there was an occasionally significant, but surprisingly small, effect of increasing the duration of the CS during extinction. For instance, by the 12th two-trial block, the 10-s and 270-s CS groups had similar nonzero levels of responding, even though they had accumulated a total of 4 and 108 min of exposure in the CS, respectively. On the other hand, responding did decline as a function of time within a single presentation of the 270-s CS, perhaps reflecting generalization decrement resulting from the increasing difference between the current CS and the 10-s CS employed in conditioning. Consistent with that view, when conditioning first occurred with a 60-s CS, extinction of responding occurred more rapidly with a 10-s CS than with a 60-s CS. Thus, either an increase or a decrease in the duration of the CS relative to conditioning accelerated the loss of responding. This effect of time was not anticipated by the rate-discrimination view (Gallistel and Gibbon, 2000).

Drew et al. (2004) reported compatible results in experiments on autoshaping in ring doves. Doubling or halving the duration of the CS from the 8-s value used in conditioning did not affect the number of trials required to stop responding. The fact that extinction was thus largely controlled by the number of CS presentations is consistent with experiments that have examined the effects of the number and duration of nonreinforced trials added to conditioning schedules (Bouton and Sunsay, 2003). On the other hand, Drew et al. found that a more extreme increase in CS duration (from 8 to 32 s) increased the rate of extinction. This was attributed to the animal learning to discriminate the longer nonreinforced CS presentations from the shorter reinforced CS presentations: When 8-s CSs were presented again after extinction, birds extinguished with 4-s and 32-s CSs responded again. Animals are sensitive to time in the CS, but the number of extinction trials appears to be an important factor.

As noted by Gallistel and Gibbon (2000), the rate discrimination theory seems especially consistent with a well-known extinction phenomenon, the partial reinforcement effect (PRE; see Mackintosh, 1974, for a review). In this phenomenon, conditioning with partial reinforcement schedules (in which nonreinforced trials are intermixed with reinforced trials) creates a slower loss of responding in extinction than does conditioning with a continuous reinforcement schedule (in which every trial is reinforced). According to a rate-discrimination hypothesis (Gallistel and Gibbon, 2000), the partially reinforced subjects have learned to expect the US after more accumulated time in the CS, and it thus takes more CS time in extinction to exceed the threshold of accumulated extinction time/expected time to each US. The more traditional approach, in contrast, has been to think that partially reinforced subjects have learned to expect the US after more trials than continuously reinforced subjects have. It therefore takes more trials to stop generalizing from conditioning to extinction (e.g., Mowrer and Jones, 1945; Capaldi, 1967, 1994).

Contrary to the rate discrimination hypothesis, Haselgrove et al. (2004) and Bouton and Woods (2004) have shown that a PRE still occurs when partially and continuously reinforced subjects expect the reinforcer after the same amount of CS time. For example, both sets of investigators showed that a group that received a 10-s CS reinforced on half its presentations (accumulated CS time of 20 s) extinguished more slowly than a continuously reinforced group that received every 20-s CS presentation reinforced. Bouton and Woods (2004) further distinguished the time-discrimination account from the traditional trial-discrimination account (e.g., Mowrer and Jones, 1945; Capaldi, 1967, 1994). Rats that had every fourth 10-s CS reinforced extinguished more slowly over a series of alternating 10-s and 30-s extinction trials than rats that had received every 10-s CS reinforced. This PRE was still observed when extinction responding was plotted as a function of time units over which the US should have been expected (every 40 s for the partially reinforced group but every 10 s for the continuously reinforced group). In contrast, the PRE disappeared when extinction responding was plotted as a function of the trials over which the US should have been expected (every fourth trial for the partially reinforced group and every trial for the continuously reinforced group). Ultimately, the PRE is better captured by trial-based theories (e.g., Capaldi, 1967, 1994; see Mackintosh, 1974, for a review of the older literature).

We have already seen that responding on a particular trial occurs in the context of memories of the outcomes of previous trials – that was the explanation provided earlier of rapid reacquisition as an ABA renewal effect (Ricker and Bouton, 1996; Bouton et al., 2004). Interestingly, the recent finding that occasional reinforced trials in extinction (partial reinforcement) can slow down the rate of reacquisition (Bouton et al., 2004; Woods and Bouton, 2007) is really just the inverse of the PRE: In the PRE, nonreinforced trials in conditioning allow more generalization from conditioning to extinction, whereas Bouton et al.'s finding suggests that reinforced trials in extinction allowed for more generalization of extinction to reconditioning. Either finding suggests the importance of considering recent trials as part of the context that controls performance in extinction.

In summary, there is little support for the idea that responding extinguishes when the US is omitted because the organism detects a lower rate of reinforcement in the CS. The number of extinction trials, rather than merely the accumulating time in the CS across trials, appears to be important to the extinction process. Time in the CS can have an effect: It appears to be another dimension over which animals generalize and discriminate (Drew et al., 2004; Haselgrove and Pearce, 2003). Explanation of the PRE, however, appears to be most consistent with a view that animals utilize their memories of the outcomes of preceding trials as a dimension over which they generalize and respond (see also Mackintosh, 1974, for an extended review).

29.2.2 Generalization Decrement

It is possible that the animal stops responding in extinction from the point at which it stops generalizing between the stimuli that prevailed in conditioning and those that prevail in extinction (e.g., Capaldi, 1967, 1994). This idea has had a long history in research on extinction, especially in research on the PRE. It is interesting to note that a generalization decrement theory of extinction does not imply destruction of the original learning in extinction, or indeed any new learning at all. However, there is still good reason to think that extinction also involves new learning. For instance, nonreinforcement of a food CS elicits measurable frustration, and this can be associated with stimuli present in the environment (Daly, 1974). Nonreinforcement of the CS in the related conditioned inhibition paradigm (in which a CS is nonreinforced in the presence of a second stimulus and that second stimulus acquires purely inhibitory properties) also generates measurable new learning in the form of conditioned inhibition. There is also evidence for new learning in the renewal effect. For example, either ABC renewal or AAB renewal (see earlier discussion) implies that the extinction context acquires an ability to modulate (suppress) performance to the CS. Such observations suggest that the animal has not merely stopped responding in extinction because of a failure to generalize. Instead, it appears to have learned that the CS means no US in the extinction context (see earlier).

29.2.3 Inhibition of the Response

Rescorla (2001) suggested that extinction might involve learning to inhibit the conditioned response. He summarized evidence from instrumental (operant) conditioning experiments indicating that the effects of extinction can be specific to the response that undergoes extinction. For example, Rescorla (1993) reinforced two operant behaviors (lever pressing and chain pulling) with food pellets and then extinguished each response in combination with a new stimulus (a light or a noise). Subsequent tests of the two responses with both light and noise indicated that each response was more depressed when it was tested in combination with the cue in which it had been extinguished (see also Rescorla, 1997a). There is thus good reason to think that the animal learns something specific about the response itself during operant extinction: It learns not to perform a particular response in a particular stimulus. One possibility is that the animal learns a simple inhibitory S–R association (Colwill, 1991). Another possibility, perhaps more consistent with the context-modulation account of extinction emphasized earlier, is that the animal learns that S sets the occasion for a response – no reinforcer relationship. Rescorla (1993: 335; 1997a: 249) has observed that the experiments do not separate the two possibilities. To our knowledge, no analogous experiments have been performed in the Pavlovian conditioning situation.

The main implication examined in Pavlovian conditioning is that extinction procedures should be especially successful at causing inhibitory S–R learning if they generate high levels of responding in extinction. This prediction may provide a reasonable rule of thumb (Rescorla, 2001). For example, when a CS is compounded with another excitatory CS and the compound is extinguished, there may be especially strong responding in extinction (due to summation between the CSs), and especially effective extinction as evidenced when the CS is tested alone (Wagner, 1969; Rescorla, 2000; Thomas and Ayres, 2004). Conversely, when the target CS is compounded with an inhibitory CS, there is relatively little responding to the compound (excitation and inhibition negatively summate), and there is also less evidence of extinction when the target is tested alone (Soltysik et al., 1983; Rescorla, 2003; Thomas and Ayres, 2004). However, although these findings are consistent with the hypothesis that the effectiveness of extinction correlates with the degree of responding, either treatment also affects the degree to which the animal's expectation of the reinforcer is violated: The stimulus compound influences the size of the error term in the Rescorla-Wagner model, and in more cognitive terms the extent to which the expectation of the US created by the compound is violated when the US does not occur. The results do not separate the response-inhibition hypothesis from an expectancy-violation hypothesis, which will be covered in the next section.

An eyeblink experiment by Krupa and Thompson (2003) manipulated the level of responding another way. During extinction, rabbits were given microinjections of the gamma-aminobutyric acid (GABA) agonist muscimol adjacent to the motor nuclei that control the conditioned response (the facial nucleus and the accessory abducens). The injection therefore eliminated the CR during extinction. However, when the subjects were then tested without muscimol, the CS evoked considerable responding, suggesting that evocation of the CR was necessary for extinction learning. Unfortunately, the muscimol microinjections also had robust stimulus effects. They caused complete inactivation of the ipsilateral facial musculature: "the external eyelids were flaccid, the left ear hung down unsupported, and no vibrissae movements were observed on the side of the infusion" (Krupa and Thompson, 2003: 10579). In effect, the rabbits received extinction in a context that was different from the one in which conditioning and testing occurred (the ordinary state without partial facial paralysis). There are thus strong grounds for expecting a renewal effect. The hypothesis that elicitation of the CR is necessary for extinction must await further tests.

There are also data suggesting that the number of responses or level of responding in extinction does not correlate with effective extinction learning. For example, Drew et al. (2004) noted that although animals given long CSs in extinction responded many more times in extinction than animals given shorter CSs, extinction was mainly a function of the number of extinction trials. In fear conditioning experiments with mice, Cain et al. (2003) reported that extinction trials that were spaced in time produced a slower loss of freezing than extinction trials that were massed in time. Nevertheless, there was less spontaneous recovery after the massed treatment, suggesting that extinction was more effective when the treatment involved less overall responding. Experiments in our own laboratory with rat appetitive conditioning (Moody et al., 2006) suggest a similar conclusion, even though the results were different. Spaced extinction trials again yielded more responding in extinction than massed trials, but the treatments caused indistinguishable amounts of extinction learning as assessed in spontaneous recovery and reinstatement tests.

In related conditioned suppression experiments, Bouton et al. (2006a) compared the effects of extinction in multiple contexts on the strength of ABA and ABC renewal effects (discussed more in the section titled 'Other behavioral techniques to optimize extinction learning'). Rats received fear conditioning with a tone CS in Context A, and then extinction of the tone for three sessions in Context B, or a session in B, then C, and then D, before final renewal tests in the original context (Context A) or a neutral fifth context (Context E). Although the successive context switches in the BCD group caused more fear responding during extinction (due to renewal effects with each context switch), the groups showed strikingly similar renewal in either Context A or Context E. Thus, higher responding in extinction does not indicate better extinction learning; in fact, the level of responding on extinction trials was positively, rather than negatively, correlated with the level of renewal (see also Moody et al., 2006). The results seem inconsistent with a response-inhibition hypothesis. Their impact on the expectancy violation hypothesis is perhaps less clear.

Rescorla (2006, Experiment 5) provided perhaps the most direct test of whether enhanced responding or enhanced associative strength is responsible for the increased extinction (loss of responding) that typically follows compound presentation of two extinguished stimuli (see also Reberg, 1972; Hendry, 1982). He studied the effects of a diffuse excitor (e.g., a noise paired with food) and a diffuse positive occasion setter (e.g., a houselight that signaled the reinforcement of a keylight CS) on extinction of autoshaped key pecking in pigeons. When combined with a target keylight CS that was undergoing extinction, the diffuse excitor failed to increase the amount of pecking at the keylight, although it theoretically increased the animal's expectation of the US. In contrast, when combined with the target keylight CS, the diffuse occasion setter increased the amount of pecking at the CS without theoretically increasing the direct expectancy of the US. Contrary to Rescorla's (2001) rule of thumb about more responding resulting in more extinction, extinction in combination with the excitor caused a more durable extinction effect (assessed in reacquisition) than did extinction in combination with the occasion setter. The occasion setter caused no more effective extinction than extinction of the target alone. This finding suggests that the actual level of responding in extinction is not as important in determining the success of extinction as the extent to which the US is predicted and thus nonreinforcement is surprising.

In summary, although animals that receive extinction after operant conditioning may in fact learn to refrain from performing a particular response in a particular context (e.g., Rescorla, 1993, 1997a), the importance of response inhibition in Pavlovian extinction is not unequivocally supported at the present time. High responding in extinction does not guarantee more effective extinction learning, and a better explanation of the results of stimulus-compounding experiments (where the level of responding does appear to predict the success of extinction) may be the violation-of-expectation hypothesis, to which we now turn.

29.2.4 Violation of Reinforcer Expectation

It is commonly thought that each CS presentation arouses a sort of expectation of the US that is disconfirmed on each extinction trial. For example, in the error-correction rule provided by Rescorla and Wagner (1972), the degree of unlearning (which we have seen can create inhibition) is provided by the difference in the overall associative strength present on a trial and the actual US that occurs on the trial. In the Pearce-Hall model (Pearce and Hall, 1980), the discrepancy was conceptualized as an event that reinforced new inhibitory learning that is overlaid on the original excitatory learning (see also Daly and Daly, 1982). Wagner's SOP ("sometimes opponent process") model (1981) accepts a similar idea. One piece of evidence that seems especially consistent with the expectation-violation view is the "overexpectation experiment," in which two CSs are separately associated with the US and then presented together in a compound that is then paired with the US. Despite the fact that the compound is paired with a US that can clearly generate excitatory learning, the two CSs undergo some extinction (e.g., Kremer, 1978; Lattal and Nakajima, 1998). The idea is that summation of the strengths of the two CSs causes a discrepancy between what the animal expects and what actually occurs, and some extinction is therefore observed. As mentioned earlier, the expectation-violation view is also consistent with the effects of compounding excitors and inhibitors with the target CS during no-US (extinction) trials (Wagner, 1969; Soltysik et al., 1983; Rescorla, 2000, 2003, 2006; Thomas and Ayres, 2004).

One theoretical challenge has been to capture the expectancy violation in real time. Gallistel and Gibbon (2000) have emphasized the fact that traditional trial-based models like the Rescorla–Wagner model have been vague about the precise point in time in a trial when the violation of expectation actually occurs. The issue is especially clear when trial-based models explain the extinction that occurs with a single extended presentation of the CS, as is the case for the context or background in conditioning protocols with very widely spaced conditioning trials. (Spaced trials are held to facilitate conditioning of the CS because long ITIs allow more context extinction and thus less blocking by context.) There is good evidence that widely spaced trials do create less contextual conditioning than massed trials (e.g., Barela, 1999). To account for contextual extinction over long ITIs, many trial-based models arbitrarily assume that the single long-context exposure is carved into many imaginary trials, and that more imaginary trials occur and create more extinction in longer-context exposures.

It is worth noting, however, that Wagner's SOP model (e.g., Wagner, 1981; Wagner and Brandon, 1989, 2001) is relatively specific about where in time the process that generates extinction occurs. According to that model, CS and US are represented as memory nodes that can become associated during conditioning. For the association between them to be strengthened, both nodes must be activated from inactivity to an active state, "A1," at the same time. Once the association has been formed, the presentation of the CS activates the US node to a secondarily active state, "A2." This in turn generates the CR. An inhibitory connection is formed between a CS and a US when the CS is activated to the A1 state and the US is activated to A2 rather than A1. This happens in simple extinction because the CS activates the US into A2. This process occurs in real time; thus, during any nonreinforced trial, inhibition will accrue to the CS from the point in time at which the US node is first activated to A2 until the CS leaves the A1 state, which may not occur until the CS is turned off at the end of the trial. Thus, extinction learning will proceed continuously as long as the CS is on and no US occurs on any extinction trial. A limiting factor, however, is the extent to which the CS itself is in the A2 state: The longer it remains on, the more likely the elements in the CS node will be in A2 rather than A1, making new learning about the CS more difficult. Nonetheless, extensions of the CS in extinction will have an effect, because elements in A2 eventually return to the inactive state, from where they will return to A1 because of the continued presence of the CS. SOP thus accounts for extinction in extended CSs without recourse to imaginary trials, and a recent extension of the model (Vogel et al., 2003) may also account for generalization decrement as a function of CS time (Haselgrove and Pearce, 2003; Drew et al., 2004). Although a complete analysis of SOP requires computer simulations that are beyond the scope of the present chapter, the principles contained in the model are consistent with many of the facts of extinction reviewed here. From the current point of view, its most significant problem is that it underestimates the role of context in extinction, and might not account for the negative occasion-setting function of context (e.g., Bouton and King, 1983; Bouton and Swartzentruber, 1986, 1989; Bouton and Nelson, 1998) that arguably provides the key to understanding the renewal, spontaneous recovery, rapid reacquisition, and reinstatement phenomena (for a start at addressing occasion-setting phenomena in terms of SOP, see Brandon and Wagner, 1998; Wagner and Brandon, 2001).

In fear extinction, at the physiological level, expectation violation may be mediated by activation of opioid receptors (see McNally and Westbrook, 2003). Fear conditioning is typically impaired by opioid receptor agonists (e.g., Fanselow, 1998) but facilitated by antagonists, such as naloxone. Extinction, in contrast, is facilitated by opioid receptor agonists and impaired by antagonists (McNally and Westbrook, 2003). According to McNally and Westbrook, opioid receptors may be involved in fear extinction because the omission of the expected US leads to a feeling of relief (Konorski, 1967; Dickinson and Dearing, 1978) that is mediated by opioid peptides; the relief associated with the absence of the US might countercondition fear responses. The idea is also captured in SOP theory's sometimes opponent process, A2. That is, activation of the US node in A2 reduces the effectiveness of the US and also constitutes the crucial event that leads to extinction. Activation of opioid receptors may thus play the physiological role of A2 in fear conditioning. A similar physiological mechanism has not yet been specified for appetitive conditioning, although the underlying basis of frustration is an obvious candidate.

29.3 Can Extinction Be Made More Permanent?

Recent research on extinction has explored several methods that might enhance extinction learning. These methods are discussed here because they provide further insight into the causes of extinction and how extinction therapies might be enhanced.

29.3.1 Counterconditioning

One way to optimize extinction learning might be to actually pair the CS with another US that evokes a qualitatively different (or opposite) response. In counterconditioning, a CS that has been associated with one US is associated with a second US, often incompatible with the first, in a second phase. Not surprisingly, performance corresponding to the second association replaces performance corresponding to the first. Clinical psychologists have incorporated this idea into therapies, such as in systematic desensitization, which involves the training of relaxation responses in the presence of a CS while fear to that CS extinguishes (e.g., Wolpe, 1958). Although counterconditioning may result in a quicker loss of phase-1 performance than simple extinction does (e.g., Scavio, 1974), it is another paradigm that, like extinction, involves a form of retroactive interference. Similar principles may therefore apply (Bouton, 1993). As with extinction, the original association remains intact despite training with a second outcome. This is true in both Pavlovian (Delamater, 1996; Rescorla, 1996a) and instrumental conditioning (Rescorla, 1991, 1995).

Equally important, counterconditioning procedures do not necessarily guarantee protection against relapse effects (the postextinction phenomena discussed earlier) (see also Rosas et al., 2001; García-Gutiérrez and Rosas, 2003, for compatible results in human causal learning). Renewal of fear occurs when rats receive CS–shock pairings in one context, then CS–food pairings in another, and are finally returned to the original context (Peck and Bouton, 1990). Complementary results were obtained when CS–food preceded CS–shock pairings. Spontaneous recovery occurs if time elapses between phase 2 and testing (Bouton and Peck, 1992; Rescorla, 1996b, 1997b). Finally, reinstatement has also been observed (Brooks et al., 1995): When CS–food follows CS–shock, noncontingent shocks delivered in the same context (but not in a different context) can reinstate the original fear performance. Counterconditioning thus supports at least three of the recovery effects suggesting that extinction involves context-dependent new learning.

29.3.2 Other Behavioral Techniques to Optimize Extinction Learning

If extinction involves new learning, then procedures that generally promote learning might also facilitate extinction. This idea has motivated recent research in several laboratories. For example, one idea is that conducting extinction in multiple contexts might connect extinction with a wider array of contextual elements and thereby increase the transfer of extinction learning to other contexts and potentially reduce the renewal effect (e.g., Bouton, 1991a). The results, however, have been mixed. Experiments in conditioned lick suppression (Gunther et al., 1998) and flavor-aversion learning with rats (Chelonis et al., 1999) have shown that extinction in multiple contexts can attenuate (but not abolish) instances of both ABC and ABA renewal relative to that observed after extinction in a single context (see also Vansteenwegen et al., 2006, for a related example). In contrast, as discussed earlier, our own experiments using a fear conditioning method (conditioned lever-press suppression) with rats found that extinction in multiple contexts had no discernible influence on either ABA or ABC renewal (Bouton et al., 2006a). Null results (in ABA renewal) have also been reported with a fear conditioning (shock expectancy) procedure in humans (Neumann et al., 2007). All results together suggest that there are important variables that modulate the positive impact of extinction in multiple contexts on the renewal effect (see Bouton et al., 2006a, for a discussion).

Another approach to optimizing extinction learning is to space extinction trials in time. This idea has been inspired by the fact that spaced trials often yield better excitatory learning than massed trials (e.g., Spence and Norris, 1950). It is worth noting, though, that the behavioral mechanisms behind trial-spacing effects on conditioning are multiple and complex (e.g., see Bouton et al., 2006b), and that many of them focus on the facilitating effects of spacing US presentations, which obviously are not involved in extinction. Nonetheless, there are still some grounds for expecting trial spacing effects in extinction, and these have been tested in several experiments. Spaced trials often cause a slower loss of responding in extinction (e.g., Cain et al., 2003; Morris et al., 2005; Moody et al., 2006), as one might expect, for example, if long intervals between successive CS presentations allow some spontaneous recovery. However, the long-term effects of spacing extinction trials have been variable and much less clear. When responding is tested after a long retention interval, spaced extinction trials have been shown to reduce responding (e.g., Westbrook et al., 1985; Morris et al., 2005), have no effect on responding (Moody et al., 2006), and create more responding than massed extinction trials (Cain et al., 2003; Rescorla and Durlach, 1987). Another complication is the results mentioned earlier, which suggest that extinction ITI can also be part of the context that controls extinction performance (Bouton and García-Gutierrez, 2006). More work will be necessary to untangle these various effects.

Another temporal manipulation has attracted recent interest. In the fear-potentiated startle paradigm in rats, extinction conducted immediately after fear acquisition leads to seemingly more durable extinction (Myers et al., 2006). In particular, rats that received extinction 10 min or 1 h (and in some cases 24 h) after a single acquisition session later failed to exhibit reinstatement, renewal, or spontaneous recovery, whereas rats tested after a longer 72-h acquisition-to-extinction interval showed all these postextinction recovery effects. Immediate extinction thus seemed to produce a more permanent form of extinction that potentially corresponds to biological depotentiation (i.e., reversal) of potentiated synapses (e.g., see Lin et al., 2003). However, once again there are complications and boundary conditions. For example, humans that have received extinction within a few minutes of fear acquisition still show reinstatement (LaBar and Phelps, 2005) and renewal (Milad et al., 2005) when these phenomena are tested later. In rat experiments that measured freezing rather than potentiated startle, Maren and Chang (2006) found that immediate fear extinction may be less effective than delayed extinction under some conditions; immediate extinction never produced a more durable loss of freezing after delayed extinction. And in several appetitive conditioning preparations, Rescorla (2004b) independently found more spontaneous recovery (less-effective extinction) in rats when extinction occurred 1 day, rather than 8 days, after acquisition. Rescorla's methods differed substantially from those in the aforementioned studies, and it is worth noting that his extinction after a 1-day interval might already be outside the temporal window in which depotentiation is possible (e.g., see Staubli and Chun, 1996; Huang et al., 2001). But it seems clear that additional research will be required to fully understand the effects of the interval between conditioning and extinction on the long-term effects of extinction.

29.3.3 Chemical Adjuncts

Research on the neurobiology of conditioning and extinction suggests that certain pharmacological agents may also be used to optimize extinction learning. For example, there has been a great deal of recent interest in D-cycloserine (DCS), a compound that is a partial agonist of the *N*-methyl-D-aspartate (NMDA) glutamate receptor. The NMDA receptor is involved in long-term potentiation, a synaptic model of learning (e.g., Fanselow, 1993), and has now been shown to be involved in several examples of learning including fear conditioning (e.g., Miserendino et al., 1990; Campeau et al., 1992, see Davis and Myers, 2002; Walker and Davis, 2002). The discovery that NMDA receptor antagonists interfere with fear extinction (e.g., Falls et al., 1992; Cox and Westbrook, 1994; Baker and Azorlosa, 1996; Lee and Kim, 1998; Santini et al., 2001) supported the idea that the NMDA receptor was also involved in extinction learning. The next step was to ask whether an NMDA agonist like DCS might correspondingly facilitate extinction. And it does; there is now evidence that administration of DCS facilitates extinction of conditioned fear in rats (Walker et al., 2002; Ledgerwood et al., 2003). And importantly, it also enhances exposure therapy in humans with acrophobia (Ressler et al., 2004) and social phobia (Hofmann et al., 2006). In each of these cases, when DCS was combined with a number of extinction trials that only partially reduced fear in a control group, it yielded more complete fear extinction as revealed during tests that were conducted without the drug.

The fact that DCS can facilitate extinction needs to be interpreted cautiously. For example, there is little in the description of how DCS works to suggest that it would do more than merely strengthen ordinary extinction learning, which, as we have shown, is relatively context specific and subject to relapse. Consistent with this possibility, although DCS facilitates the rate of fear extinction, it does not decrease the strength of the ABA renewal effect (Woods and Bouton, 2006). That is, rats for whom DCS had facilitated extinction still showed a robust return of fear when they were tested with the CS in the original conditioning context. This result indicates that DCS combined with extinction does not abolish the original learning. Woods and Bouton (2006) actually suggested that DCS might facilitate inhibitory conditioning of the context in which extinction occurs. Such a possibility is consistent with rapid extinction (enhanced contextual inhibition would decrease fear of the CS presented in it) and intact renewal (context inhibition would be gone when the CS is tested in another context). It is also consistent with other DCS effects reported in the literature. For example, DCS given during extinction can later reduce reinstatement (Ledgerwood et al., 2004); enhanced inhibition in the context would interfere with reinstatement by disrupting the development of context conditioning during US-alone presentations. DCS combined with extinction of one CS also causes less fear of a second CS tested in the same context (Ledgerwood et al., 2005); if the context were an inhibitor, it would inhibit fear of any CS tested in that context. Although DCS can have positive effects on fear extinction, it does not create unlearning.

Another compound that has been of interest is yohimbine, an alpha-2 adrenergic antagonist. This substance may cause paniclike responding when it is injected in animals or panic patients (Davis et al., 1979; Pellow et al., 1985; Johnston and File, 1989; see Stanford, 1995, for review). For that reason, it might increase the level of fear during extinction, and by thus enabling either increased response inhibition or a higher violation of reinforcer expectation (see earlier discussion), allow for better extinction learning. Consistent with this possibility, yohimbine administered before a fear extinction session can lead to better extinction learning in mice (i.e., less freezing in a subsequent test session conducted 24 hours later; Cain et al., 2003). We have replicated this effect in rats (Morris and Bouton, 2007). However, the facilitated extinction was highly context specific; rats tested in a new context or back in the original conditioning context after extinction with yohimbine still showed a strong renewal of fear. Thus, as we saw with DCS, yohimbine facilitates the rate of extinction learning without necessarily abolishing relapse. Further results suggested that presenting yohimbine on its own in a context allows that context to suppress subsequent extinguished fear performance – as if it was conditioning a form of context-specific fear inhibition. Although the exact mechanism is unclear, it seems apparent that as an adjunct to extinction, yohimbine once again may not prevent the occurrence of future relapse.

Behavioral neuroscientists have recently also become interested in memory "reconsolidation" effects (*See* Chapter 30) that might suggest a new way to modify previously learned memories. It has long been known that freshly learned memories may be labile and easily disrupted before they are consolidated into a stable long-term form (e.g., McGaugh, 2000; Dudai, 2004). The consolidation process requires synthesis of new proteins in the brain (e.g., Davis and Squire, 1984; Goelet et al., 1986) and can therefore be blocked by administration of a protein synthesis inhibitor, such as anisomycin (e.g., Schafe and LeDoux, 2000). In the case of fear memories, whose consolidation can be modulated by stress hormones, consolidation can also be hindered by administration of a β-adrenergic receptor blocker such as propranolol (Pitman et al., 2002; Vaiva et al., 2003; McGaugh, 2004; see also Pitman, 1989). Recent research suggests that an older memory that has recently been reactivated (for example) by a single exposure to the CS likewise temporarily returns to a labile state from which it needs to be reconsolidated (e.g., Nader et al., 2000; Sara, 2000; Walker et al., 2003; Lee et al., 2004; Suzuki et al., 2004; Alberini, 2005). Like consolidation, reconsolidation can be blocked by anisomycin (e.g., Nader et al., 2000), and in the case of a fear memory, by administration of propranolol (Przybyslawski et al., 1999; Debiec and LeDoux, 2004). In these experiments, memory is returned to a labile state by presenting the CS on a very small number of occasions that are insufficient to produce extinction on their own (e.g., Suzuki et al., 2004). The crucial new result is that administration of anisomycin or propranolol while the memory is in this state can reduce evidence of conditioned responding when the CS is tested later. A therapeutic implication may be that one of these drugs in combination with one or two presentations of a CS may weaken an aversive fear memory. However, more basic research is needed. For example, it is not necessarily clear that a behavioral reconsolidation result involves actual modification of the original memory or mere difficulty in retrieving it (see Duvarci and Nader, 2004, for a critical analysis of these possibilities as induced by anisomycin). It seems clear that caution is necessary in interpreting the results of any effect of a drug or chemical on learning, extinction, and therapy.

29.3.4 Summary

A variety of manipulations have been thought to hold promise in optimizing extinction learning, but their effects have been mixed and (at this point in time) are not well understood. When investigators have specifically tested their effects on the relapse effects we reviewed in the first part of this chapter, they have often provided surprisingly little protection (see Bouton et al., 2006b, for a review). In contrast, one of the most effective and durable ways to optimize extinction learning and protect against relapse seems to be with the use of techniques that bridge the extinction and testing contexts, such as retrieval cues and presentation of occasional reinforced trials during extinction (discussed earlier). Bridging treatments accept the inherent context-specificity of extinction and work by increasing the similarity between the extinction context and test contexts where lapse and relapse may be a problem.

29.4 Conclusions

Extinction is a highly complex phenomenon, even when analyzed at a purely behavioral level. It is probably multiply determined. But, according to the results reviewed here, it usually does not involve destruction of the original learning. Instead, the main behavioral factors that cause the loss of responding appear to be generalization decrement and new learning that may be initiated by the violation of an expectation of the US. In SOP (e.g., Wagner, 1981; Wagner and Brandon, 2001), perhaps the most powerful and comprehensive model of associative learning that is currently available, that expectation violation takes the form of the CS activating the US node into a secondarily active (A2) state that potentially enables new inhibitory learning as long as the CS remains on and no US is presented. Importantly, this new inhibitory learning leaves the original CS–US association intact.

Bouton (1993) has argued that the fact that extinction might leave the original learning intact means that the CS emerges from extinction with two available associations with the US. It therefore has properties analogous to those of an ambiguous word, and the current performance depends on which of two associations is retrieved. Consistent with this idea, another fact that emerges from behavioral research on extinction is that it is relatively context dependent. Given this, the CS's second (inhibitory) association is especially dependent on the context for its activation or retrieval. The role of the context is usually modulatory; it activates or retrieves the CS's second (inhibitory) association, much as a negative occasion setter might (e.g., Holland, 1992). This hypothesis begins to integrate several facts about extinction and brings relapse effects like the renewal effect, spontaneous recovery, rapid reacquisition, reinstatement, and perhaps resurgence to center stage.

The major implication of behavioral research on extinction is thus that lapse and relapse are always possibilities after exposure therapy. As just reviewed, there is substantial interest among basic researchers in discovering new ways to make extinction more permanent. To date, behavioral and pharmacological methods of enhancing or optimizing extinction learning have produced lawful effects on the rate of extinction, but their effectiveness in the long term is less clear. Treatments that increase the rate at which fear is lost in therapy may not change extinction learning's inherent context specificity. At the current time, the best way to combat the various relapse phenomena reviewed here may be to consider their behavioral causes and develop techniques that might defeat them. This perspective has led to certain bridging treatments, such as the use of reminder cues or strategies or conducting extinction in the presence of the contextual cues that can lead to particular examples of relapse, which do appear to hold some promise in maintaining extinction performance in the presence of conditions that might otherwise initiate relapse.

Acknowledgments

Preparation of this chapter was supported by Grant RO1 MH64847 from the National Institute of Mental Health.

References

Alberini CM (2005) Mechanisms of memory stabilization: Are consolidation and reconsolidation similar or distinct processes? *Trends Neurosci.* 28: 51–56.

Alessi SM, Badger GJ, and Higgins ST (2004) An experimental examination of the initial weeks of abstinence in cigarette smokers. *Exp. Clin. Psychopharmacol.* 12: 276–287.

Baker JD and Azorlosa JL (1996) The NMDA antagonist MK-801 blocks the extinction of Pavlovian fear conditioning. *Behav. Neurosci.* 110: 618–620.

Baker AG, Steinwald H, and Bouton ME (1991) Contextual conditioning and reinstatement of extinguished instrumental responding. *Q. J. Exp. Psychol.* 43B: 199–218.

Barela PB (1999) Theoretical mechanisms underlying the trial spacing effect in Pavlovian conditioning. *J. Exp. Psychol. Anim. Behav. Process* 25: 177–193.

Bouton ME (1984) Differential control by context in the inflation and reinstatement paradigms. *J. Exp. Psychol. Anim. Behav. Process* 10: 56–74.

Bouton ME (1986) Slow reacquisition following the extinction of conditioned suppression. *Learn. Motivation* 17: 1–15.

Bouton ME (1988) Context and ambiguity in the extinction of emotional learning: Implications for exposure therapy. *Behav. Res. Ther.* 26: 137–149.

Bouton ME (1991a) A contextual analysis of fear extinction. In: Martin PR (ed.) *Handbook of Behavior Therapy and Psychological Science: An Integrative Approach*, pp. 435–453. Elmsford, NY: Pergamon Press.

Bouton ME (1991b) Context and retrieval in extinction and in other examples of interference in simple associative learning. In: Dachowski L and Flaherty CF (eds.) *Current Topics in Animal Learning: Brain, Emotion, and Cognition*, pp. 25–53. Hillsdale, NJ: Erlbaum.

Bouton ME (1993) Context, time, and memory retrieval in the interference paradigms of Pavlovian learning. *Psychol. Bull.* 114: 80–99.

Bouton ME (1994) Conditioning, remembering, and forgetting. *J. Exp. Psychol. Anim. Behav. Process* 20: 219–231.

Bouton ME (2000) A learning-theory perspective on lapse, relapse, and the maintenance of behavior change. *Health Psychol.* 19: 57–63.

Bouton ME (2002) Context, ambiguity, and unlearning: Sources of relapse after behavioral extinction. *Biol. Psychiatry* 52: 976–986.

Bouton ME (2004) Context and behavioral processes in extinction. *Learn. Mem.* 11: 485–494.

Bouton ME and Bolles RC (1979a) Contextual control of the extinction of conditioned fear. *Learn. Motivation* 10: 445–466.

Bouton ME and Bolles RC (1979b) Role of conditioned contextual stimuli in reinstatement of extinguished fear. *J. Exp. Psychol. Anim. Behav. Process* 5: 368–378.

Bouton ME and Brooks DC (1993) Time and context effects on performance in a Pavlovian discrimination reversal. *J. Exp. Psychol. Anim. Behav. Process* 19: 165–179.

Bouton ME, García-Gutiérrez A, Zilski J, and Moody EW (2006a) Extinction in multiple contexts does not necessarily make extinction less vulnerable to relapse. *Behav. Res. Ther.* 44: 983–994.

Bouton ME and García-Gutiérrez A (2006) Intertrial interval as a contextual stimulus. *Behav. Processes* 71: 307–317.

Bouton ME, Kenney FA, and Rosengard C (1990) State-dependent fear extinction with two benzodiazepine tranquilizers. *Behav. Neurosci.* 104: 44–55.

Bouton ME and King DA (1983) Contextual control of the extinction of conditioned fear: Tests for the associative value of the context. *J. Exp. Psychol. Anim. Behav. Process* 9: 248–265.

Bouton ME and King DA (1986) Effect of context on performance to conditioned stimuli with mixed histories of reinforcement and nonreinforcement. *J. Exp. Psychol. Anim. Behav. Process* 12: 4–15.

Bouton ME and Nelson JB (1994) Context-specificity of target versus feature inhibition in a feature-negative discrimination. *J. Exp. Psychol. Anim. Behav. Process* 20: 51–65.

Bouton ME and Nelson JB (1998) Mechanisms of feature-positive and feature-negative discrimination learning in an appetitive conditioning paradigm. In: Schmajuk N and Holland PC (eds.) *Occasion Setting: Associative Learning and Cognition in Animals*, pp. 69–112. Washington, DC: American Psychological Association.

Bouton ME and Peck CA (1989) Context effects on conditioning, extinction, and reinstatement in an appetitive conditioning preparation. *Anim. Learn. Behav.* 17: 188–198.

Bouton ME and Peck CA (1992) Spontaneous recovery in cross-motivational transfer (counterconditioning). *Anim. Learn. Behav.* 20: 313–321.

Bouton ME and Ricker ST (1994) Renewal of extinguished responding in a second context. *Anim. Learn. Behav.* 22: 317–324.

Bouton ME, Rosengard C, Achenbach GG, Peck CA, and Brooks DC (1993) Effects of contextual conditioning and unconditional stimulus presentation on performance in appetitive conditioning. *Q. J. Exp. Psychol.* 46B: 63–95.

Bouton ME and Sunsay C (2003) Importance of trials versus accumulating time across trials in partially-reinforced appetitive conditioning. *J. Exp. Psychol. Anim. Behav. Process* 29: 62–77.

Bouton ME and Swartzentruber D (1986) Analysis of the associative and occasion-setting properties of contexts participating in a Pavlovian discrimination. *J. Exp. Psychol. Anim. Behav. Process* 12: 333–350.

Bouton ME and Swartzentruber D (1989) Slow reacquisition following extinction: Context, encoding, and retrieval mechanisms. *J. Exp. Psychol. Anim. Behav. Process* 15: 43–53.

Bouton ME and Woods AM (2004) Separating time-based and trial-based accounts of the partial reinforcement extinction effect. Presented at the meeting of the Eastern Psychological Association, Washington, DC.

Bouton ME, Woods AM, Moody EW, Sunsay C, and García-Gutiérrez A (2006b) Counteracting the context-dependence of extinction: Relapse and some tests of possible methods of relapse prevention. In: Craske MG, Hermans D, and Vansteenwegen D (eds.) *Fear and Learning: Basic Science to Clinical Application.* Washington, DC: American Psychological Association.

Bouton ME, Woods AM, and Pineño O (2004) Occasional reinforced trials during extinction can slow the rate of rapid reacquisition. *Learn. Motivation* 35: 371–390.

Brandon SE and Wagner AR (1998) Occasion setting: Influences of conditioned emotional responses and configural cues. In: Schmajuk NA and Holland PC (eds.) *Occasion Setting: Associative Learning and Cognition in Animals*, pp. 343–382. Washington, DC: American Psychological Association.

Brooks DC (2000) Recent and remote extinction cues reduce spontaneous recovery. *Q. J. Exp. Psychol.* 53B: 25–58.

Brooks DC and Bouton ME (1993) A retrieval cue for extinction attenuates spontaneous recovery. *J. Exp. Psychol. Anim. Behav. Process* 19: 77–89.

Brooks DC and Bouton ME (1994) A retrieval cue for extinction attenuates response recovery (renewal) caused by a return to the conditioning context. *J. Exp. Psychol. Anim. Behav. Process* 20: 366–379.

Brooks DC, Hale B, Nelson JB, and Bouton ME (1995) Reinstatement after counterconditioning. *Anim. Learn. Behav.* 23: 383–390.

Cain CK, Blouin AM, and Barad M (2003) Temporally massed CS presentations generate more fear extinction than spaced presentations. *J. Exp. Psychol. Anim. Behav. Process* 29: 323–333.

Campeau S, Miserendino MJD, and Davis M (1992) Intra-amygdala infusion of the N-methyl-D-aspartate receptor antagonist AP5 blocks acquisition but not expression of fear-potentiated startle to an auditory conditioned stimulus. *Behav. Neurosci.* 106: 569–574.

Capaldi EJ (1967) A sequential hypothesis of instrumental learning. In: Spence KW and Spence JT (eds.) *Psychology of Learning and Motivation,* vol. 1, pp. 67–156. New York: Academic Press.

Capaldi EJ (1994) The sequential view: From rapidly fading stimulus traces to the organization of memory and the abstract concept of number. *Psychon. Bull. Rev.* 1: 156–181.

Chelonis JJ, Calton JL, Hart JA, and Schachtman TR (1999) Attenuation of the renewal effect by extinction in multiple contexts. *Learn. Motivation* 30: 1–14.

Collins BN and Brandon TH (2002) Effects of extinction context and retrieval cues on alcohol cue reactivity among nonalcoholic drinkers. *J. Consult. Clin. Psychol.* 70: 390–397.

Colwill RW (1991) Negative discriminative stimuli provide information about the identity of omitted response-contingent outcomes. *Anim. Learn. Behav.* 19: 326–336.

Conklin C (2006) Environments as cues to smoke: Implications for human extinction-based research and treatment. *Exp. Clin. Psychopharmacol.* 14: 12–19.

Conklin CA and Tiffany ST (2002) Applying extinction research and theory to cue-exposure addiction treatments. *Addiction* 97: 155–167.

Cox J and Westbrook RF (1994) The NMDA receptor antagonist MK-801 blocks acquisition and extinction of conditioned hypoalgesia responses in the rat. *Q. J. Exp. Psychol.* 47B: 187–210.

Crombag HS and Shaham Y (2002) Renewal of drug seeking by contextual cues after prolonged extinction in rats. *Behav. Neurosci.* 116: 169–173.

Cunningham CL (1979) Alcohol as a cue for extinction: State dependency produced by conditioned inhibition. *Anim. Learn. Behav.* 7: 45–52.

Daly HB (1974) Reinforcing properties of escape from frustration aroused in various learning situations. In: Bower GH (ed.) *The Psychology of Learning and Motivation,* vol. 8, pp. 187–232. New York: Academic Press.

Daly HB and Daly JT (1982) A mathematical model of reward and aversive nonreward: Its application in over 30 appetitive learning situations. *J. Exp. Psychol. Gen.* 111: 441–480.

Danguir J and Nicolaidis S (1977) Lack of reacquisition in learned taste aversions. *Anim. Learn. Behav.* 5: 395–397.

Davis HP and Squire LR (1984) Protein synthesis and memory. *Psychol. Bull.* 96: 518–559.

Davis M, Redmund DE, and Baraban JM (1979) Noradrenergic agonists and antagonists: Effects on conditioned fear as measured by the potentiated startle paradigm. *Psychopharmacology* 65: 111–118.

Davis M and Myers KM (2002) The role of glutamate and gamma-aminobutyric acid in fear extinction: Clinical implications for exposure therapy. *Biol. Psychiatry* 52: 998–1007.

Debiec J and LeDoux JE (2004) Disruption of reconsolidation but not consolidation of auditory fear conditioning by noradrenergic blockade in the amygdala. *Neuroscience* 129: 267–272.

Delamater AR (1996) Effects of several extinction treatments upon the integrity of Pavlovian stimulus-outcome associations. *Anim. Learn. Behav.* 24: 437–449.

Delamater AR (2004) Experimental extinction in Pavlovian conditioning: Behavioural and neuroscience perspectives. *Q. J. Exp. Psychol.* 57B: 97–132.

Denniston JC, Chang RC, and Miller RR (2003) Massive extinction treatment attenuates the renewal effect. *Learn. Motivation* 34: 68–86.

Devenport L, Hill T, Wilson M, and Ogden E (1997) Tracking and averaging in variable environments: A transition rule. *J. Exp. Psychol. Anim. Behav. Process* 23: 450–460.

Dickinson A and Dearing MF (1978) Appetitive-aversion interactions and inhibitory processes. In: Dickinson A and Boakes RA (eds.) *Mechanisms of Learning and Motivation: A Memorial Volume to Jerzy Konorski*, pp. 203–231. Hillsdale, NJ: Erlbaum.

Drew MR, Yang C, Ohyama T, and Balsam PD (2004) Temporal specificity of extinction in autoshaping. *J. Exp. Psychol. Anim. Behav. Process* 30: 163–176.

Dudai Y (2004) The neurobiology of consolidations, or how stable is the engram? *Annu. Rev. Psychol.* 55: 51–86.

Duvarci S and Nader K (2004) Characterization of fear memory reconsolidation. *J. Neurosci.* 24: 9269–9275.

Epstein R (1983) Resurgence of previously reinforced behavior during extinction. *Behav. Anal. Lett.* 3: 391–397.

Epstein R (1985) Extinction-induced resurgence: Preliminary investigations and possible applications. *Psychol. Rec.* 35: 143–153.

Falls WA, Miserendino MJD, and Davis M (1992) Extinction of fear-potentiated startle: Blockade by infusion of an NMDA antagonist into the amygdale. *J. Neurosci.* 12: 854–863.

Fanselow MS (1993) Associations and memories: The role of NMDA receptors and long-term potentiation. *Curr. Dir. Psychol. Sci.* 2: 152–156.

Fanselow MS (1998) Pavlovian conditioning, negative feedback, and blocking: Mechanisms that regulate association formation. *Neuron* 20: 625–627.

Frohardt RJ, Guarraci FA, and Bouton ME (2000) The effects of neurotoxic hippocampal lesions on two effects of context after fear extinction. *Behav. Neurosci.* 114: 227–240.

Gallistel CR and Gibbon J (2000) Time, rate, and conditioning. *Psychol. Rev.* 107: 289–344.

García-Gutiérrez A and Rosas JM (2003) Context change as the mechanism of reinstatement in causal learning. *J. Exp. Psychol. Anim. Behav. Process* 29: 292–310.

Gluck M and Myers CE (1993) Hippocampal mediation of stimulus representation: A computational theory. *Hippocampus* 3: 492–516.

Goelet P, Castellucci VF, Schacher S, and Kandel ER (1986) The long and short of long-term memory – A molecular framework. *Nature* 322: 419–422.

Gunther LM, Denniston JC, and Miller RR (1998) Conducting exposure treatment in multiple contexts can prevent relapse. *Behav. Res. Ther.* 36: 75–91.

Hall G and Channell S (1985) Differential effects of contextual change on latent inhibition and on the habituation of an orienting response. *J. Exp. Psychol. Anim. Behav. Process* 11: 470–481.

Harris JA, Jones ML, Bailey GK, and Westbrook RF (2000) Contextual control over conditioned responding in an

extinction paradigm. *J. Exp. Psychol. Anim. Behav. Process* 26: 174–185.
Hart JA, Bourne MJ, and Schachtman TR (1995) Slow reacquisition of a conditioned taste aversion. *Anim. Learn. Behav.* 23: 297–303.
Haselgrove M and Pearce JM (2003) Facilitation of extinction by an increase or a decrease in trial duration. *J. Exp. Psychol. Anim. Behav. Process* 29: 153–166.
Haselgrove M, Aydin A, and Pearce JM (2004) A partial reinforcement extinction effect despite equal rates of reinforcement during Pavlovian conditioning. *J. Exp. Psychol. Anim. Behav. Process* 30: 240–250.
Hendry JS (1982) Summation of undetected excitation following extinction of the CER. *Anim. Learn. Behav.* 10: 476–482.
Hofmann SG, Meuret AE, Smits JAJ, et al. (2006) Augmentation of exposure therapy with D-cycloserine for social anxiety disorder. *Arch. Gen. Psychiatry* 63: 298–304.
Holland PC (1992) Occasion setting in Pavlovian conditioning. In: Medin DL (ed.) *The Psychology of Learning and Motivation,* vol. 28, pp. 69–125. San Diego, CA: Academic Press.
Honey RC and Hall G (1989) Acquired equivalence and distinctiveness of cues. *J. Exp. Psychol. Anim. Behav. Process* 15: 338–346.
Huang CC, Liang YC, and Hsu KS (2001) Characterization of the mechanism underlying the reversal of long-term potentiation by low frequency stimulation at hippocampal CA1 synapses. *J. Biol. Chem.* 276: 48108–48117.
Johnston AL and File SE (1989) Yohimbine's anxiogenic action: Evidence for noradrenergic and dopaminergic sites. *Pharmacol. Biochem. Behav.* 32: 151–156.
Kehoe EJ (1988) A layered network model of associative learning: Learning to learn and configuration. *Psychol. Rev.* 95: 411–433.
Kehoe EJ and Holt PE (1984) Transfer across CS-US intervals and sensory modalities in classical conditioning in the rabbit. *Anim. Learn. Behav.* 122–128.
Kehoe EJ and Macrae M (1997) Savings in animal learning: Implications for relapse and maintenance after therapy. *Behav. Ther.* 28: 141–155.
Konorski J (1967) *Integrative Activity of the Brain*. Chicago: University of Chicago Press.
Kremer EF (1978) The Rescorla-Wagner model: Losses in associative strength in compound conditioned stimuli. *J. Exp. Psychol. Anim. Behav. Process* 4: 22–36.
Krupa DJ and Thompson RF (2003) Inhibiting the expression of a classically conditioned behavior prevents its extinction. *J. Neurosci.* 23: 10577–10584.
LaBar KS and Phelps EA (2005) Reinstatement of conditioned fear in humans is context dependent and impaired in amnesia. *Behav. Neurosci.* 119: 677–686.
Lattal KM and Nakajima S (1998) Overexpectation in appetitive Pavlovian and instrumental conditioning. *Anim. Learn. Behav.* 26: 351–360.
Ledgerwood L, Richardson R, and Cranney J (2003) Effects of D-cycloserine on extinction of conditioned freezing. *Behav. Neurosci.* 117: 341–349.
Ledgerwood L, Richardson R, and Cranney J (2004) D-cycloserine and the facilitation of extinction of conditioned fear: Consequences for reinstatement. *Behav. Neurosci.* 118: 505–513.
Ledgerwood L, Richardson R, and Cranney J (2005) D-cycloserine facilitates extinction of learned fear: Effects on reacquisition and generalized extinction. *Biol. Psychiatry* 57: 841–847.
Lee H and Kim JJ (1998) Amygdalar NMDA receptors are critical for new fear learning in previously fear-conditioned rats. *J. Neurosci.* 18: 8444–8454.
Lee JL, Everitt BJ, and Thomas KL (2004) Independent cellular processes for hippocampal memory consolidation and reconsolidation. *Science* 304: 839–843.
Leitenberg H, Rawson RA, and Bath K (1970) Reinforcement of competing behavior during extinction. *Science* 169: 301–303.
Leitenberg H, Rawson RA, and Mulick JA (1975) Extinction and reinforcement of alternative behavior. *J. Comp. Physiol. Psychol.* 88: 640–652.
Lieving GA and Lattal KA (2003) Recency, repeatability, and reinforcer retrenchment: An experimental analysis of resurgence. *J. Exp. Anal. Behav.* 80: 217–233.
Lin C-H, Yeh SH, Lu H-S, and Gean P-W (2003) The similarities and diversities of signal pathways leading to consolidation of conditioning and consolidation of extinction of fear memory. *J. Neurosci.* 23: 8310–8317.
Mackintosh NJ (1974) *The Psychology of Animal Learning*. New York: Academic Press.
Maren S and Chang C (2006) Recent fear is resistant to extinction. *Proc. Natl. Acad. Sci. USA* 103: 18020–18025.
Marlatt GA and Gordon JR (1985) *Relapse Prevention: Maintenance Strategies in the Treatment of Addictive Behaviors*. New York: Guilford Press.
McClelland JL and Rumelhart DE (1985) Distributed memory and the representation of general and specific information. *J. Exp. Psychol. Gen.* 114: 159–188.
McCloskey M and Cohen NJ (1989) Catastrophic interference in connectionist networks: The sequential learning problem. In: Bower GH (ed.) *The Psychology of Learning and Motivation,* vol. 24, pp. 109–165. San Diego, CA: Academic Press.
McGaugh JL (2000) Memory – A century of consolidation. *Science* 287: 248–251.
McGaugh JL (2004) The amygdala modulates the consolidation of memories of emotionally arousing experiences. *Annu. Rev. Neurosci.* 27: 1–28.
McNally GP and Westbrook RF (2003) Opioid receptors regulate the extinction of Pavlovian fear conditioning. *Behav. Neurosci.* 117: 1292–1301.
Milad MR, Orr SP, Pitman RK, and Rauch SL (2005) Context modulation of memory for fear extinction in humans. *Psychophysiology* 42: 456–464.
Mineka S, Mystkowski JL, Hladek D, and Rodriguez BI (1999) The effects of changing contexts on return of fear following exposure therapy for spider fear. *J. Consult. Clin. Psychol.* 67: 599–604.
Miserendino MJD, Sananes CB, Melia KR, and Davis M (1990) Blocking of acquisition but not expression of conditioned fear-potentiated startle by NMDA antagonists in the amygdala. *Nature* 345: 716–718.
Moody EW, Sunsay C, and Bouton ME (2006) Priming and trial spacing in extinction: Effects on extinction performance, spontaneous recovery, and reinstatement in appetitive conditioning. *Q. J. Exp. Psychol.* 59: 809–829.
Morris RW and Bouton ME (2007) The effect of yohimbine on the extinction of conditioned fear: A role for context. *Behav. Neurosci.* 121: 501–514.
Morris RW, Furlong TM, and Westbrook RF (2005) Recent exposure to a dangerous context impairs extinction and reinstates lost fear reactions. *J. Exp. Psychol. Anim. Behav. Process* 31: 40–55.
Mowrer OH and Jones HM (1945) Habit strength as a function of the pattern of reinforcement. *J. Exp. Psychol.* 35: 293–311.
Myers KM and Davis M (2002) Behavioral and neural analysis of extinction. *Neuron* 36: 567–584.
Myers KM, Ressler KJ, and Davis M (2006) Different mechanisms of fear extinction dependent on length of time since fear acquisition. *Learn. Mem.* 13: 216–223.
Mystkowski JL, Craske MG, and Echiverri AM (2002) Treatment context and return of fear in spider phobia. *Behav. Ther.* 33: 399–416.

Mystkowski JL, Craske MG, Echiverri AM, and Labus JS (2006) Mental reinstatement of context and return of fear in spider-fearful participants. *Behav. Ther.* 37: 49–60.

Nader K, Schafe GE, and LeDoux JE (2000) Fear memories require protein synthesis in the amygdala for reconsolidation after retrieval. *Nature* 406: 722–726.

Nakajima S, Tanaka S, Urushihara K, and Imada H (2000) Renewal of extinguished lever-press responses upon return to the training context. *Learn. Motivation* 31: 416–431.

Napier RM, Macrae M, and Kehoe EJ (1992) Rapid reacquisition in conditioning of the rabbit's nictitating membrane response. *J. Exp. Psychol. Anim. Behav. Process* 18: 182–192.

Nelson JB (2002) Context specificity of excitation and inhibition in ambiguous stimuli. *Learn. Motivation* 33: 284–310.

Nelson JB and Bouton ME (1997) The effects of a context switch following serial and simultaneous feature-negative discriminations. *Learn. Motivation* 28: 56–84.

Neumann DL, Lipp OV, and Cory SE (2007) Conducting extinction in multiple contexts does not necessarily attenuate the renewal of shock expectancy in a fear-conditioning procedure with humans. *Behav. Res. Ther.* 45: 385–394.

Neuringer A, Kornell N, and Olufs M (2001) Stability and variability in extinction. *J. Exp. Psychol. Anim. Behav. Process* 27: 79–84.

Overton DA (1985) Contextual stimulus effects of drugs and internal states. In: Balsam PD and Tomie A (eds.) *Context and Learning*, pp. 357–384. Hillsdale, NJ: Erlbaum.

Pavlov IP (1927) *Conditioned Reflexes*. Oxford, UK: Oxford University Press.

Pearce JM and Hall G (1980) A model for Pavlovian conditioning: Variations in the effectiveness of conditioned but not unconditioned stimuli. *Psychol. Rev.* 87: 332–352.

Peck CA and Bouton ME (1990) Context and performance in aversive-to-appetitive and appetitive-to-aversive transfer. *Learn. Motivation* 21: 1–31.

Pellow S, Chopin P, File SE, and Briley M (1985) Validation of open:closed arm entries in an elevated plus-maze as a measure of anxiety in the rat. *J. Neurosci. Methods* 14: 149–167.

Pitman RK (1989) Post-traumatic stress disorder, hormones, and memory. *Biol. Psychiatry* 44: 221–223.

Pitman RK, Sanders KM, Zusman RM, et al. (2002) Pilot study of secondary prevention of posttraumatic stress disorder with propranolol. *Biol. Psychiatry* 51: 189–192.

Przybyslawski J, Roullet P, and Sara SJ (1999) Attenuation of emotional and nonemotional memories after their reactivation: Role of beta adrenergic receptors. *J. Neurosci.* 19: 6623–6628.

Rauhut AS, Thomas BL, and Ayres JJB (2001) Treatments that weaken Pavlovian conditioned fear and thwart its renewal in rats: Implications for treating human phobias. *J. Exp. Psychol. Anim. Behav. Process* 27: 99–114.

Rawson RA, Leitenberg H, Mulick JA, and Lefebvre MF (1977) Recovery of extinction responding in rats following discontinuation of reinforcement of alternative behavior: A test of two explanations. *Anim. Learn. Behav.* 5: 415–420.

Reberg D (1972) Compound tests for excitation in early acquisition and after prolonged extinction of conditioned suppression. *Learn. Motivation* 3: 246–258.

Reid RL (1958) The role of the reinforcer as a stimulus. *Br. J. Psychol.* 49: 202–209.

Rescorla RA (1991) Associations of multiple outcomes with an instrumental response. *J. Exp. Psychol. Anim. Behav. Process* 17: 465–474.

Rescorla RA (1993) Inhibitory associations between S and R in extinction. *Anim. Learn. Behav.* 21: 327–336.

Rescorla RA (1995) Full preservation of a response-outcome association through training with a second outcome. *Q. J. Exp. Psychol.* 48B: 235–251.

Rescorla RA (1996a) Preservation of Pavlovian associations through extinction. *Q. J. Exp. Psychol.* 49B: 245–258.

Rescorla RA (1996b) Spontaneous recovery after training with multiple outcomes. *Anim. Learn. Behav.* 24: 11–18.

Rescorla RA (1997a) Response inhibition in extinction. *Q. J. Exp. Psychol.* 50B: 238–252.

Rescorla RA (1997b) Spontaneous recovery after Pavlovian conditioning with multiple outcomes. *Anim. Learn. Behav.* 25: 99–107.

Rescorla RA (2000) Extinction can be enhanced by a concurrent exciter. *J. Exp. Psychol. Anim. Behav. Process* 26: 251–260.

Rescorla RA (2001) Experimental extinction. In: Mowrer RR and Klein SB (eds.) *Handbook of Contemporary Learning Theories*, pp. 119–154. Mahwah, NJ: Erlbaum.

Rescorla RA (2003) Protection from extinction. *Learn. Behav.* 31: 124–132.

Rescorla RA (2004a) Spontaneous recovery. *Learn. Mem.* 11: 501–509.

Rescorla RA (2004b) Spontaneous recovery varies inversely with the training-extinction interval. *Learn. Behav.* 32: 401–408.

Rescorla RA (2005) Spontaneous recovery of excitation but not inhibition. *J. Exp. Psychol. Anim. Behav. Process* 31: 277–288.

Rescorla RA (2006) Deepened extinction from compound stimulus presentation. *J. Exp. Psychol. Anim. Behav. Process* 32: 135–144.

Rescorla RA and Durlach PJ (1987) The role of context in intertrial interval effects in autoshaping. *Q. J. Exp. Psychol.* 39B: 35–48.

Rescorla RA and Heth CD (1975) Reinstatement of fear to an extinguished conditioned stimulus. *J. Exp. Psychol. Anim. Behav. Process* 1: 88–96.

Rescorla RA and Skucy JC (1969) Effect of response-independent reinforcers during extinction. *J. Comp. Physiol. Psychol.* 67: 381–389.

Rescorla RA and Wagner AR (1972) A theory of Pavlovian conditioning: Variations in the effectiveness of reinforcement and nonreinforcement. In: Black AH and Prokasy WK (eds.) *Classical Conditioning II: Current Research and Theory*, pp. 64–99. New York: Appleton-Century-Crofts.

Ressler KJ, Rothbaum BO, Tannenbaum L, et al. (2004) Cognitive enhances as adjuncts to psychotherapy: Use of D-cycloserine in phobics to facilitate extinction of fear. *Arch. Gen. Psychiatry* 61: 1136–1144.

Ricker ST and Bouton ME (1996) Reacquisition following extinction in appetitive conditioning. *Anim. Learn. Behav.* 24: 423–436.

Robbins SJ (1990) Mechanisms underlying spontaneous recovery in autoshaping. *J. Exp. Psychol. Anim. Behav. Process* 16: 235–249.

Rosas JM and Bouton ME (1997) Additivity of the effects of retention interval and context change on latent inhibition: Toward resolution of the context forgetting paradox. *J. Exp. Psychol. Anim. Behav. Process* 23: 283–294.

Rosas JM and Bouton ME (1998) Context change and retention interval can have additive, rather than interactive, effects after taste aversion extinction. *Psychon. Bull. Rev.* 5: 79–83.

Rosas JM and Callejas-Aguilera JE (2006) Context switch effects on acquisition and extinction in human predictive learning. *J. Exp. Psychol. Learn. Mem. Cogn.* 32: 461–474.

Rosas JM and Callejas-Aguilera JE (2007) Acquisition of a conditioned taste aversion becomes context dependent when it is learning after extinction. *Q. J. Exp. Psychol.* 60: 9–15.

Rosas JM, Vila NJ, Lugo M, and Lopez L (2001) Combined effect of context change and retention interval on interference in causality judgments. *J. Exp. Psychol. Anim. Behav. Process* 27: 153–164.

Santini E, Muller RU, and Quirk GJ (2001) Consolidation of extinction learning involves transfer from NMDA-independent to NMDA-dependent memory. *J. Neurosci.* 21: 9009–9017.

Sara SJ (2000) Retrieval and reconsolidation: Toward a neurobiology of remembering. *Learn. Mem.* 7: 73–84.

Scavio MJ (1974) Classical-classical transfer: Effects of prior aversive conditions upon appetitive conditioning in rabbits (*Oryctolagus cuniculus*). *J. Comp. Physiol. Psychol.* 86: 107–115.

Schafe GE and LeDoux JE (2000) Memory consolidation of auditory Pavlovian fear conditioning requires protein synthesis and protein kinase A in the amygdala. *J. Neurosci.* 20: RC96 (1–5).

Schmajuk NA and Holland PC (eds.) (1998) *Occasion-Setting: Associative Learning and Cognition in Animals*. Washington, DC: American Psychological Association.

Schreurs BG and Kehoe EJ (1987) Cross-modal transfer as a function of initial training level in classical condition with rabbit. *Anim. Learn. Behav.* 15: 47–54.

Sobell MB and Sobell LC (1973) Individualized behavior therapy for alcoholics. *Behav. Ther.* 4: 49–72.

Soltysik SS, Wolfe GE, Nicholas T, Wilson J, and Garcia-Sanchez JL (1983) Blocking of inhibitory conditioning within a serial conditioned stimulus-conditioned inhibitor compound: Maintenance of acquired behavior without an unconditioned stimulus. *Learn. Motivation* 14: 1–29.

Spence KW and Norris EB (1950) Eyelid conditioning as a function of the inter-trial interval. *J. Exp. Psychol.* 40: 716–720.

Staddon JER (1988) Learning as inference. In: Bolles RC and Beecher MD (eds.) *Evolution and Learning*, pp. 59–78. Hillsdale, NJ: Erlbaum.

Stanford SC (1995) Central noradrenergic neurones and stress. *Pharmacol. Ther.* 68: 297–342.

Staubli U and Chun D (1996) Factors regulating the reversibility of long-term potentiation. *J. Neurosci.* 16: 853–860.

Suzuki A, Josselyn SA, Frankland PW, Masushige S, Silva AJ, and Kida S (2004) Memory reconsolidation and extinction have distinct temporal and biochemical signatures. *J. Neurosci.* 24: 4787–4795.

Swartzentruber D (1995) Modulatory mechanisms in Pavlovian conditioning. *Anim. Learn. Behav.* 23: 123–143.

Swartzentruber D and Bouton ME (1992) Context sensitivity of conditioned suppression following preexposure to the conditioned stimulus. *Anim. Learn. Behav.* 20: 97–103.

Tamai N and Nakajima S (2000) Renewal of formerly conditioned fear in rats after extensive extinction training. *Int. J. Comp. Psychol.* 13: 137–147.

Thewissen R, Snijders S, Havermans RC, van den Hout M, and Jansen A (2006) Renewal of cue-elicited urge to smoke: Implications for cue exposure treatment. *Behav. Res. Ther.* 44: 1441–1449.

Thomas BL and Ayres JJB (2004) Use of the ABA fear renewal paradigm to assess the effects of extinction with co-present fear inhibitors or excitors: Implications for theories of extinction and for treating human fears and phobias. *Learn. Motivation* 35: 22–51.

Vaiva G, Ducrocq F, Jezequel K, et al. (2003) Immediate treatment with propranolol decreases posttraumatic stress disorder two months after trauma. *Biol. Psychiatry* 54: 947–949.

Vansteenwegen D, Dirikx T, Hermans D, Vervliet B, and Eelen P (2006) Renewal and reinstatement of fear: Evidence from human conditioning research. In: Craske MG, Hermans D, and Vansteenwegen D (eds.) *Fear and Learning: Basic Science to Clinical Application*, pp. 197–215. Washington, DC: American Psychological Association.

Vansteenwegen D, Hermans D, Vervliet B, et al. (2005) Return of fear in a human differential conditioning paradigm caused by a return to the original acquisition context. *Behav. Res. Ther.* 43: 323–336.

Vogel EH, Brandon SE, and Wagner AR (2003) Stimulus representation in SOP: II. An application to inhibition of delay. *Behav. Processes* 62: 27–48.

Waddell J, Morris RW, and Bouton ME (2006) Effects of bed nucleus of the stria terminalis lesions on conditioned anxiety: Aversive conditioning with long-duration conditional stimuli and reinstatement of extinguished fear. *Behav. Neurosci.* 120: 324–336.

Wagner AR (1969) Stimulus selection and a 'modified continuity theory.' In: Bower GH and Spence JT (eds.) *The Psychology of Learning and Motivation,* vol. 3, pp. 1–41. New York: Academic Press.

Wagner AR (1981) SOP: A model of automatic memory processing in animal behavior. In: Spear NE and Miller RR (eds.) *Information Processing in Animals: Memory Mechanisms*, pp. 5–47. Hillsdale, NJ: Erlbaum.

Wagner AR and Brandon SE (1989) Evolution of a structured connectionist model of Pavlovian conditioning (AESOP). In: Klein SB and Mowrer RR (eds.) *Contemporary Learning Theories: Pavlovian Conditioning and the Status of Traditional Learning Theory*, pp. 149–189. Hillsdale, NJ: Erlbaum.

Wagner AR and Brandon SE (2001) A componential theory of Pavlovian conditioning. In: Mowrer RR and Klein SB (eds.) *Handbook of Contemporary Learning Theories*, pp. 23–64. Mahwah, NJ: Erlbaum.

Walker DL and Davis M (2002) The role of amygdala glutamate receptors in fear learning, fear-potentiated startle, and extinction. *Pharmacol. Biochem. Behav.* 71: 379–392.

Walker DL, Ressler KJ, Lu, K-T, and Davis M (2002) Facilitation of conditioned fear extinction by systemic administration or intra-amygdala infusions of D-cycloserine as assessed with fear-potentiated startle in rats. *J. Neurosci.* 15: 2343–2351.

Walker DL, Toufexis DJ, and Davis M (2003) Role of the bed nucleus of the stria terminalis versus the amygdala in fear, stress, and anxiety. *Eur. J. Pharmacol.* 463: 199–216.

Walker MP, Brakefield T, Hobson JA, and Stickgold R (2003) Dissociable stages of human memory consolidation and reconsolidation. *Nature* 425: 616–620.

Westbrook RF, Smith FJ, and Charnock DJ (1985) The extinction of an aversion: Role of the interval between non-reinforced presentations of the averted stimulus. *Q. J. Exp. Psychol.* 37B: 255–273.

Wilson A, Brooks DC, and Bouton ME (1995) The role of the rat hippocampal system in several effects of context in extinction. *Behav. Neurosci.* 109: 828–836.

Weidemann G and Kehoe EJ (2003) Savings in classical conditioning in the rabbit as a function of extended extinction. *Learn. Behav.* 31: 49–68.

Weidemann G and Kehoe EJ (2004) Recovery of the rabbit's conditioned nictitating membrane response without direct reinforcement after extinction. *Learn. Behav.* 32: 409–426.

Weidemann G and Kehoe EJ (2005) Stimulus specificity of concurrent recovery in the rabbit nictitating membrane response. *Learn. Behav.* 33: 343–362.

Wolpe J (1958) *Psychotherapy by Reciprocal Inhibition*. Stanford, CA: Stanford University Press.

Woods AM and Bouton ME (2006) D-cycloserine facilitates extinction but does not eliminate renewal of the conditioned emotional response. *Behav. Neurosci.* 120: 1159–1162.

Woods AM and Bouton ME (2007) Occasional reinforced responses during extinction can slow the rate of reacquisition of an operant response. *Learn. Motivation* 38: 56–74.

30 Reconsolidation: Historical Perspective and Theoretical Aspects

S. J. Sara, Collège de France, Paris, France

> *Everything flows and nothing abides; everything gives way and nothing stays fixed.* (Heraclitus 535–475 BC)

30.1 Historical Background: Thinking About Memory

Memory is dynamic, in that it is constantly being updated as it is retrieved. Heraclitus was the first writer to insist on this dynamic nature of memory with his metaphor cited above or with the more familiar,

> You can never step twice into the same river as other waters are ever flowing on you. (Heraclitus 535–475 BC).

William James (1892) updated this view, arguing that memory was a dynamic property of the nervous system, in constant flux as a result of being retrieved within current cognitive environments. These speculations were largely supported by the seminal experiments of Bartlett (1932), showing that information was gradually biased toward the subjects' cultural expectations as it was repeatedly recalled. Extensive evidence for this comes from laboratory studies of human memory processes over the past three decades, where old memories have been shown to be profoundly influenced by information in the retrieval environment, particularly if this information is in contradiction of the old memory (see Loftus, 2005a,b for reviews; *See also* Chapter 1).

30.1.1 Reconsolidation: A Hypothetical Construct

Postretrieval retrograde amnesia was demonstrated experimentally in rats several decades ago, but the term 'reconsolidation' was introduced more recently, as a hypothetical construct to account for amnesia after cued recall (Pryzbyslawsky and Sara, 1997). Reconsolidation has attracted wide interest among contemporary neurobiologists for a number of reasons, including broad therapeutic applications (Pryzbyslawsky and Sara, 1997; Debiec and Ledoux, 2006). There has been a proliferation of papers appearing in the literature in the past decade, mostly addressed at understanding the molecular and cellular mechanisms underlying this still-hypothetical process. As with any area of scientific inquiry, as the number of investigators addressing the question increases, so do discrepancies in results, alternative explanations of the data, and definitions of constraints. Several reviews of this recent literature are available (Nader, 2003; Dudai, 2004, 2006; Alberini, 2005; Alberini et al., 2006). The purpose of this chapter is to provide a deeper historical perspective from which to understand and evaluate current issues.

30.2 The Consolidation Hypothesis

30.2.1 Origins and Fate of the Consolidation Hypothesis

To understand the significance of the growing literature and issues being raised around the reconsolidation construct requires a brief reminder concerning the origins and fate of the consolidation hypothesis (for recent, more extensive, reviews see Dudai, 2004; Sara and Hars, 2006). Scientific investigation of memory processes was initiated at the end of the nineteenth century by German psychologists, first Ebbinghaus (1885) and then Mueller and Pilzecker (1900). Their studies of verbal learning and retention in human subjects led them to suggest that a memory trace was formed gradually over time after acquisition, and they introduced the term 'consolidation.' Contemporary with this were the very influential clinical observations and theoretical elaborations of the French psychiatrist, Ribot (1882). From his studies of amnesic patients, he formulated 'La loi de regression' that simply notes that as memories age, they become more resistant to trauma-induced amnesia. The origins of the neurobiological studies of memory processes can be found in early animal models of experimental amnesia (Duncan, 1945, 1948, 1949). Based on a clear temporal gradient of efficacy of the amnestic treatment, these early investigators concluded that retrograde amnesia experiments provided direct evidence for Mueller and Pilzecker's hypothesis stating that postlearning neural perseveration was necessary for consolidating memory. Electroconvulsive shock treatments (ECS) disrupted this activity, thereby preventing postacquisition memory consolidation. In the same year, and quite independently of Duncan's results, Hebb (1949) formalized the idea that propagating or recurrent impulses of a specific spatiotemporal pattern underlie initial memory. This provided the rationale for the use of ECS as an amnesic agent to study the temporal dynamics of consolidation, since such a specific spatiotemporal pattern of neural activity could hardly survive the electrical storm induced by ECS.

Thus the study of memory became, for the most part, a study of function through dysfunction. Investigators overwhelmingly relied on amnesia – either clinical studies of amnesic patients or animal models of experimental amnesia. The protocol of retrograde amnesia, indeed, opened a door on a neurobiological approach to the study of memory, evaluating the efficacy and temporal dynamics of diverse physiological treatments to disrupt memory without interfering with acquisition. The common feature of these experiments is that amnesic agents lose their ability to respectively impair memory as the interval between memory acquisition and treatment is increased, defining a temporal gradient. This large body of data supported the consolidation hypothesis, which stipulates that (1) memories are fixated or consolidated over time; (2) once consolidated, memories are then stable; and (3) acquisition of a new memory and its consolidation together form a unique event. Consolidation happens only once (McGaugh, 1966, 2000).

30.2.2 Challenges to the Consolidation Hypothesis

Embedded in the extensive literature on memory consolidation generated during the 1970s, however, were a myriad of studies challenging the interpretation of these retrograde amnesia experiments (*See also* Chapter 31). These include scores of demonstrations of recovery from retrograde amnesia over time or after a reminder. Spontaneous recovery at various times after ECS-induced amnesia was reported by Cooper and Koppenaal (1964), Kohlenberg and Trabasso (1968), Young and Galluscio (1971), and D'Andrea and Kesner (1973). There were similar reports of spontaneous recovery after protein-synthesis-induced amnesia as well (Quartermain et al., 1970; Serota, 1971; Squire and Barondes, 1972). Moreover, reminders before the retention test in the form of exposure to the conditioned stimulus (CS) or the unconditioned stimulus (US) (Koppenaal et al., 1967; Galluscio, 1971; Miller and Springer, 1972; Quartermain et al., 1972) or to the training context (Quartermain et al., 1970; Sara, 1973; Sara and David-Remacle, 1974) could effectively promote expression of memory in rats that had been submitted to an amnestic treatment after learning. Later, pharmacological studies added particularly strong arguments for the contention that the amnesic agent did not prevent formation of a memory trace. Drug treatment given before the retention test could attenuate or reverse amnesia (Gordon and Spear, 1973; Sara and Remacle, 1977; Rigter and VanRiezen, 1979; Quartermain et al., 1988). If the animal could express memory after a drug treatment, with no further exposures to the elements of the learning situation, then the recovery could not be attributed to new learning.

This large and growing body of literature benefited from a thorough and thoughtful review by Donald Lewis as early as 1976, in a paper titled "A cognitive approach to experimental amnesia." His conclusion at that time was that memory 'fixation' was very rapid – a matter of seconds, and that the extended retrograde amnesia gradient was due to the effect of the treatments on retrieval (Lewis, 1976). Indeed, if memory disruption after ECS, hypothermia, or protein synthesis inhibition is alleviated by reminders or drugs given before the test, then the sparing of the original memory trace would be a logical imperative, requiring an alternative explanation for the behavioral deficit. Reconsolidation has awakened new interest in this literature, generated more than 30 years ago, and several reviews by those very investigators who contributed the initial studies 30 years ago have been published recently (Gold, 2006; Riccio et al., 2006; Sara and Hars, 2006).

Many clinical investigators dealing with human amnesic patients also argued convincingly that amnestic syndromes were, for the most part, due to retrieval dysfunction. This was based on experiments showing that profoundly amnesic patients were able to benefit as much as healthy volunteers from partial cuing in a memory test of previously acquired word lists. This retrieval facilitation by cuing occurred even though the patients did not remember ever having learned the list. Such a phenomenon led to the conclusion that the memory deficit was due to a retrieval dysfunction rather than a failure to consolidate the new memory (Warrington and Weiskrantz, 1970). This naturally led to a call for consideration of retrieval, itself, as an intricate part of the memory process. Warrington and Weiskrantz went on to warn against any interpretation of behavioral deficits after amnestic treatments in animals as failure to consolidate, because it was impossible to demonstrate experimentally the absence of a memory trace. On the other hand, their studies clearly demonstrated that memory traces could be revealed by appropriate retrieval cues.

30.2.3 Amnesia and Forgetting as Retrieval Failure

Norman Spear took the position, with Weiskrantz, that all memory deficits, including forgetting, should be considered as retrieval failure, since it was impossible to prove the absence of a memory trace (Spear, 1971). He argued in several monographs published in the 1970s that memory studies should focus on retrieval. Remote memory is always apprehended through its retrieval and, especially in animal studies, through its expression as adaptive behavior. Thus the context in which the retention test is administered can play a determinant role in the behavioral expression of memory (or amnesia). The retrieval context includes the learning-associated environmental cues, and also the internal state of the animal, including motivational and attentional factors (Spear, 1971, 1973, 1976, 1981; Spear and Mueller, 1984). Indeed, many studies were later to confirm this hypothesis: Spontaneous forgetting of a complex maze task could be reversed by exposure to contextual cues just before the retention test (Deweer et al., 1980; Deweer and Sara, 1984; Gisquet-Verrier and Alexinsky, 1986). Furthermore, electrical stimulation of the mesencephalic reticular formation (MRF) (Sara et al., 1980; Dekeyne et al., 1987) or the noradrenergic nucleus locus coeruleus (Sara and Devauges, 1988; Devauges and Sara, 1991) also facilitated the retrieval of the a 'forgotten' maze task when administered before the retention test. All of these experiments used the same appetitively reinforced maze task adapted from that described by Donald Lewis in his earlier 'cue-dependent amnesia' studies (see below).

While emphasizing the 'lability' of the retrieval process and its dependence on the information in the retrieval environment, Spear's main thesis was that "consolidation occurs when memory is retrieved, as well as when it was stored originally" (Spear and Mueller, 1984, p. 116; see also Spear, 1981). Nevertheless, it is nowhere specified in Spear's writings that retrieval processes trigger time-dependent neurobiological processes identical to that occurring after learning, nor does he suggest experimental protocols that would test this thesis. The experiments cited above, demonstrating a facilitation of retrieval by pretest manipulations, do not directly address the issue of consolidation occurring at retrieval, because the retention test occurs within a time frame when one would expect residual effects of the memory-modulating treatment on behavior. The adequate protocol to test treatment effects on a putative post-retrieval consolidation would be to reactivate the memory by means of a retrieval cue, administer the treatment, and then test for retention at some later time, when the effects of the treatment would have dissipated. A change in memory expression, compared with a nontreated control group, could then be attributed to reinforcement or disruption of a postretrieval consolidation process.

30.3 Cue-Dependent Amnesia

30.3.1 Seminal Studies by Donald Lewis

Such experiments, carried out independently by Donald Lewis and his colleagues, demonstrated 'cue-dependent amnesia' in the rat. These studies showed that a temporally graded retrograde amnesia could be obtained when the memory trace was activated by a reminder of the original learning event, just before the amnestic treatment. While the 'recovery' studies, discussed above, challenged the consolidation hypothesis' claim that experimental amnesia procedures block the time-dependent formation of the memory trace, the 'cue-dependent amnesia' studies challenged the corollary that consolidation occurs only once, that is, that consolidated trace is fixed and impervious to further disruption (McGaugh, 1966, 2000; Dudai, 2004).

These studies of Lewis are really at the origin of today's 'reconsolidation' hypothesis, so it is appropriate to examine these experiments in detail to determine to what extent they already addressed some of the current issues being raised. In the first series of experiments from the Lewis laboratory, rats were trained in conditioned lick-suppression protocol. Thirsty rats learned to lick a drinking spout; when this behavior was well established, a tone (conditioned stimulus, CS), followed by a footshock (unconditioned stimulus, US), was presented during the ongoing licking behavior. Subsequent presentations of the tone alone elicited suppression of licking. A day after training, when memory expression was robust and reliable in control rats, the CS was presented alone, followed by electroconvulsive shock, a treatment that produces amnesia when administered after learning. Those rats that were 'reminded' by the CS, before ECS, showed a significant behavioral deficit when tested the following day. ECS in absence of the cue had no effect on subsequent behavior. These investigators referred to the phenomenon as 'cue-dependent amnesia.' Their interpretation was that the cue reinstated the memory, putting it in an active state and making it labile, as it was immediately after acquisition (Lewis and Maher, 1965, 1966; Misanin et al., 1968; Lewis, 1969, for review). Cue-dependent amnesia was replicated by Mactutus et al. (1979), see Lewis, 1969 for review using hypothermia as the amnesic agent.

Cue-dependent amnesia could likewise be induced by protein synthesis inhibition in much the same way that newly acquired memories are. Judge and Quartermain (1982) trained mice on the conditioned lick suppression task used by Lewis. The protein synthesis inhibitor anisomycin was injected systemically at different time intervals after a single memory reactivation, consisting of a brief exposure to the training context. There was a clear renewed efficacy of the treatment after reactivation, although the temporal gradient was steeper than for that generated after initial learning. (It can be noted that the conditioned lick suppression is a Pavlovian conditioning protocol based on the tone-shock association and, as such, is perfectly analogous to the 'conditioned fear' protocol that is now almost universally used in reconsolidation studies. In both cases the response to presentation of the CS alone is behavioral inhibition; i.e., lick suppression or freezing.)

Later experiments from the Lewis laboratory showed that the phenomenon of cue-dependent amnesia was not limited to aversive Pavlovian conditioning protocols. In a series of experiments, rats were trained in a complex maze consisting of four consecutive left–right choices, using food reward as the incentive (see **Figure 1**). The training procedure

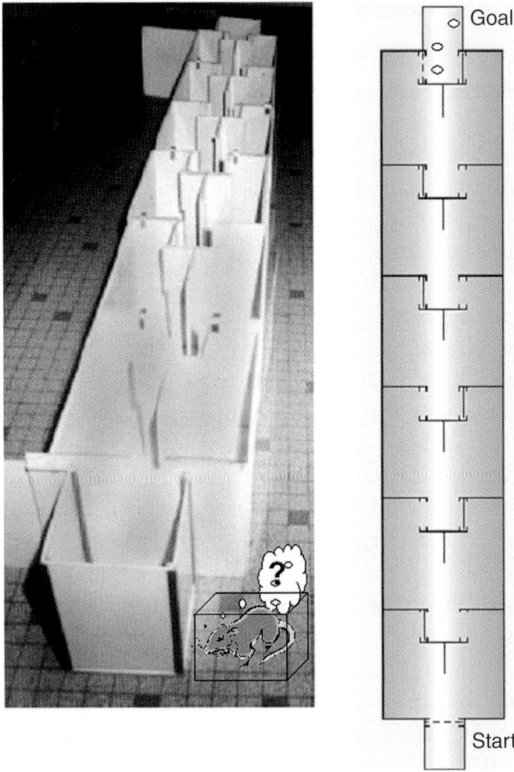

Figure 1 Krechevsky maze consisting of a series of left–right choices to reach a goal box containing palatable food. In the six-unit version, shown here, exposure to contextual cues in the experimental room, combined with stimulation of the reticular formation or the locus coeruleus just before the retention test, alleviated forgetting. A four-unit version of the task was used by Lewis to show cue-dependent amnesia. Adapted from Sara SJ (2000b) Strengthening the shaky trace through retrieval. *Nat. Rev. Neurosci.* 1: 212–213.

involved 10 days of elaborate pretraining, and then rats were trained for ten trials/day over several days until they reached the stringent behavioral criterion of 11/12 correct choices on three successive trials. During a 7-day rest period, rats were handled several times daily in order to extinguish handling-associated arousal. The following day, rats were exposed to the start box of the maze and the click of the door opening to provide reinstatement cues for the memory of the maze. This procedure was followed by electroconvulsive shock treatment. Retention was assessed 24 h later by counting the number of errors made before attaining the initial training criterion. Rats subjected to the reactivation procedure followed by ECS expressed profound amnesia compared with those subjected to ECS alone in the absence of the reactivation. A series of careful control experiments eliminated motivational and arousal confounds and explored the nature of the relevant cues in the start box. It was determined in this case that the click of the door opening in the start box was the salient feature in reinstating the memory (Lewis et al., 1972; Lewis and Bregman, 1973).

30.3.2 Behavioral Studies

Purely behavioral studies, in animals and humans, further confirmed that retrieval induces memory lability. Gordon and Spear (1973), in a series of experiments in rats, showed that reactivation of memory by various reminders makes it vulnerable to interference by another task, or to distortion by nonrelevant cues present at the moment of reactivation. This approach has been used recently with human subjects, showing that the memory for a list of junk objects can be distorted by intrusions from a second list presented right after the memory of the first list was reactivated by a reminder cue. An important observation in the latter series was that the disruption of memory was only expressed after a delay of 1 day; subjects tested right after learning the second list showed good retention (Hupbach et al., 2007). This experiment not only illustrates that memory can be distorted by intrusions but, on a more positive note, also shows how new information is integrated into an existing functional memory system when it is in an active state. This is the kind of analysis and approach advocated by Lewis several decades ago in his monograph entitled "A cognitive approach to experimental amnesia" (Lewis, 1976).

These studies are compatible with a long line of human studies suggesting that memory is substantially modified by the incorporation of new information during retrieval (Loftus, 1979, 1981). In the view of all these authors, the modulation of long-term memory is not an ongoing continuous process but occurs at transient windows of opportunity when the trace is in an active state. Reactivation can be spontaneous or triggered by external or internal events and, as discussed below, may even occur during sleep (see Sara and Hars, 2006, for review).

30.4 Cue-Dependent Amnesia: Neurobiological Hypotheses

Thus it was clearly established, by broad experimental evidence, as early as the late 1960–1970s, that well-consolidated memories are vulnerable to interference in a time-dependent manner when they were in an active state. Unfortunately, little attempt was made at the time to integrate this phenomenon of 'cue-dependent amnesia' into the rapidly developing neurobiological hypotheses of memory formation.

30.4.1 NMDA Receptors in Cue-Dependent Amnesia

In 1997, our interest in cue-dependent amnesia was rekindled by some unexpected results that would provide the opportunity for such integration. The initial purpose of our experiments had been to study the effect of *N*-methyl-D-aspartate (NMDA) receptor blockade on various stages of acquisition of a spatial reference memory task to fix a critical time point during the multisession acquisition when these receptors might play a specific role. The surprising result of the initial experiment was that not only did the NMDA receptor antagonist, MK-801, disrupt performance of a well-trained spatial task but the rats continued to show a decrement on the subsequent trial, 24 h later. Follow-up experiments showed that posttrial injections of the antagonist up to 2 h after the training trial likewise induced the performance decrement the following day. Given our long-standing interest in the dynamics of memory retrieval and recovery from amnesia, we interpreted these unexpected results within Lewis' conceptual framework of 'cue-dependent amnesia.' Since there were no previous reports of long-lasting effects of MK-801, we performed a series of experiments to confirm that a well-consolidated spatial memory, acquired over many days, reactivated by a single errorless trial, was somehow dependent upon intact NMDA receptors to maintain stability. The memory deficit was robust, in that there was no spontaneous recovery 48 h later (Przybyskawski and Sara, 1997, Exp4). Amnesia was, however, only partial, in that drug-treated rats could relearn the task and attain asymptotic levels of performance in only a few massed trials (Przybyskawski and Sara, 1997, Exp3). Extrapolating from these data, we suggested that

> memory is reconsolidated, so to speak, each time it is retrieved and these reconsolidation processes are dependent on the NMDA receptor for at least 2 h after the reactivation. (Przybyskawski and Sara, 1997, p. 245)

To our knowledge, this is the first use of the term 'reconsolidation' in the literature in relation to the well-established phenomenon of cue-dependent amnesia.

30.4.2 Role of the Noradrenergic System

We went on to investigate the role of beta-adrenergic receptors in this putative reconsolidation process and showed that postreactivation, a systemically injected beta antagonist, propranolol, induced amnesia in the spatial memory task protocol. Memory had to be reactivated by a single reminder trial for the drug to induce amnesia, expressed 24 h later.

As the spatial discrimination task is acquired over many trials, it does not lend itself to comparison of the temporal dynamics of postretrieval reconsolidation with that of postacquisition consolidation. This is an essential step in establishing that reconsolidation involves cellular processes similar to those occurring during the initial consolidation. Injection of propranolol after reactivation of a single-trial passive avoidance task also induced amnesia. In this case the effect of the beta receptor antagonist was even more robust after reactivation than after original training (Przybyskawski et al., 1999, Figs. 4 and 5).

Both the spatial memory task and passive avoidance memory formation depend upon hippocampal activity. To investigate the temporal dynamics of NMDA and beta receptors in reconsolidation in a task that does not involve the hippocampus, we used a simple, rapidly learned odor-reward association task (Tronel and Sara, 2002). Rats were extensively handled, mildly food deprived, and familiarized with the palatable reinforcement. Three sponges, each impregnated with a different odor, are arranged symmetrically within a wooden box; the spatial configuration of the sponges within the box are changed from trial to trial. Chocokrispies are hidden in the hole of the sponge with the target odor. The response is measured as a nose poke into the correct hole. Rats are very proficient at this task, learning the three-way discrimination in only three trials (for further details see Tronel and Sara, 2002). Intracerebroventricular (ICV) injections of an NMDA receptor antagonist induce amnesia not only when the injections are made immediately after learning (Tronel and Sara, 2003) but also when drug treatment is administered after a reminder cue consisting of the target odor presented in the experimental context (Torras-Garcia et al., 2005). In this task, ICV injection of beta receptor antagonists induces amnesia when the injection is made within a narrow time window around 2 h after learning, and the rat is tested 48 h later (**Figure 2**, top). Quite strikingly, the same temporal dynamic of involvement of beta receptors is seen after memory reactivation (**Figure 2**, bottom);

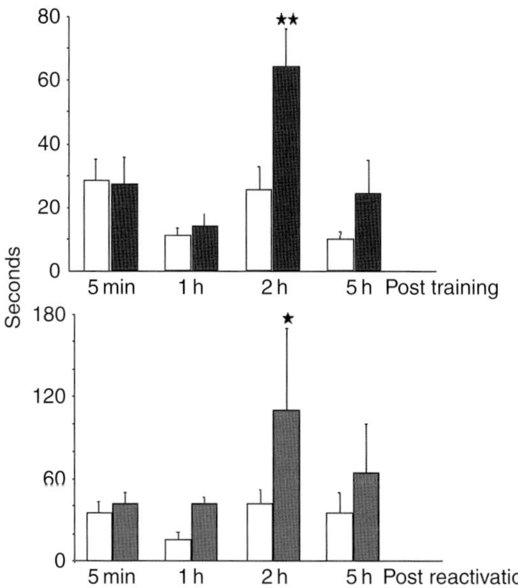

Figure 2 Retention performance in terms of latency to find the reward in an odor-reward association task 24 h after learning (top) or 24 h after memory reactivation by a brief exposure to the CS in the experimental context (bottom). Rats were injected with saline (white bars) or a beta receptor antagonist (red bars) at times indicated after training. There was a narrow time window at 2 h after training when the initial memory required beta receptors and a strikingly similar time window after reactivation when the drug treatment was effective in producing amnesia. Adapted from Tronel S, Feenstra MG, and Sara SJ (2004) Noradrenergic action in prefrontal cortex in the late stage of memory consolidation. *Learn. Mem.* 11: 453–458.

thus, the noradrenergic system appears to be involved in a late phase of memory consolidation, and again in reconsolidation (Tronel et al., 2004).

Based on the data from these studies, we proposed that treatment with propranolol in conjunction with psychotherapeutic memory reactivation could serve to attenuate the compulsive traumatic memories associated with posttraumatic stress disorder (Przybyskawski et al., 1999).

30.5 Rebirth of Reconsolidation

These pharmacological data, showing cue-dependent amnesia effects of NMDA and beta antagonists, merely confirmed and extended results obtained by many others nearly three decades earlier. Donald Lewis had proposed, in light of the large amount of data already available at this early date, to replace the consolidation paradigm by a conceptual framework of active and inactive memory in labile and stable states and to open the way for a more cognitive interpretation of amnestic syndromes (Lewis, 1979). It is truly ironic that the Lewis cue-dependent amnesia studies are at the origin of the current 'reconsolidation' hypothesis, as it is clear that the phenomenon of postreactivation lability cannot be understood by a simple extension of the consolidation concept. The problem is that cue-dependent amnesia is not predicted by the consolidation hypothesis and is, in fact, in direct contradiction of it. Neither Lewis nor his contemporaries used the term reconsolidation, and they were generally not interested in such questions as "does reconsolidation recapitulate consolidation?" Their aim had been merely to show that the amnesia gradient did not reflect the duration of a consolidation process and that consolidation was not a unique event. Memory was labile when in an active state, and lability was not time bound to acquisition. Indeed, the initial series of experiments was explicitly designed by Lewis and colleagues to challenge the interpretation of retrograde amnesia as consolidation failure and to inspire a more cognitive interpretation of memory function and dysfunction.

Nevertheless, there has been a surge of interest in 'reconsolidation' initiated by elegant experiments from the Ledoux laboratory. These investigators found that amnesia could be obtained after reactivation of conditioned fear by injecting, directly into the amygdala, the protein synthesis inhibitor anisomycin (Nader et al., 2000). The results obtained were similar to those of Judge and Quartermain (1982), except that now the protein synthesis inhibition was limited to a structure that is part of the neural circuit underlying the fear conditioning.

30.6 Neurobiological Substrates and Boundaries of Reconsolidation

The decade since this report has seen a proliferation of studies of cue-dependent amnesia that fall into two categories. One approach has been to study the cellular and molecular processes implicated in putative reconsolidation and to investigate to what extent they recapitulate consolidation processes occurring after initial learning. The second, and by far the more controversial, approach lies in an attempt to firmly establish (or repudiate) reconsolidation as a real phenomenon in memory processing by delineating the 'boundaries' within which cue-dependent amnesia can be obtained and sustained.

30.6.1 Neurobiological Substrates

The search for cellular and molecular substrates of reconsolidation has produced a myriad of results delineating neuromodulatory systems, neurotransmitters, intracellular signaling pathways, transcription factors, and brain regions that are necessary for both posttraining and postretrieval memory stabilization. Others seem to be specific to one or the other stage of memory processing. For example, NMDA receptors are necessary for both consolidation and reconsolidation across tasks and species (Pryzbyslawski and Sara, 1997; Pedreira et al., 2002; Torras-Garcia et al., 2005; Akirav and Maroun, 2006; Lee et al., 2006). The role of beta noradrenergic receptors, on the other hand, seems to be restricted to postretrieval memory processing (Roullet and Sara, 1998; Pryzbyslawski et al., 1999; Debiec and LeDoux, 2006; Diergaarde et al., 2006). Early implication of the transcription factor cAMP response element binding protein (CREB) in the stabilization of both new and reactivated fear memory was established by experiments using transgenic mice with inducible and reversible CREB repressor (Kida et al., 2002). This burgeoning literature concerning neurobiological substrates of postretrieval memory processes, focusing, for the most part, on intracellular cascades and immediate early gene expression, has been subject to several recent comprehensive reviews (Dudai and Eisenberg, 2004; Alberini, 2005; Alberini et al., 2006).

30.6.2 Boundaries of Reconsolidation

It is becoming increasingly evident, as the literature grows, that the same old questions raised during the consolidation era, concerning the nature of the memory deficit after an amnestic treatment, persist, although the discussion lacks the strong polemics of the past generation. Does the amnestic agent block consolidation, or now reconsolidation, or does it impair retrieval (*See* Chapter 31)? The single-trial inhibitory avoidance protocol that was used almost exclusively in earlier consolidation studies has been replaced by a simplified version of conditioned fear, in which a CS is associated with footshock to produce a conditioned emotional response measured as freezing behavior. The protein synthesis inhibitor, anisomycin, has largely replaced ECS as the generic amnestic agent in these reconsolidation boundary studies.

30.6.2.1 A note on the action of anisomycin

The increasing use of anisomycin as a generic amnestic agent to study boundaries and temporal dynamics of postretrieval memory processing is based on the widely held assumption that *de novo* protein synthesis is the final step of the intracellular cascade triggered by a learning or retrieval event and necessary for the consolidation or reconsolidation of long-term memory. This recent literature largely ignores the fact that caution was urged by the early users of protein synthesis inhibitors as amnestic agents in behavioral experiments, because of toxicity and ability to induce behavioral aversion. Thus, special care must be taken, especially in avoidance experiments, to dissociate aversive and amnestic effects of the drugs on behavior (Squire et al., 1975; Davis et al., 1980). Furthermore, several early investigators provided evidence that memory impairment attributed to protein synthesis inhibitors could be accounted for, at least in part, by specific effects on brain catecholamine systems (Flexner and Goodman, 1975; Quartermain et al., 1977; Flood et al., 1980; Altman and Quartermain, 1983; Davis and Squire, 1984, for review). These data take on particular importance in the light of several recent studies reporting the amnestic effects of the beta adrenergic antagonist propranolol after memory retrieval (see preceding paragraph).

More recent literature has underlined the fact that anisomycin activates the MAPkinase intracellular signaling pathway and causes apoptosis at doses lower that those that inhibit protein synthesis (Routtenberg and Rekart, 2005; Rudy et al., 2006). So, while the behavioral deficits associated with administration of anisomycin after memory reactivation are quite reliable, they may be caused by effects other than the inhibition of protein synthesis. This underlines the caveats inherent in elaborating a theory of memory function relying exclusively on a single paradigm that includes fear conditioning and anisomycin-induced amnesia.

30.6.2.2 Permanence of cue-dependent amnesia?

Is the memory deficit permanent, or is there spontaneous recovery or the possibility of recovering the memory by further treatments or reminders? Quartermain showed early on that postretrieval anisomycin-induced memory deficits in mice were less persistent than the deficits obtained by the same dose administered after training (Judge and Quartermain, 1982). They found spontaneous recovery of memory in mice 4 days after the reactivation-drug treatment, while behavioral expression of amnesia was still present in those mice receiving the anisomycin after training. In more recent studies, in mice submitted to context fear conditioning and systemic injection of anisomycin, amnesia is durable after acquisition, but after reactivation it is necessary to use repeated injections, and the amnesia is transitory (seen at 1 day but not at 21 days; Lattal and Abel, 2004; Prado-Alcala et al., 2006). Spontaneous recovery from cue-dependent amnesia has been confirmed by others using either systemic or locally injected anisomycin in rats, mice, chicks, or fish (Anokhin et al., 2002; Eisenberg and Dudai, 2004; Power et al., 2006). On the other hand, at least one group reports persistent amnesia even several weeks after retrieval and treatment by anisomycin (Duvarci and Nader, 2004). These discrepancies are similar to those reported decades ago concerning the nature and permanence of the memory dysfunction in experimental amnesia studies, as discussed above. Moreover, the same logical objection voiced by Warrington and Weiskrantz (1970) years ago can be raised here. Experimental amnesia studies are fatally flawed from the outset, since it is not possible to prove the null hypothesis (i.e., the absence of a memory trace).

30.6.2.3 Age and strength of the memory

The ease with which cue-dependent amnesia can be obtained may depend upon the age and the strength of the memory. Newer memories appear to be more susceptible to disruption after their retrieval than are older memories (Milekic and Alberini, 2002; Eisenberg and Dudai, 2004; Suzuki et al., 2004). Moreover, the strength of the memory, as revealed by the probability of its behavioral expression, also determines its vulnerability at retrieval. This has been shown by manipulating the number of unreinforced reminder trials to yield either reactivation or extinction (Eisenberg et al., 2003; Stollhoff et al., 2005). With a weak memory, resulting from a single training trial, in a conditioned taste aversion task, unreinforced presentation of the CS results in extinction. If this is followed by an amnestic treatment, extinction is blocked, and retention for initial learning is expressed at retention test. If the initial memory is strong, presentation of the CS reactivates the memory, rendering it labile, and amnesia is expressed at retention test (Eisenberg et al., 2003).

Another way to shift from retrieval to extinction in behavioral control is to modify the duration or the repetition of the cuing episode: a brief retrieval will reactivate the memory, making it labile. A long or repeated retrieval will lead to extinction (i.e., new learning, with its requirement for consolidation). Using a fear conditioning to context protocol, Suzuki et al. (2004) show that there is no amnesia with brief exposure to the CS (1 min), amnesia with a moderate exposure (3 min), or retention with a long CS exposure (30 min). This retention is interpreted as an amnesia for the extinction induced by the 30-min unreinforced CS exposure. Interestingly, they observe that the effective duration of cuing to induce lability increases with either the strength or the age of the memory.

30.6.2.4 Task- and species-related boundaries

Although most of the studies of cue-dependent amnesia use fear conditioning, the phenomenon can readily be obtained after different forms of appetitive and aversive learning in many species: rodents (Lewis et al., 1972; Lewis and Bregman, 1973; Pryzbyslawski and Sara, 1997; Pryzbyslawski et al., 1999; Torras-Garcia et al., 2005; Wang et al., 2005; *See* Chapter 29), and even in the honeybee (Stollhof et al., 2005), crab (Frenkel et al., 2005), slug (Sangha et al., 2003), and snail (Gainutdinova et al., 2005; Kemenes et al., 2006). Behavioral tasks used in these studies have included conditioned taste aversion (Eisenberg et al., 2003; Gruest et al., 2004a,b), object recognition (Kelly et al., 2003), inhibitory avoidance (Milekic and Alberini, 2002), instrumental incentive learning (Wang et al., 2005), odor reward association (Torras-Garcia et al., 2005), and eyelid conditioning (Inda et al., 2005). Moreover, at least in the case of rodents, this aspect of memorization is already present at the beginning of life, showing that it is a fundamental aspect of memory (Gruest et al., 2004a,b).

Despite generality of the cue-dependent amnesia phenomenon across species and tasks, some important constraints have recently been reported. Biedenkapp and Rudy (2004) attempted to induce amnesia by injecting anisomycin after reactivating a memory for a context. Rats received six massed exposures to a specific context in which they would be later receive tone–shock fear conditioning. In this particular protocol, the context preexposure is necessary for the rat to subsequently learn the tone–shock association. The authors clearly showed that intra-hippocampal anisomycin induces amnesia for the context when injections are made immediately after the preexposure. However, they failed to obtain cue-dependent amnesia if the injections were made after a 5-s or a 1-min reactivation of the context memory. One explanation that they offer to account for their negative findings is the 'significant event hypothesis.' A significant event is one that has been associated with a reinforcement, giving it predictive value. This hypothesis is quite appealing in light of the strong evidence for a major role for the locus-coeruleus noradrenergic system in memory retrieval and putative reconsolidation processes, as discussed above. It would take a 'significant event' to elicit the attention or arousal response associated with the activation of neuromodulatory systems (Sara, 1985, 1991; Bouret and Sara, 2004, 2006).

A related determinant of the lability of a reactivated memory is the extent to which a new encoding mode is solicited at the time of retrieval (Morris et al., 2006). These authors show that a reactivated spatial reference memory, learned in the water maze over several days, is not susceptible to amnesia induced by injection of a protein synthesis inhibitor into the hippocampus. It is only when new information must be integrated into the existing memory that amnesia follows such injections. These data fit nicely with the 'significant event' hypothesis. New information requiring behavioral adaptation should elicit attention and activate neuromodulatory systems necessary for stabilization of the reorganized memory.

30.6.2.5 A note on the problem with negative results

Cue-dependent amnesia studies lead to the conclusion that memory in an active state is labile and can be disrupted by a wide range of treatments, many of which are effective in producing amnesia when applied after new learning, as well. If an animal expresses amnesia after training and amnestic treatment, one concludes that memory consolidation was blocked by the treatment. If the memory is subsequently expressed after a reminder or a pharmacological treatment, one must conclude that the trace was there, but for some reason the animal could not express it behaviorally. What about possible outcomes of experiments evaluating the putative reconsolidation processes? There the amnestic agent is applied after a reminder that is supposed to reactivate the memory. If the rat expresses amnesia on a retention test, can it be taken as proof that the treatment erased or weakened the reactivated, labile trace by preventing reconsolidation? Suppose the memory is expressed at some later test? Or after a reminder? So, as Weiskrantz warned, we are faced with the impossible challenge of proving that the memory trace does not exist. When no cue-dependent amnesia is expressed on the retention test, there are several possible conclusions: (1) the amnestic agent was not effective in blocking reconsolidation because of, for example, inappropriate dose, (2) the reactivation treatment was not sufficient to elicit the memory to put it into an active labile state, or (3) postreactivation reconsolidation processes are not necessary.

30.7 Beyond Cue-Dependent Amnesia: Retrieval Strengthens Memory

This large body of literature concerned with cue-dependent amnesia confirms the *lability* of a memory trace after its reactivation, but it should not lead to the counterintuitive conclusion that retrieval weakens memory. Memory lability has always been easier to document behaviorally through amnesic rather than through promnesic treatments, which is why most investigators have chosen this research strategy. We know, however, that retrieval of memory does not usually result in wiping it out or even weakening it. On the contrary, a high level of attention or arousal during retrieval, a more likely real-life scenario, should *reinforce* the labile active memory. Remembering, especially when it involves effortful retrieval, usually occurs in an attentive, motivated behavioral state. During such states, neuromodulatory systems are activated (Bouret and Sara, 2004), releasing noradrenaline, dopamine, and other neuromodulators in the forebrain structures involved in the ongoing sensory processing and retrieval. These neuromodulators act to promote synaptic plasticity and trigger intracellular processes leading to new protein synthesis, upon which stable long-term memory is dependent (Sara, 2000a,b).

30.7.1 Cue-Dependent Enhancement

30.7.1.1 Enhancement by MRF stimulation

Although the strengthening of a memory trace by repeated remembering seems intuitively valid, experimental documentation of retrieval-associated memory improvement is rather sparse. There are a few reports of marked improvement of memory in the rat when retrieval is accompanied by arousal. Experiments by DeVietti et al. (1977) demonstrated that electrical stimulation of the mesencephalic reticular formation (MRF), which improves memory consolidation when administered within a short time after acquisition, improved memory for a well-consolidated conditioned fear response when it was applied after memory reactivation. The reactivation treatment consisted of a 15-s exposure to the tone in the training chamber; the rat was tested 24 h later. The shorter the interval between the reactivation and the MRF stimulation, the better the memory enhancement, the temporal gradient of efficacy being strikingly similar to the postacquisition gradient (**Figure 3**).

30.7.1.2 Enhancement by activation of the noradrenergic system

It has been shown repeatedly that stimulation of the noradrenergic system will enhance memory retrieval when given before the retention test (reviewed above), but it is only recently that the effects of pharmacologically increasing noradrenergic tonus on putative reconsolidation processes have been investigated. The alpha 2 receptor antagonist, idazoxan, increases firing of noradrenergic neurons of the locus coeruleus twofold at a dose that has no detectable effect on overt behavior such as locomotor activity (Sara, 1991). Rats were trained in the odor-reward association task used in the timolol studies described above. Forty-eight hours later, they were exposed to the odor in a neutral cage, located in the experimental room. This was followed by an injection of idazoxan; control rats were handled in the colony room before injection. Idazoxan enhanced performance when the rat was tested 48 h later, but only when the injection was given after memory reactivation (**Figure 4**). These data complement studies showing cue-dependent amnesia induced by beta adrenergic antagonists, discussed earlier. Together they lend support to the notion that the locus-coeruleus-noradrenergic system is activated by cues associated with target memories and contributes to the postreactivation stabilization or reinforcement of the memory (Sara, 2000b; see also Sara, 1985).

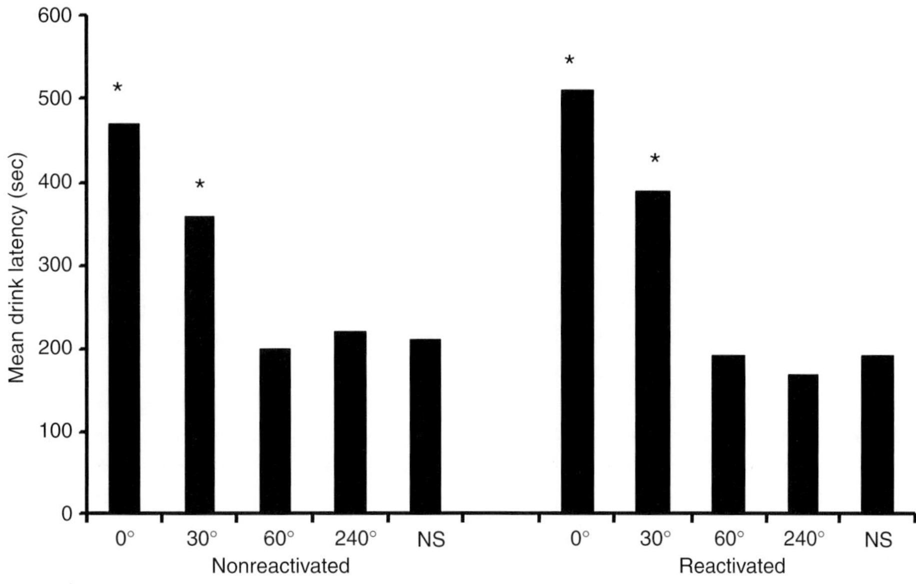

Figure 3 Retention performance in a lick suppression task after training and electrical stimulation of the mesencephalic reticular formation (MRF) (left) or after memory reactivation by the tone conditioned stimulus and (MRF) stimulation (right). In each condition one group of rats received no stimulation, to provide a baseline performance (NS). Histograms from left to right represent data from rats stimulated immediately after training or exposure to the tone or progressively longer delays. The treatment was effective in improving retention when applied up to 30 min after training; behavioral performance of rats stimulated after that was indistinguishable from that of NS rats. Note the striking similarity between the temporal gradient of efficacy after training and after reactivation. Figure adapted from Devietti TL, Conger GL, and Kirkpatrick BR (1977) Comparison of the enhancement gradients of retention obtained with stimulation of the mesencephalic reticular formation after training or memory reactivation. *Physiol. Behav.* 19: 549–554, with permission from Elsevier.

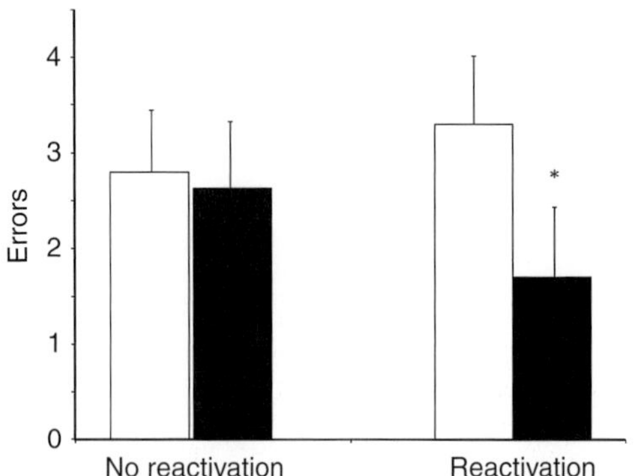

Figure 4 Retention performance in terms of errors before finding the reward in a retention test, 3 weeks after learning the odor-reward association test. Left: data from rats receiving no reactivation on the day before the test. Right: data from rats exposed for a few minutes to the target odor in the experimental room, 24 h before the retention test. White bars: saline injections after reactivation or no reactivation. Black bars: rats injected with idazoxan (an alpha 2 receptor antagonist that increases release of NE), 2 mg kg^{-1} ip, after no reactivation or reactivation.

30.7.1.3 Enhancement by activation of PKA

The beta adrenergic receptor is one of a family of receptors positively linked to G proteins that serve to activate the cyclic AMP intracellular signaling cascade, leading to gene induction by the transcription factor CREB. The resulting *de novo* protein synthesis is thought to be essential for the stabilization of long-term memory. Activation of protein kinase A (PKA) is an important step in this cyclic AMP intracellular signaling cascade. A recent study by Tronson et al. (2006) has shown that pharmacologically activating PKA within the rat amygdala can facilitate fear memory if and only if the memory has been reactivated by a reminder. These results, taken together with the studies showing enhancement of reactivated memory by beta adrenergic agonists, lend support to the notion that the noradrenergic system, activated at retrieval, serves to reinforce memories rendered labile by reactivation.

30.7.2 Clinical Significance of Cue-Dependent Enhancement

Clinical syndromes such as posttraumatic stress disorder (PTSD), phobias, obsessive compulsion, and craving in addiction share the common feature of underlying compelling, persistent memories. The possibility that memory may be rendered labile under controlled conditions has broad therapeutic applications for these disorders, accounting for the increasing number of investigators interested in this aspect of memory.

In particular, the susceptibility of reactivated memories to noradrenergic manipulation sheds some light on the underlying mechanisms of pathological persistence of memory. In the case of PTSD, it has already been established that there is greater noradrenergic (NE) activity under baseline conditions in patients with chronic PTSD than in healthy subjects, with a direct relationship of NE activity to the severity of the clinical syndrome (Geracioti et al., 2001). Further activation of this system during stress could recreate the internal state induced by the original trauma and thereby reinstate the memory (Grillon et al., 1996). The demonstrated role of the intracellular pathway activated by this system in reinforcing reactivated memories (Tronson et al., 2006) suggests that the memory recalled in the presence of a high level of NE will be reinforced each time (see also **Figure 3**).

The potential usefulness of noradrenergic receptor–blocking agents in PTSD has already been pointed out by Cahill (1997), who suggested that treatment with beta blockers as soon as possible after the traumatic event might prevent the development of PTSD. The recent 'rediscovery' of the phenomenon of lability of memory in its active state adds a new dimension to this potential use. Treatment with beta receptor antagonists, at the time of spontaneous or clinically elicited reinstatement of the traumatic memory, should serve to attenuate the active memory by blocking reconsolidation processes (Przybyskawski et al., 1999).

30.8 New Look at Retrieval and 'Reconsolidation'

Memory only lends itself to study through its retrieval; as William James underlined more than a century ago, "the only proof of there being retention is that recall actually takes place" (James, 1892). Although some memory retrieval is likely to occur spontaneously as a result of random fluctuations of network activity in the brain, retrieval is usually brought about with effort, as a result of integration of incoming environmental information with the 'memory network' driven by that information (Tulving and Thomson, 1973). It follows from this that the formation of new memories will always be made on the background of retrieved information. Recent functional imaging studies in humans are, indeed, confirming these earlier theoretical speculations (e.g., Nyberg et al., 1996a,b; Cabeza et al., 2002;). They are providing clear evidence that it is memory of the past that organizes and provides meaning to the present perceptual experience. Borrowing Tulving's terminology, new episodic memory, to be remembered in a meaningful way, must be consolidated within a preexisting semantic memory (Tulving, 2002).

This analysis does not allow a clear demarcation between consolidation and retrieval processes, and in this view, it can be assumed that every retrieval operation should trigger a reconsolidation process. This is a view similar to that of Spear, although he never used the term 'reconsolidation' (Spear and Mueller, 1984). It follows from this that retrieval will change the information content of the 'trace' such that memory can be viewed as an emergent, dynamic, adaptive property of the nervous system. It is in that sense that

> Everything flows and nothing abides; everything gives way and nothing stays fixed.

References

Akirav I and Maroun M (2006) Ventromedial prefrontal cortex is obligatory for consolidation and reconsolidation of object recognition memory. *Cereb. Cortex* 16: 1759–1765.

Alberini CM (2005) Mechanisms of memory stabilization: Are consolidation and reconsolidation similar or distinct processes? *Trends Neurosci.* 28: 51–56.

Alberini CM, Milekic MH, and Tronel S (2006) Memory: Mechanisms of memory stabilization and de-stabilization. *Cell. Mol. Life Sci.* 63: 999–1008.

Altman HJ and Quartermain D (1983) Facilitation of memory retrieval by centrally administered catecholamine stimulating agents. *Behav. Brain Res.* 7: 51–63.

Anokhin KV, Tiunova AA, and Rose SP (2002) Reminder effects – Reconsolidation or retrieval deficit? Pharmacological dissection with protein synthesis inhibitors following reminder for a passive-avoidance task in young chicks. *Eur. J. Neurosci.* 15: 1759–1765.

Bartlett FC (1932) *Remembering: A Study in Experimental and Social Psychology.* Cambridge: Cambridge University Press.

Biedenkapp JC and Rudy JW (2004) Context memories and reactivation, constraints on the reconsolidation hypothesis. *Behav. Neurosci.* 118: 956–964.

Bouret S and Sara SJ (2004) Reward expectation, orientation of attention and locus coeruleus-medial frontal cortex interplay during learning. *Eur. J. Neurosci.* 20: 791–802.

Bouret S and Sara SJ (2006) Network reset, a simplified overarching theory of locus coeruleus noradrenaline function. *Trends Neurosci.* 28: 574–582.

Cabeza R, Dolcos F, Graham R, and Nyberg L (2002) Similarities and differences in the neural correlates of episodic memory retrieval and working memory. *Neuroimage* 16: 317–330.

Cahill L (1997) The neurobiology of emotionally influenced memory. Implications for understanding traumatic memory. *Ann. N.Y. Acad. Sci.* 821: 238–246.

Cooper RM and Koppenaal RJ (1964) Suppression and recovery of a one-trial avoidance response after a single ECS. *Psychon. Sci.* 303–304.

D'Andrea J and Kesner R (1973) The effects of ECS and hypoxia on information retrieval. *Physiol. Behav.* 11: 747–752.

Davis HP, Rosenzweig MR, Bennett EL, and Squire LR (1980) Inhibition of cerebral protein synthesis, dissociation of nonspecific effects and amnesic effects. *Behav. Neural Biol.* 28: 99–104.

Davis HP and Squire LR (1984) Protein synthesis and memory, a review. *Psychol. Bull.* 96: 518–559.

Debiec J and LeDoux JE (2006) Noradrenergic signaling in the amygdala contributes to the reconsolidation of fear memory: Treatment implications for PTSD. *Ann. N.Y. Acad. Sci.* 1071: 521–524.

Dekeyne A, Deweer B, and Sara SJ (1987) Background stimuli as a reminder after spontaneous forgetting: Potentiation by stimulation of the mesencephalic reticular formation. *Psychobiology* 15: 161–166.

Devauges V and Sara SJ (1991) Memory retrieval enhancement by locus coeruleus stimulation, evidence for mediation by beta receptors. *Behav. Brain Res.* 43: 93–97.

DeVietti TL, Conger GL, and Kirkpatrick BR (1977) Comparison of the enhancement gradients of retention obtained with stimulation of the mesencephalic reticular formation after training or memory reactivation. *Physiol. Behav.* 19: 549–554.

Deweer B and Sara SJ (1984) Background stimuli as a reminder after spontaneous forgetting, Role of duration of cuing and cuing-test interval. *Anim. Learn. Behav.* 12: 238–247.

Deweer B, Sara SJ, and Hars B (1980) Contextual cues and memory retrieval in rats. Alleviation of forgetting by a pretest exposure to background stimuli. *Anim. Learn. Behav.* 8: 265–272.

Diergaarde L, Schoffelmeer AN, and De Vries TJ (2006) Beta-adrenoceptor mediated inhibition of long-term reward-related memory reconsolidation. *Behav. Brain Res.* 170: 333–336.

Dudai Y (2004) The neurobiology of consolidations, or, how stable is the engram? *Annu. Rev. Psychol.* 55: 51–86.

Dudai Y (2006) Reconsolidation, the advantage of being refocused. *Curr. Opin. Neurobiol.* 16: 174–178.

Dudai Y and Eisenberg M (2004) Rites of passage of the engram, reconsolidation and the lingering consolidation hypothesis. *Neuron* 44: 93–100.

Duncan CP (1945) The effect of electroshock convulsions on the maze habit in the white rat. *J. Exp. Psychol.* 35: 267–278.

Duncan C (1948) Habit reversal deficit induced by electroshock in the rat. *J. Comp. Physiol. Psychol.* 41: 11–16.

Duncan CP (1949) The retroactive effect of electroshock on learning. *J. Comp. Physiol. Psychol.* 42: 32–44.

Duvarci S and Nader K (2004) Characterization of fear memory reconsolidation. *J. Neurosci.* 24: 9269–9275.

Ebbinghaus H (1885) *Uber des Gedachtnis, untercuchungen zur experimentellen Psychologie.* Berlin: Dunker & Humbolt.

Eisenberg M and Dudai Y (2004) Reconsolidation of fresh, remote, and extinguished fear memory in Medaka: Old fears don't die. *Eur. J. Neurosci.* 20: 3397–3403.

Eisenberg M, Kobilo T, Berman DE, and Dudai Y (2003) Stability of retrieved memory, inverse correlation with trace dominance. *Science* 301: 1102–1104.

Flexner LB and Goodman RH (1975) Studies on memory, inhibitors of protein synthesis also inhibit catecholamine synthesis. *Proc. Natl. Acad. Sci. USA* 72: 4660–4663.

Flood JF, Smith GE, and Jarvik ME (1980) A comparison of the effects of localized brain administration of catecholamine and protein synthesis inhibitors on memory processing. *Brain Res.* 197: 153–165.

Frenkel L, Maldonado H, and Delorenzi A (2005) Memory strengthening by a real-life episode during reconsolidation, an outcome of water deprivation via brain angiotensin II. *Eur. J. Neurosci.* 22: 1757–1766.

Gainutdinova TH, Tagirova RR, Ismailova AI, et al. (2005) Reconsolidation of a context long-term memory in the terrestrial snail requires protein synthesis. *Learn. Mem.* 12: 620–625.

Galluscio E (1971) Retrograde amnesia induced by electroconvulsive shock and carbon dioxyde anesthesia in rats, an attempt to stimulate recovery. *J. Comp. Physiol. Psychol.* 75: 136–140.

Geracioti TD Jr., Baker DG, Ekhator NN, et al. (2001) CSF norepinephrine concentrations in posttraumatic stress disorder. *Am. J. Psychiatry* 158: 1227–1230.

Gisquet-Verrier P and Alexinsky T (1986) Does contextual change determine long-term forgetting? *Anim. Learn. Behav.* 14: 349–358.

Gold PE (2006) The many faces of amnesia. *Learn. Mem.* 13: 506–514.

Gordon WC and Spear NE (1973) The effects of strychnine on recently acquired and reactivated passive avoidance memories. *Physiol. Behav.* 10: 1071–1075.

Grillon C, Southwick SM, and Charney DS (1996) The psychobiological basis of posttraumatic stress disorder. *Mol. Psychiatry* 1: 278–297.

Gruest N, Richer P, and Hars B (2004a) Emergence of long-term memory for conditioned aversion in the rat fetus. *Dev. Psychobiol.* 44: 189–198.

Gruest N, Richer P, and Hars B (2004b) Memory consolidation and reconsolidation in the rat pup require protein synthesis. *J. Neurosci.* 24: 10488–10492.

Hebb DO (1949) *The Organisation of Behavior.* New York: John Wiley.

Hupbach A, Gomez R, Hardt O, and Nadel L (2007) Reconsolidation of episodic memories: A subtle reminder triggers integration of new information. *Learn. Mem.* 14: 47–53.

Inda MC, Delgado-Garcia JM, and Carrion AM (2005) Acquisition, consolidation, reconsolidation, and extinction of eyelid conditioning responses require *de novo* protein synthesis. *J. Neurosci.* 25: 2070–2080.

James W (1892) *The Principles of Psychology.* New York: Henry Holt.

Judge ME and Quartermain D (1982) Characteristics of retrograde amnesia following reactivation of memory in mice. *Physiol. Behav.* 28: 585–590.

Kelly A, Laroche S, and Davis S (2003) Activation of mitogen-activated protein kinase/extracellular signal-regulated kinase in hippocampal circuitry is required for consolidation and reconsolidation of recognition memory. *J. Neurosci.* 23: 5354–5360.

Kemenes G, Kemenes I, Michel M, Papp A, and Muller U (2006) Phase-dependent molecular requirements for memory reconsolidation: Differential roles for protein synthesis and protein kinase A activity. *J. Neurosci.* 26: 6298–6302.

Kida S, Josselyn SA, de Ortiz SP, et al. (2002) CREB required for the stability of new and reactivated fear memories. *Nat. Neurosci.* 5: 348–355.

Kohlenberg R and Trabasso T (1968) Recovery of a conditioned emotional response after one or two electroconvulsive shocks. *J. Comp. Physiol. Psychol.* 65: 270–273.

Koppenaal R, Jogoda E, and Cruce JA (1967) Recovery from ECS produced amnesia following a reminder. *Psychon. Sci.* 9: 293–294.

Lattal KM and Abel T (2004) Behavioral impairments caused by injections of the protein synthesis inhibitor anisomycin after contextual retrieval reverse with time. *Proc. Natl. Acad. Sci. USA* 101: 4667–4672.

Lee JL, Milton AL, and Everitt BJ (2006) Reconsolidation and extinction of conditioned fear: Inhibition and potentiation. *J. Neurosci.* 26: 10051–10056.

Lewis DJ (1969) Sources of experimental amnesia. *Psychol. Rev.* 76: 461–472.

Lewis DJ (1976) A cognitive approach to experimental amnesia. *Am. J. Psychol.* 89: 51–80.

Lewis DJ (1979) Psychobiology of active and inactive memory. *Psychol. Bull.* 86: 1054–1083.

Lewis DJ and Bregman NJ (1973) Source of cues for cue-dependent amnesia in rats. *J. Comp. Physiol. Psychol.* 85: 421–426.

Lewis DJ, Bregman NJ, and Mahan JJ, Jr. (1972) Cue-dependent amnesia in rats. *J. Comp. Physiol. Psychol.* 81: 243–247.

Lewis DJ and Maher BA (1965) Neural consolidation and electroconvulsive shock. *Psychol. Rev.* 72: 225–239.

Lewis DJ and Maher BA (1966) Electroconvulsive shock and inhibition, some problems considered. *Psychol. Rev.* 73: 388–392.

Loftus EF (1979) The malleability of human memory. *Am. Sci.* 67: 312–320.

Loftus EF (1981) Natural and unnatural cognition. *Cognition* 10: 193–196.

Loftus EF (2005a) Planting misinformation in the human mind: A 30-year investigation of the malleability of memory. *Learn. Mem.* 12: 361–366.

Loftus EF (2005b) Searching for the neurobiology of the misinformation effect. *Learn. Mem.* 12: 1–2.

Mactutus CF, Riccio DC, and Ferek JM (1979) Retrograde amnesia for old reactivated memory, some anomalous characteristics. *Science* 204: 1319–1320.

McGaugh JL (1966) Time dependent processes in memory storage. *Science* 153: 1351–1358.

McGaugh JL (2000) Memory – A century of consolidation. *Science* 287: 248–251.

Milekic MH and Alberini CM (2002) Temporally graded requirement for protein synthesis following memory reactivation. *Neuron* 36: 521–525.

Miller RR and Springer AD (1972) Induced recovery of memory in rats following electroconvulsive shock. *Physiol. Behav.* 8: 645–651.

Misanin JR, Miller RR, and Lewis DJ (1968) Retrograde amnesia produced by electroconvulsive shock after reactivation of a consolidated memory trace. *Science* 160: 554–555.

Morris RG, Inglis J, Ainge JA, et al. (2006) Memory reconsolidation, sensitivity of spatial memory to inhibition of protein synthesis in dorsal hippocampus during encoding and retrieval. *Neuron* 50: 479–489.

Mueller GE and Pilzecker A (1900) Experimentelle Beitrage zur Lehre vom Gedachtniss. *Z. Psychol.* 10: 388–394.

Nader K (2003) Memory traces unbound. *Trends Neurosci.* 26: 65–72.

Nader K, Schafe GE, and Le Doux JE (2000) Fear memories require protein synthesis in the amygdala for reconsolidation after retrieval. *Nature* 406: 722–726.

Nyberg L, McIntosh AR, Cabeza R, et al. (1996a) Network analysis of positron emission tomography regional cerebral blood flow data, ensemble inhibition during episodic memory retrieval. *J. Neurosci.* 16: 3753–3759.

Nyberg L, McIntosh AR, Houle S, Nilsson LG, and Tulving E (1996b) Activation of medial temporal structures during episodic memory retrieval. *Nature* 380: 715–717.

Pedreira M, Perez-Cuesta LM, and Maldonado H (2002) Reactivation and reconsolidation of long-term memory in the crab *Chasmagnathus*: Protein synthesis requirement and mediation by NMDA-type glutamate receptors. *J. Neurosci.* 22: 8305–8311.

Power AE, Berlau DJ, McGaugh JL, and Steward O (2006) Anisomycin infused into the hippocampus fails to block "reconsolidation" but impairs extinction: The role of re-exposure duration. *Learn. Mem.* 13: 27–34.
Prado-Alcala RA, Diaz Del Guante MA, Garin-Aguilar ME, Diaz-Trujillo A, Quirarte GL, and McGaugh JL (2006) Amygdala or hippocampus inactivation after retrieval induces temporary memory deficit. *Neurobiol. Learn. Mem.* 86: 144–149.
Przybyslawski J, Roullet P, and Sara SJ (1999) Attenuation of emotional and nonemotional memories after their reactivation, role of beta adrenergic receptors. *J. Neurosci.* 19: 6623–6628.
Przybyslawski J and Sara SJ (1997) Reconsolidation of memory after its reactivation. *Behav. Brain Res.* 84: 241–246.
Quartermain D, Freedman LS, Botwinick CY, and Gutwein BM (1977) Reversal of cycloheximide-induced amnesia by adrenergic receptor stimulation. *Pharmacol. Biochem. Behav.* 7: 259–267.
Quartermain D, Judge ME, and Jung H (1988) Amphetamine enhances retrieval following diverse sources of forgetting. *Physiol. Behav.* 43: 239–241.
Quartermain D, McEwen B, and Azmita E (1970) Amnesia produced by electroconvulsive shock or cycloheximide, conditions for recovery. *Science* 169: 683–686.
Quartermain D, McEwen B, and Azmita E (1972) Recovery of memory following amnesia in the rat and mouse. *J. Comp. Physiol. Psychol.* 79: 360–379.
Ribot T (1882) *Diseases of Memory.* New York: Appleton-Century Crofts.
Riccio DC, Millin PM, and Bogart AR (2006) Reconsolidation: A brief history, a retrieval view, and some recent issues. *Learn. Mem.* 13: 536–544.
Rigter H and Van Riezen H (1979) Pituitary hormones and amnesia. *Curr. Dev. Psychopharmacol.* 5: 67–124.
Roullet P and Sara S (1998) Consolidation of memory after its reactivation, involvement of beta noradrenergic receptors in the late phase. *Neural Plast.* 6: 63–68.
Routtenberg A and Rekart JL (2005) Post-translational protein modification as the substrate for long-lasting memory. *Trends Neurosci.* 28: 12–19.
Rudy JW, Biedenkapp JC, Moineau J, and Bolding K (2006) Anisomycin and the reconsolidation hypothesis. *Learn. Mem.* 13: 1–3.
Sangha S, Scheibenstock A, and Lukowiak K (2003) Reconsolidation of a long-term memory in *Lymnaea* requires new protein and RNA synthesis and the soma of right pedal dorsal 1. *J. Neurosci.* 23: 8034–8040.
Sara SJ (1973) Recovery from hypoxia and ECS-induced amnesia after a single exposure to training environment. *Physiol. Behav.* 10: 85–89.
Sara SJ (1985) Noradrenergic modulation of selective attention, its role in memory retrieval. *Ann. N.Y. Acad. Sci.* 444: 178–193.
Sara SJ (1991) Noradrenaline and memory: Neuromodulatory effects on retrieval. In: Weinman J and Hunter J (eds.) *Memory: Neurochemical and Clinical Aspects*, pp. 105–128. London: Harwood Academic.
Sara SJ (2000a) Retrieval and reconsolidation: Toward a neurobiology of remembering. *Learn. Mem.* 7: 73–84.
Sara SJ (2000b) Strengthening the shaky trace through retrieval. *Nat. Rev. Neurosci.* 1: 212–213.
Sara SJ and David-Remacle M (1974) Recovery from electroconvulsive shock-induced amnesia by exposure to the training environment, pharmacological enhancement by piracetam. *Psychopharmacologia* 36: 59–66.
Sara SJ and Devauges V (1988) Priming stimulation of locus coeruleus facilitates memory retrieval in the rat. *Brain Res.* 438: 299–303.
Sara SJ and Devauges V (1989) Idazoxan, an alpha-2 antagonist, facilitates memory retrieval in the rat. *Behav. Neural Biol.* 51: 401–411.
Sara SJ, Deweer B, and Hars B (1980) Reticular stimulation facilitates retrieval of a "forgotten" maze habit. *Neurosci. Lett.* 18: 211–217.
Sara SJ and Hars B (2006) In memory of consolidation. *Learn. Mem.* 13: 515–521.
Sara SJ and Remacle JF (1977) Strychnine-induced passive avoidance facilitation after electroconvulsive shock or undertraining, a retrieval effect. *Behav. Biol.* 19: 465–475.
Serota RG (1971) Acetoxycycloheximide and transient amnesia in the rat. *Proc. Natl. Acad. Sci. USA* 68: 1249–1250.
Spear NE (1971) *Animal Memory.* New York: Academic Press.
Spear NE (1973) Retrieval of memory in animals. *Psychol. Rev.* 80: 163–194.
Spear NE (1976) Ontogenetic factors in the retrieval of memories. *Act. Nerv. Super. Praha.* 18: 302–311.
Spear NE (1981) Extending the domain of memory retrieval. In: Spear NE and Miller RR (eds.) *Information Processing in Animals, Memory Mechanisms*, pp. 341–378. Hillsdale NJ: Lawrence Erlbaum Associates.
Spear NE and Mueller CW (1984) Consolidation as a function of retrieval. In: Weingartner H and Parker ES (eds.) *Memory Consolidation, Psychobiology of Cognition*, pp. 111–147. Hillsdale, NJ: Lawrence Erlbaum Associates.
Squire LR and Barondes SH (1972) Variable decay of memory and its recovery in cycloheximide-treated rats. *Proc. Natl. Acad. Sci. USA* 69: 1416–1420.
Squire LR, Emanuel CA, Davis HP, and Deutsch JA (1975) Inhibitors of cerebral protein synthesis, dissociation of aversive and amnesic effects. *Behav. Biol.* 14: 335–341.
Stollhoff N, Menzel R, and Eisenhardt D (2005) Spontaneous recovery from extinction depends on the reconsolidation of the acquisition memory in an appetitive learning paradigm in the honeybee *Apis Mellifera*. *J. Neurosci.* 25: 4485–4492.
Suzuki A, Josselyn SA, Frankland PW, Masushige S, Silva AJ, and Kida S (2004) Memory reconsolidation and extinction have distinct temporal and biochemical signatures. *J. Neurosci.* 24: 4787–4795.
Torras-Garcia M, Lelong J, Tronel S, and Sara SJ (2005) Reconsolidation after remembering an odor-reward association requires NMDA receptors. *Learn. Mem.* 12: 18–22.
Tronel S, Feenstra MG, and Sara SJ (2004) Noradrenergic action in prefrontal cortex in the late stage of memory consolidation. *Learn. Mem.* 11: 453–458.
Tronel S and Sara SJ (2002) Mapping of olfactory memory circuits, region-specific c-fos activation after odor-reward associative learning or after its retrieval. *Learn. Mem.* 9: 105–111.
Tronel S and Sara SJ (2003) Blockade of NMDA receptors in prelimbic cortex induces an enduring amnesia for odor-reward associative learning. *J. Neurosci.* 23: 5472–5476.
Tronson NC, Wiseman SL, Olausson P, and Taylor JR (2006) Bidirectional behavioral plasticity of memory reconsolidation depends on amygdalar protein kinase A. *Nat. Neurosci.* 9: 167–169.
Tulving E (2002) Episodic memory: From mind to brain. *Annu. Rev. Psychol.* 53: 1–25.
Tulving E and Thomson D (1973) Encoding specificity and retrieval processes in episodic memory. *Psychol. Rev.* 80: 352–372.
Wang SH, Ostlund SB, Nader K, and Balleine BW (2005) Consolidation and reconsolidation of incentive learning in the amygdala. *J. Neurosci.* 25: 830–835.
Warrington EK and Weiskrantz L (1970) Amnesic syndrome, consolidation or retrieval? *Nature* 228: 628–630.
Young AG and Galluscio EH (1971) Recovery from ECS produced amnesia. *Psychon. Sci.* 22: 149–151.

31 Retrieval from Memory

G. P. Urcelay and R. R. Miller, State University of New York at Binghamton, Binghamton, NY, USA

31.1 Retrieval from Memory

The field of learning and memory has traditionally emphasized acquisition and storage as the critical determinants of learned behavior (*See* Chapter 1). In the field of associative learning, this orientation is clearly evident in Pavlov's work, which suggested that spreading activation between nodes was necessary for memory formation (Pavlov, 1927). Similarly, Hebb (1949) proposed that experiencing a learning event temporarily activates certain neural circuits that, while active, strengthen the synaptic connections that constitute the basis for that experience becoming permanently stored in memory. This emphasis on acquisition and storage can be seen at many different levels of analysis. For instance, in the human memory literature, Craik and Lockhart (1972) proposed that the acquisition and storage of new information would create a more durable memory trace if processing during the acquisition (i.e., study) phase occurred at a relatively deep level (i.e., more integrative semantic than superficial phonetic). As another example, the Rescorla–Wagner rule for the formation of associations assumes that competition between stimuli trained together in a Pavlovian conditioning preparation occurs exclusively during the training phase (Rescorla and Wagner, 1972). All these views share the common assumption that any disruptive manipulation that occurs during training will inevitably result in that learned information being permanently lost and unavailable in future encounters within a similar situations. The influence of this view is so pervasive that the term *learning* itself for some researchers represents the totality of information processing underlying stimulus-specific changes in behavior resulting from prior experience. This use of the term discourages consideration of any of the postacquisition processing that may also be necessary to see learned behavior. By definition, learning is the process by which experience is encoded and results in stimulus-specific changes in behavior that can be observed later. By memory, we are referring to any stimulus-specific permanent change in the brain (structural and chemical) resulting from past experience that allows usage of that previous experience on future occasions. Finally, retrieval is the process of reactivating an established memory so it can influence ongoing behavior, and thus we will argue that retrieval is a key component of memory performance.

In the early 1960s, however, a number of studies showed that information thought to be lost or not encoded was still available, provided that the appropriate retrieval cues were presented at the time of testing (see Tulving and Thomson, 1973, for a review). In other words, these studies suggested that memory deficits typically thought to result from processing limitations during training could be recovered at the time of testing. These experiments, conducted primarily with human subjects, provided a strong rationale for investigating a critical stage in the information processing stream: retrieval from memory. In most of these experiments, subjects were presented with material to be learned (encoding) and subsequently evaluated to determine the conditions under which that information could be retrieved and brought to bear on response generation. As a result of this research, the emphasis on encoding that dominated the early stages of human memory research shifted to also encompass retrieval mechanisms. Interestingly, these observations with human subjects promoted changes in the study of animal memory. A vast amount of data concerning retrieval processes has been gathered from nonhumans since the late 1960s, and ever since, the notion of retrieval has proven to be a useful heuristic for the study of memory phenomena.

This chapter will focus on memory research with nonhuman animals. In the first section, we will review the empirical evidence suggesting that deficits in memory tasks do not necessarily reflect a deficit in acquisition or storage. Specifically, we will summarize representative experiments in which memory deficits are observed after changes in the internal state of the organism, or the administration of amnesic treatments such as electroconvulsive shock or protein synthesis inhibition. Moreover, we will review recent evidence suggesting that already consolidated memories, when reactivated, undergo a new period of vulnerability, so-called reconsolidation. Importantly, memory deficits can also be obtained by manipulating the amount of information presented either during training of the target memory (cue competition) or by presenting additional information at other points in the study (interference). Cue competition and memory interference experiments have also contributed evidence concerning the role of encoding and retrieval of memory and therefore will also be analyzed in this section. In the second part, we will summarize how these observations led to the development of memory models that account for a wide range of phenomena. As is the case in most scientific disciplines, there is no single approach that accounts for all the empirical evidence available. Therefore we will review three models that address the phenomena described in the first section. The first general framework is that proposed by Spear in the late 1970s that explains memory deficits induced by changes in the context or insufficient retrieval cues at the time of test. The second retrieval framework we will review is focused on associative phenomena originally thought to reflect learning deficits. As we will see, these deficits are easily anticipated in a framework that emphasizes retrieval mechanisms. The third framework is that proposed by Bouton to explain several characteristics of extinction that are important to understand some anxiety disorders in human populations (*See* Chapter 29). Lastly, we will briefly review neurobehavioral studies in which the physiological substrates of memory retrieval have been investigated. The importance of these studies lies in the fact that inquiries into the neurobiological basis of memory are inspired by behavioral models, such as the ones we describe in the section titled 'Theories of memory retrieval.'

31.2 Empirical Evidence

Several key empirical observations suggest that numerous deficits in acquired behavior result from information processing that occurs when subjects are tested rather than when they acquire or store information. Critical here is the fact that, theoretically speaking, if information is inadequately acquired or is not retained, then that information will not be available to influence the animal's behavior in any test situation. In contrast, the following observations suggest that the target information has often been sufficiently encoded and stored, but a processing deficit occurs when the information is evoked, which translates into decreased performance at the time of testing. We will review decrements in retrieval that arise from natural changes in the organism's internal state and from changes in the state of the external environment between training and testing, as well as those that arise in the laboratory as a result of programmed invasive manipulations (i.e., experimentally induced amnesia). Moreover, we will review recent evidence suggesting that memories that are retrieved from an inactive state could be subject to new consolidation processes, so-called reconsolidation (*See* Chapter 30). Finally, we will review demonstrations of recovery from performance deficits arising in situations in which multiple cues are simultaneously present during training (cue competition) and from exposing subjects to select nontarget information removed from target training (stimulus interference).

31.2.1 Changes in the Organism's Internal State

One of the earlier observations that suggested a deficit in retrieval was state-dependent learning. State-dependent learning refers to the observation that when the internal state of the organism is different at testing than it was at training, acquired performance is impaired (Overton, 1964). Operationally, state-dependent learning is observed when subjects experience training under one of two internal states (a state induced by the presence or absence of a drug in Overton's case) and tested under the opposite internal state. The common finding is that when subjects are trained in a nondrug state and tested in a nondrug state, behavior consistent with training is observed. Conversely, if subjects are trained while in a drug-induced state (e.g., amphetamine) and tested while not in a drug state, a decrement in performance is typically observed. This decrement could easily be accounted for by a deficit in learning, perhaps due to the drug-altering perceptual processes or the encoding of information. Similar decrements in performance are observed when subjects are trained while undrugged and tested while drugged. These decrements can be accounted for by perceptual processes at the time of testing. However, subjects trained under a drugged state and tested under the same drugged state do not always show a decrement in memory performance. This suggests that the observed performance decrements often result from retrieval deficits due to a change in the internal state of the organism (Spear, 1978). If the internal state of the subject during testing is the same as during training, regardless of whether it is a state induced by administration of a drug, performance consistent with training is observed. State-dependent learning has been observed in a wide range of memory tasks and with states induced by several different drugs, such as amphetamine, alcohol, and morphine (Overton, 1972, 1985), and also emotional states induced by various manipulations (for a review, see Overton, 1985). Obviously *state-dependent learning* is a misnomer; the phenomenon would more accurately be called *state-dependent retrieval.*

Another example of state-dependent learning that can be understood as a retrieval failure is the Kamin effect (Kamin, 1957, 1963). This effect typically has been observed in avoidance tasks in which subjects show poor retention of avoidance training when they are tested at intervals ranging from 1 to 6 h after training. The interesting observation is that such poor retention is not observed if subjects are tested a half hour after training or more than 24 h after training. In other words, subjects show a U-shaped retention function, with retention being good immediately after training and at later intervals, but not between 1 and 6 h after training. This U-shaped function has been viewed as the result of memory retrieval being dependent on the internal state of the organism. A more specific hypothesis was based on the fact that most of these demonstrations of the Kamin effect used aversively motivated tasks, which are known for their capacity to induce a stressful internal state. Moreover, the release of a hormone closely correlated with stress, adrenocorticotropic hormone (ACTH), is inhibited relatively soon after a stressful experience (McEwen and Weiss, 1970). Researchers reasoned that, because of ACTH inhibition, the internal state of the subjects from 1 to 6 h after training was different from the internal state during training, leading to a failure to retrieve the appropriate information required to perform in the task. Consistent with this interpretation, exposing subjects to foot shocks immediately before testing overcame the deficient retention observed at intermediate test intervals (Klein and Spear, 1970). Moreover, exposure to other stressors, such as immersion in cold water for 2 min, also alleviated the intermediate interval deficit in retention (Klein, 1972). Note that this stressor was unrelated to the training situation in terms of external, sensory attributes of the memory (other than being stressful), but it apparently restored the internal state that was temporarily inhibited after the original stressful experience. Importantly, the cold water bath had no effect at other retention intervals, suggesting that the effects are not related to overall activation or motivational effects of the stressor (Klein, 1972). Presumably, exposure to either foot shock or cold water provided subjects with an internal state (ACTH release) that corresponded to that of training and consequently alleviated the deficit observed at intermediate intervals. Moreover, this deficit in retention was also alleviated if subjects were infused with ACTH into the lateral anterior hypothalamus or if the same structure was electrically stimulated (Klein, 1972). More recently, Gisquet-Verrier and colleagues observed an alleviation of the Kamin effect when they exposed subjects simultaneously to the conditioned stimulus (CS) and the training context in a brightness-discrimination avoidance task 7.5 min before an intermediate interval test (Gisquet-Verrier et al., 1989; Gisquet-Verrier and Alexinsky, 1990). Overall, all of these demonstrations suggest that the Kamin effect can be alleviated if (a) the subject's internal state is restored (either by administration of ACTH or exposure to a stressor), or (b) the appropriate retrieval cues (such as the CS and the training context) are presented before testing.

Similar recovery effects have been found when retention deficits were induced with hypothermia. Specifically, subjects showed impaired retention if they were immersed in cold water immediately after training (Vardaris et al., 1973). However, if they were recooled before testing, no impaired retention was observed (Hinderliter et al., 1976; Mactutus and Riccio, 1978). These results have been interpreted as arising from a retrieval failure if there is a mismatch between training and testing in the subject's internal state. Consistent with this explanation, administering the recooling treatment immediately before testing presumably alleviates the effects of the hypothermic treatment by providing contextual cues that were present close to the time of training.

31.2.2 Experimentally Induced Amnesias

The notion that deficits in acquired behavior result from a processing deficit at the time of retrieval has received additional support from experimental manipulations known to induce amnesia. It is important to note that the three examples from the previous section resulted from changes in the internal state of the subject. In contrast to state-dependent learning and the Kamin effect, in the studies reviewed later, a performance deficit was induced by the administration of an amnestic agent. For example, if soon after training subjects are administered an electroconvulsive shock (hereafter ECS; Duncan, 1949), hypothermia (described earlier; Vardaris et al., 1973), or protein synthesis inhibitors (e.g., Barraco and Stettner, 1976), little behavior indicative of retention is observed. These observations have been taken by many as evidence that amnestic treatments work by disrupting memory consolidation (McGaugh, 1966, 2000; Gold and King, 1974). Memory consolidation is defined as a time-dependent process by which recent learned experiences are transformed into long-term memory, presumably by structural and chemical changes in the nervous system (e.g., the strengthening of synaptic connections between neurons). Support for this explanation comes from the fact that the effects of amnestic treatments are retrograde in nature, with recent memories being more vulnerable than earlier memories to the amnestic treatment (e.g., Duncan, 1949). The temporally graded nature of amnesia is explained by the consolidation view in the following way: After a given learning experience, memories undergo a consolidation process that leaves the memory trace more stable as time passes. Following this logic, the shorter the interval between training and the administration of the amnestic treatment, the larger the impact of the amnestic agent on the formation of the memory trace.

Since the discovery of these amnestic treatments, however, a number of observations have suggested that, instead of disrupting the consolidation process, these treatments might alter the memory's retrievability, thereby rendering it inaccessible at the time of retrieval. Evidence supporting this notion comes from studies that reminded subjects of the original episode. For example, Lewis et al. (1968) trained rats in a passive avoidance task and immediately administered amnesia-inducing ECS. They tested their subjects 20 h later and observed that subjects that received the amnestic treatment showed no behavior indicative of the passive avoidance event; that is, the amnestic treatment was effective in inducing amnesia. However, 4 h after training, they placed other rats given the amnesic treatment immediately following training in a separate compartment (different from that of training) and administered a foot shock (unconditioned stimulus – US), similar to the reinforcer used in training. When these subjects were tested 20 h later in the training compartment, they showed recovery from the amnestic treatment, as evidenced by longer avoidance latencies. In other words, when they exposed rats to a reminder of the initial training experience, subjects' performance indicated that the memory trace was not altered by the amnestic treatment. Subjects lacking original training showed no effect of such reminder shocks. Because this recovery effect could have been specific to the avoidance tasks involving stressful situations, Miller et al. (1974) conducted a similar study, but instead of using an aversive preparation, they used an appetitively motivated task with sucrose as a reinforcer. Interestingly, they reported that, after the amnestic treatment, a foot shock did not affect a recovery of memory. Moreover, they showed that exposure to the sucrose solution following the amnestic treatment reversed the retention deficit induced by the amnestic treatment. Further experiments demonstrated that exposure to the training apparatus also recovered the memory rendered silent by the amnestic treatment. Thus, exposure to any of several elements from the training task restored access to the target memory, whereas exposure to task-irrelevant stimuli, even if they were of strong affective value, did not restore memory.

31.2.3 Reconsolidation

As part of the effort to understand and contrast approaches to memory, studies of experimentally induced amnesias gained popularity during the late 1960s and 1970s. This popularity was recently reinvigorated when new findings suggested that old memories when reactivated need new (*de novo*) protein synthesis to become once again stable and permanently stored in the brain (Przybyslawski and Sara, 1997; Nader et al., 2000; *See* Chapter 30). This phenomenon has been called reconsolidation. For example, a day after Nader et al. exposed their rats to simple CS → US pairings, they presented the CS alone (which presumably reactivated the memory trace for that association) and immediately infused anisomycin (a protein synthesis inhibitor) into the lateral and basal amygdala. When they tested subjects 1 day later, they observed decreased conditioned freezing to the CS relative to anisomycin-treated rats lacking the CS exposure on day 2, suggesting that the memory trace that was activated needed new protein synthesis to become stable again. These findings brought back the question extensively debated in the 1970s: Are memories destroyed or simply made inaccessible after a retrieval manipulation followed by an amnestic agent (e.g., Miller and Springer, 1973, 1974; Gold and King, 1974)? Several recent reports suggest an answer to this question. For example, Lattal and Abel (2004) observed that after reactivating a memory of contextual fear and administrating systemic anisomycin, subjects showed decreased conditioned freezing when tested 1 day later in the training context. However, if the test was delayed by 21 days (a standard retention interval used for spontaneous recovery from extinction of fear memories), no effect of protein synthesis inhibition was observed. In fact, Lattal and Abel observed that 21 days after anisomycin treatment, response to the context was larger than that observed during immediate retrieval (1 day after training). Other recent studies also cast doubt on the generality of the reconsolidation account because similar recovery from retrieval-induced reconsolidation has been observed (Anokhin et al., 2002; Fisher et al., 2004; Power et al., 2006; but see Debiec et al., 2002; Duvarci and Nader, 2004). Moreover, some studies did not observe any immediate effect of anisomycin after retrieval-induced reconsolidation (Lattal and Abel, 2001; Vianna et al., 2001; Biedenkapp and Rudy, 2004; Cammarota et al., 2004; Hernandez and Kelley, 2004). Overall, these contradictory findings, together with demonstrations of recovery from retrieval-induced amnesia after inhibition of protein synthesis, show that further research is needed to determine whether anisomycin erases the reactivated memory or simply constrains future retrieval of the memory. More generally, it is still unclear if amnestic agents following initial training impair consolidation (storage) or subsequent retrieval (e.g., Gold and King, 1974; Miller and Matzel, 2006).

Two points deserve further discussion here. First, as recently pointed out by Rudy et al. (2006), anisomycin also has other effects beyond inhibition of protein synthesis, such as genetically programmed cell death (apoptosis). Moreover, the apoptotic cascade occurs at lower doses than those that are necessary for the inhibition of protein synthesis. Whether this is the main cause of the observed amnesia remains to be determined, but it is noteworthy that tests have not yet been conducted to determine the role of apoptosis in experimental amnesia. Second, a recent report from the same laboratory that sparked early interest in reconsolidation showed that memories activated indirectly by an associate of the target cue do not undergo reconsolidation (Debięc et al., 2006). They trained rats in a second-order conditioning preparation in which one cue was paired with the US in a first phase (CS_1 → US), and in a second phase another cue was paired with the cue trained in phase 1 ($CS_2 \rightarrow CS_1$). This procedure ordinarily results in conditioned responding to CS_2, presumably because when presented at test it retrieves a neural representation of the US through an associative chain mediated by CS_1 (or a direct CS_2 → UR link; see Rescorla, 1980, for a discussion). Notably, Debięc et al. found that responding to CS_1 was not impaired after retrieval through presentation of CS_2 and subsequent administration of anisomycin. This suggests that the reactivation treatment, at most, leaves only part of the memory in a labile state, but alternatively the entire content of the memory might not be substantially altered.

In contrast to reconsolidation accounts of the reconsolidation phenomenon, there are retrieval-focused accounts of reconsolidation such as that proposed by Millin et al. (2001). In line with Spear's (1973, 1978; see following discussion) views concerning retrieval, Riccio and his collaborators have proposed that when previously stored memories are reactivated, reprocessing of the attributes of these memories will take place for some time after the reactivation episode. As a result, the internal context provided by an amnestic treatment becomes associated with the target memory. At test, the context provided by the amnestic treatment is not ordinarily present, and thus retrieval failure occurs. Consistent with this account, amnesia induced by the administration of anisomycin has been observed to be alleviated if subjects are administered anisomycin just prior to testing (Bradley and Galal, 1988). Another explanation of this phenomenon has been advanced by Miller and Matzel (2000; also see Nadel and Land, 2000), who proposed that the amnestic treatment produces a change in the memory representation that interferes with retrieval itself, leaving the memory trace silent after the administration of the amnestic treatment. Regardless of the specific version of the retrieval explanation for the reconsolidation phenomenon put forth, these alternative views can be contrasted with reconsolidation accounts by determining the extent to which amnestic treatments really erase the memory trace or simply render it inaccessible for future use. Based on the recovery data presented earlier, the latter alternative seems to be the more plausible at this time (Prado-Alcalá et al., 2006).

Four points are important to keep in mind. (1) Recovery from amnestic treatment is often observed when subjects are exposed to a portion of the event that had been presented during training. Such reminder treatments are most effective soon before testing, but sometimes have enduring effects even when presented 24 h before testing. (2) Control groups have demonstrated that the recovery is not purely the result of altering stress levels in the subject. (3) Recovery can be obtained by reminding subjects about the training situation not only with the US, but also with other cues (such as contextual cues or sometimes even the CS) that are part of the target memory. (4) The effect of the reminder does not result from new learning concerning the cue-outcome relationship, as long as learning is defined as receiving relevant new information from events in the environment. Subjects exposed to the reminder without any prior learning experience did not show any evidence of relevant learning after the reminder experience.

So far, we have argued that most impairments in memory retention result at least in part from a retrieval failure rather than an acquisition or storage failure. We have based our assertion on studies involving changes in the state of the organism (state-dependent learning and the Kamin effect), experimentally induced amnesia (ECS, hypothermia, and antimetabolites), or reconsolidation phenomena. Next, we review evidence suggesting that decrements in learning and memory that are thought to result from processing limitations (competition) at the time of training, or from deleterious effects on learning or retention due to learning additional information (interference), could instead result from a retrieval deficit at the time of testing.

31.2.4 Cue Competition and Outcome Competition

Cue competition refers to a decrement in behavioral control by a target CS (X), which results from the addition of a nontarget stimulus to a simple CS–US learning situation. This can be observed in a number of different circumstances. For example, one can add a second CS to training and train a compound of the target cue and the added CS instead of the target cue alone (i.e., AX → US as opposed to X → US) and see less behavioral control to the target cue X (overshadowing; Pavlov, 1927). Alternatively, one can train a nontarget cue in a first phase and in a second phase train a compound of cues that contains the target cue as well as the previously trained nontarget cue (A → US in phase 1; AX → US in phase 2). This results in less behavioral control by X, the target cue, than in subjects lacking phase 1 (blocking; Kamin, 1969). A second rather different form of stimulus competition can be seen when, instead of adding a second CS, a second outcome is added. For example, one can train a cue followed by an outcome in a first phase and that same cue followed by the same outcome plus a new outcome in a second phase, and then later assess performance governed by the association between the cue and the second outcome ($X \rightarrow O_1$ in phase 1, $X \rightarrow O_1O_2$ in phase 2, test $X \rightarrow O_2$; Rescorla, 1980; Esmoris-Arranz et al., 1997). This is called blocking between outcomes. Taking these examples together, one can see that the addition of nontarget stimuli (a cue or an outcome) attenuates behavioral control by the target cue X.

Phenomena like blocking between cues gave rise to a family of models of Pavlovian conditioning that emphasized critical differences in information processing during acquisition. These models assumed that limitations in processing (e.g., attention to the CS or US) during training impeded the normal establishment of associations and consequently resulted in the observed decrements in behavioral control (e.g., Rescorla and Wagner, 1972; Mackintosh, 1975;

Pearce and Hall, 1980). Similar to consolidation theory (e.g., McGaugh, 1966, 2000), these behavioral models predict that what has not been stored due to processing constraints during learning will not be reflected in behavior simply because the information was not initially acquired.

As previously mentioned, overshadowing is observed as a response decrement that results from training a target cue (X) in the presence of another, usually more salient, cue (A). Interestingly, Kauffman and Bolles (1981; see also Matzel et al., 1985) conducted overshadowing training (AX → US) and subsequently extinguished the overshadowing cue (A) by presenting it in the absence of reinforcement. After extinguishing the overshadowing cue, they observed a recovery from overshadowing, that is, strong behavioral control by the overshadowed cue X at test. Similarly, after blocking treatment (A → US followed by AX → US), extinguishing the blocking cue (A alone presentations) can result in recovery from blocking (Blaisdell et al., 1999). However, extinction of the competing cue is not the only manipulation known to affect overshadowing and blocking. Kraemer et al. (1988) found a recovery from overshadowing training when they interposed a long retention interval between overshadowing treatment and testing, which suggests that the association between the overshadowed cue and the outcome had been established during training but was not reflected in behavior soon after training. A similar recovery from blocking has been observed after interposing a long retention interval between training and testing (Batsell, 1997; Piñeno et al., 2005).

In the same way that recovery from experimentally induced amnesia has been observed after exposing subjects to some portions of the events presented during training (CS, US, or the training context), stimulus competition phenomena have been observed to be attenuated as a result of these manipulations. For example, Kasprow et al. (1982) observed a recovery from overshadowing after they exposed subjects to two brief presentations of the overshadowed cue (the target CS). In another series of experiments, a similar recovery from blocking was observed (Balaz et al., 1982). Specifically, Balaz et al. observed a recovery from blocking after reminding subjects of the training experience either by presenting the blocked CS, the US, or the context in which subjects were trained. Additional control groups demonstrated that this recovery was specific to the blocked association and was not due to nonspecific increases in responding. All these demonstrations of recovery from cue competition are problematic for models that emphasize impaired acquisition (see earlier discussion) because, if the association between the overshadowed or blocked cue and the outcome was not learned during training, any manipulation that does not involve further training with that cue should not alter behavioral control by that cue.

Although little attention has been given to competition between outcomes, some recent studies have not only observed similar competition phenomena as those observed between cues (e.g., blocking between outcomes; Emoris-Arranz et al., 1997), but also observed that these deficits in behavioral control can be alleviated with the appropriate manipulations. For example, Wheeler and Miller (2005) observed reliable blocking between outcomes ($X \rightarrow O_1$ during phase 1; $X \rightarrow O_1O_2$ during phase 2), similar to the blocking between cues trained together originally observed by Kamin (1969). That is, responding based on the $X \rightarrow O_2$ association was weaker than in subjects that had received $X \rightarrow O_3$ in phase 1. Wheeler and Miller went on to extinguish the blocking outcome (O_1) and observed recovery from blocking between outcomes (i.e., behavioral consistent with the $X \rightarrow O_2$ association). Moreover, they observed a similar recovery when they interposed a retention interval between training and testing, and when they briefly presented the blocked outcome before testing (i.e., a reminder treatment). Overall, the results of these experiments demonstrated that blocking between outcomes can be attenuated by several manipulations similar to those that often yield recovery from blocking between cues.

31.2.5 Interference between Cues and Outcomes Trained Apart

Earlier we distinguished between impairments in acquired behavior that arise from training stimuli together (competition) and from experiencing additional training apart from training of the target stimuli (provided that the additional training includes one of the target associates). The latter deficit is called interference. We have already described how impaired performance that arises from stimulus competition can be recovered, thus suggesting that retrieval mechanisms play a fundamental role in behavioral control influenced by stimulus competition. Next we will review the basic conditions under which interference is observed and the different manipulations that often result in recovery from interference. Interference in Pavlovian conditioning is evidenced as impaired behavioral control by a target cue when it is paired with a given outcome in one phase of training and paired with another outcome in an earlier or later phase of training (e.g., X → O_1 in phase 1 and X → O_2 in phase 2). But this is not the only situation in which interference is observed. Interference is also observed when a target cue (X) is trained with an outcome in one phase of training and in a separate phase of training another cue is trained with the same outcome (e.g., X → O in phase 1 and Y → O in phase 2). A common characteristic of these two forms of interference is that there is always a common element between the two phases of training (the cue X in the case of interference between outcomes (*See* Chapter 29), and the outcome O in the case of interference between cues). The critical feature of these decrements in otherwise anticipated behavioral control by X is that the interfering cues (or outcomes) are not trained together with the target cue (or outcome).

Extinction, latent inhibition, and counterconditioning (Pavlov, 1927; Lubow, 1973; Bouton and Peck, 1992; Brooks and Bouton, 1993) are three treatments that can be viewed as forms of interference between outcomes. In simple extinction, a cue is first paired with an outcome (X → US), and in a second phase it is trained in the absence of the outcome (X-alone presentations; i.e., X → No US). As a result of these nonreinforced presentations, the cue loses behavioral control, which used to be taken as evidence of unlearning the original X → US association (e.g., Rescorla and Wagner, 1972). However, overwhelming evidence has shown that the original X → US association is not destroyed during the second phase, but rather, new learning during phase 2 interferes with the expression of the phase 1 learning. Pavlov (1927) was the first to find a [partial] recovery effect from extinction. His observation (widely replicated since then; e.g., Rescorla and Cunningham, 1978; Brooks and Bouton, 1993) was that conditioned responding soon after extinction was minimal, but if a retention interval was interposed between extinction and the test, a recovery (which Pavlov termed *spontaneous recovery*) from extinction was observed. In other words, behavior after a retention interval was relatively similar in subjects who received extinction training and those who did not receive extinction training. What was puzzling at that time (and might have encouraged Pavlov to name the effect 'spontaneous recovery') was the fact that the extinguished response was recovered despite the fact that the subjects did not undergo any treatment other than interpolation of a long retention interval. Another manipulation that also leads to recovery from extinction is a shift in context between extinction and testing. This phenomenon is called renewal. For example, one might train subjects in a distinctive context A and conduct extinction training in a different context (B). The critical determinant of renewal is that testing be conducted outside the extinction context. If subjects are tested in a different context from the one used during extinction (ABC or ABA, where the first letter denotes the training context, the second the extinction context, and the third the test context), recovery from extinction is observed (Bouton and Bolles, 1979; Bouton and King, 1983; Bouton and Swartzentruber, 1989). If subjects are tested in the same context in which extinction took place (AAA or ABB), no such recovery is observed. A similar finding is observed when the context is defined to include the internal state of the organism, which can typically be altered by administering a drug that would change the internal state. For example, renewal has been observed when the extinction context is characterized by alcohol intoxication, and subjects are tested in a sober state, which creates a different internal context (Cunningham, 1979).

Latent inhibition is observed as a retarded emergence of behavioral control due to nonreinforced presentations of the target CS prior to conditioning (X-alone presentations in phase 1; X → US in phase 2), in comparison with subjects that experience the same phase 2 training without phase 1 treatment (Lubow, 1973). Similar to extinction, in a latent inhibition treatment subjects experience the target CS alone, but before the reinforced trials rather than after. One characteristic of latent inhibition that is suggestive of the response deficit being a retrieval effect is its context specificity. Specifically, it has been observed that if subjects experience phase 1 and phase 2 training in different contexts, latent inhibition is abolished (Channell and Hall, 1983). Presumably, during phase 1 nonreinforced presentations, the CS becomes associated with the context in which it is being presented, and these associations interfere with subsequent behavioral control after reinforcement in the same context. Thus, a context switch or massive extinction of the context (Grahame et al., 1994) between phases 1 and 2 attenuates the latent inhibition effect. A recent observation that has captured researchers' attention is the super latent inhibition effect (De la Casa and Lubow, 2000,

2002; Wheeler et al., 2004). This effect is typically observed when a retention interval is interposed between phase 2 reinforced training and testing. One critical condition necessary for this effect to be observed is that subjects have to spend the retention interval in a context different from that of conditioning. Thus, the superlatent inhibition effect might be seen as a shift from behavior based on recency (phase 2 training) to behavior based on primacy (phase 1 training) after interposing a long retention interval between phase 2 training and testing.

Counterconditioning is a phenomenon similar to extinction, but during the second phase of training, the target cue is associated with a qualitatively different outcome instead of being associated with the absence of an outcome, as is the case with extinction. The phase 2 treatment radically attenuates conditioned responding based on phase 1 training (Pavlov, 1927). What distinguishes extinction from counterconditioning is the motivational nature of the outcomes, in that in counterconditioning, the outcomes of phases 1 and 2 engage different motivational systems. For example, in a counterconditioning experiment, subjects might experience a CS followed by food in the first phase (X → food) and the same CS followed by foot shock in the second phase (X → shock; this is called appetitive-aversive transfer, but counterconditioning is also observed when the two phases are reversed, which is called aversive-appetitive transfer). After this training, the CS → shock association is thought to retroactively interfere with the CS → food associations. The question of interest is whether phase 2 learning destroys the memory of phase 1 training or if it simply interferes with the expression of that association. To address this question, Peck and Bouton (1990) trained phases 1 and 2 in two physically distinct contexts and tested subjects in the phase 1 context. Consistent with an explanation in terms of retrieval disruption rather than impaired retention, subjects tested in the phase 1 context showed responding appropriate to phase 1 training, indicating that the information had not been erased (or unlearned) but rather that behavior appropriate to each phase could be observed depending on the contextual cues present at the time of testing. Similarly, Brooks et al. (1995) trained rats with X → shock pairings in phase 1 and X → food pairings in phase 2. Before testing, they exposed the critical group to six unsignaled shocks and at test (relative to appropriate control groups) found that subjects froze to the CS, consistent with the shock US, rather than approached the food hopper, which demonstrated reinstatement of original training after counterconditioning. Moreover, this reinstatement effect was dependent on the shocks being presented in the context in which testing would occur, because no reinstatement was observed when the shocks were presented in a context other than the test context.

As we mentioned earlier, interference is observed not only when a cue is associated with two outcomes (extinction and counterconditioning), but also when two cues are associated with the same outcome. For example, Escobar et al. (2001) paired a cue with an outcome (X → O) in a first phase and subsequently paired a second cue with the same outcome (A → O) and observed impaired responding to X (relative to subjects that received A and O explicitly unpaired in phase 2), thereby providing a demonstration of retroactive interference. In subsequent experiments, they showed that the retroactive interference effect could be alleviated if subjects experienced phase 1 (X → O) and phase 2 (A → O) training in different contexts and subsequently were tested in the context in which the X → O association was trained. That is, interference was affected by the context in which testing took place. Similarly, in another experiment, they presented priming stimuli (stimuli presented during phase 1 or during phase 2 sessions but far removed from presentations of the target cue or interfering cue) that distinctively signaled phase 1 or 2 of their procedure and observed retroactive interference to be dependent on which priming cue was presented immediately before the critical test. When they primed phase 2, robust retroactive interference was observed, but when they primed phase 1, an alleviation of retroactive interference was observed, relative to subjects that did not receive any priming treatment at the time of test. Similar findings were reported by Amundson et al. (2003) but in a proactive interference preparation (i.e., A → US training followed by X → US training). Specifically, they observed an attenuation of proactive interference with responding to X when they primed the second phase of their training procedure, presumably because this impaired retrieval of the competing (phase 1) association and facilitated retrieval of the second association. Moreover, they observed recovery from proactive interference when they extinguished the phase 1 association. In summary, based on these and similar findings, it is reasonable to conclude that interference is highly dependent on the cues provided at the time of testing, thus suggesting a strong role for retrieval mechanisms. Moreover, there are now several demonstrations of parallels in interference between cues and between outcomes in that both of these effects can be alleviated if the appropriate conditions prevail at the time of testing.

31.3 Theories of Memory Retrieval

There are several approaches to memory retrieval, each having been designed to explain different phenomena. However, the frameworks that we describe next point to several shared principles that have proven to be important and reliable tools for the study of retrieval from memory following learning. No single approach accounts for all the deficits in retention we have reviewed earlier. But each framework has provided an explanation of a number of observations and therefore deserves discussion.

31.3.1 Matching of Information as Critical for the Retrieval from Memory

Tulving and Thomson (1973) proposed the encoding specificity principle of retrieval that at the time accounted for many of the retrieval effects that were found with human participants. The principle states that subjects form a representation of events that encompasses not only the target events themselves but also many of the events surrounding the target event. Additionally, these episodic memories encode not only which events occurred, but where and when each event occurred relative to neighboring events. Moreover, the encoding specificity principle asserts that items (words, in the framework of the proposal) presented to aid retrieval will be effective only if they (or very similar items) were presented during training, consistent with the view that subjects encode a global representation of an item, its semantic meaning, and its content during training. Critical to this proposal is the notion that what enters into a memory representation (what it is encoded) is determined by the perceived functional meaning of an item, and this in turn determines which retrieval cues will be effective for memory retrieval.

Along similar lines, Spear (1973, 1978) has emphasized that similarity between retrieval cues and cues presented during training is critical for memory expression. He proposed the following principles as a conceptual framework for effective memory processing.

1. Attributes of memory function independently. In other words, an animal encodes a collection of separate but associated attributes that correspond to the events that form a memory episode. A constellation of attributes will be activated every time the subject experiences an event that has some similarity in attributes to the target memory. Moreover, an associated attribute might be activated when an event memory is activated. That is, some attributes might activate an event memory that in turn will activate attributes that need not have been presented but rather are associatively linked to retrieval cues presented. Additionally, attributes might activate memories of other attributes, regardless of whether they activate the full event memory representation.
2. The process of retrieval is determined by the number of retrieval cues that correspond to attributes of that memory. A memory failure is observed when an insufficient number of retrieval cues correspond at test to the memory of a given event, other things being equal. Moreover, events that are presented during testing but were not presented during training will lead to retrieval of nontarget memories that will interfere with retrieval of target memories (similar to the phenomenon of external inhibition that Pavlov, 1927, described).
3. A contextual cue is any event noticed by the organism, with the exclusion of the target stimuli that form the learning experience (e.g., the CS and US in a Pavlovian conditioning situation). Forgetting is caused in large part by a change between the context of acquisition and the context of retrieval. Context changes can result from different sources, and the differences in contextual information are more likely to increase as time passes (i.e., as the retention interval is increased; Bouton, 1993, views this as resulting from time actually being part of the context). Thus, in this framework sensory contexts from training will dissipate rapidly (soon after the stimuli are terminated), and neurochemical and hormonal states will dissipate somewhat more slowly. Importantly, contextual information here can be composed of internal stimuli (or states) and external stimuli, such as the physical attributes of the context where training or testing takes place. The internal context can also change due to preprogrammed factors such as aging or cyclical changes

in hormonal states (e.g., estrus). Contextual attributes learned during new experiences also might interfere with retrieval of the target memory if they share attributes in common.

This general framework has been one of the foundations for studying retrieval mechanisms in memory retention. For example, it easily explains state-dependent learning and the Kamin effect by assuming that the conditions at test are different than those during training. Consistent with this framework, several manipulations that recreate the training conditions at the time of testing have proven effective in restoring the deficient behavior observed due to changes in the organism's internal states or changes in the environment.

31.3.2 The Comparator Hypothesis: A Retrieval-Focused View of Cue Competition

As was mentioned in the introduction, models that emphasize processing during encoding and storage have been prevalent in the study of learned behavior in animals. One such example is the well-known Rescorla and Wagner (1972; also see Wagner and Rescorla, 1972) model. This model asserts that error correction at the time of training governs what information is acquired; that is, acquisition should be greatest when the discrepancy between the US that occurs and the US that is expected based on all cues present is largest. The model has been widely applied to Pavlovian conditioning situations in which one or more cues are concurrently paired with a given outcome. After repeated pairings, subjects emit a conditioned response when one (or more) of these cues are presented. One of the strengths of the model is that it elegantly anticipates the occurrence of cue competition (overshadowing, blocking, etc.). In fact, the model was conceived in part to account for such phenomena after Kamin's (1969) demonstration of blocking. However, one of the weaknesses of the model is that it only emphasizes processing during training, with the additional vague assumption that associative strengths map monotonically onto behavior. Given all the aforementioned examples of recovery from cue competition (see prior section on empirical evidence), it is attractive to detail here a model that also explains cue-competition phenomena but appeals centrally to a retrieval mechanism.

One such model is the comparator hypothesis of conditioned responding (Miller and Matzel, 1988). The model assumes that all pairs of stimuli, including cues, that are presented together gain associative strength with each of the other stimuli present, independent of the associative status of other cues present during training. In other words, in this model there is no competition between cues for associative strength during training – all information is stored. Associative strength between stimuli A and B depends only on their spatiotemporal contiguity and saliencies. The training context also gains associative strength, although at a much slower rate due to its lower salience than punctate stimuli. Thus, following Bush and Mosteller's (1951) error correction rule, the comparator hypothesis assumes noncompetitive learning of associations between cues and outcomes, of within-compound associations between cues trained together, and of associations between cues and the training context. What is critical in the comparator hypothesis is the process of retrieval of memories. According to this framework, responding to the presentation of a CS will be determined by a comparison between the representation of the US that is directly activated by the target CS → US association and the representation of the US that is indirectly activated conjointly by the associations between the target CS and any other cues presented during training (punctate cues or the training context) and the association between those cues and the US. In **Figure 1**, a depiction of the comparator hypothesis is provided. The

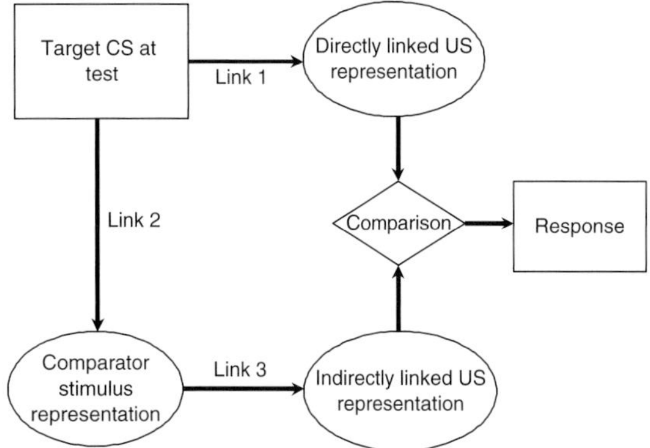

Figure 1 The original comparator hypothesis (after Miller RR and Matzel LD (1988) The comparator hypothesis: A response rule for the expression of associations. In: Bower GH (ed.) *The Psychology of Learning and Motivation, Vol. 22*, pp. 51–92. San Diego, CA: Academic Press). Rectangles represent physical events, and ovals correspond to internal representations of events that were previously associated with those physical events. The diamond represents the comparator process. Responding is directly related to the strength of link 1 and negatively related to the product of links 2 and 3.

boxes represent the external events observable in the test situation, that is, the target stimulus and the conditioned response. Ovals represent internal representations of events that were presented during training, and the diamond represents the comparator process (also internal). Direct activation of a US representation due to presentation of the target cue at test depends on the strength of the association between the target cue and the outcome, represented by link 1. Importantly, the target cue also activates a US representation mediated through other cues that were presented in the training situation, and this is represented by links 2 and 3. Responding is determined by a comparison between the directly activated representation of the US (the strength of which is determined by the target CS-US association, i.e., link 1) and the indirectly activated representation of the US (the strength of which is determined by the product of links 2 and 3). This comparison process is represented by the diamond. In an overshadowing situation (AX → US; with X being the target cue to be tested), the comparator hypothesis states that during training, subjects associate the target cue with the US (link 1 in **Figure 1**), the target cue with the overshadowing cue A (which is X's comparator cue; link 2), and A with the US (link 3). These associations are acquired independently of each other (i.e., cues do not compete during training for associative strength with the US). Critical for the comparator hypothesis is what happens when the target cue X is presented during testing. When X is presented, it directly activates a representation of the US, but it also indirectly activates a representation of the US, mediated by the overshadowing cue (which was associated during training with both the target cue and the US). This indirectly activated (competing) US representation is said to decrease (downmodulate) responding to the target cue, and thus overshadowing is observed relative to a group that experienced elemental training (X → US alone).

What differentiates the comparator hypothesis from acquisition-focused models (i.e., those that focus on limitations in processing during training) is not only the mechanism through which it explains cue competition phenomena, but also several novel predictions that have received empirical support in recent years. One such prediction is that after overshadowing training, extinguishing the overshadowing cue (that is, presenting A alone after training) should result in recovery from overshadowing. Specifically, by presenting A alone after overshadowing training, the links that mediate the indirectly activated representation of the US decrease in associative strength, and consequently the overshadowing cue should no longer interfere with the representation of the US that is directly activated by X. Importantly, here we have an example of a change in behavioral control by X as a result of conducting a posttraining manipulation that does not involve further training of X (that is, subjects have no additional experience with X after the overshadowing treatment), and still a recovery from cue competition is observed. Most models that emphasize processing during acquisition (e.g., Rescorla and Wagner, 1972; Wagner, 1981) cannot account for these results for two reasons: (1) they do not have a mechanism that allows learning about absent cues, and (2) these models state that overshadowing results from a deficit in the establishment of the X → US association during overshadowing training, so any manipulation that does not involve the presentation of X should not affect its behavioral control. In fact, recovery from overshadowing after extinguishing the overshadowing cue has been observed repeatedly (e.g., Kaufman and Bolles, 1981; Matzel et al., 1985; Urcelay and Miller, 2006), thereby lending support to a retrieval-failure account of cue competition.

A related example is recovery from blocking. After blocking treatment (A → US followed by AX → US), responding to X is usually diminished relative to a group that experienced an irrelevant cue during training of phase 1 (B → US; AX → US). According to the comparator hypothesis, acquisition of the X → US association proceeds without any competition between A and X. At the time of testing, the blocking cue is thought to decrease responding to the blocked cue through its associations with X and the US (links 2 and 3). Similar to overshadowing, the comparator hypothesis predicts that extinguishing the blocking cue should result in recovery from blocking, as has been empirically observed (e.g., Blaisdell et al., 1999).

For several years, the comparator hypothesis was unique in predicting these recovery effects that could not be explained by traditional models that emphasized acquisition processes (e.g., Rescorla and Wagner, 1972; Wagner, 1981). However, recent revision of the Rescorla–Wagner (1972) model by Van Hamme and Wasserman (1994) and of Wagner's (1981) SOP model by Dickinson and Burke (1996) introduced mechanisms that allow for learning about an absent cue provided an associate of the absent cue is present. Posttraining extinction of a companion cue (i.e., an overshadowing or blocking cue) constitutes a situation in which these models anticipate new learning about a target cue. Consequently, these two models are able to account for phenomena such as recovery from overshadowing and blocking as a result of extinction of an overshadowing or blocking cue. This prompted a revision of the comparator hypothesis, in part to differentiate this model from the revised versions of acquisition-focused models and also to account for data that were problematic for the original comparator hypothesis (Williams, 1996; Rauhut et al., 1999).

The extended comparator hypothesis (Denniston et al., 2001; also see Stout and Miller, in press, for a mathematical implementation of this model) carries the same assumptions as the original comparator hypothesis, but it further assumes that the links mediating the indirectly activated representation of the US (links 2 and 3) are also subject to a comparator process in which nontarget cues present during training can compete for roles as comparator stimuli for the target cue (see **Figure 2**). In other words, the extended version of the model is similar to the original version but allows more than one cue (comparator) to modulate conditioned responding to the target cue. If there's more than one comparator stimulus for the target, these comparator stimuli can in select situations cancel each other with respect to their capacity to modulate responding to the target cue. Thus, the extended comparator hypothesis makes a number of new predictions that allow for differentiating this retrieval-based account from models that emphasize processing during acquisition. For example, it makes the counterintuitive prediction that combining select pairs of treatments that

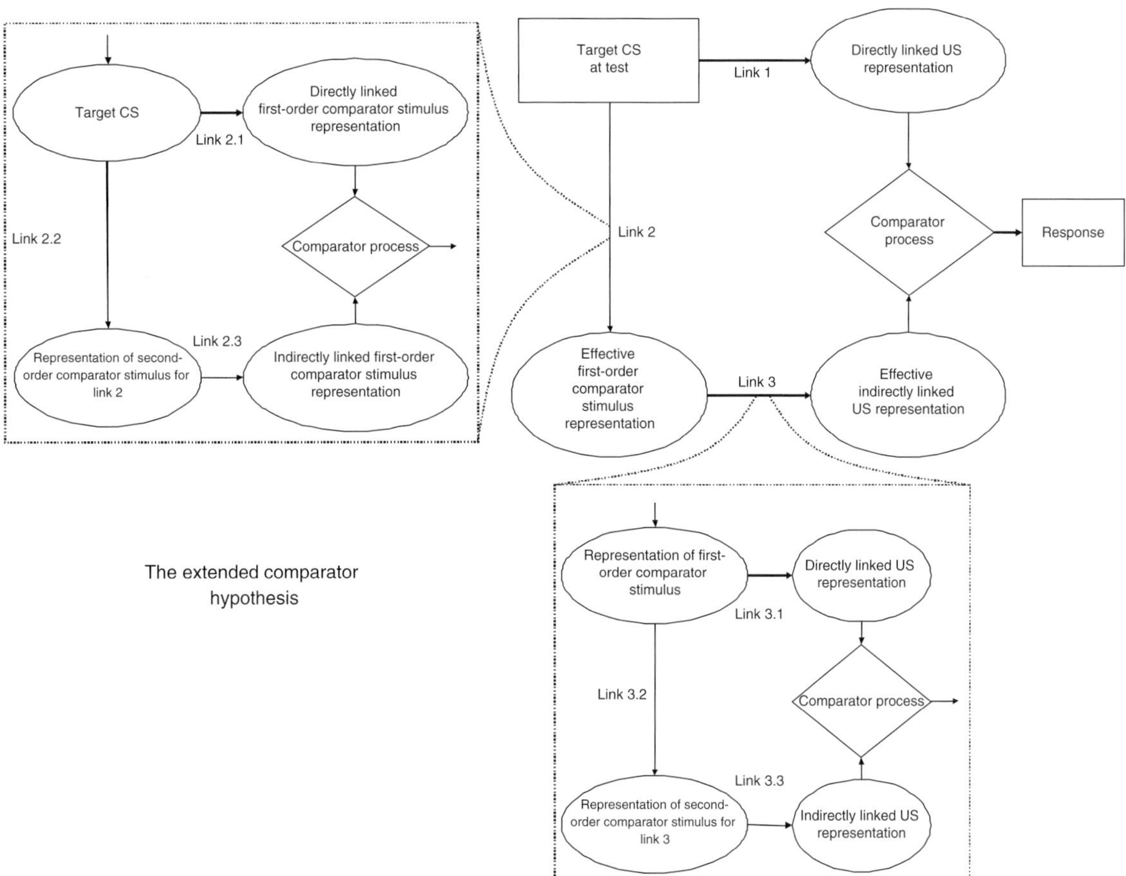

Figure 2 The extended comparator hypothesis (after Denniston JC, Savastano HI, and Miller RR (2001) The extended comparator hypothesis: Learning by contiguity, responding by relative strength. In: Mowrer RR and Klein SB (eds.) *Handbook of Contemporary Learning Theories*, pp. 65–117. Hillsdale, NJ: Erlbaum). Note principles similar to the original comparator hypothesis but with the inclusion of second-order comparator processes that operate over links 2 and 3. The magnitude of second-order comparator processes directly affects conditioned responding to the target CS, by decreasing the effectiveness of first-order comparator stimuli.

alone lead to a decrement in conditioned responding (e.g., overshadowing and the deficit seen in responding when trials are massed; see Barela, 1999, for a review of the trial massing effect) under certain circumstances can result in less (rather than more) of a decrement in behavioral control. In other words, the model predicts that the two response-degrading treatments can counteract each other, and thus less of a decrement in behavioral control should be observed during testing than with either treatment alone. How does the model anticipate this result? Because the extended comparator hypothesis allows for cues (other than the target cue) to compete with each other for comparator status provided they share a within-compound association, any treatment that establishes two comparator stimuli as potential competitors for comparator status with respect to the target cue can lead to a mutual reduction in the comparator roles of each of these stimuli and thus a reduced decrement in conditioned responding to the target cue.

As a test of this prediction, Stout et al. (2003) manipulated overshadowing and trial spacing, so that one group received elemental training with spaced trials (X → US spaced), one group received overshadowing training with spaced trials (AX → US spaced), and two more groups received identical training but with massed trials (X → US and AX → US massed). In this last group, presumably both the overshadowing cue (because of the compound training) and the training context (because of massed trials) should have been effective comparators for the target cue X, and they also should have served as comparators for each other (because A and the context should have been strongly associated). Interestingly, Stout et al. observed strong behavioral control by X in the group that experienced elemental training with spaced trials, less responding in the groups that experienced only one of the response-degrading treatments (either overshadowing or massed trials), and a recovery from these treatments (more responding) in the group that experienced both overshadowing treatment and massed trials. Similar counteractive effects have been observed when combining overshadowing with several other treatments that presumably establish the training context as a strong comparator for the target cue. These treatments include pretraining exposure to the CS alone (i.e., latent inhibition, Blaisdell et al., 1998), long CS duration during conditioning (Urushihara et al., 2004), unsignaled outcomes interspersed among the CS-outcome trials (i.e., degraded contingency, Urcelay and Miller, 2006), and unsignaled outcome alone before or after the CS → US trials (Urushihara and Miller, 2006).

In summary, the comparator hypothesis (Miller and Matzel, 1988) and its extension (Denniston et al., 2001) have proven to be powerful alternatives to associative models that emphasize acquisition processes, as evidenced by their explanatory and predictive power. However, as we shall see next, there are several effects for which the comparator model cannot account. In the next section, we detail a model that accounts for interference effects outside the domain of models of associative learning designed to explain cue competition phenomena.

31.3.3 Bouton's Retrieval Model of Outcome Interference

Perhaps one of the most intriguing findings that Pavlov (1927) documented was the occurrence of a recovery in conditioned responding after a retention interval is interposed between extinction treatment and testing. Since Pavlov's time, there have been many theoretical frameworks proposed to explain extinction and its recovery under different circumstances. One old view of extinction is that nonreinforced presentations of an already trained CS will result in a loss of the CS's associative strength with the US, leading to an irreversible loss of behavioral control. For example, the Rescorla and Wagner (1972) model explains extinction in this manner. However, as we have mentioned before, if the associative strength of an extinguished CS is reduced, there is no reason to expect that responding to the CS will ever recover without further training with the CS, which is opposite to the spontaneous recovery effect observed when a long retention interval is interposed between extinction and testing.

After conducting extensive work on extinction, Bouton (1993) proposed an alternative to the models that view extinction as unlearning of the original association between the CS and US (*See* Chapter 29). This model emphasizes retrieval mechanisms that apply to a wide range of phenomena. Bouton's model has four principles.

1. Contextual stimuli influence memory retrieval. That is, analogous to Tulving and Thomson's (1973), Spear's (1978), and Riccio's (Riccio et al., 2002, 2003) emphasis on the importance of similarity between the conditions of training and testing, Bouton proposed that retrieval of a

representation depends on the similarity between the conditions present at the time of testing with those that were present during training. Thus, as changes between the context of training and the context of testing are introduced, retrieval failure (i.e., forgetting) is more prone to occur. Furthermore, and perhaps in disagreement with Spear's elemental view, Bouton has proposed that CSs and contextual information are stored as interactive units containing information about the cues, the context, and the US. These interactive units function as an AND gate that requires activation of both the cue and the context for the activation of the representation of the US.

2. Time is part of the training context. As time elapses following training, the temporal component of the test context that is provided by external and internal cues is likely to change. In other words, the passage of time by itself will progressively result in a context change. Therefore, forgetting as a result of the passage of time is an instance of retrieval failure due to a change in the temporal context between training and testing.
3. Different memories depend differentially on the contextual information. In his 1993 seminal article, Bouton proposed that excitatory memories are relatively stable over time and do not depend on contextual information as much as do inhibitory memories (including those that represent extinction experience). Additionally he stated that a memory's sensitivity to contextual information depended on whether the training procedures promote subjects to encode and integrate contextual information with other features of the memory representation. One such procedure is when a CS takes a new meaning different from that of earlier training, as is the case when a CS is consistently followed by the US in one phase and it is no longer followed by the US (operationally, extinction) in a second phase. In this case, the second phase makes the CS an ambiguous signal for the US, and thus the model anticipates that the second-learned association will depend more on contextual information. In fact, Bouton (1997) later clarified this issue by stating that regardless of whether a memory is excitatory or inhibitory, each instance in which there is ambiguity with regard to the content of a memory (i.e., training in two sequential phases with opposing outcomes in the different phases), the second-learned meaning will be more context dependent. This later assertion has received empirical support from Nelson (2002; also see De la Casa and Lubow, 2000, 2002).
4. Interference occurs at the time of testing rather than at the time of training. This principle captures all of the previously mentioned principles by stating that interference occurs at retrieval rather than during learning. With ambiguity in the meaning of the CS, the activation of an outcome representation occurs in direct relationship to the similarity between the context at test and those during the different phases of training. Additionally, information that is similar to, but incompatible with, the target memory will compete for a limited available space in working memory (i.e., currently active memory). That is, activation of a conflicting memory could reduce activation of the target memory. Thus, forgetting can result from two sources: retrieval failure (because of a change in context) and interference due to activation of conflicting information.

Bouton's model explains spontaneous recovery from extinction by assuming that the second-learned meaning of the CS (that is, CS → no outcome or an inhibitory association between the CS and the outcome) is context dependent, based on the principle of context dependency of the second-learned meaning of a cue. Moreover, the model states that a change in temporal context is analogous to a change in spatial context. As a result, when the temporal context of the second meaning of a cue is changed between phase 2 of treatment and testing (i.e., interposing a long retention interval after extinction), the memory representation of extinction treatment cannot be as readily retrieved. Thus, a recovery from extinction is observed with a long retention interval. A similar explanation is put forth by this model to explain all forms of renewal, spatial as well as temporal. In renewal, the second-learned meaning of the CS (CS → no US) should be context dependent, so any change in the spatial attributes of the context between extinction treatment and testing will result in interference in retrieving that memory. As a result of such a context shift, a recovery from extinction should be observed.

Another finding that is problematic for models that emphasize processing during acquisition is reinstatement, which is a recovery from extinction observed when subjects experience outcome-alone presentations in the test context prior to testing. In this case, Bouton's model assumes that the test context becomes associated with the outcome so that at test it biases retrieval in favor of the memory of reinforcement. Thus, a recovery from extinction is observed. Another way by which this model has been tested is by associating a neutral cue (a priming stimulus) with the phase of treatment in which extinction occurs. If the test is conducted in a context different from that of extinction treatment, renewal typically occurs. However, if during testing subjects are presented with this neutral cue from the extinction phase soon before being tested with the target cue, renewal is attenuated, presumably because this cue retrieves the memory of extinction treatment (Brooks and Bouton, 1994). A parallel attenuation of spontaneous recovery from extinction has been observed when the temporal context, as opposed to the spatial context, is altered between extinction training and testing (i.e., interpolation of a long retention interval). That is, reduced spontaneous recovery has been observed when a retrieval cue for the memory of extinction treatment is presented before testing following a long retention interval (Brooks and Bouton, 1993).

As we previously discussed, counterconditioning is another example of the context dependency of memory. If counterconditioning training is conducted with an appetitive reinforcer given in one context and an aversive reinforcer given in a different context, conditioned responding to the CS is guided by the context in which subjects are tested (Peck and Bouton, 1990). The retrieval model outlined earlier simply states that whichever memory representation is facilitated by contextual cues will be more prone to guide behavior.

In summary, we have reviewed general models of memory that emphasize retrieval mechanisms as critical for behavioral control. In general, Spear's (1978) model emphasizes the similarity between the total information presented during training and that presented at test and by this simple principle explains memory phenomena such as state-dependent learning and the Kamin effect. The comparator hypothesis (Miller and Matzel, 1988) is an associative model that emphasizes competition between representations and explains cue-competition phenomena and recovery from cue competition that does not involve further training with the target cue. Bouton's model (1993, 1997) emphasizes the role of retrieval cues in situations in which one cue has more than one meaning, as in the cases of extinction, latent inhibition, and counterconditioning. One obvious conclusion is that each model has been designed to account for a family of phenomena at the expense of explaining other phenomena. For example, the comparator hypothesis (Miller and Matzel, 1988) accounts for cue competition phenomena and several other effects in classical conditioning, but it does not explain the recovery from extinction or counterconditioning effects that are consistently observed. Moreover, this model does not explain state-dependent learning. In contrast, Bouton's retrieval model (Bouton, 1993, 1997) accounts elegantly for interference effects, but it does not incorporate any mechanism that accounts for cue competition phenomena. Perhaps the biggest challenge these models face is to explain phenomena outside their current domain without necessarily increasing their complexity and thus losing predictive power. As we shall see in the next section, a few efforts have been made to integrate these behavioral models with the neurobiological evidence concerning the role of retrieval in memory performance.

31.4 Neurobiology of Retrieval

Recent technological advances have widened the possibilities of understanding learning and memory phenomena by studying their underlying neurophysiological basis. Interestingly, the focus on acquisition processes (e.g., Waelti et al., 2001) and memory consolidation (e.g., McGaugh, 2000) has dominated the field, perhaps because of the discovery of potential molecular mechanisms underlying long-term potentiation (Bliss and Lomo, 1973) that are thought to be the basis for the formation of memories (but see Shors and Matzel, 1997, for an alternative view). However, the neurobiological basis of retrieval mechanisms has also received some attention. But before we review some experiments that studied the role of different brain regions in retrieval, it is important that we clarify the general strategy underlying these studies. In any memory experiment, there are at least three identifiable phases amenable to study, namely acquisition, consolidation, and retrieval. As pointed out by Abel and Lattal (2001), one of the problems associated with different manipulations (pharmacological, genetic, and lesions) is that, with the exception of recently developed inactivation techniques that allow researchers to temporarily inactivate a specific anatomical area, they can affect more than one of the three stages. For example, a lesion soon after acquisition might impair not only consolidation but also retrieval. A lesion before any training might alter training, consolidation, and/or retrieval. Moreover, pharmacological manipulations might be temporary, but the effects of the mere exposure to the drug are not always completely known, as reflected earlier when we discussed the apoptotic effects of anisomycin (Rudy et al., 2006). Clearly all these considerations have to be taken into account to obtain valid information regarding the neurobiological underpinnings of memory.

Next, we briefly summarize the main findings regarding contextual determinants of memory retrieval. Notably, because of space limitations, we will only summarize a few studies that have the merit of integrating behavioral theories with neurobiological data. Studies such as these are few in number (but see, e.g., Fanselow, 1999; Waelti et al., 2001; McNally and Westbrook, 2006; for notable exceptions focused on acquisition).

The hippocampus is one of the most extensively studied brain regions with regard to retrieval mechanisms (as well as acquisition processes). In general, the hippocampus has been implicated in both the coding and retrieval of spatial information and also in relations between events in the environment (e.g., Maren, 2001; but see Wiltgen et al., 2006). In fear conditioning, the hippocampus is thought to assemble contextual representations before they reach the amygdala, which is the site in which fear-motivated information is mainly processed. As we previously mentioned, contextual information is critical for the retrieval of associations. One of the questions researchers have recently asked concerns the role of the hippocampus in the retrieval as opposed to acquisition of contextual information. For example, behavior indicative of extinction is observed when contextual cues facilitate the retrieval of the extinction memory as opposed to the acquisition memory. Based on this finding, Wilson et al. (1995) investigated the effect on context-dependent extinction of fornix (one of the two primary inputs into the dorsal hippocampus) lesions made prior to training. It is important to recall that two of these context-dependent effects are renewal and reinstatement, and in terms of Bouton's theory of retrieval, they are mediated by different mechanisms. In the case of renewal, the context seems to disambiguate the two meanings a CS has after acquisition and extinction training. In the case of reinstatement, the test context-US association facilitates retrieval of the original CS → US association. Wilson et al. (1995) observed that fornix lesions attenuated reinstatement, which depends on context-US associations, but not renewal nor spontaneous recovery which depend more on the properties of the context to disambiguate information. This outcome is surprising because it leaves no role for the hippocampus on the retrieval of ambiguous information. However, other studies using temporary reversible lesions have found that the hippocampus does in fact participate in the retrieval of information needed to disambiguate the meaning of an extinguished CS. Specifically, Corcoran and Maren (2001) used muscimol (a gamma-aminobutyric acid$_A$ ($GABA_A$) receptor agonist) infusions into the dorsal hippocampus just prior to testing (i.e., retrieval) to investigate the effect of the hippocampus on the retrieval of ambiguous memories (renewal). They found that the renewal effect was attenuated when they deactivated the dorsal hippocampus. Similar findings have been observed by Corcoran and Maren (2004; although the effect was not seen in ABA renewal). Overall, these findings raise several interesting points: (1) These results show that the hippocampus, a brain region known for its role in the encoding and retrieval of contextual information, is critical for the expression of extinction memories, which are context dependent. (2) Reversible lesions have the advantage of allowing dissection of the different processes (such as retrieval) involved in memory performance. (3) Behavioral theories (e.g., Bouton, 1993) can provide fertile grounds for research in the neurobiology of learning and memory and vice versa. Clearly, the key is to combine information from both approaches as a starting point for conducting further research.

Another recent study exemplifies context-dependent memories and the role of the hippocampus in such learning. As previously stated, latent inhibition refers to retarded emergence of behavioral control that results from CS-alone exposures prior to CS → US pairings (Lubow, 1973). A retrieval-based account such as the comparator hypothesis (Miller and Matzel, 1988) explains latent inhibition by positing that, during CS preexposure, subjects associate the CS with the context, which interferes during testing with the retrieval of the CS → US association. Consistent with this explanation, extinction of the training context abolished the latent inhibition effect (e.g., Grahame et al., 1994; Westbrook et al., 2000). Moreover, if CS preexposure is conducted in one context and reinforced training in a second context, latent inhibition is not observed (Channell and Hall, 1983). Consistent with these predictions, Talk et al. (2005) found that context extinction following the

CS-US pairings increased neural firing to the preexposed CS in the posterior cingulate cortex, a structure hypothesized to have a role in retrieval of learned behavior. Presumably, the hippocampal formation sends (through the fornix) contextual information to the posterior cingulate cortex. When the contextual information is decreased as a result of the context extinction treatment, an increase in neural responses to the CS is observed, and this is reflected in the diminished latent inhibition.

These examples have the merit of integrating retrieval-focused behavioral theories of memory and neurobiological evidence concerning the underlying mechanisms of retrieval. We believe that further understanding of the neurophysiology of learning and memory will be most fruitful when it has some relationship to behavioral models. As these examples demonstrate, research guided by knowledge obtained in behavioral experiments (and the theoretical developments that follow those results) seems to be a reliable foundation for investigation of the neural foundations of retrieval.

31.5 Concluding Remarks

In this review, we started with the premise that a vast majority of the research concerning mechanisms of learning and memory has been guided by the notion that memory depends uniquely on mechanisms of acquisition and storage. Although we should not underestimate the contribution of these processes, we pointed out numerous phenomena suggesting that retrieval mechanisms also play an important role in determining stimulus control of behavior. We reviewed various examples, ranging from forgetting due to natural changes in the environment or in the organism's internal state, through amnesia experimentally induced in the laboratory, to situations in which additional (sometimes conflicting) information decreases target behavior. In all of these examples, there was evidence that the information was not lost, but rather was present but not expressed at the time of testing. Providing conditions during testing similar to those during training strongly facilitates retrieval and, as a consequence, stimulus control of behavior. In a similar vein, facilitating retrieval by the aid of reminder cues has also proven effective for memory performance. These demonstrations imply that information was stored but not expressed at the time of testing, which suggests a strong role of retrieval mechanisms.

In the second section, we described several models that emphasize processing at the time of retrieval as being critical for memory expression. Perhaps the unsatisfying conclusion from this section is that there is not a single approach that accounts for all of the data available. Some models seem to fare well in accounting for some phenomena, but fail to explain fundamental aspects of other phenomena. As an example, we pointed out how well the comparator model accounts for cue competition phenomena, but also recognized its failure in addressing important aspects of extinction and competition between cues trained apart. Obviously, the ultimate goal of any science of behavior is not only to explain behavior but also to predict it. At least the models we reviewed provide strong foundations for future theoretical developments, and in some ways each proposal has proven its heuristic value as a tool to guide new research. Current behavioral models have stimulated research into the neurobiological underpinnings of memory. We see this avenue as perhaps the most fruitful in the future because bridging the gap that exists between behavior and its underlying neurobiological basis is an important step toward societal application.

Retrieval, the act of making stored information available for use, is as important as acquisition in terms of adaptive value. Consider, for example, what would happen if an organism faces a dangerous situation and is able to survive. If the animal does not retain that information by virtue of either acquisition failure or storage failure, memory of that experience will not be available for future use. On the contrary, if the animal stores the information, it will be available for later encounters with the dangerous situation. This brings us to the question: why does retrieval failure occur? Perhaps retrieval failures, as we have seen, arise from processing limitations. But more important, it seems plausible that retrieval failures arise from a strategy for organizing information based on how relevant this information is in the test situation. That is, leaving some information less accessible enables organisms to have access to other information that could be more important, depending on the demands imposed by the immediate environment.

Acknowledgments

Support for this research was provided by National Institute of Mental Health Grant 33881.

References

Abel T and Lattal KM (2001) Molecular mechanisms of memory acquisition, consolidation and retrieval. *Curr. Opin. Neurobiol.* 11: 180–187.

Amundson JC, Escobar M, and Miller RR (2003) Proactive interference in first-order Pavlovian conditioning. *J. Exp. Psychol. Anim. Behav. Process.* 29: 311–322.

Anokhin KV, Tiunova AA, and Rose SPR (2002) Reminder effects – reconsolidation or retrieval deficit? Pharmacological dissection with protein synthesis inhibitors following reminder for a passive-avoidance task in young chicks. *Eur. J. Neurosci.* 15: 1759–1765.

Balaz MA, Gutsin P, Cacheiro H, and Miller RR (1982) Blocking as a retrieval failure: Reactivation of associations to a blocked stimulus. *Q. J. Exp. Psychol.* 34B: 99–113.

Barela PB (1999) Theoretical mechanisms underlying the trial-spacing effect in pavlovian fear conditioning. *J. Exp. Psychol. Anim. Behav. Process.* 25: 177–193.

Barraco RA and Stettner LJ (1976) Antibiotics and memory. *Psychol. Bull.* 83: 242–302.

Batsell WR (1997) Retention of context blocking in taste-aversion learning. *Physiol. Behav.* 61: 437–446.

Biedenkapp JC and Rudy JW (2004) Context memories and reactivation: Constraints on the reconsolidation hypothesis. *Behav. Neurosci.* 118: 956–964.

Blaisdell AP, Bristol AS, Gunther LM, and Miller RR (1998) Overshadowing and latent inhibition counteract each other: Support for the comparator hypothesis. *J. Exp. Psychol. Anim. Behav. Process.* 24: 335–351.

Blaisdell AP, Gunther LM, and Miller RR (1999) Recovery from blocking achieved by extinguishing the blocking CS. *Anim. Learn. Behav.* 27: 63–76.

Bliss TV and Lomo T (1973) Long-lasting potentiation of synaptic transmission in the dentate area of the anaesthetized rabbit following stimulation of the perforant path. *J. Physiol.* 232: 331–356.

Bouton ME (1993) Context, time, and memory retrieval in the interference paradigms of Pavlovian learning. *Psychol. Bull.* 114: 80–99.

Bouton ME (1997) Signals for whether versus when an event will occur. In: Bouton ME and Fanselow MS (eds.) *Learning, Motivation and Cognition. The Functional Behaviorism of Robert C. Bolles*. Washington, DC: American Psychological Association.

Bouton ME and Bolles RC (1979) Contextual control of the extinction of conditioned fear. *Learn. Motiv.* 10: 445–466.

Bouton ME and King DA (1983) Contextual control of the extinction of conditioned fear: Tests for associative value of the context. *J. Exp. Psychol. Anim. Behav. Process.* 9: 248–265.

Bouton ME and Peck CA (1992) Spontaneous recovery in cross-motivational transfer (counterconditioning). *Anim. Learn. Behav.* 20: 313–321.

Bouton ME and Swartzentruber DE (1989) Slow reacquisition following extinction: Context, encoding, and retrieval mechanisms. *J. Exp. Psychol. Anim. Behav. Process.* 15: 43–53.

Bradley PM and Galal KM (1988) State-dependent recall can be induced by protein synthesis inhibition: Behavioural and morphological observations. *Brain Res.* 40: 243–251.

Brooks DC and Bouton ME (1993) A retrieval cue for extinction attenuates spontaneous recovery. *J. Exp. Psychol. Anim. Behav. Process.* 19: 77–89.

Brooks DC and Bouton ME (1994) A retrieval cue for extinction attenuates response recovery (renewal) caused by a return to the conditioning context. *J. Exp. Psychol. Anim. Behav. Process.* 20: 366–379.

Brooks DC, Hale B, Nelson JB, and Bouton ME (1995) Reinstatement after counterconditioning. *Anim. Learn. Behav.* 23: 383–390.

Bush RR and Mosteller F (1951) A mathematical model for simple learning. *Psychol. Rev.* 58: 313–323.

Cammarota M, Bevilaqua LRM, Medina JH, and Izquierdo I (2004) Retrieval does not induce reconsolidation of inhibitory avoidance memory. *Learn. Mem.* 11: 572–578.

Channell S and Hall G (1983) Contextual effects in latent inhibition with an appetitive conditioning procedure. *Anim. Learn. Behav.* 11: 67–74.

Corcoran KA and Maren S (2001) Hippocampal inactivation disrupts contextual retrieval of fear memory after extinction. *J. Neurosci.* 21: 1720–1726.

Corcoran KA and Maren S (2004) Factors regulating the effects of hippocampal inactivation on renewal of conditional fear after extinction. *Learn. Mem.* 11(5): 598–603.

Craik FI and Lockhart RS (1972) Levels of processing: A framework for memory research. *J. Verb. Learn. Verb. Behav.* 11: 671–684.

Cunningham CL (1979) Alcohol as a cue for extinction: State dependency produced by conditioned inhibition. *Anim. Learn. Behav.* 7: 45–52.

De la Casa LG and Lubow RE (2000) Super-latent inhibition with delayed conditioned taste aversion testing. *Anim. Learn. Behav.* 28: 389–399.

De la Casa LG and Lubow RE (2002) An empirical analysis of the super-latent inhibition effect. *Anim. Learn. Behav.* 30: 112–120.

Debięc L, LeDoux JE, and Nader K (2002) Cellular and systems reconsolidation in the hippocampus. *Neuron* 36: 527–538.

Debięc J, Doyère V, Nader K, and LeDoux JE (2006) Directly reactivated, but not indirectly reactivated, memories undergo reconsolidation in the amygdala. *Proc. Natl. Acad. Sci. USA* 103: 3428–3433.

Denniston JC, Savastano HI, and Miller RR (2001) The extended comparator hypothesis: Learning by contiguity, responding by relative strength. In: Mowrer RR and Klein SB (eds.) *Handbook of Contemporary Learning Theories*, pp. 65–117. Hillsdale, NJ: Erlbaum.

Dickinson A and Burke J (1996) Within-compound associations mediate the retrospective revaluation of causality judgments. *Q. J. Exp. Psychol. 49B,* 60–80.

Duncan CP (1949) The retroactive effect of electroshock on learning. *J. Comp. Physiol. Psychol.* 42: 32–44.

Duvarci S and Nader K (2004) Characterization of fear memory reconsolidation. *J. Neurosci.* 24: 9269–9275.

Escobar M, Matute H, and Miller RR (2001) Cues trained apart compete for behavioral control in rats: Convergence with the associative interference literature. *J. Exp. Psychol. Gen.* 130: 97–115.

Esmoris-Arranz FJ, Miller RR, and Matute H (1997) Blocking of subsequent and antecedent events: Implications for cue competition in causal judgment. *J. Exp. Psychol. Anim. Behav. Process.* 23: 145–156.

Fanselow MS (1999) Learning theory and neuropsychology: Configuring their disparate elements in the hippocampus. *J. Exp. Psychol. Anim. Behav. Process.* 25: 275–283.

Fisher A, Sananbenesi F, Schrick C, Speiss J, and Radulovic J (2004) Distinct roles of hippocampal de novo protein synthesis and actin rearrangement in extinction of contextual fear. *J. Neurosci.* 24: 1962–1966.

Gisquet-Verrier P and Alexinsky T (1990) Facilitative effect of a pretest exposure to the CS: Analysis and implications for the memory trace. *Anim. Learn. Behav.* 18: 323–331.

Gisquet-Verrier P, Dekeyne A, and Alexinsky T (1989) Differential effects of several retrieval cues over time:

Evidence for time-dependent reorganization of memory. *Anim. Learn. Behav.* 17: 394–408.
Gold PE and King RA (1974) Retrograde amnesia: Storage failure versus retrieval failure. *Psychol. Rev.* 81. 465–469.
Grahame NJ, Barnet RC, Gunther LM, and Miller RR (1994) Latent inhibition as a performance deficit resulting from CS-context associations. *Anim. Learn. Behav.* 22: 395–408.
Hebb DO (1949) *The Organization of Behavior: A Neuropsychological Theory.* Oxford, UK: Wiley.
Hernandez PJ and Kelley AE (2004) Long-term memory for instrumental responses does not undergo protein synthesis-dependent reconsolidation upon retrieval. *Learn. Mem.* 11: 748–754.
Hinderliter CF, Webster T, and Riccio DC (1976) Amnesia induced by hypothermia as a function of treatment-test interval and recooling in rats. *Anim. Learn. Behav.* 3: 257–263.
Kamin LJ (1957) The retention of an incompletely learned avoidance response. *J. Comp. Physiol. Psychol.* 50: 457–460.
Kamin LJ (1963) Retention of an incompletely learned avoidance response: Some further analyses. *J. Comp. Physiol. Psychol.* 56: 713–718.
Kamin LJ (1969) Predictability, surprise, attention, and conditioning. In: Campbell BA and Church MR (eds.) *Punishment and Aversive Behavior*, pp. 279–296. New York: Appleton-Century-Crofts.
Kasprow WJ, Cacheiro H, Balaz MA, and Miller RR (1982) Reminder induced recovery of associations to an overshadowed stimulus. *Learn. Motiv.* 13: 155–166.
Kaufman MA and Bolles RC (1981) A nonassociative aspect of overshadowing. *Bull. Psychonomic Soc.* 18: 318–320.
Klein SB (1972) Adrenal-pituitary influence in reactivation of avoidance-learning memory in the rat after intermediate intervals. *J. Comp. Physiol. Psychol.* 79: 341–359.
Klein SB and Spear NE (1970) Reactivation of avoidance-learning memory in the rat after intermediate retention intervals. *J. Comp. Physiol. Psychol.* 72: 498–504.
Kraemer PJ, Lariviere NA, and Spear NE (1988) Expression of a taste aversion conditioned with an odor taste compound: Overshadowing is relatively weak in weanlings and decreases over a retention interval in adults. *Anim. Learn. Behav.* 16: 164–168.
Lattal KM and Abel T (2001) Different requirements for protein synthesis in acquisition and extinction of spatial preferences and context-evoked fear. *J. Neurosci.* 21: 5773–5780.
Lattal KM and Abel T (2004) Behavioral impairments caused by injections of the protein synthesis inhibitor anisomycin after contextual retrieval reverse with time. *Proc. Natl. Acad. Sci. USA* 101: 4667–4672.
Lewis DJ, Misanin JR, and Miller RR (1968) Recovery of memory following amnesia. *Nature* 220: 704–705.
Lubow RE (1973) Latent inhibition. *Psychol. Bull.* 79: 398–407.
Mackintosh NJ (1975) A theory of attention: Variations in the associability of stimuli with reinforcement. *Psychol. Rev.* 82: 276–298.
Mactutus CF and Riccio DC (1978) Hypothermia-induced retrograde amnesia: Role of body temperature in memory retrieval. *Physiol. Psychol.* 6: 18–22.
Maren S (2001) Neurobiology of Pavlovian fear conditioning. *Annu. Rev. Neurosci.* 24: 897–931.
Matzel LD, Schachtman TR, and Miller RR (1985) Recovery of an overshadowed association achieved by extinction of the overshadowing stimulus. *Learn. Motiv.* 16: 398–412.
McEwen BS and Weiss JM (1970) The uptake and action of corticosterone: Regional and subcellular studies on rat brain. *Prog. Brain Res.* 32: 200–212.
McGaugh JL (1966) Time-dependent processes in memory storage. *Science* 153: 1351–1358.
McGaugh JL (2000) Memory: A century of consolidation. *Science* 287: 248–251.
McNally GP and Westbrook RF (2006) Predicting danger: The nature, consequences, and neural mechanisms of predictive fear learning. *Learn. Mem.* 13: 245–253.
Miller RR and Matute H (1998) Competition between outcomes. *Psychol. Sci.* 9: 146–149.
Miller RR and Matzel LD (1988) The comparator hypothesis: A response rule for the expression of associations. In: Bower GH (ed.) *The Psychology of Learning and Motivation, Vol. 22*, pp. 51–92. San Diego, CA: Academic Press.
Miller RR and Matzel LD (2000) Memory involves far more than 'consolidation'. *Nat. Rev. Neurosci.* 3: 214–216.
Miller RR and Matzel LD (2006) Retrieval failure vs. memory loss in experimental amnesia: Definitions and processes. *Learn. Mem.* 13: 491–497.
Miller RR, Ott CA, Berk AM, and Springer AD (1974) Appetitive memory restoration after electroconvulsive shock in the rat. *J. Comp. Physiol. Psychol.* 87: 717–723.
Miller RR and Springer AD (1973) Amnesia, consolidation, and retrieval. *Psychol. Rev.* 80: 69–79.
Miller RR and Springer AD (1974) Implications of recovery from experimental amnesia. *Psychol. Rev.* 81: 470–473.
Millin PM, Moody EW, and Riccio DC (2001) Interpretations of retrograde amnesia: Old problems redux. *Nat. Rev. Neurosci.* 2: 68–70.
Nadel L and Land C (2000) Memory traces revisited. *Nat. Rev. Neurosci.* 1: 209–212.
Nader K, Schafe GE, and Le Doux JE (2000) Fear memories require protein synthesis in the amygdala for reconsolidation after retrieval. *Nature* 406: 722–726.
Nelson JB (2002) Context specificity of excitation and inhibition in ambiguous stimuli. *Learn. Motiv.* 33: 284–310.
Overton DA (1964) State dependent or "dissociated" learning produced with pentobarbital. *J. Comp. Physiol. Psychol.* 57: 3–12.
Overton DA (1972) State-dependent learning produced by alcohol and its relevance to alcoholism. In: Kissin B and Begleiter H (eds.) *The Biology of Alcoholism.* New York: Plenum Press.
Overton DA (1985) Contextual stimulus effects of drugs and internal states. In: Balsam PD and Tomie A (eds.) *Context and Learning*, pp. 357–384. Hillsdale, NJ: Lawrence Erlbaum Associates.
Pavlov IP (1927) *Conditioned Reflexes*, Anrep GV (ed. and trans.). London: Oxford University Press.
Pearce JM and Hall G (1980) A model for Pavlovian learning: Variations in the effectiveness of conditioned but not unconditioned stimuli. *Psychol. Rev.* 82: 532–552.
Peck CA and Bouton ME (1990) Context and performance in aversive-to-appetitive and appetitive-to-aversive transfer. *Learn. Motiv.* 21: 1–31.
Power AE, Berlau DJ, McGaugh JL, and Steward O (2006) Anisomycin infused into the hippocampus fails to block "reconsolidation" but impairs extinction: The role of re-exposure duration. *Learn. Mem.* 13: 27–34.
Pineño O, Urushihara K, and Miller RR (2005) Spontaneous recovery from forward and backward blocking. *J. Exp. Psychol. Anim. Behav. Process.* 31: 172–183.
Prado-Alcalá RA, del Guante MA D, Garín-Aguilar ME, Díaz-Trujillo A, Quirarte GL, and McGaugh JL (2006) Amygdala or hippocampus inactivation after retrieval induces temporary memory deficit. *Neurobiol. Learn. Mem.* 86: 144–149.
Przybyslawski J and Sara SJ (1997) Reconsolidation of memory after its reactivation. *Behav. Brain Res.* 84: 241–246.
Rauhut AS, McPhee JE, and Ayres JB (1999) Blocked and overshadowed stimuli are weakened in their ability to serve as blockers and second-order reinforces in Pavlovian fear

conditioning. *J. Exp. Psychol. Anim. Behav. Process.* 25: 45–67.
Rescorla RA (1980) *Pavlovian Second-Order Conditioning: Studies in Associative Learning.* Hillsdale, NJ: Erlbaum.
Rescorla RA and Cunningham CL (1978) Recovery of the US representation over time during extinction. *Learn. Motiv.* 9: 373–391.
Rescorla RA and Wagner AR (1972) A theory of Pavlovian conditioning: Variations in the effectiveness of reinforcement and nonreinforcement. In: Black AH and Prokasy WF (eds.) *Classical Conditioning II: Current Research and Theory*, pp. 64–99. New York: Appleton-Century-Crofts.
Riccio DC, Millin PM, and Gisquet-Verrier P (2003) Retrograde amnesia: Forgetting back. *Curr. Dir. Psychol. Sci.* 12: 41–44.
Riccio DC, Moody EW, and Millin PM (2002) Reconsolidation reconsidered. *Integr. Physiol. Behav. Sci.* 37: 245–253.
Rudy JW, Biedenkapp JC, Moineau J, and Bolding K (2006) Anisomycin and the reconsolidation hypothesis. *Learn. Mem.* 13: 1–3.
Shors TJ and Matzel LD (1997) Long-term potentiation: What's learning got to do with it? *Behav. Brain Sci.* 20: 597–655.
Spear NE (1973) Retrieval of memories in animals. *Psychol. Rev.* 80: 163–194.
Spear NE (1978) *The Processing of Memories: Forgetting and Retention.* Hillsdale, NJ: Erlbaum.
Stout SC and Miller RR (2007) Sometimes competing retrieval (SOCR): A formalization of the comparator hypothesis. *Psychol. Rev.* 114(3): 759–783.
Stout SC, Chang R, and Miller RR (2003) Trial spacing is a determinant of cue interaction. *J. Exp. Psychol. Anim. Behav. Process.* 29: 23–38.
Talk A, Stoll E, and Gabriel M (2005) Cingulate cortical coding of context-dependent latent inhibition. *Behav. Neurosci.* 119: 1524–1532.
Tulving E and Thomson DM (1973) Encoding specificity and retrieval processes in episodic memory. *Psychol. Rev.* 80: 352–373.
Urcelay GP and Miller RR (2006) Counteraction between overshadowing and degraded contingency treatments: Support for the extended comparator hypothesis. *J. Exp. Psychol. Anim. Behav. Process.* 32: 21–32.
Urushihara K and Miller RR (2006) Overshadowing and the outcome-alone exposure effect counteract each other. *J. Exp. Psychol. Anim. Behav. Process.* 32: 253–270.
Urushihara K, Stout SC, and Miller RR (2004) The basic laws of conditioning differ for elemental cues and cues trained in compound. *Psychol. Sci.* 15: 268–271.
Van Hamme LJ and Wasserman EA (1994) Cue competition in causality judgments: The role of nonpresentation of compound stimulus elements. *Learn. Motiv.* 25: 127–151.
Vardaris RM, Gaebelein C, and Riccio DC (1973) Retrograde amnesia from hypothermia-induced brain seizures. *Physiol. Psychol.* 1: 204–208.
Vianna MR, Szapiro G, McGaugh JL, Medina JH, and Izquierdo I (2001) Retrieval of memory for fear-motivated training initiates extinction requiring protein synthesis in the rat hippocampus. *Proc. Natl. Acad. Sci. USA* 98: 12251–12254.
Waelti P, Dickinson A, and Schultz W (2001) Dopamine responses comply with basic assumptions of formal learning theory. *Nature* 412: 43–48.
Wagner AR (1981) SOP: A model of automatic memory processing in animal behavior. In: Spear NE and Miller RR (eds.) *Information Processing in Animals: Memory Mechanisms*, pp. 5–47. Hillsdale, NJ: Erlbaum.
Wagner AR and Rescorla RA (1972) Inhibition in Pavlovian conditioning: Application of a theory. In: Boakes RA and Halliday MS (eds.) *Inhibition and Learning*, pp. 301–336. London: Academic Press.
Westbrook RF, Jones ML, Bailey GK, and Harris JA (2000) Contextual control over conditioned responding in a latent inhibition paradigm. *J. Exp. Psychol. Anim. Behav. Process.* 26: 157–173.
Wheeler DS and Miller RR (2005) Recovery from blocking between outcomes. *J. Exp. Psychol. Anim. Behav. Process.* 31: 467–476.
Wheeler DS, Stout SC, and Miller RR (2004) Interaction of retention interval with CS-preexposure and extinction treatments: Symmetry with respect to primacy. *Learn. Behav.* 32: 335–347.
Williams BA (1996) Evidence that blocking is due to associative deficit: Blocking history affects the degree of subsequent associative competition. *Psychon. Bull. Rev.* 3: 71–74.
Wilson A, Brooks DC, and Bouton ME (1995) The role of the rat hippocampal system in several effects of context in extinction. *Behav. Neurosci.* 109: 828–836.
Wiltgen BJ, Sanders MJ, Anagnostaras SG, Sage JR, and Fanselow MS (2006) Context fear learning in the absence of the hippocampus. *J. Neurosci.* 26: 5484–5491.

32 False Memories

E. J. Marsh, A. N. Eslick, and L. K. Fazio, Duke University, Durham, NC, USA

Memory is impressive. People can recognize hundreds of pictures seen only once (Shepard, 1967) and recall hundreds of words in response to cues (Mäntylä, 1986). Memory's feats are not limited to short delays or to remembering simple materials in laboratory settings. People remember their high school classmates 15 years after graduation (Bahrick et al., 1975) and recall details about the German invasion of Denmark 50 years after they experienced it (Berntsen and Thomsen, 2005). This short list could easily be expanded.

And yet memory's failures can be equally impressive. For example, people's recognition memory for a penny is actually quite poor, even though they have likely handled hundreds (if not thousands) over the years (Nickerson and Adams, 1979). Similarly, the majority of people fail when asked to draw the layout of the number keys on a calculator, even though they could easily use such a device (Rinck, 1999). Memory failures are not limited to mundane objects, of course. Consider just a few examples: Parents misremember the way they raised their children (Robbins, 1963), eyewitness misidentifications occur (Wells et al., 2006), and people falsely remember being abducted by aliens (Clancy, 2005).

To understand human memory, we must understand memory's failures as well as its successes. What is more interesting than the fact that memory is fallible is that the errors are systematic. By systematic, we simply mean that the errors are not random. We understand something about the conditions under which errors are more or less likely; for example, delay is a manipulation that often increases memory errors. This systematicity occurs because errors are often byproducts of mechanisms that normally aid memory, meaning that memory errors can provide a window into the mechanisms of memory.

One of the classics in this tradition is Bartlett's 1932 study in which participants read and retold a Native American story entitled 'The War of the Ghosts.' When participants retold the story, they made systematic errors. They changed the unfamiliar Native American tale so that it made more sense to them and so that it fit better with their English culture. For example, in the retellings 'canoe' became 'boat' and the more supernatural parts of the story either disappeared or changed to be more consistent with a typical English story.

Bartlett concluded that our memories are reconstructive. We do not recall exactly what happened; rather, we reconstruct events using our knowledge, culture, and prior beliefs about what must have occurred. In other words, we use schemas to help reconstruct our memories. A schema is a knowledge structure that organizes what one knows and expects about some aspect of the world. Schemas are useful heuristics that allow us to fill in the gaps and to make predictions. Bartlett's participants possessed a schema about what happens in a typical story and they used this schema to reconstruct the atypical story that they had read.

Bartlett's ideas about reconstructive memory and the influence of one's prior knowledge have been modified only slightly through the years and are still thought to be the backbone of how our memory functions. Schemas have been repeatedly shown to have large effects on later memory. For example, consider a classic study in which participants read short passages, including one about an unruly child.

When told that the story was about Helen Keller, participants later falsely recognized sentences such as 'She was deaf, dumb, and blind.' When the protagonist was labeled as Carol Harris, however, participants rarely falsely recognized the same sentences (Dooling and Christiaansen, 1977). The familiar label presumably activated participants' prior knowledge of Helen Keller, which participants used to make sense of the passage and to fill in gaps in the story. One's schema of Helen Keller, for example, might include information about her childhood in Alabama and her disabilities, as well as how she blossomed into a successful speaker and writer with the help of her teacher Anne Sullivan. While this background knowledge is likely to aid comprehension of the passage, it also sets up the need to later discriminate between what was read in the passage versus what was inferred.

Schemas provide one example of a memory mechanism that can both help and hurt memory. Most of the time, schemas support accurate memory; however, in some instances (such as the Helen Keller example), they can lead us astray. In this chapter, we will consider several different memory mechanisms that, like schemas, can sometimes lead our memories astray. We will focus on memory errors that meet Roediger's (1996) definition of memory illusions. Specifically, the focus will be on "cases in which a rememberer's report of a past event seriously deviates from the event's actual occurrence" (Roediger, 1996: 76). We will place a particular emphasis on memory errors that are made with high confidence, are labeled as remembered, or otherwise appear phenomenologically real. To preview a few of the vivid memory errors we will discuss: they include high-confidence errors in eyewitness testimony, never-presented words 'remembered' as spoken by a specific person, and ease of processing mistaken for fame. In each case, we will describe a prototypical experiment and the results and discuss possible underlying mechanisms.

32.1 False Memory for Words: The Deese-Roediger-McDermott Paradigm

As already described, Bartlett emphasized the use of meaningful materials when examining reconstructive memory, to avoid studying memory that was "primarily or literally reduplicative, or reproductive ... I discarded nonsense material because, among other difficulties, its use almost always weights the evidence in favor of mere rote recapitulation, and for the most part I used exactly the type of material that we have to deal with in daily life" (Bartlett, 1932: 204). Consistent with Bartlett's ideas, most of the studies we will describe in this chapter involve remembering videos, stories, slide shows, or personal memories. While words and nonsense syllables were frequently used in verbal learning experiments, Bartlett did not believe they would be useful in studying reconstructive memory since they did not encourage elaboration nor the use of schemas.

However, words have many properties that make them handy tools for the experimental psychologist. Tulving (1983) has made this argument eloquently: "words to the memory researcher are what fruit flies are to the geneticist: a convenient medium through which the phenomena and processes of interest can be explored and elucidated... words are of no more intrinsic interest to the student of memory than *Drosophila* are to a scientist probing the mechanisms of heredity" (Tulving, 1983: 146). Tulving goes on to point out that words have well-defined boundaries and are easily perceived, and that memories for words can easily be checked for accuracy. The point is that using word stimuli to study false memories would be very useful, if word stimuli could be selected that would encourage elaboration and the use of schemas. The argument is that the Deese-Roediger-McDermott (DRM) stimuli fit these requirements, and allow a simple and robust paradigm for studying false memories.

In a typical DRM experiment, participants learn lists of words, each related to a central non-presented word, the critical lure. For example, participants hear or see 'nurse, sick, lawyer, medicine, health, hospital, dentist, physician, ill, patient, office, stethoscope, surgeon, clinic, cure.' Even though the critical lure 'doctor' was never presented, subjects are likely to include it when recalling the list items. They are also likely to incorrectly call it 'old' on a recognition memory test. The DRM paradigm appeals to experimenters because of the incredibly high rates of false memories observed in both free recall and on recognition measures. For example, in one of Roediger and McDermott's (1995) experiments, participants recalled the critical lures 55% of the time, a rate similar to recall of studied items presented in the middle of the list! False recognition was also very robust; Roediger and McDermott observed a false alarm rate of 76.5% for critical lures as compared to a hit rate of 72% for studied items. Similarly high levels of false memories have been observed in dozens, likely hundreds, of experiments using this methodology.

Not only are DRM errors frequent, they are also phenomenologically compelling to the rememberer. Roediger and McDermott asked participants to label each word called 'old' as either 'remembered' or 'known.' 'Remembering' was defined as vividly recollecting details associated with a word's presentation (e.g., where it occurred on the list, what it sounded like, what one was thinking during its presentation), whereas 'knowing' meant simply knowing a word had been presented even though one could not recall the details of its presentation. As shown in **Figure 1**, the proportion of remember and know responses was very similar for the studied words and for the critical lures (Roediger and McDermott, 1995). That is, people were just as likely to claim they remembered the critical nonpresented lures as the studied words. People will also describe their false memories in some detail, attributing them to locations in the study list (Read, 1996) and to a particular speaker (Payne et al., 1996). They are also willing to estimate how frequently they rehearsed each false memory (Brown et al., 2000). In general, the false memory effect is very robust, persisting even when participants have been forewarned about the nature of the illusion (McDermott and Roediger, 1998).

Given the strength of the illusion, it is intriguing that not all lists of related words yield false memories (Deese, 1959; Gallo and Roediger, 2002). Listening to 'sour, candy, sugar, bitter, good, taste, tooth, nice, honey, soda, chocolate, heart, cake, tart, pie' is likely to yield a false memory for 'sweet,' whereas listening

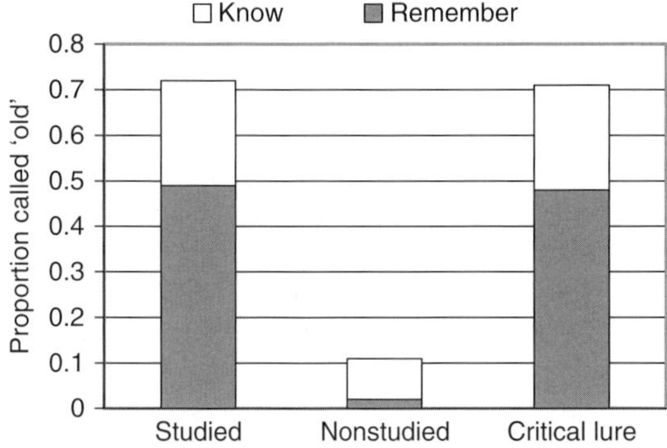

Figure 1 Recognition results for studied items and critical lures. Data from Roediger HL III and McDermott KB (1995) Creating false memories: Remembering words not presented in lists. *J. Exp. Psychol. Learn. Mem. Cogn.* 21: 803–814, Experiment 2.

to 'sweet, sour, taste, chocolate, rice, cold, lemon, angry, hard, mad, acid, almonds, herbs, grape, fruit' is very unlikely to yield a false memory for the critical lure 'bitter.' Both lists were constructed from the same free-association norms, but only one yields high levels of false memories. A key difference between the lists involves backward associative strength (BAS); this is a measure of how likely the list items are to elicit the critical item in a free association task. In other words, BAS measures how likely participants are to report the critical lure as the first word that comes to mind in response to list items. Participants are likely to respond 'sweet' but not 'bitter' in response to words like 'sugar, sour, taste,' meaning that BAS is very high for 'sweet' but very low for 'bitter.' This difference is crucial; BAS is a major predictor of false recall ($r = 0.73$, Roediger et al., 2001b).

In the activation monitoring framework's explanation of the DRM illusion, activation at encoding spreads through a preexisting semantic network of words, and the source of this activation is monitored at test. Hearing 'sour, candy, sugar' in the study list activates those nodes in the network. This activation spreads through the network (Collins and Loftus, 1975), activating related nodes. Because the critical lure is associated with so many study items (as indicated by its BAS value), it is activated from many different directions, leading to its heightened activation. If the participant fails to correctly monitor the source of that activation, a false memory will result.

According to the activation monitoring framework, manipulations that increase the amount of activation spreading to the critical lure should result in higher rates of false memories. Consistent with this, false memories increase as the study list increases in length, as longer lists mean that activation from a greater number of words spreads to the critical lure (Robinson and Roediger, 1997). Similarly, activation can spread from phonological associates. Listening to a list of words like 'bite, fight, rut, sprite, slight, rye' yields false memories for phonologically related nonpresented words such as 'right' (Sommers and Lewis, 1999). Intriguingly, lists that combine phonological and semantic associates (e.g., 'bed, rest, awake, tired, dream, scrub, weep, wane, keep') led to even higher rates of false memories than did purely semantic or purely phonological lists (Watson et al., 2003).

Activation alone cannot, however, explain all of the data. An interesting experiment on the effects of presentation rate highlights the need for both activation and monitoring components. McDermott and Watson (2001) presented DRM lists at five different presentation rates: 20, 250, 1000, 3000, and 5000 ms per word. As expected, veridical recall of list items increased with longer presentation rates. More interesting were the false recall data. When the presentation rate increased from 20 to 250 ms, false recall increased from 0.14 to 0.31. However, when the presentation rate was further increased, the rate of false memories decreased, from 0.22 at 1000 ms to 0.14 at 3000 or 5000 ms. The argument is that semantic activation is increasing as the presentation rate increases, hence the jump in false memories observed at 250 ms. However, with the longer presentation rates, participants encode more information about studied words, allowing them to invoke monitoring strategies during retrieval that help them to judge the source of the activation.

Monitoring is necessary to explain other DRM data, such as the finding that on average older adults remember fewer studied words but falsely remember just as many critical lures (or even more) as do college students (e.g., Balota et al., 1999). That is, because older adults have relatively preserved semantic memory, there should not be age differences in the activation of the critical lure. Rather, what is affected is the ability to monitor the source of activation, as older adults typically have difficulty on source-monitoring tasks (Hashtroudi et al., 1989). More direct support for the monitoring explanation comes from a study linking the age effect to problems with frontal functioning (Butler et al., 2004). In this study, older adults were classified as high versus low functioning on tasks known to require frontal functioning (e.g., the Wisconsin card sort task). Importantly, older adults who scored high on frontal tasks performed similarly to young adults in a typical DRM paradigm. Only older adults who scored poorly on frontal tasks showed reduced true recall and increased false recall. Because frontal areas are often implicated in monitoring tasks (e.g., Raz, 2000), these data suggest it is monitoring ability, not age, that is critical for avoiding false memories.

Even young adults can be placed in situations that make monitoring difficult, forcing them to rely on activation. Consider Benjamin's (2001) study in which he repeatedly presented the DRM lists. Young adults were less likely to incorrectly endorse critical lures from lists presented three times, presumably because they were able to monitor the source of that activation. However, when participants were required to respond quickly at test, they falsely recognized more critical lures from the lists presented three times. Repeating the list presumably increased the activation of the critical lures. When time was plentiful during the recognition test, participants used monitoring processes to correctly attribute the source of the activation (and thus reduce, but not eliminate, the illusion). When retrieval time was short, monitoring was not possible, and the increased activation resulted in high false alarm rates (see also Marsh and Dolan, 2007).

The distinctiveness heuristic is one monitoring strategy that has been investigated in detail. Schacter and colleagues defined the distinctiveness heuristic as "a mode of responding based on participants' metamemorial awareness that true recognition of studied items should include recollection of distinctive details" (Schacter et al., 1999: 3). Anything that makes DRM stimuli more distinctive should increase participants' standards for what they consider to be old. Thus, picture lists yield lower rates of false memories than do word lists (Israel and Schacter, 1997), and pronouncing and hearing the words at study lowers the false alarm rate as compared to only hearing the words (Dodson and Schacter, 2001).

Activation monitoring is the preferred explanation of many researchers, but certainly not all. Other explanations share in common a mechanism for the lures being encoded, and then a monitoring function at test. For example, fuzzy trace theory (Brainerd and Reyna, 2002) proposes that both verbatim and gist traces are encoded for events. Verbatim traces reflect memories of individual events, while gist traces reflect the extraction of meaning across experienced events. During the presentation of a DRM list, verbatim traces would be encoded for the individual words, while at the same time the meaning of the entire list would be extracted and encoded into a gist memory. Later, retrieval of the gist trace could drive false memory effects.

We turn now from false memories of never-presented words to errors when remembering events such as crimes or traffic accidents. More important than the switch in what is being remembered, though, is that different memory mechanisms likely underlie the two types of errors.

32.2 Eyewitness Suggestibility: The Misinformation Paradigm

Psychologists have long been interested in the reliability of witnesses. Early in the twentieth century, researchers such as Hugo Münsterberg and William Stern were publishing on the unreliability of testimony. The major methodological breakthrough in this area, though, did not appear until the 1970s when Elizabeth Loftus published her seminal work. She developed the misinformation paradigm (also known as the post-event information paradigm) that involves a twist on the basic retroactive interference paradigms that were popular during the verbal learning era (McGeoch, 1932). In retroactive interference studies, researchers examine the effect of a second, interfering event on memory for an original event (as compared to a control group that was not exposed to the interference). The typical design is shown in the top part of **Table 1**. In verbal learning terms, all participants study paired associates A – B in the first phase of the experiment (e.g., Table – Radio). Next, participants in the experimental group learn A – D associations (e.g., Table – Pencil), whereas participants in the control group rest or learn C – D (e.g., Purse – Pencil). Finally, all participants are tested on A – B (e.g., Table – ?), and memory is poorer in the group that learned two different associations in response to A. What does this have to do with eyewitness memory? The bottom portion of **Table 1** shows the connection between the standard retroactive interference design and eyewitness memory. The witness views an event (A – B), such as a traffic accident (A) occurring near a stop sign (B). After the event, the police will repeatedly interview the witness, the newspaper will publish accounts of the crime, and the witness will talk about the event with other people. All these have the potential to provide interfering information. For example, the police might erroneously suggest that the accident (A) occurred near a yield sign (D) when really it occurred near a stop sign (B). Later, when the witness tries to remember the details of the original event (A – ?), he or she may recall the interfering misinformation instead of what was actually witnessed. In contrast, misinformation production would be low for subjects in a control condition who heard a neutral reference to a traffic sign.

One of the most classic laboratory demonstrations comes from Loftus et al. (1978; see also Loftus and Palmer, 1974). All participants viewed a slide show depicting a traffic accident; in the critical slide, a red Datsun was approaching an intersection with a traffic sign. One-half of participants saw a stop sign; the other participants saw exactly the same slide except that the intersection was marked with a yield sign. After seeing the slides, all participants answered a series of questions about the accident. Embedded in one of the questions was a reference to the traffic sign; half of participants were asked 'Did another car pass the red Datsun while it was stopped at the stop sign?' whereas the others answered 'Did another car pass the red Datsun while it was stopped at the yield sign?' Twenty minutes later, participants examined pairs of slides and determined which one had been presented in the original slide show. The critical pair required participants to pick between the Datsun at a stop sign versus a yield sign. When participants had answered the question containing misinformation, they selected the correct slide 41% of the time (below chance), as compared to 75% when the question had referred to the correct sign.

Numerous studies have since replicated the basic finding: Information presented after an event can change what the eyewitness remembers. The original event may take the form of a film, slide show, staged event, written story, or a real event. The misinformation may be delivered in the form of presuppositions in questions, suggestive statements, photographs (e.g., mugshots), or narrative summaries. It can come from the experimenter, a confederate, or the witness herself. The misinformation effect qualifies as a false

Table 1 Experimental designs for studying retroactive interference (RI) and eyewitness suggestibility

	Condition	*Study target (A – B)*	*Interference (A – D) or (C – D)*	*Test target (A – B)*
RI				
	Experimental	Table – Radio	Table – Pencil	Table – ?
	Control	Table – Radio	Purse – Pencil	Table – ?
Eyewitness				
	Misled	Accident – Stop sign	Accident – Yield sign	Accident – ?
	Control	Accident – Stop sign	Accident – Traffic sign	Accident – ?

memory since participants generally endorse the misinformation quickly and with high confidence (Loftus et al., 1989). When participants described their erroneous memories, undergraduate judges were at chance at differentiating between real and suggested memories (Schooler et al., 1986).

One prerequisite for suggestibility is that participants fail to notice any problem with the misinformation when it is presented. This is called the discrepancy detection principle (Loftus, 1992). Participants are more likely to accept and reproduce misinformation about peripheral details than central characters or details (e.g., Christianson, 1992). In contrast, blatant misinformation not only is rejected, it also increases resistance to other peripheral misinformation (Loftus, 1979). Blatant misinformation may serve as a warning that the source is not to be trusted. This would be consistent with findings that warnings given before encoding of misinformation successfully reduce suggestibility, probably because warned participants read more slowly as they search for errors (Greene et al., 1982). In general, slow readers are more likely to notice (and resist) misinformation (Tousignant et al., 1986).

Given that participants do not detect the misinformation, manipulations that are generally known to enhance remembering lead to increased suggestibility, presumably because they increase memory for the misinformation. For example, suggestibility is greater if participants generate the misinformation (Roediger et al., 1996) and if the misinformation is repeated (Mitchell and Zaragoza, 1996; Zaragoza and Mitchell, 1996). Participants may also be more likely to rely on the misinformation if they have poor memory for the original events. For example, dividing attention during study (but not during the post-event information phase) increases suggestibility (Lane, 2006).

One important question is what happens to the original memory. It is easy to imagine the practical implications: If the original and post-event misinformation coexist in memory, it suggests the usefulness of developing strategies to help witnesses retrieve the original event. However, if the misinformation overwrites the original memory, it suggests that no retrieval strategy will allow access to the original event. Originally, there was much debate over this issue, but several lines of evidence suggest that the two memories may coexist. For example, consider what happens when misled participants are allowed to make a second guess after producing misinformation. If the original memories were completely unavailable, second-chance responses should be at chance (as what would they be based on?). Instead, second-chance guesses of misled participants are above chance (Wright et al., 1996), suggesting that some information about the original event is still available.

Compelling data for the coexistence hypothesis comes from experiments using source monitoring tests rather than recognition tests. Typically, in the 1970s and 1980s participants were required to make 'old/new' judgments about items. However, an 'old' judgment does not necessarily imply that participants remember seeing the misinformation in the original event. For example, participants may remember reading the misinformation in a post-event narrative and assume that remembering it from the narrative means it must have been in the video as well. To test these ideas, Lindsay and Johnson (1989) compared two groups of participants, all of whom studied the same photograph of an office. Afterward, half of participants read a narrative that mentioned eight office-related objects that were not actually in the original picture. Control participants read an accurate narrative description of the scene. The novel manipulation was at test; half of participants took a standard 'yes/no' recognition test, and half took a source monitoring test. For each item on the recognition test, participants indicated 'yes' if the object had been in the photograph and 'no' if it had not. On the source test, participants indicated whether each test object had been only in the picture, only in the text, in both the picture and the text, or in neither the picture nor the text. The results were dramatic: The misinformation effect was eliminated in the source condition! In later experiments, the advantage of the source test was replicated, although suggestibility was reduced rather than completely eliminated (Zaragoza and Lane, 1994).

Recent research on the misinformation effect has moved from the debate about the fate of the original memory trace to other interesting questions. One current trend is the examination of the effects of social context on suggestibility. This includes both the social context in which participants are exposed to misinformation, as well as the social context in which participants first intrude errors. For example, researchers are examining the effects of receiving misinformation from other people as opposed to reading it in narratives or embedded in questions (e.g., Roediger et al., 2001a; Gabbert et al., 2004; Wright et al., 2005). A related question involves the response the witness receives from other people after she (the witness) makes a mistake. The question of how feedback affects a witness' memory is an important one, as incorrectly telling the witness 'Good, you identified the suspect' can have many negative consequences (see Douglass and Steblay, 2006, for a review).

32.3 Verbal Overshadowing

Rehearsal (especially elaborative rehearsal) can be a useful mnemonic for remembering word lists and prose. But what happens when a rehearsal fails to adequately capture the original experience? For example, words rarely capture the richness of our perceptions. What are the memorial consequences of a description (a rehearsal of sorts) that is inadequate or even inaccurate?

Questions about the effects of language and memory are not new ones. Many undergraduates are familiar with a classic study in which labels influenced memory for pictures. A picture of two circles joined by a line was labeled as either 'glasses' or 'barbell,' and participants later redrew the pictures to be similar to the label (Carmichael et al., 1932). In the 1970s, there was much interest in how participants integrated verbal and visual information in memory (e.g., Pezdek, 1977; Gentner and Loftus, 1979). Depending on the study, opposite conclusions were reached. Sometimes labeling pictures and objects led to enhanced memory (e.g., Santa and Ranken, 1972), but other times labeling was associated with difficulty on later memory tests (e.g., Gentner and Loftus, 1979).

More recently, Schooler and Engstler-Schooler (1990) sparked interest in the question by contextualizing it within the eyewitness memory domain. After watching a 30-s video of a bank robbery, participants in their Face Verbalization condition wrote a description of the thief's face (participants in the control condition did an unrelated task during that time). At test, all participants saw eight similar faces (including the thief) and were asked to select the perpetrator from the video or to indicate if he was absent from the line-up. The intriguing finding was that 64% of control participants selected the target, as compared to 37% in the face verbalization condition. Schooler and Engstler-Schooler labeled their finding verbal overshadowing.

Verbal overshadowing is not limited to faces; it extends to other types of perceptual information. Describing a voice reduces the ability to later identify that voice from among six options (Perfect et al., 2002). The typical wine drinker shows verbal overshadowing for wines, as they are unable to verbalize the nuances of wine in the vocabulary of experts (Melcher and Schooler, 1996). After memorizing a map of a small town, participants who wrote about it later performed worse on distance estimation tasks than did control participants (Fiore and Schooler, 2002). That is, having described one's spatial mental model of the town led to confusion about the distances between the landmarks.

Several different explanations have been proposed. One possibility involves recoding. Specifically, when participants describe a visual stimulus from memory, they are effectively recoding it from a visual representation to a verbal one, and the more recent recoded memory then interferes with the original visual memory. Consistent with an interference account, inserting a delay between the description and the final test reduces verbal overshadowing (Finger and Pezdek, 1999), in the same way that a delayed test can reduce retrieval blocking in other interference situations (e.g., Choi and Smith, 2005).

The recoding account would predict that the quality of the new verbal representation (as measured by the description) should predict the effects of verbalization on later memory tasks. Although Schooler and Engstler-Schooler (1990) did not find a relationship between the quality of the descriptions and the ability to recognize the perpetrator, this may be because of the way the descriptions were scored. Descriptions were considered better if they described more features of the target; however, this dependent measure is not ideal, as face recognition depends on configural information rather than on recognition of individual features (e.g., Diamond and Carey, 1986). That is, while people may only be able to verbalize individual facial features (e.g., she has big eyes and she has freckles on her nose), face recognition depends upon hard-to-verbalize configural information about the relationship of features to one another (e.g., the relationship between the eyes and the nose).

Support for the recoding hypothesis comes from a meta-analysis of the literature about the type of instructions given to witnesses. Meissner and Brigham (2001) coded each study's instructions to participants as either standard or elaborative. Instructions were considered elaborative if "the authors explicitly encouraged their participants to go beyond their normal criterion of free recall and to provide more elaborative descriptions" (Meissner and Brigham, 2001: 607). Presumably, elaborative descriptions led to less accurate recodings; consistent with this, elaborative descriptions were more likely to lead to verbal overshadowing than were descriptions resulting from standard free recall instructions (Meissner and Brigham, 2001). One study published since the meta-analysis deserves mention here. MacLin (2002) compared the effects of several different types of instructions on the verbal overshadowing effect. When participants were told to describe facial features, the standard effect occurred: On a later test, participants were less likely to identify the target than were control participants who did not describe the target. However, when participants were told to write a description comparing the target to a famous person such as Julia Roberts (the exemplar condition), verbal overshadowing was reduced. The effect disappeared in a prototype condition in which participants described "what type of person you think he most looks like" (MacLin, 2002: 932) in terms of occupation and personality. Thus, verbal overshadowing was most likely in the condition in which recoding emphasized facial features rather than more holistic information about the target face.

A second explanation of verbal overshadowing also hinges on the fact that descriptions often emphasize individual facial features rather than configural information. However, rather than proposing that a feature-based description interferes with retrieval of the original memory, the argument is that verbalization induces a processing shift at test (Dodson et al., 1997; Schooler, 2002). That is, because descriptions of faces emphasize individual features (as it is hard to verbalize relations between features), the participant carries over this type of processing to test. This is considered a processing shift, as face identification is normally based on configural information rather than features; carrying over a featural orientation would constitute inappropriate processing. One interesting finding is shown in **Figure 2**. Dodson and colleagues had participants view a target face and then do one of three tasks: Describe the target face, describe a parent's face, or list U.S. states and capitals (a control condition). As shown in the figure, describing any face (e.g., a relative's) reduced participants' ability to identify the target (Dodson et al., 1997). This is hard to reconcile with the idea that a recoded representation (of the target) is interfering with access to the original memory. Rather, it suggests that anything that emphasizes featural processing will encourage that same type of processing at test.

Similar conclusions were reached by Finger (2002), who added a second factor to the typical verbal

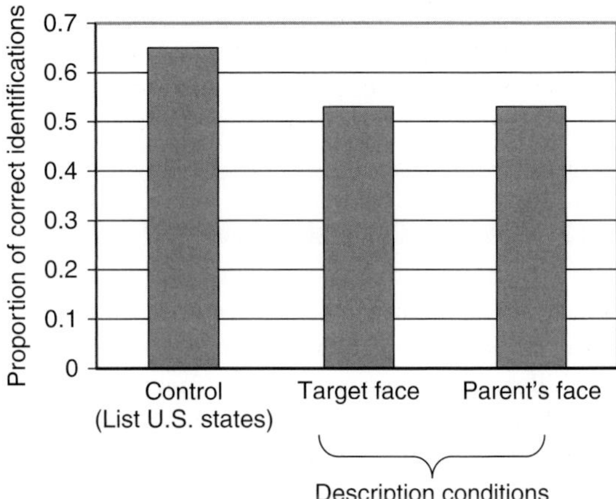

Figure 2 Recognition of target face after describing target face, parent's face, or listing U.S. states and capitals. Data from Dodson CS, Johnson MK, and Schooler JW (1997) The verbal overshadowing effect: Why descriptions impair face recognition. *Mem. Cogn.* 25: 129–139, Experiment 2.

overshadowing experiment. She crossed description (describe vs. control) with a post-description task (verbal vs. mazes). When solving mazes followed the face description, verbal overshadowing disappeared. In a second experiment, Finger replicated the effect with a second nonverbal task, namely listening to music. Engaging in holistic processing can change the processing set from one that emphasizes individual features to one that does not, with consequences for face identification.

Recent research suggests a number of relatively simple solutions to minimize the effects of verbal overshadowing of faces, such as inserting a delay between description and test (Finger and Pezdek, 1999) and preceding the test with a task that encourages configural processing (Finger, 2002). It remains to be tested whether these solutions are equally effective at reducing verbal overshadowing of other types of perceptual stimuli such as voices, wines, and maps.

32.4 Misattributions of Familiarity

Thus far, we have discussed misremembering laboratory events – be it misremembering a word that was never presented in a study list (in the DRM paradigm), incorrectly recalling a detail of a slide show (in the misinformation paradigm), or misidentifying a person from a video (in verbal overshadowing experiments). In contrast, in the next paradigm we will review, the memory error involves misattributing something learned in the laboratory to pre-experimental experience. More specifically, the paradigm is a recipe for fame; Larry Jacoby used straightforward experimental manipulations to make ordinary names appear famous.

The names Brad Pitt, Mark McGwire, and Sandra Day O'Connor are likely recognizable to you. In addition to agreeing that you have heard of these people before, you can probably justify your response by telling us Brad Pitt is an actor, Mark McGwire is an athlete, and Sandra Day O'Connor is a retired Supreme Court justice. You can also tell me whether or not other names are the names of famous people, even if you cannot say exactly why each person is famous. For example, try to identify the three famous people in the following list of six names: Zoe Flores, Minnie Pearl, Jessica Lynch, Joanna Emmons, Summer Foster, Hattie Caraway. Hopefully, at least one or two of the names will seem familiar to you, even if you do not know what accomplishments to associate with each name. Quite simply, the false fame paradigm increases the familiarity of nonfamous names (like Zoe Flores, Joanna Emmons, and Summer Foster) and places the respondent in a situation where familiarity is interpreted as fame.

In the typical paradigm, participants read a list of names explicitly labeled as nonfamous. In a second phase, participants judge the fame of each of a series of names; the test list includes moderately famous names like Minnie Pearl, new nonfamous names, and old nonfamous names that were read in the first part of the experiment. Critically, half of the participants are required to do a secondary task (e.g., monitoring an auditory stream of numbers for a series of three odd numbers in a row) at the same time as the fame judgment task. In the full-attention (control) condition, old nonfamous names are less likely to be judged famous than are new nonfamous names; in this condition, if participants can remember a name is old, then they can assume it is not famous. In contrast, in the divided-attention condition, participants are more likely to call old nonfamous names famous ($M = 0.28$) than new nonfamous names ($M = 0.14$) (Jacoby et al., 1989b). The logic is that under divided attention, participants are forced to base their judgments on the familiarity of a name, and that the cognitive load interferes with their ability to recollect whether names were presented in the first part of the experiment.

The false fame effect requires conditions that force participants to rely on familiarity rather than recollecting information about the names. For example, the false fame effect also occurs when attention is divided during encoding, as presumably that prevents encoding of item-specific information (Jacoby et al., 1989a). Similarly, under conditions of full attention, the illusion requires a delay between study of the nonfamous names and the fame judgments. Consistent with the idea that the false fame effect is familiarity driven, the effect is stronger in populations that are more likely to rely on familiarity, such as older adults (Bartlett et al., 1991; Multhaup, 1995).

This illusion is related to a more general framework on how people interpret feelings of familiarity. Vague feelings of familiarity are not specific to names; there are many situations in which familiarity is experienced and the perceiver must attribute that familiarity to something. In an impressive series of studies, Jacoby has shown that how that familiarity is interpreted depends on the experimental context. Familiarity can be interpreted as fame, but it can also lead to illusions of duration and noise level, for example. At test, previously studied words are judged to be presented longer than are new words (Witherspoon and Allan, 1985) and background noise is judged to be quieter for old sentences than for new sentences (Jacoby et al., 1988). The familiarity of the items causes them to be processed fluently, and in the context of perceptual judgments, this fluent processing is interpreted as perceptual conditions that aid identification of the items.

Familiarity may also play a role in the déjà vu experience (Brown, 2003, 2004). In the prior examples in this section, familiarity was successfully attributed to a source, albeit incorrectly: Familiarity was misinterpreted as fame and longer presentation durations, among other things. In contrast, déjà vu occurs when something feels familiar but the familiarity cannot be attributed to any prior experience. It is this unexplained familiarity with a situation that yields the puzzling déjà vu reaction. One hypothesis is that the individual previously experienced all or part of the present situation or setting, but cannot explicitly remember it. Thus implicit memory yields a familiarity response that is puzzling given the lack of episodic memory. Because déjà vu is a relatively infrequent phenomenon (Brown, 2003, 2004), it is difficult to capture in the laboratory. Some support for the implicit memory hypothesis, however, has been found in a laboratory paradigm (Brown and Marsh, in press). In this study, students from Duke University and Southern Methodist University viewed photos of the away campus in an initial exposure phase (none of these students reported having visited the other campus in real life). During the initial session, participants made a simple perceptual judgment about each of 216 photos, which included the target away-campus photos as well as many filler photos. One week later, participants made judgments about whether or not they had visited each of a series of test photos. Critically, in addition to familiar places from their home campus, participants judged photos from the prior session. Prior exposure to away-campus scenes boosted participants' beliefs that they had visited the places in real life. Intriguingly, almost half of participants reported experiencing something like déjà vu in the study. In this case, familiarity with a scene influenced belief that the place had been visited in real life, and sometimes this familiarity was puzzling enough to be labeled as déjà vu.

In this section, we described how familiarity could be interpreted as fame as well as perceptual attributes such as the volume of noise. In the next section, we will consider whether familiarity with an event can increase people's beliefs that an event happened in their pasts.

32.5 Imagination Inflation

The relationship between imagery and perception has a long intellectual history, reaching back to philosophers such as Hume and Mills. In the 1970s, the key question involved the nature of the representation underlying images. In this context, Johnson and colleagues asked how we separate memories for images from memories based on perception. More generally, reality monitoring involves deciding whether a memory originated from an internal or external source, with internal sources being cognitive processes such as imagery, thought, and dreams. Johnson argued that internally generated and externally presented memories tend to differ in prototypical ways, and that these differences in qualitative characteristics were the basis for attributing memories to thought versus perception (e.g., Johnson and Raye, 1981). Compared to memories based on perception, memories of images were postulated to be less vivid and to be associated with the cognitive operations involved in their generation. Reality monitoring errors occur when memories contain characteristics atypical of their class. For example, easily generated images are more likely to be misattributed to perception than are difficult-to-imagine objects. Easily generated images are likely atypically vivid; in addition, their easy generation means they are not associated with a record of cognitive operations (Finke et al., 1988).

Misattributions of imagined events to perception have been documented with many different kinds of stimuli, including imagined voices (Johnson et al., 1988), imagined rotations of alphanumeric characters (Kahan and Johnson, 1990), and imagined pictures (Johnson et al., 1982). But can imagery cause confusions beyond these types of simple laboratory stimuli? That is, if you imagine an event, will you later come to believe that it really happened?

Garry and colleagues (1996) created a three-stage procedure to answer this question. In the first part of the experiment, participants rated the likelihood that they had experienced each of a series of life experiences (the Life Events Inventory; LEI), including winning a stuffed animal at a fair and breaking a window with one's hand. Two weeks after reading descriptions of the target events, participants imagined both the setting and the action of events in response to specific prompts. For example, in the broken window event, participants spent 20–60 s imagining the following setting: "It is after school and you are playing in the house. You hear a strange noise outside, so you run to the window to see what made the noise. As you are running, your feet catch on something and you trip and fall" (Garry et al., 1996: 210). After the imagination phase was finished, the experimenter pretended to have lost the original LEI and asked participants to fill out the questionnaire for a second time.

There were eight critical events judged unlikely to have occurred for a majority of the participants, and each participant imagined four of those during phase 2. Of interest was whether participants were more likely to change their beliefs about events they had imagined in phase 2, as compared to the control events not imagined. Garry et al. examined the percentage of critical items that were rated as more likely to have happened at time 2 (after the imagery phase) than at time 1. Increases in likelihood ratings were more common for imagined events than for control events. For example, consider the effect of imagining on people's beliefs that as a child they broke a window with their bare hand. The likelihood ratings increased from time 1 to time 2 for 24% of participants in the imagery condition, as compared to only 12% of control participants.

It is possible, of course, that participants had actually experienced these unusual events and that imagining them helped to cue the previously forgotten memories. One solution to this criticism is to control the original events in the laboratory, to allow certainty about what actually occurred. Because this is not possible with childhood memories, Goff and Roediger (1998) brought the encoding phase into the laboratory. The experiment had three sessions; during the first session, participants enacted, heard, or imagined simple events. For example, when the experimenter read aloud the sentence 'bounce the ball,' one participant would simply listen; another would imagine bouncing the ball, and a third would actually bounce the ball. Twenty-four hours later, participants returned for a second session in which half of participants imagined events and half did math problems. In the imagery condition, participants were guided to imagine each event zero, one, three, or five times; the events included ones from the first session as well as completely new events. Participants in this condition rated the vividness of each image. Finally, 2 weeks after the initial session, participants were given recognition and source monitoring tests. Participants were explicitly told that their memory was being tested for the first day only. They were first asked if they remembered hearing certain events. If they answered no, they gave a confidence rating in their answer. If they answered yes, they specified the format of the remembered event (heard and enacted, heard and imagined, or heard only) and rated their confidence in that judgment. Of interest was whether imagining new events in session 2 would increase beliefs that the events had been performed in session 1. Replicating findings from studies using LEI measures, Goff and Roediger found that events that were only imagined during the second session were later misremembered as having been performed during the first session. Imagining a bouncing ball in the second session increased participants' beliefs that they had actually bounced a ball in the first session. Furthermore, as the number of imaginings in session 2 increased, participants were more likely to incorrectly label a never-performed action as having been performed in the first session, as shown in **Figure 3**.

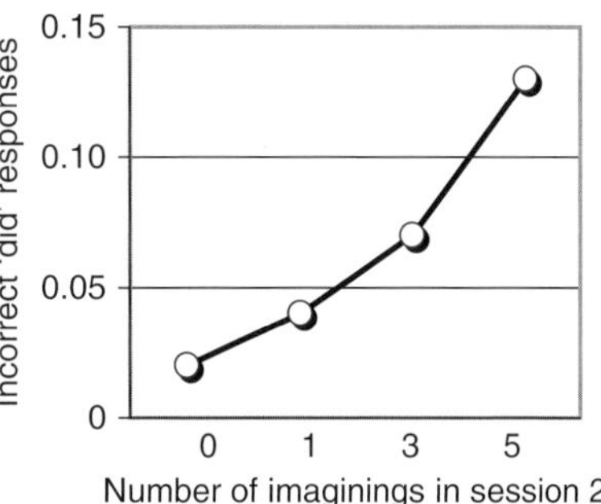

Figure 3 False 'did' judgments for never-performed actions as a function of number of imaginings in session 2. Data from Goff LM and Roediger HL III (1998) Imagination inflation for action events: Repeated imaginings lead to illusory recollections. *Mem. Cogn.* 26: 20–33.

The finding of imagination inflation for laboratory events supports the idea that imagination can yield false memories and that the effects observed with the LEI cannot be attributed solely to recovery of previously forgotten events. Why do these effects occur? In their original demonstration of imagination inflation, Garry and colleagues favored a reality monitoring explanation, whereby an imagined memory was misattributed to perception. Specifically, Garry et al. argued that imagination increased the perceptual information associated with the events, thus increasing the similarity of these imagined memories to performed events. This account predicts that imagination inflation should be greater when images are detailed, as they will be more readily confused with perception. Consistent with this hypothesis, Thomas and colleagues (2003) found that elaborative imagery instructions increased the imagination inflation effect, as compared to standard imagery instructions. Like Goff and Roediger, Thomas' participants completed an initial encoding phase and returned a day later for the imagination phase. Instructions in the simple imagery condition paralleled Goff and Roediger; for example, participants were asked to 'imagine getting up and opening the door.' Participants in the elaborative imagery condition were to imagine two additional statements, which included two sensory modalities; for example, 'Imagine getting up and opening the door. Imagine how the door handle feels in your hand. Imagine how the door sounds as you open it.' If the event was not imagined in the middle session, participants were very good at identifying new events. However, imagining events in the middle session led to imagination inflation, and this effect was bigger (12%) following elaborative imagery than simple imagery (7%).

To recap, imagining events may increase their vividness, a key characteristic of perceived memories. This is not the only explanation for the imagination inflation effect, however. Imagining events may also increase their familiarity, which can also lead to memory misattributions (as described in the previous section of this chapter). The imagination scripts used to guide the imagery also usually contain a lot of suggestive information over and above the vivid images generated by the participant. In short, does imagination underlie the effect, or is the effect at least partly driven by familiarity (as discussed in the section on false fame), as opposed to imagination?

Several data points suggest that imagining vivid details is not necessary to increase beliefs that events occurred in childhood. For example, similar effects are observed when participants paraphrase the script normally used to guide imagery (Sharman et al., 2004). The data also look similar when participants explain how the events might have happened in one's childhood (Sharman et al., 2005). Of course, in both of these cases, it is possible that participants might spontaneously generate images even though they were not explicitly directed to do so. However, Bernstein and colleagues observed inflation in a study in which spontaneous generation of images was quite unlikely. Their study extended the revelation effect to autobiographical memory (Bernstein et al., 2002). The revelation effect is the finding that requiring participants to unscramble a stimulus (to reveal it) increases the likelihood that it will be judged 'old' (Westerman and Greene, 1996). Bernstein et al. found that participants were more likely to believe childhood events had in fact occurred if they had to unscramble the events before judging them (e.g., 'broke a dwniwo playing ball'). Unscrambling presumably does not encourage imagery, and thus it suggests that LEI ratings can be based on factors other than image vividness, such as familiarity.

It should be clear that the just-described results do not negate the role of imagination in false memory creation. Finding that explaining, paraphrasing, and unscrambling events can all inflate confidence in remembered events does not preclude imagination also playing a role. Rather, such results emphasize the importance of isolating the contribution of imagination, as imagination is often combined with other factors that yield false memories.

32.6 Implanted Autobiographical Memories

It is possible to make a person remember a word that was never presented, to misjudge the fame of a name, or to misremember a detail from a witnessed event. But do people ever falsely remember entire events? The answer is yes. Consider the case of Shauna Fletcher, who came to believe her horrible memories of childhood sexual abuse were false memories (Pendergrast, 1996). How could this happen? Shauna traced her memories to several different sources, blaming her therapist for suggesting that the events occurred, and books and movies for providing the images she remembered. Shauna's experiences parallel the findings from laboratory studies: Implanting memories is possible, but not simple. A single misleading statement does not yield the kind of false memories experienced by Shauna. Correspondingly, the laboratory procedures for implanting entire memories tend to be much more complicated than those described earlier in the chapter, oftentimes combining multiple suggestive techniques.

Loftus and Pickrell (1995) demonstrated that false autobiographical memories can be implanted using laboratory techniques. The critical false memory involved being lost in a shopping mall as a child. To camouflage the purpose of the experiment, participants were also interviewed about childhood events that had actually occurred; a close relative of the participant provided the true memories. The relative also provided plausible details to aid in constructing the false memory (e.g., stores the family shopped, other family members likely to have been present, etc.) and verified that the participant had not been lost in a shopping mall around the critical time period (age 5).

Participants reviewed four events: three that were true and the critical false event. Each event was described in a booklet, and participants were instructed to remember the events and to write about the specific details of each. If participants did not remember the event, they were to indicate that on the form. Approximately 1–2 weeks later, participants were interviewed about the events. In addition to recalling details of the events, participants rated each memory for clarity (1 = not clear; 10 = extremely clear) and confidence that additional details could be remembered later (1 = not confident; 5 = extremely confident). A second interview, conducted 1–2 weeks later, was similar to the first interview.

Did participants come to remember being lost in the shopping mall at age 5? Critically, seven out of 24 participants claimed to remember the false memory (fully or partially) while writing about it in the initial booklet. Although their descriptions of the false events were shorter than those of true memories, the clarity ratings given to these false memories increased across interviews. At the end of the experiment, five participants were unable to pick out the false event and instead guessed that one of the true events had never happened.

The reader may be wondering why we consider the Loftus and Pickrell (1995) study to be an example of successful memory implantation. After all, most participants never believed the lost-in-the-mall memory and were able to identify it as the false event. What is crucial is that the implantation rate was above zero. That is, to argue that implanting false memories is possible, one only needs to show one successful implantation.

False memories are not limited to erroneous memories of being lost in the mall as a child. Experimenters have been successful at implanting many different types of events in participants. Participants have come to falsely remember participating in a religious ceremony (Pezdek et al., 1997), riding in a hot air balloon (Wade et al., 2002), putting the gooey toy Slime in an elementary school teacher's desk (Lindsay et al., 2004), and being admitted to the hospital (Hyman et al., 1995). Different approaches have been taken to ensure a false memory was in fact implanted, as opposed to a true memory being recovered. One is to confirm events with parents, as Loftus and Pickrell (1995) did. Another is to choose events that are very implausible, or even impossible. Braun and colleagues (2002) used the latter approach, implanting false memories for meeting a Warner Brothers character, Bugs Bunny, at Disneyland.

The procedures for implanting false memories are often elaborate, far beyond the simple suggestions typical of eyewitness misinformation studies. Successful studies typically follow three rules of thumb (Mazzoni et al., 2001; Lindsay et al., 2004). First, the target event must be deemed plausible. For example, it is easier to implant a false memory for being lost in the mall than it is to implant a false memory of an enema (Pezdek et al., 1997; see also Hart and Schooler, 2006). Second, the target event must be elaborated upon. For example, suggestibility was greater for participants who were required to imagine and describe the target events, probably because the guided imagery task led to more detailed memories (Hyman and Pentland, 1996). Third, the products of this elaboration must be attributed to memory, as opposed to other sources.

Although this framework is generally useful for thinking about memory implantation, one difficulty is that many manipulations likely affect more than one process. Consider, for example, Pezdek and colleagues' difficulty in implanting a false memory involving a Catholic ceremony (the Eucharist) in Jewish participants. Were the Jewish participants able to reject the event because it was implausible to them or because they were not familiar enough with the event to elaborate upon the suggestion? Similarly, consider what happens when a participant sees a doctored photograph depicting her engaged in the target false event. In this type of study, after a relative verifies that the participant has never ridden in a hot air balloon, Photoshop is used to insert a real childhood photo into a photograph depicting a hot air balloon ride (Wade et al., 2002). Such a procedure yields false memories in about half of participants (a high rate) – but is unclear at a cognitive level how the photograph has its effect on memory. The very existence of a photograph of the event increases the plausibility of the event, as well as providing vivid details about the supposed event.

The aforementioned examples illustrate the challenge of doing research in this area, namely the difficulty of linking manipulations to specific cognitive processes. We do not, however, intend to be pessimistic. The demonstrations of memory implantation were critical first steps, and they are being followed by systematic manipulations aimed at better elucidating the underlying cognitive processes. Rather than trying to equate different events with different levels of an independent variable, one approach is to try to implant the same event while experimentally manipulating a variable that affects only one possible factor, such as plausibility. Mazzoni and colleagues took this approach when examining memories for demonic possession (Mazzoni et al., 2001). Keeping the target event constant, they showed that reading articles about possession dramatically increased later beliefs that one had witnessed a demonic possession (as compared to the control group).

One of the major puzzles in this research area is why vivid false memories can be successfully implanted in some participants but not others. For example, across eight well-cited studies, Lindsay et al. (2004) observed that the implantation rate ranged from 0% to 56% of participants! We know of no study in which the false memory was successfully implanted into 100% of participants. Thus we predict one fruitful avenue for future research will be investigating individual differences in suggestibility. In the best study to date, Hyman and Billings (1998) looked for relationships between rates of false memory implantation and scores on four cognitive/personality scales. Two interesting results emerged. First, false memory scores were higher for participants who scored higher on the Creative Imagination Scale (CIS), a scale that measures imagery ability as well as suggestibility. In other words, participants who were better able to elaborate upon the suggestion were more likely to come to remember the false event. Second, false memory scores were higher for participants who scored higher on the Dissociative Experiences Scale (DES), a scale that measures both normal experiences such as distraction as well as less normal experiences such as hearing voices. Scoring higher on the DES may be related to difficulties with source monitoring.

In short, implanting detailed false memories is a complex process. It combines many of the techniques described earlier in the chapter in the context of other false memory paradigms, including imagery instructions, misleading suggestions, and a test situation that does not encourage participants to evaluate the source(s) of their memories. In this context, we turn to a discussion of how the various memory errors relate to one another.

32.7 Connections Across False Memory Paradigms

We have described six different paradigms that yield memory errors: The DRM paradigm, the eyewitness misinformation paradigm, verbal overshadowing studies, misattributions of familiarity, imagination inflation, and implanted autobiographical memories. What is the relationship between these very different paradigms?

We linked each memory error to possible mechanisms: Spreading activation (and monitoring of that activation) in the DRM paradigm, interference and failure to monitor source in the misinformation paradigm, an inappropriate shift in processing at test in the verbal overshadowing paradigm, a misattribution of familiarity in the false fame effect, increased familiarity and vividness (and possibly reality monitoring failures) in imagination inflation, and elaboration and source misattribution in the implanted memory studies. Sometimes, the same mechanism is implicated across illusions; for example, source monitoring failures are implicated in the misinformation effect and in implanting false autobiographical memories. Imagination inflation likely involves reality-monitoring errors, a specific type of source error. Misattributions of activation (in the DRM paradigm) and familiarity (as observed in the false fame paradigm) can also be interpreted as source errors. In other cases, the mechanisms appear qualitatively different, as in the case of the transfer inappropriate processing shift in verbal overshadowing studies. Of course, one issue is that likely more than one mechanism is involved in each illusion (and the convergence of mechanisms is probably why the errors are so robust). For example, imagination inflation likely depends on both vivid encoding (which may also increase familiarity) and some kind of monitoring failure at test. One other point worth noting is that even if the same mechanism is implicated in two different illusions, the instantiations of that mechanism may be quite different. For example, even though source errors are implicated in both the DRM illusion and the misinformation effect, giving participants a source test has very different effects in the two cases. As already mentioned, a source test can reduce susceptibility to post-event information (e.g., Lindsay and Johnson, 1989; Zaragoza and Lane, 1994). However, source tests yield more puzzling results when used in the DRM paradigm; depending on the features of the source test, the rate of false memories may be higher (Hicks and Marsh, 2001), lower (Multhaup and Conner, 2002), or similar (Hicks and Marsh, 1999) to that observed on item memory tests.

More generally, comparing the effects of standard manipulations on the different measures of suggestibility is a useful way of examining similarities and differences across false memory paradigms. For example, many researchers are interested in differences in suggestibility between children and college students. This comparison has been made in at least three of the six paradigms we described – DRM, eyewitness misinformation, and implanted memories – and the conclusion about age is not the same across paradigms. For example, younger children are normally more suggestible in eyewitness misinformation paradigms than are older children (Bruck and Ceci, 1999), but older children are more suggestible than younger children in the DRM paradigm (e.g., Brainerd and Reyna, 2007). That is, even though there are clear age differences in source monitoring abilities (e.g., Lindsay et al., 1991), with older children doing better than younger, older children are more suggestible in the DRM paradigm. Why is this, given that we already alluded to the role of source monitoring in the DRM paradigm? The paradox can be resolved by attributing the key age difference to encoding, rather than to retrieval-based processes such as source monitoring. Specifically, because younger children have difficulty noting semantic relations between items (Brainerd and Reyna, 2007), they may be less likely to encode the critical lure. In the terms of activation-monitoring theory, activation will be less likely to spread to the critical lure from related studied items; in the terms of fuzzy trace theory, younger children will be less likely to extract the gist of the list. By either account, the result is the same: It does not matter if younger children are poor at source monitoring if there is no trace for them to attribute to a source! Again, this example highlights the inadequacy of simply attributing DRM and eyewitness errors to difficulties with source; the full picture is more complicated.

There are at least two other approaches for connecting false memory paradigms. One is to test the same participants in multiple paradigms, and another is to link false memory in different paradigms to the same standardized measures of individual differences. The logic is that if comparable mechanisms underlie the errors, then the same individuals (or the same types of people) should perform similarly across paradigms. For example, Clancy and colleagues (2002) examined suggestibility in the DRM paradigm in control participants and in people who believed aliens had abducted them. Memories of alien abduction are of interest since the scientific community views alien abductions as impossible occurrences, leading these memories to be classified as false memories (although not implanted in the laboratory, of course). Interestingly, false recognition of nonpresented words was higher for people with alien abduction memories ($M = 0.67$) than for control participants ($M = 0.42$). In this same study, correlations between false memory and scores on individual difference scales were also observed. The rate of false memories was greater for individuals who scored highly on scales measuring absorption and dissociative experiences (DES) and reported more symptoms of post-traumatic stress disorder. The reader will recall that the DES is a scale that measures both normal experiences such as distraction as well as less normal experiences such as hearing voices, and that higher scores on the DES may be related to difficulties with source monitoring. Higher DES scores predicted implantation of a false childhood memory for spilling punch on the mother of the bride, although absorption did not (Hyman and Billings, 1998). Scores on the DES have also been related to imagination inflation (Paddock et al., 1999), and pathological scores on this scale have been linked to suggestibility in the eyewitness misinformation paradigm (Eisen et al., 2001). However, DES scores are not related to susceptibility to the false fame illusion (Peters et al., 2007). Understanding such individual differences will likely be an important part of future research on memory errors and suggestibility.

We end with a note on another approach we believe will help elucidate the relationships between different false memory paradigms: neuroimaging. Consider a study by Cabeza and colleagues (2001), in which participants watched two very different sources (a Caucasian male and an Asian female) read DRM-like lists, followed by a recognition memory test. At test, studied words and critical lures yielded similar activation in anterior medial temporal lobe (MTL) areas, but activation in posterior MTL differentiated true and false memories. Cabeza et al. associated anterior MTL with retrieval of semantic information and posterior MTL with perceptual information. What would the pattern be like for familiarity-driven illusions, such as false fame? To the extent that the same mechanisms underlie different memory errors, similar patterns of activation should occur.

32.8 Conclusions

In this chapter, we reviewed just six of the many published paradigms for creating false memories. Together, the data highlight the constructive nature of memory, as proposed by Bartlett (1932). We have also tried to stress that not all memory errors are equal. Not surprisingly, given the complexity of memory, there are many different ways that error can enter the system, from encoding to retrieval.

While we have focused on errors, we would be remiss not to point out that reconstructive memory is often very useful. For example, familiarity often is an excellent cue that something has been experienced before, and it is only in certain situations that this heuristic leads to error. More generally, errors are often the by-product of processes that support veridical memory. Memory errors are more than intriguing illusions. A thorough understanding of memory's errors will provide insight into the processes that normally aid memory.

References

Bahrick HP, Bahrick PO, and Wittlinger RP (1975) Fifty years of memory for names and faces: A cross-sectional approach. *J. Exp. Psychol. Gen.* 104: 54–75.

Balota DA, Cortese MJ, Duchek JM, et al. (1999) Veridical and false memories in healthy older adults and in dementia of the Alzheimer's type. *Cogn. Neuropsychol.* 6: 361–384.

Bartlett FC (1932) *Remembering: A Study in Experimental and Social Psychology*. Cambridge: Cambridge University Press.

Bartlett JC, Strater L, and Fulton A (1991) False recency and false fame of faces in young adulthood and old age. *Mem. Cogn.* 19: 177–188.

Benjamin AS (2001) On the dual effects of repetition on false recognition. *J. Exp. Psychol. Learn. Mem. Cogn.* 27: 941–947.

Berntsen D and Thomsen DK (2005) Personal memories for remote historical events: Accuracy and clarity of flashbulb memories related to World War II. *J. Exp. Psychol. Gen.* 134: 242–257.

Bernstein DM, Whittlesea BWA, and Loftus EF (2002) Increasing confidence in remote autobiographical memory and general knowledge: Extensions of the revelation effect. *Mem. Cogn.* 30: 432–438.

Brainerd CJ and Reyna VF (2002) Fuzzy-trace theory and false memory. *Curr. Dir. Psychol. Sci.* 11: 164–169.

Brainerd CJ and Reyna VF (2007) Explaining developmental reversals in false memory. *Psychol. Sci.* 18: 442–448.

Braun KA, Ellis R, and Loftus EF (2002) Make my memory: How advertising can change our memories of the past. *Psychol. Mark.* 19: 1–23.

Brown AS (2003) A review of the déjà vu experience. *Psychol. Bull.* 129: 394–413.

Brown AS (2004) The déjà vu illusion. *Curr. Dir. Psychol. Sci.* 13: 256–259.

Brown AS and Marsh EJ (in press) Evoking false beliefs about autobiographical experience. *Psychon. Bull. Rev.*

Brown NR, Buchanan L, and Cabeza R (2000) Estimating the frequency of nonevents: The role of recollection failure in false recognition. *Psychon. Bull. Rev.* 7: 684–691.

Bruck M and Ceci SJ (1999) The suggestibility of children's memory. *Annu. Rev. Psychol.* 50: 419–439.

Butler KM, McDaniel MA, Dornburg CC, Price AL, and Roediger HL III (2004) Age differences in veridical and false recall are not inevitable: The role of frontal lobe function. *Psychon. Bull. Rev.* 11: 921–925.

Cabeza R, Rao SM, Wagner AD, Mayer AR, and Schacter DL (2001) Can medial temporal lobe regions distinguish true from false? An event-related functional MRI study of veridical and illusory memory. *Proc. Natl. Acad. Sci. USA* 98: 4805–4810.

Carmichael L, Hogan HP, and Walter AA (1932) An experimental study of the effect of language on the reproduction of visually perceived forms. *J. Exp. Psychol.* 15: 73–86.

Choi H and Smith SM (2005) Incubation and the resolution of tip-of-the-tongue states. *J. Gen. Psychol.* 132: 365–376.

Christianson S-A (1992) Emotional stress and eyewitness memory: A critical review. *Psychol. Bull.* 112: 284–309.

Clancy SA (2005) *Abducted: How People Come to Believe They Were Kidnapped by Aliens*. Cambridge, MA: Harvard University Press.

Clancy SA, Schacter DL, Lenzenweger MF, and Pittman RK (2002) Memory distortion in people reporting abduction by aliens. *J. Abnorm. Psychol.* 111: 455–461.

Collins AM and Loftus EF (1975) A spreading-activation theory of semantic processing. *Psychol. Rev.* 82: 407–428.

Deese J (1959) On the prediction of occurrence of particular verbal intrusions in immediate recall. *J. Exp. Psychol.* 58: 17–22.

Diamond R and Carey S (1986) Why faces are and are not special: An effect of expertise. *J. Exp. Psychol. Gen.* 115: 107–117.

Dodson CS and Schacter DL (2001) If I said it I would have remembered it: Reducing false memories with a distinctiveness heuristic. *Psychon. Bull. Rev.* 8: 155–161.

Dodson CS, Johnson MK, and Schooler JW (1997) The verbal overshadowing effect: Why descriptions impair face recognition. *Mem. Cogn.* 25: 129–139.

Dooling DJ and Christiaansen RE (1977) Episodic and semantic aspects of memory for prose. *J. Exp. Psychol. Hum. Learn. Mem.* 3: 428–436.

Douglass AB and Steblay N (2006) Memory distortion in eyewitnesses: A meta-analysis of the post-identification feedback effect. *Appl. Cogn. Psychol.* 20: 859–869.

Eisen ML, Morgan DY, and Mickes L (2001) Individual differences in eyewitness memory and suggestibility: Examining relations between acquiescence, dissociation and resistance to misleading information. *Pers. Ind. Diff.* 33: 553–571.

Finger K (2002) Mazes and music: Using perceptual processing to release verbal overshadowing. *Appl. Cogn. Psychol.* 16: 887–896.

Finger K and Pezdek K (1999) The effect of the cognitive interview on face identification accuracy: Release from verbal overshadowing. *J. Appl. Psychol.* 84: 340–348.

Finke RA, Johnson MK, and Shyi GC (1988) Memory confusions for real and imagined completions of symmetrical visual patterns. *Mem. Cogn.* 16: 133–137.

Fiore SM and Schooler JW (2002) How did you get here from there? Verbal overshadowing of spatial mental models. *Appl. Cogn. Psychol.* 16: 897–910.

Gabbert F, Memon A, and Allan K (2004) Say it to my face: Examining the effects of socially encountered misinformation. *Legal Criminol. Psychol.* 9: 215–227.

Gallo DA and Roediger HL III (2002) Variability among word lists in eliciting memory illusions: Evidence for associative activation and monitoring. *J. Mem. Lang.* 47: 496–497.

Garry M, Manning CG, Loftus EF, and Sherman SJ (1996) Imagination inflation: Imagining a childhood event inflates confidence that it occurred. *Psychon. Bull. Rev.* 3: 208–214.

Gentner D and Loftus EF (1979) Integration of verbal and visual information as evidenced by distortions in picture memory. *Am. J. Psychol.* 92: 363–375.

Goff LM and Roediger HL III (1998) Imagination inflation for action events: Repeated imaginings lead to illusory recollections. *Mem. Cogn.* 26: 20–33.

Greene E, Flynn MS, and Loftus EF (1982) Inducing resistance to misleading information. *J. Verb. Learn. Verb. Behav.* 21: 207–219.

Hart RE and Schooler JW (2006) Increasing belief in the experience of an invasive procedure that never happened: The role of plausibility and schematicity. *Appl. Cogn. Psychol.* 20: 661–669.

Hashtroudi S, Johnson MK, and Chrosniak LD (1989) Aging and source monitoring. *Psychol. Aging* 4: 106–112.

Hicks JL and Marsh RL (1999) Attempts to reduce the incidence of false recall with source monitoring. *J. Exp. Psychol. Learn. Mem. Cogn.* 25: 1195–1209.

Hicks JL and Marsh RL (2001) False recognition occurs more frequently during source identification than during old-new recognition. *J. Exp. Psychol. Learn. Mem. Cogn.* 27: 375–383.

Hyman IE Jr. and Billings FJ (1998) Individual differences and the creation of false childhood memories. *Memory* 6: 1–20.

Hyman IE Jr. and Pentland J (1996) The role of mental imagery in the creation of false childhood memories. *J. Mem. Lang.* 35: 101–117.

Hyman IE Jr., Husband TH, and Billings FJ (1995) False memories of childhood experiences. *Appl. Cogn. Psychol.* 9: 181–197.

Israel L and Schacter DL (1997) Pictorial encoding reduces false recognition of semantic associates. *Psychon. Bull. Rev.* 4: 577–581.

Jacoby LL, Allan LG, Collins AM, and Larwill LK (1988) Memory influences subjective experience: Noise judgments. *J. Exp. Psychol. Learn. Mem. Cogn.* 14: 240–247.

Jacoby LL, Kelley CM, Brown J, and Jasechko J (1989a) Becoming famous overnight: Limits on the ability to avoid unconscious influences of the past. *J. Pers. Soc. Psychol.* 56(3): 326–338.

Jacoby LL, Woloshyn V, and Kelley CM (1989b) Becoming famous without being recognized: Unconscious influences of memory produced by dividing attention. *J. Exp. Psychol. Gen.* 118: 115–125.

Johnson MK and Raye CL (1981) Reality monitoring. *Psychol. Rev.* 88: 67–85.

Johnson MK, Raye CL, Foley MA, and Kim JK (1982) Pictures and images: Spatial and temporal information compared. *Bull. Psychon. Soc.* 19: 23–26.

Johnson MK, Foley MA, and Leach K (1988) The consequences for memory of imagining in another person's voice. *Mem. Cogn.* 16: 337–342.

Johnson MK, Hashtroudi S, and Lindsay DS (1993) Source monitoring. *Psychol. Bull.* 114: 3–28.

Kahan TL and Johnson MK (1990) Memory for seen and imagined rotations of alphanumeric characters. *J. Ment. Imagery* 14: 119–129.

Lane SM (2006) Dividing attention during a witnessed event increases eyewitness suggestibility. *Appl. Cogn. Psychol.* 20: 199–212.

Lindsay DS and Johnson MK (1989) The eyewitness suggestibility effect and memory for source. *Mem. Cogn.* 17: 349–358.

Lindsay DS, Johnson MK, and Kwon P (1991) Developmental changes in memory source monitoring. *J. Exp. Child Psychol.* 52: 297–318.

Lindsay DS, Hagen L, Read JD, Wade KA, and Garry M (2004) True photographs and false memories. *Psychol. Sci.* 15: 149–154.

Loftus EF (1979) Reactions to blatantly contradictory information. *Mem. Cogn.* 7: 368–374.

Loftus EF (1992) When a lie becomes memory's truth: Memory distortion after exposure to misinformation. *Curr. Dir. Psychol. Sci.* 1: 121–123.

Loftus EF and Palmer JC (1974) Reconstruction of automobile destruction: An example of the interaction between language and memory. *J. Verb. Learn. Verb. Behav.* 13: 585–589.

Loftus EF and Pickrell JE (1995) The formation of false memories. *Psychiatr. Ann.* 25: 720–725.

Loftus EF, Miller DG, and Burns HJ (1978) Semantic integration of verbal information into a visual memory. *J. Exp. Psychol. Hum. Learn. Mem.* 4: 19–31.

Loftus EF, Donders K, Hoffman HG, and Schooler JW (1989) Creating new memories that are quickly accessed and confidently held. *Mem. Cogn.* 17: 607–616.

MacLin MK (2002) The effects of exemplar and prototype descriptors on verbal overshadowing. *Appl. Cogn. Psychol.* 16: 929–936.

Mäntylä T (1986) Optimizing cue effectiveness: Recall of 500 and 600 incidentally learned words. *J. Exp. Psychol. Learn. Mem. Cogn.* 12: 66–71.

Marsh EJ and Dolan PO (2007) Test-induced priming of false memories. *Psychon. Bull. Rev.* 14: 479–483.

Mazzoni GAL, Loftus EF, and Kirsch I (2001) Changing beliefs about implausible autobiographical events: A little plausibility goes a long way. *J. Exp. Psychol. Appl.* 7: 51–59.

McDermott KB and Roediger HL III (1998) Attempting to avoid illusory memories: Robust false recognition on associates persists under conditions of explicit warnings and immediate testing. *J. Mem. Lang.* 39: 508–520.

McDermott KB and Watson JM (2001) The rise and fall of false recall: The impact of presentation duration. *J. Mem. Lang.* 45: 160–176.

McGeoch JA (1932) Forgetting and the law of disuse. *Psychol. Rev.* 39: 352–370.

Meissner CA and Brigham JC (2001) A meta-analysis of the verbal overshadowing effect in face identification. *Appl. Cogn. Psychol.* 15: 603–616.

Melcher JM and Schooler JW (1996) The misremembrance of wines past: Verbal and perceptual expertise differentially mediate verbal overshadowing of taste memory. *J. Mem. Lang.* 35: 231–245.

Mitchell KJ and Zaragoza MS (1996) Repeated exposure to suggestion and false memory: The role of contextual variability. *J. Mem. Lang.* 35: 246–260.

Multhaup KS (1995) Aging, source, and decision criteria: When false fame errors do and do not occur. *Psychol. Aging* 10: 492–497.

Multhaup KS and Conner CA (2002) The effects of considering nonlist sources on the Deese-Roediger-McDermott memory illusion. *J. Mem. Lang.* 47: 214–228.

Nickerson RS and Adams MJ (1979) Long-term memory for a common object. *Cogn. Psychol.* 11: 287–307.

Paddock JR, Noel M, and Terranova S (1999) Imagination inflation and the perils of guided visualization. *J. Psychol. Interdiscip. Appl.* 133: 581–595.

Payne DG, Elie CJ, Blackwell JM, and Neuschatz JS (1996) Memory illusions: Recalling, recognizing, and recollecting events that never occurred. *Special Issue: Illusions of Memory. J. Mem. Lang.* 35: 261–285.

Pendergrast M (1996) *Victims of Memory: Sex Abuse Accusations and Shattered Lives*. Hinesburg, VT: Upper Access.

Perfect TJ, Hunt LJ, and Harris CM (2002) Verbal overshadowing in voice recognition. *Appl. Cogn. Psychol.* 16: 973–980.

Peters MJV, Horselenberg R, and Jelicic M (2007) The false fame illusion in people with memories about a previous life. *Conscious. Cogn.* 16: 162–169.

Pezdek K (1977) Cross-modality semantic integration of sentence and picture memory. *J. Exp. Psychol. Hum. Learn. Mem.* 3: 515–524.

Pezdek K, Finger K, and Hodge D (1997) Planting false childhood memories: The role of event plausibility. *Psychol. Sci.* 8: 437–441.

Raz N (2000) Aging of the brain and its impact on cognitive performance: Integration of structural and functional findings. In: Craik FIM and Salthouse TA (eds.) *Handbook of Aging and Cognition,* 2nd edn., pp. 1–90. Mahwah, NJ: Erlbaum.

Read JD (1996) From a passing thought to a false memory in 2 minutes: Confusing real and illusory events. *Psychon. Bull. Rev.* 3: 105–111.

Rinck M (1999) Memory for everyday objects: Where are the digits on numerical keypads? *Appl. Cogn. Psychol.* 13: 329–350.

Robbins LC (1963) The accuracy of parental recall of aspects of child development and child rearing practices. *J. Abnorm. Soc. Psychol.* 66: 261–270.

Robinson KJ and Roediger HL III (1997) Associative processes in false recall and false recognition. *Psychol. Sci.* 8: 231–237.

Roediger HL III (1996) Memory illusions. *J. Mem. Lang.* 35: 76–100.

Roediger HL III and McDermott KB (1995) Creating false memories: Remembering words not presented in lists. *J. Exp. Psychol. Learn. Mem. Cogn.* 21: 803–814.

Roediger HL III, Jacoby JD, and McDermott KB (1996) Misinformation effects in recall: Creating false memories through repeated retrieval. *Special Issue: Illusions of Memory. J. Mem. Lang.* 35: 300–318.

Roediger HL III, Meade ML, and Bergman ET (2001a) Social contagion of memory. *Psychon. Bull. Rev.* 8: 365–371.

Roediger HL III, Watson JM, McDermott KB, and Gallo DA (2001b) Factors that determine false recall: A multiple regression analysis. *Psychon. Bull. Rev.* 8: 385–407.

Santa JL and Ranken HB (1972) Effects of verbal coding on recognition memory. *J. Exp. Psychol.* 93: 268–278.

Schacter DL, Israel L, and Racine C (1999) Suppressing false recognition in younger and older adults: The distinctiveness heuristic. *J. Mem. Lang.* 40: 1–24.

Schooler JW (2002) Verbalization produces a transfer inappropriate processing shift. *Appl. Cogn. Psychol.* 16: 989–997.

Schooler JW and Engstler-Schooler TY (1990) Verbal overshadowing of visual memories: Some things are better left unsaid. *Cogn. Psychol.* 22: 36–71.

Schooler JW, Gerhard D, and Loftus EF (1986) Qualities of the unreal. *J. Exp. Psychol. Learn. Mem. Cogn.* 12: 171–181.

Sharman SJ, Garry M, and Beuke CJ (2004) Imagination or exposure causes imagination inflation. *Am. J. Psychol.* 117: 157–168.

Sharman SJ, Manning CG, and Garry M (2005) Explain this: Explaining childhood events inflates confidence for those events. *Appl. Cogn. Psychol.* 19: 67–74.

Shepard RN (1967) Recognition memory for words, sentences, and pictures. *J. Verb. Learn. Verb. Behav.* 6: 151–163.

Sommers MS and Lewis BP (1999) Who really lives next door: Creating false memories with phonological neighbors. *J. Mem. Lang.* 40: 83–108.

Thomas AK, Bulevich JB, and Loftus EF (2003) Exploring the role of repetition and sensory elaboration in the imagination inflation effect. *Mem. Cogn.* 31: 630–640.

Tousignant JP, Hall D, and Loftus EF (1986) Discrepancy detection and vulnerability to misleading postevent information. *Mem. Cogn.* 14: 329–338.

Tulving E (1983) *Elements of Episodic Memory*. New York: Oxford University Press.

Wade KA, Garry M, Read JD, and Lindsay DS (2002) A picture is worth a thousand lies: Using false photographs to create false childhood memories. *Psychon. Bull. Rev.* 9: 597–603.

Watson JM, Balota DA, and Roediger HL III (2003) Creating false memories with hybrid lists of semantic and phonological associates: Over-additive false memories produced by converging associative networks. *J. Mem. Lang.* 49: 95–118.

Wells GL, Memon A, and Penrod SD (2006) Eyewitness evidence: Improving its probative value. *Psychol. Sci. Public Interest* 7: 45–75.

Westerman DL and Greene RL (1996) On the generality of the revelation effect. *J. Exp. Psychol. Learn. Mem. Cogn.* 22: 1147–1153.

Witherspoon D and Allan LG (1985) The effects of a prior presentation on temporal judgments in a perceptual identification task. *Mem. Cogn.* 13: 101–111.

Wright DB, Varley S, and Belton A (1996) Accurate second guesses in misinformation studies. *Appl. Cogn. Psychol.* 10: 13–21.

Wright DB, Mathews SA, and Skagerberg EM (2005) Social recognition memory: The effect of other people's responses for previously seen and unseen items. *J. Exp. Psychol.* 11: 200–209.

Zaragoza MS and Lane SM (1994) Source misattributions and the suggestibility of eyewitness memory. *J. Exp. Psychol. Learn. Mem. Cogn.* 20: 934–945.

Zaragoza MS and Mitchell KJ (1996) Repeated exposure to suggestion and the creation of false memories. *Psychol. Sci.* 7: 294–300.

33 Molecular Aspects of Memory Dysfunction in Alzheimer's Disease

J. Chin, E. D. Roberson, and L. Mucke, Gladstone Institute of Neurological Disease and University of California, San Francisco, CA, USA

33.1 Introduction

Alzheimer's disease (AD) is the foremost human disease of memory. Independent streams of research on the molecular mechanisms of AD and the molecular basis of memory, which historically were quite distinct, are now converging in exciting ways. The study of AD may provide novel insights into basic mechanisms of memory, and even more importantly for the over 24 million patients with AD worldwide (Ferri et al., 2005), discoveries about the molecular basis of memory are advancing our understanding of the disease and yielding new treatment targets.

AD typically begins with mild forgetfulness in the elderly. Early on, before memory problems interfere with day-to-day functioning, a diagnosis of mild cognitive impairment (MCI) is often made. As years go by, deficits become more severe and patients are forced to curtail their usual activities. Deficits in other cognitive domains become increasingly apparent, including executive dysfunction, anomia and other language problems, visuospatial dysfunction, and ultimately, global cognitive impairment. Median survival is about 12 years after first symptom onset (Roberson et al., 2005).

Although the diagnosis of probable AD is made during life, definite diagnosis is made only at autopsy. The hallmark pathological features of AD are extracellular amyloid plaques and intracellular neurofibrillary tangles (NFTs) (**Figure 1**), combined with neuronal and synaptic loss, vascular amyloidosis, astrocytosis, and microgliosis. Most of these changes occur in a stereotypical regional distribution, with medial temporal structures involved in memory affected earliest and most severely.

Biochemical and genetic studies of AD have identified several molecules that may play a causal role in its pathogenesis (**Figure 2**). For the most part, these molecules have been studied primarily in the context of AD. In the first half of this chapter, we consider the impact of these AD-related molecules on memory. In addition, many molecules that have been studied primarily in the context of synaptic plasticity and memory, including a variety of receptors, channels, second messengers, kinases, and transcription factors, are also involved in AD. In the second half of the chapter, we consider AD-related memory impairment in relation to these molecules.

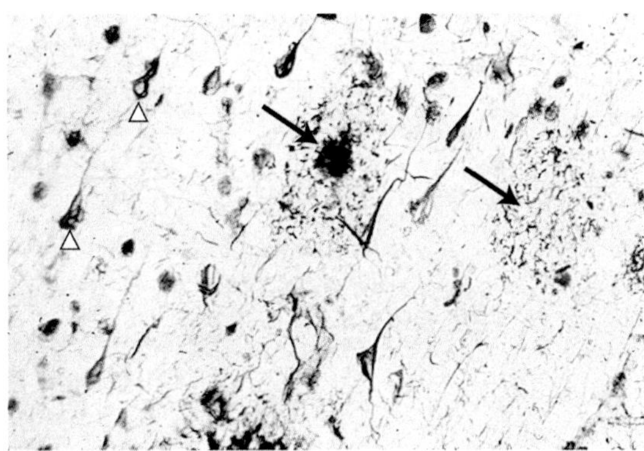

Figure 1 Plaques and tangles. This silver-stained section of cerebral cortex from a patient with Alzheimer's disease shows extracellular amyloid plaques (black arrows) and intracellular neurofibrillary tangles (white arrowheads). (Courtesy of Dr. Nitya R Ghatak, Virginia Commonwealth University Health System.)

33.2 Memory Impairment by AD-Related Molecules

In this section, we examine several molecules that likely contribute to the pathogenesis of AD, including the amyloid precursor protein (APP), amyloid-β peptide (Aβ), the β- and γ-secretases that release Aβ from APP by proteolytic cleavage, the microtubule-associated protein tau, the lipid carrier apolipoprotein E (apoE), and α-synuclein, which also plays an important role in Parkinson's disease. For each molecule, we briefly review its normal function and the evidence for its involvement in AD and then examine studies of its relationship to memory deficits in both humans and animal models.

33.2.1 APP and Aβ

APP is a ubiquitously expressed, multifunctional type I membrane protein with potential roles in signaling (Turner et al., 2003), axonal transport (Kamal et al., 2000; Satpute-Krishnan et al., 2006),

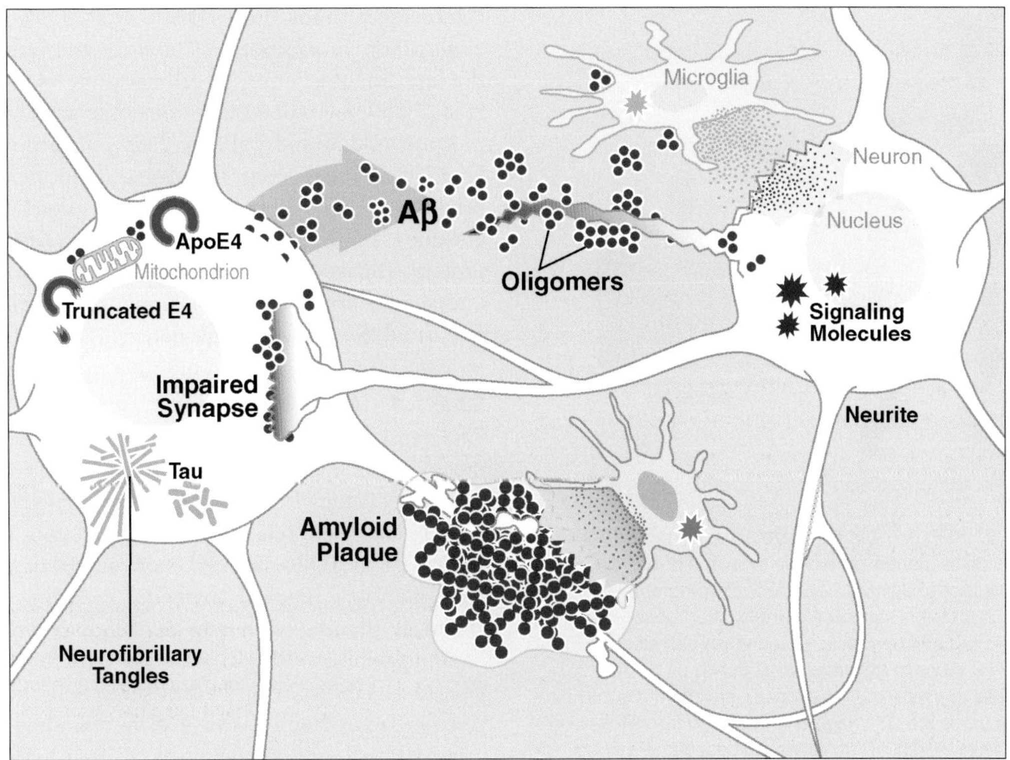

Figure 2 Key molecules involved in Alzheimer's disease pathogenesis. Aβ peptides produced by neurons and other brain cells aggregate into a variety of assemblies, including amyloid plaques containing Aβ fibrils and soluble nonfibrillar oligomers. Some of these Aβ assemblies impair synapses and neuronal dendrites, either directly or through the engagement of pathogenic glial loops. However, other glial activities protect neurons against dysfunction and degeneration. ApoE4 and tau promote Aβ-induced neuronal injury and also have independent adverse effects. (From Roberson ED and Mucke L [2006] 100 years and counting: Prospects for defeating Alzheimer's disease. *Science* 314: 781–784.)

transcriptional regulation (Cao and Südhof, 2001), neurite outgrowth (Leyssen et al., 2005), synaptogenesis (Mucke et al., 1994; Morimoto et al., 1998), and regulation of glutamate uptake (Masliah et al., 1998). APP-null mice have deficits in learning and memory, abnormal long-term potentiation (LTP), and loss of synapses (Dawson et al., 1999; Seabrook et al., 1999).

Proteolytic cleavage of APP produces several biologically active fragments. Among them are Aβ peptides, produced by the sequential action of two proteases, β- and γ-secretase, on APP (**Figure 3**). Aβ peptides of 40 (Aβ40) or 42 (Aβ42) amino acids in length are the primary species produced. Aβ42 is believed to be more pathogenic, since it is more prone to aggregation and more toxic when applied to cells than Aβ40 (Jarrett et al., 1993; Seilheimer et al., 1997). Aβ has been shown to decrease synaptic transmission (Hsia et al., 1999; Kamenetz et al., 2003; Priller et al., 2006) or LTP (Lambert et al., 1998; Walsh et al., 2002), which may represent physiological functions, pathogenic mechanisms, or both. Neuronal activity stimulates the production and release of Aβ, which in turn depresses excitatory synaptic transmission, at least at certain synapses (Kamenetz et al., 2003). Under normal circumstances, this feedback loop could help regulate synaptic activity. In AD, aberrant neuronal activity might turn this feedback loop into a vicious cycle that increases Aβ production and impairs neurotransmission (Palop et al., 2006, 2007).

A great deal of additional biochemical and genetic evidence suggests an involvement of Aβ in AD, which forms the basis of the 'amyloid hypothesis of AD pathogenesis (Hardy and Higgins, 1992; Tanzi and Bertram, 2005). Aβ is the major constituent of amyloid plaques, one of the pathological hallmarks of AD (Glenner and Wong, 1984). Mutations in APP cause autosomal dominant AD (Goate et al., 1991); AD-causing APP mutations are concentrated around the Aβ domain, and most increase the Aβ42/Aβ40 ratio or total Aβ production (Theuns et al., 2006). Presenilin mutations, the other major known cause of autosomal dominant AD, also increase the relative

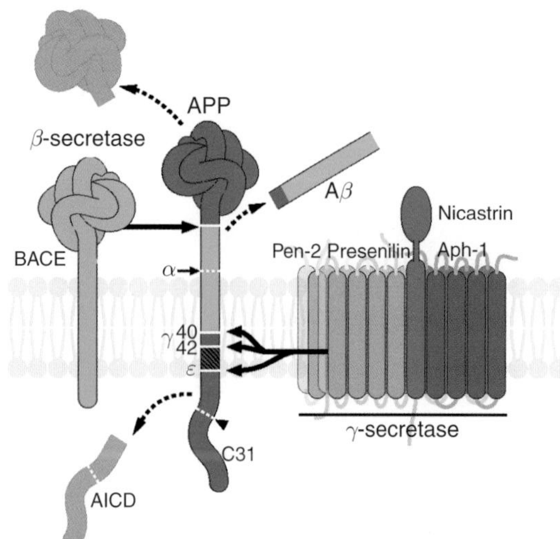

Figure 3 APP, Aβ, and the secretases. Aβ production depends on sequential proteolytic cleavage of APP by β-secretase, also known as β-site APP-cleaving enzyme 1 (BACE1), and the γ-secretase complex, composed of presenilin and other proteins. γ-Secretase can cleave APP at different locations to generate Aβ40, Aβ42, or the APP intracellular domain (AICD). Caspase cleavage at the carboxy-terminus yields the C31 fragment. (Modified from Roberson ED and Mucke L [2006] 100 years and counting: Prospects for defeating Alzheimer's disease. Science 314: 781–784.)

abundance of Aβ42 (see the section titled 'γ-Secretase') (Levy-Lahad et al., 1995; Rogaev et al., 1995; Sherrington et al., 1995). In addition, polymorphisms in the gene for insulin-degrading enzyme, which degrades Aβ, may contribute to AD risk (Ertekin-Taner et al., 2004).

The first animals with prominent AD-like pathology, and still the most widely studied, were transgenic mice with neuronal expression of human APP (hAPP) carrying familial AD mutations (Games et al., 1995; McGowan et al., 2006). These mice have high levels of Aβ and several, but not all, of the neuropathological hallmarks of AD. For example, age-dependent plaque deposition is a universal feature, whereas tangles do not develop. Because hAPP mice develop age-dependent learning and memory abnormalities (Kobayashi and Chen, 2005; McGowan et al., 2006), these models provide an opportunity to test hypotheses about how Aβ contributes to cognitive impairment in AD.

At a molecular level, there are a variety of hypotheses for how Aβ might interfere with normal neuronal function and survival. For example, Aβ can bind directly to lipid bilayers, altering membrane fluidity (Müller et al., 2001). It also forms pores or otherwise permeabilizes membranes, increasing their conductance to ion flow (Pollard et al., 1995; Kayed et al., 2004). In addition, Aβ binds to and influences the function of a variety of cellular proteins (Verdier et al., 2004), including the α7 nicotinic acetylcholine receptor (Oddo and LaFerla, 2006), integrins (Sabo et al., 1995), the receptor for advanced glycation end-products (RAGE; Yan et al., 1996), mitochondrial enzymes (Lustbader et al., 2004), and the APP holoprotein (Shaked et al., 2006). Several of these interactions are discussed in more detail in the section titled 'Memory-related molecules in AD.'

33.2.1.1 Aβ and plaques

The deposition of Aβ into amyloid plaques has been the focus of much AD research, given the prominence of plaques in AD patients and related animal models and their relative ease of detection. Plaque deposition in AD brains has historically been studied with neuropathological methods, including histochemical staining with amyloid-binding dyes and immunostaining with Aβ antibodies. It can now be imaged *in vivo* in living human subjects by positron emission tomography with a plaque-binding agent termed Pittsburgh compound B (PIB) (Klunk et al., 2004) (**Figure 4**).

The leading hypothesis for how plaques might disrupt neuronal function is by inducing changes in surrounding neurites. A subset of amyloid plaques in both AD patients and mouse models, termed neuritic plaques, are surrounded by swollen and tortuous neuronal processes (Knowles et al., 1999; Tsai et al., 2004). Plaque-associated neuritic dystrophy may alter the electrophysiological properties of the circuits involved (Knowles et al., 1999; Stern et al., 2004).

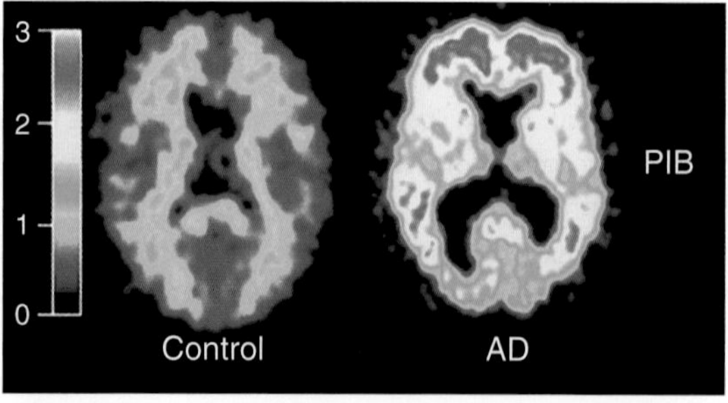

Figure 4 *In vivo* imaging of amyloid plaques with Pittsburgh compound B (PIB). PIB–positron emission tomography scan of a 79-year-old patient with AD shows a robust signal attributable to amyloid plaque binding, compared with a 67-year-old control subject. (From Klunk WE, Engler H, Nordberg A, et al. [2004] Imaging brain amyloid in Alzheimer's disease with Pittsburgh Compound-B. *Ann. Neurol.* 55: 306–319.)

However, plaque deposition does not correlate well with memory deficits in AD. Amyloid deposition tends to be an early event in AD pathogenesis that plateaus and does not worsen as cognition deteriorates throughout the disease course (Arriagada et al., 1992; Ingelsson et al., 2004; Giannakopoulos et al., 2007). Also, plaques do not have the preferential distribution in medial temporal structures involved in memory that is seen with NFTs (see the section titled 'NFTs, neuronal death, and memory loss'). Rather, plaques are seen first in the neocortex, particularly in prefrontal and posterior parietal regions (Price et al., 1991; Buckner et al., 2005; Kemppainen et al., 2006). Data from animal models also support a mechanistic dissociation between plaques and cognitive deficits (Holcomb et al., 1998; Westerman et al., 2002; Palop et al., 2003; Kobayashi and Chen, 2005; Lesné et al., 2006; Cheng et al., 2007). While neuritic dystrophy correlates with cognitive deficits better than plaque load (McKee et al., 1991), many dystrophic neurites in AD brains are not associated with plaques (Wang and Munoz, 1995). Recent findings in hAPP transgenic mice suggest that vascular amyloidosis and oxidative stress may contribute to the pathogenesis of plaque-independent neuritic dystrophy (Esposito et al., 2006).

33.2.1.2 Soluble Aβ oligomers

Because deposition of fibrillar Aβ in plaques does not correlate well with cognitive deficits, interest has grown in nonfibrillar forms of Aβ. Increasing evidence points to a pathogenic role for oligomeric Aβ assemblies that are soluble in aqueous solutions. Multiple types of Aβ oligomers have been described, including low-molecular-weight species (dimers and trimers) and larger globular species (including dodecamers and Aβ-derived diffusible ligands) (Podlisny et al., 1995; Lambert et al., 1998; Lesné et al., 2006). Putative Aβ oligomers have been detected in the cerebrospinal fluid (CSF) and brain tissue of AD patients (Podlisny et al., 1995; Kuo et al., 1996; Pitschke et al., 1998; Kayed et al., 2003; Lacor et al., 2004) and hAPP transgenic mice (Podlisny et al., 1995; Lambert et al., 1998; Lesné et al., 2006; Cheng et al., 2007). Extracellularly, oligomers seem to bind preferentially to dendritic and synaptic regions (Lacor et al., 2004; Barghorn et al., 2005). Aβ42 is more prone to oligomer formation than Aβ40 (Dahlgren et al., 2002; Bitan et al., 2003), which may relate to their relative pathogenicity (A$\beta42 > A\beta40$).

In mixed neuronal/glial cultures and brain slices, oligomeric Aβ is a potent neurotoxin, inducing neuronal death within 24 h (Roher et al., 1996; Lambert et al., 1998; Chen et al., 2005a). Direct experimental comparisons suggest that oligomeric Aβ is more toxic than fibrillar or monomeric Aβ (Klein et al., 2001; Dahlgren et al., 2002).

At physiological concentrations, Aβ oligomers interfere with synaptic plasticity, and memory. Both low-molecular-weight and larger globular oligomers interfered with LTP when acutely applied to hippocampal slices, whereas monomers did not (Lambert et al., 1998; Wang et al., 2004; Barghorn et al., 2005; Walsh et al., 2005). Injection of oligomeric Aβ into the cerebral ventricles blocked LTP *in vivo* and impaired learning and memory (Walsh et al., 2002; Cleary et al., 2005; Lesné et al., 2006). The effects of Aβ on LTP are acute and independent of neuronal death (Chen et al., 2000). Although oligomer-induced blockade of LTP in hippocampal slices could not be reversed by washing out Aβ (Townsend et al., 2006), *in vivo* impairment of LTP by oligomers could be blocked when Aβ antibodies were injected after the Aβ (Klyubin et al., 2005).

33.2.1.3 Neuronal dysfunction versus neuronal death

The ability of Aβ to induce both neuronal dysfunction and neuronal death raises the question of which effect is primarily responsible for the memory deficits in AD. Evidence from animal models points toward an important role for neuronal dysfunction. First, although hAPP mice have memory deficits, most lines do not have prominent neuron loss in the areas most affected in AD, including entorhinal cortex and hippocampal area CA1 (Irizarry et al., 1997a,b; Takeuchi et al., 2000). Also, memory impairment in hAPP mice can be rapidly reversed by treatments that lower Aβ levels but are not likely to change neuron numbers (Dodart et al., 2002; Kotilinek et al., 2002). Rather than frank neuronal loss, hAPP mice have synaptodendritic changes, including reduction of presynaptic terminals, loss of postsynaptic spines, and simplification of dendritic arborization, that may contribute to cognitive impairment (Mucke et al., 2000; Buttini et al., 2002; Lanz et al., 2003; Chin et al., 2004; Moolman et al., 2004; Wu et al., 2004; Spires et al., 2005). Whether these alterations would ultimately lead to neuronal loss if mice had a longer lifespan is unknown. It is also unknown how long it takes neurons to die in the brains of humans with AD.

Differentiating the relative contributions of neuronal dysfunction and neuronal loss to cognitive deficits in AD patients has been difficult, because neuron loss is commonly found early in the disease (Price et al., 2001). However, several observations suggest that dysfunction may at least add to the impairments that are likely to result from progressive neuronal loss. Synaptodendritic alterations similar to those observed in hAPP mice are also observed in AD (Terry et al., 1991; Masliah et al., 2001a; Shim and Lubec, 2002; Moolman et al., 2004). Synaptic loss is an early event that correlates with cognitive impairment in AD (Terry et al., 1991; Masliah et al., 2001a). In addition, synaptic failure may precede and contribute to neuronal death (Selkoe, 2002). Finally, the frequent fluctuations in cognition seen in AD patients cannot be explained by sudden changes in neuronal numbers and are likely a manifestation of neuronal dysfunction (Palop et al., 2006).

33.2.1.4 Other APP fragments

Aβ is not the only biologically active APP fragment. γ-Secretase cleavage liberates a carboxy-terminal fragment known as the APP intracellular domain (AICD). The AICD activates the adapter protein Fe65, which translocates to the nucleus and regulates gene expression (Cao and Südhof, 2001, 2004). The AICD/Fe65 pathway stimulates expression of many genes, including neprilysin, a peptidase that degrades Aβ (Pardossi-Piquard et al., 2005), the P53 tumor suppressor, which controls programmed cell death (Alves da Costa et al., 2006), and components of the cytoskeleton (Müller et al., 2006). The AICD also modulates calcium stores in the endoplasmic reticulum (Leissring et al., 2002). While AICD-dependent changes in gene expression may be a factor in patients with APP mutations (Wiley et al., 2005), their importance in sporadic AD remains unclear. AICD levels and some cytoskeletal target genes are unchanged, while others are upregulated, and neprilysin expression is decreased (Wang et al., 2005; Müller et al., 2006).

The ectodomain of APP can be shed by α- or β-secretase, generating secreted APP fragments known as sAPPα and sAPPβ, respectively. Ectodomain shedding is a prerequisite for γ-secretase cleavage and, thus, Aβ and AICD production. sAPP may have independent effects, particularly neuroprotective and neurotrophic activities (Mattson, 1997; Kerr and Small, 2005; Zheng and Koo, 2006).

Finally, APP is cleaved by caspase(s) at a site 31 amino acids from the carboxy terminus; the resulting C-terminal fragment is termed C31 (Gervais et al., 1999; Lu et al., 2000). Transgenic mice expressing hAPP with a mutation that prevents this cleavage have less pronounced cognitive impairment than mice expressing caspase-sensitive hAPP (Galvan et al., 2006). The favorable effect of this mutation may be a result of reduced generation of C31, which is neurotoxic (Lu et al., 2000; Galvan et al., 2002). It may also be caused by changes in protein–protein interactions involving the APP carboxy terminus, including APP multimerization (Lu et al., 2003) and interactions with motor proteins (Satpute-Krishnan et al., 2006).

33.2.2 BACE

The first step in production of Aβ from APP is shedding the large APP ectodomain by β-secretase (**Figure 3**). The primary β-secretase enzyme is an aspartyl protease termed β-site APP cleaving enzyme (BACE1, also known as Asp2, memapsin 2) (Hussain et al., 1999; Sinha et al., 1999; Vassar et al., 1999; Yan et al., 1999). Genetic deletion of BACE1 dramatically reduces Aβ levels (Roberds et al., 2001) and prevents Aβ-dependent cognitive deficits in hAPP mice (Ohno et al., 2006). Thus, BACE1 inhibition is an attractive potential AD therapy.

Two aspects of BACE physiology are of particular interest in relation to synaptic transmission and neuronal function. First, BACE activity, at least its cleavage of APP, is dynamically regulated and increases with neuronal activity (Kamenetz et al., 2003). This effect contributes to a putative feedback loop whereby increased neuronal activity stimulates Aβ production, which in turn can suppress synaptic transmission (Kamenetz et al., 2003). Alterations in BACE regulation may be important in AD pathogenesis, as BACE activity is increased in AD (Holsinger et al., 2002) and after other types of neuronal injury (Blasko et al., 2004). Second, BACE1 has other substrates beyond APP, many of which affect neuronal function (**Table 1**). Among these are neuregulin 1, a

Table 1 Selected BACE1 substrates

Aβ
APP
APP-like proteins
Low density lipoprotein receptor-related protein
Neuregulin-1
P-selectin glycoprotein ligand-1
ST6Gal I sialyltransferase
Voltage-gated sodium channel β subunit

Adapted from Willem M, Garratt AN, Novak B, et al. (2006) Control of peripheral nerve myelination by the β-secretase BACE1. *Science* 314: 664–666.

ligand in the ErbB signaling pathway (Willem et al., 2006). In the absence of BACE cleavage, lack of neuregulin/ErbB signaling results in peripheral nerve hypomyelination (Willem et al., 2006). Cleavage of substrates besides APP may also contribute to AD. Mice overexpressing human BACE1 have neurodegeneration and memory deficits (Rockenstein et al., 2005). However, these effects are not a result of increases in Aβ levels, which are actually lower in BACE-overexpressing mice than in mice with normal BACE levels (Lee et al., 2005; Rockenstein et al., 2005), presumably because BACE overexpression promotes APP processing in an earlier component of the secretory pathway (Lee et al., 2005).

33.2.3 Presenilins

Shortly after the discovery that mutations in the APP gene cause autosomal dominant AD, two other genes were found in other families with early-onset AD: presenilin 1 (PS1) on chromosome 14 and presenilin 2 (PS2) on chromosome 1 (Levy-Lahad et al., 1995; Rogaev et al., 1995; Sherrington et al., 1995). PS1 mutations have since proven to be the most common cause of dominantly inherited AD, responsible for more than 50% of cases. Over 150 different mutations spanning the protein have been identified. PS2 mutations are much less common and tend to produce a somewhat less severe phenotype (Bertram and Tanzi, 2004). PS1 and PS2 are 67% identical and are ubiquitously expressed in the brain and other tissues.

The normal functions of the presenilins were unknown at the time of their discovery and are still being elucidated today. Most attention has focused on presenilin's role in Aβ production as a key component of γ-secretase. However, diverse γ-secretase-independent roles of presenilins continue to emerge, and controversy remains about the degree to which these roles contribute to AD and whether the AD-linked mutations cause primarily a gain or loss of function.

33.2.3.1 γ-Secretase

The presenilins are membrane-embedded aspartyl proteases that form the catalytically active center of the γ-secretase complex, along with nicastrin, Aph-1, and Pen-2 (De Strooper et al., 1998; Edbauer et al., 2003). γ-Secretase cleaves type I membrane proteins within their transmembrane domains (reviewed in Wolfe, 2006). Its substrate selectivity is rather broad, with the main requirement being a short extracellular domain (Struhl and Adachi, 2000). Thus, γ-secretase has many substrates (**Table 2**).

Table 2 Selected γ-secretase substrates

γ-protocadherin
APLP1
APLP2
APP
CD43
CD44
DCC
Delta
E-Cadherin
ErbB-4
Jagged
LRP
Voltage-gated sodium channel β2 subunit
N-Cadherin
Nectin-1α
Notch
NRADD
P75
Syndecan-1
Tyrosinase
Tyrosinase-related proteins 1 and 2

From Vetrivel KS, Zhang YW, Xu H, et al. (2006) Pathological and physiological functions of presenilins. *Mol. Neurodegener.* 1:4.

One of these is, of course, APP. Shedding of the large extracellular domain of APP by α- or β-secretase generates carboxy-terminal fragments (CTFs) that make suitable substrates for γ-secretase (**Figure 3**). The γ-secretase complex can cleave β-CTF at different sites, generating either Aβ40 or Aβ42. PS mutations favor production of Aβ42 over Aβ40 (Borchelt et al., 1996; Scheuner et al., 1996). Given the considerable evidence that Aβ42 is more pathogenic (see the section titled 'APP and Aβ'), this effect is believed to be an important mechanism by which PS mutations lead to AD. γ-Secretase is also responsible for generation of the AICD (see the section titled 'Other APP fragments').

33.2.3.2 γ-Secretase-independent roles of presenilins

In addition to their role in Aβ production, presenilins have several other functions, many of which are independent of γ-secretase, as they are not blocked by γ-secretase inhibitors or by point mutations that abolish secretase activity.

Several of these functions relate to calcium regulation. Presenilin mutations increase calcium release from the endoplasmic reticulum induced by inositol-1,4,5-trisphosphate (IP_3) (reviewed in LaFerla, 2002). One mechanism for this effect seems to be overfilling endoplasmic reticulum (ER) Ca^{2+} stores (Leissring et al., 2000). Presenilins form calcium leak channels in the ER membrane; this function is lost in AD-associated mutants, leading to overfilling of the ER with Ca^{2+} (Tu et al., 2006). Others have pointed to an upregulation of IP_3 receptors in presenilin-deficient cells as another possible cause for increased calcium release (Kasri et al., 2006). Whatever the underlying mechanism, the resulting increases in intracellular calcium release induced by presenilin mutations are likely to contribute to neuronal dysfunction.

Presenilin also regulates intracellular signaling pathways that control tau phosphorylation. Presenilin stabilizes cadherin–cadherin complexes that interact with and activate phosphatidylinositol-3 kinase, stimulating Akt activity, which, in turn, suppresses glycogen synthase kinase (GSK) activity and tau phosphorylation (Baki et al., 2004). This γ-secretase-independent effect of presenilin in preventing tau phosphorylation is lost in AD-associated mutants and, thus, may enhance tau-mediated neurotoxicity (Baki et al., 2004).

Conditional PS1/PS2 double-knockout mice have learning and memory impairments, LTP deficits, aberrant tau phosphorylation, and neurodegeneration, although their Aβ levels are not increased (Saura et al., 2004), suggesting that mutations impairing APP-independent PS functions could also contribute to AD-related deficits.

33.2.4 Tau

Tau is a small microtubule-associated protein (MAP) and a member of the MAP2 superfamily (Weingarten et al., 1975; Cleveland et al., 1977; Dehmelt and Halpain, 2005). It has a variety of functions, including stabilizing microtubules, enabling neurite outgrowth, regulating axonal transport, and controlling neuronal susceptibility to overexcitation (Shahani and Brandt, 2002; Avila et al., 2004; Roberson et al., 2007). Tau knockout mice are surprisingly normal, with no abnormalities in general health, fertility, longevity, gross brain cytoarchitecture, or learning and memory (Harada et al., 1994; Ikegami et al., 2000; Dawson et al., 2001; Tucker et al., 2001; Roberson et al., 2007). This may be, at least in part, the result of compensation by other MAPs, since double knockouts lacking both tau and MAP1B have 80% mortality in the first few weeks postnatally (Takei et al., 2000). Microdeletions on chromosome 17q21 including the tau gene are associated with mental retardation in humans (Lupski, 2006), but these deletions also involve several other genes. The fact that tau knockout mice have a very mild phenotype suggests that the loss of other genes might underlie the deficits associated with these deletions.

Tau was first implicated in AD by the discovery that NFTs are composed of heavily phosphorylated tau forming paired helical filaments (Grundke-Iqbal et al., 1986; Kosik et al., 1986; Wood et al., 1986; Lee et al., 1991). Interestingly, mutations in tau cause frontotemporal dementia, but not AD (Rademakers et al., 2004). However, the tau gene contains several polymorphisms that are in linkage disequilibrium, creating several unique haplotypes, one of which is associated with AD (Myers et al., 2005). The high-risk haplotype, known as H1c, is associated with roughly 10% more tau expression than other haplotypes (Kwok et al., 2004). This is consistent with the observation that reducing tau expression is protective in mouse models of AD (Roberson et al., 2007). The H1c haplotype also affects splicing of tau. Transcripts of the single tau gene are alternatively spliced to generate six different isoforms in adults (**Figure 5**). The most important distinction is between those isoforms with three copies of the microtubule-binding domain (termed 3R tau) and those with four (4R). The H1c haplotype is associated with slightly higher production of 4R than 3R tau (Myers et al., 2007). The mechanism by which these differences in tau expression raise AD risk is unclear.

33.2.4.1 NFTs, neuronal death, and memory loss

The study of tau's contribution to memory dysfunction in AD has concentrated largely on NFTs. Interest in NFTs dates all the way back to Alzheimer's original report (1907), which focused more on tangles than on plaques. Two observations form the basis of the hypothesis that tangles produce memory deficits in AD. First, the regional distribution of NFTs, which evolves in a stereotypical manner over the course of the illness, begins in medial temporal structures involved in memory (Braak and Braak, 1991). Tangles first appear in the transentorhinal region (stage I), then the entorhinal cortex (stage II), hippocampus (stage III), temporal neocortex (stage IV), and eventually other neocortical areas (stages V–VI) (**Figure 6**). Second, NFT counts correlate with clinical dementia severity, unlike amyloid plaque deposition, which does not (Giannakopoulos et al., 2007; but see Näslund et al., 2000).

Neuron loss may be a key mechanism underlying the connection between tau aggregation into NFTs and memory deficits. NFT burden correlates with the severity of neuronal loss (Giannakopoulos et al., 2007). NFT counts also correlate with levels of CSF tau, which increase in AD, possibly as a result of tau release

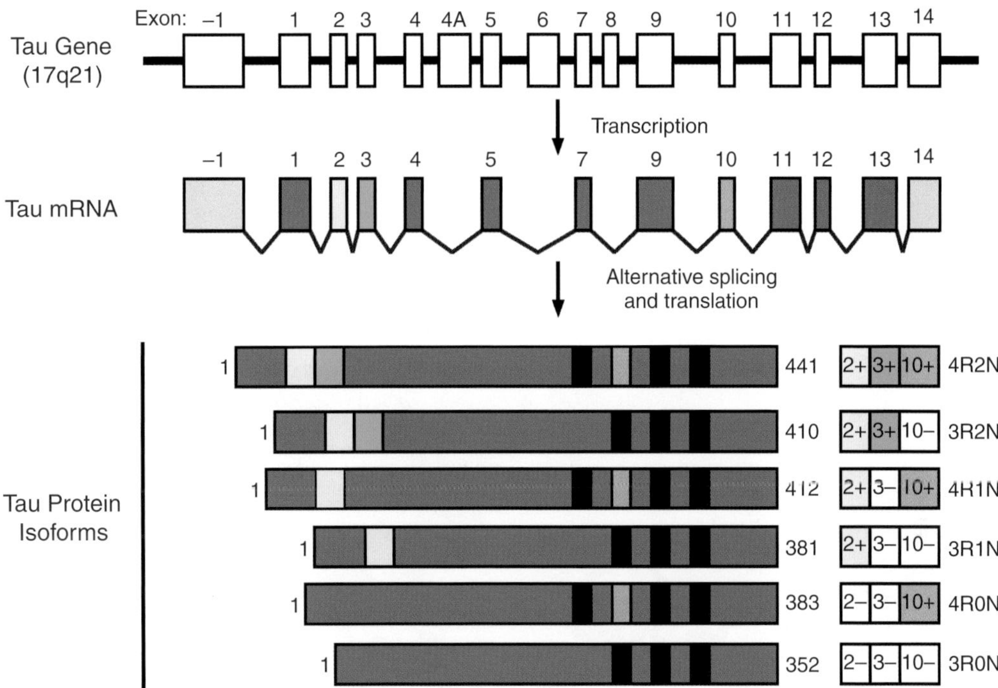

Figure 5 Alternative splicing of tau isoforms. The tau RNA can be alternatively spliced to include zero, one, or two amino-terminal inserts encoded by exons 2 and 3. Isoforms contain either three or four microtubule-binding domains, depending on whether exon 10 is included. (Modified from Buée L, Bussière T, Buée-Scherrer V, et al. [2000] Tau protein isoforms, phosphorylation and role in neurodegenerative disorders. *Brain Res. Rev.* 33: 95–130.)

from dying neurons (Arai et al., 1995; Tapiola et al., 1997; Giannakopoulos et al., 2007). Increased CSF tau is associated with poorer cognitive performance (Wallin et al., 2006) and a higher risk of progressing from MCI to AD (Blennow and Hampel, 2003).

Animal and cellular models also support a link between tau aggregation and neuron death (McGowan et al., 2006). Many transgenic mouse lines expressing human tau with mutations that favor tau aggregation display memory deficits and neuron loss (Lewis et al., 2000; Tatebayashi et al., 2002; Pennanen et al., 2004; McGowan et al., 2006). Overexpression of tau in large neurons of the lamprey leads to fibrillar tau aggregates and neuronal degeneration, an effect blocked by compounds that inhibit tau aggregation (Hall et al., 2001, 2002). Expression of aggregation-prone tau mutants in cultured neuroblastoma cells also causes toxicity that can be reversed by point mutations or small molecules that block aggregation (Khlistunova et al., 2006).

33.2.4.2 Tangle-independent roles for tau

There are limitations to the data suggesting a connection between NFTs and cognitive decline. Because much of the human data are correlational, they cannot establish causal relationships. Notably, animal model data indicate that aggregation is not the only means by which tau can impair neuronal and cognitive functions. Tau overexpression induced neurodegeneration in *Drosophila* in the absence of NFTs (Wittmann et al., 2001). Even in tau transgenic mice that have NFTs, neurodegeneration affects cells that do not have tau aggregates (Andorfer et al., 2005; Spires et al., 2006). Nonfibrillar tau might induce neuronal death by stimulating cell cycle reentry in normally postmitotic neurons (Andorfer et al., 2005; Khurana et al., 2006), although other mechanisms are possible also. The rTg4510 model has an inducible mutant tau transgene that, when turned on, causes NFT formation, severe neuronal loss, and spatial memory impairment (Ramsden et al., 2005; SantaCruz et al., 2005). However, suppressing transgene expression reverses the memory deficits, even though NFT formation continues, dissociating these processes (SantaCruz et al., 2005).

The mechanisms underlying these effects of tau on neuronal function have not yet been determined, although some leads exist. Abnormal tau can interfere with axonal transport (Ebneth et al., 1998; Ishihara et al., 1999), which seems consistent with its role as a microtubule-binding protein. Tau's influence on

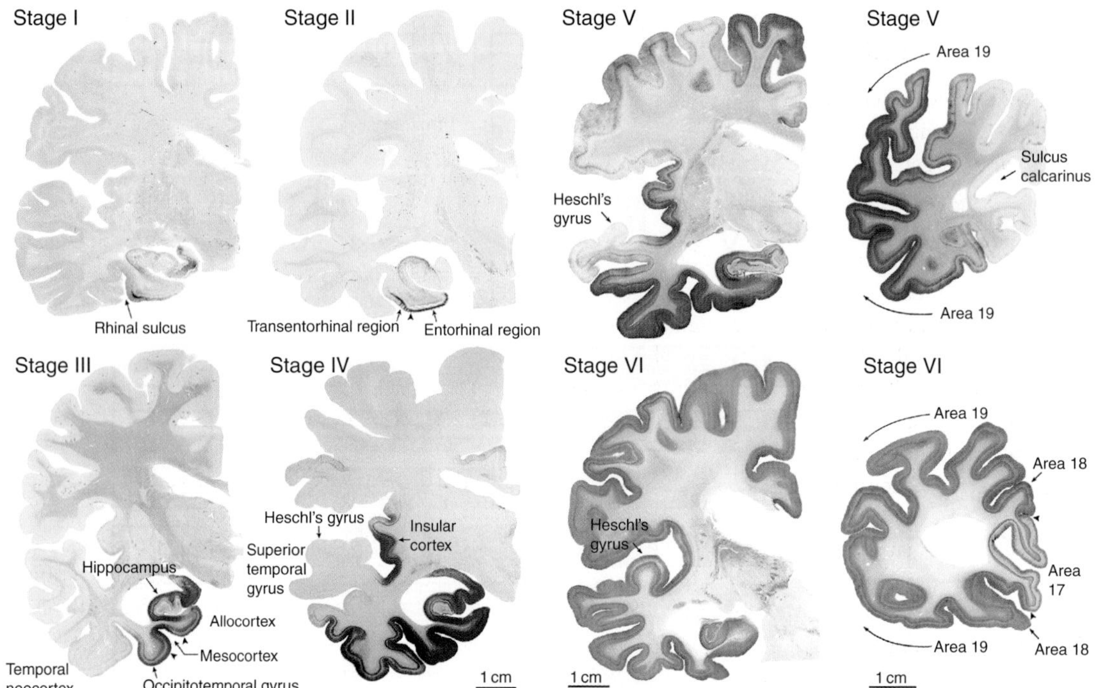

Figure 6 Stages of neurofibrillary pathology in Alzheimer's disease. Whole-brain sections were immunostained with antibody to phosphorylated tau. In stage I, involvement is limited to the transentorhinal region. Neurofibrillary pathology spreads to the entorhinal cortex in stage II. Stage III involves the hippocampus. Stage IV involves spread to the insula and inferior temporal neocortex. Finally, in stages V–VI even more neocortical areas are affected. (From Braak H, Rüb U, Schultz C, et al. [2006]. Vulnerability of cortical neurons to Alzheimer's and Parkinson's diseases. *J Alzheimers Dis* 9:35–44, with permission from IOS Press.)

microtubule stability could also affect plasticity-related structural rearrangements, and some of these effects may relate to normal tau functions. Reversible synaptic regression during hibernation in certain rodents is associated with changes in tau, especially changes in its phosphorylation (Arendt et al., 2003). At young ages, before formation of aggregates or NFTs, tau transgenic mice have better-than-normal LTP in the dentate gyrus and longer-lasting memory than nontransgenic littermates (Boekhoorn et al., 2006), suggesting a role of soluble tau in cognitive function.

33.2.4.3 Tau phosphorylation and other posttranslational modifications

Aberrant tau phosphorylation is a hallmark of AD and seems to be carried out by many of the kinases involved in learning and memory (see the section titled 'Kinases'). Fully 19% of the amino acids in tau are potential phosphorylation sites (Ser, Thr, and Tyr), and many are in fact phosphorylated in AD brains (Stoothoff and Johnson, 2005). The vast majority of the phosphorylation sites are highly conserved across species and surround tau's microtubule-binding domains (**Figure 7**). Much effort has been devoted to

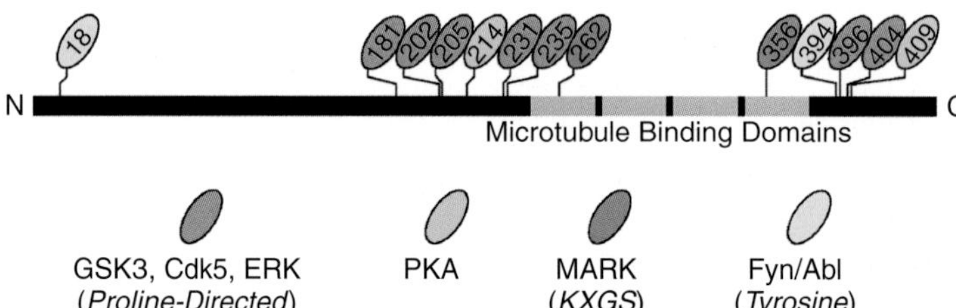

Figure 7 Tau phosphorylation sites. The four microtubule-binding domains are indicated by shading in a schematic line drawing of tau protein. Most tau phosphorylation sites surround the microtubule-binding regions.

sorting out which sites and kinases are most important in the pathogenesis of AD.

• Proline-directed kinase sites. Many tau phosphorylation sites are substrates for proline-directed kinases, which target Ser/Thr residues directly adjacent to a proline. These sites are substrates for glycogen synthase kinase 3 (GSK3), cyclin-dependent kinase 5 (Cdk5), and extracellular-signal regulated kinase (ERK), among others. Phosphorylation at these sites seems to be involved in the tau aggregation/cell death pathways mentioned above (Lucas et al., 2001; Augustinack et al., 2002; Cruz et al., 2003; Noble et al., 2003). For example, GSK3 stimulates tau aggregation (Sato et al., 2002), and GSK3 inhibition reduces tau aggregation and neurodegeneration (Noble et al., 2005).

• PKA sites. Tau is phosphorylated by cyclic AMP-dependent protein kinase (PKA), preferentially at Ser214 (Scott et al., 1993). Phosphorylation of Ser214 inhibits tau's microtubule binding and stabilizing activity (Illenberger et al., 1998). The PKA sites are near the proline-directed sites, and tau phosphorylation by PKA facilitates phosphorylation by proline-directed kinases (Singh et al., 1996; Liu et al., 2004) but may inhibit aggregation (Schneider et al., 1999).

• KXGS sites. The PKA and proline-directed sites are concentrated at both ends of the four microtubule-binding domains of tau. Within these domains are sites with a Lys-Xxx-Gly-Ser (KXGS) consensus sequence, most notably Ser262 and Ser356. These sites are phosphorylated by microtubule-affinity regulating kinase (MARK), which dramatically reduces tau's ability to stabilize microtubules (Drewes et al., 1997) and facilitates neurite outgrowth (Biernat et al., 2002). This phosphorylation may also be a prerequisite for phosphorylation at proline-directed kinase sites (Nishimura et al., 2004; but see Biernat and Mandelkow, 1999).

• Tyrosine phosphorylation. In AD brains, tau is also phosphorylated on tyrosine residues, primarily Tyr18 by Fyn and Tyr394 by Abl (Williamson et al., 2002; Lee et al., 2004; Derkinderen et al., 2005). There is considerable evidence for a role of Fyn in AD (Lambert et al., 1998; Chin et al., 2004, 2005; Lee et al., 2004), as reviewed further in the section titled 'Fyn.' Interestingly, interactions between tau and Fyn may contribute to the subcellular localization of Fyn and, thus, affect its substrate availability (Lee et al., 1998). In addition, disease-associated tau phosphorylation and mutations strongly increase Fyn binding (Bhaskar et al., 2005).

• Tau proteolysis. The carboxy terminus of tau can be cleaved by activated caspases, producing a truncated tau that aggregates more easily than full-length tau (Cotman et al., 2005). This may be an important step leading to development of tangles in AD, as tau cleavage at this site is a relatively early event in NFT formation (Rissman et al., 2004; Guillozet-Bongaarts et al., 2005). Tau is also cleaved by calpain, which produces a 17-kD tau fragment that is toxic to cultured neurons (Park and Ferreira, 2005).

33.2.4.4 Tau and Aβ

Given the prominence of Aβ and tau in AD pathology, their relationship is of considerable interest. Although expression of human Aβ does not induce NFTs in hAPP transgenic mice, it increases tangle formation in hAPP mice coexpressing mutant human tau; in contrast, expression of mutant human tau does not seem to worsen Aβ-dependent pathologies in hAPP mice (Lewis et al., 2001; Götz et al., 2001). In such multiple transgenic models, Aβ immunotherapy decreases tau pathology, further suggesting that Aβ acts upstream of tau (Oddo et al., 2004). Plausible mechanisms include Aβ-induced kinase activation and resulting tau phosphorylation (see the section titled 'Kinases'). In addition, caspase activation by Aβ may stimulate tau proteolysis that favors aggregation (Cotman et al., 2005).

Calpain-mediated tau proteolysis seems to play an important role in Aβ toxicity *in vitro*. Tau-deficient primary neurons are resistant to the rapid neurodegeneration induced by Aβ application, apparently because they lack calpain-induced tau fragments that are toxic to neurons in culture (Rapoport et al., 2002; Park and Ferreira, 2005). Reducing tau even by just 50% ameliorated Aβ-induced memory deficits in a mouse model of AD (Roberson et al., 2007). Interestingly, this effect did not seem to involve removal of a tau species with Aβ-induced posttranslational modifications. Rather, tau reduction prevented Aβ-induced epileptiform activity and compensatory inhibitory remodeling of hippocampal circuits (Palop et al., 2007; Roberson et al., 2007).

33.2.5 ApoE

ApoE is a multifunctional lipoprotein originally discovered for its role in intercellular transport and distribution of cholesterol throughout the body (Mahley, 1988). The brain is second only to the liver as a producer of apoE. In addition to mediating lipid transport within the central nervous system, apoE is involved in the response to neural injury and regulation of neurite outgrowth (Mahley and Rall, 2000).

Three main apoE isoforms are produced from different alleles ($\varepsilon2$, $\varepsilon3$, and $\varepsilon4$) of a single *APOE* gene on chromosome 19; apoE2 and apoE4 differ from each other and from the more frequent apoE3 by single amino acid substitutions, which have major effects on apoE structure and function (**Figure 8**) (Hatters et al., 2006; Mahley et al., 2006).

ApoE was implicated in AD by the near-simultaneous discoveries that it binds Aβ and colocalizes to amyloid plaques (Namba et al., 1991; Strittmatter et al., 1993) and that *APOE* genotype has dramatic effects on AD risk and onset (Corder et al., 1993). Individuals with one, and particularly those with two, $\varepsilon4$ alleles are much more likely to develop AD and have an earlier age of onset compared with $\varepsilon3$ carriers, while $\varepsilon2$ carriers are most resistant to the disease (**Figure 9**) (Corder et al., 1993). *APOE* $\varepsilon4$ appears to be the most important genetic risk factor for sporadic AD (Farrer et al., 1997; Raber et al., 2004; Bertram et al., 2007); 40–60% of all sporadic AD patients have at least one $\varepsilon4$ allele (Saunders et al., 1993).

These genetic studies established that apoE4 decreases the age at which AD becomes manifest. Interestingly, even in the absence of frank AD, individuals with apoE4 have abnormalities in cognitive performance and functional neuroimaging. In apoE4 carriers, the normal age-related decline in performance on episodic memory tasks occurs at an earlier age and progresses at a faster rate than in noncarriers, while other cognitive domains do not appear to be affected (Caselli et al., 1999, 2004). ApoE4 carriers are also more likely to develop cognitive deficits following open heart surgery or head injury (Tardiff et al., 1997; Teasdale et al., 1997). Even before cognitive impairment is detectable, apoE4 carriers have hypometabolism in the same regions affected in AD, including posterior parietal, posterior cingulate, and frontal cortex (Reiman et al.,

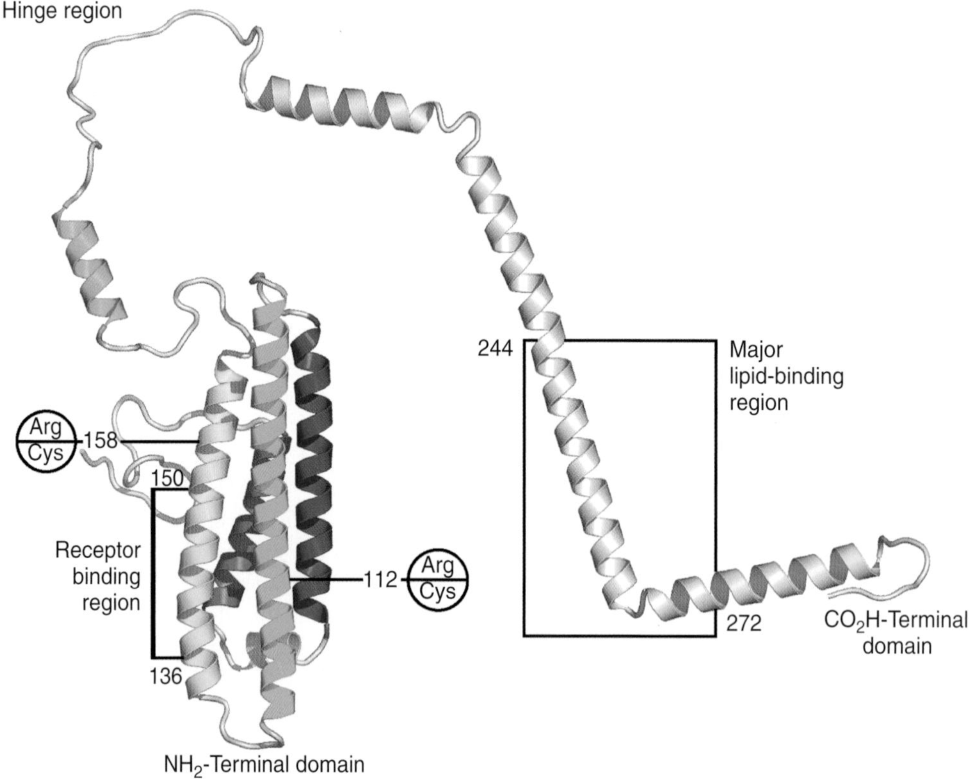

Figure 8 ApoE structure and isoforms. The apoE molecule consists of a globular amino-terminal domain that mediates receptor binding, while the lipid-binding region is in the carboxy-terminal domain. ApoE2 and apoE4 isoforms differ from the most common apoE3 by single amino acid substitutions. At amino acid positions 112 and 158, apoE3 contains Cys and Arg, whereas apoE2 contains Cys and Cys and apoE4 contains Arg and Arg. (From Hatters DM, Peters-Libeu CA, and Weisgraber KH [2006] Apolipoprotein E structure: Insights into function. *Trends Biochem. Sci.* 31: 445–454.)

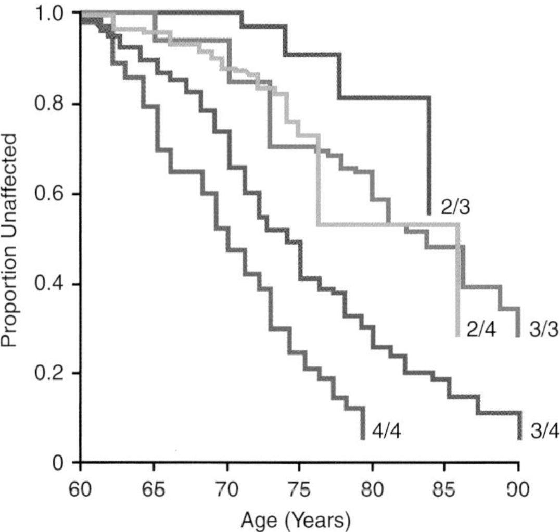

Figure 9 Effect of apoE genotype on AD risk. ApoE4 increases AD risk in a gene dose–dependent manner, while apoE2 lowers risk. (From Strittmatter WJ and Roses AD [1996] Apolipoprotein E and Alzheimer's disease. *Annu. Rev. Neurosci.* 19: 53–77.)

2004, 2005). These abnormalities are seen in apoE4 carriers as young as 20–39 years (Reiman et al., 2004).

33.2.5.1 Interactions between Aβ and apoE

ApoE4-related cognitive impairment is also seen in animal models, including mice expressing human apoE4 with or without hAPP/Aβ in neurons. ApoE3, but not apoE4, protects against hAPP/Aβ-induced cognitive deficits (Raber et al., 2000) and synaptic loss (Buttini et al., 2002). Remarkably, this effect is seen well before such mice form amyloid plaques. Consistent with these results, oligomeric Aβ impairs LTP more in slices from apoE4 knockin mice than apoE3 knockin mice (Trommer et al., 2005).

In addition, apoE has a prominent effect on Aβ aggregation and deposition. ApoE binds directly to Aβ and is a component of amyloid plaques (Namba et al., 1991; Strittmatter et al., 1993). ApoE4 is associated with increased deposition of amyloid plaques both in AD (Schmechel et al., 1993) and after head trauma (Nicoll et al., 1995). ApoE-deficient hAPP mice have almost no amyloid plaques (Bales et al., 1997). Compared with apoE3, apoE4 greatly increases amyloid plaque deposition in aged hAPP mice (Holtzman et al., 2000; Buttini et al., 2002). Given their effects on Aβ aggregation into fibrils and plaques, apoE isoforms may also have differential effects on Aβ aggregation into oligomers, although this has not yet been shown.

In addition to direct effects on Aβ aggregation, apoE4 increases Aβ production by stimulating endocytosis of APP-containing vesicles, which enter the endosomal pathway where much of Aβ is produced (Ye et al., 2005). ApoE also increases intracellular Aβ by enhancing its uptake from the extracellular space via the LDL receptor-related protein (LRP), although this effect is not isoform-dependent (Zerbinatti et al., 2006). Finally, once Aβ has been taken up into lysosomal vacuoles, apoE4 potentiates Aβ-induced lysosomal leakage and apoptosis (Ji et al., 2006).

33.2.5.2 Aβ-independent mechanisms for apoE4-induced neuronal impairments

Compared with apoE-deficient mice, female mice with neuronal expression of apoE4 develop age-dependent deficits in learning and memory even in the absence of Aβ (Raber et al., 1998, 2000), presumably because of apoE4-induced reductions in andogen receptor levels in the brain (see following). ApoE4 knockin mice also have LTP impairments not seen in apoE3 mice (Trommer et al., 2004). Neuronal expression of human apoE3, but not apoE4, protected mice lacking endogenous apoE against synaptodendritic damage elicited by excitotoxic drugs (Buttini et al., 1999). Notably, these excitoprotective effects of apoE3 were eliminated when apoE3 and apoE4 were coexpressed in the same mice, suggesting a dominant adverse effect of apoE4 (Buttini et al., 2000).

ApoE is also found in NFTs and has effects on tau (Namba et al., 1991). ApoE3 binds to tau, whereas apoE4 does not (Strittmatter et al., 1994). ε4 carriers have more NFTs than age-matched ε3 homozygotes (Ohm et al., 1999). ApoE4 also stimulates microtubule depolymerization (Nathan et al., 1995), possibly through effects on tau. Neuronal, but not astroglial, expression of apoE4 in transgenic mice increases tau phosphorylation (Tesseur et al., 2000). Neuronal expression of endogenous apoE occurs primarily after neuronal injury (Xu et al., 2006b). In neurons, apoE4 undergoes cleavage by a chymotrypsin-like protease activity, and E4 is more susceptible to cleavage than E3 (Huang et al., 2001). The resulting C-terminally truncated apoE stimulates tau phosphorylation and NFT formation (Huang et al., 2001; Brecht et al., 2004). Truncated apoE can escape the secretory pathway and enter the cytosol, where it binds to mitochondria and impairs their function (Mahley et al., 2006).

ApoE also has cerebrovascular effects that may contribute to memory dysfunction. ApoE4 carriers have higher plasma cholesterol levels (Hallman et al., 1991) and are at higher risk of carotid atherosclerosis (Terry et al., 1996), coronary artery disease (Chen et al., 2003), and ischemic stroke (McCarron et al., 1999). The overlap between these cerebrovascular risks and AD is becoming increasingly clear (Martins et al., 2006).

There are interesting gender differences in the effects of apoE that point toward important interactions with sex hormones. Among $\varepsilon 4$ carriers, women are more likely to develop AD than men (Payami et al., 1996), and female apoE4 mice are more susceptible to memory deficits than their male counterparts (Raber et al., 1998, 2000; Grootendorst et al., 2005). This difference may be the result of effects of apoE4 on androgen receptors. ApoE4 decreases androgen receptor levels in males and females, and females may be more susceptible to this effect because of their lower circulating androgen levels (Raber et al., 2002; Raber, 2004).

Last, apoE4 is intrinsically less stable than apoE3 (Morrow et al., 2002). As a result, brain apoE levels are lower in individuals with the $\varepsilon 4$ allele, an isoform difference that has also been identified in apoE4 and apoE3 knockin mice (Gregg et al., 1986; Ramaswamy et al., 2005). Thus, in addition to the adverse gain-of-function effects described above, apoE4 may contribute to neurological impairments by a loss-of-function mechanism. Consistent with this notion, ApoE-deficient mice display age-dependent synaptic loss, deficient regenerative axonal sprouting after perforant pathway transection, and greater susceptibility to diverse neural injuries (Masliah et al., 1995a, b; Buttini et al., 1999, 2000; Krzywkowski et al., 1999).

33.2.6 α-Synuclein

α-Synuclein is a small, cytosolic protein that is enriched in presynaptic terminals; it regulates presynaptic function and neurotransmitter release (Chandra et al., 2004; Fortin et al., 2005). It is also the main component of Lewy bodies, neuronal inclusions associated with most forms of Parkinson's disease (PD) and other Lewy body diseases (Spillantini et al., 1997). Mutations in α-synuclein are linked to rare forms of autosomal dominant PD (Polymeropoulos et al., 1997). α-Synuclein also seems to play a role in the intriguing clinical and neuropathological overlap between PD and AD. Many AD patients have Lewy bodies, sometimes known as the Lewy body variant of AD, and many PD patients develop AD-like dementia (Perl et al., 1998), emphasizing the fact that AD is a polyproteinopathy combining the accumulation of abnormal assemblies or fragments of Aβ, tau, apoE, and α-synuclein.

The initial link between α-synuclein and dementia was established through the discovery of a so-called 'nonamyloid component' (NAC) of plaques in AD brains, which turned out to be a fragment of α-synuclein (Uéda et al., 1993; Iwai et al., 1995). α-Synuclein promotes Aβ aggregation *in vitro* (Yoshimoto et al., 1995), although it doesn't seem to increase amyloid plaque deposition *in vivo* (Masliah et al., 2001b). α-Synuclein does, however, worsen Aβ-induced neuronal deficits independently of plaques. Doubly transgenic mice expressing hAPP/Aβ and wild-type human α-synuclein in neurons displayed more synapse loss, greater reductions in choline acetyltransferase-positive neurons, and more severe cognitive impairments than the singly transgenic parental strains, even though α-synuclein had no effect on plaque formation *in vivo* (Masliah et al., 2001b). This study also revealed that Aβ strongly promotes α-synuclein aggregation, both *in vitro* and *in vivo*. α-Synuclein concentrations are elevated in synaptic boutons in AD brains, suggesting that α-synuclein also plays a role in synaptic pathology in the human condition (Masliah et al., 1996). Whether the underlying mechanisms relate to α-synuclein's normal functions or to its abnormal aggregation remains to be determined.

33.3 Memory-Related Molecules in AD

Although some of the major players in the pathobiochemistry of AD have been identified, it is just now beginning to be understood how these molecules affect neuronal function and impair learning and memory. Mouse models of AD recapitulate many aspects of the human disease, both in terms of pathology and in relation to behavioral/memory impairments. Indeed, transgenic mouse models have provided a unique opportunity for synergy between two historically separate fields of biomedical research – AD research and the basic scientific analysis of learning and memory. As reviewed below, research in the last 15 years has revealed that AD-relevant molecules such as Aβ, tau, and apoE affect several aspects of neuronal function and cellular mechanisms of plasticity that have been implicated in the formation of long-lasting memories.

33.3.1 Neurotransmitter Release

Reliable neurotransmission requires a steady supply of synaptic vesicles filled with neurotransmitter to be ready for release at the presynaptic terminal. Since trafficking of new synaptic vesicles from the cell body can take several hours, nerve terminals are equipped with a special machinery that allows for local recycling and refilling of synaptic vesicles, a process that replenishes vesicle pools within seconds to minutes (Südhof, 2004; Fernandez-Alfonso and Ryan, 2006; Kavalali, 2006; Ryan, 2006). The number of recycling vesicles and the efficiency with which they fuse with (exocytosis) and are retrieved from (endocytosis) the presynaptic terminal plasma membrane set the boundaries on the duration and frequency of neurotransmission, particularly during repetitive stimulation. Thus, factors that affect vesicle cycling, particularly steps that are rate limiting, can have profound consequences on synaptic efficacy.

The fusion of synaptic vesicles with the presynaptic membrane and their recovery through endocytosis require a number of neuron-specific proteins. The levels of many proteins that coordinate the docking and fusion of synaptic vesicles are decreased in AD as well as in experimental models (Honer, 2003; Scheff and Price, 2003). Synaptophysin, one of the most abundant membrane proteins on synaptic vesicles, is integral to the vesicle fusion process for neurotransmitter release. Decreases in synaptophysin have been used extensively as a measure of synaptic impairments in both AD and transgenic mouse models of the disease (Masliah et al., 1993; Mucke et al., 2000; Honer, 2003; Scheff and Price, 2003). Decreased levels of proteins involved in vesicle release, such as synaptophysin, may represent decreased expression at intact synapses, synaptic degeneration, or both.

In addition, several proteins involved in the local endocytosis and recycling of vesicles, including synaptotagmin, AP2, AP180, and dynamin I, are altered in AD and in some mouse models of the disease, as illustrated in **Figure 10** (Honer, 2003; Yao, 2004; Nixon, 2005). Animal models in which any of these proteins are mutated or ablated exhibit abnormal synaptic vesicle size and number, synaptic transmission deficits, and even mortality in extreme cases (reviewed in Yao, 2004; Kavalali, 2006). For some factors, both protein and mRNA levels are decreased in AD, suggesting that the expression of the corresponding genes may be dysregulated. Other factors may be depleted by increased cleavage and degradation (Yao, 2004; Kelly et al., 2005; Kelly and Ferreira, 2006; but see Yao et al., 2005). Impaired vesicle recycling may also contribute to some of the

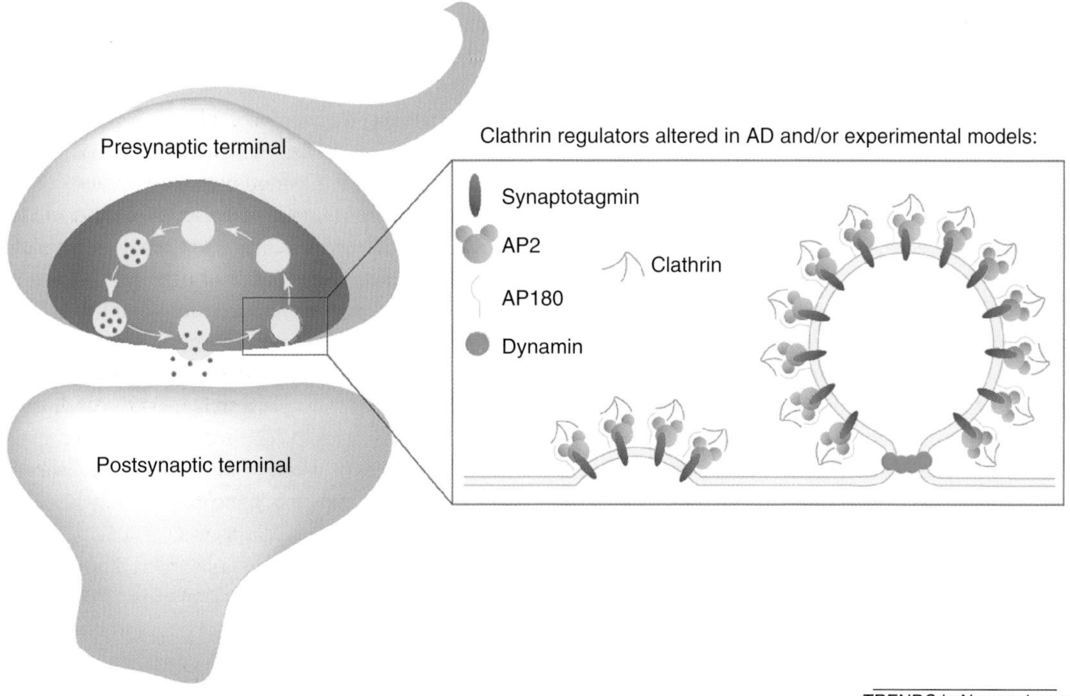

Figure 10 Alzheimer's disease (AD) affects clathrin-mediated synaptic vesicle recycling in synapses. Synaptic vesicles are recycled through clathrin-mediated endocytosis, which requires clathrin and regulatory proteins. The levels of several key regulators (see red box) of this process are decreased in AD as well as in experimental models of the disease. (From Yao P [2004] Synaptic frailty and clathrin-mediated synaptic vesicle trafficking in Alzheimer's disease. *Trends Neurosci.* 27: 24–29.)

ultrastructural changes found in AD brains and related mouse models. Decreases in synaptic density, attributed to synapse loss, are accompanied by an increase in size of the remaining synapses (reviewed in Scheff and Price, 2003). Although it has been hypothesized that such increases represent compensatory changes to maintain overall synaptic contact area, it has also been proposed that impaired endocytosis for local generation of vesicles leads to an overall accumulation of membrane and enlargement of nerve terminals (Yao, 2004).

In summary, alterations in levels of key components in synaptic vesicle trafficking may contribute to deficits in neurotransmitter release in AD.

33.3.2 Receptors and Channels

A large number of cell surface receptors and channels are located on the postsynaptic membrane, ready to receive and transduce input from presynaptic contacts. The strength of any given synapse can remain stable over time, increase, or decrease based on the number, localization, and activity of the neurotransmitter receptors and ion channels at the postsynaptic membrane. In this section, we review several receptors and channels that play important roles in synaptic plasticity and describe how alterations in their levels, localization, or function may contribute to AD-related cognitive dysfunction.

33.3.2.1 NMDA receptors

N-methyl-D-aspartate (NMDA) receptors play a critical role in the induction of LTP by acting as coincidence detectors of presynaptic glutamate release and postsynaptic depolarization (reviewed in Wang et al., 2006). Subsequent influx of calcium through the NMDA receptor triggers a series of intracellular signaling events that culminate in the induction of gene expression required for long-term changes in synaptic efficacy.

Currently approved therapies for the treatment of AD include an NMDA receptor antagonist, which is thought to protect neurons against increased calcium permeability of NMDA receptors and to increase the synaptic signal-to-noise ratio (Tariot and Federoff, 2003; Jacobsen et al., 2005). Studies in transgenic mouse models of AD and cell culture experiments are beginning to unravel the mechanisms by which AD-relevant molecules such as Aβ might alter NMDA receptor functions and impact synaptic plasticity.

As reviewed in the section titled 'Soluble Aβ oligomers,' many studies have reported that Aβ potently inhibits the induction of LTP both *in vitro* and *in vivo* (reviewed in Walsh and Selkoe, 2004). Although it is uncertain whether Aβ directly binds NMDA receptors, several lines of evidence demonstrate that at least part of Aβ's effect on LTP may be a result of alterations in the level, availability, or activity of NMDA receptors at the postsynaptic membrane.

In vitro, low concentrations of synthetic Aβ peptides acutely augment NMDA receptor–mediated calcium influx and synaptic transmission (Wu et al., 1995; Wu and Dun, 1995; Kelly and Ferreira, 2006). Furthermore, Aβ-dependent degradation of dynamin and the scaffolding protein PSD-95 can be blocked by NMDA receptor antagonists (Almeida et al., 2005; Roselli et al., 2005; Kelly and Ferreira, 2006). However, Aβ produces a delayed NMDA receptor–dependent reduction in synaptic transmission (Cullen et al., 1996). Because prolonged NMDA receptor stimulation leads to down-regulation of receptor activity through the recruitment of negative feedback loops (Oster and Schramm, 1993; Resink et al., 1995; Salter and Kalia, 2004; Braithwaite et al., 2006), it is possible that acute, Aβ facilitates glutamatergic transmission and sensitizes neurons to excitotoxic events (Mattson et al., 1993), whereas chronically, it leads to a down-regulation of NMDA receptor activity.

In vivo, hAPP transgenic mice that produce high Aβ levels have decreased levels of phosphorylation of Tyr-1472 of NR2B subunits of the NMDA receptor, particularly in the dentate gyrus (Palop et al., 2005). Phosphorylation at this residue affects the gating of the channel and is positively correlated with NMDA receptor currents (Lu et al., 1999; Alvestad et al., 2003; reviewed in Salter and Kalia, 2004), suggesting that the decreased phosphorylation found in hAPP mice may contribute to an attenuation of NMDA receptor-dependent signaling. Importantly, decreased levels of Tyr-1472 phosphorylation were associated with decreased activity of Fyn, a src-kinase family member that phosphorylates NR2B subunits at this residue, and increased expression of striatal-enriched phosphatase (STEP), a tyrosine phosphatase that negatively regulates Fyn activity (Chin et al., 2005). STEP can dampen NMDA receptor-dependent activity when engaged by high levels of stimulation (Pelkey et al., 2002; Braithwaite et al., 2006). The regulation of tyrosine kinases, such as Fyn, by Aβ is discussed in more detail in the section titled 'Kinases.'

Phosphorylation at Tyr-1472 also regulates the interaction of NMDA receptors with the scaffolding protein PSD-95 and with AP-2, an adaptor molecule that triggers clathrin-mediated endocytosis (Lavezzari et al., 2003). *In vitro* experiments demonstrate that Aβ-dependent dephosphorylation of Tyr-1472 induces endocytosis of NMDA receptors, resulting in decreased surface expression of this key regulator of LTP induction (Snyder et al., 2005). The results of this study suggested a model in which extracellular Aβ binds α7 subunit-containing nicotinic acetylcholine receptors and thereby activates the phosphatases PP2B (calcineurin) and STEP, resulting in dephosphorylation of NR2B (**Figure 11**). Thus, Aβ may impair synaptic plasticity by inducing the dephosphorylation of Tyr-1472 and attenuating NMDA receptor activity through a variety of mechanisms.

The attenuation of glutamatergic transmission by Aβ may have different consequences depending on the brain region affected. If brain regions that control neuronal excitability on a global scale are particularly susceptible to Aβ-induced impairments of glutamatergic transmission, aberrant increases in overall brain activity may result. Such a notion is supported by findings that hAPP mice with high levels of Aβ exhibit nonconvulsive seizure activity in EEG recordings, which was associated with the induction of compensatory inhibitory mechanisms and impairments in synaptic plasticity (Palop et al., 2007).

33.3.2.2 AMPA receptors

α-amino-3-hydroxy-5-methyl-4-isoxazole-proprionic acid (AMPA) receptors are glutamate-gated channels that mediate most of the fast excitatory synaptic transmission in the brain and provide the primary means of postsynaptic depolarization in glutamatergic neurotransmission. AMPA receptor localization is dynamically regulated by neuronal activity, and rapid insertion and removal of these receptors into/from the postsynaptic membrane are key mechanisms by which long-term changes in

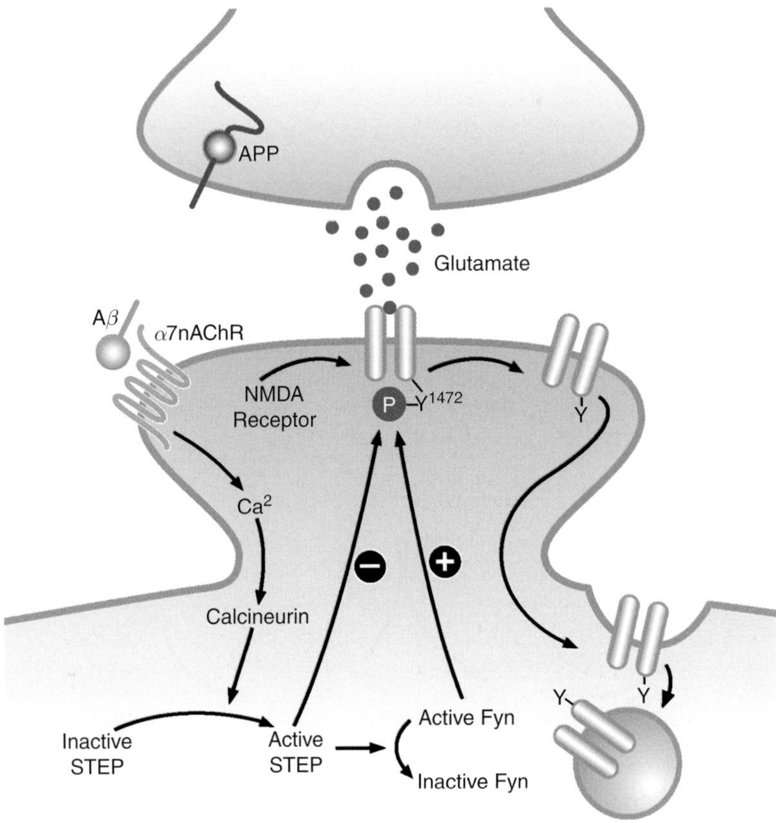

Figure 11 Aβ attenuates *N*-methyl-D-aspartate (NMDA) receptor signaling. Under normal circumstances, phosphorylation of the NMDA receptor at Tyr1472 is controlled by a balance between phosphorylation by Fyn and dephosphorylation by STEP. STEP also negatively regulates Fyn. In models of AD, Aβ activates α7 nAChRs and increases STEP activity, resulting in a net decrease in Fyn activity and Tyr1472 phosphorylation. In the absence of Fyn-mediated tyrosine phosphorylation, NMDA receptors are endocytosed.

synaptic strength (LTP and LTD) are expressed (Bredt and Nicoll, 2003; Esteban, 2003).

Such dynamic regulation of AMPA receptor density at the synapse requires that a pool of receptors be available for use at any given time. Indeed, recycling endosomes in dendritic compartments maintain a pool of AMPA receptors that can be rapidly mobilized and shuttled to the synaptic membrane in response to NMDA receptor activation to effect increases in synaptic strength (**Figure 12**) (Park et al., 2004; reviewed in Kennedy and Ehlers, 2006), whereas LTD-inducing stimuli result in endocytosis and removal of AMPA receptors from the synapse (Bredt and Nicoll, 2003).

In addition to their role in rapidly modifying synaptic strength, AMPA receptors play a critical role in another, slower form of plasticity called synaptic scaling (reviewed in Turrigiano and Nelson, 2004). In this type of homeostatic plasticity, the overall synaptic strength of a neuron is modulated to regulate its excitability depending on its history of activity. Periods of reduced activity result in increased levels of AMPA receptors at the synapse, whereas periods of increased activity lead to removal of AMPA receptors from the synapse. Moreover, regulation of AMPA receptor density at the postsynaptic membrane partly underlies distance-dependent scaling, in which synapses that lie farther from the soma are endowed with increased synaptic strength so they can transmit information with similar fidelity as synapses located closer to the soma (Andrasfalvy and Magee, 2001; Smith et al., 2003).

Several factors contribute to the ability of AMPA receptors to fulfill these critical roles in dictating synaptic strength and homeostatic control of neuronal activity, including expression levels, dendritic transport, and local synaptic trafficking within the endosomal pathway. Thus, impairments in any one of these processes may lead to deficits in synaptic plasticity and in the regulation of activity levels.

It is particularly interesting in this regard that reductions in several AMPA receptor subunits have been documented in the entorhinal cortex and hippocampus in AD and related transgenic mouse models (Yasuda et al., 1995; Chan et al., 1999; Wakabayashi et al., 1999; Carter et al., 2004; Chang et al., 2006; Palop et al., 2007). In AD, AMPA receptors also appear to be cleaved by caspases (Chan et al., 1999). In primary neurons or slices treated with Aβ or isolated from hAPP transgenic mice, surface expression of AMPA

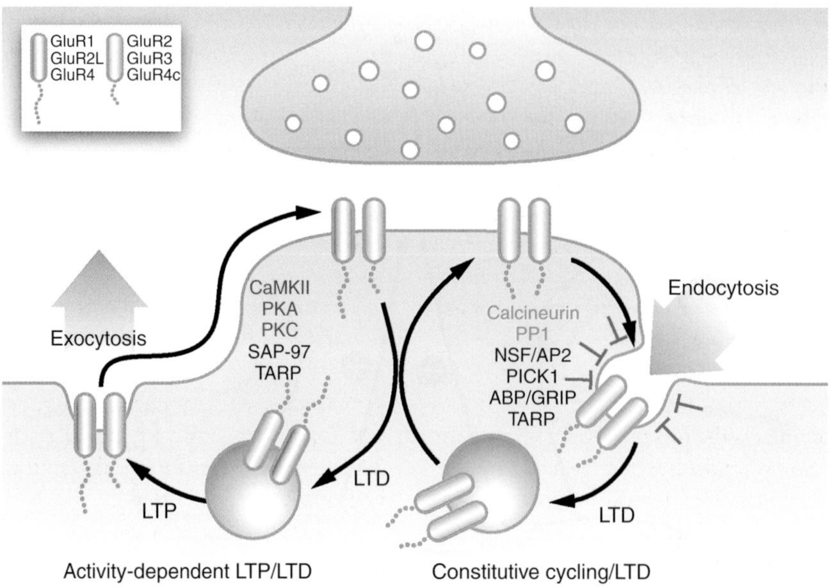

Figure 12 α-Amino-3-hydroxy-5-methyl-4-isoxazole-proprionic acid (AMPA) receptor trafficking. The trafficking of AMPA receptors between the synaptic membrane and recycling endosomes regulates synaptic strength. The insertion of AMPA receptors into the synapse (in long-term potentiation [LTP]) and the endocytosis of synaptic AMPA receptors (in long-term depression [LTD]) are governed by the activities of several kinases, phosphatases, and binding proteins. In Alzheimer's disease or related models, the activities of several kinases are decreased (red font), whereas the activities of several phosphatases are increased (green font), which may contribute to overall decreases in synaptic strength.

receptors is decreased (Almeida et al., 2005; Roselli et al., 2005; Hsieh et al., 2006). Such alterations may contribute to the decreased AMPA-mediated currents and increased NMDA/AMPA current ratios found in several *in vitro* and transgenic mouse models of AD (Hsia et al., 1999; Chang et al., 2006; Shemer et al., 2006).

Since AMPA receptors play such key roles in synaptic and homeostatic plasticity, alterations in their expression or trafficking may contribute to deficits in synaptic plasticity and learning and memory in AD and related models. As reviewed in the next section, it has been hypothesized that increased cholinergic activity in early stages of AD may be recruited to support synaptic scaling, perhaps in response to the loss of normal mechanisms underlying this homeostatic plasticity (Small, 2004).

33.3.2.3 Nicotinic acetylcholine receptors

Neuronal nicotinic acetylcholine receptors (nA ChRs) are key modulators of neurotransmission. Presynaptically localized receptors enhance neurotransmitter release, postsynaptic receptors transduce fast excitatory transmission and calcium-regulated signaling, and perisynaptic or nonsynaptic receptors modulate neuronal excitability (Dani and Bertrand, 2006).

Although cholinergic activity is increased in early stages of AD, the loss of cholinergic neurons, particularly in the basal forebrain, is a characteristic neuropathological feature of AD that is thought to contribute to cognitive decline (Auld et al., 2002). The levels of acetylcholine receptors in AD brains, particularly the primarily presynaptically localized α7 subunit–containing nAChRs, are also decreased in postmortem tissues and by *in situ* imaging of receptor binding in live patients (Burghaus et al., 2000; Guan et al., 2000; reviewed in Auld et al., 2002; and Oddo and LaFerla, 2006). It is unclear whether this decrease simply reflects the loss of neurons expressing the receptors. Some studies report that α7nAChR mRNA levels are increased in the hippocampus of AD patients (Hellstrom-Lindahl et al., 1999; but see Mousavi et al., 2003), suggesting that decreases in protein levels and receptor binding may indeed reflect synaptic loss or neuronal degeneration. The use of acetylcholinesterase inhibitors to boost cholinergic signaling has long been a standard treatment for mild to moderate AD (reviewed in Jacobsen et al., 2005; Roberson and Mucke, 2006), but these regimens do not appear to provide long-lasting benefits.

A number of studies have shed light on how Aβ peptides may alter cholinergic signaling in AD. *In vitro* evidence demonstrated that Aβ binds α7nAChRs with high affinity, although experimental conditions and cell types can determine whether Aβ inhibits or stimulates the receptor (Wang et al., 2000; Liu et al., 2001a; Dineley et al., 2001, 2002; Pettit et al., 2001). Aβ-induced stimulation of α7nAChRs can appear to block receptor function but may simply occlude the effect of other ligands such as nicotine by potently stimulating the receptor and inducing calcium influx (Dougherty et al., 2003). Unlike the majority of membrane-bound receptors, nAChR expression is increased upon receptor stimulation (Fenster et al., 1999), which may account for several reports that Aβ increases α7nAChR levels *in vitro* and in hAPP transgenic mice (Dineley et al., 2001; Chin et al., 2005; Snyder et al., 2005).

Moreover, α7nAChRs can be targeted to somatodendritic compartments and have been found in perisynaptic regions on postsynaptic membranes, where they are in a strategic position to modulate intracellular signaling processes through their high calcium permeability (Fabian-Fine et al., 2001; Xu et al., 2006a). In primary cortical neurons, Aβ activates the calcium-dependent phosphatase PP2B (calcineurin) by engaging postsynaptic α7nAChRs (Snyder et al., 2005). One consequence of this activation is activation of the phosphatase STEP and subsequent dephosphorylation of the Tyr-1472 of the NR2B subunit of the NMDA receptor, either through direct dephosphorylation by STEP or through STEP-mediated desphosphorylation and inactivation of tyrosine kinases such as Fyn that are known to phosphorylate the NMDA receptor at this residue (see **Figure 11**).

These *in vitro* findings are in line with observations in hAPP mice, in which increased levels of α7nAChRs are concomitant with increased STEP levels, Fyn suppression, and decreased phosphorylation of Tyr-1472 of NR2B subunits (Chin et al., 2005; Palop et al., 2005). It remains to be determined whether the engagement of α7nAChRs by Aβ in AD and in experimental models of the disease represent primary pathogenic mechanisms or compensatory mechanisms to boost synaptic scaling (Small, 2004; Geerts and Grossberg, 2006) or combat excitotoxicity (Palop et al., 2007).

33.3.2.4 Potassium channels

The activities of potassium (K^+) channels, which efflux K^+ and hyperpolarize cells, play an important role in neuronal survival, because they govern membrane excitability and because the intracellular potassium level is a determinant of apoptosis (Yu, 2003). New discoveries have highlighted how diverse K^+ channels in neuronal dendrites fine-tune excitability and affect neuronal information processing by regulating the induction of NMDA receptor–dependent synaptic plasticity in the hippocampus (reviewed in Yuan and Chen, 2006).

Phosphorylation-dependent modulation of K^+ channel activity, particularly of the Kv4.x family, is a major means by which synaptic plasticity is regulated and dendritic information processing is achieved (reviewed in Birnbaum et al., 2004; Yuan and Chen, 2006). Based on the kinetics of time-dependent inactivation, K^+ currents can be separated into different components. One such component, the fast-inactivating A-type K^+ current, plays a particularly important role in regulating membrane excitability, because it responds quickly to subthreshold depolarization and its activation delays the generation of action potentials (**Figure 13**). Inhibition of this current by pharmacological agents that block ion flux or stimulate phosphorylation of the channel markedly increases intracellular calcium (Hoffman et al., 1997; reviewed in Yuan and Chen, 2006).

Interestingly, Aβ inhibits A-type K^+ currents in primary hippocampal and neocortical neurons, increasing dendritic calcium influx and neuronal excitability (Good et al., 1996; Ye et al., 2003; Chen, 2005). This process may contribute to the observation that nonfibrillar Aβ assemblies increase neuronal excitability in various *in vitro* models (Hartley et al., 1999; Jhamandas et al., 2001; Turner et al., 2003; Ye et al., 2004; but see Yun et al., 2006). Aβ may inhibit K^+ currents through the aberrant engagement of tyrosine kinases, as tyrosine kinase inhibitors abrogated the ability of Aβ to increase excitability of cholinergic neurons (Jhamandas et al., 2001). Aβ treatment also induces K^+ channel abnormalities in cultured fibroblasts that are similar to K^+ channel abnormalities detected in fibroblasts isolated from AD patients (Etcheberrigaray et al., 1993, 1994). While regulated increases in intracellular calcium are important for synaptic plasticity, sustained increases in intracellular calcium through Aβ's effect on K^+ channels could impair synaptic plasticity and sensitize neurons to excitotoxic injuries (Xie, 2004).

Although A-type K^+ channel currents are generally inhibited by Aβ, the expression levels of K^+ channel subunits that contribute to the A-type current are increased in early stages of AD and in primary cerebellar neurons after treatment with Aβ (Angulo et al., 2004; Plant et al., 2006). Such increases in subunit expression may represent compensatory mechanisms aimed at restoring membrane excitability.

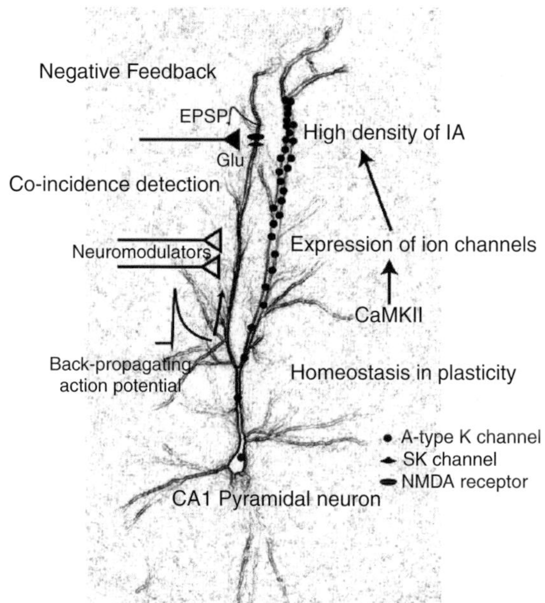

Figure 13 Dendritic K^+ channels influence neuronal information processing. SK and Kv4.2-encoded A-type K^+ channels are expressed at high levels in dendrites. Propagation of back-propagating action potentials and release of glutamate and neuromodulators within an appropriate time window ensures *N*-methyl-D-aspartate (NMDA) receptor activation through three coinciding events (as depicted in left dendrite above). Regulation of K^+ channel expression is also a homeostatic mechanism regulated by CaMKII. Activation of CaMKII promotes expression of both α-amino-3-hydroxy-5-methyl-4-isoxazole-propionic acid receptors and A-type K^+ channels, resulting in antagonizing effects on neuronal responsiveness. Alzheimer's disease–related decreases in the activity of A-type K^+ channels increase neuronal excitability and intracellular calcium and may contribute to excitotoxicity. (From Yuan L and Chen X [2006] Diversity of potassium channels in neuronal dendrites. *Prog. Neurobiol.* 78: 374–389.)

33.3.3 Calcium Signaling

Downstream of cell surface receptors and ion channels at the postsynaptic membrane, a myriad of intracellular signaling molecules await instruction. Depending on the dynamics of receptor/channel activity, local Ca^{2+} plumes of various magnitudes are generated to direct the kinase cascades and other signaling pathways that transduce signals to the nucleus or other subcellular compartments. In this section, we discuss several aspects of calcium homeostasis that impact the dynamics of postsynaptic signaling and describe kinase pathways that play key roles in the induction and maintenance of long-term changes in synaptic efficacy. Special emphasis is placed on those aspects that are altered in AD and related models and on how their dysregulation contributes to plasticity deficits. Finally, we review the mechanisms by which extracellular, neuromodulatory factors such as brain-derived neurotrophic factor (BDNF) and Reelin influence synaptic plasticity and how AD-related alterations in these factors exacerbate impairments in synaptic function.

Calcium (Ca^{2+}) plays fundamental roles in synaptic plasticity and neuronal survival. Calcium signals, either from the extracellular milieu or from intracellular stores, must be precisely regulated both temporally and spatially to achieve tight control over intracellular signaling pathways that transduce signals from extracellular sources (Yuste et al., 2000; Berridge et al., 2003). Disruptions in neuronal Ca^{2+} homeostasis and calcium-regulated signaling likely play important roles in normal aging and AD, impairing synaptic plasticity and cognitive function, and contributing to neuronal loss in vulnerable regions (Mattson and Chan, 2003; Xie, 2004; Smith et al., 2005a; Kelly et al., 2006). Acute treatment of primary neurons and cell lines of neuronal origin with Aβ induces rapid, transient increases in intracellular calcium levels, whereas chronic exposure to Aβ leads to slower, more progressive increases in resting calcium levels (Xie, 2004; Kelly and Ferreira, 2006). Aβ peptides, particularly oligomeric assemblies, have been suggested to insert into neuronal cell membranes and form calcium-fluxing pores (reviewed in Pollard et al., 1995; Glabe and Kayed, 2006). Alternatively, such assemblies may increase intracellular calcium levels by increasing influx through calcium channels, releasing calcium from intracellular stores, or modulating intracellular calcium dynamics through alterations in endogenous calcium binding proteins (**Figure 14**).

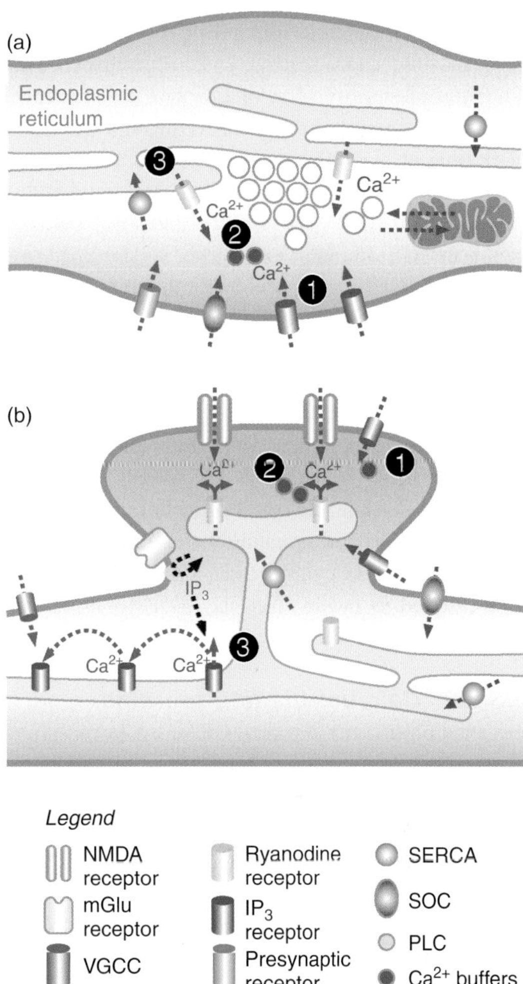

Figure 14 Ca^{2+} dysregulation in AD. Intracellular Ca^{2+} levels in the presynaptic terminal (top) and postsynaptic spine (bottom) are regulated by the influx of Ca^{2+} through Ca^{2+} channels (1), the buffering of free Ca^{2+} by Ca^{2+}-binding proteins (2), and the release of Ca^{2+} from intracellular Ca^{2+} stores (3). AD-related alterations in the levels and/or activities of Ca^{2+} channels, receptors, and Ca^{2+}-binding proteins perturb calcium homeostasis and may contribute to deficits in synaptic plasticity as well as increase susceptibility to excitotoxicity. (Modified from Bardo S, Cavazzini MG, and Emptage N [2006] The role of the endoplasmic reticulum Ca^{2+} store in the plasticity of central neurons. *Trends Pharmacol. Sci.* 27: 78–84).

33.3.3.1 Calcium channels

Ca^{2+} channels play diverse roles in synaptic transmission, on both the presynaptic and the postsynaptic side (Augustine et al., 2003). Presynaptic N- and P/Q-type voltage-sensitive Ca^{2+} channels are primarily involved in triggering synaptic vesicle exocytosis, whereas postsynaptic L-type voltage-sensitive Ca^{2+} channels contribute to the integration of synaptic activity and the transduction of signals that trigger a transcriptional response. Synaptic activity induces Ca^{2+} entry through NMDA receptors and L-type channels. The magnitude and temporal dynamics of the combined calcium influx determine which signaling pathways become engaged (Bradley and Finkbeiner, 2002; Deisseroth et al., 2003; Thiagarajan et al., 2006).

Aβ potentiates currents through L-type voltage-sensitive Ca^{2+} channels in primary neurons (Brorson et al., 1995; Ueda et al., 1997; Ekinci et al., 1999; Fu et al., 2006). Although the underlying mechanisms have not been fully characterized, one possibility is Aβ-stimulated phosphorylation of L-type Ca^{2+} channels, which would increase conductance through the channel (Ekinci et al., 1999). In addition, because L-type Ca^{2+} channels are voltage sensitive, Aβ could indirectly modulate Ca^{2+} currents by blocking voltage-gated potassium channels (see earlier section), altering neuronal excitability and prolonging membrane depolarization (Good et al., 1996; Birnbaum et al., 2004). Finally, Aβ exposure leads to increased expression of particular L-type Ca^{2+} channel subunits on surface membranes in neuronal cell lines (Scragg et al., 2005; Chiou, 2006), which may contribute to long-term changes in Ca^{2+} homeostasis. Because Ca^{2+} influx through L-type channels could contribute to deranged Ca^{2+} homeostasis and signaling, L-type Ca^{2+} channel blockers are now in clinical trials for the treatment of AD (reviewed in Jacobsen et al., 2005; Roberson and Mucke, 2006).

33.3.3.2 Calcium-binding proteins

The level of intracellular free Ca^{2+} is governed by a balance between the entry of Ca^{2+} into the cytoplasm, either from extracellular sources or from intracellular stores, and the removal of Ca^{2+} by buffers, pumps, and exchangers (reviewed in Berridge et al., 2003). Many cell types contain particular calcium-binding proteins that act as buffers by rapidly binding and sequestering free Ca^{2+}. The primary cytosolic calcium-buffering proteins include calbindin-D_{28K}, calretinin, and parvalbumin, which are differentially expressed in various populations of neurons and play important regulatory roles in the maintenance of Ca^{2+} homeostasis (Hof et al., 1999). Parvalbumin is expressed in interneurons that modulate local circuitry in the neocortex and hippocampus, whereas calbindin and calretinin are expressed by both interneurons and pyramidal cells in the neocortex and hippocampus. Since disruption of neuronal Ca^{2+} homeostasis appears to contribute to AD pathogenesis, the levels and distribution of these types of calcium buffers in various areas of the AD brain and AD models have been the focus of a rapidly increasing number of studies.

Neuronal populations that express the calcium buffers calretinin and parvalbumin appear to be relatively preserved in AD (Hof et al., 1993; Fonseca and Soriano, 1995; Sampson et al., 1997). Losses of parvalbumin-expressing neurons have been documented in the entorhinal cortex and hippocampus of AD brains, but this loss appears to occur at late stages of the disease and may be secondary to degeneration of principal neurons in the same region (Solodkin et al., 1996; Brady and Mufson, 1997; Mikkonen et al., 1999). Such findings supported the hypothesis that neurons containing high levels of calcium-buffering proteins, and presumably a high calcium-buffering capacity, are relatively resistant to AD-related neurotoxicity (Hof et al., 1993). Late-stage loss of calcium-binding proteins was related to loss of neurons producing these proteins (Solodkin et al., 1996).

The calcium-binding protein calbindin is expressed in local circuit interneurons and pyramidal cells of the neocortex. In addition, it is very highly expressed in granule cells of the dentate gyrus and in Purkinje cells of the cerebellum (Celio, 1990). Calbindin regulates intracellular Ca^{2+} levels and is important for synaptic plasticity and learning and memory (Molinari et al., 1996). Calbindin levels in dentate granule cells are depleted in hAPP mice with high hippocampal levels of Aβ, and the magnitude of this depletion correlates tightly with cognitive deficits (Palop et al., 2003). Transgenic mice expressing the carboxy terminus of hAPP also exhibit depletions of calbindin in the dentate gyrus (Lee et al., 2006). Similar calbindin depletions occur in the dentate gyrus of AD patients, in whom the greatest depletions were seen in individuals with the most severe dementia (Palop et al., 2003). Moreover, calbindin mRNA levels in the hippocampus are also reduced in AD and in hAPP mice, supporting the hypothesis that calbindin depletions result from decreased expression of the calbindin gene rather than from loss of dentate granule cells (Iacopino and Christakos, 1990; Sutherland et al., 1993; Palop et al., 2003).

Similar calbindin depletions in the dentate gyrus have been observed after chronic neuronal overexcitation, for example, in human temporal lobe epilepsy, $GABA_B$ receptor-deficient mice, and models of kindling or kainate-induced chronic excitotoxicity (Tonder et al., 1994; Magloczky et al., 1997; Nägerl et al., 2000; Ruttimann et al., 2004; Palop et al., 2007). Calbindin reductions in the dentate gyrus of hAPP mice and in AD brains may also result from an imbalance between excitatory and inhibitory inputs (Palop et al., 2003, 2006, 2007). The ability of granule cells to downmodulate calbindin over a wide dynamic range may explain, at least in part, why these neurons are relatively resistant to degeneration in AD (West et al., 1994; Irizarry et al., 1997b; Palop et al., 2003), since calbindin reduction can lead to an inactivation of voltage-gated calcium channels, limiting calcium entry and protecting against excitotoxicity (Nägerl et al., 2000).

33.3.3.3 Intracellular stores

In addition to influx from the extracellular compartment, the release of Ca^{2+} from intracellular stores in the ER is a major source of free Ca^{2+} that is available for signaling and synaptic plasticity (Rose and Konnerth, 2001; Berridge et al., 2003; Bardo et al., 2006). To maintain such a supply of Ca^{2+}, the ER faces the daunting task of sustaining an immense concentration gradient of Ca^{2+} across its membrane: The concentration of free Ca^{2+} in the ER lumen is about one thousand times greater than resting levels in the cytosol. Sarco-ER Ca^{2+} ATPases (SERCAs) actively transport Ca^{2+} into the ER to clear Ca^{2+} from the cytosol and fill ER stores. The liberation of Ca^{2+} from these internal stores is regulated by two types of channels in the ER membrane: the ryanodine receptor (RyR) and the inositol triphosphate receptor (IP_3R).

RyRs are activated by cytosolic Ca^{2+}, and their sensitivity is modulated by several factors: caffeine binding, oxidation, and high luminal Ca^{2+} levels increase sensitivity, whereas phosphorylation (by PKA) and calmodulin binding decrease activity (reviewed in Berridge et al., 2003; Bardo et al., 2006). IP_3Rs must be activated by the second messenger IP_3, which is generated upon stimulation of Gq-coupled receptors on the plasma membrane, such as metabotropic glutamate receptor types 1 and 5 ($mGluR_{1,5}$), serotonin receptors ($5\text{-}HT_2$), and muscarinic receptors (M1–3). The binding of IP_3 to IP_3Rs then sensitizes the receptors to Ca^{2+}, which increases receptor activity at low concentrations but inhibits it at high concentrations, such as those reached after release of Ca^{2+} from the ER (Berridge et al., 2003). IP_3Rs are often tethered to IP_3-producing cell surface receptors by scaffolding proteins such as Homer, linking the source of IP_3-production to its site of action (Ehrengruber et al., 2004). IP_3R activity can also be influenced by phosphorylation, which modulates the sensitivity of IP_3Rs in different directions, depending on the kinase involved. For example, phosphorylation by Ca^{2+}/calmodulin-dependent protein kinase II (CaMKII) decreases activity, whereas phosphorylation by Fyn kinase increases activity (Cui et al., 2004; Bare et al., 2005). Together, the activities of SERCAs, RyRs, and IP_3Rs monitor intracellular Ca^{2+} levels and regulate release of Ca^{2+} from the ER in a process called Ca^{2+}-induced Ca^{2+} release (CICR).

Several aspects of Ca^{2+} dysregulation in AD and AD mouse models have been linked to alterations in ER Ca^{2+} signaling. AD-related mutations in presenilin 1, presenilin 2, and APP increase cellular sensitivities to IP_3, caffeine activation of RyRs, and blockade of SERCA pumps, enhancing Ca^{2+} liberation from the ER (Smith et al., 2005a; Stutzmann, 2005). Overfilling of ER stores or excess phosphorylation of IP_3Rs or RyRs through aberrant activation of kinases by $A\beta$ or other AD-related molecules may result in ER hypersensitivity and exaggerated Ca^{2+} release upon physiological stimulation of these receptors (discussed in the section titled 'Intracellular calcium stores'). As a result, even normal stimuli, such as synaptic activity and activation of mGluRs, could disrupt the intracellular Ca^{2+} homeostasis.

Mutations in presenilin 1 have been particularly linked to dysregulation of ER Ca^{2+} signaling by mechanisms that are unrelated to γ-secretase activity. As mentioned in Section 33.2.3.2, wild-type, but not AD-mutant, presenilin 1 and 2 can act as low-conductance Ca^{2+}-permeable ion channels, which may account for the majority of passive Ca^{2+} leaks from the ER (Tu et al., 2006). This Ca^{2+}-fluxing activity is important for maintaining normal steady-state intraluminal levels of Ca^{2+} and is exhibited by the unprocessed, holoprotein form of presenilin in the ER (Tu et al., 2006). In contrast, the secretase activity of presenilin emerges only in later compartments (trans-Golgi network, endosome) after assembly with other components of the γ-secretase complex (Tandon and Fraser, 2002). AD-related mutations in PS1 (PS1-M146V) or PS2 (PS2-N141I) abrogate the Ca^{2+} fluxing properties of the presenilins and abolish the passive efflux of Ca^{2+} out of the ER, overloading the ER with Ca^{2+}.

AD-related increases in levels of RyRs may also contribute to ER hypersensitivity and exaggerated Ca^{2+} release. RyR binding is increased in the entorhinal cortex and hippocampus in early stages of AD, suggesting increased levels of RyRs in these areas (Kelliher et al., 1999). Presenilin mutations are associated with increased levels of RyRs in transgenic mice and cell culture models (Chan et al., 2000; Smith et al., 2005b; Stutzmann et al., 2006). hAPP mice and primary cortical neurons treated with $A\beta$ also show increases in RyRs (Supnet et al., 2006), suggesting that increased levels of $A\beta$ are the unifying mechanism.

Together, these studies indicate that dysregulation of ER Ca^{2+} dynamics may contribute to impairments in synaptic plasticity and cognitive function associated with AD.

33.3.4 Kinases

Kinase activity is often coupled to the activity of receptors and channels at the plasma membrane and is crucial to the transduction of extracellular signals to cytosolic or nuclear targets. Signaling specificity is conferred by the type of receptor activated by synaptic activity, the dynamics and distribution of the ensuing Ca^{2+} influx, and the scaffolding of particular kinases to receptors/channels. Phosphorylation events triggered by active kinases can alter enzymatic activities or protein conformations of target molecules, setting in motion molecular cascades that culminate in cytoplasmic changes or nuclear events including gene transcription. Over the years, researchers have uncovered important roles for many kinases in synaptic plasticity and demonstrated how the orchestration of their activities leads to the induction, expression, and maintenance of long-term changes in synaptic efficacy. Notably, the levels, localization, or activities of many of these kinases are disrupted in AD, providing clues into the mechanisms by which AD impairs synaptic and cognitive function. In this section, we discuss several kinases whose roles in synaptic plasticity have been well characterized and how AD-related alterations in these kinases or associated signaling pathways may contribute to synaptic dysfunction.

33.3.4.1 MAPKs

The mitogen-activated protein kinase (MAPK) superfamily comprises three major subclasses of Ser/Thr kinases that are involved in the regulation of growth, differentiation, and cellular responses to stress and/or inflammatory cytokines. The extracellular signal-regulated kinases (ERKs) regulate growth, proliferation, and differentiation in many cell types and are essential for short-term increases in synaptic efficacy and for the expression and maintenance of LTP (Pearson et al., 2001; Thomas and Huganir, 2004; Davis and Laroche, 2006). The p38 branch of the MAPK family was originally characterized as key transducers of stress and inflammatory responses to cytokines but has recently been discovered to also mediate the induction and expression of LTD (Pearson et al., 2001; Thomas and Huganir, 2004). The activity or localization of ERK and p38 family members are altered in AD and related models, and their misregulation has been implicated in impairments of synaptic plasticity (Johnson and Bailey, 2003; Haddad, 2004). The third branch of the MAPK family is made up of the c-Jun N-terminal kinase/stress-activated protein kinases (JNK/SAPKs), which transduce stress signals, including oxidation and DNA damage, as well as growth and differentiation signals (Raivich and Behrens, 2006). Aβ-induced generation of reactive oxygen species activates JNK/SAPK, and such activation has been documented in AD and in AD models (reviewed in Zhu et al., 2004; Smith et al., 2006). Aβ-related engagement of JNK/SAPKs has been associated with overt cell death rather than more subtle effects on synaptic/neuronal functions. We will thus focus our discussion of MAPKs in AD-related synaptic impairments on ERK and p38.

ERK1/2 is activated rapidly after the induction of LTP. Although ERK1/2 activity is not necessary for the induction of LTP, it is critical for its maintenance and for learning and memory (English and Sweatt, 1997; reviewed in Thomas and Huganir, 2004; Davis and Laroche, 2006). In combination with other signaling pathways, LTP-induced ERK1/2 activation increases the expression of proteins necessary for long-term changes in synaptic efficacy, including the activity-regulated cytoskeletal protein (Arc/Arg3.1) (Roberson et al., 1999; Waltereit et al., 2001; Ying et al., 2002). Additional targets of ERK1/2 that are important for the expression or maintenance of LTP include cytoskeletal proteins such as MAP-2 and Tau, which modulate the structural organization of neurites; Kv4.2 potassium channels, which control dendritic depolarization and neuronal excitability; AMPA receptors, which are inserted into the membrane and increase synaptic strength; and mTOR, a component of the ribosomal machinery that controls synthesis of new proteins (reviewed in Haddad, 2004; Birnbaum et al., 2004; Kelleher et al., 2004; Sweatt, 2004). Clearly, tight regulation of ERK1/2 activity, dynamics, and localization is necessary to orchestrate its many effects on synaptic efficacy (**Figure 15**).

Increased levels of active ERK1/2 in AD brains are typically associated with neurofibrillary tangles and amyloid plaques (Trojanowski et al., 1993; Pei et al., 2002; Haddad, 2004; Webster et al., 2006). ERK1/2 phosphorylation of tau, described above in the section titled 'Tau phosphorylation and other posttranslational modifications,' has been well documented as a means by which hyperphosphorylated tau is generated in AD (reviewed in Haddad, 2004). In addition, the dysregulation of ERK1/2 activity may contribute in other ways to synaptic dysfunction, as indicated by studies in animal and *in vitro* models of AD. ERK1/2 activity has been shown to mediate the effects of Aβ on synaptic plasticity, including Aβ's effect on L-type calcium channels

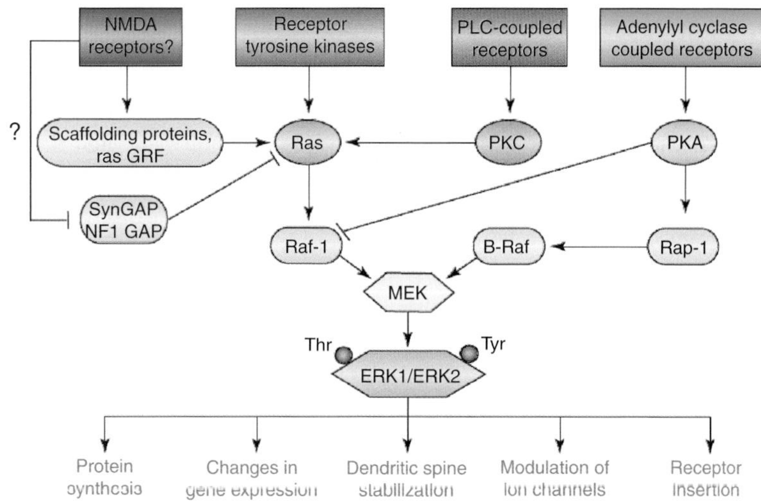

Figure 15 Regulation and targets of extracellular signal-regulated kinase (ERK)1/2 signaling in neurons. The ERK/mitogen-activated protein kinase cascade is activated by a number of receptors and pathways, and therefore plays a critical role in the integration of a wide variety of signals. The targets of ERK1/2 modulate processes that are crucial for synaptic plasticity (red font), all of which are impaired in Alzheimer's disease and experimental models. (From Sweatt JD [2004] Mitogen-activated protein kinases in synaptic plasticity and memory. *Curr. Opin. Neurobiol.* 14: 311–317.)

(reviewed in the section titled 'Calcium channels'). Interestingly, the kinetics of ERK1/2 activity depend on the duration of Aβ exposure and on Aβ's assembly state. Exposure of primary neurons or hippocampal slices to oligomeric Aβ acutely activated ERK1/2, but chronically decreased ERK1/2 activity, while exposure to fibrillar Aβ progressively increased ERK1/2 activity (Rapoport and Ferreira, 2000; Bell et al., 2004). Similarly, young hAPP transgenic mice exhibit increased ERK1/2 activity, whereas older hAPP mice exhibit decreased ERK1/2 activity, in particular in hippocampal subregions (Dineley et al., 2001; Chin et al., 2005; Palop et al., 2005). Certain brain regions may be able to downregulate ERK1/2 activity through compensatory mechanisms. For example, the phosphatase STEP dephosphorylates and inactivates ERK1/2 and is increased by Aβ *in vitro* and in the hippocampus of hAPP mice (Chin et al., 2005; Snyder et al., 2005; Braithwaite et al., 2006). Although the downregulation of aberrant ERK1/2 activity may be neuroprotective, it may also increase Aβ production (Kim et al., 2006) and decrease the expression of gene products required for the formation of long-term memories.

Although much emphasis has been placed on p38-mediated phosphorylation of tau, this process does not contribute greatly to the hyperphosphorylation of tau in AD (reviewed in Johnson and Stoothoff, 2004). p38 signaling also regulates synaptic plasticity by mediating long-term depression (LTD) of synaptic strength (reviewed in Thomas and Huganir, 2004). Inhibitors of p38 activity block LTD mediated by mGluRs or NMDARs (Bolshakov et al., 2000; Zhu et al., 2002), and inhibition of either p38 or mGluR activity prevents Aβ-induced LTP deficits in hippocampal slices (Wang et al., 2004). Furthermore, levels of phosphorylated, active p38 are increased in AD brains and related mouse models (Hensley et al., 1999; Zhu et al., 2000; Savage et al., 2002; reviewed in Johnson and Bailey, 2003; Hwang et al., 2005). Thus, Aβ-induced neuronal p38 activation may impair synaptic function in AD by promoting LTD.

33.3.4.2 CaMKII

Calcium/calmodulin-dependent protein kinase II is a major constituent of the postsynaptic density (PSD) that interacts with NMDA receptors and the cytoskeletal protein α-actinin. When activated by calcium influx during high-frequency stimulation, CaMKII translocates to the PSD and undergoes autophosphorylation at Thr286 of the αCaMKII subunit, resulting in prolonged calcium/calmodulin-independent CaMKII activity. This process is thought to underlie, at least in part, the conversion of a transient calcium signal to long-lasting enhancement of synaptic strength. Genetic or pharmacological manipulations that decrease levels of CamKII or prevent its autophosphorylation abolish

LTP and impair learning and memory (reviewed in Colbran and Brown, 2004).

In addition to its influence on gene transcription, CaMKII's cytoplasmic targets have also received great attention for their roles in the expression and maintenance of LTP. CaMKII promotes the insertion of alpha-amino-3-hydroxyl-5-methyl-4-isoxazolepropionate receptors (AMPARs) into the synapse, surface expression of Kv4.2 potassium channels, and activity of R-type calcium channels (reviewed in Colbran and Brown, 2004). Moreover, CaMKII-dependent modulation of cytoskeletal proteins regulates modifications of dendritic spine morphology associated with LTP (reviewed in Carlisle and Kennedy, 2005).

Although levels of CaMKII are relatively preserved in AD brains, levels of active, autophosphorylated CaMKII are significantly decreased (Mah et al., 1992; Simonian et al., 1994; Amada et al., 2005). These changes may be subregion specific, as decreases in autophorylated CaMKII were found in the hippocampus, but not in the amygdala (Amada et al., 2005). Consistent with these findings, Aβ acutely inhibits the ability of high-frequency stimuli to induce αCaMKII autophosphorylation and subsequent LTP in hippocampal slices (Zhao et al., 2004).

Autophosphorylation of αCaMKII, and thus CaMKII activity, are negatively regulated by the phosphatase PP1, which acts downstream of the calcium-dependent phosphatase calcineurin (Blitzer et al., 1998; Hedou and Mansuy, 2003). Particularly interesting in this regard are the findings by multiple groups that Aβ activates calcineurin *in vitro* and in transgenic mouse models of AD (Chen et al., 2002; reviewed in Xie, 2004; Cardoso and Oliveira, 2005; Snyder et al., 2005). Calcineurin levels and activity are also increased in AD (Hata et al., 2001; Liu et al., 2005; but see Lian et al., 2001). Together, these results suggest that enhanced negative regulation of CaMKII may diminish its activity in AD and impair synaptic plasticity.

33.3.4.3 PKC

Considerable evidence indicates that protein kinase C (PKC) is critical for long-term synaptic plasticity (Hvalby et al., 1994; Bortolotto and Collingridge, 2000). Indeed, ablation of PKC or inhibition of its activity impairs LTP as well as learning and memory (reviewed in Battaini and Pascale, 2005). Part of PKC's role in LTP may relate to its actions on AMPARs (Chung et al., 2000; Boehm et al., 2006). In addition, crosstalk between the PKC and PKA pathways can amplify ERK1/2 signaling (Roberson et al., 1999).

PKC is kept in a folded, inactive conformation by the binding of its pseudosubstrate domain to the substrate-binding site in the catalytic domain. Activation of the conventional, calcium-dependent isoforms of PKC, which are highly expressed in the brain, is regulated by binding to the second messengers calcium and diacylglycerol (DAG, reviewed in Battaini and Pascale, 2005). Upon binding and activation by second messengers, PKC translocates to the membrane via interactions with the scaffolding protein RACK1, which stands for receptor for activated C kinase (reviewed in Sklan et al., 2006). Interactions with RACK1 therefore aid in localizing PKC to its substrates.

Decreased activity of PKC has been implicated in the pathogenesis of AD. PKC levels are reduced in AD brains (Cole et al., 1988). In addition to deficits in PKC activation, which may result from decreased synaptic transmission and depletion of growth factors, PKC does not translocate effectively from the cytosolic to the membrane fraction in samples from AD brains, possibly because of decreased levels of RACK1 (Wang et al., 1994; Battaini et al., 1999).

Increased PKC immunoreactivity has been found in some AD cases and in hAPP transgenic mice at the beginning stages of amyloid deposition (Saitoh et al., 1993; Rossner et al., 2001), suggesting an early hyperactivation of PKC by Aβ, which may be followed by chronic suppression. Indeed, chronic activation is known to downregulate PKC activity (reviewed in Battaini and Pascale, 2005).

The consequences of reduced PKC activity are several-fold. In addition to decreasing the potential for synaptic plasticity, reduction of PKC activity may enhance the production of neurotoxic Aβ peptides. PKC increases the processing of APP by α-secretase in the nonamyloidogenic pathway, releasing the neurotrophic sAPPα fragment and precluding Aβ production (reviewed in Olariu et al., 2005). Treatment of APP/PS1 transgenic mice with small molecule activators of PKC significantly increased sAPPα, decreased Aβ levels, and reduced premature mortality (Etcheberrigaray et al., 2004). In addition, PKC regulates Aβ levels by increasing its clearance. Overexpression of the epsilon isoform of PKC activated endothelin-converting enzyme, an Aβ-degrading enzyme, and decreased Aβ levels, plaque deposition, neuritic dystrophy, and reactive astrocytosis in hAPP transgenic mice (Choi et al., 2006).

Together, these results suggest that enhancement of PKC activity may provide some benefit in AD.

33.3.4.4 PKA

Since the discovery in the 1980s that activation of cyclic AMP-dependent PKA increases synaptic efficacy in *Aplysia* neurons, numerous roles for PKA have been described in both short-term and long-term plasticity (reviewed in Nguyen and Woo, 2003; Waltereit and Weller, 2003). PKA is activated rapidly by calcium influx, which leads to increased synthesis of cyclic adenosine monophosphate (cAMP) by calcium/calmodulin-sensitive adenyl cyclases. Short-term actions of PKA include phosphorylation of potassium channels, to acutely increase excitability, and phosphorylation of synaptic vesicle proteins, to increase neurotransmitter release.

LTP-inducing stimuli lead to the degradation of the regulatory subunits of PKA, resulting in sustained activity of the catalytic subunits, which translocate to the nucleus and phosphorylate the transcription factor cAMP response element binding protein (CREB) to initiate gene transcription (reviewed in Kandel, 2001). Activity of PKA is necessary for long-lasting LTP in the hippocampus: it initiates gene transcription by direct phosphorylation of transcription factors and synergizes with other kinases, such as PKC, to activate ERK1/2 signaling (Roberson et al., 1999; Impey et al., 1998; reviewed in Waltereit and Weller, 2003). The combined actions of PKA and ERK1/2 are necessary for the transcription of immediate-early genes such as Arc/Arg3.1 that are critical to memory consolidation (Waltereit et al., 2001). PKA also increases current conductance and synaptic strength via phosphorylation of synaptic AMPA receptors (reviewed in Nguyen and Woo, 2003).

Alterations in PKA signaling have been implicated in several aspects of AD. PKA contributes to tau hyperphosphorylation by direct phosphorylation and by rendering tau susceptible to phosphorylation by GSK-3 (Liu et al., 2004; reviewed in Gong et al., 2005). Although PKA is responsible for a large proportion of tau hyperphosphorylation in AD, PKA activity is decreased in AD as well as in animal and cell culture models of the disease (Kim et al., 2001; Vitolo et al., 2002; Gong et al., 2006), possibly because Aβ inhibits the proteasomal degradation of PKA's regulatory subunits (**Figure 16**) (Vitolo et al., 2002). Increasing cAMP levels by inhibition of phosphodiesterases that break down cAMP ameliorates Aβ-induced deficits in synaptic plasticity and

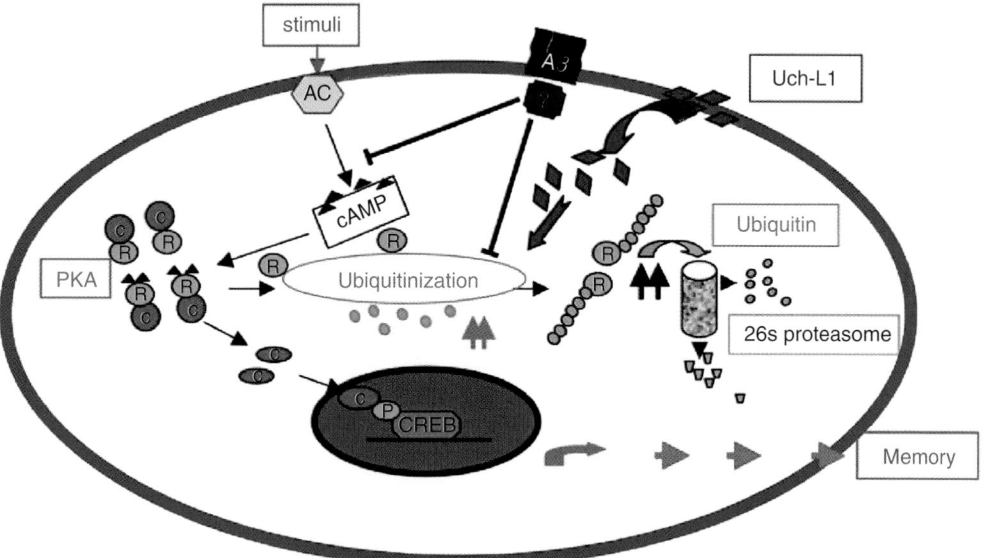

Figure 16 Aβ modulation of the ubiquitin-proteasome-protein kinase A (PKA)-cyclic adenosine monophosphate response element binding protein (CREB) pathway. Aβ inhibits adenylate cyclase activity and proteasomal degradation of the regulatory subunits of PKA, resulting in their accumulation and a shift in the PKA complex toward the inactive tetramer. Consequently, CREB phosphorylation and initiation of transcription is impaired. Transduction of Uch-L1 promotes proteasomal activity, normalizing levels of the PKA regulatory subunit and freeing the active catalytic subunit. (From Gong B, Cao Z, Zheng P, et al. [2006] Ubiquitin hydrolase Uch-L1 rescues β-amyloid-induced decreases in synaptic function and contextual memory. *Cell* 126: 775–788.)

learning and memory (Vitolo et al., 2002; Gong et al., 2004). Exogenous ubiquitin C-terminal hydrolase L1 (Uch-L1), which boosts proteasome activity, reversed Aβ-induced LTP deficits in hippocampal slices (Gong et al., 2006). Moreover, endogenous Uch-L1 activity was decreased in APP/PS1 transgenic mice, and treatment of these mice with exogenous Uch-L1 restored PKA activity and contextual memory (Gong et al., 2006).

33.3.4.5 Fyn

The tyrosine kinase Fyn can be activated through diverse receptors and participates in signaling pathways that control a broad spectrum of biological activities, including long-term changes in synaptic efficacy (Thomas and Brugge, 1997; Roskoski, 2004; Salter and Kalia, 2004). Ablation of Fyn abolishes LTP and impairs spatial learning and memory (Grant et al., 1992). Postnatal overexpression of Fyn can restore LTP, indicating that Fyn is a critical modulator of long-term synaptic efficacy (Kojima et al., 1997). Anchored to NMDA receptor complexes through interactions with PSD-95, Fyn phosphorylates the NR2B subunit at tyrosine residue 1472 (Tyr1472), which increases calcium conductance by altering channel gating properties and controls the internalization of the receptors by preventing AP-2 binding, a signal for endocytosis (reviewed in Salter and Kalia, 2004; Prybylowski et al., 2005). In addition, Fyn can modulate cytoskeletal dynamics by altering the phosphorylation and/or localization of cytoskeletal elements such as tau, adducin, and β-catenin (Williamson et al., 2002; Lilien and Balsamo, 2005; Gotoh et al., 2006). Moreover, phosphorylation by Fyn influences the integrity of synaptic AMPA receptors by rendering them less susceptible to proteolytic cleavage (Rong et al., 2001).

A number of findings suggest that misregulation of Fyn activity may play a role in AD. The distribution and levels of Fyn are altered in AD brains (Shirazi and Wood, 1993; Ho et al., 2005), and the toxic effects of Aβ oligomers on hippocampal slices can be blocked by the genetic ablation of Fyn (Lambert et al., 1998). Ablation of Fyn decreases – whereas overexpression of Fyn increases – Aβ-induced synaptotoxicity and premature mortality in hAPP transgenic mice (Chin et al., 2004). In addition, Fyn phosphorylates tau and binds it in a manner that is modulated both by AD-related hyperphosphorylation and by disease-related mutations in tau (Bhaskar et al., 2005; Lee, 2005). Together with *in vitro* studies demonstrating that acute application of Aβ leads to activation of Fyn signaling pathways and increased interactions with binding partners, these results suggested that Aβ may derange synaptic functions by aberrantly engaging Fyn-related pathways (Zhang et al., 1996; Williamson et al., 2002). Indeed, the overexpression of Fyn in hAPP mice with moderate levels of Aβ rendered the mice as severely impaired, with respect to biochemical and behavioral alterations, as hAPP mice with high levels of Aβ (Chin et al., 2005). These results suggest that Fyn activity sensitizes neurons to Aβ-induced neuronal impairments. Fyn also exacerbates Aβ-induced aberrant increases in neuronal activity (Palop et al., 2007).

Interestingly, aberrant engagement of Fyn activity also appears to trigger compensatory mechanisms that limit Fyn activity in the presence of elevated Aβ levels. hAPP transgenic mice exhibit significant increases in levels of the phosphatase STEP, which dephosphorylates and inactivates Fyn, and have corresponding decreases in levels of active Fyn (see **Figure 11**) (Chin et al., 2005). The increase in STEP and decrease in Fyn activity are most prominent in the dentate gyrus, a region particularly susceptible to Aβ-related synaptic dysfunction. The compensatory downregulation of Fyn activity in this region has consequences on NMDA receptor phosphorylation, calcium gating, and receptor internalization that likely further contribute to deficits in synaptic plasticity and learning and memory (Chin et al., 2005; Palop et al., 2005; Snyder et al., 2005).

33.3.4.6 Cdk5

Cyclin-dependent kinase 5 is an unusual Cdk that lacks a role in the cell cycle and is activated by two noncyclin activators, p35 and p39. With an extensive list of substrates, the primarily neuronal Cdk5 regulates cell death and survival, as well as a variety of specific cellular functions (reviewed in Cheung and Ip, 2004; Cruz and Tsai, 2004). Cdk5 activity is increased in AD brains and in neurons and cell lines treated with Aβ and mediates tau hyperphosphorylation (reviewed in Giese et al., 2005). It also modulates synaptic plasticity, with consequences on learning and memory (reviewed in Cruz and Tsai, 2004; Cheung et al., 2006; Angelo et al., 2006).

Presynaptic roles for Cdk5 that influence synaptic transmission include the regulation of synaptic vesicle exocytosis through phosphorylation of P/Q-type calcium channels and synapsin 1, which increases calcium influx and releases synapsin's tethering of synaptic vesicles in a reserve pool (reviewed in Angelo et al., 2006). Cdk5 also modulates endocytosis for the recycling of synaptic vesicles by phosphorylating dynamin

I and amphiphysin I, proteins necessary for clathrin-mediated endocytosis (reviewed in Angelo et al., 2006).

Postsynaptic roles for Cdk5 in synaptic plasticity include phosphorylation of PSD-95, which suppresses its multimerization and decreases PSD-95-dependent clustering of NMDA receptors and Kv1.4 potassium channels (Morabito et al., 2004). Cdk5 also phosphorylates NR2A subunits of NMDA receptors and increases calcium conductance (Li et al., 2001). Moreover, Cdk5 activity regulates dendritic spine remodeling through actions on proteins that modulate cytoskeletal dynamics, including Rho GTPases and PAK1 (Nikolic et al., 1998).

Direct evidence for a role of Cdk5 in learning and memory has come from studies of transgenic mice expressing p25, a truncated form of the Cdk5 activator p35 that results in constitutive activation of Cdk5. Transient expression of p25 led to improved synaptic plasticity and learning in hippocampus-dependent tasks (Fischer et al., 2005). These improvements were accompanied by increased spine density and synapse formation.

Thus, Cdk5 activity must be well regulated in order to maintain control over the numerous aspects of neuronal function that it modulates. p25 levels are higher in AD brains than in normal controls (Lee et al., 1999; Patrick et al., 1999; reviewed in Giese et al., 2005). Although transient expression of p25 increases synaptic plasticity, prolonged neuronal expression of p25 in transgenic mice leads to synaptic impairments, learning and memory deficits, neurofibrillary tangle formation, and neurodegeneration (Cruz and Tsai, 2004; Fischer et al., 2005). In addition, sustained Cdk5 activity increases Aβ production (Cruz et al., 2006). Thus, the generation of p25 may be initiated in early stages of AD as a compensatory mechanism to support waning plasticity and memory, but its continued presence and the resulting overactivation of Cdk5 may eventually contribute to synaptic impairments and other neuronal deficits.

33.3.5 Neurotrophic and Neuromodulatory Factors

During development of the nervous system, secreted neurotrophic and neuromodulatory factors regulate axonal outgrowth, dendritic maturation, synapse formation, and synaptic strength. These processes overlap widely with those necessary for synaptic plasticity and the maintenance of long-term changes in synaptic function. Therefore, it is not surprising that nature has recycled many of these same neurotrophic and neuromodulatory factors to effect synaptic plasticity in adult organisms. Two such neuromodulatory factors are brain-derived neurotrophic factor (BDNF) and Reelin. We discuss their roles in synaptic plasticity and how AD-related alterations in their levels may contribute to synaptic and cognitive dysfunction.

33.3.5.1 BDNF

BDNF belongs to the neurotrophin family of signaling proteins that also includes nerve growth factor (NGF), neurotrophin 3 (NT-3), and neurotrophins 4/5(NT-4/5), all of which participate in regulating the survival and differentiation of specific neuronal populations during development. However, BDNF is unique among its family members in its ability to modulate activity-dependent synaptic plasticity in the developing and the adult brain (reviewed in Lu, 2003).

The actions of BDNF have long been studied in the context of learning and memory in animal models, but the recent discovery that a Val→Met mutation in the prodomain of BDNF is linked to memory impairment and susceptibility to neuropsychiatric disorders in humans has fueled additional research (reviewed in Bath and Lee, 2006). This mutation affects the trafficking of BDNF to the secretory pathway, resulting in reduced secretion of BDNF in target regions. Moreover, BDNF mRNA and protein levels are decreased in brain regions that are vulnerable in AD, suggesting that alterations in BDNF may reflect or contribute to cognitive impairments in AD (reviewed in Murer et al., 2001; Allen and Dawbarn, 2006).

BDNF has multiple distinct functions in synaptic plasticity that can be divided into two broad categories: permissive and instructive (reviewed in Schinder and Poo, 2000; Bramham and Messaoudi, 2005). Permissive actions of BDNF prepare synapses to be LTP-competent but do not actually generate LTP. Such actions include the maintenance of the presynaptic release machinery (vesicle docking and vesicle pool dynamics), which allows neurons to follow high-frequency stimuli.

Instructive signals from BDNF are initiated in response to high-frequency stimuli that induce LTP and result in the activity-dependent expression and release of BDNF. Some of these signals modulate postsynaptic calcium influx through voltage-gated sodium channels, reducing the amount of stimulation necessary for LTP induction (gating) (reviewed in Blum and Konnerth, 2005). The majority of BDNF's effects are mediated by TrKB receptors and subsequent signaling events that engage ERK1/2 and regulate the expression of genes, including the immediate-early gene Arc/Arg3.1 (reviewed in Blum and Konnerth, 2005; Bramham and Messaoudi, 2005). BDNF also regulates the translation of dendritically localized mRNAs associated with synapse-specific LTP (reviewed in Schuman et al., 2006). Together, BDNF's actions lead to long-lasting increases in synaptic strength.

Regulated BDNF expression also plays a central role in homeostatic synaptic scaling, through which the overall activity of a neuronal network is maintained over time (reviewed in Turrigiano and Nelson, 2004). As mentioned above, BDNF expression is activity dependent. Under situations of reduced activity, BDNF expression is reduced. GABA expression in inhibitory interneurons is then reduced, diminishing inhibition and promoting the firing rate of pyramidal neurons (Rutherford et al., 1997, 1998; reviewed in Turrigiano and Nelson, 2004).

The role of BDNF in scaling is particularly interesting in light of the decreased levels of BDNF observed in vulnerable brain regions in AD. Does the decrease in BDNF result from a primary insult and exacerbate synaptic deficits and plasticity in AD, or does it represent the attempts of an impaired network to increase neuronal activity and maintain synaptic connections? Answers to these questions are pending.

An additional complexity in considering the role of BDNF in AD is that the regulation and effects of BDNF have different outcomes depending on the state of the neuronal network on which it acts (Turrigiano and Nelson, 2004). The role of BDNF reductions in homeostatic scaling described above is evident in conditions in which normal activity has been abolished. However, in situations containing normal levels of background activity, BDNF's potentiating activity prevails. Transgenic mice overexpressing BDNF have increased seizure severity after kainic acid challenge and develop hyperexcitability in the entorhinal cortex and the CA regions of the hippocampus (Croll et al., 1999). Transgenic mice overexpressing BDNF's receptor TrKB also have a reduced threshold for kainate-induced seizures (Lahteinen et al., 2003). These studies suggest that a reduction of BDNF in AD may represent a compensatory mechanism against hyperexcitability. Consistent with this idea, removal of one BDNF allele in mice leads to increased synaptic inhibition (Olofsdotter et al., 2000).

33.3.5.2 Reelin

Reelin is a large glycoprotein of the extracellular matrix involved in neuronal migration and positioning during development (Tissir and Goffinet, 2003). In the mature brain, it modulates neuronal function and synaptic plasticity and regulates tau phosphorylation as well as axonal growth and dendritic spine morphology (Hiesberger et al., 1999; Liu et al., 2001b; Fatemi, 2005; Herz and Chen, 2006; Qiu et al., 2006b).

In most of the brain, Reelin is expressed by GABAergic interneurons that regulate the activity and function of neighboring glutamatergic neurons (Pesold et al., 1998; Ramos-Moreno et al., 2006). Interestingly, Reelin is also expressed highly by glutamatergic pyramidal neurons in layer II of the entorhinal cortex (Pesold et al., 1998; Perez-Garcia et al., 2001; Ramos-Moreno et al., 2006), a population of neurons that is affected early and severely by AD (Blennow et al., 2006). These neurons project primarily to the dentate gyrus and area CA1 of the hippocampus (Ramos-Moreno et al., 2006; van Groen et al., 2003), which are also vulnerable to AD (Blennow et al., 2006; Palop et al., 2003). Although Reelin does not appear to undergo calcium-dependent exocytosis (Lacor et al., 2000), its localization in secretory vesicles, axons, and dendritic spine-rich neuropils suggests that it may be released from both the cell soma and synaptic terminals (Pesold et al., 1998; Lacor et al., 2000; Pappas et al., 2001; Ramos-Moreno et al., 2006). Reelin immunoreactivity is also present in the axonal projections of glutamatergic pyramidal neurons in layer II of the entorhinal cortex (Ramos-Moreno et al., 2006), suggesting that Reelin produced by these cells is transported down axons and may impact neuronal function in target regions such as the dentate gyrus and CA1.

Two neuronal cell surface receptors that bind apoE and transport cholesterol into neurons, very low density lipoprotein receptor (VLDLR) and apolipoprotein E receptor 2 (ApoER2), bind Reelin and cooperate to transduce its signals (reviewed in Herz and Chen, 2006). The close proximity between Reelin receptors and NMDA receptors allows crosstalk between the two signaling pathways: Through a series of phosphorylation events, Reelin increases NMDA receptor function and thereby enhances the induction of LTP (**Figure 17**) (Weeber et al., 2002; Beffert et al., 2005; Chen et al., 2005b). Reelin also enhances synaptic function by stimulating the translation of dendritically expressed mRNAs, such as Arc/Arg3.1 mRNA (Dong et al., 2003). Reelin-deficient mice have a diminished capacity for hippocampus-dependent memory, indicating that Reelin is necessary for normal plasticity and memory formation (Qiu et al., 2006a).

The localization of Reelin expression and its roles in regulating synaptic plasticity as well as tau phosphorylation suggest that decreases in Reelin might exacerbate synaptic impairments in AD. In addition to memory deficits, Reelin-deficient mice exhibit robust increases in levels of hyperphosphorylated tau (Hiesberger et al., 1999; reviewed in Herz and Chen, 2006), suggesting a role for Reelin in the generation of tau pathology in AD. Furthermore, apoE competes with Reelin for binding to VLDLR/ApoER2 receptors and decreases Reelin signaling (D'Arcangelo et al., 1999; Herz and Bock, 2002). It has been suggested that apoE4 competes more efficiently than apoE3 (reviewed in Herz and Bock, 2002), providing yet another mechanism by which apoE4 may increase the susceptibility to AD (**Figure 17**; see also the section titled 'Aβ-Independent mechanisms for apoE-induced neuronal impairments').

A few recent studies have begun to examine whether AD is associated with Reelin alterations hAPP transgenic mice with high levels of Aβ were found to have significantly fewer Reelin-expressing

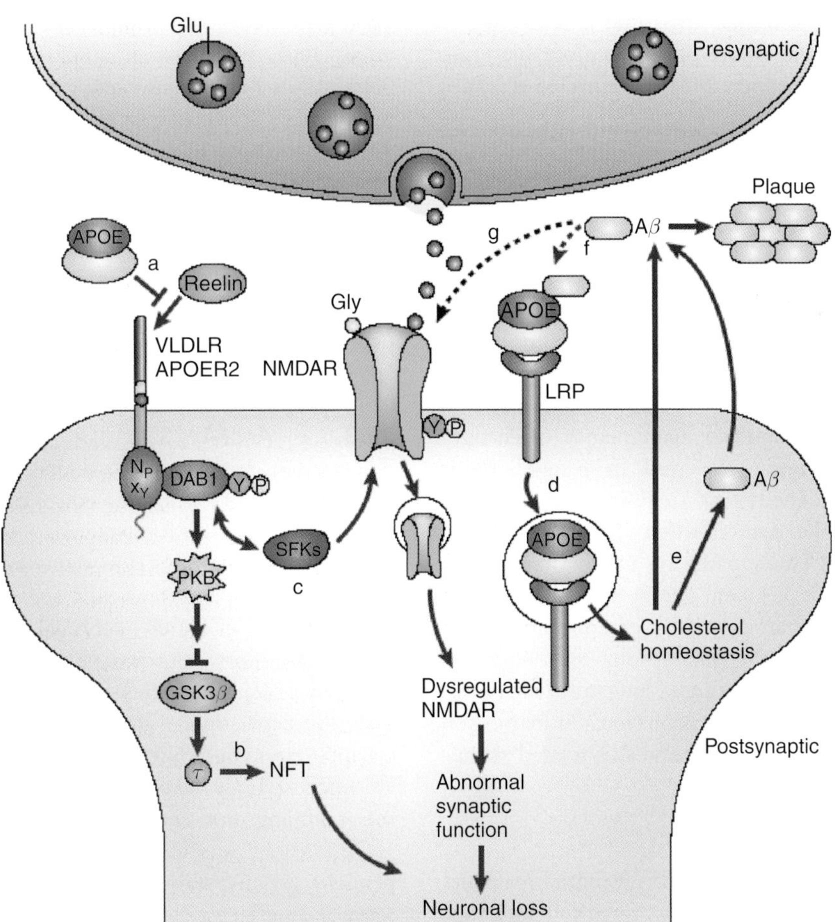

Figure 17 Reelin and ApoE signaling – implications for AD. Binding of Reelin to VLDLR and ApoER2 receptors initiates a cascade of events that leads to modulation of NMDA receptor function and enhanced long-term potentiation. ApoE can impede Reelin signaling by competing for receptor binding. Impaired Reelin signaling results in impaired synaptic plasticity as well as in elevated tau phosphorylation, which could contribute to neurofibrillary tangles associated with AD. In addition, binding of ApoE to the LRP lipoprotein receptor results in internalization of the ligand-bound receptor. Cholesterol homeostasis modulates the production and trafficking of Aβ. Secreted Aβ can bind apoE and be cleared through receptor-mediated endocytosis, promote the internalization of NMDA receptors, and deposit into plaques (From Herz J and Chen Y [2006] Reelin, lipoprotein receptors and synaptic plasticity. *Nat. Rev. Neurosci.* 7: 850–859.)

pyramidal cells in the entorhinal cortex and corresponding reductions in Reelin levels in the hippocampus relative to nontransgenic mice (Chin et al., 2007). In contrast, the number of Reelin-expressing GABAergic interneurons was not altered in either the entorhinal cortex or the hippocampus. Underscoring the relevance of these findings, qualitatively similar reductions of Reelin-expressing pyramidal neurons were found in the entorhinal cortex of AD brains (Chin et al., 2007). Increased fragments of Reelin were found in the CSF of AD patients, suggesting altered processing of Reelin (Saez-Valero et al., 2003). Increased levels of Reelin were found in the frontal cortex of AD brains (Botella-López et al., 2006). Conceivably, increases in Reelin in frontal brain regions reflect the kind of hyperactivation of frontal areas that is presumed to compensate for the failure of more vulnerable brain regions in AD (Buckner, 2004; Pariente et al., 2005; Palop et al., 2006).

33.3.6 Gene Expression

Short-term synaptic plasticity is effected by noncovalent modifications of existing proteins, such as ion channels, receptors, or components of the vesicle-release machinery that lead to acute modulation of synaptic strength. Long-lasting synaptic plasticity, however, requires protein synthesis and structural changes for the long-term maintenance of changes in synaptic strength (reviewed in Kandel, 2001; Carlisle and Kennedy, 2005). It is clear from the discussion in the section titled 'Kinases' that the derangement of kinase pathways in AD may disrupt the expression of pertinent genes. We consider here two proteins that play particularly important roles in gene transcription necessary for long-term plasticity (CREB) and in consolidation of long-term memories (Arc/Arg3.1), and how alterations in their expression or localization may contribute to AD-related synaptic and cognitive impairments.

33.3.6.1 CREB

The transcription factor CREB is essential for many forms of learning and memory (reviewed in Lonze and Ginty, 2002; and Tully et al., 2003). CREB is a nuclear protein that modulates the transcription of genes containing cAMP-responsive elements (CREs). Phosphorylation of CREB at Ser133 leads to the recruitment of other components of the transcription machinery to CREs. Both PKA and Ca^{2+}/calmodulin kinase type IV (CaMKIV) can phosphorylate CREB at Ser133 and are responsible for rapid initial increases in CREB phosphorylation in response to neuronal activity, whereas ERK1/2-dependent phosphorylation of Ser 133 occurs with slower kinetics, involves an intermediate such as RSK or MSK family kinases, and leads to prolonged phosphorylation of CREB.

CREB target genes encompass diverse proteins, ranging from proteins involved in neurotransmission, the transcriptional machinery, or signal transduction to growth factors such as BDNF, structural proteins, channels, and transporters (reviewed in Lonze and Ginty, 2002). Consequently, disruptions in CREB activation impair numerous neurological functions.

Decreased activity of PKA and ERK1/2 in AD and related experimental models is accompanied by decreased levels of phosphorylated CREB (Dineley et al., 2001; Vitolo et al., 2002; Gong et al., 2004, 2006). Efforts are being made to determine whether promoting CREB activity is an effective means to enhance memory in normal aging and in AD (Tully et al., 2003). Indeed, treatment of transgenic mouse models of AD with agents that boost cAMP levels (and thus PKA activity) do restore PKA/CREB signaling and are associated with an amelioration of deficits in synaptic plasticity and hippocampus-dependent memory (Vitolo et al., 2002; Gong et al., 2004, 2006).

33.3.6.2 Arc/Arg3.1

The activity-regulated cytoskeletal protein/activity-regulated gene 3.1 is an immediate early gene (IEG) that is critical for LTP maintenance and for the consolidation of memories (Tzingounis and Nicoll, 2006). IEGs are rapidly and transiently activated at the transcriptional level after neuronal stimulation by neurotransmitters or growth factors. Some IEGs, for example, c-fos, encode transcription factors that modulate the expression of genes for proteins that affect synaptic strength, while others, such as Arc/Arg3.1, are effector IEGs whose products directly effect or maintain long-term changes in synaptic strength.

Arc/Arg3.1 was identified in 1995 by two independent groups searching for an IEG that might serve as an effector of long-term changes in synaptic strength (Link et al., 1995; Lyford et al., 1995). Both groups posited that the expression of such an effector should be (1) rapidly stimulated by neuronal activity, (2) blocked by NMDA receptor antagonists, and (3) localized to dendritic compartments. Using these criteria, both groups identified the same IEG, now known by the combined name of Arc/Arg3.1.

Arc/Arg3.1 is rapidly activated by patterned synaptic activity, including seizure activity, LTP, exploration of a novel environment, and memory-inducing behavioral paradigms (reviewed in Guzowski, 2002; Tzingounis and Nicoll, 2006). Newly synthesized Arc/Arg3.1 mRNA is rapidly transported to dendrites and accumulates in the particular synapses that were previously activated (Steward and Worley, 2001a,b). Because of these properties, the expression of Arc/Arg3.1 has been used to image behaviorally relevant activity in neuronal networks (Guzowski et al., 1999; Temple et al., 2003; Burke et al., 2005; Tagawa et al., 2005; Zou and Buck, 2006). For example, the sequential exposure of rats to two different environments results in the activation of distinct patterns of Arc/Arg3.1 expression in the hippocampus, particularly in the dentate gyrus, suggesting that Arc/Arg3.1 represents the activity of neuronal ensembles involved in the encoding of contextual information (Guzowski et al., 1999; reviewed in Guzowski et al., 2005).

Arc/Arg3.1 expression has also been used to examine the susceptibility of particular neuronal populations to Aβ-induced impairments in transgenic mouse models of AD (**Figure 18**). The induction of Arc/Arg3.1 after various stimuli is diminished in hAPP mice and hAPP/PS1 mice (Dickey et al., 2004; Chin et al., 2005; Palop et al., 2005). After exploration of a novel environment, Arc/Arg3.1 expression is reliably induced in the dentate gyrus of nontransgenic rodents (reviewed in Guzowski et al., 2005), but not in hAPP transgenic mice (Chin et al., 2005; Palop et al., 2005). Basal levels of Arc/Arg3.1 were also markedly reduced in the dentate gyrus. These alterations in Arc/Arg3.1 expression were accompanied by

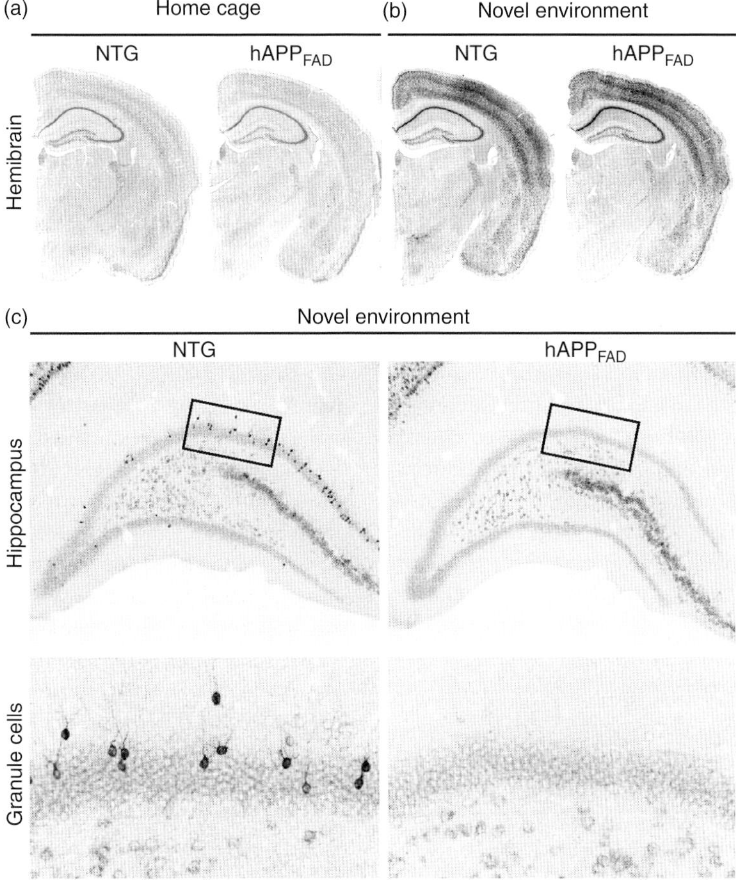

Figure 18 Imaging neuronal network activity using Arc/Arg3.1 expression. (a, b) After exploration of a novel environment, Arc/Arg3.1 expression is reliably induced in nontransgenic (NTG) mice in several brain regions including neocortex and hippocampus. hAPP transgenic mice show normal induction in the neocortex and CA1, but a striking lack of induction in the dentate granule cells of the hippocampus (a–c). (From Palop JJ, Chin J, Bien-Ly N, et al. [2005] Vulnerability of dentate granule cells to disruption of Arc/Arg3.1 expression in human amyloid precursor protein transgenic mice. *J. Neurosci.* 25: 9686–9693. Copyright 2005 by the Society for Neuroscience.)

decreased activities of NMDA receptors and ERK1/2, which regulate Arc/Arg3.1 expression. Other calcium-regulated proteins, for example, Fos and calbindin, are also depleted in the dentate gyrus of hAPP mice, and these depletions correlate well with deficits in learning and memory (Palop et al., 2003). Together, these studies indicate that the dentate gyrus is particularly vulnerable to Aβ-induced deficits in synaptic function, encoding of spatial information, and learning and memory.

Recent work by several groups has begun to shed light on Arc/Arg3.1 activities that may be particularly relevant to the synaptic and cognitive deficits observed in AD. Arc/Arg3.1 regulates AMPA receptor trafficking through interactions with endophilin and dynamin, proteins critically involved in the endocytotic recycling of synaptic vesicles (Chowdhury et al., 2006). Overexpression of Arc/Arg3.1 increases recycling rates and decreases surface expression of AMPA receptors, with corresponding decreases in AMPA receptor-mediated currents (Chowdhury et al., 2006; Rial Verde et al., 2006). In contrast, ablation of Arc/Arg3.1 increases surface expression of AMPA receptors and impairs long-term memory (Plath et al., 2006; Shepherd et al., 2006). Notably, the regulation of Arc/Arg3.1 and AMPA receptors is bidirectional, as AMPA receptor activity downregulates Arc/Arg3.1 expression (Rao et al., 2006).

The dynamic interactions between Arc/Arg3.1 and AMPA receptors may play a critical role in homeostatic scaling of synaptic strength (reviewed in Turrigiano and Nelson, 2004; Davis, 2006). Synaptic scaling is an important mode of plasticity by which neuronal networks maintain an optimal equilibrium of activity over time, and impairments of this plasticity may exacerbate synaptic and cognitive deficits in AD (Small, 2004; Palop et al., 2006).

33.4 Conclusions

We have surveyed here a multitude of molecules whose functions are perturbed in AD and animal models of the disease. The complexity of the pathways and interactions involved can be overwhelming, and it may be tempting to ask whether any molecule in the brain is left unaffected by the disease. Such a question has several potential answers.

Perhaps not coincidentally, this situation evokes similarities to LTP and the molecular basis of synaptic plasticity, where an equally long (and largely overlapping) list of molecules is involved (Roberson et al., 1996; Sanes and Lichtman, 1999; Malenka and Bear, 2004). This parallel highlights the fact that AD is a disease of memory not just in terms of neuropsychology but also at the molecular level, and that addressing AD may be one of the most critical applications of basic knowledge about the molecular basis of synaptic plasticity.

Second, the molecular changes in AD are not unlimited and are, in fact, bounded by multiple levels of specificity. Many are restricted to specific anatomic structures (e.g., hippocampus vs. neocortex) or even to specific subregions (e.g., CA1 vs. CA3). It is increasingly apparent that this specificity extends to the level of individual cells (e.g., principal cells vs. interneurons), an observation with important implications. Aβ-induced activation of a neurotransmitter receptor on an excitatory principal neuron might result in overexcitation of its circuit, whereas activating the same receptor on inhibitory interneurons could shut the network down (Palop et al., 2006) (**Figure 19**). Even at the molecular level, AD-related changes can be quite specific; among the important neurotrophic factors, BDNF seems to play an important role in AD, whereas in NT3 does not appear to be involved (Hock et al., 2000).

Finally, there is at least one great boon to the long list of molecules involved in AD: a surfeit of potential targets for treating the disease. Indeed, treatments aimed at many of the molecules discussed here are now in trials for AD (Jacobsen et al., 2005; Roberson and Mucke, 2006). In terms of the AD-associated molecules in the section titled 'Memory impairment by AD-related molecules,' diverse approaches are under study, including (1) reducing the production or speeding the removal of potentially toxic proteins, for example, with β- or γ-secretase inhibitors or via immune-mediated clearance (Citron, 2004; Weiner and Frenkel, 2006); (2) preventing unwanted post-translational processing or aggregation of Aβ, tau, and apoE into particularly toxic forms (Harris et al., 2003; Khlistunova et al., 2006; McLaurin et al., 2006); (3) restoring normal functions lost by AD-related modifications, such as the microtubule-stabilizing effect of tau (Zhang et al., 2005); and (4) in the case of apoE, forcing apoE4 to adopt more apoE3-like structure and function (Mahley et al., 2006). The plasticity-related molecules highlighted in the section titled 'Memory-related molecules in AD' may provide good complementary targets. Here, the goal is to restore plasticity, boost related memory mechanisms, and protect neurons against aberrant network

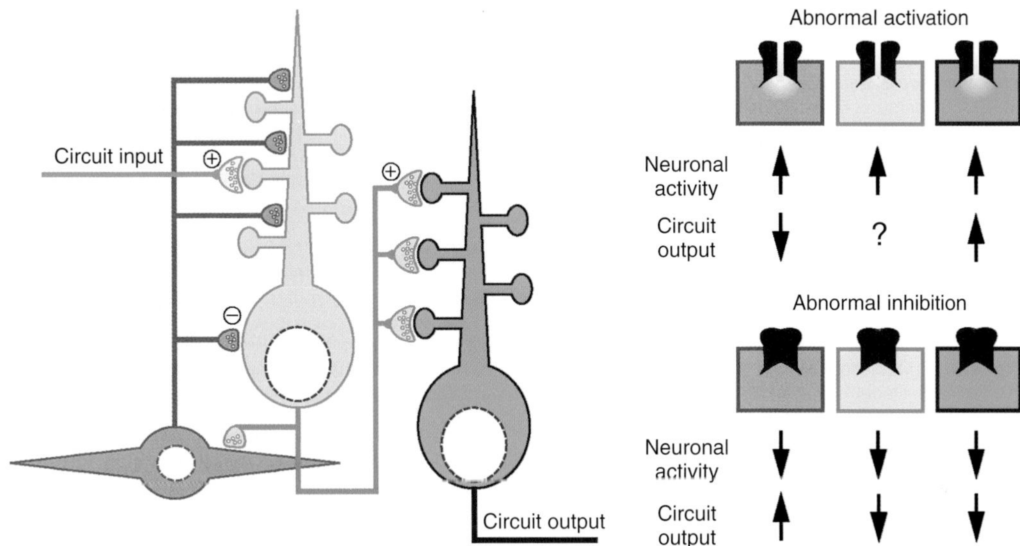

Figure 19 Consequences of the same molecular process on different cell types. The same molecular process can have a very different effect on circuit output depending on whether the cell it affects is an excitatory principal neuron (shades of green) or an inhibitory interneuron (red). Abnormal activation of an excitatory principal neuron will lead to overexcitation of the circuit, whereas abnormal activation of an inhibitory interneuron will shut the circuit down.

activities, even in the presence of pathogenic protein assemblies (Palop et al., 2006).

Thus, while complexity is certainly a feature of our current molecular understanding of AD, such issues pose exciting opportunities for neuroscientists working at the interface between AD and plasticity research, which is rapidly becoming one of the most active fronts in the battle against AD.

Acknowledgments

We thank J. Palop and J. Carroll for graphics. This work was supported by National Institutes of Health grants AG011385, AG022074, AG023501 (L.M) and NS054811 (E.D.R.), and by S.D. Bechtel, Jr. (E.D.R.).

References

Allen SJ and Dawbarn D (2006) Clinical relevance of the neurotrophins and their receptors. *Clin. Sci. (Lond.)* 110: 175–191.

Almeida CG, Tampellini D, Takahashi RH, et al. (2005) β-amyloid accumulation in APP mutant neurons reduces PSD-95 and GluR1 in synapses. *Neurobiol. Dis.* 20: 187–198.

Alves da Costa C, Sunyach C, Pardossi-Piquard R, et al. (2006) Presenilin-dependent γ-secretase-mediated control of p53-associated cell death in Alzheimer's disease. *J. Neurosci.* 26: 6377–6385.

Alvestad RM, Grosshans DR, Coultrap SJ, Nakazawa T, Yamamoto T, and Browning MD (2003) Tyrosine dephosphorylation and ethanol inhibition of N-methyl-D-aspartate receptor function. *J. Biol. Chem.* 278: 11020–11025.

Alzheimer A (1907) Über eine eigenartige Erkrankung der Hirnrinde. *Allg. Z. Psychiatr.* 64: 146–148.

Alzheimer Disease & Frontotemporal Dementia Mutation Database. http://www.molgen.ua.ac.be/ADMutations

Alzheimer Research Forum. http://www.alzforum.org

Amada N, Aihara K, Ravid R, and Horie M (2005) Reduction of NR1 and phosphorylated Ca^{2+}/calmodulin-dependent protein kinase II levels in Alzheimer's disease. *Neuroreport* 16: 1809–1813.

Andorfer C, Acker CM, Kress Y, Hof PR, Duff K, and Davies P (2005) Cell-cycle reentry and cell death in transgenic mice expressing nonmutant human tau isoforms. *J. Neurosci.* 25: 5446–5454.

Andrasfalvy BK and Magee JC (2001) Distance-dependent increase in AMPA receptor number in the dendrites of adult hippocampal CA1 pyramidal neurons. *J. Neurosci.* 21: 9151–9159.

Angelo M, Plattner F, and Giese KP (2006) Cyclin-dependent kinase 5 in synaptic plasticity, learning and memory. *J. Neurochem.* 99: 353–370.

Angulo E, Noe V, Casado V, et al. (2004) Up-regulation of the Kv3.4 potassium channel subunit in early stages of Alzheimer's disease. *J. Neurochem.* 91: 547–557.

Arai H, Terajima M, Miura M, et al. (1995) Tau in cerebrospinal fluid: A potential diagnostic marker in Alzheimer's disease. *Ann. Neurol.* 38: 649–652.

Arendt T, Stieler J, Strijkstra AM, et al. (2003) Reversible paired helical filament-like phosphorylation of tau is an adaptive process associated with neuronal plasticity in hibernating animals. *J. Neurosci.* 23: 6972–6981.

Arriagada PV, Growdon JH, Hedley-Whyte ET, and Hyman BT (1992) Neurofibrillary tangles but not senile plaques parallel duration and severity of Alzheimer's disease. *Neurology* 42: 631–639.

Augustinack JC, Schneider A, Mandelkow EM, and Hyman BT (2002) Specific tau phosphorylation sites correlate with severity of neuronal cytopathology in Alzheimer's disease. *Acta Neuropathol. (Berl.)* 103: 26–35.

Augustine GJ, Santamaria F, and Tanaka K (2003) Local calcium signaling in neurons. *Neuron* 40: 331–346.

Auld DS, Kornecook TJ, Bastianetto S, and Quirion R (2002) Alzheimer's disease and the basal forebrain cholinergic system: Relations to β-amyloid peptides, cognition, and treatment strategies. *Prog. Neurobiol.* 68: 209–245.

Avila J, Lucas JJ, Pérez M, and Hernández F (2004) Role of tau protein in both physiological and pathological conditions. *Physiol. Rev.* 84: 361–384.

Baki L, Shioi J, Wen P, et al. (2004) PS1 activates PI3K thus inhibiting GSK-3 activity and tau overphosphorylation: Effects of FAD mutations. *EMBO J.* 23: 2586–2596.

Bales KR, Verina R, Dodel RC, et al. (1997) Lack of apolipoprotein E dramatically reduces amyloid β-peptide deposition. *Nat. Genet.* 17: 263–264.

Bardo S, Cavazzini MG, and Emptage N (2006) The role of the endoplasmic reticulum Ca^{2+} store in the plasticity of central neurons. *Trends Pharmacol. Sci.* 27: 78–84.

Bare DJ, Kettlun CS, Liang M, Bers DM, and Mignery GA (2005) Cardiac type 2 inositol 1,4,5-trisphosphate receptor: Interaction and modulation by calcium/calmodulin-dependent protein kinase II. *J. Biol. Chem.* 280: 15912–15920.

Barghorn S, Nimmrich V, Striebinger A, et al. (2005) Globular amyloid β-peptide$_{1-42}$ oligomer – A homogenous and stable neuropathological protein in Alzheimer's disease. *J. Neurochem.* 95: 834–847.

Bath KG and Lee FS (2006) Variant BDNF (Val66Met) impact on brain structure and function. *Cogn. Affect. Behav. Neurosci.* 6: 79–85.

Battaini F and Pascale A (2005) Protein kinase C signal transduction regulation in physiological and pathological aging. *Ann. N.Y. Acad. Sci.* 1057: 177–192.

Battaini F, Pascale A, Lucchi L, Pasinetti GM, and Govoni S (1999) Protein kinase C anchoring deficit in postmortem brains of Alzheimer's disease patients. *Exp. Neurol.* 159: 559–564.

Beffert U, Weeber EJ, Durudas A, et al. (2005) Modulation of synaptic plasticity and memory by Reelin involves differential splicing of the lipoprotein receptor Apoer2. *Neuron* 47: 567–579.

Bell KA, O'Riordan KJ, Sweatt JD, and Dineley KT (2004) MAPK recruitment by β-amyloid in organotypic hippocampal slice cultures depends on physical state and exposure time. *J. Neurochem.* 91: 349–361.

Berridge MJ, Bootman MD, and Roderick HL (2003) Calcium signalling: Dynamics, homeostasis and remodelling. *Nat. Rev. Mol. Cell Biol.* 4: 517–529.

Bertram L, McQueen MB, Mullin K, Blacker D, and Tanzi RE (2007) Systematic meta-analyses of Alzheimer disease genetic association studies: The AlzGene database. *Nat. Genet.* 39: 17–23.

Bertram L and Tanzi RE (2004) The current status of Alzheimer's disease genetics: What do we tell the patients? *Pharmacol. Res.* 50: 385–396.

Bhaskar K, Yen SH, and Lee G (2005) Disease-related modifications in tau affect the interaction between Fyn and Tau. *J. Biol. Chem.* 280: 35119–35125.

Biernat J and Mandelkow E-M (1999) The development of cell processes induced by tau protein requires phosphorylation of serine 262 and 356 in the repeat domain and is inhibited by phosphorylation in the proline-rich domains. *Mol. Biol. Cell* 10: 727–740.

Biernat J, Wu Y-Z, Timm T, et al. (2002) Protein kinase MARK/PAR-1 is required for neurite outgrowth and establishment of neuronal polarity. *Mol. Biol. Cell* 13: 4013–4028.

Birnbaum SG, Varga AW, Yuan LL, Anderson AE, Sweatt JD, and Schrader LA (2004) Structure and function of Kv4-family transient potassium channels. *Physiol. Rev.* 84: 803–833.

Bitan G, Vollers SS, and Teplow DB (2003) Elucidation of primary structure elements controlling early amyloid β-protein oligomerization. *J. Biol. Chem.* 278: 34882–34889.

Blasko I, Beer R, Bigl M, et al. (2004) Experimental traumatic brain injury in rats stimulates the expression, production and activity of Alzheimer's disease β-secretase (BACE-1). *J. Neural Transm.* 111: 523–536.

Blennow K, de Leon MJ, and Zetterberg H (2006) Alzheimer's disease. *Lancet* 368: 387–403.

Blennow K and Hampel H (2003) CSF markers for incipient Alzheimer's disease. *Lancet Neurol.* 2: 605–613.

Blitzer RD, Connor JH, Brown GP, et al. (1998) Gating of CaMKII by cAMP-regulated protein phosphatase activity during LTP. *Science* 280: 1940–1942.

Blum R and Konnerth A (2005) Neurotrophin-mediated rapid signaling in the central nervous system: Mechanisms and functions. *Physiology (Bethesda)* 20: 70–78.

Boehm J, Kang MG, Johnson RC, Esteban J, Huganir RL, and Malinow R (2006) Synaptic incorporation of AMPA receptors during LTP is controlled by a PKC phosphorylation site on GluR1. *Neuron* 51: 213–225.

Boekhoorn K, Terwel D, Biemans B, et al. (2006) Improved long-term potentiation and memory in young tau-P301L transgenic mice before onset of hyperphosphorylation and tauopathy. *J. Neurosci.* 26: 3514–3523.

Bolshakov VY, Carboni L, Cobb MH, Siegelbaum SA, and Belardetti F (2000) Dual MAP kinase pathways mediate opposing forms of long-term plasticity at CA3-CA1 synapses. *Nat. Neurosci.* 3: 1107–1112.

Borchelt DR, Thinakaran G, Eckman CB, et al. (1996) Familial Alzheimer's disease-linked presenilin 1 variants elevate Aβ 1-42/1-40 ratio *in vitro* and *in vivo*. *Neuron* 17: 1005–1013.

Bortolotto ZA and Collingridge GL (2000) A role for protein kinase C in a form of metaplasticity that regulates the induction of long-term potentiation at CA1 synapses of the adult rat hippocampus. *Eur. J. Neurosci.* 12: 4055–4062.

Botella-López A, Burgaya F, Gavin R, et al. (2006) Reelin expression and glycosylation patterns are altered in Alzheimer's disease. *Proc. Natl. Acad. Sci. USA* 103: 5573–5578.

Braak H and Braak E (1991) Neuropathological stageing of Alzheimer-related changes. *Acta Neuropathol.* 82: 239–259.

Bradley J and Finkbeiner S (2002) An evaluation of specificity in activity-dependent gene expression in neurons. *Prog. Neurobiol.* 67: 469–477.

Brady DR and Mufson EJ (1997) Parvalbumin-immunoreactive neurons in the hippocampal formation of Alzheimer's diseased brain. *Neuroscience* 80: 1113–1125.

Braithwaite SP, Paul S, Nairn AC, and Lombroso PJ (2006) Synaptic plasticity: One STEP at a time. *Trends Neurosci.* 29: 452–458.

Bramham CR and Messaoudi E (2005) BDNF function in adult synaptic plasticity: The synaptic consolidation hypothesis. *Prog. Neurobiol.* 76: 99–125.

Brecht WJ, Harris FM, Chang S, et al. (2004) Neuron-specific apolipoprotein E4 proteolysis is associated with increased tau phosphorylation in brains of transgenic mice. *J. Neurosci.* 24: 2527–2534.

Bredt DS and Nicoll RA (2003) AMPA receptor trafficking at excitatory synapses. *Neuron* 40: 361–379.

Brorson JR, Bindokas VP, Iwama T, Marcuccilli CJ, Chisholm JC, and Miller RJ (1995) The Ca2+ influx induced by β-amyloid peptide 25–35 in cultured hippocampal neurons results from network excitation. *J. Neurobiol.* 26: 325–338.

Buckner RL (2004) Memory and executive function in aging and AD: Multiple factors that cause decline and reserve factors that compensate. *Neuron* 44: 195–208.

Buckner RL, Snyder AZ, Shannon BJ, et al. (2005) Molecular, structural, and functional characterization of Alzheimer's disease: Evidence for a relationship between default activity, amyloid, and memory. *J. Neurosci.* 25: 7709–7717.

Burghaus L, Schutz U, Krempel U, et al. (2000) Quantitative assessment of nicotinic acetylcholine receptor proteins in the cerebral cortex of Alzheimer patients. *Brain Res. Mol. Brain Res.* 76: 385–388.

Burke SN, Chawla MK, Penner MR, et al. (2005) Differential encoding of behavior and spatial context in deep and superficial layers of the neocortex. *Neuron* 45: 667–674.

Buttini M, Akeefe H, Lin C, et al. (2000) Dominant negative effects of apolipoprotein E4 revealed in transgenic models of neurodegenerative disease. *Neuroscience* 97: 207–210.

Buttini M, Orth M, Bellosta S, et al. (1999) Expression of human apolipoprotein E3 or E4 in the brains of *Apoe*$^{-/-}$ mice: Isoform-specific effects on neurodegeneration. *J. Neurosci.* 19: 4867–4880.

Buttini M, Yu G-Q, Shockley K, et al. (2002) Modulation of Alzheimer-like synaptic and cholinergic deficits in transgenic mice by human apolipoprotein E depends on isoform, aging, and overexpression of amyloid β peptides but not on plaque formation. *J. Neurosci.* 22: 10539–10548.

Cao XW and Südhof TC (2001) A transcriptively active complex of APP with Fe65 and histone acetyltransferase Tip60. *Science* 293: 115–120.

Cao X and Südhof TC (2004) Dissection of amyloid-β precursor protein-dependent transcriptional transactivation. *J. Biol. Chem.* 279: 24601–24611.

Cardoso SM and Oliveira CR (2005) The role of calcineurin in amyloid-β-peptides-mediated cell death. *Brain Res. Mol. Brain Res.* 1050: 1–7.

Carlisle HJ and Kennedy MB (2005) Spine architecture and synaptic plasticity. *Trends Neurosci.* 28: 182–187.

Carter TL, Rissman RA, Mishizen-Eberz AJ, et al. (2004) Differential preservation of AMPA receptor subunits in the hippocampi of Alzheimer's disease patients according to Braak stage. *Exp. Neurol.* 187: 299–309.

Caselli RJ, Graff-Radford NR, Reiman M, et al. (1999) Preclinical memory decline in cognitively normal apolipoprotein E-ε4 homozygotes. *Neurology* 53: 201–207.

Caselli RJ, Reiman EM, Osborne D, et al. (2004) Longitudinal changes in cognition and behavior in asymptomatic carriers of the APOE ε4 allele. *Neurology* 62: 1990–1995.

Celio MR (1990) Calbindin D-28k and parvalbumin in the rat nervous system. *Neuroscience* 35: 375–475.

Chan SL, Griffin WST, and Mattson MP (1999) Evidence for caspase-mediated cleavage of AMPA receptor subunits in neuronal apoptosis and Alzheimer's disease. *J. Neurosci. Res.* 57: 315–323.

Chan SL, Mayne M, Holden CP, Geiger JD, and Mattson MP (2000) Presenilin-1 mutations increase levels of ryanodine receptors and calcium release in PC12 cells and cortical neurons. *J. Biol. Chem.* 275: 18195–18200.

Chandra S, Fornai F, Kwon H-B, et al. (2004) Double-knockout mice for α- and β-synucleins: Effect on synaptic functions. *Proc. Natl. Acad. Sci. USA* 101: 14966–14971.

Chang EH, Savage MJ, Flood DG, et al. (2006) AMPA receptor downscaling at the onset of Alzheimer's disease pathology in double knockin mice. *Proc. Natl. Acad. Sci. USA* 103: 3410–3415.

Cheng IH, Scearce-Levie K, Legleiter J, Palop JJ, Gerstein H, Bien-Ly N, Puolivali J, Lesné S, Ashe KH, Muchowski PJ, Mucke L. (2007) Accelerating amyloid-beta fibrillization reduces oligomer levels and functional deficits in Alzheimer disease mouse models. *J. Biol. Chem.* 282(33): 23818–28.

Chen C (2005) β-Amyloid increases dendritic Ca^{2+} influx by inhibiting the A-type K^+ current in hippocampal CA1 pyramidal neurons. *Biochem. Biophys. Res. Commun.* 338: 1913–1919.

Chen J, Zhou Y, Mueller-Steiner S, et al. (2005a) SIRT1 protects against microglia-dependent amyloid-β toxicity through inhibiting NF-κB signaling. *J. Biol. Chem.* 280: 40364–40374.

Chen Q, Reis SE, Kammerer CM, et al. WISE Study Group (2003) APOE polymorphism and angiographic coronary artery disease severity in the Women's Ischemia Syndrome Evaluation (WISE) study. *Atherosclerosis* 169: 159–167.

Chen QS, Kagan BL, Hirakura Y, and Xie CW (2000) Impairment of hippocampal long-term potentiation by Alzheimer amyloid β-peptides. *J. Neurosci. Res.* 60: 65–72.

Chen QS, Wei WZ, Shimahara T, and Xie CW (2002) Alzheimer amyloid β-peptide inhibits the late phase of long-term potentiation through calcineurin-dependent mechanisms in the hippocampal dentate gyrus. *Neurobiol. Learn. Mem.* 77: 354–371.

Chen Y, Beffert U, Ertunc M, et al. (2005b) Reelin modulates NMDA receptor activity in cortical neurons. *J. Neurosci.* 25: 8209–8216.

Cheung ZH, Fu AK, and Ip NY (2006) Synaptic roles of Cdk5: Implications in higher cognitive functions and neurodegenerative diseases. *Neuron* 50: 13–18.

Cheung ZH and Ip NY (2004) Cdk5: Mediator of neuronal death and survival. *Neurosci. Lett.* 361: 47–51.

Chin J, Massaro C, Palop J, Thwin M, et al. (2007) Reelin depletion in the entorhinal cortex of human amyloid precursor protein transgenic mice and humans with Alzheimer's disease. *J. Neurosci.* 27: 2727–2733.

Chin J, Palop JJ, Puoliväli J, et al. (2005) Fyn kinase induces synaptic and cognitive impairments in a transgenic mouse model of Alzheimer's disease. *J. Neurosci.* 25: 9694–9703.

Chin J, Palop JJ, Yu G-Q, Kojima N, Masliah E, and Mucke L (2004) Fyn kinase modulates synaptotoxicity, but not aberrant sprouting, in human amyloid precursor protein transgenic mice. *J. Neurosci.* 24: 4692–4697.

Chiou WF (2006) Effect of Aβ exposure on the mRNA expression patterns of voltage-sensitive calcium channel α_1 subunits (α_{1A}-α_{1D}) in human SK-N-SH neuroblastoma. *Neurochem. Int.* 49: 256–261.

Choi D-S, Wang D, Yu G-Q, et al. (2006) PKC epsilon increases endothelin converting enzyme activity and reduces amyloid plaque pathology in transgenic mice. *Proc. Natl. Acad. Sci. USA* 103: 8215–8220.

Chowdhury S, Shepherd JD, Okuno H, et al. (2006) Arc/Arg3.1 interacts with the endocytic machinery to regulate AMPA receptor trafficking. *Neuron* 52: 445–459.

Chung HJ, Xia J, Scannevin RH, Zhang X, and Huganir RL (2000) Phosphorylation of the AMPA receptor subunit GluR2 differentially regulates its interaction with PDZ domain-containing proteins. *J. Neurosci.* 20: 7258–7267.

Citron M (2004) Strategies for disease modification in Alzheimer's disease. *Nat. Rev. Neurosci.* 5: 677–685.

Cleary JP, Walsh DM, Hofmeister JJ, et al. (2005) Natural oligomers of the amyloid-β protein specifically disrupt cognitive function. *Nat. Neurosci.* 8: 79–84.

Cleveland DW, Hwo SY, and Kirschner MW (1977) Purification of tau, a microtubule-associated protein that induces assembly of microtubules from purified tubulin. *J. Mol. Biol.* 116: 207–225.

Colbran RJ and Brown AM (2004) Calcium/calmodulin-dependent protein kinase II and synaptic plasticity. *Curr. Opin. Neurobiol.* 14: 318–327.

Cole G, Dobkins KR, Hansen LA, Terry RD, and Saitoh T (1988) Decreased levels of protein kinase C in Alzheimer brain. *Brain Res.* 452: 165–174.

Corder EH, Saunders AM, Strittmatter WJ, et al. (1993) Gene dose of apolipoprotein E type 4 allele and the risk of Alzheimer's disease in late onset families. *Science* 261: 921–923.

Cotman CW, Poon WW, Rissman RA, and Blurton-Jones M (2005) The role of caspase cleavage of tau in Alzheimer disease neuropathology. J. Neuropathol. *Exp. Neurol.* 64: 104–112.

Croll SD, Suri C, Compton DL, et al. (1999) Brain-derived neurotrophic factor transgenic mice exhibit passive avoidance deficits, increased seizure severity and *in vitro* hyperexcitability in the hippocampus and entorhinal cortex. *Neuroscience* 93: 1491–1506.

Cruz JC, Kim D, Moy LY, et al. (2006) p25/cyclin-dependent kinase 5 induces production and intraneuronal accumulation of amyloid β *in vivo*. *J. Neurosci.* 26: 10536–10541.

Cruz JC and Tsai LH (2004) Cdk5 deregulation in the pathogenesis of Alzheimer's disease. *Trends Mol. Med.* 10: 452–458.

Cruz JC, Tseng HC, Goldman JA, Shih H, and Tsai LH (2003) Aberrant Cdk5 activation by p25 triggers pathological events leading to neurodegeneration and neurofibrillary tangles. *Neuron* 40: 471–483.

Cui J, Matkovich SJ, deSouza N, Li S, Rosemblit N, and Marks AR (2004) Regulation of the type 1 inositol 1,4,5-trisphosphate receptor by phosphorylation at tyrosine 353. *J. Biol. Chem.* 279: 16311–16316.

Cullen WK, Wu JQ, Anwyl R, and Rowan MJ (1996) beta-amyloid produces a delayed NMDA receptor-dependent reduction in synaptic transmission in rat hippocampus. *Neuroreport* 8: 87–92.

D'Arcangelo G, Homayouni R, Keshvara L, Rice DS, Sheldon M, and Curran T (1999) Reelin is a ligand for lipoprotein receptors. *Neuron* 24: 471–479.

Dahlgren KN, Manelli AM, Stine WB, Jr., Baker LK, Krafft GA, and LaDu MJ (2002) Oligomeric and fibrillar species of amyloid-β peptides differentially affect neuronal viability. *J. Biol. Chem.* 277: 32046–32053.

Dani JA and Bertrand D (2006) Nicotinic acetylcholine receptors and nicotinic cholinergic mechanisms of the central nervous system. *Annu. Rev. Pharmacol. Toxicol.* 47: 699–729.

Davis GW (2006) Homeostatic control of neural activity: From phenomenology to molecular design. *Annu. Rev. Neurosci.* 29: 307–323.

Davis S and Laroche S (2006) Mitogen-activated protein kinase/ extracellular regulated kinase signalling and memory stabilization: A review. *Genes Brain Behav.* 5(supplement 2): 61–72.

Dawson GR, Seabrook GR, Zheng H, et al. (1999) Age-related cognitive deficits, impaired long-term potentiation and reduction in synaptic marker density in mice lacking the β-amyloid precursor protein. *Neuroscience* 90: 1–13.

Dawson HN, Ferreira A, Eyster MV, Ghoshal N, Binder LI, and Vitek MP (2001) Inhibition of neuronal maturation in primary hippocampal neurons from tau deficient mice. *J. Cell Sci.* 114: 1179–1187.

De Strooper B, Saftig P, Craessaerts K, et al. (1998) Deficiency of presenilin-1 inhibits the normal cleavage of amyloid precursor protein. *Nature* 391: 387–390.

Dehmelt L and Halpain S (2005) The MAP2/Tau family of microtubule-associated proteins. *Genome Biol.* 6: 204.

Deisseroth K, Mermelstein PG, Xia H, and Tsien RW (2003) Signaling from synapse to nucleus: The logic behind the mechanisms. *Curr. Opin. Neurobiol.* 13: 354–365.

Derkinderen P, Scales TME, Hanger DP, et al. (2005) Tyrosine 394 is phosphorylated in Alzheimer's paired helical filament tau and in fetal tau with c-Abl as the candidate tyrosine kinase. *J. Neurosci.* 25: 6584–6593.

Dickey CA, Gordon MN, Mason JE, et al. (2004) Amyloid suppresses induction of genes critical for memory consolidation in APP + PS1 transgenic mice. *J. Neurochem.* 88: 434–442.

Dineley KT, Bell KA, Bui D, and Sweatt JD (2002) β-amyloid peptide activates α7 nicotinic acetylcholine receptors expressed in *Xenopus* oocytes. *J. Biol. Chem.* 277: 25056–25061.

Dineley KT, Westerman M, Bui D, Bell K, Ashe KH, and Sweatt JD (2001) β-Amyloid activates the mitogen-activated protein kinase cascade via hippocampal α7 nicotinic acetylcholine receptors: *In vitro* and *in vivo* mechanisms related to Alzheimer's disease. *J. Neurosci.* 21: 4125–4133.

Dodart JC, Bales KR, Gannon KS, et al. (2002) Immunization reverses memory deficits without reducing brain Aβ burden in Alzheimer's disease model. *Nat. Neurosci.* 5: 452–457.

Doglio LE, Kanwar R, Jackson GR, et al. (2006) γ–Cleavage-independent functions of presenilin, nicastrin, and Aph-1 regulate cell-junction organization and prevent tau toxicity *in vivo*. *Neuron* 50: 359–375.

Dong E, Caruncho H, Liu WS, et al. (2003) A reelin-integrin receptor interaction regulates Arc mRNA translation in synaptoneurosomes. *Proc. Natl. Acad. Sci. USA* 100: 5479–5484.

Dougherty JJ, Wu J, and Nichols RA (2003) beta;-amyloid regulation of presynaptic nicotinic receptors in rat hippocampus and neocortex. *J. Neurosci.* 23: 6740–6747.

Drewes G, Ebneth A, Preuss U, Mandelkow E-M, and Mandelkow E (1997) MARK, a novel family of protein kinases that phosphorylate microtubule-associated proteins and trigger microtubule disruption. *Cell* 89: 297–308.

Ebneth A, Godemann R, Stamer K, et al. (1998) Overexpression of tau protein inhibits kinesin-dependent trafficking of vesicles, mitochondria, and endoplasmic reticulum: Implications for Alzheimer's disease. *J. Cell Biol.* 143: 777–794.

Edbauer D, Winkler E, Regula JT, Pesold B, Steiner H, and Haass C (2003) Reconstitution of γ-secretase activity. *Nat. Cell Biol.* 5: 486–488.

Ehrengruber MU, Kato A, Inokuchi K, and Hennou S (2004) Homer/Vesl proteins and their roles in CNS neurons. *Mol. Neurobiol.* 29: 213–227.

Ekinci FJ, Malik KU, and Shea TB (1999) Activation of the L voltage-sensitive calcium channel by mitogen-activated protein (MAP) kinase following exposure of neuronal cells to beta-amyloid – Map kinase mediates beta-amyloid-induced neurodegeneration. *J. Biol. Chem.* 274: 30322–30327.

English JD and Sweatt JD (1997) A requirement for the mitogen-activated protein kinase cascade in hippocampal long term potentiation. *J. Biol. Chem.* 272: 19103–19106.

Ertekin-Taner N, Allen M, Fadale D, et al. (2004) Genetic variants in a haplotype block spanning IDE are significantly associated with plasma Aβ42 levels and risk for Alzheimer disease. *Hum. Mutat.* 23: 334–342.

Esposito L, Raber J, Kekonius L, et al. (2006) Reduction in mitochondrial superoxide dismutase modulates Alzheimer's disease-like pathology and accelerates the onset of behavioral changes in human amyloid precursor protein transgenic mice. *J. Neurosci.* 26: 5167–5179.

Esteban JA (2003) AMPA receptor trafficking: A road map for synaptic plasticity. *Mol. Interv.* 3: 375–385.

Etcheberrigaray R, Ito E, Kim CS, and Alkon DL (1994) Soluble β-amyloid induction of Alzheimer's phenotype for human fibroblast K+ channels. *Science* 264: 276–279.

Etcheberrigaray R, Ito E, Oka K, Tofel-Grehl B, Gibson GE, and Alkon DL (1993) Potassium channel dysfunction in fibroblasts identifies patients with Alzheimer disease. *Proc. Natl. Acad. Sci. USA* 90: 8209–8213.

Etcheberrigaray R, Tan M, Dewachter I, et al. (2004) Therapeutic effects of PKC activators in Alzheimer's disease transgenic mice. *Proc. Natl. Acad. Sci. USA* 101: 11141–11146.

Fabian-Fine R, Skehel P, Errington ML, et al. (2001) Ultrastructural distribution of the α7 nicotinic acetylcholine receptor subunit in rat hippocampus. *J. Neurosci.* 21: 7993–8003.

Farrer LA, Cupples LA, Haines JL, et al. (1997) Effects of age, sex, and ethnicity on the association between apolipoprotein E genotype and Alzheimer disease. A meta-analysis. *JAMA* 278: 1349–1356.

Fatemi SH (2005) Reelin glycoprotein: Structure, biology and roles in health and disease. *Mol. Psychiatry* 10: 251–257.

Fenster CP, Whitworth TL, Sheffield EB, Quick MW, and Lester RA (1999) Upregulation of surface $\alpha 4\beta 2$ nicotinic receptors is initiated by receptor desensitization after chronic exposure to nicotine. *J. Neurosci.* 19: 4804–4814.

Fernandez-Alfonso T and Ryan TA (2006) The efficiency of the synaptic vesicle cycle at central nervous system synapses. *Trends Cell Biol.* 16: 413–420.

Ferri CP, Prince M, Brayne C, et al. (2005) Global prevalence of dementia: A Delphi consensus study. *Lancet* 366: 2112–2117.

Fischer A, Sananbenesi F, Pang PT, Lu B, and Tsai LH (2005) Opposing roles of transient and prolonged expression of p25 in synaptic plasticity and hippocampus-dependent memory. *Neuron* 48: 825–838.

Fonseca M and Soriano E (1995) Calretinin-immunoreactive neurons in the normal human temporal cortex and in Alzheimer's disease. *Brain Res.* 691: 83–91.

Fortin DL, Nemani VM, Voglmaier SM, Anthony MD, Ryan TA, and Edwards RH (2005) Neural activity controls the synaptic accumulation of α-synuclein. *J. Neurosci.* 25: 10913–10921.

Fu H, Li W, Lao Y, et al. (2006) Bis(7)-tacrine attenuates β amyloid-induced neuronal apoptosis by regulating L-type calcium channels. *J. Neurochem.* 98: 1400–1410.

Galvan V, Chen S, Lu D, et al. (2002) Caspase cleavage of members of the amyloid precursor family of proteins. *J. Neurochem.* 82: 283–294.

Galvan V, Gorostiza OF, Banwait S, et al. (2006) Reversal of Alzheimer's-like pathology and behavior in human APP transgenic mice by mutation of Asp664. *Proc. Natl. Acad. Sci. USA* 103: 7130–7135.

Games D, Adams D, Alessandrini R, et al. (1995) Alzheimer-type neuropathology in transgenic mice overexpressing V717F β-amyloid precursor protein. *Nature* 373: 523–527.

Geerts H and Grossberg GT (2006) Pharmacology of acetylcholinesterase inhibitors and *N*-methyl-D-aspartate receptors for combination therapy in the treatment of Alzheimer's disease. *J. Clin. Pharmacol.* 46: 8S–16S.

Gervais FG, Xu D, Robertson GS, et al. (1999) Involvement of caspases in proteolytic cleavage of Alzheimer's amyloid-β precursor protein and amyloidogenic Aβ peptide formation. *Cell* 97: 395–406.

Giannakopoulos P, Gold G, Kövari E, et al. (2007) Assessing the cognitive impact of Alzheimer disease pathology and vascular burden in the aging brain: The Geneva experience. *Acta Neuropathol. (Berl.)* 113: 1–12.

Giese KP, Ris L, and Plattner F (2005) Is there a role of the cyclin-dependent kinase 5 activator p25 in Alzheimer's disease? *Neuroreport* 16: 1725–1730.

Glabe CG and Kayed R (2006) Common structure and toxic function of amyloid oligomers implies a common mechanism of pathogenesis. *Neurology* 66: S74–78.

Glenner GG and Wong CW (1984) Alzheimer's disease: Initial report of the purification and characterization of a novel cerebrovascular amyloid protein. *Biochem. Biophys. Res. Commun.* 120: 885–890.

Goate A, Chartier-Harlin M-C, Mullan M, et al. (1991) Segregation of a missense mutation in the amyloid precursor protein gene with familial Alzheimer's disease. *Nature* 349: 704–706.

Gong B, Cao Z, Zheng P, et al. (2006) Ubiquitin hydrolase Uch-L1 rescues β-amyloid-induced decreases in synaptic function and contextual memory. *Cell* 126: 775–788.

Gong B, Vitolo OV, Trinchese F, Liu S, Shelanski M, and Arancio O (2004) Persistent improvement in synaptic and cognitive functions in an Alzheimer mouse model after rolipram treatment. *J. Clin. Invest.* 114: 1624–1634.

Gong CX, Liu F, Grundke-Iqbal I, and Iqbal K (2005) Post-translational modifications of tau protein in Alzheimer's disease. *J. Neural Transm.* 112: 813–838.

Good TA, Smith DO, and Murphy RM (1996) Beta-amyloid peptide blocks the fast-inactivating K^+ current in rat hippocampal neurons. *Biophys. J.* 70: 296–304.

Gotoh H, Okumura N, Yagi T, Okumura A, Shima T, and Nagai K (2006) Fyn-induced phosphorylation of β-adducin at tyrosine 489 and its role in their subcellular localization. *Biochem. Biophys. Res. Commun.* 346: 600–605.

Götz J, Chen F, van Dorpe J, and Nitsch RM (2001) Formation of neurofibrillary tangles in P301L tau transgenic mice induced by Aβ42 fibrils. *Science* 293: 1491–1495.

Grant SGN, O'Dell TJ, Karl KA, Stein PL, Soriano P, and Kandel ER (1992) Impaired long-term potentiation, spatial learning, and hippocampal development in *fyn* mutant mice. *Science* 258: 1903–1910.

Gregg RE, Zech LA, Schaefer EJ, Stark D, Wilson D, and Brewer HB, Jr. (1986) Abnormal *in vivo* metabolism of apolipoprotein E4 in humans. *J. Clin. Invest.* 78: 815–821.

Grootendorst J, Bour A, Vogel E, et al. (2005) Human apoE targeted replacement mouse lines: H-apoE4 and h-apoE3 mice differ on spatial memory performance and avoidance behavior. *Behav. Brain Res.* 159: 1–14.

Grundke-Iqbal I, Iqbal K, Quinlan M, Tung YC, Zaidi MS, and Wisniewski HM (1986) Microtubule-associated protein tau. A component of Alzheimer paired helical filaments. *J. Biol. Chem.* 261: 6084–6089.

Guan ZZ, Zhang X, Ravid R, and Nordberg A (2000) Decreased protein levels of nicotinic receptor subunits in the hippocampus and temporal cortex of patients with Alzheimer's disease. *J. Neurochem.* 74: 237–243.

Guillozet-Bongaarts AL, Garcia-Sierra F, Reynolds MR, et al. (2005) Tau truncation during neurofibrillary tangle evolution in Alzheimer's disease. *Neurobiol. Aging* 26: 1015–1022.

Guzowski JF (2002) Insights into immediate-early gene function in hippocampal memory consolidation using antisense oligonucleotide and fluorescent imaging approaches. *Hippocampus* 12: 86–104.

Guzowski JF, McNaughton BL, Barnes CA, and Worley PF (1999) Environment-specific expression of the immediate-early gene Arc in hippocampal neuronal ensembles. *Nat. Neurosci.* 2: 1120–1124.

Guzowski JF, Timlin JA, Roysam B, McNaughton BL, Worley PF, and Barnes CA (2005) Mapping behaviorally relevant neural circuits with immediate-early gene expression. *Curr. Opin. Neurobiol.* 15: 599–606.

Haddad JJ (2004) Mitogen-activated protein kinases and the evolution of Alzheimer's: A revolutionary neurogenetic axis for therapeutic intervention? *Prog. Neurobiol.* 73: 359–377.

Hall GF, Lee S, and Yao J (2002) Neurofibrillary degeneration can be arrested in an *in vivo* cellular model of human tauopathy by application of a compound which inhibits tau filament formation *in vitro*. *J. Mol. Neurosci.* 19: 251–260.

Hall GF, Lee VM, Lee G, and Yao J (2001) Staging of neurofibrillary degeneration caused by human tau overexpression in a unique cellular model of human tauopathy. *Am. J. Pathol.* 158: 235–246.

Hallman DM, Boerwinkle E, Saha N, et al. (1991) The apolipoprotein E polymorphism: A comparison of allele frequencies and effects in nine populations. *Am. J. Hum. Genet.* 49: 338–349.

Harada A, Oguchi K, Okabe S, et al. (1994) Altered microtubule organization in small-calibre axons of mice lacking *tau* protein. *Nature* 369: 488–491.

Hardy JA and Higgins GA (1992) Alzheimer's disease: The amyloid cascade hypothesis. *Science* 256: 184–185.

Harris F, Brecht WJ, Xu Q, et al. (2003) Carboxyl-terminal-truncated apolipoprotein E4 causes Alzheimer's disease-like neurodegeneration and behavioral deficits in transgenic mice. *Proc. Natl. Acad. Sci. USA* 100: 10966–10971.

Hartley DM, Walsh DM, Ye CP, et al. (1999) Protofibrillar intermediates of amyloid β-protein induce acute electrophysiological changes and progressive neurotoxicity in cortical neurons. *J. Neurosci.* 19: 8876–8884.

Hata R, Masumura M, Akatsu H, et al. (2001) Up-regulation of calcineurin Aβ mRNA in the Alzheimer's disease brain: Assessment by cDNA microarray. *Biochem. Biophys. Res. Commun.* 284: 310–316.

Hatters DM, Peters-Libeu CA, and Weisgraber KH (2006) Apolipoprotein E structure: Insights into function. *Trends Biochem. Sci.* 31: 445–454.

Hedou G and Mansuy IM (2003) Inducible molecular switches for the study of long-term potentiation. *Philos. Trans. R. Soc. Lond. B. Biol. Sci.* 358: 797–804.

Hellstrom-Lindahl E, Mousavi M, Zhang X, Ravid R, and Nordberg A (1999) Regional distribution of nicotinic receptor subunit mRNAs in human brain: Comparison between Alzheimer and normal brain. *Brain Res. Mol. Brain Res.* 66: 94–103.

Hensley K, Floyd RA, Zheng NY, et al. (1999) p38 kinase is activated in the Alzheimer's disease brain. *J. Neurochem.* 72: 2053–2058.

Herz J and Bock HH (2002) Lipoprotein receptors in the nervous system. *Annu. Rev. Biochem.* 71: 405–434.

Herz J and Chen Y (2006) Reelin, lipoprotein receptors and synaptic plasticity. *Nat. Rev. Neurosci.* 7: 850–859.

Hiesberger T, Trommsdorff M, Howell BW, et al. (1999) Direct binding of Reelin to VLDL receptor and ApoE receptor 2 induces tyrosine phosphorylation of disabled-1 and modulates tau phosphorylation. *Neuron* 24: 481–489.

Ho GJ, Hashimoto M, Adame A, et al. (2005) Altered p59Fyn kinase expression accompanies disease progression in Alzheimer's disease: Implications for its functional role. *Neurobiol. Aging* 26: 625–635.

Hock C, Heese K, Hulette C, Rosenberg C, and Otten U (2000) Region-specific neurotrophin imbalances in Alzheimer disease decreased levels of brain-derived neurotrophic factor and increased levels of nerve growth factor in hippocampus and cortical areas. *Arch. Neurol.* 57: 846–851.

Hof PR, Glezer II, Conde F, et al. (1999) Cellular distribution of the calcium-binding proteins parvalbumin, calbindin, and calretinin in the neocortex of mammals: Phylogenetic and developmental patterns. *J. Chem. Neuroanat.* 16: 77–116.

Hof PR, Nimchinsky EA, Celio MR, Bouras C, and Morrison JH (1993) Calretinin-immunoreactive neocortical interneurons are unaffected in Alzheimer's disease. *Neurosci. Lett.* 152: 145–148.

Hoffman DA, Magee JC, Colbert CM, and Johnston D (1997) K^+ channel regulation of signal propagation in dendrites of hippocampal pyramidal neurons. *Nature* 387: 869–875.

Holcomb L, Gordon MN, McGowan E, et al. (1998) Accelerated Alzheimer-type phenotype in transgenic mice carrying both mutant amyloid precursor protein and presenilin 1 transgenes. *Nat. Med.* 4: 97–100.

Holsinger RM, McLean CA, Beyreuther K, Masters CL, and Evin G (2002) Increased expression of the amyloid precursor β-secretase in Alzheimer's disease. *Ann. Neurol.* 51: 783–786.

Holtzman DM, Bales KR, Tenkova T, et al. (2000) Apolipoprotein E isoform-dependent amyloid deposition and neuritic degeneration in a mouse model of Alzheimer's disease. *Proc. Natl. Acad. Sci. USA* 97: 2892–2897.

Honer WG (2003) Pathology of presynaptic proteins in Alzheimer's disease: More than simple loss of terminals. *Neurobiol. Aging* 24: 1047–1062.

Hsia A, Masliah E, McConlogue L, et al. (1999) Plaque-independent disruption of neural circuits in Alzheimer's disease mouse models. *Proc. Natl. Acad. Sci. USA* 96: 3228–3233.

Hsieh H, Boehm J, Sato C, et al. (2006) AMPAR removal underlies Aβ-induced synaptic depression and dendritic spine loss. *Neuron* 52: 831–843.

Huang Y, Liu XQ, Wyss-Coray T, Brecht WJ, Sanan DA, and Mahley RW (2001) Apolipoprotein E fragments present in Alzheimer's disease brains induce neurofibrillary tangle-like intracellular inclusions in neurons. *Proc. Natl. Acad. Sci. USA* 98: 8838–8843.

Hussain I, Powell D, Howlett DR, et al. (1999) Identification of a novel aspartic protease (Asp 2) as β-secretase. *Mol. Cell. Neurosci.* 14: 419–427.

Hvalby O, Hemmings HC, Jr., Paulsen O, et al. (1994) Specificity of protein kinase inhibitor peptides and induction of long-term potentiation. *Proc. Natl. Acad. Sci. USA* 91: 4761–4765.

Hwang DY, Cho JS, Oh JH, et al. (2005) Early changes in behavior deficits, amyloid β-42 deposits and MAPK activation in doubly transgenic mice co-expressing NSE-controlled human mutant PS2 and APPsw. Cell. *Mol. Neurobiol.* 25: 881–898.

Iacopino AM and Christakos S (1990) Specific reduction of calcium-binding protein (28-kilodalton calbindin-D) gene expression in aging and neurodegenerative diseases. *Proc. Natl. Acad. Sci. USA* 87: 4078–4082.

Ikegami S, Harada A, and Hirokawa N (2000) Muscle weakness, hyperactivity, and impairment in fear conditioning in tau-deficient mice. *Neurosci. Lett.* 279: 129–132.

Illenberger S, Zheng-Fischhöfer Q, Preuss U, et al. (1998) The endogenous and cell cycle-dependent phosphorylation of tau protein in living cells: Implications for Alzheimer's disease. *Mol. Biol. Cell* 9: 1495–1512.

Impey S, Obrietan K, Wong ST, et al. (1998) Cross talk between ERK and PKA is required for Ca^{2+} stimulation of CREB-dependent transcription and ERK nuclear translocation. *Neuron* 21: 869–883.

Ingelsson M, Fukumoto H, Newell KL, et al. (2004) Early Abeta accumulation and progressive synaptic loss, gliosis, and tangle formation in AD brain. *Neurology* 62: 925–931.

Irizarry MC, McNamara M, Fedorchak K, Hsiao K, and Hyman BT (1997a) APP_{Sw} transgenic mice develop age-related Aβ deposits and neuropil abnormalities, but no neuronal loss in CA1. J. Neuropathol. *Exp. Neurol.* 56: 965–973.

Irizarry MC, Soriano F, McNamara M, et al. (1997b) Aβ deposition is associated with neuropil changes, but not with overt neuronal loss in the human amyloid precursor protein V717F (PDAPP) transgenic mouse. *J. Neurosci.* 17: 7053–7059.

Ishihara T, Hong M, Zhang B, et al. (1999) Age-dependent emergence and progression of a tauopathy in transgenic mice overexpressing the shortest human tau isoform. *Neuron* 24: 751–762.

Iwai A, Masliah E, Yoshimoto M, et al. (1995) The precursor protein of non-Aβ component of Alzheimer's disease amyloid is a presynaptic protein of the central nervous system. *Neuron* 14: 467–475.

Jacobsen JS, Reinhart P, and Pangalos MN (2005) Current concepts in therapeutic strategies targeting cognitive decline and disease modification in Alzheimer's disease. *NeuroRx* 2: 612–626.

Jarrett JT, Berger EP, and Lansbury JPT (1993) The carboxy terminus of the β amyloid protein is critical for the seeding of amyloid formation: Implications for the pathogenesis of Alzheimer's disease. *Biochemistry* 32: 4693–4697.

Jhamandas JH, Cho C, Jassar B, Harris K, MacTavish D, and Easaw J (2001) Cellular mechanisms for amyloid β-protein activation of rat cholinergic basal forebrain neurons. *J. Neurophysiol.* 86: 1312–1320.

Ji ZS, Mullendorff K, Cheng IH, Miranda RD, Huang Y, and Mahley RW (2006) Reactivity of apolipoprotein E4 and amyloid β peptide: Lysosomal stability and neurodegeneration. *J. Biol. Chem.* 281: 2683–2692.

Johnson GV and Bailey CD (2003) The p38 MAP kinase signaling pathway in Alzheimer's disease. *Exp. Neurol.* 183: 263–268.

Johnson GV and Stoothoff WH (2004) Tau phosphorylation in neuronal cell function and dysfunction. *J. Cell Sci.* 117: 5721–5729.

Kamal A, Stokin GB, Yang ZH, Xia CH, and Goldstein LSB (2000) Axonal transport of amyloid precursor protein is mediated by direct binding to the kinesin light chain subunit of kinesin-I. *Neuron* 28: 449–459.

Kamenetz F, Tomita T, Hsieh H, et al. (2003) APP processing and synaptic function. *Neuron* 37: 925–937.

Kandel ER (2001) Neuroscience – The molecular biology of memory storage: A dialogue between genes and synapses. *Science* 294: 1030–1038.

Kasri NN, Kocks SL, Verbert L, et al. (2006) Up-regulation of inositol 1,4,5-trisphosphate receptor type 1 is responsible for a decreased endoplasmic-reticulum Ca^{2+} content in presenilin double knock-out cells. *Cell Calcium* 40: 41–51.

Kavalali ET (2006) Synaptic vesicle reuse and its implications. *Neuroscientist* 12: 57–66.

Kayed R, Head E, Thompson JL, et al. (2003) Common structure of soluble amyloid oligomers implies common mechanism of pathogenesis. *Science* 300: 486–489.

Kayed R, Sokolov Y, Edmonds B, et al. (2004) Permeabilization of lipid bilayers is a common conformation-dependent activity of soluble amyloid oligomers in protein misfolding diseases. *J. Biol. Chem.* 279: 46363–46366.

Kelleher RJ, Govindarajan A, Jung HY, Kang H, and Tonegawa S (2004) Translational control by MAPK signaling in long-term synaptic plasticity and memory. *Cell* 116: 467–479.

Kelliher M, Fastbom J, Cowburn RF, et al. (1999) Alterations in the ryanodine receptor calcium release channel correlate with Alzheimer's disease neurofibrillary and β-amyloid pathologies. *Neuroscience* 92: 499–513.

Kelly BL and Ferreira A (2006) β-Amyloid-induced dynamin 1 degradation is mediated by *N*-methyl-D-aspartate receptors in hippocampal neurons. *J. Biol. Chem.* 281: 28079–28089.

Kelly BL, Vassar R, and Ferreira A (2005) β-amyloid-induced dynamin 1 depletion in hippocampal neurons. A potential mechanism for early cognitive decline in Alzheimer disease. *J. Biol. Chem.* 280: 31746–31753.

Kelly KM, Nadon NL, Morrison JH, Thibault O, Barnes CA, and Blalock EM (2006) The neurobiology of aging. *Neuroscientist* 68(supplement 1): S5–20.

Kemppainen NM, Aalto S, Wilson IA, et al. (2006) Voxel-based analysis of PET amyloid ligand [^{11}C]PIB uptake in Alzheimer disease. *Neurology* 67: 1575–1580.

Kennedy MJ and Ehlers MD (2006) Organelles and trafficking machinery for postsynaptic plasticity. *Annu. Rev. Neurosci.* 29: 325–362.

Kerr ML and Small DH (2005) Cytoplasmic domain of the β-amyloid protein precursor of Alzheimer's disease: Function, regulation of proteolysis, and implications for drug development. *J. Neurosci. Res.* 80: 151–159.

Khlistunova I, Biernat J, Wang Y, et al. (2006) Inducible expression of Tau repeat domain in cell models of tauopathy: Aggregation is toxic to cells but can be reversed by inhibitor drugs. *J. Biol. Chem.* 281: 1205–1214.

Khurana V, Lu Y, Steinhilb ML, Oldham S, Shulman JM, and Feany MB (2006) TOR-mediated cell-cycle activation causes neurodegeneration in a *Drosophila* tauopathy model. *Curr. Biol.* 16: 230–241.

Kim SH, Nairn AC, Cairns N, and Lubec G (2001) Decreased levels of ARPP-19 and PKA in brains of Down syndrome and Alzheimer's disease. *J. Neural Transm.* supplement: 263–272.

Kim SK, Park HJ, Hong HS, Baik EJ, Jung MW, and Mook-Jung I (2006) ERK1/2 is an endogenous negative regulator of the γ-secretase activity. *FASEB J.* 20: 157–159.

Klein WL, Krafft GA, and Finch CE (2001) Targeting small Aβ oligomers: The solution to an Alzheimer's disease conundrum. *Trends Neurosci.* 24: 219–224.

Klunk WE, Engler H, Nordberg A, et al. (2004) Imaging brain amyloid in Alzheimer's disease with Pittsburgh Compound-B. *Ann. Neurol.* 55: 306–319.

Klyubin I, Walsh DM, Lemere CA, et al. (2005) Amyloid β protein immunotherapy neutralizes Aβ oligomers that disrupt synaptic plasticity *in vivo*. *Nat. Med.* 11: 556–561.

Knowles RB, Wyart C, Buldyrev SV, et al. (1999) Plaque-induced neurite abnormalities: Implications for disruption of neural networks in Alzheimer's disease. *Proc. Natl. Acad. Sci. USA* 96: 5274–5279.

Kobayashi DT and Chen KS (2005) Behavioral phenotypes of amyloid-based genetically modified mouse models of Alzheimer's Disease. *Genes Brain Behav.* 4: 173–196.

Kojima N, Wang J, Mansuy IM, Grant SGN, Mayford M, and Kandel ER (1997) Rescuing impairment of long-term potentiation in fyn-deficient mice by introducing Fyn transgene. *Proc. Natl. Acad. Sci. USA* 94: 4761–4765.

Kosik KS, Joachim CL, and Selkoe DJ (1986) Microtubule-associated protein tau (τ) is a major antigenic component of paired helical filaments in Alzheimer disease. *Proc. Natl. Acad. Sci. USA* 83: 4044–4048.

Kotilinek LA, Bacskai B, Westerman M, et al. (2002) Reversible memory loss in a mouse transgenic model of Alzheimer's disease. *J. Neurosci.* 22: 6331–6335.

Krzywkowski P, Ghribi O, Gagné J, et al. (1999) Cholinergic systems and long-term potentiation in memory-impaired apolipoprotein E-deficient mice. *Neuroscience* 92: 1273–1286.

Kuo Y, Emmerling MR, Vigo-Pelfrey C, et al. (1996) Water-soluble Aβ (N–40, N–42) oligomers in normal and Alzheimer disease brains. *J. Biol. Chem.* 271: 4077–4081.

Kwok JB, Teber ET, Loy C, et al. (2004) Tau haplotypes regulate transcription and are associated with Parkinson's disease. *Ann. Neurol.* 55: 329–334.

Lacor PN, Buniel MC, Chang L, et al. (2004) Synaptic targeting by Alzheimer's-related amyloid beta oligomers. *J. Neurosci.* 24: 10191–10200.

Lacor PN, Grayson DR, Auta J, Sugaya I, Costa E, and Guidotti A (2000) Reelin secretion from glutamatergic neurons in culture is independent from neurotransmitter regulation. *Proc. Natl. Acad. Sci. USA* 97: 3556–3561.

LaFerla FM (2002) Calcium dyshomeostasis and intracellular signalling in Alzheimer's disease. *Nat. Rev. Neurosci.* 3: 862–872.

Lahteinen S, Pitkanen A, Koponen E, Saarelainen T, and Castren E (2003) Exacerbated status epilepticus and acute cell loss, but no changes in epileptogenesis, in mice with increased brain-derived neurotrophic factor signaling. *Neuroscience* 122: 1081–1092.

Lambert MP, Barlow AK, Chromy BA, et al. (1998) Diffusible, nonfibrillar ligands derived from $A\beta_{1-42}$ are potent central nervous system neurotoxins. *Proc. Natl. Acad. Sci. USA* 95: 6448–6453.

Lanz TA, Carter DB, and Merchant KM (2003) Dendritic spine loss in the hippocampus of young PDAPP and Tg2576 mice and its prevention by the ApoE2 genotype. *Neurobiol. Dis.* 13: 246–253.

Lavezzari G, McCallum J, Lee R, and Roche KW (2003) Differential binding of the AP-2 adaptor complex and PSD-95 to the C-terminus of the NMDA receptor subunit NR2B regulates surface expression. *Neuropharmacology* 45: 729–737.

Lee EB, Zhang B, Liu K, et al. (2005) BACE overexpression alters the subcellular processing of APP and inhibits Aβ deposition *in vivo*. *J. Cell Biol.* 168: 291–302.

Lee G (2005) Tau and src family tyrosine kinases. Biochim. *Biophys. Acta* 1739: 323–330.

Lee G, Newman ST, Gard DL, Band H, and Panchamoorthy G (1998) Tau interacts with src-family non-receptor tyrosine kinases. *J. Cell Sci.* 111(Pt 21): 3167–3177.

Lee G, Thangavel R, Sharma VM, et al. (2004) Phosphorylation of tau by fyn: Implications for Alzheimer's disease. *J. Neurosci.* 24: 2304–2312.

Lee KW, Im JY, Song JS, et al. (2006) Progressive neuronal loss and behavioral impairments of transgenic C57BL/6 inbred mice expressing the carboxy terminus of amyloid precursor protein. *Neurobiol. Dis.* 22: 10–24.

Lee KY, Clark AW, Rosales JL, Chapman K, Fung T, and Johnston RN (1999) Elevated neuronal Cdc2-like kinase activity in the Alzheimer disease brain. *Neurosci. Res.* 34: 21–29.

Lee VM, Balin BJ, Otvos L, Jr., and Trojanowski JQ (1991) A68: A major subunit of paired helical filaments and derivatized forms of normal Tau. *Science* 251: 675–678.

Leissring MA, Akbari Y, Fanger CM, Cahalan MD, Mattson MP, and LaFerla FM (2000) Capacitative calcium entry deficits and elevated luminal calcium content in mutant presenilin-1 knockin mice. *J. Cell Biol.* 149: 793–798.

Leissring MA, Murphy MP, Mead TR, et al. (2002) A physiologic signaling role for the γ-secretase-derived intracellular fragment of APP. *Proc. Natl. Acad. Sci. USA* 99: 4697–4702.

Lesné S, MTK, and Kotilinek L, et al. (2006) A specific amyloid-β protein assembly in the brain impairs memory. *Nature* 440: 352–357.

Levy-Lahad E, Wasco W, Poorkaj P, et al. (1995) Candidate gene for the chromosome 1 familial Alzheimer's disease locus. *Science* 269: 973–977.

Lewis J, Dickson DW, Lin WL, et al. (2001) Enhanced neurofibrillary degeneration in transgenic mice expressing mutant tau and APP. *Science* 293: 1487–1491.

Lewis J, McGowan E, Rockwood J, et al. (2000) Neurofibrillary tangles, amyotrophy and progressive motor disturbance in mice expressing mutant (P301L) tau protein. *Nat. Genet.* 25: 402–405.

Leyssen M, Ayaz D, Hébert SS, Reeve S, De Strooper B, and Hassan BA (2005) Amyloid precursor protein promotes post-developmental neurite arborization in the *Drosophila* brain. *EMBO J.* 24: 2944–2955.

Li BS, Sun MK, Zhang L, et al. (2001) Regulation of NMDA receptors by cyclin-dependent kinase-5. *Proc. Natl. Acad. Sci. USA* 98: 12742–12747.

Lian Q, Ladner CJ, Magnuson D, and Lee JM (2001) Selective changes of calcineurin (protein phosphatase 2B) activity in Alzheimer's disease cerebral cortex. *Exp. Neurol.* 167: 158–165.

Lilien J and Balsamo J (2005) The regulation of cadherin-mediated adhesion by tyrosine phosphorylation/dephosphorylation of β-catenin. *Curr. Opin. Cell Biol.* 17: 459–465.

Link W, Koniezko U, Kauselmann G, et al. (1995) Somatodendritic exprsesion of an immediate early gene is regulated by synaptic activity. *Proc. Natl. Acad. Sci. USA* 92: 5734–5738.

Liu F, Grundke-Iqbal I, Iqbal K, Oda Y, Tomizawa K, and Gong CX (2005) Truncation and activation of calcineurin A by calpain I in Alzheimer disease brain. *J. Biol. Chem.* 280: 37755–37762.

Liu Q-S, Kawai H, and Berg DK (2001a) Beta-amyloid peptide blocks the response of α7-containing nicotinic receptors on hippocampal neurons. *Proc. Natl. Acad. Sci. USA* 98: 4734–4739.

Liu SJ, Zhang JY, Li HL, et al. (2004) Tau becomes a more favorable substrate for GSK-3 when it is prephosphorylated by PKA in rat brain. *J. Biol. Chem.* 279: 50078–50088.

Liu WS, Pesold C, Rodriguez MA, et al. (2001b) Down-regulation of dendritic spine and glutamic acid decarboxylase 67 expressions in the reelin haploinsufficient heterozygous reeler mouse. *Proc. Natl. Acad. Sci. USA* 98: 3477–3482.

Lonze BE and Ginty DD (2002) Function and regulation of CREB family transcription factors in the nervous system. *Neuron* 35: 605–623.

Lu B (2003) BDNF and activity-dependent synaptic modulation. *Learn. Mem.* 10: 86–98.

Lu DC, Rabizadeh S, Chandra S, et al. (2000) A second cytotoxic proteolytic peptide derived from amyloid β-protein precursor. *Nat. Med.* 6: 397–404.

Lu DC, Shaked GM, Masliah E, Bredesen DE, and Koo EH (2003) Amyloid β protein toxicity mediated by the formation of amyloid-β protein precursor complexes. *Ann. Neurol.* 54: 781–789.

Lu WY, Xiong ZG, Lei S, et al. (1999) G-protein-coupled receptors act via protein kinase C and Src to regulate NMDA receptors. *Nat. Neurosci.* 2: 331–338.

Lucas JJ, Hernández F, Gómez-Ramos P, Morán MA, Hen R, and Avila J (2001) Decreased nuclear β-catenin, tau hyperphosphorylation and neurodegeneration in GSK-3β conditional transgenic mice. *EMBO J.* 20: 27–39.

Lupski JR (2006) Genome structural variation and sporadic disease traits. *Nat. Genet.* 38: 974–976.

Lustbader JW, Cirilli M, Lin C, et al. (2004) ABAD directly links Aβ to mitochondrial toxicity in Alzheimer's disease. *Science* 304: 448–452.

Lyford GL, Yamagata K, Kaufmann WE, et al. (1995) *Arc,* a growth factor and activity-regulated gene, encodes a novel cytoskeleton-associated protein that is enriched in neuronal dendrites. *Neuron* 14: 433–445.

Magloczky Z, Halasz P, Vajda J, Czirjak S, and Freund TF (1997) Loss of Calbindin-D_{28K} immunoreactivity from dentate granule cells in human temporal lobe epilepsy. *Neuroscience* 76: 377–385.

Mah VH, Eskin TA, Kazee AM, Lapham L, and Higgins GA (1992) In situ hybridization of calcium/calmodulin dependent protein kinase II and tau mRNAs; species differences and relative preservation in Alzheimer's disease. *Brain Res. Mol. Brain Res.* 12: 85–94.

Mahley RW (1988) Apolipoprotein E: Cholesterol transport protein with expanding role in cell biology. *Science* 240: 622–630.

Mahley RW and Rall SC, Jr. (2000) Apolipoprotein E: Far more than a lipid transport protein. *Annu. Rev. Genomics Hum. Genet.* 1: 507–537.

Mahley RW, Weisgraber KH, and Huang Y (2006) Apolipoprotein E4: A causative factor and therapeutic target in neuropathology, including Alzheimer's disease. *Proc. Natl. Acad. Sci. USA* 103: 5644–5651.

Malenka RC and Bear MF (2004) LTP and LTD: An embarrassment of riches. *Neuron* 44: 5–21.

Martins IJ, Hone E, Foster JK, et al. (2006) Apolipoprotein E, cholesterol metabolism, diabetes, and the convergence of risk factors for Alzheimer's disease and cardiovascular disease. *Mol. Psychiatry* 11: 721–736.

Masliah E, Abraham CR, Johnson W, et al. (1993) Synaptic alterations in the cortex of APP transgenic mice. *J. Neuropathol. Exp. Neurol.* 52: 307.

Masliah E, Iwai A, Mallory M, Uéda K, and Saitoh T (1996) Altered presynaptic protein NACP is associated with plaque formation and neurodegeneration in Alzheimer's disease. *Am. J. Pathol.* 148: 201–210.

Masliah E, Mallory M, Alford M, et al. (2001a) Altered expression of synaptic proteins occurs early during progression of Alzheimer's disease. *Neurology* 56: 127–129.

Masliah E, Mallory M, Alford M, Ge N, and Mucke L (1995a) Abnormal synaptic regeneration in hAPP695 transgenic and apoE knockout mice. In: Iqbal K, Mortimer J, Winblad B, and Wisniewski H (eds.) *Research Advances in Alzheimer's Disease and Related Disorders*, pp. 405–414. New York: John Wiley & Sons.

Masliah E, Mallory M, Ge N, Alford M, Veinbergs I, and Roses AD (1995b) Neurodegeneration in the central nervous system of apoE-deficient mice. *Exp. Neurol.* 136: 107–122.

Masliah E, Raber J, Alford M, et al. (1998) Amyloid protein precursor stimulates excitatory amino acid transport: Implications for roles in neuroprotection and pathogenesis. *J. Biol. Chem.* 273: 12548–12554.

Masliah E, Rockenstein E, Veinbergs I, et al. (2001b) β-Amyloid peptides enhance α-synuclein accumulation and neuronal deficits in a transgenic mouse model linking Alzheimer's disease and Parkinson's disease. *Proc. Natl. Acad. Sci. USA* 98: 12245–12250.

Mattson MP (1997) Cellular actions of β-amyloid precursor protein and its soluble and fibrillogenic derivatives. *Physiol. Rev.* 77: 1081–1132.

Mattson MP, Barger SW, Cheng B, Lieberburg I, Smith-Swintosky VL, and Rydel RE (1993) β-amyloid precursor protein metabolites and loss of neuronal Ca^{2+} homeostasis in Alzheimer's disease. *TINS* 16: 409–414.

Mattson MP and Chan SL (2003) Neuronal and glial calcium signaling in Alzheimer's disease. *Cell Calcium* 34: 385–397.

McCarron MO, Delong D, and Alberts MJ (1999) APOE genotype as a risk factor for ischemic cerebrovascular disease: A meta-analysis. *Neurology* 53: 1308–1311.

McGowan E, Eriksen J, and Hutton M (2006) A decade of modeling Alzheimer's disease in transgenic mice. *Trends Genet.* 22: 281–289.

McKee AC, Kosik KS, and Kowall NW (1991) Neuritic pathology and dementia in Alzheimer's disease. *Ann. Neurol.* 30: 156–165.

McLaurin J, Kierstead ME, Brown ME, et al. (2006) Cyclohexanehexol inhibitors of Aβ aggregation prevent and reverse Alzheimer phenotype in a mouse model. *Nat. Med.* 12: 801–808.

Mikkonen M, Alafuzoff I, Tapiola T, Soininen H, and Miettinen R (1999) Subfield- and layer-specific changes in parvalbumin, calretinin and calbindin-D28k immunoreactivity in the entorhinal cortex in Alzheimer's disease. *Neuroscience* 92: 515–532.

Molinari S, Battini R, Ferrari S, et al. (1996) Deficits in memory and hippocampal long-term potentiation in mice with reduced calbindin D_{28K} expression. *Proc. Natl. Acad. Sci. USA* 93: 8028–8033.

Moolman DL, Vitolo OV, Vonsattel JP, and Shelanski ML (2004) Dendrite and dendritic spine alterations in Alzheimer models. *J. Neurocytol.* 33: 377–387.

Morabito MA, Sheng M, and Tsai LH (2004) Cyclin-dependent kinase 5 phosphorylates the N-terminal domain of the postsynaptic density protein PSD-95 in neurons. *J. Neurosci.* 24: 865–876.

Morimoto I, Ohsawa I, Takamura C, Ishiguro M, and Kohsaka S (1998) Involvement of amyloid precursor protein in functional synapse formation in cultured hippocampal neurons. *J. Neurosci. Res.* 51: 185–195.

Morrow JA, Hatters DM, Lu B, et al. (2002) Apolipoprotein E4 forms a molten globule. A potential basis for its association with disease. *J. Biol. Chem.* 277: 50380–50385.

Mousavi M, Hellstrom-Lindahl E, Guan ZZ, Shan KR, Ravid R, and Nordberg A (2003) Protein and mRNA levels of nicotinic receptors in brain of tobacco using controls and patients with Alzheimer's disease. *Neuroscience* 122: 515–520.

Mucke L, Masliah E, Johnson WB, et al. (1994) Synaptotrophic effects of human amyloid β protein precursor in the cortex of transgenic mice. *Brain Res.* 666: 151–167.

Mucke L, Masliah E, Yu G-Q, et al. (2000) High-level neuronal expression of A$\beta_{1\text{-}42}$ in wild-type human amyloid protein precursor transgenic mice: Synaptotoxicity without plaque formation. *J. Neurosci.* 20: 4050–4058.

Müller T, Concannon CG, Ward MW, W, et al. (2006) Modulation of gene expression and cytoskeletal dynamics by the APP intracellular domain (AICD). *Mol. Biol. Cell* 18: 201–210.

Müller WE, Kirsch C, and Eckert GP (2001) Membrane-disordering effects of β-amyloid peptides. *Biochem. Soc. Trans.* 29: 617–623.

Murer MG, Yan Q, and Raisman-Vozari R (2001) Brain-derived neurotrophic factor in the control human brain, and in Alzheimer's disease and Parkinson's disease. *Prog. Neurobiol.* 63: 71–124.

Myers AJ, Kaleem M, Marlowe L, et al. (2005) The H1c haplotype at the MAPT locus is associated with Alzheimer's disease. *Hum. Mol. Genet.* 14: 2399–2404.

Myers AJ, Pittman AM, Zhao AS, et al. (2007) The MAPT H1c risk haplotype is associated with increased expression of tau and especially of repeat containing transcripts. *Neruobiol. Dis.* 25: 561–570.

Nägerl UV, Mody I, Jeub M, Lie AA, Elger CE, and Beck H (2000) Surviving granule cells of the sclerotic human hippocampus have reduced Ca^{2+} influx because of a loss of calbindin-D_{28K} in temporal lobe epilepsy. *J. Neurosci.* 20: 1831–1836.

Namba Y, Tomonaga M, Kawasaki H, Otomo E, and Ikeda K (1991) Apolipoprotein E immunoreactivity in cerebral amyloid deposits and neurofibrillary tangles in Alzheimer's disease and kuru plaque amyloid in Creutzfeldt-Jakob disease. *Brain Res.* 541: 163–166.

Näslund J, Haroutunian V, Mohs R, et al. (2000) Correlation between elevated levels of amyloid β-peptide in the brain and cognitive decline. *JAMA* 283: 1571–1577.

Nathan BP, Chang K-C, Bellosta S, et al. (1995) The inhibitory effect of apolipoprotein E4 on neurite outgrowth is associated with microtubule depolymerization. *J. Biol. Chem.* 270: 19791–19799.

Nguyen PV and Woo NH (2003) Regulation of hippocampal synaptic plasticity by cyclic AMP-dependent protein kinases. *Prog. Neurobiol.* 71: 401–437.

Nicoll JAR, Roberts GW, and Graham DI (1995) Apolipoprotein E ε4 allele is associated with deposition of amyloid β-protein following head injury. *Nat. Med.* 1: 135–137.

Nikolic M, Chou MM, Lu W, Mayer BJ, and Tsai LH (1998) The p35/Cdk5 kinase is a neuron-specific Rac effector that inhibits Pak1 activity. *Nature* 395: 194–198.

Nishimura I, Yang Y, and Lu B (2004) PAR-1 kinase plays an initiator role in a temporally ordered phosphorylation process that confers tau toxicity in *Drosophila*. *Cell* 116: 671–682.

Nixon RA (2005) Endosome function and dysfunction in Alzheimer's disease and other neurodegenerative diseases. *Neurobiol. Aging* 26: 373–382.

Noble W, Planel E, Zehr C, et al. (2005) Inhibition of glycogen synthase kinase-3 by lithium correlates with reduced tauopathy and degeneration *in vivo*. *Proc. Natl. Acad. Sci. USA* 102: 6990–6995.

Noble W, Olm V, Takata K, et al. (2003) Cdk5 is a key factor in tau aggregation and tangle formation *in vivo*. *Neuron* 38: 555–565.

Oddo S, Billings L, Kesslak JP, Cribbs DH, and LaFerla FM (2004) Aβ immunotherapy leads to clearance of early, but not late, hyperphosphorylated tau aggregates via the proteasome. *Neuron* 43: 321–332.

Oddo S and LaFerla FM (2006) The role of nicotinic acetylcholine receptors in Alzheimer's disease. *J. Physiol. Paris* 99: 172–179.

Ohm TG, Scharnagl H, März W, and Bohl J (1999) Apolipoprotein E isoforms and the development of low and high Braak stages of Alzheimer's disease-related lesions. *Acta Neuropathol. (Berl.)* 98: 273–280.

Ohno M, Chang L, Tseng W, et al. (2006) Temporal memory deficits in Alzheimer's mouse models: Rescue by genetic deletion of BACE1. *Eur. J. Neurosci.* 23: 251–260.

Olariu A, Yamada K, and Nabeshima T (2005) Amyloid pathology and protein kinase C (PKC): Possible therapeutics effects of PKC activators. *J. Pharmacol. Sci.* 97: 1–5.

Olofsdotter K, Lindvall O, and Asztely F (2000) Increased synaptic inhibition in dentate gyrus of mice with reduced levels of endogenous brain-derived neurotrophic factor. *Neuroscience* 101: 531–539.

Oster Y and Schramm M (1993) Down-regulation of NMDA receptor activity by NMDA. *Neurosci. Lett.* 163: 85–88.

Palop JJ, Chin J, Bien-Ly N, et al. (2005) Vulnerability of dentate granule cells to disruption of Arc expression in human amyloid precursor protein transgenic mice. *J. Neurosci.* 25: 9686–9693.

Palop JJ, Chin J, and Mucke L (2006) A network dysfunction perspective on neurodegenerative diseases. *Nature* 443: 768–773.

Palop JJ, Chin J, Roberson ED, Wang J, Thwin MT, Bien-Ly N, Yoo J, Ho KO, Yu GQ, Kreitzer A, Finkbeiner S, Noebels JL, and Mucke L (2007) Aberrant excitatory neuronal activity and compensatory remodeling of inhibitory hippocampal circuits in mouse models of Alzheimer's disease. *Neuron* 55(5): 697–711.

Palop JJ, Jones B, Kekonius L, et al. (2003) Neuronal depletion of calcium-dependent proteins in the dentate gyrus is tightly linked to Alzheimer's disease-related cognitive deficits. *Proc. Natl. Acad. Sci. USA* 100: 9572–9577.

Pappas GD, Kriho V, and Pesold C (2001) Reelin in the extracellular matrix and dendritic spines of the cortex and hippocampus: A comparison between wild type and heterozygous *reeler* mice by immunoelectron microscopy. *J. Neurocytol.* 30: 413–425.

Pardossi-Piquard R, Petit A, Kawarai T, et al. (2005) Presenilin-dependent transcriptional control of the Aβ-degrading enzyme neprilysin by intracellular domains of βAPP and APLP. *Neuron* 46: 541–554.

Pariente J, Cole S, Henson R, et al. (2005) Alzheimer's patients engage an alternative network during a memory task. *Ann. Neurol.* 58: 870–879.

Park M, Penick EC, Edwards JG, Kauer JA, and Ehlers MD (2004) Recycling endosomes supply AMPA receptors for LTP. *Science* 305: 1972–1975.

Park SY and Ferreira A (2005) The generation of a 17 kDa neurotoxic fragment: An alternative mechanism by which tau mediates β-amyloid-induced neurodegeneration. *J. Neurosci.* 25: 5365–5375.

Patrick GN, Zukerberg L, Nikolic M, de la Monte S, Dikkes P, and Tsai L-H (1999) Conversion of P35 to P25 deregulates Cdk5 activity and promotes neurodegeneration. *Nature* 402: 615–622.

Payami H, Zareparsi S, Montee KR, et al. (1996) Gender difference in apolipoprotein E-associated risk for familial Alzheimer disease: A possible clue to the higher incidence of Alzheimer disease in women. *Am. J. Hum. Genet.* 58: 803–811.

Pearson G, Robinson F, Beers Gibson T, et al. (2001) Mitogen-activated protein (MAP) kinase pathways: Regulation and physiological functions. *Endocr. Rev.* 22: 153–183.

Pei JJ, Braak H, An WL, et al. (2002) Up-regulation of mitogen-activated protein kinases ERK1/2 and MEK1/2 is associated with the progression of neurofibrillary degeneration in Alzheimer's disease. *Brain Res. Mol. Brain Res.* 109: 45–55.

Pelkey KA, Askalan R, Paul S, et al. (2002) Tyrosine phosphatase STEP is a tonic brake on induction of long-term potentiation. *Neuron* 34: 127–138.

Pennanen L, Welzl H, D'Adamo P, Nitsch RM, and Götz J (2004) Accelerated extinction of conditioned taste aversion in P301L tau transgenic mice. *Neurobiol. Dis.* 15: 500–509.

Perez-Garcia CG, Gonzalez-Delgado FJ, Suarez-Sola ML, et al. (2001) Reelin-immunoreactive neurons in the adult vertebrate pallium. *J. Chem. Neuroanat.* 21: 41–51.

Perl DP, Olanow CW, and Calne D (1998) Alzheimer's disease and Parkinson's disease: Distinct entities or extremes of a spectrum of neurodegeneration? *Ann. Neurol.* 44: S19–31.

Pesold C, Impagnatiello F, Pisu MG, et al. (1998) Reelin is preferentially expressed in neurons synthesizing γ-aminobutyric acid in cortex and hippocampus of adult rats. *Proc. Natl. Acad. Sci. USA* 95: 3221–3226.

Pettit DL, Shao Z, and Yakel JL (2001) β-Amyloid$_{1\text{-}42}$ peptide directly modulates nicotinic receptors in the rat hippocampal slice. *J. Neurosci.* 21: 1–5.

Pitschke M, Prior R, Haupt M, and Riesner D (1998) Detection of single amyloid β-protein aggregates in the cerebrospinal fluid of Alzheimer's patients by fluorescence correlation spectroscopy. *Nat. Med.* 4: 832–834.

Plant LD, Webster NJ, Boyle JP, et al. (2006) Amyloid β peptide as a physiological modulator of neuronal 'A'-type K^+ current. *Neurobiol. Aging* 27: 1673–1683.

Plath N, Ohana O, Dammermann B, et al. (2006) Arc/Arg3.1 is essential for the consolidation of synaptic plasticity and memories. *Neuron* 52: 437–444.

Podlisny MB, Ostaszewski BL, Squazzo SL, et al. (1995) Aggregation of secreted amyloid β-protein into sodium dodecyl sulfate-stable oligomers in cell culture. *J. Biol. Chem.* 270: 9564–9570.

Pollard HB, Arispe N, and Rojas E (1995) Ion channel hypothesis for Alzheimer amyloid peptide neurotoxicity. Cell. *Mol. Neurobiol.* 15: 513–526.

Polymeropoulos MH, Lavedan C, Leroy E, et al. (1997) Mutation in the α-synuclein gene identified in families with Parkinson's disease. *Science* 276: 2045–2047.

Price JL, Davis PB, Morris JC, and White DL (1991) The distribution of tangles, plaques and related immunohistochemical markers in healthy aging and Alzheimer's disease. *Neurobiol. Aging* 12: 295–312.

Price JL, Ko AI, Wade MJ, Tsou SK, McKeel DW, and Morris JC (2001) Neuron number in the entorhinal cortex and CA1 in preclinical Alzheimer disease. *Arch. Neurol.* 58: 1395–1402.

Priller C, Bauer T, Mitteregger G, Krebs B, Kretzschmar HA, and Herms J (2006) Synapse formation and function is modulated by the amyloid precursor protein. *J. Neurosci.* 26: 7212–7221.

Prybylowski K, Chang K, Sans N, Kan L, Vicini S, and Wenthold RJ (2005) The synaptic localization of NR2B-containing NMDA receptors is controlled by interactions with PDZ proteins and AP-2. *Neuron* 47: 845–857.

Qiu S, Korwek KM, Pratt-Davis AR, Peters M, Bergman MY, and Weeber EJ (2006a) Cognitive disruption and altered hippocampus synaptic function in Reelin haploinsufficient mice. *Neurobiol. Learn. Mem.* 85: 228–242.

Qiu S, Korwek KM, and Weeber EJ (2006b) A fresh look at an ancient receptor family: Emerging roles for low density lipoprotein receptors in synaptic plasticity and memory formation. *Neurobiol. Learn. Mem.* 85: 16–29.

Raber J (2004) Androgens, apoE, and Alzheimer's disease. *Sci. Aging Knowledge Environ.* 2004: re2.

Raber J, Huang Y, and Ashford JW (2004) ApoE genotype accounts for the vast majority of AD risk and AD pathology. *Neurobiol. Aging* 25: 641–650.

Raber J, LeFevour A, Buttini M, and Mucke L (2002) Androgens protect against Apolipoprotein E4-induced cognitive deficits. *J. Neurosci.* 22: 5204–5209.

Raber J, Wong D, Buttini M, et al. (1998) Isoform-specific effects of human apolipoprotein E on brain function revealed in *ApoE* knockout mice: Increased susceptibility of females. *Proc. Natl. Acad. Sci. USA* 95: 10914–10919.

Raber J, Wong D, Yu G-Q, et al. (2000) Alzheimer's disease: Apolipoprotein E and cognitive performance. *Nature* 404: 352–354.

Rademakers R, Cruts M, and van Broeckhoven C (2004) The role of tau (*MAPT*) in frontotemporal dementia and related tauopathies. *Hum. Mutat.* 24: 277–295.

Raivich G and Behrens A (2006) Role of the AP-1 transcription factor c-Jun in developing, adult and injured brain. *Prog. Neurobiol.* 78: 347–363.

Ramaswamy G, Xu Q, Huang Y, and Weisgraber KH (2005) Effect of domain interaction on apolipoprotein E levels in mouse brain. *J. Neurosci.* 25: 10658–10663.

Ramos-Moreno T, Galazo MJ, Porrero C, Martinez-Cerdeno V, and Clasca F (2006) Extracellular matrix molecules and synaptic plasticity: Immunomapping of intracellular and secreted Reelin in the adult rat brain. *Eur. J. Neurosci.* 23: 401–422.

Ramsden M, Kotilinek L, Forster C, et al. (2005) Age-dependent neurofibrillary tangle formation, neuron loss, and memory impairment in a mouse model of human tauopathy (P301L). *J. Neurosci.* 25: 10637–10647.

Rao VR, Pintchovski SA, Chin J, Peebles CL, Mitra S, and Finkbeiner S (2006) AMPA receptors regulate transcription of the plasticity-related immediate-early gene Arc. *Nat. Neurosci.* 9: 887–895.

Rapoport M, Dawson HN, Binder LI, Vitek MP, and Ferreira A (2002) Tau is essential to β-amyloid-induced neurotoxicity. *Proc. Natl. Acad. Sci. USA* 99: 6364–6369.

Rapoport M and Ferreira A (2000) PD98059 prevents neurite degeneration induced by fibrillar β-amyloid in mature hippocampal neurons. *J. Neurochem.* 74: 125–133.

Reiman EM, Chen K, Alexander GE, et al. (2004) Functional brain abnormalities in young adults at genetic risk for late-onset Alzheimer's dementia. *Proc. Natl. Acad. Sci. USA* 101: 284–289.

Reiman EM, Chen K, Alexander GE, et al. (2005) Correlations between apolipoprotein E ε4 gene dose and brain-imaging measurements of regional hypometabolism. *Proc. Natl. Acad. Sci. USA* 102: 8299–8302.

Resink A, Villa M, Boer GJ, Mohler H, and Balazs R (1995) Agonist-induced down-regulation of NMDA receptors in cerebellar granule cells in culture. *Eur. J. Neurosci.* 7: 1700–1706.

Rial Verde EM, Lee-Osbourne J, Worley PF, Malinow R, and Cline HT (2006) Increased expression of the immediate-early gene arc/arg3.1 reduces AMPA receptor-mediated synaptic transmission. *Neuron* 52: 461–474.

Rissman RA, Poon WW, Blurton-Jones M, et al. (2004) Caspase-cleavage of tau is an early event in Alzheimer disease tangle pathology. *J. Clin. Invest.* 114: 121–130.

Roberds SL, Anderson J, Basi G, et al. (2001) BACE knockout mice are healthy despite lacking the primary β-secretase activity in brain: Implications for Alzheimer's disease therapeutics. *Hum. Mol. Genet.* 10: 1317–1324.

Roberson ED, English JD, Adams JP, Selcher JC, Kondratick C, and Sweatt JD (1999) The mitogen-activated protein kinase cascade couples PKA and PKC to cAMP response element binding protein phosphorylation in area CA1 of hippocampus. *J. Neurosci.* 19: 4337–4348.

Roberson ED, English JD, and Sweatt JD (1996) A biochemist's view of long-term potentiation. *Learn. Mem.* 3: 1–24.

Roberson ED, Hesse JH, Rose KD, et al. (2005) Frontotemporal dementia progresses to death faster than Alzheimer disease. *Neurology* 65: 719–725.

Roberson ED and Mucke L (2006) 100 years and counting: Prospects for defeating Alzheimer's disease. *Science* 314: 781–784.

Roberson ED, Scearce-Levie K, Palop JJ, et al. (2007) Reducing endogenous tau ameliorates amyloid β-induced deficits in an Alzheimer's disease mouse model. *Science* 316: 750–754.

Rockenstein E, Mante M, Alford M, et al. (2005) High β-Secretase activity elicits neurodegeneration in transgenic mice despite reductions in amyloid-β levels: Implications for the treatment of Alzheimer's disease. *J. Biol. Chem.* 280: 32957–32967.

Rogaev EI, Sherrington R, Rogaeva EA, et al. (1995) Familial Alzheimer's disease in kindreds with missense mutations in a gene on chromosome 1 related to the Alzheimer's disease type 3 gene. *Nature* 376: 775–778.

Roher AE, Chaney MO, Kuo Y-M, et al. (1996) Morphology and toxicity of Aβ-(1–42) dimer derived from neuritic and vascular amyloid deposits of Alzheimer's disease. *J. Biol. Chem.* 271: 20631–20635.

Rong Y, Lu X, Bernard A, Khrestchatisky M, and Baudry M (2001) Tyrosine phosphorylation of ionotropic glutamate receptors by Fyn or Src differentially modulates their susceptibility to calpain and enhances their binding to spectrin and PSD-95. *J. Neurochem.* 79: 382–390.

Rose CR and Konnerth A (2001) Stores not just for storage. Intracellular calcium release and synaptic plasticity. *Neuron* 31: 519–522.

Roselli F, Tirard M, Lu J, et al. (2005) Soluble β-amyloid$_{1-40}$ induces NMDA-dependent degradation of postsynaptic density-95 at glutamatergic synapses. *J. Neurosci.* 25: 11061–11070.

Roskoski R Jr. (2004) Src protein-tyrosine kinase structure and regulation. *Biochem. Biophys. Res. Commun.* 324: 1155–1164.

Rossner S, Mehlhorn G, Schliebs R, and Bigl V (2001) Increased neuronal and glial expression of protein kinase C isoforms in neocortex of transgenic Tg2576 mice with amyloid pathology. *Eur. J. Neurosci.* 13: 269–278.

Rutherford LC, DeWan A, Lauer HM, and Turrigiano GG (1997) Brain-derived neurotrophic factor mediates the activity-dependent regulation of inhibition in neocortical cultures. *J. Neurosci.* 17: 4527–4535.

Rutherford LC, Nelson SB, and Turrigiano GG (1998) BDNF has opposite effects on the quantal amplitude of pyramidal neuron and interneuron excitatory synapses. *Neuron* 21: 521–530.

Ruttimann E, Vacher CM, Gassmann M, Kaupmann K, Van der Putten H, and Bettler B (2004) Altered hippocampal expression of calbindin-D-28k and calretinin in GABA(B(1))-deficient mice. *Biochem. Pharmacol.* 68: 1613–1620.

Ryan TA (2006) A pre-synaptic to-do list for coupling exocytosis to endocytosis. *Curr. Opin. Cell Biol.* 18: 416–421.

Sabo S, Lambert MP, Kessey K, Wade W, Krafft G, and Klein WL (1995) Interaction of β-amyloid peptides with integrins in a human nerve cell line. *Neurosci. Lett.* 184: 25–28.

Saez-Valero J, Costell M, Sjogren M, Andreasen N, Blennow K, and Luque JM (2003) Altered levels of cerebrospinal fluid reelin in frontotemporal dementia and Alzheimer's disease. *J. Neurosci. Res.* 72: 132–136.

Saitoh T, Horsburgh K, and Masliah E (1993) Hyperactivation of signal transduction systems in Alzheimer's disease. *Ann. N.Y. Acad. Sci.* 695: 34–41.

Salter MW and Kalia LV (2004) Src kinases: A hub for NMDA receptor regulation. *Nat. Rev. Neurosci.* 5: 317–328.

Sampson VL, Morrison JH, and Vickers JC (1997) The cellular basis for the relative resistance of parvalbumin and calretinin immunoreactive neocortical neurons to the pathology of Alzheimer's disease. *Exp. Neurol.* 145: 295–302.

Sanes JR and Lichtman JW (1999) Can molecules explain long-term potentiation? *Nat. Neurosci.* 2: 597–604.

SantaCruz K, Lewis J, Spires T, et al. (2005) Tau suppression in a neurodegenerative mouse model improves memory function. *Science* 309: 476–481.

Sato S, Tatebayashi Y, Akagi T, et al. (2002) Aberrant tau phosphorylation by glycogen synthase kinase-3β and JNK3 induces oligomeric tau fibrils in COS-7 cells. *J. Biol. Chem.* 277: 42060–42065.

Satpute-Krishnan P, Degiorgis JA, Conley MP, Jang M, and Bearer EL (2006) A peptide zipcode sufficient for anterograde transport within amyloid precursor protein. *Proc. Natl. Acad. Sci. USA* 103: 16532–16537.

Saunders AM, Strittmatter WJ, Schmechel D, et al. (1993) Association of apolipoprotein E allele ε4 with late-onset familial and sporadic Alzheimer's disease. *Neurology* 43: 1467–1472.

Saura CA, Choi SY, Beglopoulos V, et al. (2004) Loss of presenilin function causes impairments of memory and synaptic plasticity followed by age-dependent neurodegeneration. *Neuron* 42: 23–36.

Savage MJ, Lin YG, Ciallella JR, Flood DG, and Scott RW (2002) Activation of c-Jun N-terminal kinase and p38 in an Alzheimer's disease model is associated with amyloid deposition. *J. Neurosci.* 22: 3376–3385.

Scheff SW and Price DA (2003) Synaptic pathology in Alzheimer's disease: A review of ultrastructural studies. *Neurobiol. Aging* 24: 1029–1046.

Scheuner D, Eckman C, Jensen M, et al. (1996) Secreted amyloid β-protein similar to that in the senile plaques of Alzheimer's disease is increased *in vivo* by the presenilin 1 and 2 and APP mutations linked to familial Alzheimer's disease. *Nat. Med.* 2: 864–870.

Schinder AF and Poo M (2000) The neurotrophin hypothesis for synaptic plasticity. *Trends Neurosci.* 23: 639–645.

Schmechel DE, Saunders AM, Strittmatter WJ, et al. (1993) Increased amyloid β-peptide deposition in cerebral cortex as a consequence of apolipoprotein E genotype in late-onset Alzheimer disease. *Proc. Natl. Acad. Sci. USA* 90: 9649–9653.

Schneider A, Biernat J, von Bergen M, Mandelkow E, and Mandelkow E-M (1999) Phosphorylation that detaches tau protein from microtubules (Ser262, Ser214) also protects it against aggregation into Alzheimer paired helical filaments. *Biochemistry* 38: 3549–3558.

Schuman EM, Dynes JL, and Steward O (2006) Synaptic regulation of translation of dendritic mRNAs. *J. Neurosci.* 26: 7143–7146.

Scott CW, Spreen RC, Herman JL, et al. (1993) Phosphorylation of recombinant tau by cAMP-dependent protein kinase. Identification of phosphorylation sites and effect on microtubule assembly. *J. Biol. Chem.* 268: 1166–1173.

Scragg JL, Fearon IM, Boyle JP, Ball SG, Varadi G, and Peers C (2005) Alzheimer's amyloid peptides mediate hypoxic up-regulation of L-type Ca^{2+} channels. *FASEB J.* 19: 150–152.

Seabrook GR, Smith DW, Bowery BJ, et al. (1999) Mechanisms contributing to the deficits in hippocampal synaptic plasticity in mice lacking amyloid precursor protein. *Neuropharmacology* 38: 349–359.

Seilheimer B, Bohrmann B, Bondolfi L, Müller F, Stüber D, and Döbeli H (1997) The toxicity of the Alzheimer's β-amyloid peptide correlates with a distinct fiber morphology. *J. Struct. Biol.* 119: 59–71.

Selkoe DJ (2002) Alzheimer's disease is a synaptic failure. *Science* 298: 789–791.

Shahani N and Brandt R (2002) Functions and malfunctions of the tau proteins. *Cell. Mol. Life Sci.* 59: 1668–1680.

Shaked GM, Kummer MP, Lu DC, Galvan V, Bredesen DE, and Koo EH (2006) Aβ induces cell death by direct interaction with its cognate extracellular domain on APP (APP 597–624). *FASEB J.* 20: 1254–1256.

Shemer I, Holmgren C, Min R, et al. (2006) Non-fibrillar β-amyloid abates spike-timing-dependent synaptic potentiation at excitatory synapses in layer 2/3 of the neocortex by targeting postsynaptic AMPA receptors. *Eur. J. Neurosci.* 23: 2035–2047.

Shepherd JD, Rumbaugh G, Wu J, et al. (2006) Arc/Arg3.1 Mediates Homeostatic Synaptic Scaling of AMPA Receptors. *Neuron* 52: 475–484.

Sherrington R, Rogaev EI, Liang Y, et al. (1995) Cloning of a gene bearing missense mutations in early-onset familial Alzheimer's disease. *Nature* 375: 754–760.

Shim KS and Lubec G (2002) Drebrin, a dendritic spine protein, is manifold decreased in brains of patients with Alzheimer's disease and Down syndrome. *Neurosci. Lett.* 324: 209–212.

Shirazi SK and Wood JG (1993) The protein tyrosine kinase, fyn, in Alzheimer's disease pathology. *Neuroreport* 4: 435–437.

Simonian NA, Elvhage T, Czernik AJ, Greengard P, and Hyman BT (1994) Calcium/calmodulin-dependent protein kinase II immunostaining is preserved in Alzheimer's disease hippocampal neurons. *Brain Res.* 657: 294–299.

Singh TJ, Zaidi T, Grundke-Iqbal I, and Iqbal K (1996) Non-proline-dependent protein kinases phosphorylate several sites found in tau from Alzheimer disease brain. *Mol. Cell. Biochem.* 154: 143–151.

Sinha S, Anderson JP, Barbour R, et al. (1999) Purification and cloning of amyloid precursor protein β-secretase from human brain. *Nature* 402: 735–741.

Sklan EH, Podoly E, and Soreq H (2006) RACK1 has the nerve to act: Structure meets function in the nervous system. *Prog. Neurobiol.* 78: 117–134.

Small DH (2004) Do acetylcholinesterase inhibitors boost synaptic scaling in Alzheimer's disease? *Trends Neurosci.* 27: 245–249.

Smith IF, Green KN, and LaFerla FM (2005a) Calcium dysregulation in Alzheimer's disease: Recent advances gained from genetically modified animals. *Cell Calcium* 38: 427–437.

Smith IF, Hitt B, Green KN, Oddo S, and LaFerla FM (2005b) Enhanced caffeine-induced Ca^{2+} release in the 3xTg-AD mouse model of Alzheimer's disease. *J. Neurochem.* 94: 1711–1718.

Smith MA, Ellis-Davies GC, and Magee JC (2003) Mechanism of the distance-dependent scaling of Schaffer collateral synapses in rat CA1 pyramidal neurons. *J. Physiol.* 548: 245–258.

Smith WW, Gorospe M, and Kusiak JW (2006) Signaling mechanisms underlying Aβ toxicity: Potential therapeutic targets for Alzheimer's disease. *CNS Neurol. Disord. Drug Targets* 5: 355–361.

Snyder EM, Nong Y, Almeida CG, et al. (2005) Regulation of NMDA receptor trafficking by amyloid-β. *Nat. Neurosci.* 8: 1051–1058.

Solodkin A, Veldhuizen SD, and Van Hoesen GW (1996) Contingent vulnerability of entorhinal parvalbumin-containing neurons in Alzheimer's disease. *J. Neurosci.* 16: 3311–3321.

Spillantini MG, Schmidt ML, Lee VM-Y, Trojanowski JQ, Jakes R, and Goedert M (1997) α-Synuclein in Lewy bodies. *Nature* 388: 839–840.

Spires TL, Meyer-Luehmann M, Stern EA, et al. (2005) Dendritic spine abnormalities in amyloid precursor protein transgenic mice demonstrated by gene transfer and intravital multiphoton microscopy. *J. Neurosci.* 25: 7278–7287.

Spires TL, Orne JD, SantaCruz K, et al. (2006) Region-specific dissociation of neuronal loss and neurofibrillary pathology in a mouse model of tauopathy. *Am. J. Pathol.* 168: 1598–1607.

Stern EA, Bacskai BJ, Hickey GA, Attenello FJ, Lombardo JA, and Hyman BT (2004) Cortical synaptic integration *in vivo* is disrupted by amyloid-β plaques. *J. Neurosci.* 24: 4535–4540.

Steward O and Worley PF (2001a) Selective targeting of newly synthesized *Arc* mRNA to active synapses requires NMDA receptor activation. *Neuron* 30: 227–240.

Steward O and Worley PF (2001b) A cellular mechanism for targeting newly synthesized mRNAs to synaptic sites on dendrites. *Proc. Natl. Acad. Sci. USA* 98: 7062–7068.

Stoothoff WH and Johnson GV (2005) Tau phosphorylation: Physiological and pathological consequences. *Biochim. Biophys. Acta* 1739: 280–297.

Strittmatter WJ, Saunders AM, Schmechel D, et al. (1993) Apolipoprotein E: High-avidity binding to β-amyloid and increased frequency of type 4 allele in late-onset familial Alzheimer's disease. *Proc. Natl. Acad. Sci. USA* 90: 1977–1981.

Strittmatter WJ, Weisgraber KH, Goedert M, et al. (1994) Microtubule instability and paired helical filament formation in the Alzheimer disease brain are related to apolipoprotein E genotype. *Exp. Neurol.* 125: 163–171.

Struhl G and Adachi A (2000) Requirements for presenilin-dependent cleavage of notch and other transmembrane proteins. *Mol. Cell* 6: 625–636.

Stutzmann GE (2005) Calcium dysregulation, IP3 signaling, and Alzheimer's disease. *Neuroscientist* 11: 110–115.

Stutzmann GE, Smith I, Caccamo A, Oddo S, Laferla FM, and Parker I (2006) Enhanced ryanodine receptor recruitment contributes to Ca^{2+} disruptions in young, adult, and aged Alzheimer's disease mice. *J. Neurosci.* 26: 5180–5189.

Südhof TC (2004) The synaptic vesicle cycle. *Annu. Rev. Neurosci.* 27: 509–547.

Supnet C, Grant J, Kong H, Westaway D, and Mayne M (2006) Aβ 1–42 increases ryanodine receptor-3 expression and function in TgCRND8 mice. *J. Biol. Chem.* 281: 38440–38447.

Sutherland MK, Wong L, Somerville MJ, et al. (1993) Reduction of calbindin-28k mRNA levels in Alzheimer as compared to Huntington hippocampus. *Brain Res. Mol. Brain Res.* 18: 32–42.

Sweatt JD (2004) Mitogen-activated protein kinases in synaptic plasticity and memory. *Curr. Opin. Neurobiol.* 14: 311–317.

Tagawa Y, Kanold PO, Majdan M, and Shatz CJ (2005) Multiple periods of functional ocular dominance plasticity in mouse visual cortex. *Nat. Neurosci.* 8: 380–388.

Takei Y, Teng J, Harada A, and Hirokawa N (2000) Defects in axonal elongation and neuronal migration in mice with disrupted *tau* and *map1b* genes. *J. Cell Biol.* 150: 989–1000.

Takeuchi A, Irizarry MC, Duff K, et al. (2000) Age-related amyloid β deposition in transgenic mice overexpressing both Alzheimer mutant presenilin 1 and amyloid beta precursor protein Swedish mutant is not associated with global neuronal loss. *Am. J. Pathol.* 157: 331–339.

Tandon A and Fraser P (2002) The presenilins. *Genome Biol.* 3: 3014.3011–3014.3019.

Tanzi R and Bertram L (2005) Twenty years of the Alzheimer's disease amyloid hypothesis: A genetic perspective. *Cell* 120: 545–555.

Tapiola T, Overmyer M, Lehtovirta M, et al. (1997) The level of cerebrospinal fluid tau correlates with neurofibrillary tangles in Alzheimer's disease. *Neuroreport* 8: 3961–3963.

Tardiff BE, Newman MF, Saunders AM, et al. (1997) The Neurologic Outcome Research Group of the Duke Heart Center. Preliminary report of a genetic basis for cognitive decline after cardiac operations. *Ann. Thorac. Surg.* 64: 715–720.

Tariot PN and Federoff HJ (2003) Current treatment for Alzheimer disease and future prospects. *Alzheimer Dis. Assoc. Disord.* 17(supplement 4): S105–S113.

Tatebayashi Y, Miyasaka T, Chui DH, et al. (2002) Tau filament formation and associative memory deficit in aged mice expressing mutant (R406W) human tau. *Proc. Natl. Acad. Sci. USA* 99: 13896–13901.

Teasdale GM, Nicoll JAR, Murray G, and Fiddes M (1997) Association of apolipoprotein E polymorphism with outcome after head injury. *Lancet* 350: 1069–1071.

Temple MD, Worley PF, and Steward O (2003) Visualizing changes in circuit activity resulting from denervation and reinnervation using immediate early gene expression. *J. Neurosci.* 23: 2779–2788.

Terry JG, Howard G, Mercuri M, Bond MG, and Crouse JR (1996) Apolipoprotein E polymorphism is associated with segment-specific extracranial carotid artery intima-media thickening. *Stroke* 27: 1755–1759.

Terry RD, Masliah E, Salmon DP, et al. (1991) Physical basis of cognitive alterations in Alzheimer's disease: Synapse loss is the major correlate of cognitive impairment. *Ann. Neurol.* 30: 572–580.

Tesseur I, Van Dorpe J, Spittaels K, Van den Haute C, Moechars D, and Van Leuven F (2000) Expression of human apolipoprotein E4 in neurons causes hyperphosphorylation of protein tau in the brains of transgenic mice. *Am. J. Pathol.* 156: 951–964.

Theuns J, Marjaux E, Vandenbulcke M, et al. (2006) Alzheimer dementia caused by a novel mutation located in the APP C-terminal intracytosolic fragment. *Hum. Mutat.* 27: 888–896.

Thiagarajan TC, Lindskog M, Malgaroli A, and Tsien RW (2006) LTP and adaptation to inactivity: Overlapping mechanisms and implications for metaplasticity. *Neuropharmacology* 52: 156–175.

Thomas GM and Huganir RL (2004) MAPK cascade signalling and synaptic plasticity. *Nat. Rev. Neurosci.* 5: 173–183.

Thomas SM and Brugge JS (1997) Cellular functions regulated by src family kinases. *Cell Dev. Biol.* 13: 513–609.

Tissir F and Goffinet AM (2003) Reelin and brain development. *Nat. Rev. Neurosci.* 4: 496–505.

Tonder N, Kragh J, Finsen BR, Bolwig TG, and Zimmer J (1994) Kindling induces transient changes in neuronal expression of somatostatin, neuropeptide Y, and calbindin in adult rat hippocampus and fascia dentata. *Epilepsia* 35: 1299–1308.

Townsend M, Shankar GM, Mehta T, Walsh DM, and Selkoe DJ (2006) Effects of secreted oligomers of amyloid β-protein on hippocampal synaptic plasticity: A potent role for trimers. *J. Physiol.* 572: 477–492.

Trojanowski JQ, Mawal-Dewan M, Schmidt ML, Martin J, and Lee VM (1993) Localization of the mitogen activated protein kinase ERK2 in Alzheimer's disease neurofibrillary tangles and senile plaque neurites. *Brain Res.* 618: 333–337.

Trommer BL, Shah C, Yun SH, et al. (2004) ApoE isoform affects LTP in human targeted replacement mice. *Neuroreport* 15: 2655–2658.

Trommer BL, Shah C, Yun SH, et al. (2005) ApoE isoform-specific effects on LTP: Blockade by oligomeric amyloid-β1–42. *Neurobiol. Dis.* 18: 75–82.

Tsai J, Grutzendler J, Duff K, and Gan WB (2004) Fibrillar amyloid deposition leads to local synaptic abnormalities and breakage of neuronal branches. *Nat. Neurosci.* 7: 1181–1183.

Tu H, Nelson O, Bezprozvanny A, et al. (2006) Presenilins form ER Ca^{2+} leak channels, a function disrupted by familial Alzheimer's disease-linked mutations. *Cell* 126: 981–993.

Tucker KL, Meyer M, and Barde YA (2001) Neurotrophins are required for nerve growth during development. *Nat. Neurosci.* 4: 29–37.

Tully T, Bourtchouladze R, Scott R, and Tallman J (2003) Targeting the CREB pathway for memory enhancers. *Nat. Rev. Drug Discov.* 2: 267–277.

Turner PR, O'Connor K, Tate WP, and Abraham WC (2003) Roles of amyloid precursor protein and its fragments in regulating neural activity, plasticity and memory. *Prog. Neurobiol.* 70: 1–32.

Turrigiano GG and Nelson SB (2004) Homeostatic plasticity in the developing nervous system. *Nat. Rev. Neurosci.* 5: 97–107.

Tzingounis AV and Nicoll RA (2006) Arc/Arg3.1: Linking gene expression to synaptic plasticity and memory. *Neuron* 52: 403–407.

Uéda K, Fukushima H, Masliah E, et al. (1993) Molecular cloning of cDNA encoding an unrecognized component of amyloid in Alzheimer disease. *Proc. Natl. Acad. Sci. USA* 90: 11282–11286.

Ueda K, Shinohara S, Yagami T, Asakura K, and Kawasaki K (1997) Amyloid β protein potentiates Ca2+ influx through L-type voltage-sensitive Ca2+ channels: A possible involvement of free radicals. *J. Neurochem.* 68: 265–271.

van Groen T, Miettinen P, and Kadish I (2003) The entorhinal cortex of the mouse: Organization of the projection to the hippocampal formation. *Hippocampus* 13: 133–149.

Vassar R, Bennett BD, Babu-Khan S, et al. (1999) β-secretase cleavage of Alzheimer's amyloid precursor protein by the transmembrane aspartic protease BACE. *Science* 286: 735–741.

Verdier Y, Zarándi M, and Penke B (2004) Amyloid β-peptide interactions with neuronal and glial cell plasma membrane: Binding sites and implications for Alzheimer's disease. *J. Pept. Sci.* 10: 229–248.

Vitolo OV, Sant'Angelo A, Costanzo V, Battaglia F, Arancio O, and Shelanski M (2002) Amyloid β-peptide inhibition of the PKA/CREB pathway and long-term potentiation: Reversibility by drugs that enhance cAMP signaling. *Proc. Natl. Acad. Sci. USA* 99: 13217–13221.

Wakabayashi K, Narisawa-Saito M, Iwakura Y, et al. (1999) Phenotypic down-regulation of glutamate receptor subunit GluR1 in Alzheimer's disease. *Neurobiol. Aging* 20: 287–295.

Wallin AK, Blennow K, Andreasen N, and Minthon L (2006) CSF biomarkers for Alzheimer's Disease: Levels of β-amyloid, tau, phosphorylated tau relate to clinical symptoms and survival. *Dement. Geriatr. Cogn. Disord.* 21: 131–138.

Walsh DM, Klyubin I, Fadeeva JV, et al. (2002) Naturally secreted oligomers of amyloid β protein potently inhibit hippocampal long-term potentiation *in vivo*. *Nature* 416: 535–539.

Walsh DM and Selkoe DJ (2004) Deciphering the molecular basis of memory failure in Alzheimer's disease. *Neuron* 44: 181–193.

Walsh DM, Townsend M, Podlisny MB, et al. (2005) Certain inhibitors of synthetic amyloid β-peptide (Aβ) fibrillogenesis block oligomerization of natural Aβ and thereby rescue long-term potentiation. *J. Neurosci.* 25: 2455–2462.

Waltereit R, Dammermann B, Wulff P, et al. (2001) Arg3.1/Arc mRNA induction by Ca^{2+} and cAMP requires protein kinase A and mitogen-activated protein kinase/extracellular regulated kinase activation. *J. Neurosci.* 21: 5484–5493.

Waltereit R and Weller M (2003) Signaling from cAMP/PKA to MAPK and synaptic plasticity. *Mol. Neurobiol.* 27: 99–106.

Wang D and Munoz DG (1995) Qualitative and quantitative differences in senile plaque dystrophic neurites of Alzheimer's disease and normal aged brain. J. Neuropathol. *Exp. Neurol.* 54: 548–556.

Wang DS, Lipton RB, Katz MJ, et al. (2005) Decreased neprilysin immunoreactivity in Alzheimer disease, but not in pathological aging. J. Neuropathol. *Exp. Neurol.* 64: 378–385.

Wang H, Hu Y, and Tsien JZ (2006) Molecular and systems mechanisms of memory consolidation and storage. *Prog. Neurobiol.* 79: 123–135.

Wang H-Y, Pisano MR, and Friedman E (1994) Attenuated protein kinase C activity and translocation in Alzheimer's disease brain. *Neurobiol. Aging* 15: 293–298.

Wang HY, Lee DHS, Davis CB, and Shank RP (2000) Amyloid peptide A$\beta_{1\text{-}42}$ binds selectively and with picomolar affinity to α7 nicotinic acetylcholine receptors. *J. Neurochem.* 75: 1155–1161.

Wang Q, Walsh DM, Rowan MJ, Selkoe DJ, and Anwyl R (2004) Block of long-term potentiation by naturally secreted and synthetic amyloid β-peptide in hippocampal slices is mediated via activation of the kinases c-Jun N-terminal kinase, cyclin-dependent kinase 5, and p38 mitogen-activated protein kinase as well as metabotropic glutamate receptor type 5. *J. Neurosci.* 24: 3370–3378.

Webster B, Hansen L, Adame A, et al. (2006) Astroglial activation of extracellular-regulated kinase in early stages of Alzheimer disease. *J. Neuropathol. Exp. Neurol.* 65: 142–151.

Weeber EJ, Beffert U, Jones C, et al. (2002) Reelin and ApoE receptors cooperate to enhance hippocampal synaptic plasticity and learning. *J. Biol. Chem.* 277: 39944–39952.

Weiner HL and Frenkel D (2006) Immunology and immunotherapy of Alzheimer's disease. *Nat. Rev. Immunol.* 6: 404–416.

Weingarten MD, Lockwood AH, Hwo SY, and Kirschner MW (1975) A protein factor essential for microtubule assembly. *Proc. Natl. Acad. Sci. USA* 72: 1858–1862.

West MJ, Coleman PD, Flood DG, and Troncoso JC (1994) Differences in the pattern of hippocampal neuronal loss in normal ageing and Alzheimer's disease. *Lancet* 344: 769–772.

Westerman MA, Cooper-Blacketer D, Mariash A, et al. (2002) The relationship between Aβ and memory in the Tg2576 mouse model of Alzheimer's disease. *J. Neurosci.* 22: 1858–1867.

Wiley JC, Hudson M, Kanning KC, Schecterson LC, and Bothwell M (2005) Familial Alzheimer's disease mutations inhibit γ-secretase-mediated liberation of β-amyloid precursor protein carboxy-terminal fragment. *J. Neurochem.* 94: 1189–1201.

Willem M, Garratt AN, Novak B, et al. (2006) Control of peripheral nerve myelination by the β-secretase BACE1. *Science* 314: 664–666.

Williamson R, Scales T, Clark BR, et al. (2002) Rapid tyrosine phosphorylation of neuronal proteins including tau and focal adhesion kinase in response to amyloid-β peptide exposure: Involvement of Src family protein kinases. *J. Neurosci.* 22: 10–20.

Wittmann CW, Wszolek MF, Shulman JM, et al. (2001) Tauopathy in *Drosophila*: Neurodegeneration without neurofibrillary tangles. *Science* 293: 711–714.

Wolfe MS (2006) The γ-secretase complex: Membrane-embedded proteolytic ensemble. *Biochemistry* 45: 7931–7939.

Wood JG, Mirra SS, Pollock NJ, and Binder LI (1986) Neurofibrillary tangles of Alzheimer disease share antigenic determinants with the axonal microtubule-associated protein tau (τ). *Proc. Natl. Acad. Sci. USA* 83: 4040–4043.

Wu CC, Chawla F, Games D, et al. (2004) Selective vulnerability of dentate granule cells prior to amyloid deposition in PDAPP mice: Digital morphometric analyses. *Proc. Natl. Acad. Sci. USA* 101: 7141–7146.

Wu JQ, Anwyl R, and Rowan MJ (1995) β-Amyloid selectively augments NMDA receptor-mediated synaptic transmission in rat hippocampus. *Neuroreport* 6: 2409–2413.

Wu SY and Dun NJ (1995) Calcium-activated release of nitric oxide potentiates excitatory synaptic potentials in immature rat sympathetic preganglionic neurons. *J. Neurophysiol.* 74: 2600–2603.

Xie CW (2004) Calcium-regulated signaling pathways: Role in amyloid β-induced synaptic dysfunction. *Neuromolecular Med.* 6: 53–64.

Xu J, Zhu Y, and Heinemann SF (2006a) Identification of sequence motifs that target neuronal nicotinic receptors to dendrites and axons. *J. Neurosci.* 26: 9780–9793.

Xu Q, Bernardo A, Walker D, Kanegawa T, Mahley RW, and Huang Y (2006b) Profile and regulation of apolipoprotein E

(ApoE) expression in the CNS in mice with targeting of green fluorescent protein gene to the ApoE locus. *J. Neurosci.* 26: 4985–4994.

Yan R, Bienkowski MJ, Shuck ME, et al. (1999) Membrane-anchored aspartyl protease with Alzheimer's disease β-secretase activity. *Nature* 402: 533–537.

Yan SD, Chen X, Fu J, et al. (1996) RAGE and amyloid-β peptide neurotoxicity in Alzheimer's disease. *Nature* 382: 685–691.

Yao PJ (2004) Synaptic frailty and clathrin-mediated synaptic vesicle trafficking in Alzheimer's disease. *Trends Neurosci.* 27: 24–29.

Yao PJ, Bushlin I, and Furukawa K (2005) Preserved synaptic vesicle recycling in hippocampal neurons in a mouse Alzheimer's disease model. *Biochem. Biophys. Res. Commun.* 330: 34–38.

Yasuda RP, Ikonomovic MD, Sheffield R, Rubin RT, Wolfe BB, and Armstrong DM (1995) Reduction of AMPA-selective glutamate receptor subunits in the entorhinal cortex of patients with Alzheimer's disease pathology: A biochemical study. *Brain Res.* 678: 161–167.

Ye C, Walsh DM, Selkoe DJ, and Hartley DM (2004) Amyloid β–protein induced electrophysiological changes are dependent on aggregation state: *N*-methyl-D-aspartate (NMDA) versus non-NMDA receptor/channel activation. *Neurosci. Lett.* 366: 320–325.

Ye CP, Selkoe DJ, and Hartley DM (2003) Protofibrils of amyloid β-protein inhibit specific K^+ currents in neocortical cultures. *Neurobiol. Dis.* 13: 177–190.

Ye S, Huang Y, Mullendorff K, et al. (2005) Apolipoprotein (apo) E4 enhances amyloid β peptide production in cultured neuronal cells: ApoE structure as a potential therapeutic target. *Proc. Natl. Acad. Sci. USA* 102: 18700–18705.

Ying SW, Futter M, Rosenblum K, et al. (2002) Brain-derived neurotrophic factor induces long-term potentiation in intact adult hippocampus: Requirement for ERK activation coupled to CREB and upregulation of *Arc* synthesis. *J. Neurosci.* 22: 1532–1540.

Yoshimoto M, Iwai A, Kang D, Otero DAC, Xia Y, and Saitoh T (1995) NACP, the precursor protein of the non-amyloid β/A4 protein (Aβ) component of Alzheimer disease amyloid, binds Aβ and stimulates Aβ aggregation. *Proc. Natl. Acad. Sci. USA* 92: 9141–9145.

Yu SP (2003) Regulation and critical role of potassium homeostasis in apoptosis. *Prog. Neurobiol.* 70: 363–386.

Yuan LL and Chen X (2006) Diversity of potassium channels in neuronal dendrites. *Prog. Neurobiol.* 78: 374–389.

Yun SH, Gamkrelidze G, Stine WB, et al. (2006) Amyloid-beta$_{1-42}$ reduces neuronal excitability in mouse dentate gyrus. *Neurosci. Lett.* 403: 162–165.

Yuste R, Majewska A, and Holthoff K (2000) From form to function: Calcium compartmentalization in dendritic spines. *Nat. Neurosci.* 3: 653–659.

Zerbinatti CV, Wahrle SE, Kim H, et al. (2006) Apolipoprotein E and low density lipoprotein receptor-related protein facilitate intraneuronal Aβ42 accumulation in amyloid model mice. *J. Biol. Chem.* 281: 36180–36186.

Zhang B, Maiti A, Shively S, et al. (2005) Microtubule-binding drugs offset tau sequestration by stabilizing microtubules and reversing fast axonal transport deficits in a tauopathy model. *Proc. Natl. Acad. Sci. USA* 102: 227–231.

Zhang C, Qiu HE, Krafft GA, and Klein WL (1996) Aβ peptide enhances focal adhesion kinase/Fyn association in a rat CNS nerve cell line. *Neurosci. Lett.* 211: 187–190.

Zhao D, Watson JB, and Xie CW (2004) Amyloid β prevents activation of calcium/calmodulin-dependent protein kinase II and AMPA receptor phosphorylation during hippocampal long-term potentiation. *J. Neurophysiol.* 92: 2853–2858.

Zheng H and Koo EH (2006) The amyloid precursor protein: Beyond amyloid. *Mol. Neurodegener.* 1: 5.

Zhu JJ, Qin Y, Zhao M, Van Aelst L, and Malinow R (2002) Ras and Rap control AMPA receptor trafficking during synaptic plasticity. *Cell* 110: 443–455.

Zhu X, Raina AK, Lee HG, Casadesus G, Smith MA, and Perry G (2004) Oxidative stress signalling in Alzheimer's disease. *Brain Res.* 1000: 32–39.

Zhu XW, Rottkamp CA, Boux H, Takeda A, Perry G, and Smith MA (2000) Activation of p38 kinase links tau phosphorylation, oxidative stress, and cell cycle-related events in Alzheimer disease. *J. Neuropathol. Exp. Neurol.* 59: 880–888.

Zou Z and Buck LB (2006) Combinatorial effects of odorant mixes in olfactory cortex. *Science* 311: 1477–1481.

34 Developmental Disorders of Learning*

E. L. Grigorenko, Yale University, New Haven, CT, USA

34.1 Developmental Disorders of Learning: What Do They Actually Mean?

Phenomenologically, the category of developmental disorders of learning refers to children who, for one reason or another, differ from their peers in acquisition of developmentally appropriate skills (e.g., speaking, counting, reading).

Conceptually, the category of developmental disorders of learning refers to deviations from typical development (1) that are substantial enough to qualify as disorders and (2) that affect learning. However, there is no single nosological category that brings these disorders together, and the two most established diagnostic manuals, the *Diagnostic and Statistical Manual of Mental Disorders* (DSM-IV, published by the American Psychiatric Association, 1994) and the *International Classification of Diseases and Related Health Problems* (IDC-10, published by the World Health Organization, 2005), present only a partial overlap in how these disorders are classified.

The diversity of the disorders commonly viewed as developmental disorders of learning is captured in the following paragraphs. This list is presented here not to overwhelm the reader (and the information is quite daunting!), but rather to demonstrate a lack of agreement of what disorders of learning actually are.

Specifically, DSM-IV distinguishes a large category of Disorders Usually First Diagnosed in Infancy, Childhood, or Adolescence. This category includes, among other subcategories, the disorders that directly involve and affect learning, specifically, Mental Retardation; Learning Disorders (Reading Disorder, Mathematics Disorder, Disorder of Written Expression, and Learning Disorder Not Otherwise Specified, NOS); Motor Skills Disorders; Communication Disorders (Expressive Language Disorder, Mixed Receptive-Expressive Language Disorder, Phonological Disorder, Stuttering, and Communication Disorder NOS); Pervasive Developmental Disorders (Autistic Disorder, Rett's Disorder, Childhood Disintegrative Disorder, Asperger's Disorder, and Pervasive Developmental Disorder NOS); and Attention-Deficit and Disruptive Behavior Disorders (Attention-Deficit/Hyperactivity Disorder (ADHD), Conduct Disorder, Oppositional Defiant Disorder, and Disorders in Both Categories NOS).

ICD-10's Chapter V presents Mental and Behavioural Disorders with subcategories referred to as (1) Disorders of Psychological Development and (2) Mental and Behavioural Disorders. The former category is subdivided into Specific Developmental Disorder of

* With permission from the publishers, the content of this chapter partially overlaps with Grigorenko EL (2007) Learning disabilities. In: Martin A and Volkmar F (eds.) *Lewis's Child and Adolescent Psychiatry: A Comprehensive Textbook,* 4th edn. Baltimore, MD: Lippincott Williams and Wilkins; and Grigorenko EL (2007) Triangulating developmental dyslexia: Behavior, brain, and genes. In: Coch D, Dawson G, and Fischer K (eds.) *Human Behavior and the Developing Brain.* New York: Guilford Press.

Speech and Language (Specific Speech Articulation Disorder, Expressive Language Disorder, Receptive Language Disorder, Acquired Aphasia with Epilepsy, Other Developmental Disorders of Speech and Language, and Developmental Disorder of Speech and Language, Unspecified); Specific Developmental Disorders of Scholastic Skills (Specific Reading Disorder, Specific Spelling Disorder, Specific Disorder of Arithmetic Skills, Mixed Disorder of Scholastic Skills, Other Developmental Disorder of Scholastic Skills, Developmental Disorder of Scholastic Skills, Unspecified); Specific Develop-mental Disorder of Motor Function; Mixed Specific Developmental Disorders; Pervasive Developmental Disorders (Pervasive Developmental Disorders, Child-hood Autism, Atypical Autism, Rett's Syndrome, Other Childhood Disintegrative Disorder, Overactive Disorder Associated with Mental Retardation and Stereotyped Movements, Asperger's Syndrome, Other Pervasive Developmental Disorders, Pervasive Developmental Disorder, Unspecified), among other disorders. The latter category includes a cluster of disorders associated with hyperactivity and conduct problems (e.g., Hyperkinetic Disorder and Conduct Disorder), separating attention problems from problems of hyperactivity (with attention problems listed in the first category as a psychological problem) and including stuttering in this category, rather than as a disorder of speech and language.

To restate, there is no uniformly accepted approach in how developmental disorders of learning should be referred to or classified. Correspondingly, in staging the discussion that unfolds in this chapter, it is important to comment on the following three issues. First, it is clear that no single nosological category captures all developmental disorders of learning. There are many developmental disorders where learning is disrupted. Second, many of these developmental disorders are comorbid, that is, co-occur in the same individual. Thus, which disorder is diagnosed as primary and what other disorders are codiagnosed is variable. Third, although there are many disorders in which learning is disrupted, the 'label' that typically denotes challenged learning is Learning Disability (LD). As mentioned earlier, this category is not used as a diagnostic category. Yet, there is a mountain (or rather a mountain chain) of literature on this category. For the ensuing discussion, it is important to differentiate nonspecific (or general) and specific LDs. Conventionally, the term nonspecific LD is used to refer to generalized problems of learning, such as mental retardation, and the term specific LD (SLD) is used to refer to disorders in a particular domain of acquisition or learning, such as reading, writing, or mathematics.

In this chapter, I use the concept of LD even though, as mentioned earlier, it does not correspond directly to any particular nosological category in the two predominant diagnostic schemes of the developed world. Throughout the chapter, I argue that LD best captures the common thread of all developmental disorders of learning.

34.2 The Concept of Learning Disabilities

Fundamentally, the concept of LD encompasses society's capacity

> . . . to monitor (and recruit) children for unexplained school failure in a way that was not possible before the LD category was reified and passed into law in 1969. (Reid and Valle, 2004: 467)

The LD category replaced a variety of 'loose' definitional references to previously used qualifiers such as 'slow learner,' 'backward children' (Franklin, 1987), and 'minimal brain dysfunction' (Fletcher et al., 2002).

In terms of its 'realization' in the context of current practices, the LD label typically assumes the presence of the following process. Under normal circumstances, LDs are not diagnosable prior to a child's engagement with schooling and the opportunity to master key academic competencies. While in school, a child is assumed to be assigned grade-appropriate tasks. These tasks assume some degree of variability in children's performance; these theoretical ranges constrain the definitions of acceptable and worrisome variability in performance. It is when the child's performance consistently falls out of the acceptable range in one or more academic subjects that the child becomes the focus of intense observation and documentation and is referred for evaluation to appropriate professionals (e.g., educational psychologists, neuropsychologists, and clinicians such as pediatricians, clinical psychologists, or psychiatrists). An important qualifier here is that such observation, documentation, and evaluation are considered only for children whose performance is below that expected based on their general capacity to learn; thus, the concept of 'unexpected' school failure is central to the definition of LD. When reports on the child's performance in the classroom, testing results, and clinical evaluations are compiled, the child and his or her family are referred to a special education committee, which determines eligibility for individualized special education services. If eligibility is established, an Individualized Education Program (IEP) is created. The IEP refers to a specific diagnostic label carried by the child and cites the proper category of public laws that guarantees services for an individual with such a diagnosis.

34.3 Definition

The definition that currently drives federal regulations was produced by the National Advisory Committee on Handicapped Children in 1968 and subsequently adopted by the U.S. Office of Education in 1977 (Mercer et al., 1996). According to this definition,

> Specific learning disability means a disorder in one or more of the basic psychological processes involved in understanding or in using language, spoken or written, which may manifest itself in an imperfect ability to listen, think, speak, read, write, spell, or to do mathematical calculations. The term includes such conditions as perceptual handicaps, brain injury, minimal brain dysfunction, dyslexia, and developmental aphasia. The term does not include children who have learning problems which are primarily the result of visual, hearing, or motor handicaps, of mental retardation, or emotional disturbance, or of environmental, cultural, or economic disadvantage. (U.S. Office of Education, 1977: 65083)

Again, neither DSM-IV nor ICD-10 uses the term learning disabilities. DSM-IV makes a reference to learning disorders (American Psychiatric Association, 1994), which, according to DSM-IV, can be diagnosed,

> ...when the individual's achievement on individually administered, standardized tests in reading, mathematics, or written expression is substantially below that expected for age, schooling, and level of intelligence. (American Psychiatric Association, 1994: 46)

Of interest here is that this is one of the very few categories of DSM-IV where a reference is made explicitly to psychological tests, although DSM-IV does not provide specific guidelines as to what 'substantially below' means. Thus, DSM-IV implicitly refers to evidence-based practices (Fletcher et al., 2002) in the field. The problem, of course, is that there are multiple interpretations of these best practices (see discussion to follow). Yet, assuming there are consistent and coherent guidelines in place for establishing a diagnosis of LD, DSM-IV classifies types of LDs by referencing the primary academic areas of difficulty. The classification includes three specific categories and a residual diagnosis: Reading Disorder, Mathematics Disorder, Disorder of Written Expression, and Learning Disorder NOS. A common practice in the field is to view a diagnosis of a learning disorder as established by DSM-IV as an equivalent to 'specific learning disability,' which qualifies a child for special services under federal regulations (House, 2002).

34.4 History

The introduction of the concept of LD is typically credited to Samuel Kirk (then a professor of special education at the University of Illinois), who, while presenting at a parent meeting in Chicago on April 6, 1963, proposed the term learning disabled to refer to "children who have disorders in development of language, speech, reading, and associated communication skills" (Strydom and du Plessis, 2000). The category was well received by parents and promoted shortly thereafter by an established parent advocacy group known as the Association for Children with Learning Disabilities. Prior to the formal introduction of this concept, the literature had accumulated numerous descriptions of isolated cases and group analyses of children with specific deficits in isolated domains of academic performance (e.g., reading and math) whose profiles were later reinterpreted as those of individuals with specific LDs (e.g., specific reading and math disabilities). It is those examples in the literature and the experiences of many distressed parents who could not find adequate educational support for their struggling children that, in part, resulted in the creation of the field of LDs as a social reality and professional practice (Hallahan and Mercer, 2002). Subsequent accumulation of research evidence and experiential pressure led to the formulation of legislation protecting the rights of children with LDs.

Congress enacted the Education for All Handicapped Children Act (Public Law 94-142) in 1975 to support states and educational institutions in protecting the rights of, meeting the individual needs of, and improving the results of schooling for infants, toddlers, children, and youth with disabilities and their families. This landmark law is currently enacted as the Individuals with Disabilities Education Act (IDEA, Public Law 105-17; although the precise title of the law in its 2004 amendment is Individuals with Disabilities Education Improvement Act, it is still referred to as IDEA), as amended in 2004. The importance of this law is difficult to overstate: In 1970, U.S. schools provided education to only one in five children with disabilities (U.S. Office of Special Education Programs, 2000). By 2003–2004, the number of children aged 3–21 served under IDEA was more than 6.6 million (National Center for Education Statistics, 2005b).

SLDs make up 50% of all special education students served under IDEA. The term has proliferated very successfully and very quickly within the last two decades. There are multiple reasons why the concept of LD has enjoyed such success, among which are a lack of social stigma (i.e., parents are much more comfortable with the label of LD than with categories such as minimal brain dysfunction or brain injury), absence of implication of low intelligence or behavioral problems, and access to services (Zigmond, 1993).

In its 2004 amendment, IDEA recognized 13 categories under which a child can be identified as having a disability: autism; deaf–blindness; deafness; emotional disturbance; hearing impairment; mental retardation; multiple disabilities; orthopedic impairment; other health impairment; specific learning disability; speech or language impairment; traumatic brain injury; and visual impairment including blindness. It is notable that LDs as described in IDEA are referred to as 'specific learning disabilities' to emphasize the difference between children with SLDs and those with general learning difficulties characteristic of other IDEA categories (e.g., autism and mental retardation). The consensus in the field is that children with LDs possess average to above-average levels of intelligence across many domains of functioning but demonstrate specific deficits within a narrow range of academic skills. Finally, as stated earlier, exclusionary factors have been central to diagnoses of LDs since the authoritative definition of LD was introduced in 1977. As per these exclusionary criteria, a child cannot be diagnosed with an LD unless factors such as other disorders or lack of exposure to high-quality age-, language-, and culture-appropriate educational environments have been ruled out. It is the desire to rule out the exclusionary factor of lack of exposure to high-quality environments that prompted the introduction of the concept of Response to Treatment Intervention (RTI) (Deshler et al., 2005) in the 2004 amendment of IDEA. RTI signifies

> . . . individual, comprehensive student-centered assessment models that apply a problem-solving framework to identify and address a student's learning difficulties. (Deshler et al., 2005: 483)

It is important to note that RTI might appear counterintuitive at first: How can a disorder be defined through treatment if treatment is prescribed for a particular disorder? This 'circularity' of RTI, however, is only superficial. An implicit assumption behind RTI is that teaching is inadequate, and that is why schools 'produce' such a high level of LDs. A closer analogy would not be with treatment, but with prevention with vitamins; if vitamins are delivered properly, then many deficiencies can be avoided. Thus, if all children get extensive preventive instruction, the frequencies of LDs will diminish (see more detail on RTI in the section titled 'Presentation and diagnoses').

34.5 Epidemiology

Since the 1968 statutory introduction of LD as a legislated disability (i.e., within ~35 years of its existence as a category), approximately 50% of all students receiving special educational services across the nation have received them under the category of LD (Donovan and Cross, 2002). Among these students, the majority (80–90%) demonstrate substantial difficulties in reading (Kavale and Reese, 1992), and two of every five were identified because of persistent difficulties in reading acquisition (President's Commission on Excellence in Special Education, 2002).

There are two main sources for estimates of prevalence rates of LDs.

The first and most obvious one is linked to the number of children served under this category of IDEA. When this number is mapped on the total number of school-age children in the United States, although the number fluctuates from year to year, the average estimates of prevalence rates for LDs are around 5–6% of the total school-age population. To illustrate, in 2003, 2.72 million children were identified as having LDs. This represents a 150–200% increase in the number of students aged 6–17 with LDs compared with that number in 1975.

Yet, it is important to note that prevalence rates vary substantially from district to district and from state to state. For example, in 2004, under the SLD category, in Kentucky, 1.8% of all students aged 6–21 received special education services, compared with 5.9% in Iowa. Thus, based on these numbers, the prevalence rates of LDs in Iowa are about 3.3 times as high as in Kentucky, two states in close geographic proximity! This observation stresses the mosaic-like situation of LD diagnosis – there is no unified approach to these diagnoses across different local education agencies in the United States.

When IDEA-related prevalence rates are considered, LDs are observed more frequently in boys than in girls (64.5% vs. 33.5% for boys and girls aged 6–17, respectively) and more frequently in underrepresented minority groups than in Asian Americans or Whites. Risk ratios (which compare the proportion of a particular racial/ethnic group served to the proportion of all other racial/ethnic groups combined) are 1.5, 0.4, 1.3, 1.1, and 0.9 for American Indian, Asian American, African American, Hispanic American, and White students, respectively. A risk ratio of 1.0 indicates no difference between the racial/ethnic groups.

The second source for these rates is research studies. Per results from these studies, it is assumed that, although 10–12% of school-age children show specific deficits in selected academic domains, high-quality classroom instruction and supplemental intensive small-group activities can reduce this number to ~6% of children. It is assumed that these 6% will meet strict criteria for LDs and require special education intervention.

It is important to note that most of the research in the field of LDs is currently conducted with reading and, correspondingly, Specific Reading Disability (SRD). There is little established evidence that reliably points to prevalence rates of disorders of math and writing.

To illustrate, according to the results of current research on early reading acquisition, 2–6% of children do not show expected progress even in the context of the highest quality evidence-based reading instructions. Based on U.S. national data, the risk for reading problems as defined through failure to reach age- and grade-adequate milestones ranges from 20–80%. Specifically, data from the 2005 National Assessment of Educational Progress show that 36% of fourth graders do not possess the adequate reading skills required for completion of grade-appropriate educational tasks (National Center for Education Statistics, 2005a). However, it is clear that far from all of these children have SRD. The majority of these children mostly likely underachieve because of inadequate educational experiences and causes other than SRD.

Some changes in the 2004 version of IDEA were invoked directly because of concerns regarding the overidentification of students as learning disabled. The category of LDs has often been the largest single category of children served under IDEA (for latest relevant statistics, see IDEA Data, 2006). The reality of everyday practices in school districts was such that most diagnoses prior to the 2004 reauthorization were based on so-called aptitude–achievement discrepancy criteria, which required a severe discrepancy between IQ and achievement scores (e.g., two standard deviations, 2 years of age equivalence), although IDEA had never specifically required a discrepancy formula (Mandlawitz, 2006). Correspondingly, it has been argued that these discrepancy-based approaches are flawed (Francis et al., 2005) and might have led to overidentification. In light of this hypothesis, IDEA 2004 emphasizes that there is no explicit IQ–achievement discrepancy requirement for diagnosis of LDs. As a possible alternative approach for identification and diagnosis, IDEA 2004 states that local educational agencies may use a child's RTI in lieu of classification processes (Council of Parent Attorneys and Advocates, 2004). A local educational agency (e.g., a school) may choose to administer to the child in question an evidence-based intervention program to determine his or her eligibility for special education services under IDEA based on the child's response to this program.

Specifically, the statutory language of IDEA 2004 (Public Law 108-446) states:

> (6) Specific Learning Disabilities.
> (A) In general.
> Notwithstanding section 607(b), when determining whether a child has a specific learning disability as defined in section 602, a local educational agency shall not be required to take into consideration whether a child has a severe discrepancy between achievement and intellectual ability in oral expression, listening comprehension, written expression,

> basic reading skill, reading comprehension, mathematical calculation, or mathematical reasoning.
> (B) Additional authority.
> In determining whether a child has a specific learning disability, a local educational agency may use a process that determines if the child responds to scientific, research-based intervention as a part of the evaluation procedures described in paragraphs (2) and (3). (§614(b) (6))

As a consequence of this language, although aptitude–achievement discrepancy has been and continues to remain the common, although not required, practice for local educational agencies, there is a new 'entry point' for RTI. Needless to say, these changes are of great theoretical and practical importance. The tradition and system of specific LD identification in the United States are now fluid, and rather few specific recommendations exist to help local educational agencies smoothly transition into the implementation of IDEA 2004.

34.6 Presentation and Diagnoses

As stated earlier, it is crucially important in a diagnosis of LD to establish a child's 'typical' intellectual performance and to document that the child's performance in the area of difficulty (e.g., reading or mathematics) does not correspond to what would be expected, given average intellectual functioning. Although this general principle is relatively easy to grasp, the field of LDs has struggled since its inception in the early 1960s to establish specific steps that should lead to the establishment of the diagnosis.

Prior to the 2004 reauthorization of IDEA, the most common way of establishing an LD diagnosis was the discrepancy criterion. The introduction of the discrepancy between ability and achievement criteria in the 1977 law was not based on empirical research, but rather driven by a need for a more objective approach to the diagnoses than those commonly used and largely discredited at the time (Gresham et al., 2004). Two decades of research and practical explorations of the discrepancy model resulted in its discreditation from points of view of theory (Sternberg and Grigorenko, 2002), reliability of diagnosis and classification (Francis et al., 2005), robustness of implementation (Haight et al., 2002), and treatment validity (Aaron, 1997). In response to the overwhelming amount of evidence for the inadequacy of the discrepancy model, however realized (through psychometric indices, age equivalences, regression approaches, or expert opinions), a number of alternative models have been proposed. The major dividing line between these new models and previous discrepancy-based models is in their theoretical orientation. Previous diagnostic models attempted to identify children diagnosable with LDs by looking for characteristic cognitive deficits, so that an intervention could be delivered to children with such deficits (Reschly, 1996), whereas the modern models argue for the need to deliver best pedagogical practices to all children and then best remediational-intervention approaches to those children who do not respond as well to good teaching (Reschly and Ysseldyke, 2002).

As per the 2004 reauthorization of IDEA, local educational agencies have some choice in selecting diagnostic models. At this point, the most widely discussed and evidence-supported model of LD identification is the Responsiveness/Response to Intervention (RTI) model (Vaughn and Fuchs, 2003). The RTI model has a number of features. First, the performance of the student in question is compared with the performance of his/her immediate peers on academic tasks. Specifically, RTI assumes tracking the academic performance and rate of its growth for all students within a given class, with a goal of identifying those students in a class whose performance differs from that of their peers both in absolute (i.e., level) and relative (i.e., rate of growth) terms. Second, the model is structured primarily by intervention, so students identified by these means are offered individualized accommodations and interventions with a goal of maximizing the effectiveness of the learning environment for a given student in need. Third, the model is multilayered, so that each layer offers an opportunity for further differentiation and individualization of education for students who need it. Typically, three layers are recommended: The first tier covers regular classroom environment; the second tier is characterized as 'supplemental' to tier 1; and the third tier is 'intensive,' 'individualized,' and 'strategic.' Fourth, only if these multilayered attempts to modify the regular classroom pedagogical environment are unsuccessful is the prospect of an LD diagnosis considered. In summary, a child could be identified as having an LD if he or she consistently failed to perform at a level and progress at a rate comparable with the child's peers in general education after having participated in an evidence-based intervention.

Although there is considerable agreement in the field on the promise of RTI as a diagnostic paradigm, there are a variety of opinions regarding how, specifically, RTI should be quantified. Currently, the following paradigms are on trial: (1) Administer norm-referenced assessment batteries at the beginning and end of every school year to quantify the growth in response to intervention – students whose growth rate is below 'appropriate' should receive additional intervention, and (2) administer norm-referenced assessment batteries with a particular performance threshold (i.e., 25th percentile) – students whose performance is below this threshold should receive intensive interventions, and their performance should be monitored at least four times a year. There is also significant theoretical and experimental evidence suggesting the need for and importance of continuous progress monitoring with frequent (e.g., weekly) assessments of improvement. Currently, however, there are concerns about both approaches because of a lack of trained educational and practical professionals equipped to translate and implement research-based interventions into the everyday life of American schools. Since the 2004 reauthorization of IDEA, local education agencies have been in search of new robust solutions for identifying LDs that will meet the regulations of federal laws. RTI-based approaches to LD diagnosis present considerable challenges for all professionals involved in the realization of IDEA: general and special education teachers, diagnosticians (psychologists and psychiatrists), and school psychologists. The heart of this challenge is the lack of operationalization and practical guidelines that can be easily implemented at the 'frontiers' of diagnosing and treating children with LDs.

The majority of students with LDs are identified in middle and high school: Early years of schooling might simply be insufficient for exposing and making evident a deficit in a particular academic domain. As mentioned, the core conceptual piece of the LD definition is that the deficit could have not been predicted reliably prior to the child's school entry because a child with LDs demonstrates otherwise typical levels of cognitive functioning.

Previously when the discrepancy criteria were applied, the diagnosis of LD was different from other forms of learning difficulties because of its stress on the specificity of the deficit (i.e., a discrepancy was expected not in all academic domains, but in a specific academic domain). The introduction of RTI-based approaches to diagnosis makes the question of differential diagnosis somewhat difficult to address. In fact, students with mental retardation, emotional or behavior disorders, ADHD, and other childhood and adolescent disorders might also exhibit low responsiveness to intervention. Yet, their nonresponsiveness will occur for reasons very different from those of students with LDs. In other words, if RTI cannot differentiate LDs from other diagnoses where learning difficulties are present but nonspecific, can RTI even be considered as a classification/diagnostic instrument (Mastropieri and Scruggs, 2005)?

Although this question has been raised, it has not yet been answered. The pre-2004 conceptualization of LDs assumed that the texture of LDs was in deficient (or different, atypical) psychological processing of information. In other words, the field was driven by the assumption that LDs were likely to represent a dysfunction in one or more basic psychological processes (e.g., phonological processing, sustained attention, different types of memory, executive functioning). These deficient processes in turn can slow down or inhibit mastery of a particular academic domain (e.g., reading or mathematics). Under this assumption, intensive academic instruction could improve performance in specific academic domains but could not treat the disorder. Even if reading improves as a result of intervention, in this paradigm the disorder might remanifest as a deficiency in a bordering domain (e.g., writing). In other words, although reading skills might be enhanced, the deficient psychological skills might impede some other academic domain of functioning.

Throughout the existence of the category of specific LDs, there has been a consistent and strong drive from parents, researchers, and educators for differentiating these disorders from generic learning difficulties. In its current iteration, RTI does not differentiate nonspecific and specific learning difficulties, because nonresponsiveness to intervention can occur with a variety of developmental disorders. In sum, because IDEA preserved the category of SLDs, there is a new huge task to differentiate specific and nonspecific learning difficulties by means of RTI and possibly other methods in the field.

One of these 'other' methods has to do, of course, with psychological testing. Many researchers argue for the necessity of maintaining the role of psychoeducational and neuropsychological tests on a variety of indicators, including IQ, in establishing LD diagnosis (Mastropieri and Scruggs, 2005; Semrud-Clikeman, 2005).

34.7 Etiology

There is a consensus in the field that LDs arise from intrinsic factors and have neurobiological bases, specifically atypicalities of brain maturation and function. There is a substantial body of literature convincingly supporting this consensus and pointing to genetic factors as major etiological factors of LDs. The working assumption in the field is that these genetic factors affect the development, maturation, and functional structure of the brain and in turn influence cognitive processes associated with LDs. Yet the field is acutely aware that a number of external risk factors, such as poverty and lack of educational opportunities, affect patterns of brain development and function and, correspondingly, might worsen the prognosis for biological predisposition for LDs or act as a trigger in LD manifestation.

Although this model, in main strokes, appears to be relevant to all LDs, far more research on relevant genes and brain structure and function is available for children with SRD than for any other LD. Thus, illustrative findings are presented here from SRD (for a more comprehensive review, see Grigorenko, 2007).

Multiple methodological techniques, such as electroencephalograms, event-related potentials, functional resonance imaging, magnetoencephalography, positron emission tomography, and transcranial magnetic stimulation, have been used to elicit brain–reading relationships (for recent reviews, see Price and Mechelli, 2005; Shaywitz and Shaywitz, 2005; Simos et al., in press). When data from multiple sources are combined, it appears that a developed, automatized skill of reading engages a wide bilateral (but predominantly left-hemispheric) network of brain areas passing activation from occipitotemporal, through temporal (posterior), toward frontal (precentral and inferior frontal gyri) lobes. Clearly, the process of reading is multifaceted and involves evocation of orthographical, phonological, and semantic representations that in turn call for the activation of brain networks participating in visual, auditory, and conceptual processing. Correspondingly, it is expected that the areas of activation serve as anatomic substrates supporting all these types of representation and processing.

Somewhat surprisingly, per recent reviews, there appear to be only four areas of the brain of particular, specific interest with regard to reading. These areas are the fusiform gyrus (i.e., the occipitotemporal cortex in the ventral portion of Brodmann's area 37, BA 37), the posterior portion of the middle temporal gyrus (roughly BA 21, but possibly more specifically, the ventral border with BA 37 and the dorsal border of the superior temporal sulcus), the angular gyrus (BA 39), and the posterior portion of the superior temporal gyrus (BA 22).

It is also important to note the developmental changes in patterns of brain functioning that occur with increased mastery of reading skill: progressive, behaviorally modulated development of left-hemispheric 'versions' of these areas and progressive disengagement of right-hemispheric areas. In addition, there appears to be a shift of regional activation preferences. The frontal regions are used by fluent more than by beginning readers, and readers with difficulties activate the parietal and occipital regions more than the frontal regions.

In an attempt to understand the mechanism of the 'deficient' pattern of brain activation while engaged in reading, researchers are looking for genes that might be responsible, at least partially, for these observed differences in functional brain patterns. This search is supported by a set of convergent lines of evidence (for reviews, see Fisher and DeFries, 2002; Grigorenko, 2005; Barr and Couto, in press). First, SRD has been considered a familial disorder since the late nineteenth century. This consideration is grounded in years of research into the familiality of SRD (i.e., similarity on the skill of reading among relatives of different degree), characterized by studies that have engaged multiple genetic methodologies, specifically twin (Cardon et al., 1994, 1995; Byrne et al., 2005), family (Wolff and Melngailis, 1994; Grigorenko et al., 1997; Cope et al., 2005) and sib-pair designs (Francks et al., 2004; Ziegler et al., 2005). Although each of these methodologies has its own resolution power to explain similarities among relatives by referring to genes and environments as sources of these similarities and obtaining corresponding estimates of relative contributions of genes and environments, all methodologies have produced data that unanimously point to genetic similarities as the main source of familiality of SRD.

Today, it is assumed that multiple genes contribute to the biological risk factor that runs in families and forms the foundation for the development of SRD. Specifically, nine candidate regions of the human genome have been implicated (Grigorenko, 2005). These regions are recognized as SRD candidate regions; they are abbreviated as *DYX1–9*

(DYX for dyslexia, a term often used to refer to SRD) and refer to the regions on chromosomes 15q, 6p, 2p, 6q, 3cen, 18p, 11p, 1p, and Xq, respectively. Each of these regions harbors dozens of genes, so clearly, the field offers empirical validation that multiple genes contribute to the manifestation of SRD. A number of different research groups are actively at work on these genetic regions in an attempt to identify plausible candidate genes. Four successful attempts have been announced in the literature: one for the 15q region, the candidate gene known as *DYX1C1* (Taipale et al., 2003); two for the 6p region, the candidate gene known as *KIAA0319* (Francks et al., 2004; Cope et al., 2005) and the candidate gene knows as *DCDC2* (Meng et al., 2005; Schumacher et al., 2006); and one for the 3cen region, *ROBO1* (Hannula-Jouppi et al., 2005). Although the field has not yet converged on 'firm' candidates, it is remarkable and of great scientific interest that all four current candidate genes for SRD are involved with biological functions of neuronal migration and axonal crossing. Thus, all these genes are plausible candidates for understanding the pattern of brain functioning in SRD described earlier.

34.8 Relevant Theoretical Models and Considerations

As mentioned earlier, the literature on LDs is uneven, with the vast majority relating to SRD. Correspondingly, here I summarize the so-referred overarching model of LDs (Fletcher et al., 2007). Subsequently, I illustrate this model with detailed references to SRD. The overarching LD model delineates multiple levels of analyses and evidence.

According to this general model, LDs are anchored in a domain of particular academic difficulties (e.g., reading, spelling, computing, and writing). Correspondingly, the identification of an LD assumes that a diagnosis can be validly and reliably established on the basis of observed repeated patterns of weaknesses in a particular academic domain in the presence of strengths in all or some other academic domains. Thus, concerns, referrals, and diagnostic assessments are always centered on a particular academic domain that defines the content of LD. Correspondingly, the first step in LD identification is documenting the presence of a consistent failure or academic skill deficits, when compared with peer performance, on a set of specific tasks. Thus, behavioral presentation in a particular academic domain is the first level of analysis in the pyramid of LD diagnoses. However, the presence of an academic deficit is a necessary but insufficient condition for establishing an LD diagnosis.

The second level of analysis pertains to capturing individual characteristics of the child for whom an LD diagnosis is considered. Specifically, at this level, clusters of child characteristics are considered within the paradigm of inclusion and exclusion criteria of the LD category. Typically, at this level, the information is gathered in four directions: (1) pertaining to the academic domain of concern and cognitive processing known to be relevant to this particular domain, (2) pertaining to other academic domains in which the child demonstrates average or above-average levels of performance, (3) indicators of general cognitive functioning, and (4) other noncognitive and nonacademic domains of child's functioning (e.g., motivation, neurological and psychiatric indicators). Obviously, the information gathered at (1) is used within the context of inclusion and the information gathered in (2)–(4) within the context of exclusion criteria. It is critically important that there are well-developed psychological models available both for (1) and (2). For example, to identify LD in reading (SRD), it is important to know what cognitive processes constitute the texture of this academic skill. Similarly, since academic skills tend to correlate substantially in typically developing children, it is important to know what SRD and, for example, specific math disability (SMD) have in common and how they differ in terms of overlapping and specific psychological processes. To illustrate this level of analysis, I discuss modern psychological models of SRD below.

The third level of analysis involves both causal and associated etiological factors of LD. Specifically, a number of risk and protective factors rooted in the child's biology (e.g., gene and brain factors) and environment (e.g., school, neighborhood, and family environment factors) are considered at this level. The point here is to capitalize on the evidence in the field to differentiate LDs and underachievement, specific and nonspecific LDs, and specific LDs and comorbid conditions.

It is important to note that this model allows a diagnostician to move both up and down. The expectation is that the information converges across all three levels of analysis, and the diagnosis of LD is reliably established. However, it is possible, especially with young children, that the first 'level of entry' into the model is through cognitive processes that constitute the texture of the skill and thus emerge prior to the acquisition of the skill; for example, a child having difficulty mastering rhymes and letters might be identified as at risk for reading failure prior to entering formal reading instruction (Lonigan, 2003). Similarly, it is possible to enter the model through the level of biological risk factors; for example, given that SRD appears to be genetic, a child whose parents both have difficulty reading is at higher risk for SRD than is a child from a risk-free family (Gallagher et al., 2000; Lyytinen and Lyytinen, 2004). But, again, no matter what level of analysis this overarching model is entered through, it is very important that there are evidence-based models of acquisition of a particular skill (e.g., reading or mathematics) that is challenged in an LD.

Although psychological models of other LDs have been developed, here only those for SRD are exemplified for illustration purposes.

So far, there have been only generic references to the disruption of both the acquisition and mastery of reading skills that constitute the texture of SRD. When this generic reference is closely considered, another massive body of literature materializes: (1) cognitive psychology literature on types of representation of information involved in reading (i.e., reading involves the translation of meaningful symbolic visual codes (orthographical representation) into pronounceable and distinguishable sounds of language (phonological representation) so a meaning (semantic representation) arises) (Harm and Seidenberg, 2004); (2) developmental psychology literature on when these representations develop and what might cause the development of a dysfunctional representational system (Karmiloff-Smith, 1998); and (3) educational psychology literature on how the formation of functional representations can be aided or corrected when at risk for malfunction (Blachman et al., 2004).

Here only brief commentaries relevant to these literatures are offered. Today, given the predominance of the phonology-based connectionist account of SRD, behavioral manifestation of SRD is captured through a collection of highly correlated psychological traits. Although different researchers use different terms for specific traits, these can be loosely structured into groups aimed at capturing different types of information representation, for example: (1) performance on orthographic choice or homonym choice judgment tasks for quantifying parameters of orthographical representation; (2) phonemic awareness, phonological decoding, and phonological memory for quantifying phonological representation; and (3) vocabulary and indices of comprehension at different levels of linguistic processing for quantifying semantic representation. Correspondingly, in studies of the etiology, development, and educational malleability of SRD, the quantification of the disorder is carried out through these various traits (or components of SRD). Thus, many studies attempt to subdivide SRD into its components and explore their etiological bases, developmental trajectories, and susceptibility to pedagogical interventions separately as well as jointly.

Of note is that similar developments with regard to dissection of an academic skill and differentiation of componential psychological processes contributing to this skill have been taking place in the studies of acquisition of other academic skills, for example, mathematics (Butterworth, 2005; Geary, 2005; Fuchs et al., 2006; Fletcher et al., 2007).

34.9 Manifestation and Life Course

There is an accepted understanding in the field that LDs are typically lifelong disorders, although their manifestations might and often do vary depending on developmental stage and demands of the environment (e.g., school, work, retirement) imposed on an individual at a particular time. This understanding assumes that LDs do not manifest themselves exclusively in academic settings. In fact, although it might be successfully remediated during schooling, a particular LD might need further assistance and remediation in later years (e.g., as a part of the workforce). Although the literature on adults with LDs is still somewhat limited, there is an accumulation of evidence that LDs constitute a serious public health problem even after schooling. Such evidence is particularly rich in the field of studies of SRD.

LDs are comorbid with a number of other disorders typically diagnosed in childhood or adolescence, especially attention deficit (Semrud-Clikeman et al., 1992) and disruptive behavior disorders (Grigorenko, 2006). LDs also often co-occur with anxiety and depression (Martinez and Semrud-Clikeman, 2004). Correspondingly, individuals with LDs are at higher risk for developing other mental health problems.

Yet, the main drawback for individuals with specific LDs has to do with their educational achievement. On average, only ~50% of students aged 14 and older diagnosed with LDs graduate with regular high school diplomas. The dropout rate among these students is very high (~45%), and it is even higher for underrepresented minority students. The employment prospects of these students are also troublesome – only about 60% of student ages 14 and older diagnosed with LDs have paid jobs outside the home.

Thus, it is important to realize that the impact of LDs is not limited to any one academic domain (e.g., reading or mathematics); these are lifetime disorders with wide-ranging consequences.

34.10 Treatment, Remediation, Intervention, and Prevention

Currently, there are no approved medical treatments for children with LDs. There is a consensus in the field that children with LDs should be provided special education and related services upon establishment of their eligibility and determination of the necessity, content, duration, and desired outcomes of such education and services.

Yet, in much of the literature, many educators have expressed concern with the possible presence of faulty identification procedures in states and districts across the country, which has resulted in the possible abuse of the classification and service systems. The ever-growing number of children identified with LDs might indicate that this category has become a 'trap' for lower-performing students, irrespective of an LD diagnosis.

In response to this concern, the 2004 reauthorization of IDEA makes reference to a set of prevention mechanisms intended to establish a better classification strategy for identifying children with LDs. By law, schools need to implement systemic models of prevention that address (1) primary prevention: the provision of high-quality education for all children; (2) secondary prevention: targeted, scientifically based interventions for children who do not respond to primary prevention; and (3) tertiary prevention: the provision of intensive individualized services and interventions for those children who have not responded to high-quality instruction or subsequent intervention efforts. As per new regulations, it is assumed that this third group of children, namely those children who have failed to respond to age-, language-, and culture-appropriate, evidence-based, domain-specific instruction (e.g., in reading or mathematical cognition), can be identified as eligible for special education services. These prevention mechanisms are also assumed to be used as diagnostic mechanisms (see earlier discussion of RTI). This circular system of an outcome of intervention being also an entry point to diagnosis is currently creating significant turmoil in the literature and in practice.

In general, RTI approaches are conceived as a twofold simultaneous realization of high-quality, domain-specific instruction and continuous formative evaluation of students' performance and learning (Mellard et al., 2004a,b). In other words, RTI refers to ongoing assessment of students' response to evidence-based pedagogical interventions in particular academic domains. Thus, it is assumed that LDs can be identified only when underachievement related to poor instruction is ruled out. (It is also important to note that the primary diagnosis of LD is established only in the absence of other neuropsychaitric conditions.) Although it exists in a number of alternative forms, RTI includes eight central features and six common attributes. Among the central features linking all forms of RTI are: (1) high-quality classroom instruction, (2) research-based instruction, (3) classroom performance measures, (4) universal screening, (5) continuous progress monitoring, (6) research-based intervention, (7) progress monitoring during intervention, and (8) fidelity measures. Among common attributes of different RTI models, there are concepts of (1) multiple tiers; (2) transition from instruction for all to increasingly intense interventions; (3) implementation of differentiated curricula; (4) instruction delivered by staff other than the classroom teacher; (5) varied duration, time, and frequency of intervention; and (6) categorical or noncategorical placement decisions (Graner et al., 2005). Clearly, the concept of RTI is centered on the field's definition of high-quality research-validated instruction. It is important to note that, although there is growing consensus on the critical elements for effective reading instruction (e.g., Foorman et al., 2003), other domains of teaching for academic competencies are far from consensus-driven.

There are numerous examples of RTI-based treatment of LDs; two often-cited ones are the Minneapolis Public School's Problem Solving Model, in action since 1994 (Marston et al., 2003), and the Heartland (Iowa) Area Education Association's Model, implemented in 1986 (Ikeda and Gustafson, 2002). The Minneapolis model is a three-tier intervention model where the referral to special education is made only after consecutive failures to benefit from instruction throughout all three tiers of pedagogical efforts. The Iowa model originally included four tiers, where the third tier was subdivided into two related steps, but it was then collapsed into one tier, similar to the

Minneapolis model. Unfortunately, neither model has published empirical data on its effectiveness. Yet, years of implementation have resulted in appreciation from the communities they serve and in a stable, relatively small special education population.

Currently, the concept of RTI is under careful examination by researchers supported by both the U.S. Department of Education and the National Institute of Child Health and Development. The future of RTI and its role in diagnosing and treating specific LDs is dependent on answers to critical questions: (1) whether an RTI model can be implemented on a large scale; (2) how an RTI model can be used for LD eligibility determination; (3) whether an RTI is an effective prevention system; and (4) whether RTI enhances LD determination and minimizes the number of false positives.

34.11 Conclusion

I began this chapter with a brief discussion of the concept of developmental disorders of learning and with the concern that there is no single definition of this concept. In fact, the discussion of the 'multi-representativeness' of this concept in the two main diagnostic schemes (DSM-IV and ICD-10) led me to substitute it with the concept of LD. The discussion of the category of LD in this chapter hopefully stresses the importance of this concept and, indirectly, the concept of developmental disorders of learning. The LD concept is important because of its (1) prevalence, (2) implications for countless school-age students and adults, and (3) importance for the development of fundamental models of acquisition of cognitive skills and strategies of prevention and remediation of failure of acquisition.

Currently, students with specific LDs constitute about half of all students served under IDEA. Effective identification of such students and their efficacious and efficient remediation are crucial steps to address their individual educational needs and to provide them with adequate and equal life opportunities.

Given changes in IDEA 2004, it is no surprise that RTI is been central to current discourse on specific LDs. RTI is essential to the professional discussions of educators, diagnosticians, and policy makers because of its promise to alleviate many long-standing concerns with the IQ/aptitude–achievement discrepancy model predominant in the field of LDs for the last 30 years. At this point, however, RTI has yet to deliver on its promise. If RTI succeeds, numerous benefits to educational systems and individuals might be realized (Graner et al., 2005). Specifically, as for the system, many inappropriate referrals might be eliminated to increase the legitimacy and fair nature of 'true' referrals; the costs of special education services might be reduced; various gender and ethnicity biases might be minimized; and accountability for student learning might increase. As for individuals, because the 'labeling' criteria will change, there will be less time for a student to demonstrate a 'true' failure in achieving the stipulated discrepancy value – prevention and remediation efforts are expected to start as early as possible; instruction will be individualized; identification will be focused on achievement rather than on aptitude–achievement discrepancy; and minimized labeling should result in less social stigma.

Yet, these are only expectations for now, and the immediate future will show whether RTI is a viable replacement to the discrepancy criteria.

Acknowledgment

Preparation of this chapter was supported by grants R206R00001 from the Javits Act Program administered by the Institute for Educational Sciences, U.S. Department of Education, and TW006764 and DC007665 from the National Institutes of Health (PI: Grigorenko). Grantees undertaking such projects are encouraged to express freely their professional judgment. This chapter, therefore, does not necessarily represent the position or policies of the IES or the NIH, and no official endorsement should be inferred.

References

Aaron PG (1997) The impending demise of the discrepancy formula. *Rev. Educ. Res.* 67: 461–502.

American Psychiatric Association (1994) *Diagnostic and Statistical Manual of Mental Disorders,* 4th edn. Washington, DC: American Psychiatric Association.

Barr CL and Couto JM (in press) Molecular genetics of reading. In: Grigorenko EL and Naples A (eds.) *Single-Word Reading: Cognitive, Behavioral and Biological Perspectives.* Mahwah, NJ: Lawrence Erlbaum.

Blachman BA, Schatschneider C, Fletcher JM, et al. (2004) Effects of intensive reading remediation for second and third graders and a 1-year follow-up. *J. Educ. Psychol.* 96: 444–461.

Butterworth B (2005) Developmental dyscalculia. In: Campbell JID (ed.) *Handbook of Mathematical Cognition*, pp. 455–467. New York: Psychology Press.

Byrne B, Wadsworth S, Corley R, et al. (2005) Longitudinal twin study of early literacy development: Preschool and kindergarten phases. *Sci. Stud. Reading* 9: 219–235.

Cardon LR, Smith SD, Fulker DW, Kimberling WJ, Pennington BF, and DeFries JC (1994) Quantitative trait locus for reading disability on chromosome 6. *Science* 226: 276–279.

Cardon LR, Smith SD, Fulker DW, Kimberling WJ, Pennington BF, and DeFries JC (1995) Quantitative trait locus for reading disability: Correction. *Science* 268: 1553.

Cope N, Harold D, Hill G, et al. (2005) Strong evidence that KIAA0319 on chromosome 6p is a susceptibility gene for developmental dyslexia. *Am. J. Hum. Genet.* 76: 581–591.

Council of Parent Attorneys and Advocates (2004) *H. R. 1350 Individuals with Disabilities Education Improvement Act of 2004 Compared to IDEA 97*. Warrenton, VA: Council of Parent Attorneys and Advocates, Inc.

Deshler DD, Mellard DF, Tollefson JM, and Byrd SE (2005) Research topics in responsiveness to intervention: Introduction to the special series. *J. Learn. Disabil.* 38: 483–484.

Donovan MS and Cross CT (2002) *Minority Students in Special and Gifted Education*. Washington, DC: National Academy Press.

Fisher SE and DeFries JC (2002) Developmental dyslexia: Genetic dissection of a complex cognitive trait. *Nat. Rev. Neurosci.* 3: 767–780.

Fletcher JM, Lyon GR, Barnes M, et al. (2002) Classification of learning disabilities: An evidence-based evaluation. In: Bradley R, Danielson L, and Hallahan DP (eds.) *Identification of Learning Disabilities: Research to Practice*, pp. 185–250. Mahwah, NJ: Lawrence Erlbaum.

Fletcher JM, Lyon GR, Fuchs LS, and Barnes MA (2007) *Learning Disabilities*. New York: Guilford.

Foorman BR, Breier JI, and Fletcher JM (2003) Interventions aimed at improving reading success: An evidence-based approach. *Dev. Neuropsychol.* 24: 613–639.

Francis DJ, Fletcher JM, Stuebing KK, Lyon GR, Shaywitz BA, and Shaywitz SE (2005) Psychometric approaches to the identification of LD: IQ and achievement scores are not sufficient. *J. Learn. Disabil.* 38: 98–108.

Francks C, Paracchini S, Smith SD, et al. (2004) A 77-kilobase region on chromosome 6p22.2 is associated with dyslexia in families from the United Kingdom and from the United States. *Am. J. Hum. Genet.* 75: 1046–1058.

Franklin BM (1987) The first crusade for learning disabilities: The movement for the education of backward children. In: Popkewitz T (ed.) *The Foundation of the School Subjects*, pp. 190–209. London: Falmer.

Fuchs LS, Fuchs D, Compton DL, et al. (2006) The cognitive correlates of third-grade skill in arithmetic, algorithmic computation, and arithmetic word problems. *J. Educ. Psychol.* 98: 29–43.

Gallagher AM, Frith U, and Snowling MJ (2000) Precursors of literacy delay among children at genetic risk of dyslexia. *J. Child Psychol. Psychiatry* 4: 202–213.

Geary DC (2005) Role of cognitive theory in the study of learning disability in mathematics. *J. Learn. Disabil.* 38: 305–307.

Graner PS, Faggetta-Luby MN, and Fritschmann NS (2005) An overview of responsiveness to intervention: What practitioners ought to know. *Top. Lang. Disord.* 25: 93–105.

Gresham FM, Reschly DJ, Tilly WD, et al. (2004) Comprehensive evaluation of learning disabilities: A response to intervention perspective. *Sch. Psychol.* 59: 26–29.

Grigorenko EL (2005) A conservative meta-analysis of linkage and linkage-association studies of developmental dyslexia. *Sci. Stud. Reading* 9: 285–316.

Grigorenko EL (2006) Learning disabilities in juvenile offenders. *Child Adolesc. Psychiatr. Clin. N. Am.* 15: 353–371.

Grigorenko EL (2007) Triangulating developmental dyslexia: Behavior, brain, and genes. In: Coch D, Dawson G, and Fischer K (eds.) *Human Behavior and the Developing Brain*, pp. 117–144. New York, NY: Guilford Press.

Grigorenko EL, Wood FB, Meyer MS, et al. (1997) Susceptibility loci for distinct components of developmental dyslexia on chromosomes 6 and 15. *Am. J. Hum. Genet.* 60: 27–39.

Haight SL, Patriarca LA, and Burns MK (2002) A statewide analysis of eligibility criteria and procedures for determining learning disabilities. *Learn. Disabil. Multidisciplinary J.* 11: 39–46.

Hallahan DP and Mercer CR (2002) Learning disabilities: Historical perspectives. In: Bradley R, Danielson L, and Hallahan DP (eds.) *Identification of Learning Disabilities: Research to Practice*, pp. 1–67. Mahwah, NJ: Lawrence Erlbaum.

Hannula-Jouppi K, Kaminen-Ahola N, Taipale M, et al. (2005) The axon guidance receptor gene *ROBO1* is a candidate dene for developmental dyslexia. *PLoS Genet.* 1: e50.

Harm MW and Seidenberg MS (2004) Computing the meanings of words in reading: Cooperative division of labor between visual and phonological processes. *Psychol. Rev.* 111: 662–720.

House AE (2002) *DSM-IV Diagnosis in the Schools*. New York: Guilford Press.

IDEA Data (2006) Part B Annual Report Tables. IDEA Data Website. https://www.ideadata.org/PartBReport.asp (accessed May 2007).

Ikeda MJ and Gustafson JK (2002) *Heartland AEA 11's Problem Solving Process: Impact on Issues Related to Special Education* (No. 2002–01). Johnston, IA: Heartland Area Educational Agency 11.

Karmiloff-Smith A (1998) Development itself is the key to understanding developmental disorders. *Trends Cogn. Sci.* 2: 389–398.

Kavale KA and Reese JH (1992) The character of learning disabilities: An Iowa profile. *Learn. Disabil. Q.* 15: 74–94.

Lonigan CJ (2003) Development and promotion of emergent literacy skills in children at-risk of reading difficulties. In: Foorman BR (ed.) *Preventing and Remediating Reading Difficulties*, pp. 23–50. Baltimore, MD: York Press.

Lyytinen P and Lyytinen H (2004) Growth and predictive relations of vocabulary and inflectional morphology in children with and without familial risk for dyslexia. *Appl. Psycholinguist.* 25: 397–411.

Mandlawitz M (2006) *What Every Teacher Should Know about IDEA 2004*. Boston: Allyn and Bacon.

Marston D, Muyskens P, Lau MY-Y, and Canter A (2003) Problem-solving model for decision making with high-incidence disabilities: The Minneapolis experience. *Learn. Disabil. Res. Pract.* 18: 187–200.

Martinez RS and Semrud-Clikeman M (2004) Emotional adjustment and school functioning of young adolescents with multiple versus single learning disabilities. *J. Learn. Disabil.* 37: 411–420.

Mastropieri MA and Scruggs TE (2005) Feasibility and consequences of response to intervention: Examination of the issues and scientific evidence as a model for the identification of individuals with learning disabilities. *J. Learn. Disabil.* 38: 525–531.

Mellard DF, Byrd SE, Johnson E, Tollefson JM, and Boesche L (2004a) Foundations and research on identifying model responsiveness-to-intervention sites. *Learn. Disabil. Q.* 27: 243–256.

Mellard DF, Deshler DD, and Barth A (2004b) LD identification: It's not simply a matter of building a better mousetrap. *Learn. Disabil. Q.* 274: 229–242.

Meng H, Smith SD, Hager K, et al. (2005) DCDC2 is associated with reading disability and modulates neuronal development in the brain. *Proc. Natl. Acad. Sci. USA* 102: 17053–17058.

Mercer CD, Jordan L, Allsopp DH, and Mercer AR (1996) Learning disabilities definitions and criteria used by state education departments. *Learn. Disabil. Q.* 19: 217–232.

National Center for Education Statistics (2005a) *National Assessment of Educational Progress: The Nation's Report Card: Reading (2005).* National Center for Education Statistics, U.S. Department of Education, Institute of Education Sciences. http://nces.ed.gov/nationsreportcard/pdf/main2005/2006451.pdf (accessed May 2007).

National Center for Education Statistics (2005b) Number and percent of children served under Individuals with Disabilities Education Act, Part B, by age group and state or jurisdiction: Selected years, 1990–91 to 2003–04. National Center for Education Statistics, Institute of Education Sciences, U.S. Department of Education. http://nces.ed.gov/programs/digest/d04/tables/dt04_054.asp (accessed May 2007).

President's Commission on Excellence in Special Education (2002) *A New Era: Revitalizing Special Education for Children and Their Families.* Washington, DC: U.S. Department of Education.

Price CJ and Mechelli A (2005) Reading and reading disturbance. *Curr. Opin. Neurobiol.* 15: 231–238.

Reid DK and Valle JW (2004) The discursive practice of learning disability. *J. Learn. Disabil.* 37: 466–481.

Reschly DJ (1996) Functional assessment and special education eligibility. In: Stainback W and Stainback S (eds.) *Controversial Issues Confronting Special Education: Divergent Perspective,* 2nd edn., pp. 115–128. Boston: Allyn and Bacon.

Reschly DJ and Ysseldyke JE (2002) Paradigm shift: The past is not the future. In: Thomas A and Grimes J (eds.) *Best Practices in School Psychology,* 4th edn., pp. 3–20. Bethesda, MD: National Association of School Psychologists.

Schumacher J, Anthoni H, Dahdouh F, et al. (2006) Strong genetic evidence of *DCDC2* as a susceptibility gene for dyslexia. *Am. J. Hum. Genet.* 78: 52–62.

Semrud-Clikeman M (2005) Neuropsychological aspects for evaluating learning disabilities. *J. Learn. Disabil.* 38: 563–568.

Semrud-Clikeman M, Biederman J, Sprich-Buckminster S, Lehman BK, Faraone SV, and Norman D (1992) Comorbidity between ADDH and learning disability: A review and report in a clinically referred sample. *J. Am. Acad. Child Adolesc. Psychiatry* 31: 439–448.

Shaywitz SE and Shaywitz BA (2005) Dyslexia (specific reading disability). *Biol. Psychiatry* 57: 1301–1309.

Simos PG, Billingsley-Marshall B, Sarkari S, and Papanicolaou AC (in press). Single-word reading: Perspectives from magnetic source imaging. In: Grigorenko EL and Naples A (eds.) *Single-Word Reading: Cognitive, Behavioral and Biological Perspectives.* Mahwah, NJ: Lawrence Erlbaum.

Sternberg RJ and Grigorenko EL (2002) Difference scores in the identification of children with learning disabilities: It's time to use a different method. *J. Sch.Psychol.* 40: 65–83.

Strydom J and du Plessis S (2000) Birth of a syndrome. In: *The Right to Read: Beating Dyslexia and Other Learning Disabilities.* Audiblox. http://www.audiblox2000.com/book2.htm (accessed May 2007).

Taipale M, Kaminen N, Nopola-Hemmi J, et al. (2003) A candidate gene for developmental dyslexia encodes a nuclear tetratricopeptide repeat domain protein dynamically regulated in brain. *Proc. Natl. Acad. Sci. USA* 100: 11553–11558.

U.S. Office of Education (1977) Assistance to states for education for handicapped children: Procedures for evaluating specific learning disabilities. *Fed. Regist.* 42: 65082–65085.

U.S. Office of Special Education Programs (2000) *History: Twenty-Five Years of Progress in Educating Children with Disabilities through IDEA.* Washington, DC: U.S. Department of Education.

Vaughn S and Fuchs LS (2003) Redefining learning disabilities as inadequate response to instruction: The promise and potential problems. *Learn. Disabil. Res. Pract.* 18: 137–146.

Wolff PH and Melngailis I (1994) Family patterns of developmental dyslexia. *Am. J. Med. Genet. B Neuropsychiatr. Genet.* 54: 122–131.

World Health Organization (2005) *International Statistical Classification of Diseases and Related Health Problems (The) ICD-10*, 2nd edn. Geneva: World Health Organization.

Ziegler A, Konig IR, Deimel W, et al. (2005) Developmental dyslexia – recurrence risk estimates from a German bi-center study using the single proband sib pair design. *Hum. Hered.* 59: 136–143.

Zigmond N (1993) Learning disabilities from an educational perspective. In: Lyon GR, Gray DB, Kavanagh JF, and Krasnegor NA (eds.) *Better Understanding Learning Disabilities: New Views from Research and Their Implications for Education and Public Policies*, pp. 251–272. Baltimore, MD: Paul H. Brookes Publishing.

35 Angelman Syndrome

J. L. Banko and E. J. Weeber, Vanderbilt University Medical Center, Nashville, TN, USA

35.1 Introduction

The ability to perceive our environment, store information about our experiences, and retrieve that information when needed is a fundamental necessity for human cognition. Neuroscience research has only recently begun to unravel the mysteries of learning and memory by identifying the elemental molecules, important proteins, and signal transduction pathways that underlie the formation of long-lasting memories. The identification of specific genes and their products involved in disorders associated with human mental retardation has greatly facilitated our overall understanding of the mechanisms underlying human cognition. Recent research of Angelman Syndrome (AS) represents a quintessential example of this process at work.

Angelman syndrome is a devastating human mental retardation condition that affects specific areas of the central nervous system, including the hippocampus. The discovery of this brain region–specific disorder and subsequent production of a mouse model has allowed researchers the unique opportunity to explore the molecular mechanisms at work in the adult hippocampus that directly underlie human memory processes. This chapter recounts the important discoveries surrounding this disorder and the implications of these discoveries for our current knowledge of the molecular players present in the hippocampus that are thought to facilitate learning and memory.

35.2 Understanding the Genetics of AS

35.2.1 The Prevalence of AS

The prevalence of AS among children and young adults is between 1/10 000 and 1/20 000 and is commonly accompanied by severe mental retardation, epilepsy, a puppet-like gait, dysmorphic facial features, a happy disposition with bouts of inappropriate laughter, hyperactivity, sleep disorders, and lack of speech. The etiology of AS arises from an absence of genetic contribution from a localized region on chromosome 15. Nearly 70% of AS cases involve cytogenetic deletion of q11-q13 (~4 Mb) on the maternally inherited chromosome 15 (15_{mat}).

Interestingly, 15q11 deletions also occur in Prader-Willi syndrome (PWI); however, the deletion is found on the paternally inherited chromosome 15 (15_{pat}), and the two disorders are characterized by distinct phenotypic differences (Cassidy et al., 2000). This suggests that there is differential expression of the genes in the homologous chromosome 15 and that the etiology of AS is specifically the consequence of cytogenetic disruption of the maternal chromosome (first to postulate this were Magenis in 1990 and Williams in 1990).

Understanding the genetic anomaly that defines AS begins in understanding how genes can be inherited in an active state from one parent and, alternatively, in an inactive state from the other parent. This phenomenon, referred to as genomic imprinting, is a poorly understood epigenetic mechanism affecting a relatively few known autosomal mammalian genes (Redei et al., 2006). Usually, autosomal genes are present in duplicate (i.e., two alleles), with one inherited from the father and one from the mother. For the majority of genes, both alleles are transcribed (or expressed) equally. However, for a small subset of genes, known as imprinted genes, only one allele is expressed in a parent-of-origin-dependent manner. Note that the 'imprint' here refers to the epigenetic mechanism through which one allele is silenced and is completely unrelated to the classical 'filial imprinting' manifest at the behavioral level.

35.2.2 Maternal Imprinting and AS

The mechanism of imprinting involves the biochemical marking of DNA by methylation of CpG-rich domains in association with particular chromatin conformations. This epigenetic mark allows the molecular machinery of each cell in the progeny to recognize and appropriately express only one allele at a particular locus. For example, during maternal expression, paternally allelic DNA methylation silences the paternal transcript, and the remaining functional genes in the locus are exclusively expressed maternally. Chromosome 15 contains a cluster of imprinted genes in the q11-q13 region, many of which are involved in brain development and function and normally undergo exclusively maternal expression. Therefore, if cytogenetic deletion of q11-q13 occurs on 15_{mat}, none of the imprinted gene products are expressed. There are additional genetic mutations that can occur to produce null expression of these imprinted genes. For example, 7–9% of AS cases are the result of imprinting mutations in which both the maternal and paternal copies undergo paternal-like methylation, and 2–3% show paternal unpaired disomy (UPD), whereby two copies of the paternal chromosome region are inherited with no maternal copies present (**Figure 1**). Finally, there is a subpopulation of patients with clinically diagnosable AS who do not fall into the aforementioned three groups but, rather, represent familial-derived mutations of one or more genes in the maternal 15q11-q13 critical region.

The discovery that 15q11-q13 represents the AS critical region narrowed the search for candidate genes that give rise to AS. In 1997, a gene within the AS critical region named *Ube3a* was found to be mutated in approximately 5% of AS individuals. These mutations can be as small as 1 base pair. The product of the *Ube3a* gene was initially identified following viral studies of p53 tumor suppressor protein degradation by the oncogenic human papilloma virus (HPV). Researchers interested in HPV *E6* gene expression following infection found that the HPV E6 protein alone had no effect on p53; however, in the presence of an associated protein p53, degradation was observed (Huibregtse et al., 1991). This associated protein, referred to as E6-associated protein, or E6-AP, was found to be the 100-kDa protein encoded by the *Ube3a* gene. The *Ube3a* gene has a spatially restricted imprinted expression pattern.

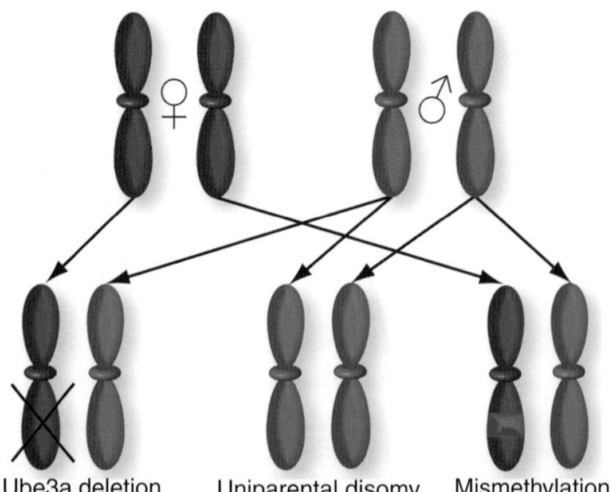

Figure 1 Maternal imprinting disorders resulting in Angelman Syndrome (AS). Genomic imprinting results in parent-specific epigenetic differentiation and monoallelic gene expression. Parental imprints are established during gametogenesis, where alleles of imprinted genes are maintained as either paternal or maternal origin. AS can arise from maternal deletion, uniparental disomy, or mismethylation of the AS critical region.

Ube3a shows imprinted expression in the brain but biallelic expression in other tissues. Each of the four genetic mechanisms described above that cause AS – large deletion, imprinting mutation, UPD, and point mutation – also cause inactivation or absence of the *Ube3a* gene.

35.2.3 The Ubiquitin Ligase Pathway

E6-AP is an enzymatic component of a complex protein degradation system termed the ubiquitin-proteosome pathway. This pathway is located in the cytoplasm of all cells. The pathway involves a small molecule, ubiquitin, which can be attached to proteins causing them to be degraded. Multiple steps are involved in the ubiquitination process (**Figure 2**). In the initial enzymatic step, the ubiquitin-activating enzyme E1 activates ubiquitin in an ATP-dependent reaction that links the E1 with the C terminus of a ubiquitin molecule. The ubiquitin-conjugating E2 enzymes then accept and transfer the activated ubiquitin moiety from E1 either to an E3 ligase or directly to a target substrate. The E3 ligase confers specificity to substrate recognition for ubiquitination. E6-AP ubiquitin ligase falls into the E3 category of ubiquitin lipases; therefore, it was believed that identifying the protein target(s) of E6-AP would unlock the mystery surrounding the AS disorder. To date, only four proteins have been identified as targets of E6-AP-dependent ubiquitination. These include the p53 tumor suppressor protein; the HHR23A protein, a human homolog to the yeast DNA repair protein Rad23 (Kumar et al., 1999); the multicopy maintenance protein (Mcm) 7 subunit involved in the initiation of DNA replication (Kuhne and Banks, 1998); and E6-AP, which is a target for itself (Nuber et al., 1998). Unfortunately, no obvious connection can be made between these identified targets and the etiology of AS.

35.3 Modeling AS in a Mouse

35.3.1 Production of the AS Mouse Model

The lack of a clear connection between E6-AP function and AS, coupled with the scarce availability of

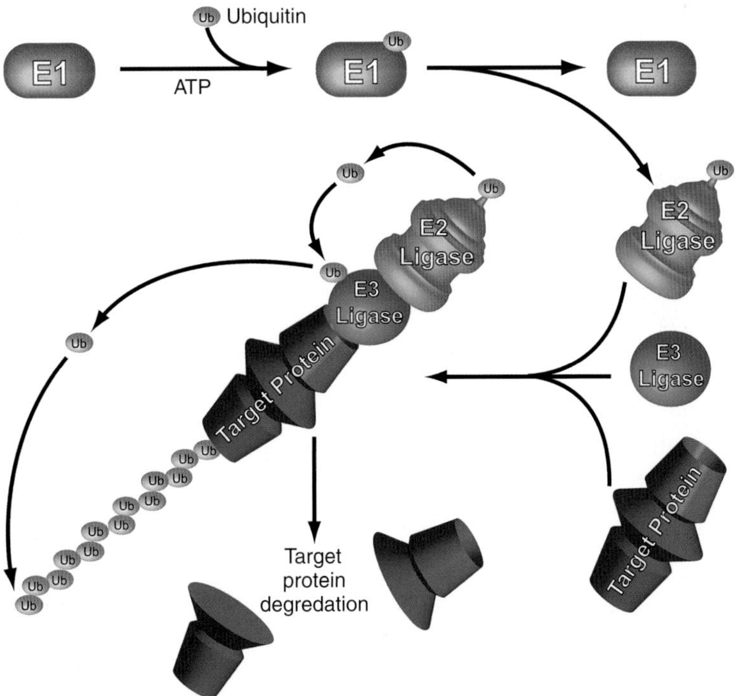

Figure 2 Ubiquitin ligase pathway. Association of an E1 ubiquitin ligase with a single ubiquitin (Ub) molecule results in an ATP-dependent manner. Ub is subsequently transferred to an E2 ligase. The E2 then associates with the E3, in this case Ube3a, and the target protein specified by the E3 ligase. The E3 ligase transfers successive Ub molecules to the target protein forming poly-Ub chains. When a critical length of the Ub chain is reached, the targeted protein associates with the proteosome and undergoes degradation.

AS postmortem brain tissue, necessitated the production of a mouse model for AS. Two mouse models were developed, each with a different strategy to disrupt the murine homolog of *Ube3a*. The mouse chromosome 7 contains a region exhibiting a similar gene compliment to the human AS critical region. The first mouse line, created by Gabriel and colleagues, utilized an Epstein-Barr virus latent membrane protein 2A (LMP2A) transgenic insertion that resulted in the deletion of the entire murine equivalent AS critical region. The rational for this method lies in mimicking what is seen in humans that exhibit the most common genetic defect leading to AS: an approximately 4-Mb deletion in the 15_{mat}q11-q13 region. Alternatively, the mouse model developed by Jiang and colleagues utilized a null mutation in *Ube3a* via a single gene knockout (Jiang et al., 1998). While both of these mouse models effectively disrupt *Ube3a*, there exists some controversy over whether *Ube3a* deficiency in and of itself is responsible for the manifestation of AS, or if the full phenotype is due to the combined affect of disrupting several genes in the human chromosome 15_{mat}q11-q13 critical region (Lee and Wevrick, 2000).

A phenotypic assessment in patients with the cytogenetic deletion (class I) exhibit a profile more true to what is commonly considered to be clinically classical AS. These patients show the full realm of AS characteristics including microcephaly and hypopigmentation. In contrast, patients for whom AS arises from specific *Ube3a* mutation (class II) or *Ube3a* mismethylation (class III) result in patients with fewer instances of hypopigmentation, microcephaly, and seizure. This indicates that AS caused by *Ube3a* disruption is exacerbated by the disruption of additional genes located at the same locus. Among these genes is the $GABA_A$ receptor $\beta3$ subunit (*GABRB3*). There is evidence that the inhibitory neurotransmitter GABA is involved in the suppression of seizures, which may explain why class II and III AS patients experience fewer occurrences of seizure. In support of this hypothesis, a lower instance of seizure activity in the Jiang et al. mouse model compared to the other mouse model was observed. Because nearly all available evidence points to *Ube3a* as the locus for AS, and given the inherent difficulties in interpreting the effects of multiple gene deletions in mice, the consensus was that the single *Ube3a*-null mutation mouse would provide a better instrument to investigate the molecular mechanisms underlying the AS etiology. The following section discusses experiments conducted using the Jiang et al. AS mouse model and relates the results to the human condition.

35.3.2 Characterization of the AS Mouse Model

The initial characterization of the maternal deficient *Ube3a*-null mouse mutant (*Ube3a* m^-/p^+) revealed striking similarities to the human phenotype (Jiang et al., 1998). These phenotypic similarities are more easily discernible when they are subdivided into categories of physical and physiologic characteristics.

35.3.2.1 Physical Similarities of AS and the Maternal Deficient Ube3a-Null Mouse

The brains of *Ube3a*-m^-/p^+ mice showed an overall normal morphology, with no obvious abnormalities in any particular brain regions, suggesting that maternal E6-AP deficiency does not effect neuronal development or organization. However, by 18 days of age *Ube3a*-m^-/p^+ mice were observed to have smaller bodies and brains than wild-type mice. This size difference was seen in both the cortex and cerebellum of the brain. Imprinted expression analysis revealed that, similar to the human *Ube3a* gene, the murine *Ube3a* gene also exhibited a spatially restricted imprinted expression pattern in which exclusively maternal expression was observed in the brain. In adult wild-type mice, the detection of *Ube3a* mRNA revealed high expression levels in areas CA1 and CA3 of the hippocampus, basal ganglia, cerebellum, and cerebral cortex and the periglomerular, granual and mitral cells of the olfactory bulb. This was compared to maternal deficient mice that showed no detectable hippocampal expression, reduced cerebellar expression with no detectable expression in the Purkinje cell layer, and an overall reduced expression in the olfactory region associated with a lack of detectable expression in the mitral cell layer.

Motor function and coordination was assessed using hind-paw footprint analysis, the bar crossing test and the accelerating Rotorod test. Each of these tests confirmed a distinct and significant motor deficit in the *Ube3a*-m^-/p^+ mice, which mimics the tremor, ataxia and motor coordination defect described in human AS patients. In addition, seizure in AS patients is very prominent and found to affect greater than 90% of diagnosed AS patients. Likewise, seizures in *Ube3a*-m^-/p^+ mice could easily be induced through audiogenic means by simply running an object vigorously over the metal grate lid of the mouse's home cage. Physical changes are more easily quantifiable and tend to be a more convincing argument for the recapitulation of a human mouse model. However, there are several ways to measure the behavioral correlates to human cognitive ability in the mouse by assessing its learning ability through behavioral testing and its function at a synaptic level through electrophysiologic techniques.

35.3.2.2 Cognitive Similarities of AS and the Maternal Deficient Ube3a-Null Mouse

The hippocampus is intimately involved in spatial memory processes and is linked to numerous cortical regions. Acquisition of explicit memory involves the hippocampus as part of a polymodal sensory integration scheme that processes visual, auditory, and somatosensory inputs. A great deal of evidence now implicates the hippocampus as an important brain structure involved in cognitive processing in humans. Although determining cognition is less straightforward in mice than it is in humans, we can call upon Pavlovian conditioning paradigms to asses the associative learning ability of *Ube3a*-m$^-$/p$^+$ mice.

The cognitive ability of the *Ube3a*-m$^-$/p$^+$ mice was assessed with the fear conditioning learning paradigm. The training paradigm consisted of an auditory conditioned stimulus (CS) paired twice with an unconditioned aversive stimulus (US: a mild foot shock) (*See* Chapter 21). The mice demonstrated their ability to associate the CS as a cue for the US or the training chamber context and the US by exhibiting a freezing behavior when re-presented with the CS or the training chamber. Although both contextual and cued fear-conditioned learning is dependent on the proper function of the amygdala, only the contextual learning is hippocampus dependent. The *Ube3a*-m$^-$/p$^+$ mutant mice exhibited robust freezing when re-presented with the CS 24 h after training, but significantly less freezing when reintroduced to the training chamber. These results indicate that hippocampus-dependent associative learning is disrupted in the *Ube3a*-m$^-$/p$^+$ mutant mice and is concordant with the imprinted expression pattern of *Ube3a*.

35.3.2.3 Physiologic Similarities of AS and the Maternal Deficient Ube3a-Null Mouse

The lack of hippocampal *Ube3a* expression coupled with the severe hippocampus-dependent learning deficit made the characterization of hippocampal synaptic function essential. The hippocampus is separated into three distinct synaptic pathways: the perforant path, the mossy fiber synapse, and the Schaffer collateral synapses. Of these three major synaptic connections, the Schaffer collaterals in area CA1 of the hippocampus are by far the most well characterized. It is in this region that synaptic transmission and plasticity were characterized in the *Ube3a*-m$^-$/p$^+$ mice. Jiang and colleagues found that basal synaptic transmission was unaltered in the AS mouse. This indicated that overall connectivity and single-stimulus synaptic function were essentially normal. Next, synaptic plasticity induced with high-frequency stimulation (HFS) was tested. It was shown that *Ube3a*-m$^-$/p$^+$ mice exhibited a severe deficit in long-term potentiation (LTP) induction. Although controversial, parallels can be drawn between the mechanisms of synaptic strengthening that occur during hippocampal LTP and those postulated to occur during hippocampus-dependent learning and memory events. Thus, a deficit in hippocampal LTP is consistent with a deficit in learning and memory. Perhaps most importantly, these studies were the first to implicate a deficit in hippocampal LTP in a human learning disability.

35.3.3 AS Mouse Hippocampal Physiology

It took nearly 3 years to identify a specific biochemical alteration in the AS mouse. Initially, the strategy employed identification of proteins that exhibited (1) a lack of ubiquitination in the AS mouse compared to normal mouse brain protein complement and (2) increased levels due to lack of degradation through the ubiquitin proteosome pathway. Although sound in design, identifying short-lived ubiquitinated proteins is problematic, and no gross changes in protein levels were observed in the AS mouse imprinted brain regions. It was not until a more in-depth analysis of hippocampal synaptic plasticity was performed that new and interesting implications of maternal Ube3a deficiency in the hippocampus were revealed.

Multiple stimulation patterns will elicit LTP in area CA1 of the hippocampus. To better understand the basis of the LTP deficit in the AS mouse, it is prudent to consider the LTP response to different patterns of stimulation (*See* Chapter 11). A standard LTP-inducing stimulation consisting of a 1-s, 100-Hz stimulation elicits a long-lasting increase in synaptic plasticity. Alternatively, increasing the number of high-frequency trains of stimulation can produce a potentiation that is both substantially higher in magnitude and longer lasting. Manipulating these variables in the LTP induction protocol is often used to determine the efficacy or potency of an applied drug or, as in this case, to evaluate the severity or penetrance of the Ube3a deficiency. In order to test the possibility that the LTP deficits in *Ube3a*-m^{-}/p^{+} mutants were due to an increase in the threshold of LTP induction, LTP was induced with a saturating amount of HFS designed to give the maximum potentiation in a given hippocampal slice. It was found that the saturating HFS could rescue the LTP deficit in the AS mouse.

What was the mechanism by which the LTP deficit could be overcome? The induction of LTP is highly dependent upon an influx of postsynaptic Ca^{2+}. Increasing the number of stimulations would increase the amount of Ca^{2+} influx significantly and could explain the LTP rescue. The question then would be whether the derangement of LTP induction was upstream (receptor activation) or downstream of calcium influx. The major neurotransmitter-activated calcium channel at the CA1 hippocampal synapse is the *N*-methyl-D-aspartate receptor (NMDAR). Slices stimulated with repeated very high frequency stimulation in the presence of the NMDA receptor antagonist DL-2-Amino-5-phosphonopentanoic acid (AP5) would determine whether the increase in LTP threshold observed in *Ube3a*-m^{-}/p^{+} mutants was due to insufficient postsynaptic NMDAR-dependent Ca^{2+} influx. Under these conditions, the LTP deficit in the *Ube3a*-m^{-}/p^{+} mice remained. The inability of *Ube3a*-m^{-}/p^{+} mutants to achieve NMDAR-independent LTP induction suggested that the LTP deficit, and importantly, the potential site of hippocampal synaptic dysfunction, resided downstream of calcium influx. The studies described earlier set the stage for the investigation into the molecular derangements that could be responsible for the cognitive loss in AS patients.

35.4 Molecular Changes in the AS Mouse

It has been hypothesized that the deficit in LTP and learning was biochemical in origin. The lack of any morphological changes in the CNS, coupled with the ability to rescue LTP, suggested that a disruption in a biochemical signal transduction pathway was the explanation. The rescue of LTP also suggested that the mechanisms responsible for proper synaptic function were present but that the system needed to be pushed, (i.e., during repeated HFS) in order for the system to function at a level for LTP induction to occur. More importantly, the in-depth electrophysiology described earlier reduced the number of proteins to be examined from the greater than 10 000 present in the central nervous system to just a handful. The proteins chosen to be examined closer had to meet the following specific criteria: (1) known to be involved in LTP induction processes, (2) known to be involved in learning and memory processes, and (3) known to be activated or modified in the presence of Ca^{2+}. Extensive research showed no changes in the major synaptic-associated protein kinases including the phosphorylation levels of PKC, PKA, or ERK (P42) isolated from hippocampal homogenates of *Ube3a*-m^{-}/p^{+} mice. However, a significant increase was detected in phospho-αCaMKII at the autophosphorylation site threonine 286 (Thr^{286}) (**Figure 3**) and threonine 305/306 (Thr^{305}/Thr^{306}). This single observation represented the first identified biochemical alteration in the AS mouse model that could potentially explain the learning and LTP deficits in the mouse and the cognitive deficits in human AS (Weeber et al., 2003). To help explain the implications of CaMKII misregulation, the next section addresses what is currently known about CaMKII regulation and its importance in normal signaling in the mammalian CNS.

35.5 CaMKII in Synaptic Plasticity and Memory Formation

35.5.1 Activation and Regulation of CaMKII

Initial studies of CaMKII's involvement in memory formation were conducted using an *in vitro* model for memory formation: LTP of the Schaffer-collateral synapses in area CA1 of the hippocampus. The Schaffer-collateral synapses are excitatory and use L-glutamate as their excitatory neurotransmitter. It has long been appreciated that induction of LTP requires high-frequency synaptic activity (Bliss and Lomo, 1973; Alger and Teyler, 1976) that results in activation of two types of glutamate receptors on postsynaptic CA1 pyramidal neurons: alpha-amino-3-hydroxy-

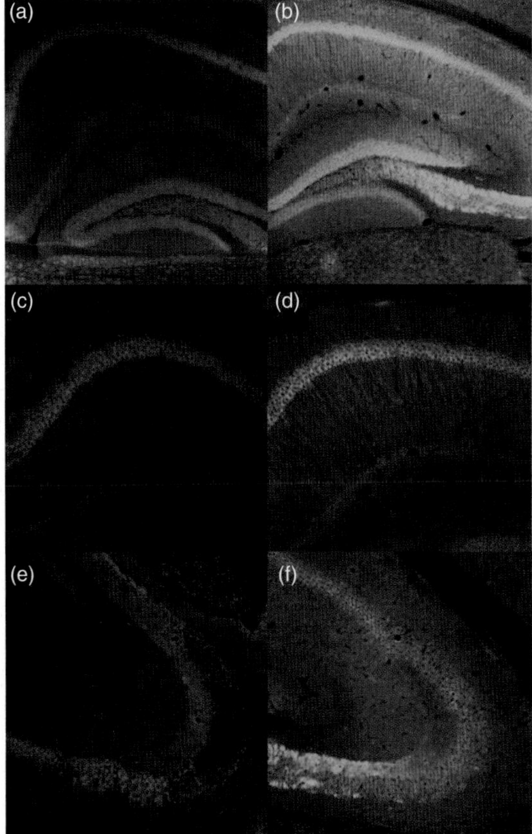

Figure 3 Increased threonine 286 Thr^{286} CaMKII phosphorylation in the Angelman Syndrome mouse model. Increased immunoreactivity to phosphorylated CaMKII at Thr^{286} in Angelman mouse hippocampus. Phosphorylated CaMKII at Thr^{286} was detected immunohistochemically in the hippocampi of wild type (a, c, e) and Angelman (b, d, f) mice. Increases in immunoreactivity are seen in the stratum pyramidale, stratum oriens, and stratum radiatum of CA1 and CA3 as well as the molecular layer and granule cell layer of the dentate gyrus. a, b, 100× magnification of the hippocampus. c, d, 200× magnification of area CA1. e, f, 200× magnification of area CA3.

5-methyl-4-isoxazole propionic acid (AMPA) and NMDA receptors. AMPA receptors have an ion channel that, when activated by glutamate, allows Na^{+} to enter the cell, resulting in depolarization of the postsynaptic membrane. NMDARs are also coupled to an ion channel; however, under resting conditions this ion channel is blocked by a molecule of Mg^{2+}. Once the membrane is depolarized, the Mg^{2+} block is removed and Ca^{2+} ions flow through the NMDAR ion channel into the cytoplasm. The resulting increase in intracellular Ca^{2+} mediated by the NMDAR is the primary signal for induction of LTP (Lynch et al., 1983; Harris et al., 1984; Morris et al., 1986; Malenka et al., 1988). The increase in cytoplasmic Ca^{2+} concentration mediated by NMDARs is relatively short-lived, and therefore it cannot account for the long-term increase in synaptic efficacy observed after induction of LTP. Therefore, it has been proposed that the initial increase in Ca^{2+} leads to the activation of several downstream kinases, which modify the function of the various synaptic proteins and induce long-lasting changes in synaptic efficacy. This intimate relationship between NMDAR-mediated Ca^{2+} influx and CaMKII activation brings us back to the LTP deficit seen in the AS mouse. Saturating amounts of high-frequency stimulation, causing an optimum amount of Ca^{2+} influx, were used to overcome the LTP deficit. The signaling and autoregulatory aspects of Ca^{2+} on CaMKII will become more apparent in the following section.

The regulation of CaMKII through autophosphorylation mechanisms is extraordinarily dynamic. Briefly, Ca^{2+}-calmodulin activates CaMKII by disrupting the association between the catalytic and inhibitory domains (Colbran et al., 1989) (**Figure 4**). Once bound to Ca^{2+}-calmodulin, CaMKII undergoes autophosphorylation at amino acid residue Thr^{286}, a residue located within the inhibitory domain. Phosphorylation of Thr^{286} has three consequences for CaMKII function: the kinase becomes autonomously active (Saitoh and Schwartz, 1985), the affinity of Ca^{2+}-calmodulin for CaMKII increases 1000-fold, and a site becomes exposed, allowing CaMKII to bind NMDA glutamate receptors (Strack and Colbran, 1998; Leonard et al., 1999; Bayer et al., 2001). There exists another autophosphorylation site within the regulatory domain of the enzyme at threonine 305 and 306 ($Thr^{305/306}$) of the alpha and beta subunits, respectively. The potential functional consequences of phosphorylation at $Thr^{305/306}$ are poorly understood. However, it has been shown that $Thr^{305/306}$ phosphorylation can render the CaMKII enzyme inactive (Colbran, 1993). In addition, the $Thr^{305/306}$ resides in the Ca^{2+}-calmodulin binding site of CaMKII and inhibits subsequent binding of Ca^{2+}-calmodulin to CaMKII. Phosphorylation of $Thr^{305/306}$ can also occur in the absence of activation of CaMKII and possibly prevents subsequent activation by Ca^{2+}-calmodulin. This management of activation, alterations in Ca^{2+} and calmodulin sensitivity, and autophosphorylation is highly orchestrated. Thus, even slight disruptions of this process can have devastating affects on synaptic function and cognitive ability (Colbran and Brown, 2004).

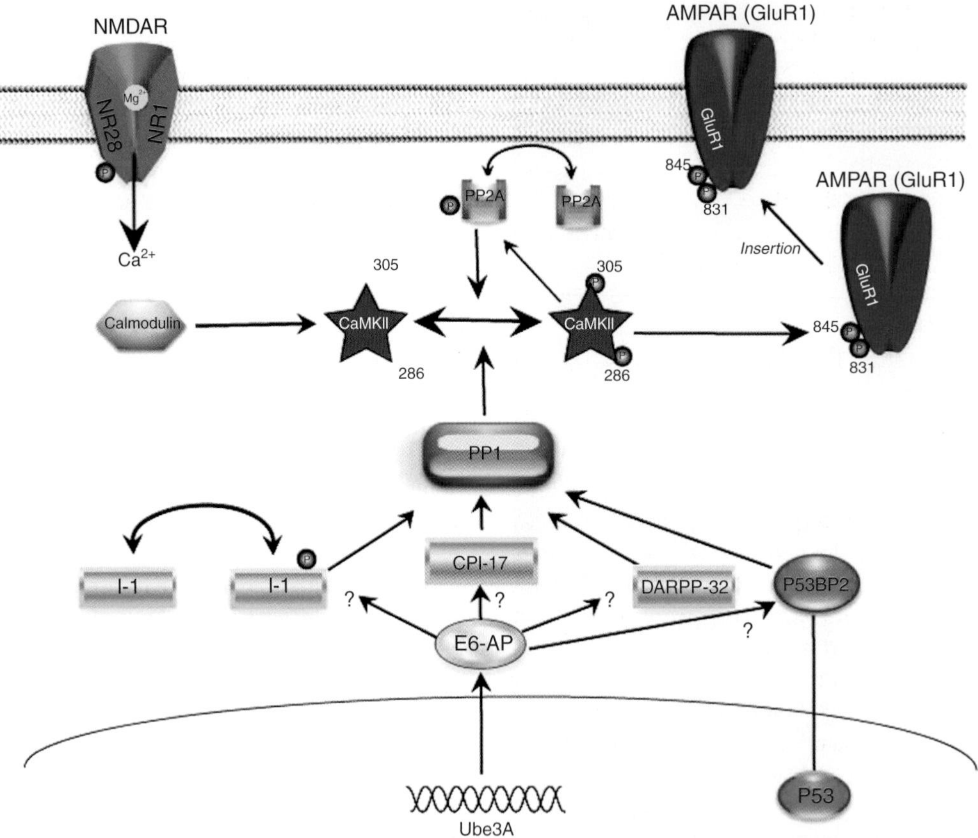

Figure 4 Schematic model of CaMKII regulation in the hippocampus. Inactivated CaMKII is located in the cytoplasm. Once activated by calcium-calmodulin and phosphorylated at threonine 286 (Thr^{286}), CaMKII translocates to the postsynaptic density, where it associates with *N*-methyl-D-aspartate receptors and is involved in alpha-amino-3-hydroxy-5-methyl-4-isoxazole propionic acid receptor insertion. Autophosphorylation at $Thr^{305/306}$ decreases the affinity of CaMKII for *N*-methyl-D-aspartate receptors and signals for CaMKII translocation away from the postsynaptic density. Dephosphorylation of CaMKII by phosphatase activity once again allows sensitivity of CaMKII to future signaling via calcium influx.

35.5.2 Regulation of CaMKII Activity in Synaptic Plasticity and Memory Formation

How is autophosphorylation tied to the regulation of synaptic plasticity? Recent studies have examined the role of the Thr^{286} and $Thr^{305/306}$ autophosphorylation in CaMKII-dependent synaptic function. Genetically modifying the Thr^{286} site to an alanine (T286A), which prevents phosphorylation at the Thr^{286} site, results in complete loss of LTP induction. Genetically modifying the Thr^{286} site to an aspartate (T286D), which mimics phosphorylation, also leads to impairment of LTP induction. More refined studies suggest that low levels of the autonomously active kinase facilitate, while high levels of autonomously active kinase inhibit, LTP induction. Alternatively, mutating the $Thr^{305/306}$ sites from a threonine to an alanine (T305/306A) increases the amount of CaMKII in the postsynaptic density (PSD) and enhances LTP induction (Elgersma et al., 2002). Furthermore, mutating the threonine to an aspartate (T305/306D) decreases the amount of CaMKII in the PSD and blocks induction of LTP (Elgersma et al., 2002). Together, these results indicate that CaMKII is critical in the induction of LTP and must be active in a precise spatiotemporal pattern. Synaptic plasticity in the hippocampus is believed to be involved in the formation of spatial memories. Disruption of CaMKII function has profound effects on hippocampal LTP; therefore, one would expect disruption of CaMKII to have dramatic effects on long-term memory formation. Animals lacking the CaMKII gene show profound deficits in spatial learning tasks (Silva et al., 1992; Bach et al., 1995). In addition, both sites of autophosphorylation appear to be involved in the formation of long-term memory. Deficits in spatial learning tasks are observed in animals that have either the T286A or T286D mutation. Moreover, animals possessing the T305/6A mutation exhibited enhanced spatial learning, while animals with the T305D mutation had severe deficits in spatial learning. All of these observations indicate that CaMKII is critical for the proper formation of hippocampus-dependent spatial memory.

35.6 Genetic Rescue of the AS Phenotype

The identified alterations in CaMKII raise the question of which alteration in phosphorylation, Thr^{286}, $Thr^{305/306}$, or both, is responsible for the observed AS phenotype. Due to the severe detrimental effects of CaMKII $Thr^{305/306}$ phosphorylation on synaptic plasticity and memory formation, as well as the similarities in the phenotypes with the AS mouse, the $Thr^{305/306}$ site was hypothesized to be responsible for the major phenotypes seen in AS. Studies in the laboratories of Weeber and Elgersma utilized female AS mice crossed with heterozygous αCaMKII males that carried the targeted *αCaMKII-T305V/T306A* mutation (CaMKII-TT305/6AV). This point mutation essentially prevents CaMKII inhibitory phosphorylation, but the use of heterozygotes allows a subset of endogenous CaMKII to be present without the mutation. Thus, the resulting F1 offspring yielded mutants with four different genotypes: wild-type (WT) mice, mutants carrying the single *αCaMKII-305/*$6^{+/-}$ or AS mutation, and mice carrying the double AS/CaMKII-305/$6^{+/-}$ mutation. Hippocampal-dependent learning was assessed using the contextual fear-conditioning paradigm (*See* Chapter 21), utilizing the same protocol of two US–CS pairings employed in the original AS mouse characterization. The genetic prevention of $Thr^{305/306}$ phosphorylation is sufficient to rescue the defect in learning and memory. The CaMKII-305/$6^{+/-}$ mice can learn to associate the context and the foot shock to the same extent as wild-type littermates tested 24 h or 7 days following training (**Figure 5**). These results support the hypothesis that the underlying hippocampal learning deficit is due primarily to αCaMKII inhibitory phosphorylation.

Interestingly, αCaMKII inhibitory phosphorylation can influence the threshold for the induction of LTP. This is nicely demonstrated in the homozygous CaMKII-TT305/6AV mouse that exhibits increased LTP induction when a subthreshold stimulation is given, but in which normal LTP is induced when a strong stimulation is applied (*See* Chapter 11). In contrast, AS mice exhibit a significant LTP deficit utilizing a modest stimulation protocol, which is rescued using multiple trains of HFS. Consistent with the associative learning rescue experiments, AS mice showed a severe LTP deficit compared to wild-type mice and CaMKII-305/$6^{+/-}$ mice. However, the AS/CaMKII-305/$6^{+/-}$ double mutants show comparable LTP to that of wild-type mice and lack the LTP deficit seen in their AS mouse littermates (**Figure 5**). These studies dramatically show that the synaptic plasticity deficits established in the AS mice are the result of increased CaMKII inhibitory phosphorylation. Thus, genetic manipulation of the phosphorylation state of the inhibitory site of CaMKII effectively rescues both the synaptic plasticity deficit and cognitive disruption in the *Ube3a*-null mutation mouse model of AS.

The studies described here strongly suggest that the increased inhibitory phosphorylation of CaMKII is the site of molecular dysfunction underlying the cognitive and synaptic plasticity deficits associated with AS. This validates the great amount of research showing CaMKII dependence for normal synaptic plasticity and memory formation. Astonishingly, AS represents the lone human disorder that to date presents with a disruption in cognition that is associated with CaMKII dysfunction. This is likely attributed to both the importance of CaMKII substrates in peripheral cellular function and the number of developmental pathways in which CaMKII is enlisted. If not for the limited region-specific deletion of Ube3a, it is likely AS would result in embryonic lethality. This consideration raises the obvious question of whether the genetic rescue with the CaMKII-305/$6^{+/-}$ mutation is due to the normalization of the CaMKII signaling capacity in the adult, the ability for normal CaMKII-dependent development of the central nervous system, or both. The observation of occasional abnormalities in AS patients including scoliosis, hyperreflexia, hypopigmentation, strabismus, myopia or hypermetropia, and nystagmus would suggest a development component resulting from a CaMKII dysfunction.

35.7 Proposed Mechanisms Underlying CaMKII Misregulation

The genetic rescue of the AS phenotype is a tremendous step forward, but the molecular connection between ubiquitin deficiency and alterations in

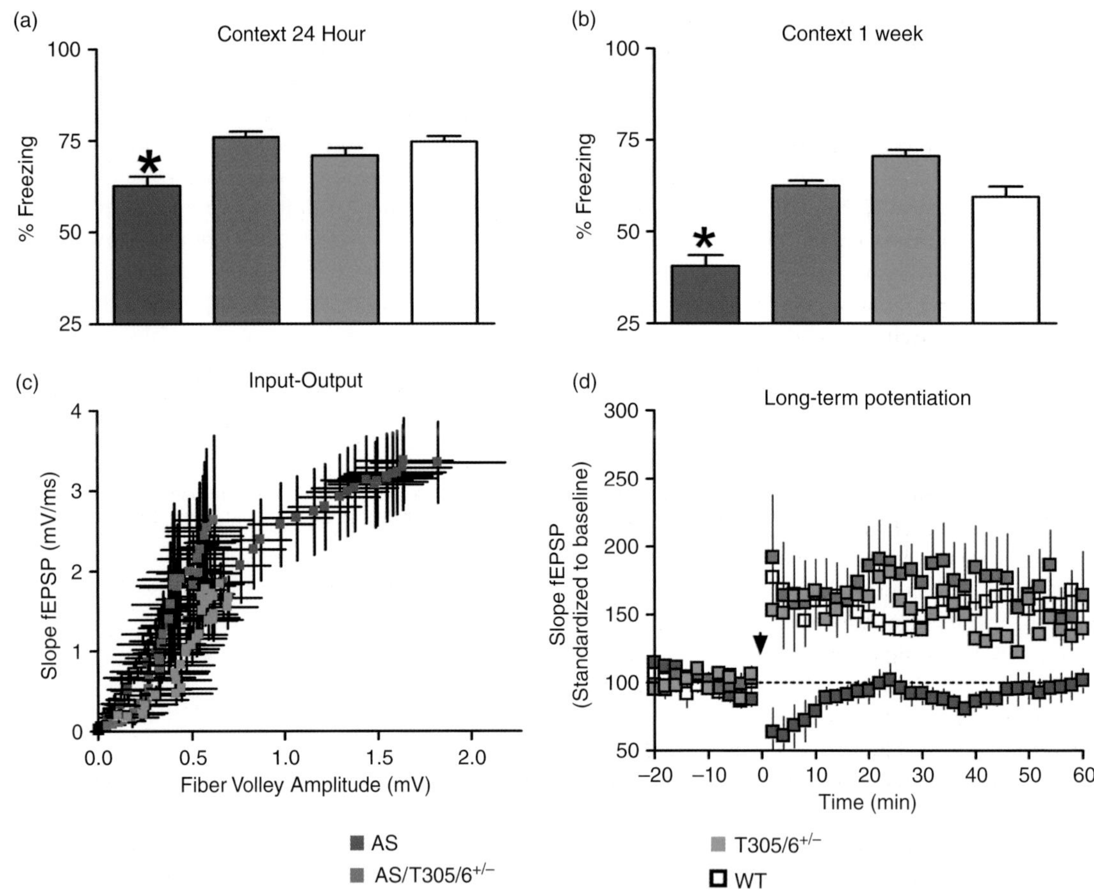

Figure 5 Hippocampal learning and synaptic plasticity in AS mice is rescued by the T305/6-CaMKII mutation. Mice trained in a conditioning chamber through the association with the context and two mild foot shocks were later reintroduced to the context. Freezing was assessed during a 3-min time period, and the amount of freezing represents the strength of the associative memory formed. Angelman Syndrome (AS) mutants show impaired contextual conditioning 24 h (a) and 1 week (b) after training, which is rescued in the AS/T305/6-CaMKII$^{+/-}$ mutants. Increased synaptic transmission (c) and disruption of LTP (d) is rescued in *Ube-3a*-m^{-}/p^{+}/T305/6-CaMKII$^{+/-}$ double mutants compared to AS mice. LTP was induced with two trains of 100-Hz stimulation delivered 20 s apart (represented by arrow) in hippocampus area CA1.

CaMKII phosphorylation remains unclear. As discussed above, CaMKII cycles between phosphorylated and nonphosphorylated states. The cycling state of CaMKII is not unlike many other proteins involved in signal transduction processes that undergo endless cycles of phosphorylation and dephosphorylation. Evolution has perfected this process in the CNS in order to provide an exceptionally rapid and potent mechanism for the regulation of protein function. The phosphorylation of numerous proteins is kept in check by three major protein phosphatases (PP) found in the brain: PP1, PP2A, and PP2B (calcineurin). PP1 and PP2A appear to be primarily responsible for dephosphorylation of CaMKII at Thr^{286}, with PP2A regulating CaMKII phosphorylation in the cytoplasm and PP1 in the postsynaptic density (Mansuy, 2003) (**Figure 4**). Through the actions of PP1 and PP2A, the activity of CaMKII is held in check and allows the enzyme to return to a state where Ca^{2+} influx can again activate the proper signal transduction cascades involving CaMKII. The presence of PP1 and PP2A causes an apparent conundrum in the regulation of CaMKII. CaMKII is a Ca^{2+}-dependent kinase; however, under conditions conducive to induction of long-term synaptic plasticity or memory formation, CaMKII undergoes autophosphorylation and becomes a Ca^{2+}-independent autonomous enzyme. How does this occur in the presence of PP1 and PP2A? Several proteins have been identified that act as inhibitors of

PP activity. One example is the Inhibitor 1 (I1) protein (Huang and Glinsmann, 1976). When phosphorylated via protein kinase A, I1 can bind to and inhibit the activity of PP1. Inhibition of PP1 via I1 facilitates the transition of CaMKII from a Ca^{2+}-dependent to an autonomous state. The functional consequences of PPs on CaMKII activity are not solely negative. As noted above, CaMKII contains an inhibitory autophosphorylation site at $Thr^{305/306}$. Phosphorylation at this site downregulates CaMKII activity and prevents binding by Ca^{2+}-calmodulin. PP1 can dephosphorylate $Thr^{305/306}$, which then allows for reactivation of CaMKII by Ca^{2+}-calmodulin (Patton et al., 1990). **Figure 4** shows the highly regulated action of protein phosphatases, and the proteins that control their activity as well. Thus, the changes in the phosphorylation state of AS mouse hippocampal CaMKII could be due to changes in protein levels in one or more of these proteins. Interestingly, PP1 and/or PP2A phosphatase activity is significantly reduced in the AS mutants by a prodigious 2.5-fold decrease (Weeber et al., 2003). This finding strongly suggests that the aberrant state of P-Thr^{286} and P-Thr^{305} αCaMKII phosphorylation is due to changes in the activity of one or both of these important phosphatases. This also suggests that the increase in Thr^{305} αCaMKII is due to both the increase in P-Thr^{286} αCaMKII, since phosphorylation at Thr^{286} precedes phosphorylation at Thr^{305} (Colbran and Soderling, 1990; Hanson and Schulman, 1992), and reduced PP1 and/or PP2A activity, which are known to dephosphorylate P-Thr^{305} αCaMKII *in vitro* (Patton et al., 1990).

35.8 Concluding Remarks

The studies discussed here have set the stage for the next phase of research that will work toward uncovering the molecular pathways and mechanisms linking Ube3a maternal deficiency and CaMKII regulation. Future discoveries of E6-AP targets will likely shed the most light on this puzzling connection. Regardless, important lessons have been learned from the discovery of AS allele and its regulation. First, the production of the AS mouse model re-emphasizes the utility and importance of mouse models for human disorders (*See* Chapter 36). Second, AS was one of the first human mental retardation disorders to bring to light the potential deleterious effects of epigenetic changes. The identification that the AS gene expresses a housekeeping-type protein dramatically illustrates the unexpected importance of proteins such as ubiquitin ligases once considered minor for normal synaptic function. Finally, these studies illustrate a compelling example of a human learning and memory disorder associated with deficits in hippocampal synaptic plasticity and CaMKII function.

References

Alger BE and Teyler TJ (1976) Long-term and short-term plasticity in the CA1, CA3, and dentate regions of the rat hippocampal slice. *Brain Res.* 110: 463–480.

Bach ME, Hawkins RD, Osman M, Kandel ER, and Mayford M (1995) Impairment of spatial but not contextual memory in CaMKII mutant mice with a selective loss of hippocampal LTP in the range of the theta frequency. *Cell* 81: 905–915.

Bayer KU, De Koninck P, Leonard AS, Hell JW, and Schulman H (2001) Interaction with the NMDA receptor locks CaMKII in an active conformation. *Nature* 411: 801–805.

Bliss TV and Lomo T (1973) Long-lasting potentiation of synaptic transmission in the dentate area of the anaesthetized rabbit following stimulation of the perforant path. *J. Physiol.* 232: 331–356.

Cassidy SB, Dykens E, and Williams CA (2000) Prader-Willi and Angelman syndromes: Sister imprinted disorders. *Am. J. Med. Genet.* 97: 136–146.

Colbran RJ (1993) Inactivation of Ca2+/calmodulin-dependent protein kinase II by basal autophosphorylation. *J. Biol. Chem.* 268: 7163–7170.

Colbran RJ and Brown AM (2004) Calcium/calmodulin-dependent protein kinase II and synaptic plasticity. *Curr. Opin. Neurobiol.* 14: 318–327.

Colbran RJ and Soderling TR (1990) Calcium/calmodulin-independent autophosphorylation sites of calcium/calmodulin-dependent protein kinase II. Studies on the effect of phosphorylation of threonine 305/306 and serine 314 on calmodulin binding using synthetic peptides. *J. Biol. Chem.* 265: 11213–11219.

Colbran RJ, Smith MK, Schworer CM, Fong YL, and Soderling TR (1989) Regulatory domain of calcium/calmodulin-dependent protein kinase II. Mechanism of inhibition and regulation by phosphorylation. *J. Biol. Chem.* 264: 4800–4804.

Elgersma Y, Fedorov NB, Ikonen S, et al. (2002) Inhibitory autophosphorylation of CaMKII controls PSD association, plasticity, and learning. *Neuron* 36: 493–505.

Hanson PI and Schulman H (1992) Inhibitory autophosphorylation of multifunctional Ca2+/calmodulin-dependent protein kinase analyzed by site-directed mutagenesis. *J. Biol. Chem.* 267: 17216–17224.

Harris EW, Ganong AH, and Cotman CW (1984) Long-term potentiation in the hippocampus involves activation of N-methyl-D-aspartate receptors. *Brain Res.* 323: 132–137.

Huang FL and Glinsmann WH (1976) Separation and characterization of two phosphorylase phosphatase inhibitors from rabbit skeletal muscle. *Eur. J. Biochem.* 70: 419–426.

Huibregtse JM, Scheffner M, and Howley PM (1991) A cellular protein mediates association of p53 with the E6 oncoprotein of human papillomavirus types 16 or 18. *EMBO J.* 10: 4129–4135.

Jiang YH, Armstrong D, Albrecht U, et al. (1998) Mutation of the Angelman ubiquitin ligase in mice causes increased

cytoplasmic p53 and deficits of contextual learning and long-term potentiation. *Neuron* 21: 799–811.
Kuhne C and Banks L (1998) E3-ubiquitin ligase/E6-AP links multicopy maintenance protein 7 to the ubiquitination pathway by a novel motif, the L2G box. *J. Biol. Chem.* 273: 34302–34309.
Kumar S, Talis AL, and Howley PM (1999) Identification of HHR23A as a substrate for E6-associated protein-mediated ubiquitination. *J. Biol. Chem.* 274: 18785–18792.
Lee S and Wevrick R (2000) Identification of novel imprinted transcripts in the Prader-Willi syndrome and Angelman syndrome deletion region: Further evidence for regional imprinting control. *Am. J. Hum. Genet.* 66: 848–858.
Leonard AS, Lim IA, Hemsworth DE, Horne MC, and Hell JW (1999) Calcium/calmodulin-dependent protein kinase II is associated with the N-methyl-D-aspartate receptor. *Proc. Natl. Acad. Sci. USA* 96: 3239–3244.
Lynch G, Larson J, Kelso S, Barrionuevo G, and Schottler F (1983) Intracellular injections of EGTA block induction of hippocampal long-term potentiation. *Nature* 305: 719–721.
Malenka RC, Kauer JA, Zucker RS, and Nicoll RA (1988) Postsynaptic calcium is sufficient for potentiation of hippocampal synaptic transmission. *Science* 242: 81–84.
Mansuy IM (2003) Calcineurin in memory and bidirectional plasticity. *Biochem. Biophys. Res. Commun.* 311: 1195–1208.
Morris RG, Anderson E, Lynch GS, and Baudry M (1986) Selective impairment of learning and blockade of long-term potentiation by an N-methyl-D-aspartate receptor antagonist, AP5. *Nature* 319: 774–776.
Nuber U, Schwarz SE, and Scheffner M (1998) The ubiquitin-protein ligase E6-associated protein (E6-AP) serves as its own substrate. *Eur. J. Biochem.* 254: 643–649.
Patton BL, Miller SG, and Kennedy MB (1990) Activation of type II calcium/calmodulin-dependent protein kinase by Ca2+/calmodulin is inhibited by autophosphorylation of threonine within the calmodulin-binding domain. *J. Biol. Chem.* 265: 11204–11212.
Redei GP, Koncz C, and Phillips JD (2006) Changing images of the gene. *Adv. Genet.* 56: 53–100.
Saitoh T and Schwartz JH (1985) Phosphorylation-dependent subcellular translocation of a Ca2+/calmodulin-dependent protein kinase produces an autonomous enzyme in Aplysia neurons. *J. Cell Biol.* 100: 835–842.
Silva AJ, Paylor R, Wehner JM, and Tonegawa S (1992) Impaired spatial learning in alpha-calcium-calmodulin kinase II mutant mice. *Science* 257: 206–211.
Strack S and Colbran RJ (1998) Autophosphorylation-dependent targeting of calcium/calmodulin-dependent protein kinase II by the NR2B subunit of the N-methyl-D-aspartate receptor. *J. Biol. Chem.* 273: 20689–20692.
Weeber EJ, Jiang YH, Elgersma Y, et al. (2003) Derangements of hippocampal calcium/calmodulin-dependent protein kinase II in a mouse model for Angelman mental retardation syndrome. *J. Neurosci.* 23: 2634–2644.

36 Epigenetics – Chromatin Structure and Rett Syndrome

J. M. Levenson, University of Wisconsin School of Medicine and Public Health, Madison, WI, USA

M. A. Wood, University of California–Irvine, Irvine, CA, USA

36.1 Introduction

Much scientific effort over the last three decades has focused on understanding the molecular basis of memory formation. A great deal of progress has been made, and we have a very comprehensive understanding of the molecules and signaling pathways engaged during the early stages of memory formation. Despite the wealth of knowledge that exists about the molecular basis for memory formation, we have an incipient understanding of how a memory persists in the brain for the lifetime of an organism. For instance, what molecules are used to actually store the memory of your first kiss, or your first car accident?

A major question that will drive the next three decades of research into the molecular mechanisms of information storage in the brain is what are the molecular substrates for 'lifetime' memory storage? This question is particularly intriguing when one considers that nearly every molecule in the brain has a lifetime that is measured in minutes to hours. It has been estimated that the molecular composition of the brain is renewed every 2 months. How can information persist in the face of constant molecular renewal?

The answer to the question of how information is stored in the nervous system for the lifetime of an organism might not lie in the classic mechanisms identified as important for information storage in the brain thus far. Every cell in a metazoan must 'remember' at least one complex piece of information for the lifetime of the organism: cellular phenotype.

Early in development, stem cells are induced to differentiate into phenotypically distinct tissues. Once differentiated, the memory for cellular phenotype must endure in the face of molecular turnover and even mitosis. Is it possible that the nervous system has co-opted this ancient and evolutionarily conserved form of cellular memory for use in lifelong storage of memory?

Cell phenotype is due, in large part, to epigenetic marking of the genome. Recent studies have demonstrated that epigenetic gene regulation has a critical role in neuronal cell fate specification, synaptic development, and synaptic function (reviewed in Hsieh and Gage, 2004, 2005). These epigenetic marks induce lifelong changes in gene expression that reside in the cell and determine its phenotype. Epigenetics and its associated terminology have several different connotations, and specific terms need to be defined before we can discuss them in detail. We define the genome as a complete set of haploid DNA and the functional units that it encodes. In the nucleus, DNA exists as a highly compressed structure known as chromatin. The epigenome is the sum of both chromatin structure and the pattern of DNA methylation, which is the result of an interaction between the genome and the environment. There are three commonly used definitions for the term 'epigenetic' in the literature currently.

The broadest definition of epigenetics includes the transmission and perpetuation of information through meiosis or mitosis that is not based on the sequence of DNA. This process is not restricted to DNA-based transmission and can also be protein-based. This definition is broadly used in the yeast literature, wherein phenotypes that can be inherited by daughter cells are perpetuated past cell division using protein-based mechanisms (Si et al., 2003a,b; Pray, 2004). A second definition of epigenetics has arisen from the field of developmental biology that posits some meiotically and mitotically heritable changes in *gene expression* are not coded in the DNA sequence itself. The altered patterns of gene expression can occur through several mechanisms that are based on DNA, RNA, or proteins (see below) (Egger et al., 2004). A third definition of epigenetics is the mechanism for stable maintenance of gene expression that involves physically 'marking' DNA or its associated proteins, which allow genotypically identical cells to be phenotypically distinct. The molecular and physical basis for this type of change in DNA or chromatin structure is the focus of this review (Rakyan et al., 2001). By this definition, the regulation of chromatin structure is equivalent to epigenetics.

Epigenetics is an attractive candidate molecular mechanism for lifetime storage of memory. DNA and chromatin are relatively constant molecular substrates in neurons and most other cell types. DNA and chromatin are not continually degraded and resynthesized as all other molecular constituents of a neuron are. Thus, the half-life of epigenetic marks is not affected by the lifetime of the molecule. Therefore, epigenetic marks are a more direct reflection of the ongoing state of the neuron, or any other cell (**Figure 1**(**a**)). This positions chromatin as an ideal molecular substrate for long-term signal integration and information storage (**Figure 1**(**a**)).

36.2 Mechanisms of Epigenetic Marking

There are several mechanisms whereby epigenetic marks can be placed on chromatin. Each mark has been associated with distinct effects on transcription and chromatin structure. We will briefly review several of the most commonly studied epigenetic marks.

36.2.1 Epigenetic Marking of Histones

Histones are highly basic proteins that comprise the major protein component of chromatin. Histones are some of the most evolutionarily conserved proteins but among the most variable with respect to posttranslational modifications, which include acetylation, phosphorylation, methylation, ubiquitination, and sumoylation (reviewed in Thiagalingam et al., 2003). One function of histones is structural; DNA is tightly packaged into chromatin through interactions with histone octamers, referred to as nucleosomes. Interaction between histones and DNA is mediated in part by the N-terminal tail of histone proteins. The primary interface between histone and DNA is believed to be an electrostatic interaction between positively charged lysine residues within the N-terminal tails of histones and the negatively charged sugar-phosphate backbone of DNA. Interestingly, structural studies indicate that the N-terminal tails of histones protrude beyond the chromosomes (Luger et al., 1997), where they could potentially serve as signal integration platforms. Posttranslational modification of

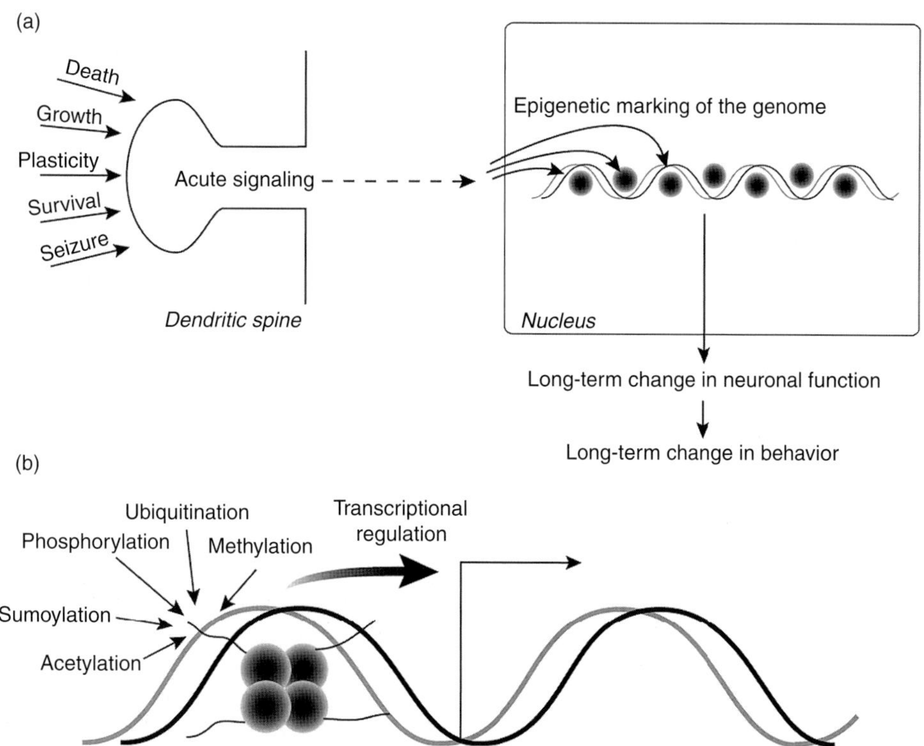

Figure 1 Chromatin as a substrate for signal integration. We propose that epigenetic marking of the genome represents a form of cellular memory utilized by neurons to subserve information storage. (a) Dendritic spines receive several distinct extracellular signals. These signals activate a variety of intracellular signaling cascades that ultimately lead to epigenetic marking of the genome. The half-life of these epigenetic marks is much longer than traditional posttranslational modifications, and so their effects on gene expression persist for much longer periods of time. Therefore, as a consequence of epigenetically modifying the genome, neuronal function and ultimately behavior of the animal are modified for very long periods of time. (b) Histone tails and cytosine residues of DNA can receive a variety of distinct epigenetic marks. Each mark has a different effect on transcription. The functional consequence of epigenetically marking the genome is ultimately precise modulation of transcription.

histones, either on their N-terminal tail or within the globular domain (van Leeuwen et al., 2002), represents one mechanism for epigenetic marking of the genome. Current hypotheses posit that post-translational modifications along the N-terminal tails are combined in a 'histone code' that ultimately directs the activity of numerous transcription factors, cofactors, and the transcriptional machinery in general (Strahl and Allis, 2000). The histone code is the specific pattern of posttranslational modifications of a given histone octamer in chromatin (**Figure 1**(**b**)). This code, or pattern, is read out as an influence on the specific level of expression of the associated gene(s). We have chosen to focus on N-terminal–directed posttranslation modifications because of the rapidly growing literature describing these different modifications, their associated effects on transcription, and their interdependence.

36.2.2 Histone Acetylation

Several specific sites of posttranslational modification exist within the N-terminal tails of histone proteins, and modifications of these sites can modulate the overall structure of chromatin. Currently, five post-translational modifications of histone tails have been characterized: acetylation, methylation, ubiquitination, sumoylation, and phosphorylation. Acetylation is the best characterized of the posttranslational modifications on histones to date. Acetylation of histones occurs on lysine residues, effectively neutralizing their positive charge and interfering with the electrostatic interaction between histone and nucleotide. Acetylation is catalyzed by histone acetyltransferases (HATs), which transfer an acetyl group from acetyl-CoA to the ε-NH^{+} group of a lysine residue within a histone (Tanner et al., 1999, 2000a,b; Lau et al., 2000). Histone acetylation is reversed via the action of histone deacetylases (HDACs).

36.2.3 Histone Methylation

Histone methylation is another histone-directed epigenetic tag. Like acetylation, methylation of histones occurs on ε-NH^+ groups of lysine residues, and it is mediated by histone methyltransferases (HMTs). Unlike acetylation, lysines can accept up to three methyl groups, and methylation does not affect the positive charge of lysine residues. Thus, methylation of histones on lysine residues does not interfere with the electrostatic histone–DNA interaction. Methylation of histones can also occur on arginine residues, catalyzed by protein arginine methyltransferases (PRMTs). Arginines can be either mono- or dimethylated on their guanidine nitrogen.

36.2.4 Histone Ubiquitination

Ubiquitination of histones has only recently begun to be characterized in detail. Ubiquitin, a protein with 76 amino acids that is named for its ubiquitous distribution in all cell types and high degree of conservation across species, is a posttranslational modification usually used as a signal for degradation by the proteasome when substrates are polyubiquitinated (Pickart, 2001). Interestingly, most histones appear to be monoubiquitinated (reviewed in Hicke, 2001). Monoubiquitination has been shown to be involved in a range of cellular functions distinct from proteasome-dependent proteolysis (reviewed in Pickart, 2001; Murphey and Godenschwege, 2002). Histones, like other proteins, are ubiquitinated through attachment of a ubiquitin to the ε-NH^+ group of a lysine (Nickel and Davie, 1989). Ubiquitination of histones H2A, H2B, H3, and H1 has been observed (Goldknopf et al., 1975; West and Bonner, 1980; Chen et al., 1998; Pham and Sauer, 2000). Although sites of ubiquitination have been identified on histones, the function of histone ubiquitination remains unclear.

36.2.5 Histone Sumoylation

There are several ubiquitin-like posttranslational modifications that proteins can undergo. One example is the small ubiquitin-related modifier (SUMO) (Melchior, 2000; Hay, 2001; Johnson and Gupta, 2001). SUMO modifications are attached to proteins in a manner similar to the mechanisms involved in ubiquitination. Although SUMO is related to ubiquitination, sumoylation of proteins does not result in their degradation, suggesting that sumoylation of proteins has relevance in other signaling cascades. Initial studies suggested that histone H4 can be sumoylated, and that sumoylation of histone H4 is associated with transcriptional repression (Shiio and Eisenman, 2003). In yeast, the SUMO-conjugating enzyme Hus5 is highly enriched in heterochromatic regions, and knockout of SUMO results in loss of heterochromatic silencing, providing direct evidence that, at least in simple eukaryotes, SUMO modification of chromatin results in transcriptional silencing (Shin et al., 2005).

36.2.6 Histone Phosphorylation

Phosphorylation of histones H1 and H3 was first discovered in the context of chromosome condensation during mitosis (Bradbury et al., 1973; Gurley et al., 1974). Phosphorylation of histone H3 has since been associated with activation of mitogenic signaling pathways (Mahadevan et al., 1991). Phosphorylation of serine 10 on H3 is mediated by Rsk2, Msk1, and the aurora kinase family member Ipl1 (Sassone-Corsi et al., 1999; Thomson et al., 1999; Hsu et al., 2000; Di Agostino et al., 2002). Recent evidence also implicates aurora kinases in the phosphorylation of serine 28 in histone H3 (Goto et al., 2002). As with other proteins, phosphatases are responsible for catalyzing the removal of phosphate groups from histones (Mahadevan et al., 1991; Ajiro et al., 1996). To date, the phosphatases PP1 and PP2A have been shown to regulate levels of phosphorylation on H3 (Hsu et al., 2000; Nowak et al., 2003).

36.2.7 Other Histone Modifications

While a great deal of attention has been given to the N-termini of the histones, there is increasing evidence suggesting that other histone regions are targeted for modulation. For example, dot1p has been shown to methylate histone H3 on lysine 79, a residue that lies within the globular domain (van Leeuwen et al., 2002). Additionally, higher-order folding of chromatin is also undoubtedly involved in the regulation of gene expression. In this regard, there is increasing evidence that the linker histone H1 plays a role in modulation of chromatin structure (Brown, 2003).

36.2.8 DNA (Cytosine-5) Methylation

In addition to posttranslational modification of histones, DNA itself can be directly modified via methylation. Methylation of DNA is catalyzed by a class of enzymes known as DNA (cytosine-5) methyltransferases (DNMTs) (Bestor et al., 1988; Yen et al., 1992; Okano et al., 1998; Lyko et al., 1999; Okano et al., 1999). DNMTs transfer methyl groups to cytosine (C) residues within a continuous stretch of DNA, specifically at the 5-position of the pyrimidine ring (Chen et al., 1991). Not all cytosines can be methylated; usually cytosines must be immediately followed by a guanine (G) to be methylated (Bird, 1978; Cedar et al., 1979). These 'CpG' dinucleotide sequences are highly underrepresented in the genome relative to what would be predicted by random chance; however, about 70% of the existing CpG dinucleotides are methylated (Cooper and Krawczak, 1989). The rest of the normally unmethylated CpG dinucleotides occur in small clusters, known as 'CpG islands' (Bird, 1986).

DNA methylation leads to marked changes in the structure of chromatin that ultimately result in significant downregulation of transcription. It can directly interfere with the ability of transcription factors to bind to regulatory elements. The transcription factor Ets-1 and the boundary element CCCTC binding factor (CTCF) can efficiently bind to nonmethylated, but not methylated DNA (Bell and Felsenfeld, 2000; Maier et al., 2003). Moreover, several proteins recognize and bind to methylated CpG residues independent of DNA sequence. The five proteins that are known to bind to methylated CpGs are MeCP2, MBD1, MBD2, MBD4, and Kaiso (Hendrich and Bird, 1998; Prokhortchouk et al., 2001). These proteins mediate transcriptional repression by recruiting chromatin remodeling enzymes. For example, MeCP2 directly associates with the transcriptional corepressor Sin3A and HDAC (Jones et al., 1998; Nan et al., 1998).

36.2.9 Epigenetic Modulation of Transcription

Several hypotheses have been put forth to explain how the many modifications made on histone proteins are interpreted to extend the information potential of the genetic (DNA) code. The most popular of these hypotheses is the histone code initially described by B. M. Turner (1993) and more recently elaborated and popularized by C. D. Allis and colleagues (Strahl and Allis, 2000; Jenuwein and Allis, 2001). Distinct histone posttranslational modifications can generate synergistic or antagonistic interaction sites for transcription factors and associated chromatin remodeling enzyme complexes. The combinatorial nature of these histone modifications may be thought of as a histone code that extends the information potential of the genetic code (Jenuwein and Allis, 2001). However, a very different hypothesis suggests that it is not combinatorial complexity, but rather a simple net charge effect. Genetic experiments, microarray analysis, and hierarchical cluster analysis were used to demonstrate that the interchangeability of acetylation sites on histone H4 provides support for a charge neutralization model (Dion et al., 2005; reviewed in Henikoff, 2005). Lastly, histone modifications have been related to signal-transducing modifications, and histone modifications provide switch-like properties and ensure robustness of the signal (Schreiber and Bernstein, 2002). This idea has been termed the signaling network model. These three hypotheses for how histone modifications direct transcriptional activation are not mutually exclusive, and thus, it will be interesting to see how future studies into chromatin regulation and information storage regulate cell fate, cellular memory, and as we propose below, long-term memory storage at the behavioral level.

36.3 Epigenetic Mechanisms in Synaptic Plasticity

Synaptic plasticity, defined as the activity-dependent change in synaptic strength, is currently viewed as a widely accepted hypothesis to explain the underlying cellular mechanisms of memory processes. The discovery of two forms of synaptic plasticity, long-term facilitation in *Aplysia,* where brief exposure to the neuromodulator serotonin induces a persistent enhancement of neurotransmitter release (Kandel and Tauc, 1964; Brunelli et al., 1976), and long-term potentiation (LTP), a form of synaptic plasticity whereby high-frequency stimulation of a neuronal pathway induces long-lasting increases in synaptic efficacy (*See* Chapter 11) (Bliss and Lomo, 1973), sparked decades of research into the role of synaptic plasticity in learning and memory. A recent review by Martin and Morris (2002) elegantly discusses the validity of synaptic plasticity as a cellular mechanism for memory formation. In the previous section of this chapter, we introduced the intriguing idea that epigenetic regulation of transcription may provide a mechanism for cellular memory in a neuron. This cellular memory may be involved in maintaining the long-lasting neuronal changes required for long-term synaptic plasticity changes. In this next section, we discuss the recent evidence that epigenetic regulation of transcription may be required for certain forms of long-lasting synaptic plasticity.

36.3.1 Transcription and Chromatin Structure

Transcriptional activation is required for certain long-lasting forms of synaptic plasticity and memory storage (Nguyen et al., 1994; Korzus, 2003). Activation of transcription factors in neurons can occur via several mechanisms. In relation to activity-dependent synaptic plasticity and memory formation, it is generally accepted that increased neuronal activity engages a wide variety of intracellular signaling cascades including PKC, PKA, Ca,$^{++}$ PI3-K, and ERK (Adams and Sweatt, 2002). Once engaged, these signaling pathways activate several distinct transcription factors, ultimately leading to the expression of gene products required for maintenance of synaptic plasticity and consolidation of long-term memory. For many actively transcribed genes, it is necessary to overcome the repressive chromatin structure surrounding the gene, especially in the promoter region. Genomic DNA is tightly packaged into chromatin, the major protein component of which is composed of nucleosomes that are octamers of core histone proteins. DNA is wrapped around the nucleosomes (~146 bp) and is then subjected to higher-order folding, resulting in a chromatin structure that is highly inhibitory to transcription. As described earlier, histone acetylation has been shown to alter chromatin structure (Norton et al., 1989), which can result in increased accessibility for transcriptional regulatory proteins to chromatin templates (Vettese-Dadey et al., 1996). The identification of transcriptional cofactors with HAT and HDAC activity has strengthened the relationship between histone acetylation and gene expression. Recently, several studies examining the role of HAT and HDAC enzymes in long-term synaptic plasticity demonstrated that there is a correlation between changes in synaptic plasticity and corresponding modifications of chromatin structure.

36.3.2 Chromatin Remodeling Enzymes and Synaptic Plasticity

One of the first demonstrations that chromatin remodeling enzymes are involved in synaptic plasticity came from a study in *Aplysia*. Several different forms of transcription-dependent synaptic plasticity have been identified in *Aplysia*, including long-term facilitation (LTF, characterized by enhanced synaptic transmission) and long-term depression (LTD, characterized by decreased synaptic transmission) (Montarolo et al., 1986, 1988; Hammer et al., 1989; Dale and Kandel, 1990). To understand the changes in chromatin structure that affect transcription required for LTF and LTD, Guan et al. (2002) examined the chromatin surrounding the promoter of ApC/EBP. ApC/EBP is an immediate early response gene critical for induction of LTF (Alberini et al., 1994) and is a downstream target of the transcription factor ApCREB1. Guan et al. (2002) showed that induction of LTF by treatment with serotonin activates ApCREB1, which recruits the transcriptional coactivator CREB binding protein (CBP, a potent HAT) to the ApC/EBP promoter (i.e., **Figure 2(a)**). Recruitment of cAMP response element binding protein (CREB) and CBP correlates with increased histone H4 acetylation and ApC/EBP expression (Guan et al., 2002). In contrast, induction of LTD by treatment with neuropeptide FMRFamide resulted in the recruitment of ApCREB2, an inhibitory form ApCREB that lacks a transcription activation domain, and an HDAC5-like molecule to the ApC/EBP promoter decreasing histone H4 acetylation and ApC/EBP expression (Guan et al., 2002). These two results suggest that, in *Aplysia* sensory neurons, the genome serves as a substrate for signal integration upon which long-term neuronal state is encoded. In support of this hypothesis, increasing levels of histone acetylation with the HDAC inhibitor trichostatin A (TSA) and mimicking the epigenetic state of the genome normally seen after induction of LTF transforms short-term synaptic facilitation into LTF (Guan et al., 2002). These results demonstrate that enzymes such as HATs and HDACs are actively involved in regulating chromatin structure at specific gene promoters relevant for induction of long-term synaptic plasticity.

Recently, several studies have demonstrated that CBP is involved in specific forms of hippocampal synaptic plasticity and hippocampus-dependent long-term memory formation (**Figure 2(a)**) (Oike et al., 1999; Bourtchouladze et al., 2003; Alarcon et al., 2004; Korzus et al., 2004; reviewed in Josselyn, 2005; Wood et al., 2005, 2006). These six studies utilized five different *cbp* genetically modified mice in which the activity of CBP was specifically impaired to investigate the role of CBP in synaptic plasticity and memory storage. With respect to synaptic

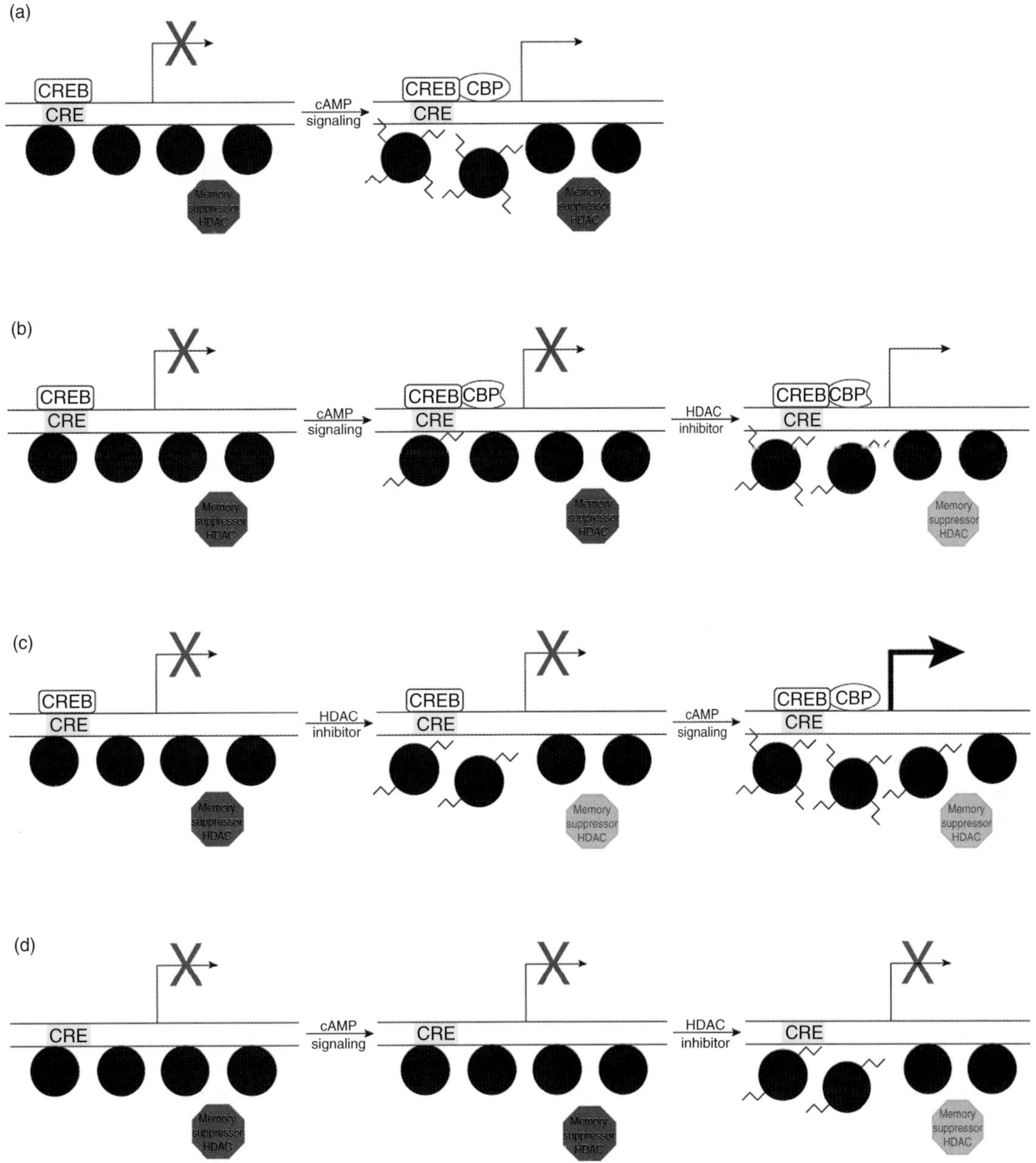

Figure 2 Epigenetics in synaptic plasticity and memory formation. Long-term forms of synaptic plasticity and memory require transcription for consolidation and maintenance. The diagrams indicate many aspects where epigenetics are involved in synaptic plasticity and long-term memory formation. (a) Induction of synaptic plasticity or formation of long-term memory requires the transcription factor CREB and the coactivator CBP. CBP is a HAT that acetylates histones and facilitates transcription of consolidation-associated genes. (b) Loss of CBP function, either through truncation mutations that eliminate the HAT domain or through haploinsufficiency, prevents CREB-mediated transcription of consolidation-associated genes. Addition of an HDAC inhibitor ameliorates the inability to induce long-term synaptic plasticity or form long-term memory. (c) Administration of HDAC inhibitors alone does not affect the expression of memory-associated genes. However, HDAC inhibitor preadministration facilitates the induction of synaptic plasticity and long-term memory. (d) Loss of CREB function, such as in CREB $\alpha\Delta$ mice, prevents induction of synaptic plasticity or formation of long-term memory. Administration of HDAC inhibitors does not restore plasticity or memory formation in these mice.

plasticity, *cbp*$^{+/-}$ heterozygous mice that lack one allele of *cbp* were found to have impairments in long-lasting LTP (L-LTP, a form of synaptic plasticity requiring transcription and translation), but normal early-phase LTP (E-LTP, a form of synaptic plasticity that is independent of transcription; *See* Chapter 11) (Alarcon et al., 2004). Similarly, transgenic mice expressing an inhibitory truncation mutant of CBP in forebrain neurons also exhibited deficits in L-LTP, with normal E-LTP (**Figure 2**(**b**)) (Wood et al., 2005). To overcome the deficits in histone acetylation and synaptic plasticity, mutant *cbp* mice were treated with HDAC inhibitors to induce a hyperacetylated genomic state. HDAC inhibition by suberoylanilide hydroxamic acid (SAHA) ameliorated impairments in hippocampal LTP in *cbp*$^{+/-}$ heterozygous mice (**Figure 2**(**b**)) (Alarcon et al., 2004). These results demonstrate that synaptic plasticity deficits in *cbp* mutant mice may be overcome by increasing histone acetylation via HDAC inhibition. However, the effect of modifying chromatin structure on synaptic plasticity and memory storage was not specifically addressed by these studies.

36.3.3 Histone Acetylation and Synaptic Plasticity

To directly examine the effect of increasing histone acetylation on synaptic plasticity, a recent study showed that the HDAC inhibitors TSA and sodium butyrate enhance LTP at Schaffer-collateral synapses in area CA1 of the hippocampus (**Figure 2**(**c**)) (Levenson et al., 2004b). Further, the authors demonstrated that the HDAC inhibitor–enhanced LTP is dependent on transcription. A similar result was observed in a study examining the effects of HDAC inhibition on E-LTP in the CA1 region of hippocampal slices from C57BL/6 mice. In this study, synaptic efficacy at both the collateral and commissural pathways was monitored simultaneously. Both pathways received baseline stimulation, but LTP was only induced in the collateral pathway, with the commissural fibers serving as a control. TSA had no effect on baseline responses in the commissural pathway as compared to vehicle, similar to other observations in TSA-treated slices (Alarcon et al., 2004; Levenson et al., 2004b). However, in the collateral pathways where E-LTP was induced, treatment with TSA converted transcription-independent E-LTP to L-LTP (Vecsey et al., in press). Other studies in the amygdala have shown that TSA can enhance forskolin-induced LTP at the sensory input synapses (**Figure 2**(**c**)) (Yeh et al., 2004). Together, these studies demonstrate that increasing histone acetylation via HDAC inhibitors can enhance synaptic plasticity in the hippocampus and amygdala.

What is the molecular mechanism whereby HDAC inhibitors enhance synaptic plasticity? A clue to answering this question came from examining the molecular mechanism underlying TSA-dependent enhancement of E-LTP. This form of E-LTP is independent of transcription, translation, protein kinase A (PKA), and CREB (reviewed in Nguyen and Woo, 2003; Pittenger and Kandel, 2003). This allowed Vecsey et al. (in press) to specifically examine whether the TSA-dependent enhancements in E-LTP were dependent on CREB function. CREB is thought to activate transcription through the coactivator CBP and its associated HAT activity. In addition, the significant phenotypic overlap between memory and synaptic plasticity deficits exhibited by transgenic mice expressing dominant negative inhibitors of CREB or CBP suggests that they function together during memory processes (Pittenger et al., 2002; Wood et al., 2005). Mice with targeted deletions of two *creb* isoforms (α and Δ; CREB $\alpha\Delta$ mice) on a defined F1 hybrid genetic background of C57BL/6 and 129/SvEvTac strains were used to investigate the role of CREB in TSA-dependent enhancement of E-LTP (Walters and Blendy, 2001; Graves et al., 2002). Hippocampal slices from CREB $\alpha\,\Delta$ mice did not exhibit the TSA-dependent enhancement of E-LTP observed in wild-type littermates, suggesting that a CREB-dependent process is involved in regulating the transcription of genes sensitive to histone hyperacetylation required for TSA-dependent enhancement of E-LTP. Further, genetically modified *cbp* mutant mice carrying a triple point mutation in the CREB-binding (KIX) domain of CBP (*CBP*$^{KIX/KIX}$ knockin mice) failed to exhibit TSA-dependent enhancement of E-LTP as well, specifically implicating the CREB:CBP complex in enhancement of LTP by HDAC inhibitors (Vecsey et al., in press). Together with the observations made concerning the effects of HDAC inhibitors on CBP-deficient and normal animals (Korzus et al., 2004; Levenson et al., 2004b; Yeh et al., 2004; Vecsey et al., in press), these results also suggest that HDAC inhibitors reduce the signaling threshold required for engagement of CREB-dependent maintenance of plasticity, but that these treatments by themselves do not induce expression of CRE-containing genes.

36.3.4 Histone Acetylation and Seizure

As reviewed at the beginning of this section, different patterns of synaptic activity can lead to differential regulation of gene expression and ultimately a change in synaptic efficacy. A particularly dramatic example is seizure, which is a widespread burst of abnormal excitatory synaptic activity in the central nervous system (CNS). Seizure induces many changes in gene expression in the nervous system, which can lead to the development of chronic epilepsy and/or neurodegeneration. Early studies revealed that transcription of the immediate early gene *c-Fos* was upregulated in many regions of the brain after seizure (Morgan et al., 1987). Electron microscopy studies showed that c-Fos protein is preferentially localized to the euchromatic regions of chromosomes, which suggests that part of the transcriptional response to seizure involves changes in chromatin structure (Mugnaini et al., 1989).

Other studies have shown that expression of the glutamate receptor 2 (GluR2) alpha-amino-3-hydroxy-5-methyl-4-isoxazole propionic acid (AMPA) receptor subunit and brain-derived neurotrophic factor (BDNF) are also regulated by seizure (Ernfors et al., 1991; Isackson et al., 1991; Timmusk et al., 1993; Kokaia et al., 1995; Nibuya et al., 1995; Binder et al., 1999; Grooms et al., 2000; Sanchez et al., 2001). Expression of GluR2 mRNA is downregulated by seizure, whereas expression of BDNF mRNA is upregulated (Ernfors et al., 1991; Timmusk et al., 1993; Nibuya et al., 1995; Grooms et al., 2000). If seizure-induced changes in gene expression are due to changes in chromatin structure, then changes in chromatin structure should occur around the genes that are regulated by seizure. Recent studies have used the chromatin immunoprecipitation (ChIP) approach to monitor posttranslational modifications of histones that are located in the promoters of the BDNF and GluR2 genes. The first study to characterize the epigenetic regulation of GluR2 and BDNF demonstrated that pilocarpine-induced seizure significantly decreased acetylation of histone H4 in the GluR2 promoter, whereas acetylation of H4 in the P2 promoter of BDNF was significantly increased (Huang et al., 2002). The GluR2 promoter contains a repressor element-1 (RE1)-like silencer element in its promoter, and a recent study demonstrated that treatment of cultured neurons with kainic acid, an *in vitro* model for induction of seizures, resulted in increased binding of the transcriptional corepressor REST (RE1 silencer transcription factor), suggesting one possible mechanism for the downregulation of histone H4 acetylation (Jia et al., 2006). In another line of experiments, Tsankova et al. (2004) investigated changes in chromatin structure after electroconvulsive seizures (ECS), a form of human antidepressant therapy. ECS increased the acetylation of H4 at the P2 promoter of BDNF, and acetylation and phosphoacetylation of H3 were regulated within the P2 and P3 promoters of BDNF (Tsankova et al., 2004). These results indicate that ECS induces complex regulation of the epigenetic state of the BDNF promoters. ECS also had significant effects on the acetylation of H4 and phosphoacetylation of H3 within the *c-Fos* promoter and on the acetylation of H3 and H4 in the CREB promoter (Tsankova et al., 2004). Together, these data indicate that the synaptic activity and/or action potential firing that occurs during seizure results in complex regulation of the epigenetic state of chromatin.

36.3.5 Epigenetics in Plasticity and Seizure – Conclusions

Observations made regarding the role of epigenetics in plasticity and seizure strongly support a role for chromatin remodeling enzymes and histone acetylation in activity-dependent changes in synaptic and neuronal function. Moreover, all of these results support the hypothesis that epigenetic changes in chromatin structure are the basis of a cellular form of memory that influences neuronal state. Further examination of additional chromatin remodeling enzymes, as well as the analysis of additional histone modifications and their coregulation, will undoubtedly expand our understanding of the transcriptional profiles regulated by chromatin structure that are involved in long-term memory processes.

36.4 Epigenetics in Memory Formation

There are numerous studies indicating that many of the molecules necessary for induction of LTP are also required for normal long-term memory storage (reviewed by Malenka, 2003; Lynch, 2004). In light of the relationship between LTP and long-term memory formation, we next review the evidence associating epigenetic changes in chromatin structure with long-term memory storage. We will focus on the chromatin remodeling enzymes that appear to be involved, the specific chromatin modifications that correlate with memory storage, and what chromatin remodeling may provide in terms of mechanistic advantage for long-term memory storage processes.

36.4.1 Chromatin Remodeling Enzymes and Memory Storage

Rubinstein-Taybi syndrome (RTS), a human disease characterized by developmental abnormalities and mental retardation, is caused by translocations, deletions, and point mutations of the *cbp* gene (Petrij et al., 1995; Coupry et al., 2004). As discussed above, CREB and CBP are critical for successful induction of synaptic plasticity in species ranging from flies and slugs to rodents. Considering the role of CREB in learning, memory, and synaptic plasticity that has emerged from studies in *Aplysia, Drosophila,* and mice (Silva et al., 1998), it was reasonable to hypothesize that the cognitive impairments observed in RTS patients may be due directly to alterations in CBP activity in the brain. In a screen designed to identify genes involved in developmental regulation in mice, Oike et al. (1999) isolated a truncation mutation of CBP that lacks the HAT domain. These mice, which have one wild-type allele of *cbp* and one truncated allele, phenocopied many aspects of RTS quite well, with mice even exhibiting memory impairments (Oike et al., 1999). More recently, these animals were used in a study by Bourtchouladze et al. (2003) in which mice possessing the truncated CBP exhibited long-term memory deficits but normal learning and short-term memory in an object-recognition task (Bourtchouladze et al., 2003). Interestingly, inhibitors of phosphodiesterase 4, which enhance CREB-dependent gene expression, ameliorate memory deficits for object recognition in a dose-dependent manner in the mice containing the truncated form of CBP (Bourtchouladze et al., 2003). This suggests that pharmacologically enhancing cAMP-mediated signaling can compensate for the disruptions caused by the inhibitory truncated-CBP mutant expressed in these mice. Together, these results suggest that CBP, a potent HAT and chromatin remodeling enzyme, is involved in formation of long-term memory. However, this interpretation must be viewed with the caveat that the mice generated by Oike et al. (1999) have severe growth and developmental abnormalities, suggesting the alternative hypothesis that the memory impairments in these CBP-deficient mice are secondary to a neurodevelopmental abnormality.

To more directly study the effect of altering CBP activity on memory storage, two recent studies generated mice carrying spatially and temporally restricted expression of CBP mutants. Korzus et al. (2004) generated conditional transgenic mice expressing a HAT-deficient CBP transgene. The CaMKIIα promoter was used to spatially restrict transgene expression to forebrain neurons (Mayford et al., 1996) and the tetracycline system to temporally restrict transgene expression. These mice exhibited impaired memory for spatial and object recognition tasks that were ameliorated by intraperitoneal administration of the HDAC inhibitor TSA (Korzus et al., 2004). Thus, inducing a hyperacetylated histone state was able to compensate for the lack of HAT activity in these HAT-deficient CBP transgenic mice (i.e., **Figure 2**(**b**)). In a second study, Wood et al. (2005) generated transgenic mice expressing an inhibitory truncation mutant of CBP that contains the CREB-binding domain but lacks the HAT domain. The CaMKIIα promoter was used to spatially restrict transgene expression to forebrain neurons (Mayford et al., 1996), and this promoter does not activate transcription until 10–21 days postpartum (Kojima et al., 1997). These mice exhibited long-term memory deficits when assessed with hippocampus-dependent tasks such as contextual fear conditioning and the spatial water maze, but not in amygdala-dependent cued-fear conditioning (Wood et al., 2005). Together, these results demonstrate that more spatially restricted and temporally restricted alterations of CBP activity affect long-term memory storage (**Figure 2**(**b**)). Further, Korzus et al. (2004) were able to ameliorate long-term memory deficits by increasing histone acetylation using HDAC inhibitors. Similarly, HDAC inhibitors ameliorate long-term memory deficits for contextual fear in CBP heterozygous mice (non-regionally restricted deletion of one endogenous *cbp* allele) that exhibit long-term memory deficits for contextual fear and object recognition (Alarcon et al., 2004). Together, these studies demonstrate that brain-specific reduction of CBP activity results in long-term memory impairments and that these impairments may be ameliorated by increasing histone acetylation in general via administration of HDAC inhibitors (**Figure 2**(**b**)).

36.4.2 Histone Acetylation and Memory Storage

If a reduction of CBP activity results in memory deficits, and increasing histone acetylation via HDAC inhibitors can overcome these memory deficits, then an intriguing hypothesis arises suggesting that increasing histone acetylation might be a mechanism to enhance cognitive ability in general. Even more fundamental is the question: how do specific forms of memory formation affect histone acetylation? And lastly, what signaling cascades are involved in the transduction of information from the synapse to chromatin? Levenson et al. (2004b) addressed these questions in a set of experiments that were the first to demonstrate that chromatin structure modifications are involved in long-term memory formation. First, the authors examined histone acetylation in hippocampal area CA1 of rats subjected to contextual fear conditioning or latent inhibition (when an animal is preexposed to a novel context before receiving the shock in that context). They found that contextual fear conditioning correlated with increased acetylation of histone H3, whereas latent inhibition correlated with increased acetylation of histone H4 (Levenson et al., 2004b). These results demonstrate that differential regulation of hippocampal histone acetylation may be induced by specific forms of memory formation. Second, after demonstrating that fear conditioning correlates with increases in histone acetylation, the authors continued by examining the signaling cascades involved in histone acetylation changes. Using acute hippocampal slice preps, they found that *N*-methyl-D-aspartate receptor (NMDAR)-dependent synaptic transmission and signaling via the ERK-MAPK pathway were essential for acetylation of histone H3, but not acetylation of histone H4 (Levenson et al., 2004b). These results suggest that signaling pathways involved in the acetylation of H3 are different from those required for the acetylation of H4. Third, the authors showed that rats treated with HDAC inhibitors via intraperitoneal injection exhibited enhanced long-term memory for contextual fear conditioning when tested 24 h postconditioning, but normal short-term memory when tested 1 h postconditioning (**Figure 2(c)**) (Levenson et al., 2004b). Importantly, control experiments demonstrated that the HDAC inhibitors did not have an indirect effect on performance (Levenson et al., 2004b). Together, the study by Levenson et al. (2004b) demonstrated that changes in chromatin structure correlated with long-term memory formation and activation of second messenger signaling pathways that are known to be involved in memory processes.

In a similar study, Vecsey et al. (in press) found that delivering HDAC inhibitors directly to the hippocampus in mice via intrahippocampal cannulae enhanced long-term memory for contextual fear conditioning (**Figure 2(c)**). Interestingly, the authors found that delivery of the HDAC inhibitors during memory consolidation, but not during retrieval, enhanced memory. These results suggest that increasing histone acetylation during the consolidation stage of memory is involved in memory enhancement, a stage of memory formation that has been shown to be dependent on transcription (Abel and Lattal, 2001). The authors investigated the underlying molecular mechanism for HDAC inhibitor–dependent enhanced memory formation by examining the effect of HDAC inhibitors in CREB $\alpha\Delta$ knockout mice. These mice carry a targeted deletion of the α and Δ isoforms of CREB, the two most abundant isoforms of CREB (Hummler et al., 1994). CREB $\alpha\Delta$ knockout mice failed to exhibit enhanced memory for contextual fear after intrahippocampal administration of an HDAC inhibitor. These results suggest that the TSA-enhanced memory for contextual fear conditioning requires the transcription factor CREB (**Figure 2(d)**). As mentioned earlier in the synaptic plasticity section, the authors also demonstrated that HDAC inhibitor–dependent enhancement of LTP required CREB as well. Finally, the authors showed using quantitative real-time reverse transcriptase polymerase chain reaction that only a subset of CREB-target genes is affected by HDAC inhibition following contextual fear conditioning. Thus, CREB:CBP-mediated transcription appears to be essential for HDAC inhibitor enhanced memory and synaptic plasticity, which seems reasonable considering that CREB is a transcription factor that recruits CBP, a potent HAT, for transcriptional activation of memory-associated target genes.

36.4.3 Factor Acetylation and Memory Storage

Acetylation is a posttranslational modification that can occur on lysine residues in general. Therefore, acetylation can occur on non-histone (factor) proteins. For example, the histone acetyltransferase CBP acetylates several factors including the transcription factors p53, CREB, and NF-κB (Gu and Roeder, 1997; Furia et al., 2002; Kiernan et al., 2003; Yeh et al., 2004; Hassa et al., 2005). Thus, although HDAC inhibitor–dependent enhancement of memory and synaptic plasticity most likely occurs through histone acetylation that directly facilitates transcriptional activation, it is possible that this process may also be regulated by factor acetylation. For example, p65 (an NF-κB subunit also known as Rel-A) acetylation increases in the amygdala of rats subject to a fear-potentiated startle paradigm (Yeh et al., 2004). Increases in p65 acetylation correlate with increased

CBP interaction, whereas decreases in p65 acetylation correlate with increased HDAC3 interaction (Yeh et al., 2004). Interestingly, the HDAC inhibitor TSA blocks the interaction between HDAC3 and p65, suggesting that TSA may be able to increase NF-κB-mediated transcription in a manner that does not involve histone acetylation. Finally, the authors demonstrated that TSA injections directly to the amygdala enhanced fear-potentiated startle (Yeh et al., 2004). These results open the possibility that factor acetylation may also be involved in the mechanism by which HDAC inhibitors enhance memory storage. This idea is further supported by studies showing that the HDAC inhibitor TSA disrupts interactions between CREB and HDAC1/PP1, and Akt and HDAC1&6/PP1 (PP1 is a protein phosphatase that regulates CREB and other factors), thus increasing phosphorylation of CREB and Akt, directly regulating their function (Canettieri et al., 2003; Brush et al., 2004; Chen et al., 2005). An important distinction to make here is that acetylation of a factor will be transient. In contrast, histone acetylation establishes a pattern of histone modifications that may be much more stable, resulting in a long-term transcriptional profile required to maintain a cellular memory for memory storage. This idea is discussed in detail in the first section of this chapter.

36.4.4 DNA Methylation and 'Lifetime' Memory Storage

All of the studies discussed thus far have investigated the role of epigenetic marking of the genome in an early and acute phase of memory formation. A recent study published from the Meaney laboratory (Weaver et al., 2004) suggests that DNA methylation patterns of specific genes in the brain are used as part of the mechanisms for storing early childhood experiences. Mother rats exhibit strong nurturing behaviors toward their pups, most notably in the form of licking and grooming their offspring. Patterns of DNA methylation in the glucocorticoid receptor gene are directly correlated with the quality of maternal care, and these patterns of DNA methylation persist into adulthood (Weaver et al., 2004). Moreover, these changes in DNA methylation patterns result in decreased anxiety and a strong maternal nurturing instinct in the adult offspring (Weaver et al., 2004). Therefore, alterations in DNA methylation result in a 'learned' and persistent change in adult behavior. Interestingly, maternally induced patterns of DNA methylation can be altered by central infusion of either an HDAC inhibitor or L-methionine, a precursor in the synthesis of the methyl donor S-adenosyl-methionine, suggesting that learning-induced changes in patterns of DNA methylation are dynamic and can exhibit plasticity during the lifetime of the animal (Meaney and Szyf, 2005; Szyf et al., 2005; Weaver et al., 2005). It is important to note that disruption of the epigenetic state of neurons did not result in a loss of neuronal phenotype, as might be expected if the same kind of cellular memory were used to store long-term memory of phenotype and childhood experience. Moreover, persistence of neonatally acquired patterns of DNA methylation in the mature CNS is consistent with our hypothesis that epigenetic mechanisms contribute to persistent changes in neural function. Interestingly, this study suggests a unique mechanism whereby the status of at least one component of the epigenome is transmitted across generations using the basic mechanisms in place for information storage in the nervous system.

36.4.5 Epigenetics in Memory Formation – Conclusions

Formation of several different types of memory appears to be dependent upon some of the molecular machinery involved in chromatin structure remodeling; specifically HATs. Formation of some types of long-term memory is correlated with epigenetic tagging of the genome. Finally, treatment with HDAC inhibitors can compensate for loss of HAT function and even enhance normal long-term memory formation. All of these observations indicate that the processes involved in induction of long-term memory formation utilize epigenetic mechanisms. Future experiments should begin to investigate the role of epigenetics in other phases of long-term memory formation, including consolidation and lifetime or remote (see Frankland et al., 2004) storage.

36.5 Epigenetics in Cognition: Rett Syndrome

As reviewed, there is considerable evidence implicating epigenetic mechanisms in neural function and memory formation. Moreover, even though epigenetic regulation of chromatin structure is a vital step in cellular differentiation, the studies published to date indicate an active and ongoing role for epigenetic regulation of chromatin structure in the nervous system as it relates to plasticity and memory formation. Thus, postdevelopmental regulation of chromatin structure in the nervous system appears to be an important component of cognition. This suggests that derangement of the mechanisms responsible for regulation of chromatin structure would lead to severe cognitive impairment. Rett syndrome (RS) represents one disease of cognition where a specific molecule important for regulation of chromatin structure is mutated, resulting in severe cognitive impairments.

RS, first described by Austrian pediatrician Andreas Rett (1966), is an inherited, X-linked disease that afflicts about 1 in 15 000 females by 2 to 18 years of age and is estimated to be the second leading cause of mental retardation in women (Ellaway and Christodoulou, 2001). Development during the first 3 to 6 months of life is normal in RS patients; symptoms of RS first appear between 3 months and 3 years of age. The trademark of RS is a display of continuous, stereotypical hand movements, such as wringing, washing, clapping, and/or patting, which appear after the loss of purposeful hand movement. Other signs of RS include decreased growth (including microcephaly), abnormal respiration, gait ataxia, autism, seizures, and other neurological dysfunctions. Mapping studies identified a putative RS locus at Xq28 (Sirianni et al., 1998). Recent studies indicate that, in a percentage of patients, a mutation of the methyl CpG binding protein 2 (MeCP2) located in Xq28 is correlated with Rett syndrome (Sirianni et al., 1998; Amir et al., 1999; Ellaway and Christodoulou, 2001).

MeCP2 is a member of a family of methyl CpG binding proteins that function to link DNA (cytosine-5) methylation with gene silencing. As discussed earlier, DNMTs catalyze the methylation of cytosines at the 5-position of the pyrimidine ring. Once methylated, 5mCpG is bound by MeCP2, which then recruits a complex of proteins including histone deacetylases and transcriptional corepressors such as Sin3A (**Figure 3**(**a**)) (Roopra et al., 2000). The histones associated with the 5mCpG become hypoacetylated, promoting tight association between DNA and histones, ultimately resulting in formation of a transcriptionally repressive heterochromatin complex (**Figure 3**(**a**)).

The role that MeCP2 might play in the memory deficits observed in RS is still unclear. DNA methylation is thought to be involved in genomic imprinting and dosage compensation. Therefore, MeCP2 could play a prominent role during development. Indeed, MeCP2 appears to be critically involved in neuronal maturation, and not surprisingly, early attempts to create mouse models lacking MeCP2 resulted in embryonic lethality (Tate et al., 1996; Cohen et al., 2003; Matarazzo et al., 2004; Matarazzo and Ronnett, 2004; Fukuda et al., 2005). However, RS is a progressive disease that does not result in symptoms until early childhood. More recent attempts to create MeCP2-deficient mice have succeeded (Chen et al., 2001; Guy et al., 2001). These mice display several of the characteristics of human RS; however, no studies of cognitive performance in these mouse models have been published to date (Chen et al., 2001; Guy et al., 2001). To more closely approximate the mutations commonly found in RS patients, another strain of mouse was developed where the last one-third of MeCP2 was removed ($MeCP2^{308/y}$) (Shahbazian et al., 2002). $MeCP2^{308/y}$ mice share phenotypic similarities with human RS, including stereotypy, spontaneous seizures, increased anxiety, altered diurnal activity levels, and abnormal social interaction (Shahbazian et al., 2002; Moretti et al., 2005). Initial studies of $MeCP2^{308/y}$ animals suggested that long-term memory formation was normal (Shahbazian et al., 2002); however, further studies of these mice have revealed significant deficits in formation of hippocampus-dependent long-term memory and induction of synaptic plasticity in the sensory-motor cortex and hippocampus (**Figure 3**(**b**)) (Moretti et al., 2006). The derangements observed in $MeCP2^{308/y}$ animals do not appear to be due to aberrant development, as mice where MeCP2 was removed from forebrain neurons postnatally display many of the same social and memory impairments (Gemelli et al., 2006).

Several recent studies have begun to explore the function of MeCP2 in neurons and have identified a few mechanisms by which loss of MeCP2 could result in the cognitive derangements observed in RS model mice and human patients. One study demonstrated that a truncated form of MeCP2 protein, which mimics the most common mutation observed in human RS patients, tightly associates with methylated DNA in *Xenopus* embryos, suggesting that mutated MeCP2 protein can have profound effects on early developmental processes and possibly also interfere with normal regulation of chromatin structure and gene expression in the adult (Stancheva et al., 2003). Morphological studies have revealed that MeCP2 is expressed in excitatory cortical

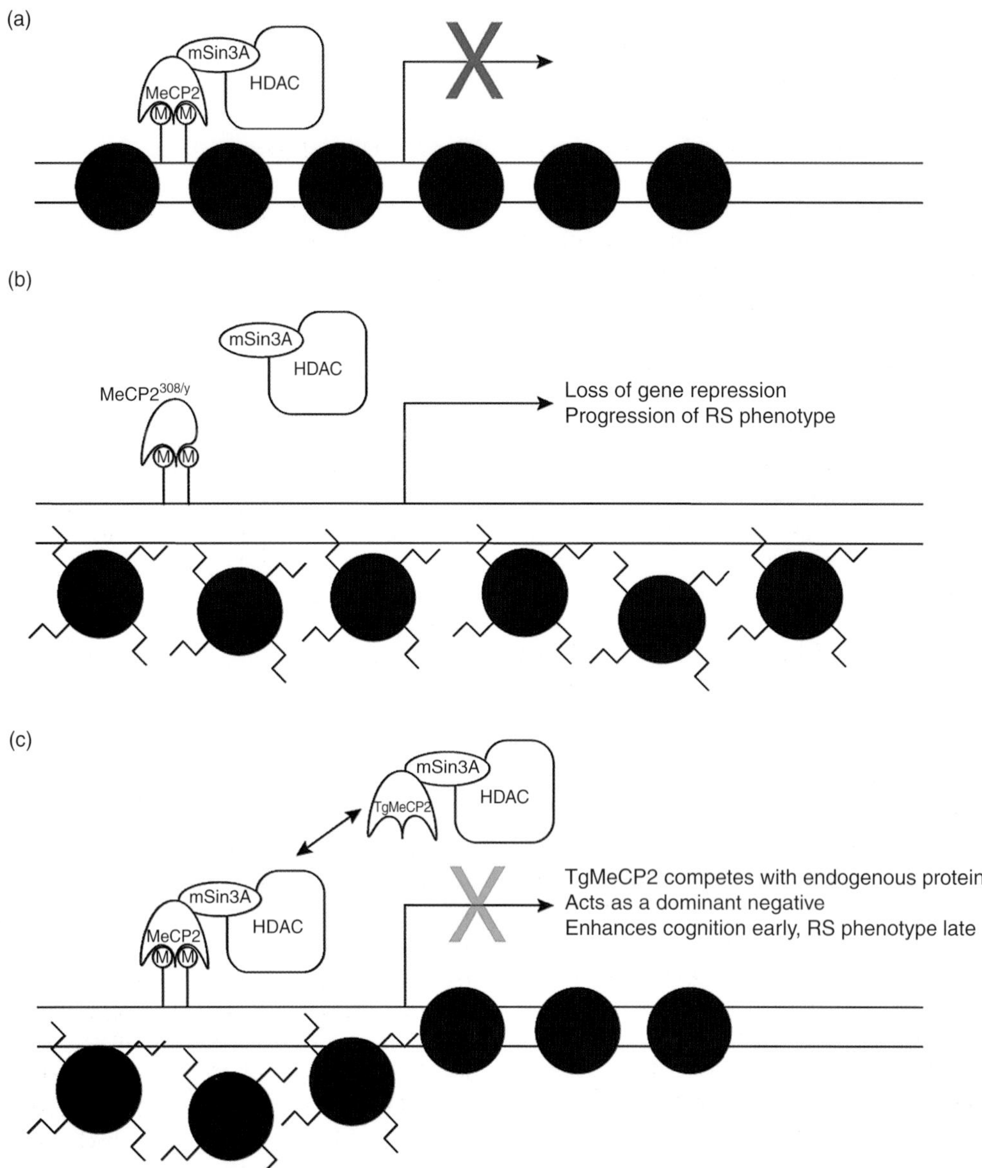

Figure 3 Role of MeCP2 in Rett syndrome, synaptic plasticity, and memory formation. MeCP2 is a member of the family of methyl CpG binding proteins. (a) MeCP2 binds to methylated cytosines and recruits the adapter protein mSin3A and HDAC to repress gene expression. (b) Loss of MeCP2 function through truncation mutations is thought to underlie RS. Truncation of MeCP2 results in loss of gene silencing, aberrant gene expression, and progression of the RS phenotype. (c) Overexpression of MeCP2 represents one possible therapeutic approach for treatment of RS. MeCP2 overexpression appears to have a dominant negative effect on normal MeCP2 function as determined through measures of synaptic plasticity and cognitive performance. Excess MeCP2 may sequester mSin3A and HDAC, limiting the ability of MeCP2 to repress gene expression. The early effects of MeCP2 overexpression lead to enhancement of synaptic plasticity and cognition. Continuous overexpression of MeCP2 eventually results in progression of a RS-like phenotype and death.

neurons and GABAergic interneurons, with little to no expression in glial cells (Akbarian et al., 2001; LaSalle et al., 2001; Adachi et al., 2005; Pelka et al., 2005). Restriction of MeCP2 expression to excitatory and inhibitory neurons in the cortex is consistent with the observations that expression of *dlx5*, a gene responsible for the regulation of GABA-synthesizing enzymes, is increased due to a loss of MeCP2-mediated imprinting in human fibroblasts (Horike et al., 2005), and cortical inhibitory tone is enhanced in one strain of MeCP2-null mice (Dani et al., 2005). Investigating possible causes of the aberrant social behavior, several studies indicate that expression of stress-related genes is increased and levels of nor-epinephrine, dopamine, and serotonin were decreased in MeCP2-null mice (Ide et al., 2005; Nuber et al., 2005). Additionally, loss of MeCP2 leads to aberrations in chromatin structure around the Prader Willi and Angelman loci, two regions of the genome implicated in autism (Makedonski et al., 2005; Samaco et al., 2005). It is interesting to note that all of these aberrations observed in the context of loss of MeCP2 function are due to dysfunction of chromatin structure and gene expression (Tudor et al., 2002).

As detailed earlier, several studies indicate that loss of MeCP2 function leads to severe alterations in chromatin structure, gene expression, and neuronal function. Several labs have begun to explore the efficacy of overexpression of normal MeCP2 as a potential therapy to treat RS patients. In one study, overexpression of MeCP2 was shown to enhance long-term memory formation and the induction of hippocampal LTP in young mice (**Figure 3(c)**) (Collins et al., 2004). However, as the mice aged, overexpression of MeCP2 led to impairments in motor function and a decrease in longevity (Collins et al., 2004; Luikenhuis et al., 2004). Interestingly, overexpression of MeCP2 in mice that lack MeCP2 rescues the RS phenotype, suggesting that genetic replacement of MeCP2 expression is sufficient to rescue some of the RS-associated phenotypes (Luikenhuis et al., 2004). Moreover, these results suggest that levels of MeCP2 are coupled to cognitive performance, and suggest the broader implication that methyl-DNA binding protein function, and possibly DNA (cytosine-5) methylation itself, plays a significant role in induction of plasticity and memory formation in the adult CNS.

In support of an active role for DNA (cytosine-5) methylation in plasticity, a recent study by Levenson et al. (2006) demonstrated that inhibition of DNMT activity blocks induction of LTP in the hippocampus. Moreover, activation of PKC through the use of phorbol esters significantly increased expression of DNMT3A, suggesting that DNMT expression and activity is regulated by a signaling pathway that is crucial for the induction of synaptic plasticity and memory formation (Lovinger et al., 1987; Abeliovich et al., 1993; Weeber et al., 2000). Collectively, these results are consistent with the observations made in MeCP2 model mice and suggest an active role for DNMT activity and DNA (cytosine-5) methylation in synaptic plasticity and long-term memory formation.

36.6 Conclusions

Epigenetic cellular memory is an ancient and evolutionarily conserved form of lifetime memory. Every cell in a metazoan relies on cellular memory to exist and function normally in its environment. A common theme emerging in the field of learning and memory is that the nervous system has co-opted several evolutionarily conserved processes to subserve long-term information storage. Some examples include molecules relevant for immune system function, such as class I major histocompatibility complex proteins and the NF-κB family of transcription factors (Meberg et al., 1996; Corriveau et al., 1998; Albensi and Mattson, 2000; Huh et al., 2000; Kassed et al., 2002; Yeh et al., 2002; Meffert et al., 2003; Levenson et al., 2004a; Oliveira et al., 2004) and signaling pathways involved in early development, such as the ras-MEK-ERK MAPK signaling pathway (English and Sweatt, 1996, 1997; Atkins et al., 1998; Silva et al., 1998; Selcher et al., 1999; Schafe et al., 2000; Giese et al., 2001). The realization that the processes involved in forming epigenetic cellular memory have been co-opted by the nervous system for induction of long-term memory and storage of some forms of lifetime memory has brought the field of neuroscience to an exciting juncture. For example, therapies based on modulation of epigenetic states could be used to treat a host of neurological conditions potentially including Huntington's disease, Alzheimer's disease, schizophrenia, and Rubinstein-Taybi syndrome (Kimberly et al., 2001; Steffan et al., 2001; Ferrante et al., 2003; Hockly et al., 2003; Kim et al., 2004; Numachi et al., 2004; Rouaux et al., 2004; Von Rotz et al., 2004; Grayson et al., 2005; Tremolizzo et al., 2005). Perhaps most relevant for the general population is the exciting possibility that, as we gain a deeper understanding of how epigenetics factors into cognition, novel drugs could be developed to enhance memory formation in otherwise normal individuals (Levenson et al., 2004b).

References

Abel T and Lattal KM (2001) Molecular mechanisms of memory acquisition, consolidation and retrieval. *Curr. Opin. Neurobiol.* 11: 180–187.

Abeliovich A, Paylor R, Chen C, Kim JJ, Wehner JM, and Tonegawa S (1993) PKC gamma mutant mice exhibit mild deficits in spatial and contextual learning. *Cell* 75: 1263–1271.

Adachi M, Keefer EW, and Jones FS (2005) A segment of the Mecp2 promoter is sufficient to drive expression in neurons *Hum. Mol. Genet*. 14(23): 3709–3702.

Adams JP and Sweatt JD (2002) Molecular psychology: Roles for the ERK MAP kinase cascade in memory. *Annu. Rev. Pharmacol. Toxicol*. 42: 135–163.

Ajiro K, Yoda K, Utsumi K, and Nishikawa Y (1996) Alteration of cell cycle-dependent histone phosphorylations by okadaic acid. Induction of mitosis-specific H3 phosphorylation and chromatin condensation in mammalian interphase cells. *J. Biol. Chem*. 271: 13197–13201.

Akbarian S, Chen RZ, Gribnau J, et al. (2001) Expression pattern of the Rett syndrome gene MeCP2 in primate prefrontal cortex. *Neurobiol. Dis*. 8: 784–791.

Alarcon JM, Malleret G, Touzani K, et al. (2004) Chromatin acetylation, memory, and LTP are impaired in CBP+/– mice: A model for the cognitive deficit in Rubinstein-Taybi syndromeand its amelioration. *Neuron*. 42: 947–959.

Albensi BC and Mattson MP (2000) Evidence for the involvement of TNF and NF-kappaB in hippocampal synaptic lasticity. *Synapse*. 35: 151–159.

Alberini CM, Ghirardi M, Metz R, and Kandel ER (1994) C/EBP is an immediate-early gene required for the consolidation of long-term facilitation in *Aplysia*. *Cell* 76: 1099–1114.

Amir RE, Van den Veyver IB, Wan M, Tran CQ, Francke U, and Zoghbi HY (1999) Rett syndrome is caused by mutations in X-linked MECP2, encoding methyl-CpG-binding protein 2. *Nat. Genet*. 23: 185–188.

Atkins CM, Selcher JC, Petraitis JJ, Trzaskos JM, and Sweatt JD (1998) The MAPK cascade is required for mammalian associative learning. *Nat. Neurosci*. 1: 602–609.

Bell AC and Felsenfeld G (2000) Methylation of a CTCF-dependent boundary controls imprinted expression of the Igf2 gene. *Nature* 405: 482–485.

Bestor T, Laudano A, Mattaliano R, and Ingram V (1988) Cloning and sequencing of a cDNA encoding DNA methyltransferase of mouse cells. The carboxyl-terminal domain of the mammalian enzymes is related to bacterial restriction methyltransferases. *J. Mol. Biol*. 203: 971–983.

Binder DK, Routbort MJ, Ryan TE, Yancopoulos GD, and McNamara JO (1999) Selective inhibition of kindling development by intraventricular administration of TrkB receptor body. *J. Neurosci*. 19: 1424–1436.

Bird AP (1978) Use of restriction enzymes to study eukaryotic DNA methylation: II. The symmetry of methylated sites supports semi-conservative copying of the methylation pattern. *J. Mol. Biol*. 118: 49–60.

Bird AP (1986) CpG-rich islands and the function of DNA methylation. *Nature* 321: 209–213.

Bliss TV and Lomo T (1973) Long-lasting potentiation of synaptic transmission in the dentate area of the anaesthetized rabbit following stimulation of the perforant path. *J. Physiol*. 232: 331–356.

Bourtchouladze R, Lidge R, Catapano R, et al. (2003) A mouse model of Rubinstein-Taybi syndrome: Defective long-term memory is ameliorated by inhibitors of phosphodiesterase 4. *Proc. Natl. Acad. Sci. USA* 100: 10518–10522.

Bradbury EM, Inglis RJ, Matthews HR, and Sarner N (1973) Phosphorylation of very-lysine-rich histone in *Physarum polycephalum*. Correlation with chromosome condensation. *Eur. J. Biochem*. 33: 131–139.

Brown DT (2003) Histone H1 and the dynamic regulation of chromatin function. *Biochem. Cell Biol*. 81: 221–227.

Brunelli M, Castellucci V, and Kandel ER (1976) Synaptic facilitation and behavioral sensitization in *Aplysia*: Possible role of serotonin and cyclic AMP. *Science* 194: 1178–1181.

Brush MH, Guardiola A, Connor JH, Yao TP, and Shenolikar S (2004) Deactylase inhibitors disrupt cellular complexes containing protein phosphatases and deacetylases. *J. Biol. Chem*. 279: 7685–7691.

Canettieri G, Morantte I, Guzman E, et al. (2003) Attenuation of a phosphorylation-dependent activator by an HDAC-PP1 complex. *Nat. Struct. Biol*. 10: 175–181.

Cedar H, Solage A, Glaser G, and Razin A (1979) Direct detection of methylated cytosine in DNA by use of the restriction enzyme MspI. *Nucleic Acids Res*. 6: 2125–2132.

Chen CS, Weng SC, Tseng PH, and Lin HP (2005) Histone acetylation-independent effect of histone deacetylase inhibitors on Akt through the reshuffling of protein phosphatase 1 complexes. *J. Biol. Chem*. 280: 38879–38887.

Chen HY, Sun JM, Zhang Y, Davie JR, and Meistrich ML (1998) Ubiquitination of histone H3 in elongating spermatids of rat testes. *J. Biol. Chem*. 273: 13165–13169.

Chen L, MacMillan AM, Chang W, Ezaz-Nikpay K, Lane WS, and Verdine GL (1991) Direct identification of the active-site nucleophile in a DNA (cytosine-5)-methyltransferase. *Biochemistry* 30: 11018–11025.

Chen RZ, Akbarian S, Tudor M, and Jaenisch R (2001) Deficiency of methyl-CpG binding protein-2 in CNS neurons results in a Rett-like phenotype in mice. *Nat. Genet*. 27: 327–331.

Cohen DR, Matarazzo V, Palmer AM, et al. (2003) Expression of MeCP2 in olfactory receptor neurons is developmentally regulated and occurs before synaptogenesis. *Mol. Cell. Neurosci*. 22: 417–429.

Collins AL, Levenson JM, Vilaythong AP, et al. (2004) Mild overexpression of MeCP2 causes a progressive neurological disorder in mice. *Hum. Mol. Genet*. 13: 2679–2689.

Cooper DN and Krawczak M (1989) Cytosine methylation and the fate of CpG dinucleotides in vertebrate genomes. *Hum. Genet*. 83: 181–188.

Corriveau RA, Huh GS, and Shatz CJ (1998) Regulation of class I MHC gene expression in the developing and mature CNS by neural activity. *Neuron* 21: 505–520.

Coupry I, Monnet L, Attia AA, Taine L, Lacombe D, and Arveiler B (2004) Analysis of CBP (CREBBP) gene deletions in Rubinstein-Taybi syndrome patients using real-time quantitative PCR. *Hum. Mutat*. 23: 278–284.

Dale N and Kandel ER (1990) Facilitatory and inhibitory transmitters modulate spontaneous transmitter release at cultured *Aplysia* sensorimotor synapses. *J. Physiol*. 421: 203–222.

Dani VS, Chang Q, Maffei A, Turrigiano GG, Jaenisch R, and Nelson SB (2005) Reduced cortical activity due to a shift in the balance between excitation and inhibition in a mouse model of Rett syndrome. *Proc. Natl. Acad. Sci. USA* 102: 12560–12565.

Di Agostino S, Rossi P, Geremia R, and Sette C (2002) The MAPK pathway triggers activation of Nek2 during chromosome condensation in mouse spermatocytes. *Development* 129: 1715–1727.

Dion MF, Altschuler SJ, Wu LF, and Rando OJ (2005) Genomic characterization reveals a simple histone H4 acetylation code. *Proc. Natl. Acad. Sci. USA* 102: 5501–5506.

Egger G, Liang G, Aparicio A, and Jones PA (2004) Epigenetics in human disease and prospects for epigenetic therapy. *Nature* 429: 457–463.

Ellaway C and Christodoulou J (2001) Rett syndrome: Clinical characteristics and recent genetic advances. *Disabil. Rehabil*. 23: 98–106.

English JD and Sweatt JD (1996) Activation of p42 mitogen-activated protein kinase in hippocampal long term potentiation. *J. Biol. Chem*. 271: 24329–24332.

English JD and Sweatt JD (1997) A requirement for the mitogen-activated protein kinase cascade in hippocampal long term potentiation. *J. Biol. Chem.* 272: 19103–19106.

Ernfors P, Bengzon J, Kokaia Z, Persson H, and Lindvall O (1991) Increased levels of messenger RNAs for neurotrophic factors in the brain during kindling epileptogenesis. *Neuron* 7: 165–176.

Ferrante RJ, Kubilus JK, Lee J, et al. (2003) Histone deacetylase inhibition by sodium butyrate chemotherapy ameliorates the neurodegenerative phenotype in Huntington's disease mice. *J. Neurosci.* 23: 9418–9427.

Frankland PW, Bontempi B, Talton LE, Kaczmarek L, and Silva AJ (2004) The involvement of the anterior cingulate cortex in remote contextual fear memory. *Science* 304: 881–883.

Fukuda T, Itoh M, Ichikawa T, Washiyama K, and Goto Y (2005) Delayed maturation of neuronal architecture and synaptogenesis in cerebral cortex of Mecp2-deficient mice. *J. Neuropathol. Exp. Neurol.* 64: 537–544.

Furia B, Deng L, Wu K, et al. (2002) Enhancement of nuclear factor-kappa B acetylation by coactivator p300 and HIV-1 Tat proteins. *J. Biol. Chem.* 277: 4973–4980.

Gemelli T, Berton O, Nelson ED, Perrotti LI, Jaenisch R, and Monteggia LM (2006) Postnatal loss of methyl-CpG binding protein 2 in the forebrain is sufficient to mediate behavioral aspects of Rett syndrome in mice. *Biol. Psychiatry.* 59: 468–476.

Giese KP, Friedman E, Telliez JB, et al. (2001) Hippocampus-dependent learning and memory is impaired in mice lacking the Ras-guanine-nucleotide releasing factor 1 (Ras-GRF1). *Neuropharmacology* 41: 791–800.

Goldknopf IL, Taylor CW, Baum RM, et al. (1975) Isolation and characterization of protein A24, a "histone-like" non-histone chromosomal protein. *J. Biol. Chem.* 250: 7182–7187.

Goto H, Yasui Y, Nigg EA, and Inagaki M (2002) Aurora-B phosphorylates histone H3 at serine28 with regard to the mitotic chromosome condensation. *Genes Cells* 7: 11–17.

Graves L, Dalvi A, Lucki I, Blendy JA, and Abel T (2002) Behavioral analysis of CREB alphadelta mutation on a B6/129 F1 hybrid background. *Hippocampus* 12: 18–26.

Grayson DR, Jia X, Chen Y, et al. (2005) Reelin promoter hypermethylation in schizophrenia. *Proc. Natl. Acad. Sci. USA* 102: 9341–9346.

Grooms SY, Opitz T, Bennett MV, and Zukin RS (2000) Status epilepticus decreases glutamate receptor 2 mRNA and protein expression in hippocampal pyramidal cells before neuronal death. *Proc. Natl. Acad. Sci. USA* 97: 3631–3636.

Gu W and Roeder RG (1997) Activation of p53 sequence-specific DNA binding by acetylation of the p53 C-terminal domain. *Cell* 90: 595–606.

Guan Z, Giustetto M, Lomvardas S, et al. (2002) Integration of long-term-memory-related synaptic plasticity involves bidirectional regulation of gene expression and chromatin structure. *Cell* 111: 483–493.

Gurley LR, Walters RA, and Tobey RA (1974) Cell cycle-specific changes in histone phosphorylation associated with cell proliferation and chromosome condensation. *J. Cell Biol.* 60: 356–364.

Guy J, Hendrich B, Holmes M, Martin JE, and Bird A (2001) A mouse Mecp2-null mutation causes neurological symptoms that mimic Rett syndrome. *Nat. Genet.* 27: 322–326.

Hammer M, Cleary LJ, and Byrne JH (1989) Serotonin acts in the synaptic region of sensory neurons in *Aplysia* to enhance transmitter release. *Neurosci. Lett.* 104: 235–240.

Hassa PO, Haenni SS, Buerki C, et al. (2005) Acetylation of poly(ADP-ribose) polymerase-1 by p300/CREB-binding protein regulates coactivation of NF-kappaB-dependent transcription. *J. Biol. Chem.* 280: 40450–40464.

Hay RT (2001) Protein modification by SUMO. *Trends Biochem. Sci.* 26: 332–333.

Hendrich B and Bird A (1998) Identification and characterization of a family of mammalian methyl-CpG binding proteins. *Mol. Cell. Biol.* 18: 6538–6547.

Henikoff S (2005) Histone modifications: Combinatorial complexity or cumulative simplicity? *Proc. Natl. Acad. Sci. USA* 102: 5308–5309.

Hicke L (2001) Protein regulation by monoubiquitin. *Nat. Rev. Mol. Cell Biol.* 2: 195–201.

Hockly E, Richon VM, Woodman B, et al. (2003) Suberoylanilide hydroxamic acid, a histone deacetylase inhibitor, ameliorates motor deficits in a mouse model of Huntington's disease. *Proc. Natl. Acad. Sci. USA* 100: 2041–2046.

Horike S, Cai S, Miyano M, Cheng JF, and Kohwi-Shigematsu T (2005) Loss of silent-chromatin looping and impaired imprinting of DLX5 in Rett syndrome. *Nat. Genet.* 37: 31–40.

Hsieh J and Gage FH (2004) Epigenetic control of neural stem cell fate. *Curr. Opin. Genet. Dev.* 14: 461–469.

Hsieh J and Gage FH (2005) Chromatin remodeling in neural development and plasticity. *Curr. Opin. Cell Biol.* 17: 664–671.

Hsu JY, Sun ZW, Li X, et al. (2000) Mitotic phosphorylation of histone H3 is governed by Ipl1/aurora kinase and Glc7/PP1 phosphatase in budding yeast and nematodes. *Cell* 102: 279–291.

Huang Y, Doherty JJ, and Dingledine R (2002) Altered histone acetylation at glutamate receptor 2 and brain-derived neurotrophic factor genes is an early event triggered by status epilepticus. *J. Neurosci.* 22: 8422–8428.

Huh GS, Boulanger LM, Du H, Riquelme PA, Brotz TM, and Shatz CJ (2000) Functional requirement for class I MHC in CNS development and plasticity. *Science* 290: 2155–2159.

Hummler E, Cole TJ, Blendy JA, et al. (1994) Targeted mutation of the CREB gene: Compensation within the CREB/ATF family of transcription factors. *Proc. Natl. Acad. Sci. USA* 91: 5647–5651.

Ide S, Itoh M, and Goto Y (2005) Defect in normal developmental increase of the brain biogenic amine concentrations in the mecp2-null mouse. *Neurosci. Lett.* 386: 14–17.

Isackson PJ, Huntsman MM, Murray KD, and Gall CM (1991) BDNF mRNA expression is increased in adult rat forebrain after limbic seizures: Temporal patterns of induction distinct from NGF. *Neuron* 6: 937–948.

Jenuwein T and Allis CD (2001) Translating the histone code. *Science* 293: 1074–1080.

Jia YH, Zhu X, Li SY, Ni JH, and Jia HT (2006) Kainate exposure suppresses activation of GluR2 subunit promoter in primary cultured cerebral cortical neurons through induction of RE1-silencing transcription factor. *Neurosci. Lett.* 403: 103–108.

Johnson ES and Gupta AA (2001) An E3-like factor that promotes SUMO conjugation to the yeast septins. *Cell* 106: 735–744.

Jones PL, Veenstra GJ, Wade PA, et al. (1998) Methylated DNA and MeCP2 recruit histone deacetylase to repress transcription. *Nat. Genet.* 19: 187–191.

Josselyn SA (2005) What's right with my mouse model? New insights into the molecular and cellular basis of cognition from mouse models of Rubinstein-Taybi Syndrome. *Learn. Mem.* 12: 80–83.

Kandel ER and Tauc L (1964) Mechanism of prolonged hetero-synaptic facilitation. *Nature* 202: 145–147.

Kassed CA, Willing AE, Garbuzova-Davis S, Sanberg PR, and Pennypacker KR (2002) Lack of NF-kappaB p50 exacerbates degeneration of hippocampal neurons after chemical exposure and impairs learning. *Exp. Neurol.* 176: 277–288.

Kiernan R, Bres V, Ng RW, et al. (2003) Post-activation turn-off of NF-kappa B-dependent transcription is regulated by acetylation of p65. *J. Biol. Chem.* 278: 2758–2766.

Kim HS, Kim EM, Kim NJ, et al. (2004) Inhibition of histone deacetylation enhances the neurotoxicity induced by the C-terminal fragments of amyloid precursor protein. *J. Neurosci. Res.* 75: 117–124.

Kimberly WT, Zheng JB, Guenette SY, and Selkoe DJ (2001) The intracellular domain of the beta-amyloid precursor protein is stabilized by Fe65 and translocates to the nucleus in a notch-like manner. *J. Biol. Chem.* 276: 40288–40292.

Kojima N, Wang J, Mansuy IM, Grant SG, Mayford M, and Kandel ER (1997) Rescuing impairment of long-term potentiation in fyn-deficient mice by introducing Fyn transgene. *Proc. Natl. Acad. Sci. USA* 94: 4761–4765.

Kokaia M, Ernfors P, Kokaia Z, Elmer E, Jaenisch R, and Lindvall O (1995) Suppressed epileptogenesis in BDNF mutant mice. *Exp. Neurol.* 133: 215–224.

Korzus E (2003) The relation of transcription to memory formation. *Acta Biochim. Pol.* 50: 775–782.

Korzus E, Rosenfeld MG, and Mayford M (2004) CBP histone acetyltransferase activity is a critical component of memory consolidation. *Neuron* 42: 961–972.

LaSalle JM, Goldstine J, Balmer D, and Greco CM (2001) Quantitative localization of heterogeneous methyl-CpG-binding protein 2 (MeCP2) expression phenotypes in normal and Rett syndrome brain by laser scanning cytometry. *Hum. Mol. Genet.* 10: 1729–1740.

Lau OD, Courtney AD, Vassilev A, et al. (2000) p300/CBP-associated factor histone acetyltransferase processing of a peptide substrate. Kinetic analysis of the catalytic mechanism. *J. Biol. Chem.* 275: 21953–21959.

Levenson JM, Choi S, Lee SY, et al. (2004a) A bioinformatics analysis of memory consolidation reveals involvement of the transcription factor c-rel. *J. Neurosci.* 24: 3933–3943.

Levenson JM, O'Riordan KJ, Brown KD, Trinh MA, Molfese DL, and Sweatt JD (2004b) Regulation of histone acetylation during memory formation in the hippocampus. *J. Biol. Chem.* 279: 40545–40559.

Levenson JM, Roth TL, Lubin FD, et al. (2006) Evidence that DNA (cytosine-5) methyltransferase regulates synaptic plasticity in the hippocampus. *J. Biol. Chem.* 281: 15763–15773.

Lovinger DM, Wong KL, Murakami K, and Routtenberg A (1987) Protein kinase C inhibitors eliminate hippocampal long-term potentiation. *Brain Res.* 436: 177–183.

Luger K, Mader AW, Richmond RK, Sargent DF, and Richmond TJ (1997) Crystal structure of the nucleosome core particle at 2.8 A resolution. *Nature* 389: 251–260.

Luikenhuis S, Giacometti E, Beard CF, and Jaenisch R (2004) Expression of MeCP2 in postmitotic neurons rescues Rett syndrome in mice. *Proc. Natl. Acad. Sci. USA* 101: 6033–6038.

Lyko F, Ramsahoye BH, Kashevsky H, et al. (1999) Mammalian (cytosine-5) methyltransferases cause genomic DNA methylation and lethality in *Drosophila*. *Nat. Genet.* 23: 363–366.

Lynch MA (2004) Long-term potentiation and memory. *Physiol. Rev.* 84: 87–136.

Mahadevan LC, Willis AC, and Barratt MJ (1991) Rapid histone H3 phosphorylation in response to growth factors, phorbol esters, okadaic acid, and protein synthesis inhibitors. *Cell* 65: 775–783.

Maier H, Colbert J, Fitzsimmons D, Clark DR, and Hagman J (2003) Activation of the early B-cell-specific mb-1 (Ig-alpha) gene by Pax-5 is dependent on an unmethylated Ets binding site. *Mol. Cell. Biol.* 23: 1946–1960.

Makedonski K, Abuhatzira L, Kaufman Y, Razin A, and Shemer R (2005) MeCP2 deficiency in Rett syndrome causes epigenetic aberrations at the PWS/AS imprinting center that affects UBE3A expression. *Hum. Mol. Genet.* 14: 1049–1058.

Malenka RC (2003) The long-term potential of LTP. *Nat. Rev. Neurosci.* 4: 923–926.

Martin SJ and Morris RG (2002) New life in an old idea: The synaptic plasticity and memory hypothesis revisited. *Hippocampus* 12: 609–636.

Matarazzo V, Cohen D, Palmer AM, et al. (2004) The transcriptional repressor Mecp2 regulates terminal neuronal differentiation. *Mol. Cell. Neurosci.* 27: 44–58.

Matarazzo V and Ronnett GV (2004) Temporal and regional differences in the olfactory proteome as a consequence of MeCP2 deficiency. *Proc. Natl. Acad. Sci. USA* 101: 7763–7768.

Mayford M, Bach ME, Huang YY, Wang L, Hawkins RD, and Kandel ER (1996) Control of memory formation through regulated expression of a CaMKII transgene. *Science* 274: 1678–1683.

Meaney MJ and Szyf M (2005) Environmental programming of stress responses through DNA methylation: Life at the interface between a dynamic environment and a fixed genome. *Dialogues Clin. Neurosci.* 7: 103–123.

Meberg PJ, Kinney WR, Valcourt EG, and Routtenberg A (1996) Gene expression of the transcription factor NF-kappa B in hippocampus: Regulation by synaptic activity. *Brain Res. Mol. Brain Res.* 38: 179–190.

Meffert MK, Chang JM, Wiltgen BJ, Fanselow MS, and Baltimore D (2003) NF-kappa B functions in synaptic signaling and behavior. *Nat. Neurosci.* 6: 1072–1078.

Melchior F (2000) SUMO – nonclassical ubiquitin. *Annu. Rev. Cell Dev. Biol.* 16: 591–626.

Montarolo PG, Goelet P, Castellucci VF, Morgan J, Kandel ER, and Schacher S (1986) A critical period for macromolecular synthesis in long-term heterosynaptic facilitation in *Aplysia*. *Science* 234: 1249–1254.

Montarolo PG, Kandel ER, and Schacher S (1988) Long-term heterosynaptic inhibition in *Aplysia*. *Nature* 333: 171–174.

Moretti P, Bouwknecht JA, Teague R, Paylor R, and Zoghbi HY (2005) Abnormalities of social interactions and home-cage behavior in a mouse model of Rett syndrome. *Hum. Mol. Genet.* 14: 205–220.

Moretti P, Levenson JM, Battaglia F, et al. (2006) Learning and memory and synaptic plasticity are impaired in a mouse model of Rett syndrome. *J. Neurosci.* 26: 319–327.

Morgan JI, Cohen DR, Hempstead JL, and Curran T (1987) Mapping patterns of c-fos expression in the central nervous system after seizure. *Science* 237: 192–197.

Mugnaini E, Berrebi AS, Morgan JI, and Curran T (1989) Fos-like immunoreactivity induced by seizure in mice is specifically associated with euchromatin in neurons. *Eur. J. Neurosci.* 1: 46–52.

Murphey RK and Godenschwege TA (2002) New roles for ubiquitin in the assembly and function of neuronal circuits. *Neuron* 36: 5–8.

Nan X, Ng HH, Johnson CA, et al. (1998) Transcriptional repression by the methyl-CpG-binding protein MeCP2 involves a histone deacetylase complex. *Nature* 393: 386–389.

Nguyen PV, Abel T, and Kandel ER (1994) Requirement of a critical period of transcription for induction of a late phase of LTP. *Science* 265: 1104–1107.

Nguyen PV and Woo NH (2003) Regulation of hippocampal synaptic plasticity by cyclic AMP-dependent protein kinases. *Prog. Neurobiol.* 71: 401–437.

Nibuya M, Morinobu S, and Duman RS (1995) Regulation of BDNF and trkB mRNA in rat brain by chronic electroconvulsive seizure and antidepressant drug treatments. *J. Neurosci.* 15: 7539–7547.

Nickel BE and Davie JR (1989) Structure of polyubiquitinated histone H2A. *Biochemistry* 28: 964–968.

Norton VG, Imai BS, Yau P, and Bradbury EM (1989) Histone acetylation reduces nucleosome core particle linking number change. *Cell* 57: 449–457.

Nowak SJ, Pai CY, and Corces VG (2003) Protein phosphatase 2A activity affects histone H3 phosphorylation and transcription in *Drosophila melanogaster*. *Mol. Cell. Biol.* 23: 6129–6138.

Nuber UA, Kriaucionis S, Roloff TC, et al. (2005) Up-regulation of glucocorticoid-regulated genes in a mouse model of Rett syndrome. *Hum. Mol. Genet.* 14: 2247–2256.

Numachi Y, Yoshida S, Yamashita M, et al. (2004) Psychostimulant alters expression of DNA methyltransferase mRNA in the rat brain. *Ann. N. Y. Acad. Sci.* 1025: 102–109.

Oike Y, Hata A, Mamiya T, et al. (1999) Truncated CBP protein leads to classical Rubinstein-Taybi syndrome phenotypes in mice: Implications for a dominant-negative mechanism. *Hum. Mol. Genet.* 8: 387–396.

Okano M, Bell DW, Haber DA, and Li E (1999) DNA methyltransferases Dnmt3a and Dnmt3b are essential for de novo methylation and mammalian development. *Cell* 99: 247–257.

Okano M, Xie S, and Li E (1998) Cloning and characterization of a family of novel mammalian DNA (cytosine-5) methyltransferases. *Nat. Genet.* 19: 219–220.

Oliveira AL, Thams S, Lidman O, et al. (2004) A role for MHC class I molecules in synaptic plasticity and regeneration of neurons after axotomy. *Proc. Natl. Acad. Sci. USA* 101: 17843–17848.

Pelka GJ, Watson CM, Christodoulou J, and Tam PP (2005) Distinct expression profiles of Mecp2 transcripts with different lengths of 3′UTR in the brain and visceral organs during mouse development. *Genomics* 85: 441–452.

Petrij F, Giles RH, Dauwerse HG, et al. (1995) Rubinstein-Taybi syndrome caused by mutations in the transcriptional co-activator CBP. *Nature* 376: 348–351.

Pham AD and Sauer F (2000) Ubiquitin-activating/conjugating activity of TAFII250, a mediator of activation of gene expression in *Drosophila*. *Science* 289: 2357–2360.

Pickart CM (2001) Mechanisms underlying ubiquitination. *Annu. Rev. Biochem.* 70: 503–533.

Pittenger C, Huang YY, Paletzki RF, et al. (2002) Reversible inhibition of CREB/ATF transcription factors in region CA1 of the dorsal hippocampus disrupts hippocampus-dependent spatial memory. *Neuron* 34: 447–462.

Pittenger C and Kandel ER (2003) In search of general mechanisms for long-lasting plasticity: *Aplysia* and the hippocampus. *Philos. Trans. R. Soc. Lond. B Biol. Sci.* 358: 757–763.

Pray L (2004) Epigenetics: Genome, meet your environment. *The Scientist*. 18.

Prokhortchouk A, Hendrich B, Jorgensen H, et al. (2001) The p120 catenin partner Kaiso is a DNA methylation-dependent transcriptional repressor. *Genes Dev.* 15: 1613–1618.

Rakyan VK, Preis J, Morgan HD, and Whitelaw E (2001) The marks, mechanisms and memory of epigenetic states in mammals. *Biochem. J.* 356: 1–10.

Rett A (1966) Uber ein eigenartiges hirnatrophisches Syndrom bei Hyperammonamie im Kindesalter. *Wien. Med. Wochenschr.* 116: 723–726.

Roopra A, Sharling L, Wood IC, et al. (2000) Transcriptional repression by neuron-restrictive silencer factor is mediated via the Sin3-histone deacetylase complex. *Mol. Cell. Biol.* 20: 2147–2157.

Rouaux C, Loeffler JP, and Boutillier AL (2004) Targeting CREB-binding protein (CBP) loss of function as a therapeutic strategy in neurological disorders. *Biochem. Pharmacol.* 68: 1157–1164.

Samaco RC, Hogart A, and LaSalle JM (2005) Epigenetic overlap in autism-spectrum neurodevelopmental disorders: MECP2 deficiency causes reduced expression of UBE3A and GABRB3. *Hum. Mol. Genet.* 14: 483–492.

Sanchez RM, Koh S, Rio C, et al. (2001) Decreased glutamate receptor 2 expression and enhanced epileptogenesis in immature rat hippocampus after perinatal hypoxia-induced seizures. *J. Neurosci.* 21: 8154–8163.

Sassone-Corsi P, Mizzen CA, Cheung P, et al. (1999) Requirement of Rsk-2 for epidermal growth factor-activated phosphorylation of histone H3. *Science* 285: 886–891.

Schafe GE, Atkins CM, Swank MW, Bauer EP, Sweatt JD, and LeDoux JE (2000) Activation of ERK/MAP kinase in the amygdala is required for memory consolidation of pavlovian fear conditioning. *J. Neurosci.* 20: 8177–8187.

Schreiber SL and Bernstein BE (2002) Signaling network model of chromatin. *Cell* 111: 771–778.

Selcher JC, Atkins CM, Trzaskos JM, Paylor R, and Sweatt JD (1999) A necessity for MAP kinase activation in mammalian spatial learning. *Learn. Mem.* 6: 478–490.

Shahbazian M, Young J, Yuva-Paylor L, et al. (2002) Mice with truncated MeCP2 recapitulate many Rett syndrome features and display hyperacetylation of histone H3. *Neuron* 35: 243.

Shiio Y and Eisenman RN (2003) Histone sumoylation is associated with transcriptional repression. *Proc. Natl. Acad. Sci. USA* 100: 13225–13230.

Shin JA, Choi ES, Kim HS, et al. (2005) SUMO modification is involved in the maintenance of heterochromatin stability in fission yeast. *Mol. Cell* 19: 817–828.

Si K, Giustetto M, Etkin A, et al. (2003a) A neuronal isoform of CPEB regulates local protein synthesis and stabilizes synapse-specific long-term facilitation in aplysia. *Cell* 115: 893–904.

Si K, Lindquist S, and Kandel ER (2003b) A neuronal isoform of the aplysia CPEB has prion-like properties. *Cell* 115: 879–891.

Silva AJ, Elgersma Y, Friedman E, Stern J, and Kogan J (1998) A mouse model for learning and memory defects associated with neurofibromatosis type I. *Pathol. Biol. (Paris)* 46: 697–698.

Sirianni N, Naidu S, Pereira J, Pillotto RF, and Hoffman EP (1998) Rett syndrome: Confirmation of X-linked dominant inheritance, and localization of the gene to Xq28. *Am. J. Hum. Genet.* 63: 1552–1558.

Stancheva I, Collins AL, Van den Veyver IB, Zoghbi H, and Meehan RR (2003) A mutant form of MeCP2 protein associated with human Rett syndrome cannot be displaced from methylated DNA by notch in *Xenopus* embryos. *Mol. Cell* 12: 425–435.

Steffan JS, Bodai L, Pallos J, et al. (2001) Histone deacetylase inhibitors arrest polyglutamine-dependent neurodegeneration in *Drosophila*. *Nature* 413: 739–743.

Strahl BD and Allis CD (2000) The language of covalent histone modifications. *Nature* 403: 41–45.

Szyf M, Weaver IC, Champagne FA, Diorio J, and Meaney MJ (2005) Maternal programming of steroid receptor expression and phenotype through DNA methylation in the rat. *Front. Neuroendocrinol.* 26: 139–162.

Tanner KG, Langer MR, and Denu JM (2000a) Kinetic mechanism of human histone acetyltransferase P/CAF. *Biochemistry* 39: 11961–11969.

Tanner KG, Langer MR, Kim Y, and Denu JM (2000b) Kinetic mechanism of the histone acetyltransferase GCN5 from yeast. *J. Biol. Chem.* 275: 22048–22055.

Tanner KG, Trievel RC, Kuo MH, et al. (1999) Catalytic mechanism and function of invariant glutamic acid 173 from the histone acetyltransferase GCN5 transcriptional coactivator. *J. Biol. Chem.* 274: 18157–18160.

Tate P, Skarnes W, and Bird A (1996) The methyl-CpG binding protein MeCP2 is essential for embryonic development in the mouse. *Nat. Genet.* 12: 205–208.

Thiagalingam S, Cheng KH, Lee HJ, Mineva N, Thiagalingam A, and Ponte JF (2003) Histone deacetylases: Unique players in shaping the epigenetic histone code. *Ann. N. Y. Acad. Sci.* 983: 84–100.

Thomson S, Clayton AL, Hazzalin CA, Rose S, Barratt MJ, and Mahadevan LC (1999) The nucleosomal response associated with immediate-early gene induction is mediated via alternative MAP kinase cascades: MSK1 as a potential histone H3/HMG-14 kinase. *EMBO J.* 18: 4779–4793.

Timmusk T, Palm K, Metsis M, et al. (1993) Multiple promoters direct tissue-specific expression of the rat BDNF gene. *Neuron* 10: 475–489.

Tremolizzo L, Doueiri MS, Dong E, et al. (2005) Valproate corrects the schizophrenia-like epigenetic behavioral modifications induced by methionine in mice. *Biol. Psychiatry* 57: 500–509.

Tsankova NM, Kumar A, and Nestler EJ (2004) Histone modifications at gene promoter regions in rat hippocampus after acute and chronic electroconvulsive seizures. *J. Neurosci.* 24: 5603–5610.

Tudor M, Akbarian S, Chen RZ, and Jaenisch R (2002) Transcriptional profiling of a mouse model for Rett syndrome reveals subtle transcriptional changes in the brain. *Proc. Natl. Acad. Sci. USA* 99: 15536–15541.

Turner BM (1993) Decoding the nucleosome. *Cell* 75: 5–8.

van Leeuwen F, Gafken PR, and Gottschling DE (2002) Dot1p modulates silencing in yeast by methylation of the nucleosome core. *Cell* 109: 745–756.

Vecsey CG, Hawk JD, Lattal KM, et al. (in press) Histone deacetylase inhibitors enhance memory and synaptic plasticity via CREB:CBP-dependent transcriptional activation. *J. Neurosci.*

Vettese-Dadey M, Grant PA, Hebbes TR, Crane-Robinson C, Allis CD, and Workman JL (1996) Acetylation of histone H4 plays a primary role in enhancing transcription factor binding to nucleosomal DNA in vitro. *EMBO J.* 15: 2508–2518.

Von Rotz RC, Kohli BM, Bosset J, et al. (2004) The APP intracellular domain forms nuclear multiprotein complexes and regulates the transcription of its own precursor. *J. Cell Sci.* 117: 4435–4448.

Walters CL and Blendy JA (2001) Different requirements for cAMP response element binding protein in positive and negative reinforcing properties of drugs of abuse. *J. Neurosci.* 21: 9438–9444.

Weaver IC, Cervoni N, Champagne FA, et al. (2004) Epigenetic programming by maternal behavior. *Nat. Neurosci.* 7: 847–854.

Weaver IC, Champagne FA, Brown SE, et al. (2005) Reversal of maternal programming of stress responses in adult offspring through methyl supplementation: Altering epigenetic marking later in life. *J. Neurosci.* 25: 11045–11054.

Weeber EJ, Atkins CM, Selcher JC, et al. (2000) A role for the beta isoform of protein kinase C in fear conditioning. *J. Neurosci.* 20: 5906–5914.

West MH and Bonner WM (1980) Histone 2B can be modified by the attachment of ubiquitin. *Nucleic Acids Res.* 8: 4671–4680.

Wood MA, Attner MA, Oliveira AM, Brindle PK, and Abel T (2006) A transcription factor-binding domain of the coactivator CBP is essential for long-term memory and the expression of specific target genes. *Learn Mem.* 13: 609–617.

Wood MA, Kaplan MP, Park A, et al. (2005) Transgenic mice expressing a truncated form of CREB-binding protein (CBP) exhibit deficits in hippocampal synaptic plasticity and memory storage. *Learn. Mem.* 12: 111–119.

Yeh SH, Lin CH, and Gean PW (2004) Acetylation of nuclear factor-kappaB in rat amygdala improves long-term but not short-term retention of fear memory. *Mol. Pharmacol.* 65: 1286–1292.

Yeh SH, Lin CH, Lee CF, and Gean PW (2002) A requirement of nuclear factor-kappaB activation in fear-potentiated startle. *J. Biol. Chem.* 277: 46720–46729.

Yen RW, Vertino PM, Nelkin BD, et al. (1992) Isolation and characterization of the cDNA encoding human DNA methyltransferase. *Nucleic Acids Res.* 20: 2287–2291.

37 Neurogenesis

S. Jessberger, J. B. Aimone, and F. H. Gage, Salk Institute for Biological Studies, La Jolla CA, USA

37.1 Introduction

During the development of the central nervous system (CNS), neural stem cells give rise to neurons, oligodendrocytes, and astrocytes, the three major lineages that constitute the brain. Although a fundamental dogma of neuroscience predicted that neurogenesis ceases with the end of development, as early as 40 years ago studies by Altman and Das showed that dividing cells persist throughout life in the mammalian

CNS (Altman and Das, 1965). Indeed, Altman and colleagues' data suggested that not only glial cells but also new neurons are continuously added into the adult brain circuitry. Despite confirming reports by other groups (Hinds, 1968; Kaplan and Hinds, 1977), the finding that neural stem cells persist and can give rise to new neurons even in the adult brain remained a subject of great controversy. Nevertheless, improved techniques to identify newborn cells and their respective neural phenotype within the adult tissue finally led to the acceptance of the fact that (1) neural stem cells persist in the adult brain and (2) new neurons are continuously generated in the adult CNS in two restricted areas: the hippocampal dentate gyrus (DG) and the subventricular zone (SVZ) of the lateral ventricle (Ming and Song, 2005). In the meantime, adult neurogenesis was found to exist in all mammals, including humans (Eriksson et al., 1998). In this chapter, we mainly focus on adult neurogenesis in the hippocampal dentate gyrus and present recent advances in the understanding of the biology of adult neural stem cells, the maturation of new neurons into the preexisting circuitry, and the potential significance of adult neurogenesis in hippocampal function.

37.2 Stem Cells in the Adult Brain

37.2.1 Neural Stem Cells *in vitro*

Despite the early reports by Altman and colleagues in the 1960s, it took almost another three decades to successfully grow neural stem cells that were isolated from the adult brain in the culture dish (Reynolds and Weiss, 1992). The *in vitro* characterization of proliferative cells that were isolated from adult brain tissue was crucial to identifying a subpopulation of them as stem cells. Even though the consensus definition of a stem cell has been modified several times (Smith, 2006), two characteristics are generally required for a cell to be identified as a true stem cell: (1) the capacity for theoretically unlimited self-renewal and (2) the ability to generate cells different from themselves through asymmetric cell division. In general, stem cells can be divided into several levels of potency: (1) the 'totipotent' zygote capable of generating a complete organism when implanted into the uterus of a living animal; (2) the 'pluripotent' embryonic stem cell, which can give rise to all body tissues except the trophoblasts of the placenta and, perhaps, the gonads; and (3) the 'multipotent' stem cell that self-renews but gives rise to only tissue-specific cell types. Even though there is recent evidence that neural stem cells (NSCs) can give rise to tissue types other than CNS tissue under *in vitro* conditions (Wurmser et al., 2004), they are still mainly classified as multipotent stem cells (Gage, 2000).

37.2.1.1 Culturing of neural stem cells

The neurosphere assay is the most commonly used technique to analyze the stem cell capacity of isolated brain cells (**Figure 1(a)**) (Reynolds and Weiss, 1992; Lie et al., 2004). In this preparation, the brain area of interest is dissected and plated as a single-cell suspension that is propagated as floating aggregates. The addition of

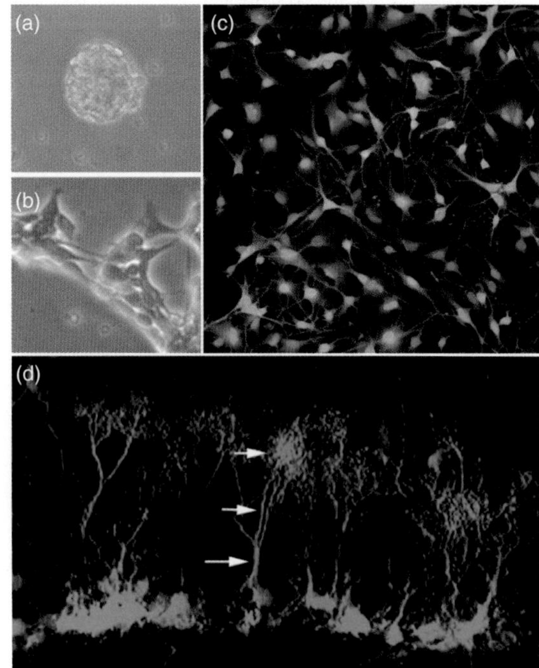

Figure 1 Neural stem cells (NSCs) *in vitro* and *in vivo.* NSCs can be grown as free-floating cell aggregates, so called neurospheres (a), or under adherent culture conditions forming monolayers (b). In both conditions strong mitogens such as EGF and/or FGF-2 are added (for details see Ray and Gage, 2006). *In vitro* propagated stem cells retain the capacity to differentiate into all three neural lineages. (c) Rat NSCs (expressing green fluorescent protein, green) that were differentiated into neuronal cells expressing MAP2ab (red) with the addition of retinoic acid and forskolin in the culture medium for 4 days. Nuclei were counterstained with 4′,6-diamidino-2-phenylindole (DAPI) (blue). (d) A population of NSCs residing in the adult brain is expressing nestin. Shown is the dentate area of an adult transgenic mouse expressing green fluorescent protein under the control of the nestin promoter. Note the typical morphology of type 1 nestin cells with a tree-like process that branches in the inner molecular layer (arrow). In contrast to this morphology, type 2 cells are small, rounded cells that show a higher proliferative activity *in vivo* than type 1 cells (for details see Kempermann et al., 2004).

strong mitogens such as epidermal growth factor (EGF) and fibroblast growth factor 2 (FGF-2) allows the propagation of endogenous proliferative cells (the putative NSCs). The forming spheres, referred to as neurospheres, can be propagated over many passages and have the potential to differentiate into all three neural lineages after the withdrawal of mitogens and/or addition of differentiating factors. Even though it appears that neurospheres do not grow clonally (Jessberger et al., 2006; Singec et al., 2006), self-renewal can be tested by the formation of secondary or tertiary spheres; a single cell is grown in a miniwell until the sphere reaches a certain size, after which the sphere is again dissociated into single cells that can give rise to a new, and thus secondary, multipotent neurosphere. An alternative method to grow adult NSCs is the so-called monolayer assay, where multipotent cells grow adherent to the dish surface (**Figure 1(b)**) (Ray et al., 1993; Gage et al., 1995; Palmer et al., 1995). Using these culturing techniques, NSCs can be isolated and propagated from many species, including humans (Palmer et al., 2001). Using the neurosphere assay, several laboratories have tried to identify differences in the potency of NSCs derived from different regions of the adult brain. Due to conflicting *in vitro* results, which might be due to differences in dissection and culturing methods, there is an ongoing controversy about whether the hippocampus contains true stem cells with theoretically unlimited self-renewal, or whether hippocampus-derived neurosphere cultures have only limited proliferative and differentiating capacities (Seaberg and van der Kooy, 2002).

37.2.1.2 Proliferation and differentiation of NSCs

The *in vitro* propagation of adult NSCs allowed the extensive biochemical and molecular characterization of fate choice, proliferative capacity, and cellular potency. *In vitro* studies identified a variety of factors and mechanisms that regulate cell proliferation and instruct NSCs to adopt a neuronal or glial fate (**Figure 1(c)**) (Lie et al., 2004; Ming and Song, 2005). Subsequent studies showed an *in vivo* role for most of those factors as well, thus confirming the *in vitro* NSC model system. New mechanisms that affect proliferation and/or differentiation of NSCs are constantly being discovered; the regulation of proliferation and differentiation clearly occurs on multiple molecular levels. We and others have shown that epigenetic mechanisms, growth factors such as brain-derived neurotrophic factor (BDNF) and vascular endothelial growth factor (VEGF), sonic hedgehog signaling, WNT signaling, small double-stranded RNAs, retrotransposition, transcription factor expression such as E2F, cyclin-D2 expression, and cell-cycle inhibitors such as p27kip1 (Lie et al., 2004; Ming and Song, 2005; Cao et al., 2006) are among important regulators of proliferation and/or neuronal differentiation. Considerably less is known regarding differentiation toward glial cells, though several important signaling pathways have been identified that induce NSCs to differentiate into oligodendrocytes, such as insulin-like growth factor (IGF) signaling (Hsieh et al., 2004), or astrocytes, such as bone morphogenetic protein (BMP) and leukemia inhibitory factor (LIF) signaling (Bonaguidi et al., 2005).

Despite the great utility of *in vitro* assays in the biochemical and molecular characterization of NSCs, there are several important caveats about using them to study NSCs. Isolated cells must be exposed to high levels of mitogens that potentially induce cellular changes different from those seen in an *in situ* stem cell. Furthermore, NSCs in culture are 'naked' and may not receive the same factors as those that are embedded in their respective cellular niche. Importantly, cells with stem cell capacity can be easily isolated from almost all areas of the adult brain and the spinal cord, even though only two areas in the adult brain are capable of generating new neuronal cells.

37.2.2 Neural Stem Cells *in vivo*

The adult DG continuously produces new neuronal cells. Neurons born in the adult hippocampus are glutamatergic granule cells, the principal cell type of the DG. Granule cells reside in the densely packed granule cell layer (GCL), receive their main excitatory input from layer II of the entorhinal cortex (EC), and largely project toward area 3 of the cornu ammonis (CA3) via the mossy fiber tract. The DG is a very densely packed structure: a single mouse DG consists of approximately 300,000 granule cells, rat DG about 1 million, and human DG between 15 and 20 million (Simic et al., 1997). These cell numbers are very large relative to the DG's input (EC) and output (CA3) structures, both of which have an order of magnitude fewer neurons.

37.2.2.1 The hippocampal neurogenic niche

Proliferative activity within the dentate area occurs largely in the zone just below the GCL and the hilus. This area, called the subgranular zone (SGZ), does not have strict boundaries and is commonly defined as an intermediate region about two cell layers deep into the hilus below the GCL (corresponding to approximately 20–30 μm). Significant research has been devoted to determining how to identify dividing cells in the SGZ morphologically and whether they can be classified using differential gene expression. Acutely dividing cells can be visualized by the detection of cell cycle–associated genes such as Ki-67, PCNA, and phospho-histone H3.

Whether or not those proliferating cells in the DG are true NSCs *in vivo* is still unknown. This categorization requires the observation of self-renewal and multipotency, and neither has been definitively shown due to the technical difficulties in following single cells and their lineages over time *in vivo.* Several labeling techniques have been used to label proliferating populations of cells in the DG and track their progeny, including bromo-deoxyuridine (BrdU) and tritiated (^{3}H)-thymidine (nucleotide analogues) and marker-expressing retroviruses (**Figure 2(a)**).

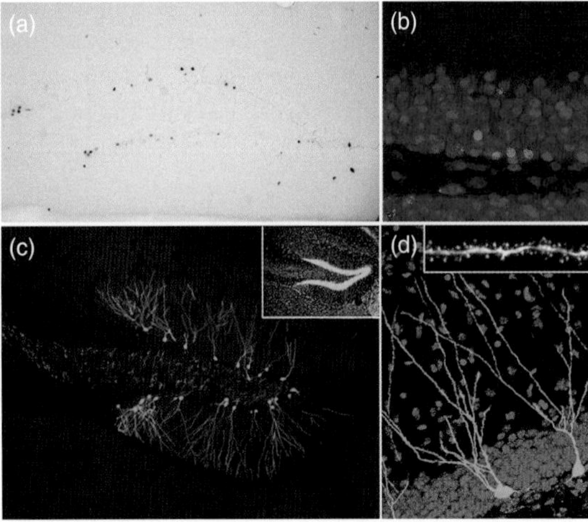

Figure 2 Labeling of newborn cells *in vivo.* The thymidine analogue bromo-deoxyuridine (BrdU) is integrated into the DNA of proliferating cells during S-phase. (a) BrdU-labeled cells can be visualized in the adult dentate gyrus with specific antibodies. The example shows a section of an adult mouse that received five consecutive BrdU injections and was sacrificed 4 weeks after the last injection. (b) The phenotype of the BrdU-positive cells (red) can be reliably analyzed by confocal microscopy using, for example, neuronal markers such as NeuN (blue), again 4 weeks after BrdU injection. Dividing cells and their progeny can also be visualized with retroviruses expressing green fluorescent protein (or any other label that can be later visualized), allowing the direct detection of newborn cells without the need for *post hoc* detection methods. (c) A 40-μm section of an adult mouse that was injected 4 weeks earlier with a retrovirus expressing green fluorescent protein under the control of the CAG promoter. (d) Retroviral labeling visualizes the whole cell (including dendritic and axonal processes) and even allows the analysis of neuronal fine structures such as dendritic spines (inset in (d); for details see Zhao et al., 2006).

The most commonly used label is BrdU, a thymidine analogue that becomes integrated into the DNA during the S-phase of the cell cycle. BrdU-labeled cells can be visualized with a specific antibody and then analyzed histologically to determine their neural phenotype (**Figure 2(b)**). The major advantage of BrdU labeling is the easy and reliable quantification of new cells. There are several drawbacks to BrdU, however. Because BrdU incorporates into newly formed DNA, several successive rounds of DNA replication after BrdU administration will dilute the signal. Furthermore, the BrdU signal is restricted to the nucleus and thus does not show the morphology of newborn cells. Given these limitations, the use of retroviral vectors expressing green fluorescent (GFP) or red fluorescent protein (RFP) to visualize the whole cell morphology opened up a completely new level of analysis (**Figures 2(c)** and **2(d)**) (van Praag et al., 2002). Because retroviruses require the breakdown of the nuclear membrane for genomic integration, only dividing cells are transduced. Retrovirus infection and delivery are not as ubiquitous as BrdU uptake, limiting their value as quantification tools; however, the transduction of progenitors results in a stable and robust expression of a marker protein that is detectable in both fixed and live tissue.

Using these markers, it has been shown that proliferating cells that can generate all three lineages exist in the DG (Kempermann et al., 2004). As it is unclear that these cells are individually multipotent and self-renewing, they are referred to as neural progenitor cells (NPCs). Accumulating evidence suggests that there are actually several types of dividing cells within the adult hippocampus, and their relationship to one another remains somewhat elusive (Kempermann et al., 2004). One type of NSC within the hippocampal DG appears to be very similar to a mature astrocyte (**Figure 1(d)**). These cells express glial fibrillary acidic protein (GFAP) (Seri et al., 2001), have the electrophysiological properties of astrocytes, and possess astrocytic vascular end feet (Filippov et al., 2003). Depending on the nomenclature used, these cells are referred to as type 1 or B-cells. Type 1 cells also express the intermediate filament protein nestin, and a subpopulation of type 1 cells also colabels with the HMG-transcription factor Sox-2. The low proliferative activity of type 1 cells may indicate that these cells represent a largely quiescent, true stem cell within the hippocampus, but this hypothesis remains to be proven. In contrast to the slowly dividing type 1 cells, type 2 cells exhibit a much higher proliferative activity. Type

2 cells are negative for GFAP but still express nestin and Sox-2, and a fraction of type 2 cells expresses early neuronal markers such as doublecortin (DCX) and the bHLH transcription factor Prox-1. One theory is that the expression of these neuronal markers in a subset of dividing cells indicates that type 2 cells (and type 3 cells that divide but are negative for nestin and Sox-2 and positive for DCX) represent committed neuroblasts that have lost their multipotentiality (Kempermann et al., 2004).

The rate at which neurons are born in the adult hippocampus is not fixed but is instead dynamically regulated by a variety of factors. Despite increasing knowledge about how progenitor cells 'translate' signals such as local network activity into altered cell division or differentiation, the exact mechanisms remain unclear. Recent reports have shown that depolarizing events trigger NSCs to initiate neuronal differentiation (Deisseroth et al., 2004; Tozuka et al., 2005), providing an explanation for how network activity within the dentate gyrus may shape the cellular composition of the area itself. Furthermore, elegant *in vivo* studies have shown the synaptic integration of nestin-expressing cells in the SGZ and their functional GABAergic input (Tozuka et al., 2005). Those reports have led to the hypothesis that dentate NSCs may 'sense' the activity of surrounding mature, neuronal networks and respond with a distinct action, such as increased or decreased cell proliferation and/or differentiation. The regulation of adult neurogenesis on a systems level will be extensively discussed in the section titled "Systems regulation of adult neurogenesis."

As stated earlier, NSCs can be isolated and grown *in vitro* from almost all brain areas. Furthermore, Sox-2, nestin, and dividing GFAP-positive cells are scattered throughout the adult brain. One major question is what allows the DG and SVZ to be unique in permitting the generation of new neurons in the adult. Most likely, there is something in the microenvironmental niche that surrounds NSC *in vivo* that permits and/or supports neuronal differentiation and maturation. A detailed study by Seri and colleagues (2004) showed a close association of hippocampal NSCs with the vasculature, a proximity that might be a critical factor in the distribution of trophic support for not only NSCs but also immature neurons (Palmer et al., 2000). Importantly, hippocampal astrocytes also play a pivotal role in making the DG a neurogenic area (Song et al., 2002). While astrocytes from nonneurogenic regions such as the spinal cord appear to inhibit neurogenesis, hippocampal astrocytes appear to be the source of important differentiation and/or stem cell maintenance factors, such as WNT proteins (Lie et al., 2005).

37.2.3 Neurogenesis in Nonneurogenic Areas Following Manipulation

Although the DG and SVZ are the only brain regions that undergo continual neurogenesis in the healthy adult, it appears that endogenous NSCs throughout the nervous system maintain the capability to become neurons. When grown *in vitro*, NSCs from nonneurogenic areas can be induced to differentiate into neurons, and when transplanted into a neurogenic area they will differentiate into neurons. The exciting possibility also exists that nonneurogenic brain areas can be manipulated by traumatic insults or other means to induce the production of new neurons. A recent report showed that the production of new neurons in the hypothalamus could be induced by injection of ciliary neurotrophic factor (CTNF), which is critically involved in feeding behavior (Kokoeva et al., 2005). Thus, new neurons in the hypothalamus feeding centers may be involved in regulating the energy balance in rodents. The potential to produce new neurons apparently also holds true for the striatum and cornu ammonis area 1 (CA1) following ischemic stroke and for the cortex following targeted cellular ablation (Abrous et al., 2005). However, the numbers of new neurons produced following strokes, for example, are extremely low, and it is not clear what their functional impact may be. Nevertheless the potential for endogenous repair has sparked high levels of excitement, and future studies will have to determine the feasibility of neuronal repair from endogenous NSCs following brain injury.

37.3 Maturation of Adult-Born Granule Cells

37.3.1 Molecular Maturation and Identification of Adult-Born Granule Cells

As described earlier, the availability of robust and reliable methods to label cells and/or their progeny enabled the identification of genes expressed during the maturation of adult-born granule cells (AGCs). Importantly, and in striking contrast to neuronal maturation during embryonic development, all stages of maturation coexist in the adult DG at any given time point. Therefore, every observation has to focus on a single cell and is a mere snapshot of neuronal development in the adult brain. This heterogeneity of adult neurogenesis has complicated large-scale approaches to identifying specific gene expression patterns of AGCs at a certain stage of maturation. Moreover, the development of new neurons is accompanied by gliogenesis (Kempermann et al., 2004), and if the current assumption of a common precursor for all three neural lineages holds true, the decisive branching point between neuronal and glial development has not yet been identified. Finally, only a subset of the AGCs that are born and are clearly classifiable as neuronal cells eventually becomes stably integrated into the dentate circuitry (Kempermann et al., 2004). However, the work of several laboratories has generated an astoundingly clear picture of the molecular maturation of AGCs (Brandt et al., 2003; Fukuda et al., 2003; Kempermann et al., 2004; Gleiberman et al., 2005). Much of this information has been generated by characterizing the molecular makeup of BrdU-positive cells at different time points after the injection of the thymidine analogue.

The molecular characteristics of adult progenitors were described in the earlier section covering NSCs. **Figure 3** shows examples of several immature neuron–specific markers. The first gene considered to be neuronal is expressed in dividing cells: DCX. DCX is a microtubule-associated protein that is critically involved in neuronal migration during development; mutations in the DCX gene cause lissencephalic malformations in humans. Even though DCX is expressed in acutely dividing cells, expression persists for approximately 3 weeks after BrdU injection. Thus, the DCX-expressing cell population consists of a very heterogeneous population of newborn cells. The functional importance of DCX in AGC maturation remains unclear. Comparable to the timing of DCX expression is the expression of the polysialylated form of the neural cell adhesion molecule (PSA-NCAM) – a protein that appears to be involved in cell migration, axonal fasciculation, and neurite outgrowth. The proneural basic helix-loop-helix transcription factor NeuroD1 is expressed early after cell division and tapers off approximately 7 days after BrdU. NeuroD1 has been found to be critically involved in neuronal fate instruction, particularly for granule cells, as *NeuroD1 −/−* mice fail to ever develop a DG. Expression of Prox-1, the mammalian homologue of the transcription factor prospero that is critically involved in cell cycle regulation, appears together with DCX and PSA-NCAM in newborn cells. In contrast to DCX and PSA-NCAM, prox-1 remains expressed throughout the life of a granule cell. This expression pattern is similar to the pan-neuronal protein NeuN, which can be detected as early as 3 days after BrdU injection but remains expressed later on. The expression of the Ca^{2+}-binding protein Calretinin marks the definite exit from cell cycle. Calretinin is replaced approximately 3 weeks later by calbindin, the Ca^{2+}-binding protein of mature granule cells (Kempermann et al., 2004). As described later, the regulation of the survival and integration of AGCs seemingly occurs during many, if not all, stages of neuronal maturation.

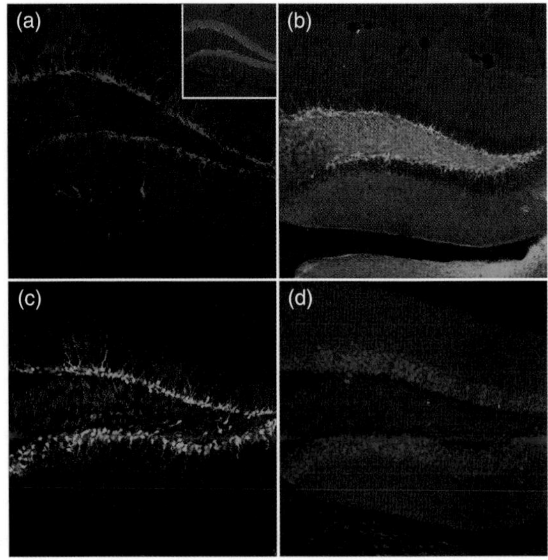

Figure 3 Endogenous and transgenic markers of adult neurogenesis. There are numerous endogenous proteins that are expressed during specific stages of neuronal maturation in the adult dentate gyrus. (a) Doublecortin (DCX) labeling of immature neurons lining the inner granule cell layer (visualized by prox-1 staining, blue in inset). (b) polysialylated neural cell adhesion molecule labeling of immature neurons, which includes staining of axons. (c) The dentate gyrus from a *POMC*-driven green fluorescent protein transgenic mouse (green) that was generated by Overstreet-Wadiche and colleagues. (4) Calbindin, the mature granule cell Ca^{2+}-binding protein, is only expressed in granule cells after 3–4 weeks of maturation.

37.3.2 Electrophysiology of Maturing AGCs

Critical to our understanding of the role adult neurogenesis has in cognition is the functional maturation of these neurons. Increasingly, it appears that these new neurons become functional parts of the DG circuit, passing through several maturation

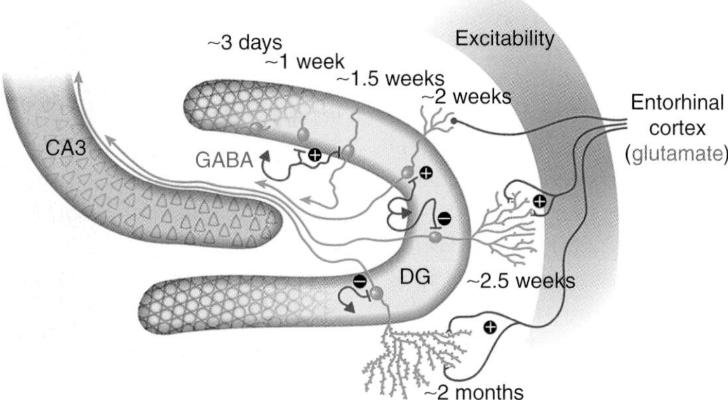

Figure 4 Maturation of newborn neurons. Adult-born granule cells progress through several states before they reach full maturity. Early in maturation, the neurons have limited processes and receive only GABA inputs from local interneurons. By 2 weeks, the neuron's dendrite protrudes into the molecular layer. Soon thereafter, spine formation begins, indicating the onset of glutamatergic input. After several months of maturation, the newborn neuron becomes indistinguishable from other granule cells. The bar labeled "excitability" indicates a period in which immature neurons may be more responsive to the network due to depolarizing GABA, depolarized resting potentials, and increased LTP. Figure from Aimone JB, Wiles J, and Gage FH (2006) Potential role for adult neurogenesis in the encoding of time in new memories. *Nat. Neurosci.* 9: 723–727, with permission.

stages and ultimately developing a cellular physiology indistinguishable from that of embryonic-born neurons (**Figure 4**). This section reviews the maturation process of newborn granule cells.

37.3.2.1 Techniques used in characterizing maturation stages of AGCs

Following the characterization of the critical steps leading to the molecular maturation of AGCs, several laboratories have made significant strides in characterizing the physiological maturation of AGCs using several different approaches to labeling and recording from specific ages of new neurons. One approach has been to segregate cells based on location and passive membrane properties (i.e., membrane resistance) and to use *post hoc* histological and morphological observations to confirm maturation state. While this approach has proven effective at distinguishing between mature and immature neurons, it is difficult to *a priori* identify neurons of a specific age or maturation state. Because early cell division markers such as ^{3}H-Thy and BrdU only label nuclei, studies investigating the maturation of AGCs were limited until the development of more sophisticated labeling techniques using fluorescent genetic markers. Two approaches in particular have boosted research in this area: GFP retrovirus and GFP driven by immature granule cell–specific promoters. By using a retroviral vector that only incorporates itself into dividing neurons to deliver GFP, researchers can identify and observe the morphology of cells that divide at a known time. This process allows the determination of the actual 'age' of the neuron. On the other hand, GFP driven by promoters that specifically label immature neurons or NPCs, such as *Pomc,* allows the identification of a group of cells at a similar maturation state (Overstreet et al., 2004). Importantly, since not all AGCs mature at the same rate, the retrovirus-GFP and cell-specific GFP labeling approaches are not immediately comparable, and care must be taken when interpreting data across experiments.

37.3.2.2 Depolarizing GABA input

Using retrovirus labeling, neurons – as defined by the ability to fire an action potential – can be observed as 1 day postinjection (dpi) in slice (Esposito et al., 2005). These early neurons have little distinguishing morphology beyond possibly a few small nonoriented projections. These young neurons lack synaptic inputs, though it appears that even at this young age there is a tonic GABA input, suggesting the presence of nonsynaptic somatic receptors that are sensitive to levels of local interneuron activity.

By around 1 week of age, these neurons begin to take on a neuronal morphology. Although at this age most neurons still lack a robust dendritic arborization, oriented processes extending to the molecular layer can be seen. It is at this stage in development that these young neurons begin to receive synaptic GABAergic inputs from the local interneuron population. The fact that GABA-releasing axons are the first to contact the young neurons is important for several reasons. First, having GABA synapses preceding glutamate synapses is similar to the order seen during embryonic development. Like in development, this early GABA has a depolarizing impact on the neuron. Second, this depolarizing GABA appears to have long-lasting implications for the neurons' development, suggesting the onset of activity-dependent maturation.

By 2 weeks postinjection, there appears to be a substantial amount of depolarizing GABA input. A similar group of neurons has also been identified by Overstreet-Wadiche and colleagues (2005) by using GFP driven by the *Pomc* promoter. These GABA-only neurons have identifiable dendrites, but they barely extend into the molecular layer with limited branching. Despite not receiving glutamatergic inputs, they can be depolarized by perforant path stimulation, presumably via polysynaptic activation of GABAergic basket cells.

Although 1- to 2-week-old neurons receive depolarizing synaptic inputs, it is not clear at what point they begin to communicate with other neurons. While these GABA-excited neurons are capable of exhibiting action potentials, their spiking is not typical of mature granule cells' bursting patterns. The extent to which GABA can induce action potentials *in vivo* remains to be seen. GFP-labeled axonal processes do not appear in the CA3 until about 11 or 12 dpi and do not reach the CA3/CA2 boundary until 16 dpi.

37.3.2.3 Spine formation and the onset of glutamatergic inputs

According to several studies (Esposito et al., 2005; Zhao et al., 2006), spine formation begins just after 2 weeks and continues beyond 1 month of age. This time frame is consistent with electrophysiology studies, which show the onset of weak glutamatergic inputs at around 2 weeks of age (Esposito et al., 2005; Ge et al., 2006). The earliest stages of glutamate inputs are characterized by a high *N*-methyl-D-aspartate (NMDA) dependence; the blockade of NR1 receptors has been shown to kill most immature neurons between 2 and 3 weeks of age (Tashiro et al., 2006). Spine formation is rapid, increasing from about 0.43 spines/μm to 1.95 spines/μm between 21 and 28 dpi.

It is at these early glutamate stages that synaptic plasticity has been best characterized. Numerous studies have observed a difference in long-term potentiation (LTP) between immature and mature DG granule cells. Schmidt-Hieber and colleagues (2004) showed that high-resistance, PSA-NCAM+ neurons (corresponding to between 1 and 3 weeks of age) experienced associative LTP more readily than mature neurons (Schmidt-Hieber et al., 2004). Similarly, Wang et al. (2000) showed, using several paradigms, that medial perforant path stimulation did not induce LTP in mature neurons unless GABA was blocked with bicucilline, whereas immature neurons had robust LTP regardless of GABA blockade (Wang et al., 2000). Consistent with this increased propensity for LTP, Zhao et al. (2006) showed that immature neurons had higher levels of spine motility and a lower proportion of large mushroom spines.

By around 1 month of age, the neurons are similar to fully mature neurons, but not yet identical. Electrophysiologically, there are few significant differences at this stage, though it appears that some differences in plasticity remain when compared to fully mature neurons (van Praag et al., 2002). Morphologically, the dendritic arborizations appear roughly similar, but there are still morphological differences. Overall spine density continues to increase until about 2 months of age, after which the density remains relatively constant. Likewise, spine motility at 28 dpi is still higher than that seen in fully mature neurons. Furthermore, Toni et al. (in press) show that spines on new neurons preferentially form connections on already existing synaptic sites.

37.3.2.4 Timeline of projections to CA3

All indications suggest that AGCs project axons to the same neurons to which embryonic and postnatal granule cells project, specifically the CA3 and interneurons in the hilus, although these studies are limited. Markakis and Gage (1999) and Hastings and Gould (1999) both showed that fluorescent retrograde tracers injected into the CA3 colocalized with BrdU cells in the DG (Hastings and Gould, 1999; Markakis and Gage, 1999). Colabeling can be seen in some cells as early as 10 days after BrdU was first administered. This finding is consistent with observations using GFP retrovirus. Zhao et al. (2006) showed that GFP driven by the CAG promoter is present in the axons of immature neurons (Zhao et al., 2006). At 10 dpi, axons are restricted to the hilus, but they reach the CA3/CA2 boundary by 16 dpi.

Although the inputs to AGCs have been well characterized electrophysiologically, the physiology of newborn axonal projections to the CA3 has not been studied. The mossy fiber projection of dentate granule cells has several unique characteristics, including its sparse topography – one granule cell connects to only about a dozen CA3 pyramidal neurons – and the ability of a single active mossy terminal to fire its downstream target. It will be interesting to see whether the unusual properties of DG mossy fibers are also found in adult-born neurons.

37.3.2.5 Regulation of maturation process

Although the phases of AGC maturation mimic those of the embryonic and early postnatal granule cells, the network into which they are maturing is unique in that it is a real-time functioning network. Not surprisingly, the maturation of AGCs is a tightly regulated process at each stage. Increasingly more is being learned about what regulates the way in which these new neurons integrate into the network.

Experience-dependent regulation of maturation appears to begin very soon after differentiation. Ge and colleagues (2006) have demonstrated that 3-dpi neurons receive tonic GABA depolarization several days before the appearance of synapses, and the depolarizing nature of this input is important for further development (Ge et al., 2006). Their data suggest that the depolarizing effects of GABA in very immature neurons are regulated by a tight balance between NKCCl and KCC2 transporters, and the disruption of this balance results in dramatically underdeveloped dendritic arborizations by 2 weeks.

After this GABA-dependent phase of maturation, the neuron appears to enter an NMDA-dependent maturation phase. A study by Tashiro et al. (2006) demonstrated that immature neurons deficient in the NR1 subunit of the NMDA receptor develop normally for the first 2 weeks, but by 3 weeks most are dead. Furthermore, this required NMDA activation is relative to the local network; if NMDA is globally blocked using AP5, the *NR1–/–* neurons survive more successfully.

In summary, the maturation of new neurons appears to take a course similar to that seen during development, but over a more extended time scale. Importantly, at each stage of development, the efficacy of integration appears to be critical for further maturation and ultimate survival. Consistent with this dependence on activity, these neurons appear to be much more responsive to the network, in terms of both synaptic plasticity (spinogenesis, LTP) and basic physiological states (more depolarized resting potentials, higher input resistances, longer membrane time constant, higher E_{GABA}). Their excitable state stands out in contrast to mature granule cells, which are characterized by very low activity due to high levels of tonic inhibition.

37.4 Systems Regulation of Adult Neurogenesis

37.4.1 Physiological Regulators of Adult Neurogenesis

The amount of progenitor cell division and the subsequent numbers of new neurons that are born in the adult DG are dynamically regulated by a variety of both physiological and pathological factors. The finding that adult neurogenesis is a highly dynamic feature of adult brain plasticity challenged our understanding of how the mature brain responds to its environment and showed that the cellular composition in the adult dentate area is subject to constant change. How adult neurogenesis is regulated and what factors influence the number of adult-generated neurons have been important questions in the field.

The number of new granule cells can be changed by two mechanisms: (1) an increase in progenitor cell proliferation and (2) an increase in newborn neuron survival. Regulators of adult neurogenesis often have an effect on both proliferation and survival, and currently there is no easy way to completely separate these two mechanisms. However, some regulators act more strongly on proliferation than on survival and vice versa. The regulators discussed here and in the next section represent only the major factors that influence adult hippocampal neurogenesis, and the list of manipulations that enhance or abate adult neurogenesis is growing constantly (Ming and Song, 2005). These results are summarized in **Table 1**.

37.4.1.1 Natural variation in adult neurogenesis

Without a doubt there is a very strong genetic impact on the number of adult-born neurons. Inbred mice strains can differ 10-fold or more in the number of new granule cells, either by dramatically decreased/elevated levels of cell proliferation or by low/high levels of cell survival, respectively. Using quantitative trait loci analyses of inbred mice strains, several genetic loci have been identified that appear to be critically involved in the regulation of adult neurogenesis (Kempermann et al., 2006). Further studies are designed to narrow the identified loci down to single genes.

Table 1 Regulation of adult neurogenesis

Regulator	*Proliferation*	*Survival*	*Neuronal differentiation*
Physiological Regulators of Adult Neurogenesis			
Genetic background	+/−	+/−	+/−
Enriched environment	?	+	+
Physical exercise	+	no change	+
Learning	no change	+	?
Aging	−	?	−
Dietary restriction	no change	+	?
Neurotransmitters	see text		
Pathological Regulators of Adult Neurogenesis			
Stress	−	no change	?
Seizure activity	+	+ (?)	+
Ischemia	+	+ (?)	+
Irradiation	−	−	−
Neurodegenerative Diseases			
Alzheimer's disease	+/−	?	?/−
Huntington's disease	−	no change	no change
Parkinson's disease	−	?	?
Drugs			
Opiates	−	?	?
Antidepressants	+	+	+
Ethanol	no change/−	−	?

37.4.1.2 Environmental enrichment

Genetic background is not alone in having a powerful influence on adult hippocampal neurogenesis. It has been known for a long time that housing laboratory animals in an enriched environment exerts positive effects on the animals' behavior (van Praag et al., 2000), even though the structural correlate of this improvement remained unclear. Kempermann and colleagues found that housing adult mice for several weeks together in a large cage with toys and a changing environment had strong effects on their performance in hippocampus-dependent learning tasks (Kempermann et al., 1997). In addition to improving learning, environmental enrichment doubled the number of new neurons in the DG. This dramatic effect on hippocampal neurogenesis appeared to be mainly due to an increased survival of the new neurons, preventing the apoptotic death of immature neurons. Later studies showed that the effects of environmental enrichment on adult neurogenesis are mediated by VEGF signaling in the dentate area (Cao et al., 2004). Recent work has shown that 2- to 3-week-old neurons appear to be the most affected by an enriched environment, as cells labeled that far ahead of enrichment are substantially more likely to survive and respond to that environment at a later date (Tashiro et al., 2007).

37.4.1.3 Physical exercise

After the robust effects of environmental enrichment on adult neurogenesis were discovered, it remained unclear which of the multimodal effects of enrichment on the animals' life was responsible for the enrichment-induced increase in neurogenesis: larger cages may result in more physical activity, and bigger housing groups increase social interaction (to prevent the strong formation of social dominance, all initial experiments were performed using female mice). van Praag and colleagues tried to dissect out those factors and found that the physical activity itself – in contrast to the survival-promoting effect of enrichment – had a very potent effect on progenitor cell division, subsequently leading to an increased net number of newborn neurons (van Praag et al., 1999b). The exercise-induced increase in newborn neurons in the dentate area also correlated with improved performance in learning tasks and facilitated the induction of LTP on perforant path/granule cell layer synapses (van Praag et al., 1999a).

37.4.1.4 Learning

Hippocampus-dependent learning itself can increase the number of surviving neurons, even though the survival-increasing effect of learning on immature neurons appears to be restricted to a limited stage of neuronal development (Gould et al., 1999).

Supporting the finding of learning-enhanced neurogenesis are reports that the *in vivo* induction of LTP elevates the number of newborn neurons (Bruel-Jungerman et al., 2006). Recent experiments suggest that this effect on the hippocampal structure may also occur in humans (Draganski et al., 2006). However, it remains unclear whether the observed changes in hippocampal volume are indeed causally related to increased neurogenesis.

37.4.1.5 Aging

The age of the animal also has a dramatic influence on the number of adult-generated neurons. According to van Praag et al. (2005), the number of AGCs surviving for a month is estimated to be between 500 and 1000 per week in young adult mice (between 2 and 6 months of age) but drops to about 100 per week in aged animals. The reasons for this strong decrease are both low levels of progenitor cell proliferation and low levels of neuronal differentiation compared to young animals. An elegant study by Cameron and colleagues indicated that corticosteroids play a pivotal role in the age-related decline of adult neurogenesis (Cameron and McKay, 1999). However, it is important to notice that even in old age, both environmental enrichment and physical activity are still powerful tools to increase the number of newborn neurons (Kempermann et al., 2002; van Praag et al., 2005). To date it is still unclear whether decreased neurogenesis in aged animals is caused by an intrinsic progenitor cell failure or by changes in the neurogenic environment, but studies are under way that will address this critical question.

37.4.1.6 Neurotransmitters

Most neurotransmitters that have been studied appear to have an influence on the number of new neurons formed, although in most cases it has been technically very difficult to distinguish whether their effects on NPCs are direct or occur through the transmitters' effects on the surrounding network. For example, the direct roles of glutamate and GABA are still unclear. The principal input to the DG is glutamate from the EC. Disruption of the perforant path in the rat results in an increase in cell proliferation, suggesting that excitatory input might inhibit neurogenesis. Similarly, systemic NMDA receptor blockade enhances proliferative activity (Nacher and McEwen, 2006). However, as discussed in the following text, the activation of kainic acid glutamate receptors dramatically increases cell proliferation, and depolarization of progenitor cells appears to facilitate neurogenesis. Given these findings, the simple assumption that glutamatergic excitation generally downregulates neurogenesis might be too simple, especially considering that glutamate is rarely released in the DG without simultaneous release of GABA from interneurons. GABA signaling is not only involved in maturation – as outlined in earlier sections – but is also critically involved in proliferation (Tozuka et al., 2005; Ge et al., 2006). Therefore, it is probable that a delicate balance between excitation and inhibition is responsible for modulating the levels of neurogenesis (Deisseroth et al., 2004).

In addition to the glutamatergic EC input and internal circuitry, the DG receives inputs from a variety of different brain regions carrying a wide range of neurotransmitters. Cholinergic (as well as GABAergic and glutamatergic) fibers from the septum and nucleus basalis terminate throughout the DG, and particularly at the SGZ. Selective lesions of cholinergic neurons in the forebrain revealed a survival-promoting effect of acetylcholine, as lesions increased apoptotic cells' deaths and lowered neurogenesis levels (Cooper-Kuhn et al., 2004). Likewise, there is a strong serotonergic innervation of the SGZ from the raphe nuclei, and gain- and loss-of-function studies showed that release of serotonin strongly increased the numbers of newborn neurons (Gould, 1999). It has also been shown that drugs increasing serotonin levels such as fluoxetine upregulate adult neurogenesis (see following section for more details).

The DG also receives norepinephrine from the locus coereleus and dopamine from the ventral tegmental area. Less is known regarding the overall role of these neurotransmitters in the adult DG, but there are indications that both transmitters influence the levels of adult neurogenesis (Abrous et al., 2005). Furthermore, a wide range of neuropeptides and other molecules are released by axons in the DG, and several of these, including endocannabinoids, NPY, and endogenous opiates, appear to have effects on the proliferation of NPCs.

37.4.1.7 Additional regulators of adult neurogenesis

Another strong modulator of adult neurogenesis is dietary restriction, which increases the number of newborn granule cells by increased proliferation (Prolla and Mattson, 2001). Dietary intake may strongly influence the hormonal state, and several hormones have been shown to have a strong effect on the number of newborn neurons in the dentate area. Both positive (e.g., dehydroepiandrosterone,

DHEA) and negative (e.g., corticosterone) hormonal regulators could be identified (Abrous et al., 2005). Another modulator of adult neurogenesis is sleep deprivation. Interestingly, a single night of sleep deprivation appears to increase adult neurogenesis, whereas more chronic forms of sleep restriction had the opposite effect (Guzman-Marin et al., 2005; Grassi Zucconi et al., 2006). It is important to note that the number of physiological modulators is constantly growing, and the list described here is not complete (Abrous et al., 2005).

37.4.2 Pathological Regulators of Adult Neurogenesis

The previous section indicated the enormous degree of regulation that adult neurogenesis undergoes under normal conditions. Thus, it is not surprising that a long list of pathological conditions also have an effect on the number of newborn neurons in the DG.

37.4.2.1 Stress and depression

One very prominent negative regulator of adult neurogenesis is stress. Pioneering work by Gould and colleagues showed that psychosocial stress leads to a strong decrease in progenitor cell proliferation and new neuron numbers (Abrous et al., 2005). Mechanistically, the negative effects of stress on neurogenesis appear to be largely mediated by corticosteroids; adrenalectomy has been shown to prevent the stress-induced decline in new neuron production in rodents. Importantly, very similar results were obtained using primates (Abrous et al., 2005). The finding that stress has a strong, negative effect on adult neurogenesis lead to the hypothesis that hippocampal neurogenesis may also be critically involved in the disease process of depressive disorders. Interestingly, many human patients suffering from major depression have elevated serum levels of corticosteroids as well as reduced hippocampal volume, as measured by MRI (Sapolsky, 2000). Furthermore, it has been shown that several antidepressive drugs, such as fluoxetine, which belongs to the class of selective serotonin reuptake inhibitors (SSRIs), have a positive impact on adult neurogenesis. In addition, electroconvulsive seizures, which are a powerful clinical tool used to treat certain forms of major depression, increase the number of newborn neurons (Warner-Schmidt and Duman, 2006; and see following). The delay in the effectiveness of a variety of antidepressants for several weeks nicely fits with the idea that new neurons may be partially responsible for the drug's efficacy. In fact, Santarelli and colleagues showed that the inhibition of adult neurogenesis abolished the behavioral effects of fluoxetine on certain aspects of anxiety and stress (Santarelli et al., 2003). The link between adult neurogenesis and emotions will be discussed in more detail in the next section.

37.4.2.2 Seizures

Compared to stress and depression, seizure activity has the opposite effect on adult neurogenesis within the hippocampal circuitry. Epileptic discharges lead to a massive increase in cell proliferation and subsequent integration of new neurons into the dentate area (Parent, 2002). The exact mechanisms of how seizures result in increased numbers of new neurons is not fully understood, but it seems that cell death following seizure activity is not a critical factor. Even though the number of new neurons is dramatically upregulated within the first several days following seizures, recent data suggest that, after the initial insult, numbers drop below controls (Hattiangady et al., 2004). Whether this decrease is due to an 'exhaustion' of the progenitor population or to environmental changes in the neurogenic niche remains unclear.

Notably, a significant fraction of seizure-generated neurons either has aberrant basal dendrites (Shapiro and Ribak, 2006) or is ectopically located at the hilar/CA3 border (Parent et al., 1997; Scharfman et al., 2000). These basal dendrites reach deep into the hilus and, as observed with DCX analyses, have immature synapses that appear to integrate into the circuitry. However, little is known about the stability of these aberrant connections and what their functional impact on synaptic transmission through the dentate circuitry might be. Besides having abnormal dendritic processes, many seizure-generated granule cells ectopically migrate into the hilus toward area CA3. Studies by Scharfman provided evidence that these aberrant granule cells show synchronous firing patterns with CA3 pyramidal cells and may initiate recurrent excitation onto granule cells (Scharfman et al., 2000). These abnormal features of seizure-generated granule cells have led to the hypothesis that seizure-induced neurogenesis might be responsible for certain aspects of the epileptogenic disease process (Parent, 2002). However, it may also be true that seizure-induced neurogenesis is instead an attempt by the injured brain to replace lost cells and to rebuild damaged hippocampal structure (Bjorklund and Lindvall, 2000).

37.4.2.3 Ischemia

Similar to seizure activity, though less dramatic, ischemic insults to the adult brain increase the number of new neurons (Zhang et al., 2005). Unlike ischemia-induced neurogenesis in the SVZ, where newborn cells appear to migrate toward the lesion and possibly participate in repair function, the cause or value for increased neurogenesis within the hippocampus following ischemia remains unclear. Importantly, short ischemic episodes that do not result in measurable cell death still affect neurogenesis (Zhang et al., 2005). There are certain types of ischemic stroke induction, such as the four-vessel occlusion, that specifically target the hippocampal area in rodents. Experiments from the Nakafuku laboratory showed that poststroke infusion of the growth factors EGF and FGF-2 led to a robust repopulation of the damaged CA1 area with functional pyramidal neurons (Nakatomi et al., 2002), suggesting that endogenous progenitors are capable of repopulating substantial lesions in the adult brain. Further studies will have to determine the feasibility of this approach and what the actual benefit of endogenous neuronal replacement in injured subjects is.

37.4.2.4 Irradiation and inflammation

Brain irradiation is often used clinically to control tumorous growth within the CNS, especially in children. Palmer and colleagues showed that brain irradiation almost completely abolished cell proliferation within the SGZ, resulting in a lasting decrease in neurogenesis (Monje et al., 2002). Interestingly, the depletion of neurogenesis following irradiation was not entirely due to the radiation effect alone. Rather, the inflammatory response that accompanies irradiation strongly decreases the number of new neurons, and anti-inflammatory treatment augmented neurogenesis in radiated animals (Monje et al., 2003). The detrimental role of inflammation regarding neurogenesis was confirmed by studies showing that the decrease in neurogenesis following endotoxin-induced neuroinflammation was blocked by anti-inflammatory treatment (Hagberg and Mallard, 2005).

37.4.2.5 Neurodegenerative diseases and drugs

Clearly, the above-mentioned pathological regulators are not a complete list of disease states that influence the number of newborn neurons. If anything, people have sought unsuccessfully for a disease or pathological state that does not affect adult neurogenesis. There are reports that neurogenesis appears to be disturbed in animal models of Alzheimer's disease and in specimens from human Alzheimer's patients (Jin et al., 2004a,b). However, these findings remain controversial (Donovan et al., 2006). In addition, several other neurodegenerative disorders, such as Huntington's and Parkinson's diseases, have been shown to affect the number of newborn neurons in the dentate area (Abrous et al., 2005). The number of new neurons is also greatly influenced by abuse of substances such as ethanol, opioids, cannabionoids, barbiturates, nicotine, and benzodiazepines (Abrous et al., 2005).

Adult hippocampal neurogenesis is highly responsive and vulnerable to a variety of pathologies affecting the CNS. In most cases, however, the underlying cause or consequence of altered neurogenesis levels in the disease process of many neurological disorders remains unclear and may simply be epiphenomenological. Nevertheless, the finding that neurogenesis in the adult hippocampus is misregulated in many diseases has opened up several new approaches to understanding and ultimately curing human neurological disease.

37.5 Function of Neurogenesis

Two theories of hippocampal function have developed in parallel over the past 50 years, and both have been considered in the search for possible roles for neurogenesis. The first, originating in the 1950s from human amnesia studies, is that the hippocampus plays a critical role in the formation of episodic memories. Medial temporal lobe patients – the most famous being H.M. – display a robust, temporally graded retrograde amnesia (Milner et al., 1998). Hippocampal lesion patients, as well as monkeys and rodents, display difficulties in the recall of declarative memories (Squire et al., 2004). The second theory of hippocampal function originated in the 1970s from studies showing that hippocampal neurons in rats have strong place fields (O'Keefe and Conway, 1978; Jung and McNaughton, 1993; Best et al., 2001). This spatial map theory has been very well supported by the use of *in vivo* recordings of hippocampal and entorhinal cortex neurons. Despite these distinct theories, there is increasingly a consensus that the hippocampus has roles in both types of processing.

Although the precise function of granule cell neurogenesis in cognition is still not clear, computational and behavioral studies have led to more sophisticated ideas of what the addition of new neurons would mean to this well-studied circuit. This section describes the progress of both computational approaches and knock-down behavioral experiments.

37.5.1 Hippocampal Circuit Function and the Role of the DG

One reason that the hippocampus has been one of the more well-studied regions of the mammalian brain over the past century has been its seemingly simple neural circuitry. Although an oversimplification, the idea of a trisynaptic excitatory circuit (DG → CA3 → CA1) has proven very accessible to both electrophysiology and theoretical work. In particular, the recurrent connectivity of the CA3 region and the presence of strong place fields in CA1 have led to numerous theoretical ideas about the different hippocampal subregions.

Despite the lack of a consensus on the function of the hippocampus as a whole and for its subregions, a general agreement exists that the DG is most probably responsible for separating inputs presented to the hippocampus. This agreement has been based on the anatomy of the DG (Patton and McNaughton, 1995) and on *in vivo* electrophysiology studies (Jung and McNaughton, 1993), behavioral lesion studies (Kesner et al., 2004), and computational models (Rolls and Kesner, 2006). The region receives a very divergent projection from the EC (~200,000 cells project to >1 million granule cells in the rat) while having a very sparse projection onto the CA3. Within the network, granule cells receive strong tonic inhibition from local interneurons, and they are rarely active during behavior. However, when they are active, they have a potent effect on downstream CA3 neurons (Henze et al., 2002). These properties were used, and in some cases even predicted, by computational models describing the computational need for the DG in the production of sparse codes to facilitate memory formation (Rolls and Kesner, 2006).

37.5.2 Theoretical Functions of Adult Neurogenesis

Like most theories of hippocampal computation, most neurogenesis theories and network models have focused on a role in memory formation. However, as mentioned before, the DG's presumed role in pattern separation is similar in both mnemonic and spatial processing, suggesting that several of these conclusions are relevant for both general hippocampal functions.

Early theoretical and computational considerations of adult neurogenesis focused on the idea that neurogenesis might be a real-time regulator of memory capacity (Schinder and Gage, 2004). Indeed, several neural network studies demonstrated exactly this. Chambers et al. (2004) and Deisseroth et al. (2004) showed that a simple, three-layer neural network experiencing cell death and neurogenesis is capable of learning more information than a fixed-layer network. Although these models were only conceptual models of hippocampal circuitry and did not explicitly investigate pattern separation, their conclusions are still relevant to this theory of DG function. By replacing neurons in an input layer, they showed that the number of possible states of the output layer increases considerably, indicating increased memory capacity regardless of where the storage occurs.

Becker (2005) was one of the first to consider the effects of neurogenesis in a full hippocampal model and to limit the role of the DG to the encoding phase of learning, a hypothesis that has been the developing consensus in the hippocampal literature (Becker, 2005). The key result of this model was that DG size directly affects the storage capacity of the hippocampus, supporting the idea that neurogenesis facilitates the formation of new memories by permitting more network states. However, contrary to earlier models that involved the DG in the retrieval phase, Becker's model suggests that neural turnover actually reduces possible interference between memory traces in the CA3. The idea that neurogenesis keeps old and new memories separated was examined in detail by the network model of Wiskott et al. (2006). The Wiskott model suggests that interference between memories in the hippocampus is reduced by only permitting new neurons to adapt to new memories, consistent with physiological data showing increased LTP in immature neurons (Wiskott et al., 2006).

Most of these computational theories of neurogenesis have sought a role for new neurons in the framework of functions already considered for the hippocampus. Another view proposes that neurogenesis may have a function that is distinct from those traditionally assigned to the DG. The rationale behind this view is that most current hippocampal theories were derived without regard for adult neurogenesis.

For example, Aimone et al. (2006) described how increased excitability in immature neurons may contribute to the formation of temporal linkages between memories, a function that had not previously been attributed to the DG.

It is likely that any additional functions that neurogenesis contributes (beyond simply improving the DG's function) would be hippocampus dependent as well, just as linking memories in time would still be categorized as a type of declarative memory. However, without the benefit of the existing paradigms used to test memory, such novel functions will likely be difficult to investigate and will present additional challenges to behavioral scientists seeking evidence of a neurogenesis function in rodents. Despite the potential difficulties, it would not be surprising for neurogenesis to have several effects on cognition, as it increasingly appears that the hippocampus serves several functions in the brain.

37.5.3 Experimental Evidence for Functional Significance of Adult Neurogenesis

As outlined above, the hippocampus is critically involved in a variety of processes underlying certain forms of learning and memory. New neurons in the dentate area represent only a very small part of the hippocampal structure. As a result, a conclusive answer regarding the function of adult-born neurons is not easy to obtain experimentally. The difficulty in analyzing the functional significance of adult neurogenesis begins in choosing the right test. As mentioned above, the exact function of new neurons might be best appreciated in tests specifically designed to challenge new neurons. Furthermore, there might be species-dependent differences in the use for neurogenesis. Nevertheless, it appears to be mandatory to characterize a potential contribution of new neurons in standard hippocampus-dependent tasks to reach the goal of designing adult neurogenesis–specific tests.

The gold standard of testing hippocampal function remains the Morris water maze (MWM), which is highly sensitive to hippocampal lesions. Many of the behavioral data discussed below are indeed derived from using this test. Recent studies have provided evidence that newborn neurons functionally respond to the acquisition and recall phase during water maze testing (Jessberger and Kempermann, 2003; Kee et al., 2007). However, it is crucial to keep in mind that even the very standardized MWM tasks have an endless list of variations that may utilize newborn neurons differently. The following section will discuss correlational evidence and emerging causal evidence for a role for adult neurogenesis in hippocampal function.

37.5.3.1 Correlational evidence

Because the number of neurons born in the adult DG is highly dynamic, an extensive number of studies have been conducted correlating adult neurogenesis with hippocampus-dependent behavior. Kempermann and colleagues used a large set of recombinant inbred (RI) mice and found that the number of new neurons correlates with certain aspects of the MWM (Kempermann and Gage, 2002). Even though the findings using RI mice are still correlational, they are especially valuable because the number of strains analyzed was very large. Reduced latencies for the RI mice to reach the hidden platform in the water maze compared to standard housed control animals were also found when the net number of newborn granule cells was increased with environmental enrichment or physical exercise in animals with identical genetic backgrounds (Kempermann et al., 1997; van Praag et al., 1999a). The same was true when aged animals that show an age-dependent decline in adult neurogenesis were housed in the enriched environment or had access to a running wheel: both numbers of newborn neurons and performance in the Morris water maze were enhanced (Kempermann et al., 2002; van Praag et al., 2005). However, it is obvious that alterations induced by enrichment or physical exercise may not be exclusive to adult neurogenesis. Thus, additional changes within the hippocampal formation that are different from increased neurogenesis may also be partially responsible for the observed behavioral effects.

In addition to these positive correlations, there are also several studies that showed a relationship between low levels of neurogenesis and poor performance in hippocampus-dependent learning tasks. The low levels of neurogenesis in aged animals showing an age-related memory decline correlated well with the performance in the MWM (Zyzak et al., 1995). Furthermore, the age-dependent decline in neurogenesis was also associated with high levels of serum corticosteroids, confirming a potential mechanism explaining how aging may affect neurogenesis (Montaron et al., 2006).

Correlations between neurogenesis and performance in hippocampus-dependent memory tasks were also found in a variety of transgenic mice. The genetic deletion of methyl-CpG binding protein results in low levels of neurogenesis and is also associated with impaired MWM performance (Zhao et al., 2003). The same is true for NT-3 mutant mice and neuropeptide Y mutant mice, both showing reduced numbers of new neurons in the adult hippocampus and impaired learning and memory (Howell et al., 2005). Using a conditional knock-out of the *presenelin* gene, Tsien and his laboratory found decreased numbers of newborn neurons, whereas the acquisition of hippocampus-dependent learning was normal (Feng et al., 2001). However, the mutant animals showed apparent deficits in the clearance of older memories, suggesting that new neurons might be important not only for the acquisition but also for the clearance of memory traces (Feng et al., 2001).

37.5.3.2 'Causal' evidence

The correlative nature of the above-mentioned studies implies several caveats regarding the specificity of the manipulation of neurogenesis or genetic mutations. Therefore, current endeavors in the field aim to specifically knock down hippocampal neurogenesis without affecting other neural structures. To date, there is no widely accepted technical approach that is devoid of any unwanted side effects. This section discusses current strategies as well as the advantages and potential disadvantages of three experimental approaches: cytostatic drugs, irradiation, and molecular knock-downs.

An early study that was designed to reduce neurogenesis and analyze its impact on hippocampus-dependent learning was a report by Shors and colleagues (Shors et al., 2001). In this study, the cytostatic drug toxin methylazoxymethanol acetate (MAM) was used to block cell division and subsequent neurogenesis in the adult rat DG. Rats treated with MAM were found to be impaired in a trace eyeblink-conditioning paradigm that was associated with a decrease in dentate synaptic plasticity. When the treatment was discontinued and neurogenesis was allowed to recover, performance in the trace eyeblink-conditioning was normal. Similar results were obtained when testing the animals in a trace fear-conditioning test, whereas other hippocampal memory tasks, such as the MWM and contextual fear conditioning, appeared to be unaffected by MAM treatment (Shors et al., 2002). MAM was also found to block the beneficial effects of environmental enrichment in an object recognition task (Bruel-Jungerman et al., 2005). Notably, in each of these experiments MAM was injected systemically and potentially resulted in secondary effects on the animals' health that might account for some of the observed behavioral deficits (Dupret et al., 2005). Furthermore, MAM has been shown to interfere with protein synthesis, a crucial requirement for long-term memory (Grab et al., 1979).

Another approach to knock-down cell proliferation has been to use X-ray irradiation, which results in a robust and lasting reduction of neurogenesis in the adult brain (Parent et al., 1999; Monje et al., 2002). Whole-brain irradiation of adult rats left the acquisition phase of the MWM unaffected but impaired the long-term retention (over 14 days after the last training trial) of the platform location, which is suggestive of a functional role of new neurons in spatial memory (Snyder et al., 2005). Furthermore, the performance in a non-matching-to-sample (NMTS) task was impaired when the delays between sample and test trials were relatively long (Winocur et al., 2006). In contrast to MAM-treated animals (Shors et al., 2002), irradiation also led to memory deficits in contextual fear conditioning (Winocur et al., 2006). Studies by the Hen laboratory have selectively targeted the hippocampus instead of using whole-brain irradiation to determine the contribution of newborn neurons in cognitive improvement following environmental enrichment. Irradiated mice showed no impairment in the water maze, and enriched housing was effective at improving the acquisition of the hidden platform location, even in the absence of new neurons (Meshi et al., 2006). These findings indicate that certain aspects of the beneficial effects of enrichment may not depend on adult neurogenesis.

As outlined in an earlier section, adult neurogenesis might be also associated with anxiety and depression, and targeted irradiation of the hippocampus was used to address the relationship between new neurons and antidepressant treatment. Indeed, intact hippocampal neurogenesis appears to be required for the effectiveness of the antidepressant fluoxetine (Santarelli et al., 2003). However, it seems that neurogenesis is not a critical component *per se* in emotional control, because the anxiolytic effects of environmental enrichment were completely unaffected by the ablation of new neurons (Meshi et al., 2006). Despite the robust and complete ablation of new neurons in the adult hippocampus following irradiation, this approach also implies some unwanted side effects, such as ablation of all dividing cells (including glial progenitors outside the dentate gyrus), inflammation, and potential radiation-induced damage of mature neurons.

The existing causal evidence regarding a functional role for new neurons in hippocampal function allows one to speculate that newborn neurons are required for certain aspects of learning and memory and might also be involved in emotional behavior. However, the available data remain inconclusive. The hope for identifying the functional significance of adult neurogenesis unambiguously lies in the development of specific behavioral tests and new strategies to knock down neurogenesis as specifically and gently as possible. These new strategies will likely include the use of neural progenitor and immature neuron-specific promoters to drive the expression of suicide genes and the virus-mediated inhibition (or enhancement) of adult neurogenesis.

37.6 Conclusions

The discovery of ongoing neurogenesis throughout adulthood has undoubtedly challenged our understanding of neuronal development and adult hippocampal function. Even though our understanding of fate instruction, neuronal maturation, and integration is quickly growing, several key questions remain unanswered. From a cellular and molecular standpoint, it will be very important to understand the *in vivo* potency of NSCs and why neurogenesis only occurs in two restricted areas of the adult brain under normal conditions. Furthermore, little is known about which signaling pathways are involved in the extension and pathfinding of axonal and dendritic processes arising from newborn neurons.

Finally, the ultimate challenge will be to truly decode the functional role of adult neurogenesis. Defining that role might not only fundamentally change current concepts regarding hippocampal function but could also help us to understand and eventually improve treatment of human neurological disease.

Acknowledgments

Supported by grants from Lookout Fund, NIA, NINDS, and DARPA.

References

Abrous DN, Koehl M, and Le Moal M (2005) Adult neurogenesis: From precursors to network and physiology. *Physiol. Rev.* 85: 523–569.

Aimone JB, Wiles J, and Gage FH (2006) Potential role for adult neurogenesis in the encoding of time in new memories. *Nat. Neurosci.* 9: 723–727.

Altman J and Das GD (1965) Autoradiographic and histologic evidence of postnatal neurogenesis in rats. *J. Comp. Neurol.* 124: 319–335.

Becker S (2005) A computational principle for hippocampal learning and neurogenesis. *Hippocampus* 15: 722–738.

Best PJ, White AM, and Minai A (2001) Spatial processing in the brain: The activity of hippocampal place cells. *Annu. Rev. Neurosci.* 24: 459–486.

Bjorklund A and Lindvall O (2000) Cell replacement therapies for central nervous system disorders. *Nat. Neurosci.* 3: 537–544.

Bonaguidi MA, McGuire T, Hu M, Kan L, Samanta J, and Kessler JA (2005) LIF and BMP signaling generate separate and discrete types of GFAP-expressing cells. *Development* 132: 5503–5514.

Brandt MD, Jessberger S, Steiner B, et al. (2003) Transient caltetinin expression defines early postmitotic step of neuronal differentiation in adult hippocampal neurogenesis of mice. *Mol. Cell. Neurosci.* 24: 603–613.

Bruel-Jungerman E, Davis S, Rampon C, and Laroche S (2006) Long-term potentiation enhances neurogenesis in the adult dentate gyrus. *J. Neurosci.* 26: 5888–5893.

Bruel-Jungerman E, Laroche S, and Rampon C (2005) New neurons in the dentate gyrus are involved in the expression of enhanced long-term memory following environmental enrichment. *Eur. J. Neurosci.* 21: 513–521.

Cameron HA and McKay RD (1999) Restoring production of hippocampal neurons in old age. *Nat. Neurosci.* 2: 894–897.

Cao L, Jiao X, Zuzga DS, et al. (2004) VEGF links hippocampal activity with neurogenesis, learning and memory. *Nat. Genet.* 36: 827–835.

Cao X, Yeo G, Muotri AR, Kuwabara T, and Gage FH (2006) Noncoding RNAs in the mammalian central nervous system. *Annu. Rev. Neurosci.* 29: 77–103.

Chambers RA, Potenza MN, Hoffman RE, and Miranker W (2004) Simulated apoptosis/neurogenesis regulates learning and memory capabilities of adaptive neural networks. *Neuropsychopharmacology* 29: 747–758.

Cooper-Kuhn CM, Winkler J, and Kuhn HG (2004) Decreased neurogenesis after cholinergic forebrain lesion in the adult rat. *J. Neurosci. Res.* 77: 155–165.

Deisseroth K, Singla S, Toda H, Monje M, Palmer TD, and Malenka RC (2004) Excitation-neurogenesis coupling in adult neural stem/progenitor cells. *Neuron* 42: 535–552.

Donovan MH, Yazdani U, Norris RD, Games D, German DC, and Eisch AJ (2006) Decreased adult hippocampal neurogenesis in the PDAPP mouse model of Alzheimer's disease. *J. Comp. Neurol.* 495: 70–83.

Draganski B, Gaser C, Kempermann G, et al. (2006) Temporal and spatial dynamics of brain structure changes during extensive learning. *J. Neurosci.* 26: 6314–6317.

Dupret D, Montaron MF, Drapeau E, et al. (2005) Methylazoxymethanol acetate does not fully block cell genesis in the young and aged dentate gyrus. *Eur. J. Neurosci.* 22: 778–783.

Eriksson PS, Perfilieva E, Björk-Eriksson T, et al. (1998) Neurogenesis in the adult human hippocampus. *Nat. Med.* 4: 1313–1317.

Esposito MS, Piatti VC, Laplagne DA, et al. (2005) Neuronal differentiation in the adult hippocampus recapitulates embryonic development. *J. Neurosci.* 25: 10074–10086.

Feng R, Rampon C, Tang YP, et al. (2001) Deficient neurogenesis in forebrain-specific presenilin-1 knockout mice is associated with reduced clearance of hippocampal memory traces. *Neuron* 32: 911–926.

Filippov V, Kronenberg G, Pivneva T, et al. (2003) Subpopulation of nestin-expressing progenitor cells in the adult murine hippocampus shows electrophysiological and morphological characteristics of astrocytes. *Mol. Cell. Neurosci.* 23: 373–382.

Fukuda S, Kato F, Tozuka Y, Yamaguchi M, Miyamoto Y, and Hisatsune T (2003) Two distinct subpopulations of nestin-positive cells in adult mouse dentate gyrus. *J. Neurosci.* 23: 9357–9366.

Gage F (2000) Mammalian neural stem cells. *Science* 287: 1433–1438.

Gage FH, Coates PW, Palmer TD, et al. (1995) Survival and differentiation of adult neuronal progenitor cells transplanted to the adult brain. *Proc. Natl. Acad. Sci. USA* 92: 11879–11883.

Ge S, Goh EL, Sailor KA, Kitabatake Y, Ming GL, and Song H (2006) GABA regulates synaptic integration of newly generated neurons in the adult brain. *Nature* 439: 589–593.

Gleiberman AS, Encinas JM, Mignone JL, Michurina T, Rosenfeld MG, and Enikolopov G (2005) Expression of nestin-green fluorescent protein transgene marks oval cells in the adult liver. *Dev. Dyn.* 234: 413–421.

Gould E (1999) Serotonin and hippocampal neurogenesis. *Neuropsychopharmacology* 21(supplement 2): 46S–51S.

Gould E, Beylin A, Tanapat P, Reeves A, and Shors TJ (1999) Learning enhances adult neurogenesis in the hippoampal formation. *Nat. Neurosci.* 2: 260–265.

Grab DJ, Pavlovec A, Hamilton MG, and Zedeck MS (1979) Mechanism of inhibition of hepatic protein synthesis in rats by the carcinogen, methylazoxymethanol acetate. *Biochim. Biophys. Acta* 563: 240–252.

Grassi Zucconi G, Cipriani S, Balgkouranidou I, and Scattoni R (2006) 'One night' sleep deprivation stimulates hippocampal neurogenesis. Brain Res Bull 69: 375–381.

Guzman-Marin R, Suntsova N, Methippara M, Greiffenstein R, Szymusiak R, McGinty D (2005) Sleep deprivation suppresses neurogenesis in the adult hippocampus of rats. *Eur. J. Neurosci.* 22: 2111–2116.

Hagberg H and Mallard C (2005) Effect of inflammation on central nervous system development and vulnerability. *Curr. Opin. Neurol.* 18: 117–123.

Hastings NB and Gould E (1999) Rapid extension of axons into the CA3 region by adult-generated granule cells. *J. Comp. Neurol.* 413: 146–154.

Hattiangady B, Rao MS, and Shetty AK (2004) Chronic temporal lobe epilepsy is associated with severely declined dentate neurogenesis in the adult hippocampus. *Neurobiol. Dis.* 17: 473–490.

Henze DA, Wittner L, and Buzsaki G (2002) Single granule cells reliably discharge targets in the hippocampal CA3 network *in vivo*. *Nat. Neurosci.* 5: 790–795.

Hinds JW (1968) Autoradiographic study of histogenesis in the mouse olfactory bulb. II. Cell proliferation and migration. *J. Comp. Neurol.* 134: 305–322.

Howell OW, Doyle K, Goodman JH, et al. (2005) Neuropeptide Y stimulates neuronal precursor proliferation in the post-natal and adult dentate gyrus. *J. Neurochem.* 93: 560–570.

Hsieh J, Aimone JB, Kaspar BK, Kuwabara T, Nakashima K, and Gage FH (2004) IGF-I instructs multipotent adult neural progenitor cells to become oligodendrocytes. *J. Cell Biol.* 164: 111–122.

Jessberger S, Clemenson GD Jr., and Gage FH (2006) Spontaneous fusion and non-clonal growth of adult neural stem cells. *Stem Cells* DOI: 10. 1634 stem cells. 2006 - 0620.

Jessberger S and Kempermann G (2003) Adult-born hippocampal neurons mature into activity-dependent responsiveness. *Eur. J. Neurosci.* 18: 2707–2712.

Jin K, Galvan V, Xie L, et al. (2004a) Enhanced neurogenesis in Alzheimer's disease transgenic (PDGF-APPSw,Ind) mice. *Proc. Natl. Acad. Sci. USA* 101: 13363–13367.

Jin K, Peel AL, Mao XO, et al. (2004b) Increased hippocampal neurogenesis in Alzheimer's disease. *Proc. Natl. Acad. Sci. USA* 101: 343–347.

Jung MW and McNaughton BL (1993) Spatial selectivity of unit activity in the hippocampal granular layer. *Hippocampus* 3: 165–182.

Kaplan MS and Hinds JW (1977) Neurogenesis in the adult rat: Electron microscopic analysis of light radioautographs. *Science* 197: 1092–1094.

Kee N, Teixeira CM, Wang AH, and Frankland PW (2007) Preferential incorporation of adult-generated granule cells into spatial memory networks in the dentate gyrus. *Nat. Neurosci.* 10: 355–362.

Kempermann G, Chesler EJ, Lu L, Williams RW, and Gage FH (2006) Natural variation and genetic covariance in adult hippocampal neurogenesis. *Proc. Natl. Acad. Sci. USA* 103: 780–785.

Kempermann G and Gage FH (2002) Genetic determinants of adult hippocampal neurogenesis correlate with acquisition, but not probe trial performance, in the water maze task. *Eur. J. Neurosci.* 16: 129–136.

Kempermann G, Gast D, and Gage FH (2002) Neuroplasticity in old age: Sustained fivefold induction of hippocampal neurogenesis by long-term environmental enrichment. *Ann. Neurol.* 52: 135–143.

Kempermann G, Kuhn HG, and Gage FH (1997) More hippocampal neurons in adult mice living in an enriched environment. *Nature* 386: 493–495.

Kempermann G, Jessberger S, Steiner B, and Kronenberg G (2004) Milestones of neuronal development in the adult hippocampus. *Trends Neurosci.* 27: 447–452.

Kesner RP, Lee I, and Gilbert P (2004) A behavioral assessment of hippocampal function based on a subregional analysis. *Rev. Neurosci.* 15: 333–351.

Kokoeva MV, Yin H, and Flier JS (2005) Neurogenesis in the hypothalamus of adult mice: Potential role in energy balance. *Science* 310: 679–683.

Lie DC, Colamarino SA, Song HJ, et al. (2005) Wnt signalling regulates adult hippocampal neurogenesis. *Nature* 437: 1370–1375.

Lie DC, Song H, Colamarino SA, Ming GL, and Gage FH (2004) Neurogenesis in the adult brain: New strategies for central nervous system diseases. *Annu. Rev. Pharmacol. Toxicol.* 44: 399–421.

Markakis E and Gage FH (1999) Adult-generated neurons in the dentate gyrus send axonal projections to the field CA3 and are surrounded by synaptic vesicles. *J. Comp. Neurol.* 406: 449–460.

Meshi D, Drew MR, Saxe M, et al. (2006) Hippocampal neurogenesis is not required for behavioral effects of environmental enrichment. *Nat. Neurosci.* 9: 729–731.

Milner B, Squire LR, and Kandel ER (1998) Cognitive neuroscience and the study of memory. *Neuron* 20: 445–468.

Ming GL and Song H (2005) Adult neurogenesis in the mammalian central nervous system. *Annu. Rev. Neurosci.* 28: 223–250.

Monje ML, Mizumatsu S, Fike JR, and Palmer TD (2002) Irradiation induces neural precursor-cell dysfunction. *Nat. Med.* 8: 955–962.

Monje ML, Toda H, and Palmer TD (2003) Inflammatory blockade restores adult hippocampal neurogenesis. *Science* 302: 1760–1765.

Montaron MF, Drapeau E, Dupret D, et al. (2006) Lifelong corticosterone level determines age-related decline in neurogenesis and memory. *Neurobiol. Aging* 27: 645–654.

Nacher J and McEwen BS (2006) The role of N-methyl-D-asparate receptors in neurogenesis. *Hippocampus* 16: 267–270.

Nakatomi H, Kuriu T, Okabe S, et al. (2002) Regeneration of hippocampal pyramidal neurons after ischemic brain injury by recruitment of endogenous neural progenitors. *Cell* 110: 429–441.

O'Keefe J and Conway DH (1978) Hippocampal place units in the freely moving rat: Why they fire where they fire. *Exp. Brain Res.* 31: 573–590.
Overstreet LS, Hentges ST, Bumaschny VF, et al. (2004) A transgenic marker for newly born granule cells in dentate gyrus. *J. Neurosci.* 24: 3251–3259.
Overstreet-Wadiche L, Bromberg DA, Bensen AL, and Westbrook GL (2005) GABAergic signaling to newborn neurons in dentate gyrus. *J. Neurophysiol.* 94: 4528–4532.
Palmer TD, Ray J, and Gage FH (1995) FGF-2-responsive neuronal progenitors reside in proliferative and quiescent regions of the adult rodent brain. *Mol. Cell. Neurosci.* 6: 474–486.
Palmer TD, Schwartz PH, Taupin P, Kaspar B, Stein SA, and Gage FH (2001) Cell culture. Progenitor cells from human brain after death. *Nature* 411: 42–43.
Palmer TD, Willhoite AR, and Gage FH (2000) Vascular niche for adult hippocampal neurogenesis. *J. Comp. Neurol.* 425: 479–494.
Parent JM (2002) The role of seizure-induced neurogenesis in epileptogenesis and brain repair. *Epilepsy Res.* 50: 179–189.
Parent JM, Tada E, Fike JR, and Lowenstein DH (1999) Inhibition of dentate granule cell neurogenesis with brain irradation does not prevent seizure-induced mossy fiber synaptic reorganization in the rat. *J. Neurosci.* 19: 4508–4519.
Parent JM, Yu TW, Leibowitz RT, Geschwind DH, Sloviter RS, and Lowenstein DH (1997) Dentate granule cell neurogenesis is increased by seizures and contributes to aberrant network reorganization in the adult rat hippocampus. *J. Neurosci.* 17: 3727–3738.
Patton PE and McNaughton B (1995) Connection matrix of the hippocampal formation: I. The dentate gyrus. *Hippocampus* 5: 245–286.
Prolla TA and Mattson MP (2001) Molecular mechanisms of brain aging and neurodegenerative disorders: Lessons from dietary restriction. *Trends Neurosci.* 24: S21–31.
Ray J and Gage FH (2006) Differential properties of adult rat and mouse brain derived stem/progenitor cells. *Mol. Cell. Neurosci.* 31: 560–573.
Ray J, Peterson DA, Schinstine M, and Gage FH (1993) Proliferation, differentiation, and long-term culture of primary hippocampal neurons. *Proc. Natl. Acad. Sci. USA* 90: 3602–3606.
Reynolds BA and Weiss S (1992) Generation of neurons and astrocytes from isolated cells of the adult mammalian central nervous system [see comments]. *Science* 255: 1707–1710.
Rolls ET and Kesner RP (2006) A computational theory of hippocampal function, and empirical tests of the theory. *Prog. Neurobiol.* 79: 1–48.
Santarelli L, Saxe M, Gross C, et al. (2003) Requirement of hippocampal neurogenesis for the behavioral effects of antidepressants. *Science* 301: 805–809.
Sapolsky RM (2000) Glucocorticoids and hippocampal atrophy in neuropsychiatric disorders. *Arch. Gen. Psychiatry* 57: 925–935.
Scharfman HE, Goodman JH, and Sollas AL (2000) Granule-like neurons at the hilar/CA3 border after status epilepticus and their synchrony with area CA3 pyramidal cells: Functional implications of seizure-induced neurogenesis. *J. Neurosci.* 20: 6144–6158.
Schinder AF and Gage FH (2004) A hypothesis about the role of adult neurogenesis in hippocampal function. *Physiology (Bethesda)* 19: 253–261.
Schmidt-Hieber C, Jonas P, and Bischofberger J (2004) Enhanced synaptic plasticity in newly generated granule cells of the adult hippocampus. *Nature* 429: 184–187.
Seaberg RM and van der Kooy D (2002) Adult rodent neurogenic regions: The ventricular subependyma contains neural stem cells, but the dentate gyrus contains restricted progenitors. *J. Neurosci.* 22: 1784–1793.
Seri B, Garcia-Verdugo JM, Collado-Morente L, McEwen BS, and Alvarez-Buylla A (2004) Cell types, lineage, and architecture of the germinal zone in the adult dentate gyrus. *J. Comp. Neurol.* 478: 359–378.
Seri B, Garcia-Verdugo JM, McEwen BS, and Alvarez-Buylla A (2001) Astrocytes give rise to new neurons in the adult mammalian hippocampus. *J. Neurosci.* 21: 7153–7160.
Shapiro LA and Ribak CE (2006) Newly born dentate granule neurons after pilocarpine-induced epilepsy have hilar basal dendrites with immature synapses. *Epilepsy Res.* 69: 53–66.
Shors TJ, Miesegaes G, Beylin A, Zhao M, Rydel T, and Gould E (2001) Neurogenesis in the adult is involved in the formation of trace memories. *Nature* 410: 372–376.
Shors TJ, Townsend DA, Zhao M, Kozorovitskiy Y, and Gould E (2002) Neurogenesis may relate to some but not all types of hippocampal-dependent learning. *Hippocampus* 12: 578–584.
Simic G, Kostovic I, Winblad B, and Bogdanovic N (1997) Volume and number of neurons of the human hippocampal formation in normal aging and Alzheimer's disease. *J. Comp. Neurol.* 379: 482–494.
Singec I, Knoth R, Meyer RP, et al. (2006) Defining the actual sensitivity and specificity of the neurosphere assay in stem cell biology. *Nat. Methods* 3: 801–806.
Smith A (2006) A glossary for stem-cell biology. *Nature* 441, 1060.
Snyder JS, Hong NS, McDonald RJ, and Wojtowicz JM (2005) A role for adult neurogenesis in spatial long-term memory. *Neuroscience* 130: 843–852.
Song H, Stevens CF, and Gage FH (2002) Astroglia induce neurogenesis from adult neural stem cells. *Nature* 417, 39–44.
Squire LR, Stark CE, and Clark RE (2004) The medial temporal lobe. *Annu. Rev. Neurosci.* 27: 279–306.
Tashiro A, Makino H and Gage FH (2007) Experience-specific functional modification of the dentate gyrus through adult neurogenesis: A critical period during an immature stage. *J. Neurosci.* 27: 3252–3259.
Tashiro A, Sandler VM, Toni N, Zhao C, and Gage FH (2006) NMDA receptor-mediated, cell-specific integration of new neurons in adult dentate gyrus, *Nature* 442: 929–933.
Toni N, Teng EM, Bushong EA, et al. Synapse formation in press on neurons born in the adult hippocampus. Nat. Neurosci.
Tozuka Y, Fukuda S, Namba T, Seki T, and Hisatsune T (2005) GABAergic excitation promotes neuronal differentiation in adult hippocampal progenitor cells. *Neuron* 47: 803–815.
van Praag H, Christie BR, Sejnowski TJ, and Gage FH (1999a) Running enhances neurogenesis, learning and long-term potentiation in mice. *Proc. Natl. Acad. Sci. USA* 96: 13427–13431.
van Praag H, Kempermann G, and Gage FH (1999b) Running increases cell proliferation and neurogenesis in the adult mouse dentate gyrus. *Nat. Neurosci.* 2: 266–270.
van Praag H, Kempermann G, and Gage FH (2000) Neural consequences of environmental enrichment. Nat. *Rev. Neurosci.* 1: 191–198.
van Praag H, Schinder AF, Christie BR, Toni N, Palmer TD, and Gage FH (2002) Functional neurogenesis in the adult hippocampus. *Nature* 415: 1030–1034.
van Praag H, Shubert T, Zhao C, and Gage FH (2005) Exercise enhances learning and hippocampal neurogenesis in aged mice. *J. Neurosci.* 25: 8680–8685.
Wang S, Scott BW, and Wojtowicz JM (2000) Heterogenous properties of dentate granule neurons in the adult rat. *J. Neurobiol.* 42: 248–257.

Warner-Schmidt JL and Duman RS (2006) Hippocampal neurogenesis: Opposing effects of stress and antidepressant treatment. *Hippocampus* 16: 239–249.

Winocur G, Wojtowicz JM, Sekeres M, Snyder JS, and Wang S (2006) Inhibition of neurogenesis interferes with hippocampus-dependent memory function. *Hippocampus* 16: 296–304.

Wiskott L, Rasch MJ, and Kempermann G (2006) A functional hypothesis for adult hippocampal neurogenesis: Avoidance of catastrophic interference in the dentate gyrus. *Hippocampus* 16: 329–343.

Wurmser AE, Nakashima K, Summers RG, et al. (2004) Cell fusion-independent differentiation of neural stem cells to the endothelial lineage. *Nature* 430: 350–356.

Zhang RL, Zhang ZG, and Chopp M (2005) Neurogenesis in the adult ischemic brain: Generation, migration, survival, and restorative therapy. *Neuroscientist* 11: 408–416.

Zhao C, Teng EM, Summers RG, Jr., Ming GL, and Gage FH (2006) Distinct morphological stages of dentate granule neuron maturation in the adult mouse hippocampus. *J. Neurosci.* 26: 3–11.

Zhao X, Ueba T, Christie BR, et al. (2003) Mice lacking methyl-CpG binding protein 1 have deficits in adult neurogenesis and hippocampal function. *Proc. Natl. Acad. Sci. USA* 100: 6777–6782.

Zyzak DR, Otto T, Eichenbaum H, and Gallagher M (1995) Cognitive decline associated with normal aging in rats: A neuropsychological approach. *Learn. Mem.* 2: 1–16.

Subject Index

Arrangement:, This index is in word-by-word order, whereby hyphens are treated as spaces (e.g. 'multi-trial' precedes 'multiple'). Prefixes and terms in parentheses are excluded from the initial alphabetization.

Cross-reference terms in italics are general cross-references, or refer to subentry terms within the main entry (the main entry is not repeated to save space). Readers are also advised to refer to the end of each article for additional cross-references - not all of these cross-references have been included in the index cross-references.

Major discussion of a subject is indicated by bold page numbers. Page numbers suffixed by T and F refer to Tables and Figures respectively. *vs.* indicates a comparison.

Subentries listed under a main entry with the same page numbers were included to illustrate the breadth of the coverage of the topic.

To save space in the index, the following abbreviations have been used:

BrdU - bromo-deoxyuridine
CREB - cAMP response element binding protein
CS - conditioned stimulus (stimuli)
ECT - electroconvulsive shock treatment
ERPs - event-related potentials
fMRI - functional magnetic resonance imagery
LTD - long-term depression
LTM - long-term memory
LTP - long-term potentiation
MEG - magnetoencephalography
MS/VDB - medial septum/vertical limb of the diagonal band
MTL - medial temporal lobe
NBM/SI - nucleus basalis magnocellularis/substantia innominata
PSC - primary sensory cortex
SD - semantic dementia
S–R - stimulus–response
S–Rf - stimulus–reinforcer
SRTT - serial reaction time task
S–S - stimulus–stimulus
STD - short-term depression
STM - short-term memory
US - unconditioned stimulus (stimuli)
VBM - voxel-based morphometry
VOR - vestibulo-ocular reflex

A

B

C

D

E

F

G

H

I

J

K

L

M

N

O

P

Q

R

S

T

U

V

W

X

Y